Success in the Classroom, in Clinicals, and o... W9-AKX-015

Classroom

- Detailed lecture notes organized by learning outcome
- Suggestions for classroom activities
- Guide to relevant additional resources
- Comprehensive PowerPoint™ presentations integrating lecture, images, animations, and videos
- Classroom Response questions
- Image Gallery
- Video and Animation Gallery
- Online course management systems complete with instructor tools and student activities available in a variety of formats

PEARSON mynursinglab

- Saves instructors time by providing quality feedback, ongoing formative assessments and customized remediation for students.
- Provides easy, one-stop access to a wealth of teaching resources, such as test item files, PowerPoint™ slides, and video suggestions.
- A built-in electronic gradebook tracks students' progress on assessment and remediation activities.

Clinical

- Suggestions for Clinical Activities and other clinical resources organized by learning outcome

Real Nursing Simulations Facilitator's Guide: Institutional Edition

- 25 simulation scenarios that span the nursing curriculum
- Consistent format includes learning objectives, case flow, instructions for set up, student debriefing questions and more!
- Companion online course cartridge with student exercises, activities, videos, skill checklists, and reflective questions also available for adoption

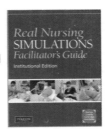

NCLEX-RN®

- Test Item Files with NCLEX®-style questions and complete rationales for correct and incorrect answers mapped to learning outcomes. *available in TestGen, Par Test, and MS Word*

Instructor Resources

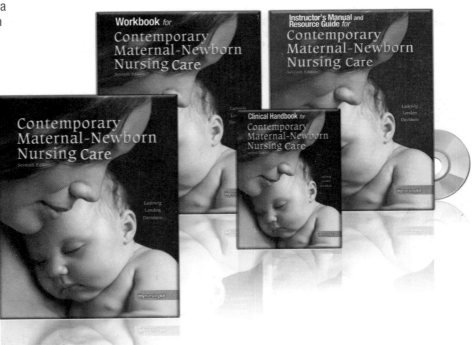

More information and instructor resources **visit** www.mynursingkit.com

Brief Contents

Contemporary Maternal-Newborn Nursing Care

Seventh Edition

Patricia A. Wieland Ladewig, PhD, RN
PROFESSOR AND ACADEMIC DEAN; RUECKERT-HARTMAN COLLEGE FOR HEALTH PROFESSIONS
Regis University
Denver, Colorado

Marcia L. London, RN, MSN, APRN, CNS, NNP-BC
SENIOR CLINICAL INSTRUCTOR AND RET. DIRECTOR OF NEONATAL NURSE PRACTITIONER PROGRAM
Beth-El College of Nursing and Health Sciences—University of Colorado
Colorado Springs, Colorado
STAFF CLINICAL NURSE
Urgent Care and After Hours Clinic
Colorado Springs, Colorado

Michele R. Davidson, PhD, RN, CNM
EXECUTIVE DIRECTOR
Smith Island Foundation
Smith Island, Virginia

Pearson
New York   Boston   San Francisco
London   Toronto   Sydney   Tokyo   Singapore   Madrid
Mexico City   Munich   Paris   Cape Town   Hong Kong   Montreal

Library of Congress Cataloging-in-Publication Data
Ladewig, Patricia W.
  Contemporary maternal-newborn nursing care / Patricia A. Wieland Ladewig,
Marcia L. London, Michele R. Davidson. — 7th ed.
    p. ; cm.
  Includes bibliographical references and index.
  ISBN 978-0-13-502585-7
  1. Maternity nursing.   I. London, Marcia L.   II. Davidson, Michele R.   III. Title.
  [DNLM: 1. Maternal-Child Nursing. WY 157.3 L154c 2009]
  RG951.L33 2009
  618.2'0231—dc22
                                                              2008043256

Publisher: Julie Levin Alexander
Assistant to Publisher: Regina Bruno
Editor-in-Chief: Maura Connor
Assistant to the Editor-in-Chief: Marion Gottlieb
Executive Acquisitions Editor: Pamela Fuller
Assistant to the Executive Acquisitions Editor: Sarah Wrocklage
Development Editor: iD8 Publishing Services, Inc., Marion Waldman, Jill Rembetski
Media Product Manager: Travis Moses-Westphal
Director of Marketing: Karen Allman
Senior Marketing Manager: Francisco del Castillo
Marketing Specialist: Michael Sirinides
Managing Editor, Production: Patrick Walsh
Production Editor: Lynn Steines, S4Carlisle Publishing Services
Production Liaison: Anne Garcia
Media Project Manager: Lorena Cerisano
Manufacturing Manager: Ilene Sanford
Manager, Rights and Permissions: Zina Arabia
Manager, Visual Research: Beth Brenzel
Senior Image Permission Coordinator: Cynthia Vincenti
Cover Permission Coordinator: Rita Wenning
Senior Design Coordinator: Maria Guglielmo-Walsh
Interior Design: Jill Lehan
Cover Design: Lisa Delgado
Composition: S4Carlisle Publishing Services
Printer/Binder: RR Donnelley
Cover Printer: Lehigh-Phoenix Color/Hagerstown

DEDICATION

We dedicate this book to parents—
*Who love, cherish, and protect their children;
Who guide, nurture, and shape them
So that they grow to be compassionate, loving,
responsible adults.
Such parents know that the reward comes when
The children you love become adults you also like
and enjoy as people!
And, as always, we dedicate our work to our beloved
families
To Tim Ladewig; Ryan, Amanda, Reed, and
Addison Grace; Erik, Kedri, and Emma
To David London, Craig, and Matthew
To Nathan Davidson, Hayden, Chloe, Caroline,
and Grant*

Notice: Care has been taken to confirm the accuracy of information presented in this book. The authors, editors, and the publisher, however, cannot accept any responsibility for errors or omissions or for consequences from application of the information in this book and make no warranty, express or implied, with respect to its contents.

The authors and publisher have exerted every effort to ensure that drug selections and dosages set forth in this text are in accord with current recommendations and practice at time of publication. However, in view of ongoing research, changes in government regulations, and the constant flow of information relating to drug therapy and reactions, the reader is urged to check the package inserts of all drugs for any change in indications or dosage and for added warning and precautions. This is particularly important when the recommended agent is a new and/or infrequently employed drug.

Pearson Education Ltd., London
Pearson Education Singapore, Pte. Ltd
Pearson Education Canada, Inc.
Pearson Education—Japan
Pearson Education Australia PTY, Limited

Pearson Education North Asia, Ltd., Hong Kong
Pearson Educación de Mexico, S.A. de C.V.
Pearson Education Malaysia, Pte. Ltd.
Pearson Education Upper Saddle River, New Jersey

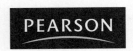

www.pearsonhighered.com

10 9 8 7 6 5 4 3

ISBN-13:   978-0-13-502585-7
ISBN-10:   0-13-502585-0

Patricia A. Wieland Ladewig

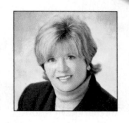

received her BS from the College of Saint Teresa in Winona, Minnesota; her MSN from Catholic University of America in Washington, D.C.; and her PhD in higher education administration from the University of Denver in Colorado. She served as an Air Force nurse and discovered her passion for teaching as a faculty member at Florida State University. Over the years, she taught at several schools of nursing. In addition, she became a women's health nurse practitioner and maintained a part-time clinical practice. In 1988, Dr. Ladewig became the first director of the nursing program at Regis College in Denver. In 1991, when the college became Regis University, she be-came academic dean of the Rueckert-Hartman College for Health Professions. Under her guidance, the School of Nursing has added a graduate program. In addition, the College has added a School of Physical Therapy and is in the process of developing a School of Pharmacy. Dr. Ladewig and her husband, Tim, enjoy skiing, baseball games, and traveling. However, their greatest pleasure comes from their family: son, Ryan, his wife, Amanda, and grandchildren, Reed and Addison Grace; and son, Erik, his wife, Kedri, and granddaughter, Emma.

Marcia L. London

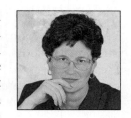

received her BSN and School Nurse Certificate from Plattsburgh State University in Plattsburgh, New York, and her MSN in pediatrics as a clinical nurse specialist from the University of Pittsburgh in Pennsylvania. She worked as a pediatric nurse and began her teaching career at Pittsburgh Children's Hospital Affiliate Program. Mrs. London began teaching at Beth-El School of Nursing and Health Science in 1974 (now part of the University of Colorado, Colorado Springs) after opening the first intensive care nursery at Memorial Hospital of Colorado Springs. She has served in many faculty positions at Beth-El, including assistant director of the School of Nursing. Mrs. London obtained her postmaster's Neonatal Nurse Practitioner certificate and subsequently developed the Neonatal Nurse Practitioner (NNP) certificate and the master's NNP program at Beth-El. She is active nationally in neonatal nursing and was involved in the development of National Neonatal Nurse Practitioner educational program guidelines. Mrs. London and her husband, David, enjoy reading, travel, and hockey games. They have two sons. Craig, who lives in Florida, works with Internet companies. Matthew works in computer teleresearch. Both are more than willing to give Mom helpful hints about computers.

Michele R. Davidson

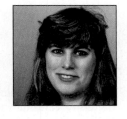

received an ADN degree from Marymount University in 1990 and, upon graduation, began working in postpartum and the newborn nursery in Washington, D.C. She obtained a BSN from George Mason University and then earned her MSN and a nurse-midwifery certificate at Case Western Reserve University. She worked as a nurse-midwife at Columbia Hospital for Women in Washington, D.C., while completing her PhD in nursing administration and healthcare policy from George Mason University (GMU). Dr. Davidson began teaching at GMU in 1999. She is a member of the American College of Nurse Midwives Certification Council, the body that writes the national certification examination for certified nurse-midwives. Dr. Davidson has developed an immersion clinical experience for GMU students on a remote island in the Chesapeake Bay where she teaches community health nursing to students who reside in the community. In 2003, she founded the Smith Island Foundation, a nonprofit organization in which she serves as executive director. In her free time, Michele enjoys spending time with her mother, gardening, reading, and camping with her nurse practitioner husband, Nathan, and their four young children, Hayden, Chloe, Caroline, and Grant.

Thank You

CONTRIBUTORS

We extend a sincere thank you to our contributors, who gave their time, effort, and expertise so tirelessly to develop and write resources that help provide students with the latest information by extending our content beyond the book.

Barbara Cheuvront, BSN, MS
Evidence-in-Action boxes
Regis University
Denver, Colorado

Janet Houser, PhD, RN
Evidence-Based-Practice boxes
Regis University
Denver, Colorado

Barbara McClaskey, PhD, MN, ARNP
Pittsburgh State University
Department of Nursing
Pittsburg, Kansas

Traci Moore, RN, MSN
Nursing Faculty
Caldwell Community College
Hudson, North Carolina

REVIEWERS

With each revision, our goal remains constant—to ensure that our text reflects the most current research and the latest information about nursing. This would not be possible without the support of our colleagues in clinical practice and nursing education. Their suggestions, contributions, and words of encouragement help us achieve this goal. In publishing, as in health care, quality assurance is an essential part of this process—and this is the dimension that reviewers add. We extend a sincere thanks to all those who reviewed the manuscript for this text.

Dwayne Accardo, CRNA, MSNA
University of Tennessee
Memphis, Tennessee

Janice M. Ambrose
York College of Pennsylvania
York, Pennsylvania

Jan Andrews, PhD, RNC, WHNP
Macon State College
Macon, Georgia

Samantha H. Bishop, MN, RN, CPNP
Gordon College
Barnesville, Georgia

Kathleen E. Borcherding, PhD, RN
University of Missouri at St. Louis
St. Louis, Missouri

Julia A. Campbell, RN, MSN
University of Missouri at St. Louis
St. Louis, Missouri

Shelia F. Catlett, MSN, ARNP, IBCLC
Western Kentucky University
Bowling Green, Kentucky

Barbara A. Caton, MSN, RN
Missouri State University–West Plains
West Plains, Missouri

Lynn B. Clutter, MSN, RN, BC, CNS, CNE, IBCLC
Langston University, Tulsa
Tulsa, Oklahoma

Marie A. Cobb, RNC, MSN, CNS, IBCLC
The University of Akron
Akron, Ohio

Kelley Connor, MS, RNC
Boise State University
Boise, Idaho

Teri D. Crawford, RNC, MSN, WHNP
Macon State College
Macon, Georgia

Margot R. De Sevo, PhD, RNC, LCCE, IBCLC
Adelphi University
Garden City, New York

Linda L. Dunn, DSN, RN, CCE
The University of Alabama
Tuscaloosa, Alabama

Susan M. Ellerbee, PhD, RNC, IBCLC
University of Oklahoma,
Oklahoma City, Oklahoma

Christi Emerson, RN, MSN
University of Mary Hardin–Baylor
Belton, Texas

Michele Z. Enlow, RNC, DNP
University of Akron
Akron, Ohio

Karen Ferguson, PhD, RNC
Martin Methodist College
Pulaski, Tennessee

Julia M. Fine, RN, PhD, FNP-BC
Indiana State University
Terre Haute, Indiana

Stacy E. Garrity, RNC, MS, WHNP
Boston College
Chestnut Hill, Massachusetts

Susan Golden, MSN, RN
Eastern New Mexico University –Roswell
Roswell, New Mexico

Sharon Hadenfeldt, PhD, CRNA
BryanLGH Medical Center School of Nurse Anesthesia
Lincoln, Nebraska

Lisa Haynie, PhD, RN, CFNP
University of Mississippi Medical Center
Jackson, Mississippi

Pamela Hetrick, CNM, MSN
University Hospitals Case Medical Center
Cleveland, Ohio

Rita Horgos, BSN, MSN, MEd, RN, CPN
Community College of Allegheny County, South Campus
West Mifflin, Pennsylvania

Debra Hrelic, PhD, RNC
Mount Saint Mary College
Newburgh, New York

Nancy V. Jackson, RN, EdD, C-PNP
New York University
New York, New York

Linda Johnson, MS, RN
Sinclair Community College
Dayton, Ohio

Deborah Hill Ketner, RNC, MSN, CNM
Winston Salem State University
Winston Salem, North Carolina

Kathleen N. Krov, RN, CNM, MSN
Raritan Valley Community College
Somerville, New Jersey

Patricia S. Kupina, RN, MSN, EdD
Joliet Junior College
Joliet, Illinois

Sister Corinne M. Lemmer, PhD, RN
Mount Marty College
Yankton, South Dakota

Lynne Porter Lewallen, PhD, RN, CNE
The University of North Carolina, Greensboro
Greensboro, North Carolina

Karen Lincoln, RNC, MSN
Montcalm Community College
Sidney, Michigan

Jeanne Linhart, RN, MS, FNP-C
Rockland Community College
Suffern, New York

Maria A. Marconi, RN, MS
University of Rochester
Rochester, New York

Denise Marshall, BSN, MEd, EdD
Wor-Wic Community College
Salisbury, Maryland

Kathleen Masters, MS, RN
Monroe Co. Community College
Monroe, Michigan

Magda Sandra McCarthy, MSN, RN
Houston Community College
Houston, Texas

Barbara McClaskey, PhD, MN, ARNP
Pittsburg State University
Pittsburg, Kansas

Dennis J. McKenna, CRNA, MHA
Medical University of South Carolina
Charleston, South Carolina

Jill A. Mishkel, MS, RNC, WHNP
Hampton University
Hampton, Virginia

Traci Moore, RN, MSN
Caldwell Community College
Hudson, North Carolina

Daniel D. Moos, CRNA, MS
BryanLGH College
Lincoln, Nebraska

Mary O'Connor, PhD, RN, BSN, MS
University of Missouri–Kansas City
Kansas City, Missouri

Ellen O'Rourke, MSN, RN
Southeast Missouri State University
Cape Girardeau, Missouri

Tina Paulk, RN, MSN
Gordon College
Wenham, Massachusetts

Melodie Rowbotham, PhD, RN
University of Missouri–St. Louis
St. Louis, Missouri

Ann Schide, MSN, RN, MS, LCCE, CLNC, BSC
Chattanooga State Technical Community College
Chattanooga, Tennessee

Cordia Starling, RN, BSN, MS, EdD
Dalton State College
Dalton, Georgia

Sue G. Thacker, RNC, BSN, MS, PhD
Wytheville Community College
Wytheville, Virginia

Bobbie Walker, MSN, RNC, IBCLC
Montgomery College
Takoma Park, Maryland

Gerry Walker, MSN, RN
Park University
Parkville, Missouri

Robin Wilson, RNC, MSN
Lincoln Memorial University
Harrogate, Tennessee

Michele Woodbeck, MS, RN
Hudson Valley Community College
Troy, New York

Preface

Maternal-newborn nursing is multifaceted, challenging, rewarding, and endlessly varied. Opportunities abound to touch lives and to make a difference. Many nurses opt for a career in mother-baby care and clinic or office nursing so that they can work closely with childbearing families. As these nurses continue their education, they may embrace the role of nurse practitioner, nurse-midwife, genetic counselor, lactation consultant, or childbirth educator. Those nurses who find the most reward by working in intense, highly technical situations are often drawn to the neonatal intensive care unit, to high-risk pregnancy units, or to work with laboring families. As these nurses advance their education, they often choose the clinical specialist role. Some nurses become enthralled by the possibility of shaping the profession for years to come, and so they become nurse managers or administrators, nursing faculty, advocates, influential leaders in national associations such as AWHONN, or even authors. We applaud them, too!

Because of the varied and rich opportunities for nurses, the theme we emphasize in this edition is the many facets of maternal-newborn nursing. This thread is subtly woven throughout the book. You will find it in the chapter opening quotes from nurses in a variety of roles and settings, in the photographs on the cover and part openers, and in the text itself. As authors and educators, it is our hope that we can encourage and inspire students to consider a rewarding career in maternal-newborn nursing.

As always, the underlying philosophy of *Contemporary Maternal-Newborn Nursing Care* remains unchanged. We see pregnancy and childbirth as normal life processes with the family members as co-participants in care. We remain committed to providing a text that is accurate and readable, a text that helps students develop the skills and abilities they need now and in the future in an ever-changing healthcare environment.

ORGANIZATION—A NURSING CARE MANAGEMENT FRAMEWORK

Nurses today must be able to think critically and to solve problems effectively. For these reasons, we begin with an introductory unit to set the stage by providing information about maternal-newborn nursing and important related concepts. Subsequent units progress in a way that closely reflects the steps of the nursing process. We clearly delineate the nurse's role within this framework. Thus, the units related to pregnancy, labor and birth, the newborn period, and postpartum care begin with a discussion of basic theory followed by chapters on nursing assessment and nursing care for essentially healthy women or infants. Within the nursing care chapters and content areas, we use the heading **Nursing Care Management** and the subheadings **Nursing Assessment and Diagnosis, Planning and Implementation**, and **Evaluation**.

Complications of a specific period appear in the last chapter or chapters of each unit. The chapters also use the nursing process as an organizational framework. We believe that students can more clearly grasp the complicated content of the high-risk conditions once they have a good understanding of the normal processes of pregnancy, birth, and postpartal and newborn care. However, to avoid overemphasizing the prevalence of complications in such a wonderfully normal process as pregnancy and birth, we avoid including an entire unit that focuses only on complications. To aid student study we have developed a new chapter, **Childbirth at Risk: Pre-Labor Complications (Chapter 21)**, which focuses on content that impacts both pregnancy and labor and birth. We think you will find the new approach very helpful.

More specialized or distinctive material is sometimes focused in a single chapter, such as the chapters on maternal nutrition, adolescent pregnancy, special diagnostic procedures, and newborn nutrition. For faculty, we provide detailed syllabus suggestions and reading assignments for your course, whether you teach high-risk conditions at the end of the course or integrate them throughout the course. We include this guide in the **Instructor's Resource Manual** and other resources developed specifically for instructors.

THEMES FOR THE SEVENTH EDITION

Evidence-Based Practice

Healthcare professionals are increasingly aware of the importance of using reliable information as the basis for planning and providing effective care. This approach, referred to as evidence-based practice, draws on information from a variety of sources including nursing research. To help nurses become more comfortable in using evidence-based practice, we include a brief discussion of it in Chapter 1, "Complementary Maternal-Newborn Care," and then provide examples of evidence-based practice as it relates to maternal-newborn nursing throughout the textbook. A new feature in this edition, the **Evidence in Action** box, provides a quick "clinical pearl" for effective nursing practice.

Community-Based Nursing Care

Although pregnancy, birth, and the postpartal period cover a period of many months, in reality most women spend only 2 to 3 days, if any, in the hospital. Thus, by its very nature, maternal-newborn nursing is primarily community-based nursing care. This emphasis on nursing care provided in community-based settings is a driving force in health care today and, consequently, forms a dominant theme through this edition. We address this topic in focused, user-friendly ways. For example, **Community-Based Nursing Care** is a special heading used throughout this text. Because we consider home care to be one form of community-based care, it often has a separate heading under Community-Based Nursing Care. Even more important, Chapter 32, "Home Care of the Postpartal Family," provides a thorough explanation of home care, both from a theoretical perspective and as a significant tool in caring for childbearing families.

Emphasis on Client and Family Teaching

Client and family teaching remains a critical element of effective nursing care, one that we continue to emphasize. Our focus is on the teaching that nurses do at all stages of pregnancy and the childbearing process—including the important postpartum teaching that is done before and after families are discharged from the hospital. **Teaching Tips** are included throughout the book. These brief tips provide helpful hints instructing the nurse on how to teach specific items to clients and their families. Also, more detailed discussions of client and family teaching are summarized in **Client Teaching** guides, such as the one on sexual activity during pregnancy. These Client Teaching guides help students plan and organize their thoughts for preparing to teach women and their families. The tearout

Client-Family Teaching Cards in the center of the text are also handy tools for the student to use while studying or as a quick reference in the clinical setting. In addition, a foldout, full-color **Fetal Development Chart** depicts maternal and fetal development by month and provides specific teaching guidelines for each stage of pregnancy. Students can use this chart as another study tool or as a quick clinical reference.

Commitment to Cultural Competence

As nurses and educators, we feel a strong commitment to the importance of acknowledging and respecting diversity and multiculturalism. Thus, we strive continually to make our textbook ever more inclusive, integrating diversity in our photographs, illustrations, case scenarios, and content. Chapter 2, "Culture and the Childbearing Family," lays the foundational concepts for students to develop cultural competence, whereas **Cultural Perspectives** carries the concept forward by providing insights into specific issues related to culture. In addition, integrated into our narrative are a variety of issues and scenarios affecting maternal-newborn nursing care.

Complementary and Alternative Therapies

Nurses and other healthcare professionals recognize that today, more than ever, complementary and alternative therapies have become a credible component of holistic care. To help nurses become more familiar with these therapies, Chapter 2, "Culture and the Childbearing Family," provides basic information on some of the more commonly used therapies. Then, throughout the text, we expand the topic by providing a boxed feature that highlights specific therapies.

Women's Health Care

Women's health care is specifically addressed in Chapter 5, "Health Promotion for Women," and Chapter 6, "Common Gynecologic Problems." Because of the nature of this textbook, we do not address gynecologic cancers. However, we are delighted to announce that you can find information on these disorders in great detail on the book-specific website at MyNursingKit.com.

Features That Help You Use This Textbook Successfully

Instructors and students alike value the in-text learning aids that we include in our textbooks. With this edition, we developed a textbook that is easy to learn from and easy to use as a reference. The following guide will help you use the features and resources from **Contemporary Maternal-Newborn Nursing Care, Seventh Edition** to be successful in the classroom, in the clinical setting, on the NCLEX-RN® examination, and in nursing practice.

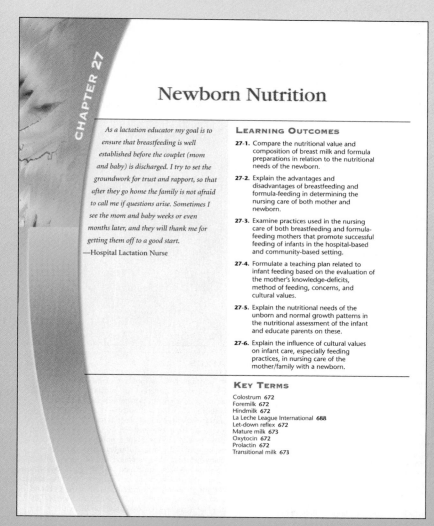

CHAPTER 27

Newborn Nutrition

As a lactation educator my goal is to ensure that breastfeeding is well established before the couplet (mom and baby) is discharged. I try to set the groundwork for trust and rapport, so that after they go home the family is not afraid to call me if questions arise. Sometimes I see the mom and baby weeks or even months later, and they will thank me for getting them off to a good start.
—Hospital Lactation Nurse

LEARNING OUTCOMES

27-1. Compare the nutritional value and composition of breast milk and formula preparations in relation to the nutritional needs of the newborn.

27-2. Explain the advantages and disadvantages of breastfeeding and formula-feeding in determining the nursing care of both mother and newborn.

27-3. Examine practices used in the nursing care of both breastfeeding and formula-feeding mothers that promote successful feeding of infants in the hospital-based and community-based setting.

27-4. Formulate a teaching plan related to infant feeding based on the evaluation of the mother's knowledge-deficits, method of feeding, concerns, and cultural values.

27-5. Explain the nutritional needs of the unborn and normal growth patterns in the nutritional assessment of the infant and educate parents on these.

27-6. Explain the influence of cultural values on infant care, especially feeding practices, in nursing care of the mother/family with a newborn.

KEY TERMS

Colostrum 672
Foremilk 672
Hindmilk 672
La Leche League International 688
Let-down reflex 672
Mature milk 673
Oxytocin 672
Prolactin 672
Transitional milk 673

▲ Each chapter begins with **Learning Outcomes** and a list of **Key Terms**. Page numbers are included with each key term to identify the place where the term first appears in the chapter. New chapter opening **Vignettes** from nurses in a variety of maternal, newborn, and women's health roles illustrate the diversity of career options and settings available in this field. These vignettes reflect the deep satisfaction that these nurses experience in their profession.

h Special Reproductive Concerns **149**

required biologic window of time
ryopreservation.

netic disorders before implantation
the option of forgoing the attempt
cy and thereby avoiding a difficult
ating an affected pregnancy (Simp-
). This technology also raises several
g the following:

ples at risk. There is a need for crite-
les at risk for diseases that constitute
b and suffering so that "wrongful
voided.

access to centers providing PGD.
vide access for those at risk for ge-
sease but without the financial re-
he services?

neres for sex chromosome testing
order carried on the sex chromo-

MyNursingKit | Resolve: The National Infertility Association

▲ **MyNursingKit** tabs appear in the outer margins of the textbook to indicate topics that refer students to specific videos, animations, or website links provided in the accompanying MyNursingKit. For example, students can watch an animation of embryonic heart formation and fetal circulation in Chapter 4.

▶ **Cultural Perspectives** expose students to cultural factors that influence a family's expectations of and responses to their health care provider and their experiences with the health care system.

CULTURAL PERSPECTIVES

Middle East Initial Postpartum Experience

In many countries in the Middle East that follow a patriarchal system, the new mother and her infant stay with the husband's family following the birth of the infant. Frequent visits from the woman's family are discouraged and may even be viewed as burdensome by the husband's family. Typically, only women visit the new mother during the postpartum period. For the birth of the first baby, the wife's parents are expected to purchase all of the baby's supplies and clothing.

EVIDENCE-BASED PRACTICE

Breastfeeding for Low-Birth-Weight and Premature Newborns

Clinical Question

Does breastfeeding low-birth-weight and premature newborns while they are in the NICU demonstrate improved outcomes for the baby?

The Evidence

The benefits of breastfeeding for newborns up to 6 months of age are well documented. However, when these babies require treatment in the Neonatal Intensive Care Unit (NICU), breastfeeding presents challenges for mothers, newborns, and nurses. Research shows that it is possible to successfully establish breastfeeding in more than 90% of preterm and low-birth-weight babies. Several authors in both the United States and internationally used various experimental designs to determine if the efforts made to provide breastfeeding to babies in the NICU resulted in improved outcomes over babies who were not afforded this type of nutrition. Several randomized trials have focused on the outcomes of breastfed high-risk newborns, and one longitudinal study followed a group of 50 breastfed low-birth-weight premature infants to determine if there were long-term benefits of breast milk feeding. The replication of these experiments across settings represents strong evidence for nursing practice.

What Is Effective?

These studies revealed that more than half of the babies who receive breast milk in the NICU will continue breastfeeding after discharge. Premature and low-birth-weight newborns who were fed breast milk in the NICU and continued breastfeeding after discharge had higher scores on a measure of mental development and an index of physical development at 6 months of age. The infants with the higher scores were not necessarily exclusively fed breast milk, but were consistently receiving human milk in some amount from [...] 6 months corrected age. Family support, timely b[...] ing information, and a supportive and encouraging [...]

intensive care unit environment are needed for women to succeed in breastfeeding their hospitalized newborns. The NICU is an ideal environment to instruct and support mothers about human milk feeding because of low nurse/patient-family ratios that allow the nurse to have extended contact with the family. The NICU provides opportunities for teaching and instruction about the health benefits of human milk. Getting started with breastfeeding soon after birth is a critical point.

What Is Inconclusive?

The amount of breast milk needed to achieve these outcomes is unclear; these studies did not measure the quantity of milk but rather whether any breast milk was given at all. Alternatives for the nearly 10% of NICU babies for whom breast milk is not an option were not explored.

Best Practice

You can help mothers of premature and low-birth-weight babies in the NICU to breastfeed to achieve optimal outcomes for the baby. To promote breastfeeding in vulnerable infants, help the mother make an informed decision, establish and maintain her milk supply, feed the baby breast milk that has been pumped, and prepare both the mother and baby for a transition to breastfeeding after discharge.

References

Akerstrom, S., Asplund, I., & Norman, M. (2007). Successful breastfeeding after discharge of preterm and sick newborn infants. *Acta Paediatrica, 96*(10), 1450–1454.

Lessen, R., & Crivelli-Kovach, A. (2007). Prediction of initiation and duration of breastfeeding for neonates admitted to the neonatal intensive care unit. *Journal of Perinatal and Neonatal Nurses, 21*(3), 256–266.

Zukowsky, K. (2007). Breast-fed low-birth-weight premature

◀ **Evidence-Based Practice** boxes relate research evidence to maternal-newborn nursing. These boxes pose a clinical question, offer the research evidence, and ask what is the best practice. Each box includes a critical-thinking activity asking students to apply the evidence to their own practice or to a scenario.

▶ In addition to an introduction in Chapter 2, **Complementary and Alternative Therapies** boxes inform students about therapies their clients might be using or therapies the nurse might safely suggest. In all cases, research is cited for safe practice of these therapies.

COMPLEMENTARY AND ALTERNATIVE THERAPIES

Pain Relief in the NICU

The newborn relies on the nurse's observational, assessment, and interventional skills for anticipation and prevention of pain if possible and then prompt, safe, and effective pain relief. It is vital that the nurse assist infants to cope with and recover from necessary painful clinical procedures (Saniski, 2005). A variety of nonpharmacologic pain-prevention and relief techniques have been shown to be effective in reducing pain from minor procedures in newborns.

Pain can be managed effectively by limiting or avoiding noxious stimuli and by providing analgesia. Any unnecessary stimuli (i.e., noise, visual, tactile, and vestibular) of the newborn should be avoided, if possible (AAP & ACOG, 2007). Developmental care, which includes limiting environmental stimuli, lateral positioning, the use of supportive bedding, and attention to behavioral cues, assists the newborn to cope with painful procedures (AAP & CPS, 2006).

Containment with swaddling or facilitated tucking (holding the arms and legs in a flexed position) is effective in reducing excessive immature motor responses. Swaddling also may provide comfort through other senses, such as thermal, tactile, and proprioceptive senses. Breastfeeding and skin-to-skin contact with the mother during the painful procedure may help to relieve pain. Nonnutritive sucking (NNS) refers to the provision of a pacifier into the infant's mouth to promote sucking without the provision of breast milk or for-

mula for nutrition. NNS is thought to produce analgesia through stimulation of orotactile and mechanoreceptors when the pacifier is placed into the infant's mouth. Allowing nonnutritive sucking with a pacifier aids in the reduction of procedural pain and stress. Unfortunately a rebound in distress occurs when the NNS pacifier is removed from the infant's mouth (Walden, 2007).

A wide range of oral sucrose doses have been used for procedural pain relief (heel sticks, venipuncture, IM injections); but no optimal dose has been established (AAP & CPS, 2006). The sweetness of the sucrose, a disaccharide, elevates the pain threshold through endogenous opioid release in the CNS and produces a calming effect (AAP & CPS, 2006). A range of 0.05 to 0.5 mL of 24% sucrose is administered on the anterior part of the tongue via a syringe or nipple approximately 2 minutes before the procedure (Walden & Jorgensen, 2004). Some authors have suggested that multiple doses, such as giving a dose 2 minutes before and 1 to 2 minutes after a procedure, is more effective. It is important to be careful with repeated doses of sucrose, as the concern for hyperglycemia may arise. Also, repeated use of sucrose analgesia in preterm infants may affect their neurologic development and behavioral outcomes. Until further research is done, repeated doses of sucrose are not recommended (AAP & CPS, 2006). Because oral sucrose reduces but does not eliminate pain, it should be used with other nonpharmacologic measures to enhance effectiveness.

◀ **Teaching Tips** are brief pearls offered from experts to students on how to teach clients and families about specific topics or procedures.

Clinical Pathway — NEWBORN CARE

FIRST 4 HOURS	4 TO 8 HOURS PAST BIRTH	8 TO 24 HOURS PAST BIRTH
REFERRAL		
Review labor/birth record Review transitional nursing record Check ID bands and security alarms if present Consult prn: orthopedics, genetics, infectious disease	Check ID bands and security alarms Transfer to mother-baby care at 4 to 6 hours of age if stable As parents desire, obtain circumcision permit after their discussion with physician Lactation consult prn	Check ID bands and security alarm q shift **Expected Outcomes** Mother/baby ID bands correlate at time of discharge, security alarms in place at all times; consults completed prn
ASSESSMENTS		
Continue assessments begun first hour after birth Vital sign: TPR, BP prn, q1h × 4 (skin temp 36°C to 36.5°C [96.8°F to 97.7°F], resp may be irregular but within 30 to 60 per min) **Newborn Assessments** • Respiratory status with resp. distress scale × 1 then prn. If resp. distress, assess q5–15 min • Cord: bluish white color, clamp in place and free from skin • Color: skin, mucous membranes, extremities, trunk pink with slight acrocyanosis of hands and feet • Wt (5 lb. 8 oz to 8 lb. 13 oz) 2500 to 4000 g, length (18 to 22 in.) 46 to 56 cm, HC (12.5 to 14.5 in.) 32 to 37 cm, CC (32.5 cm, 1 to 2 cm less than head) • Extremity movement—may be jerky or brief twitches • Gestational age classification—term AGA • Anomalies (cong. anomalies can interfere with normal extrauterine adaptation)	Assess newborn's progress through periods of reactivity Vital signs: TPR q8h and prn, or per agency protocol, BP prn **Newborn Assessments** • Skin color q4h prn (circulatory system stabilizing, acrocyanosis decreased) • Eyes for drainage, redness, hemorrhage • Auscultate lungs q4h (noisy, wet breath sounds clear and equal) • Increased mucus production (normal in second period of reactivity) • Check apical pulse q4h • Check umbilical cord base for redness, drainage, foul odor, drying, clamp in place • Extremity movements q4h • Check for expected reflexes (suck, rooting, Moro, grasp, blink, yawn, sneeze, tonic neck, Babinski) • Note common normal variations • Assess suck and swallow during feeding • Note behavioral characteristics • Check temp before and after admission bath	VS q8h; normal ranges: T, 36.4°C to 37.2°C (97.5°F to 99°F) P, 120 to 160; R, 30 to 60; BP, 90–60/50–40 mm Hg **Continue Newborn Assessments** • Skin color q4h • Signs of drying or infection in cord area • Check that clamp is in place until removed before discharge • Check circ. for bleeding after procedure, then q30min × 2, then q4h and prn Observe for jaundice. Obtain serum bili (TsB) if infant visibly jaundiced before 24 hours of age. Obtain transcutaneous bili on all infants not previously tested before discharge. **Expected Outcomes** Vital signs medically acceptable, color pink, assessments WNL, circ. site without s/s infection, cord site without s/s of infection and clamp removed; newborn behavior WNL
TEACHING/PSYCHOSOCIAL		
Admission activities performed at mother's bedside if possible, orient to nursery prn, handwashing, assess teaching needs Teach parents use of bulb syringe, signs of choking, positioning, and when to call for assistance Teach reasons for use of radiant warmer, infant hat, and warmed blankets when out of warmer Discuss/teach infant security, identification	Reinforce teaching about choking, bulb syringe use, positioning, temperature maintenance with clothing and blankets Teach infant positioning to facilitate breathing and digestion Teach new parents holding and feeding skills Teach parents soothing and calming techniques Teach parents [...] newborn to sib[...]	Final discharge teaching: diapering, normal void and stool patterns, bathing, nail and cord care, circumcision/uncircumcised penis/genital care and normal characteristics, rashes, jaundice, sleep-wake cycles, soothing activities, taking temperatures, thermometer reading Explain s/s of illness and when to call

◀ In keeping with the changing approaches to nursing care management, we feature **Clinical Pathways** throughout the text. Four clinical pathways— intrapartal, newborn, postpartal, and cesarean birth—are designed to help students plan and manage care within normally anticipated time frames.

Client Teaching — NEWBORN BATHING

Content	**Teaching Method**
Describe the proper timing and environment (including safety factors) for sponge and tub bathing for newborns.	Clarify information related to sponge bathing and the proper timing of tub baths for safe newborn bathing. Explain that the proper environment is needed for newborn safety and comfort.
Identify proper bathing supplies that are needed for both sponge and tub baths.	Encourage the family to assemble supplies before beginning the newborn bath to avoid cold exposure and ensure that proper supplies are being used.
Demonstrate sponge bathing.	Demonstrate proper technique and encourage the family to ask questions as they arise. Help instill confidence in new parents.
Discuss and demonstrate tub bathing using an infant model. Explain the need for neutral pH, fragrance-free, and dye-free cleansing products for newborn use.	Clarify the need for appropriate cleansing agents for newborns.

▶ **Client Teaching Guides** provide students with a teaching plan to use when educating the client and family about any aspect of self-care or a special healthcare issue.

► To help students hone their critical-thinking skills, **Critical Thinking Case Studies** ask students to consider a brief scenario and to determine the appropriate response in that situation. Suggested answers to the case studies are provided in Appendix H so that students will have immediate feedback on their decision-making skills.

CRITICAL THINKING

You are caring for baby girl Linn, who is a 39-week, AGA female born by repeat cesarean birth to a 34-year-old G3, now P3 mother. Baby Linn's Apgar scores were 7 at 1 minute and 9 at 5 minutes. At 2 hours of age, you note an elevated respiratory rate of 70 to 80 and mild cyanosis. The infant is now receiving 30% oxygen and has a respiratory rate of 100 to 120. The baby's clinical course, chest X-ray examination, and lab work are all consistent with transient tachypnea of the newborn. Her mother calls you to ask about her baby. She tells you that her last child was born at 30 weeks' gestation, had respiratory distress syndrome requiring ventilator support, and was hospitalized for 6 weeks. She asks you, "Is this the same respiratory distress?" What will you tell her?

Answers can be found in Appendix F ∞.

Nursing Care Plan — Care of Newborn with Respiratory Distress

CLIENT SCENARIO

Baby boy Ryan, 3 hours old, born at 36 weeks' gestation weighs 6 lb, 12 oz. Ryan was born by cesarean section to a 26-year-old G1P0 mother. Apgars at birth were 6 at 1 min and 7 at 5 min. (normal range 7–10). On admission to the nursery Ryan's respirations were 80 breaths per minute with noticeable expiratory grunting and suprasternal retractions. The skin was pale and slightly cyanotic. Arterial blood gases showed a Pao_2 of 40 mm Hg and a Pco_2 of 70 mm Hg. Assessment data are consistent with respiratory distress syndrome (RDS). The nurse administers surfactant via endotracheal tube. Ryan was placed under an oxygen hood and continues to remain in the radiant warmer.

ASSESSMENT

Subjective: N/A

Objective: Respirations 80, expiratory grunting, cyanosis, nasal flaring, visible suprasternal retractions, oxygenation saturation 84%, ABGs: Pao_2 of 40 mm Hg and a Pco_2 of 70 mm Hg

► We also provide **Nursing Care Plans** that address nursing care for women who have complications, such as preeclampsia or diabetes mellitus, as well as for high-risk newborns. We designed this information to help prepare students better for the clinical setting.

Nursing Diagnosis #1	Impaired Gas Exchange related to inadequate lung surfactant*
Client Goal	The client will maintain adequate oxygenation and ventilation.
AEB:	• Vital signs within normal limits • No signs of suprasternal retractions, expiratory grunting, or nasal flaring

NURSING INTERVENTIONS

1. Administer surfactant replacement therapy as ordered.

2. Monitor respiratory rate every 2 hours and prn.

3. Assess chest wall movement.

4. Observe newborn for labored respirations.

5. Administer warmed, humidified oxygen to newborn as ordered.

6. Monitor arterial blood gases every 8 hours and prn.

RATIONALES

Rationale: Surfactant improves lung compliance; therefore the need for ventilatory support may be decreased. Surfactant provides alveolar stability by decreasing the alveoli's surface tension and tendency to collapse. Alterations in surfactant quantity, composition, function, or production results in respiratory distress syndrome. Surfactant replacement therapy may be administered via endotracheal tube either in the birthing room or in the nursery.

Rationale: Normal newborn respiratory rate is 30 to 60 breaths per minute. Elevations above 60 breaths per minute may be indicative of respiratory distress. The most frequent and easily detectable sign of respiratory distress is an increased respiratory rate.

Rationale: Respiratory movements that are asymmetrical may reflect pathology such as a pneumothorax or diaphragmatic hernia. Inspection of the chest wall for breathing effort should reflect symmetrical and diaphragmatic respiratory movements.

Rationale: The Silverman-Andersen index may be used to evaluate respiratory distress. Retractions, nasal flaring, and grunting indicate an increase in breathing effort. The Silverman-Andersen index grades retractions, nasal flaring, and grunting according to severity.

Rationale: Oxygenation and ventilatory therapy may prevent hypoventilation and hypoxia. Mild cases of respiratory distress may only require increased humidified oxygen concentrations whereas more severe cases may require continuous positive airway pressure. The nurse may administer oxygen to the newborn experiencing mild respiratory distress via nasal cannula or oxygen hood. With severe respiratory distress mechanical ventilatory assistance from a respirator may be necessary.

Rationale: A failure to synthesize surfactant increases atelectasis which causes hypoxia and acidosis caused by lack of gas exchange. Lung compliance will deteriorate and result in difficulty of inflation, labored respirations, and increased work of breathing. Progressive hypoxia may be seen when arterial blood gas levels are compared and evaluated.

Physical Assessment/ Normal Findings	Alterations and Possible Causes*	Nursing Responses to Data†
Vital Signs		
Blood pressure (BP) At birth: 70–50/ 45–30 mm Hg Day 10: 90/50 mm Hg (may be unable to measure diastolic pressure with standard sphygmomanometer)	Low BP (hypovolemia, shock)	Monitor BP in all cases of distress, prematurity, or suspected anomaly. Low BP: Refer to physician immediately so measures to improve circulation are begun.
Pulse: 120 to 160 bpm (if asleep, as low as 100 bpm; if crying, up to 180 bpm)	Weak pulse (decreased cardiac output) Bradycardia (severe asphyxia) Tachycardia (over 160 bpm at rest) (infection, CNS problems, arrhythmia, stress, hypovolemia)	Assess skin perfusion by blanching (capillary refill test-normal 2-3 sec.). Correlate finding with BP assessments; refer to physician. Carry out neurologic and thermoregulation assessments. Check blood pressure and Hct.
Respirations: 30 to 60 breaths/minute Synchronization of chest and abdominal movements Diaphragmatic and abdominal breathing	Tachypnea (pneumonia, respiratory distress syndrome [RDS]) Rapid, shallow breathing (hypermagnesemia caused by large doses given to mothers with preeclampsia) Respirations below 30 breaths/minute (maternal anesthesia or analgesia)	Identify sleep-wake state; correlate with respiratory pattern. Evaluate for all signs of respiratory distress; report findings to physician.
Transient tachypnea	Expiratory grunting, subcostal and substernal retractions; flaring of nares (respiratory distress); apnea (cold stress, respiratory disorder)	Evaluate for cold stress. Report findings to physician/neonatal nurse practitioner.
Crying: Strong and lusty Moderate tone and pitch	High pitched, shrill (neurologic disorder, hypoglycemia)	Discuss newborn's use of cry for communication.
Cries vary in length from 3 to 7 minutes after consoling measures are used	Weak or absent (CNS disorder, laryngeal problem)	Assess and record abnormal cries. Reduce environmental noises.
Temperature: Axilla 36.4°C to 37.2°C (97.5°F to 99°F)	Elevated temperature (room too warm, too much clothing or covers, dehydration, sepsis, brain damage) Subnormal temperature (brainstem involvement, cold, sepsis)	Notify physician of elevation or drop. Counsel parents on possible causes of elevated or low temperatures, appropriate home-care measures, when to call physician.
Heavier newborns tend to have higher body temperatures	Swings of more than 2°F from one reading to next or subnormal temperature (infection)	Teach parents how to take rectal and/or axillary temperature; assess parents' information regarding use of thermometer; provide teaching as needed.
Weight: 2500 to 4000 g (5 lb. 8 oz to 8 lb. 13 oz)	Less than 2748 g (less than 6 lb) = SGA or preterm infant greater than 4050 g (greater than 9 lb) = LGA or infants of diabetic mothers	Plot weight and gestational age on growth chart to identify high-risk infants. Ascertain body build of parents. Counsel parents regarding appropriate caloric intake.
Within first 3 to 4 days, normal weight loss of 5% to 10% Large babies tend to lose more because of greater fluid loss in proportion to birth weight except infants of diabetic mother	Loss grea loss of m difficultie	
Length: 46 to 56 cm (18 to 22 in.) Grows 10 cm (3 in.) during first 3 months	Less than Short/lor (achondr Short/lor Creveld s	
	*Possible parenthes	

The **Assessment Guides** incorporate physical assessment and normal findings, alterations and possible causes, and guidelines for nursing interventions. These guides prepare students for performing critical assessments on real clients.

Where appropriate, we include **Drug Guides** for those medications commonly used in maternal-newborn nursing. These charts guide students in correctly administering medications.

Drug Guide   Naloxone Hydrochloride (Narcan)

Overview of Neonatal Action   Naloxone hydrochloride (Narcan) is used to reverse respiratory depression caused by acute narcotic toxicity when the mother received a narcotic within 4 hours of birth. It displaces morphine-like drugs from receptor sites on the neurons; therefore the narcotics can no longer exert their depressive effects. It is essentially a pure opioid antagonist. Naloxone reverses narcotic-induced respiratory depression, analgesia, sedation, hypotension, and pupillary constriction.

Route, Dosage, Frequency   Intravenous dose is 0.1 mg/kg (0.25 mL/kg of 0.4 mg/mL concentration) at birth, including for premature infants. This drug is usually given through the umbilical vein or endotracheal tube (ET), although naloxone can be given intramuscularly (delays onset of action) if adequate perfusion exists. For IV push, infuse over at least 1 minute; for ET administration dilute in 1 to 2 milliliters of normal saline (NS).

Reversal of drug depression occurs within 1 to 2 minutes after IV administration and within 15 minutes of IM administration. The duration of action is variable (minutes to hours) and depends on the amount of the drug present and the rate of excretion. Duration of narcotic action often exceeds that of the naloxone. The dose may be repeated in 3 to 5 minutes. If there is no improvement after two or three doses, discontinue naloxone administration. If the initial reversal occurs, repeat the dose as needed (Young & Mangum, 2007).

Neonatal Contraindications   Naloxone should not be administered to infants of mothers who chronically use narcotics or those on methadone maintenance because it may precipitate acute withdrawal syndrome (increased heart rate and blood pressure, vomiting, seizures, tremors).

Respiratory depression may result from nonmorphine drugs, such as sedatives, hypnotics, anesthetics, or other nonnarcotic central nervous system (CNS) depressants.

Neonatal Side Effects   Excessive doses may result in irritability, increased crying, and possible prolongation of partial thromboplastin time (PTT).

Tachycardia may occur.

Nursing Considerations

- Monitor respirations—rate and depth—closely for improved respiratory effort.
- Assess for return of respiratory depression when naloxone effects wear off and effects of longer-acting narcotics reappear.
- Assess continued respiratory depression after positive-pressure ventilation has restored normal heart rate and color.
- Have resuscitative equipment, O₂, and ventilatory equipment available.
- Note that naloxone is incompatible with alkaline solutions such as sodium bicarbonate.
- Store at room temperature and protect from light.
- Remember that naloxone is compatible with heparin.

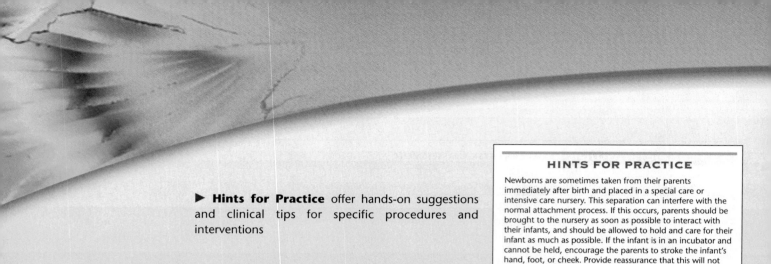

Clinical Skill Performing a Heel Stick on a Newborn

NURSING ACTION	RATIONALE
Preparation	
• Explain to parents what will be done.	
• Select a clear, previously unpunctured site.	*The selection of a previously unpunctured site minimizes the risk of infection and excessive scar formation.*
• The infant's lateral heel is the site of choice because it precludes damaging the posterior tibial nerve and artery, plantar artery, and the important longitudinally oriented fat pad of the heel, which in later years could impede walking (Figure 29–10 ■). This is especially important for infants undergoing multiple heel stick procedures. Toes are acceptable sites if necessary.	
Equipment and Supplies	
• Microlancet (do not use a needle)	
• Alcohol swabs	
• 2 × 2 sterile gauze squares	*A needle may nick the periosteum.*
• Small bandage	
• Transfer pipette or capillary tubes	
• Glucose reagent strips and reflectance meters	
• Gloves	
Procedure	
1. Apply gloves.	*Gloves are used to implement standard precautions and prevent nosocomial infections.*
2. May try warm wet wrap or specially designed chemical heat pad to warm the infant's heel for 5 to 10 seconds to facilitate blood flow.	
Performing the Heel Stick	
1. Grasp the infant's lower leg and foot so as to impede venous return slightly. This will facilitate extraction of the blood sample (Figure 29–11 ■).	

Puncture sites

FIGURE 29–10 Potential sites for heel sticks. Avoid shaded areas to prevent injury to arteries and nerves in the foot.

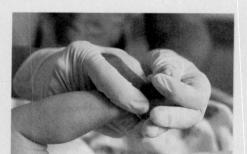

FIGURE 29–11 Heel stick.

- The overall goal of newborn nursing care is to provide comprehensive care while promoting the establishment of a well-functioning family unit.
- In the period immediately after birth, during which adaptation to extrauterine life occurs, the newborn requires close monitoring to identify any deviations from normal.
- Nursing goals during the first 4 hours after birth (admission and transitional period) are to maintain a clear airway, maintain a neutral thermal environment, prevent hemorrhage and infection, initiate oral feedings, and facilitate attachment.
- The newborn is routinely given prophylactic vitamin K to prevent possible hemorrhagic disease of the newborn.
- Prophylactic eye treatment for *Neisseria gonorrhoeae* is legally required for all newborns.
- Nursing goals for ongoing newborn care include maintenance of cardiopulmonary function, maintenance of neutral thermal environment, promotion of adequate hydra-

tion and nutrition, prevention of complications, promotion of safety, and enhancement of attachment and family knowledge of child care.
- Essential daily care includes assessing vital signs, weight, overall color, intake, output, umbilical cord and circumcision, newborn nutrition, parent education, and attachment.
- Following a circumcision, the newborn must be observed closely for signs of bleeding, inability to void, and signs of infection and pain.
- Signs of illness in newborns include temperature above 38°C (100.4°F) axillary or below 36.6°C (97.8°F) axillary, more than one episode of forceful vomiting, refusal of two feedings in a row, lethargy, cyanosis with or without a feeding, and absence of breathing for longer than 20 seconds.
- Newborn screening for congenital hypothyroidism and phenylketonuria may be done on all newborns in the first 1 to 3 days.

◄ Each chapter ends with a chapter review that consists of a summary of **Chapter Highlights**, a list of **References**, and **directions to link to MyNursingKit for additional resources**.

EXPLORE **mynursingkit** PEARSON

MyNursingKit is your one stop for online chapter review materials and resources. Prepare for success with additional NCLEX®-style practice questions, interactive assignments and activities, web links, animations and videos, and more!

Register your access code from the front of your book at
www.mynursingkit.com

American Academy of Pediatrics (AAP). (2008). Car safety seats: A guide for families 2008. Retrieved April 20, 2008, from www.aap.org/family/carseatguide

American Academy of Pediatrics (AAP) & Canadian Paediatric Society (CPS). (2006). Prevention and management of pain in the neonate: An update. *Pediatrics, 118*(5), 2231–2241.

American Academy of Pediatrics (AAP), Committee on Fetus and Newborn & American College of Obstetricians and Gynecologists (ACOG) Committee on Obstetrics. (2007). *Guidelines for perinatal care* (6th ed.). Evanston, IL: Author.

American Academy of Pediatrics (AAP), Newborn Screening Authoring Committee. (2008). Newborn screening expands: Recommendations for pediatricians and medical homes—implications for the system. *Pediatrics, 121*(1), 192–217.

American Academy of Pediatrics (AAP). Task Force on Sudden Infant Death Syndrome. (2005). The changing concept of sudden infant death syndrome: Diagnostic coding shifts, controversies regarding the sleeping environment, and new variables to consider in reducing risk. *Pediatrics, 116*(5), 1245–1255.

American College of Obstetricians and Gynecologists (ACOG), Committee on Genetics. (2003). Newborn screening (ACOG Committee Opinion No. 287). *Obstetric Gynecology, 102,* 887–889.

Andrews, M. M. (2008). Transcultural perspectives in the nursing care of children and adolescents.

In M. M. Andrews & J. S. Boyle (Eds.), *Transcultural concepts in nursing care* (5th ed., pp. 116–145). Philadelphia: Lippincott.

Askin, D. (2008). Newborn adaptations to extrauterine life. In K. R. Simpson & P. A. Creehan, *Perinatal nursing* (3rd ed., pp. 527–545). Philadelphia: Lippincott Williams & Wilkins.

Association of Women's Health, Obstetric and Neonatal Nurses (AWHONN). (2001). *Evidence-based clinical practice guideline: Neonatal skin care.* Washington, DC: Author.

Blackburn, S. T. (2007). *Maternal, fetal, & neonatal physiology: A clinical perspective* (3rd ed.). St. Louis: Saunders.

Creehan, P. A. (2008). Newborn physical assessment. In K. R. Simpson & P. A. Creehan, *Perinatal nursing.* (3rd ed., pp. 546–574). Philadelphia: Lippincott Williams & Wilkins.

D'Avanzo, C. E., & Geissler, E. M. (2008). *Pocket guide to cultural assessment* (4th ed.). St. Louis, MO: Mosby.

Green-Hernandez, G., Quinne, A., Falkenstern, S., Denman-Vitale, S., & Judge-Ellis, T. (2004). Making nursing care culturally competent. *Holistic Nursing Practice,* July/August, 215–218.

Hedayat, K. M. (2001). Issues in Islamic biomedical ethics: A primer for the pediatrician. *Pediatrics, 108*(4), 965–971.

Karl, D. J. (2004). Using principles of newborn behavioral state organization to facilitate breastfeeding. *MCN American Journal of Maternal Child Nursing, 29*(5), 292–298.

Klaus, M., & Klaus, P. (1985). *The amazing newborn.* Menlo Park, CA: Addison-Wesley.

Lipson, J. G., & Dibble, S. L. (2008). Culture & Clinical Care. (7th ed.). San Francisco, CA: The Regents, University of California.

Medves, J. M., & O'Brien, B. (2004). The effect of bather and location of first bath on maintaining thermal stability in newborns. *Journal of Obstetric, Gynecologic, and Neonatal Nursing, 33*(2), 175–182.

Ott, B., Al-Khadhuri, J., & Al-Junaibi, S. (2003). Preventing ethical dilemmas: Understanding Islamic health care practices. *Pediatrics, 29*(3), 227–230.

Roach, J. A. (2004). Newborn stimulation: Preventing over-stimulation is key for optimal growth & well-being. *AWHONN Lifelines, 7*(6), 531–535.

Thureen, P. J., Deacon, J., Hernandez, J. A., & Hall, D. M. (2005). *Assessment and care of the well newborn.* (2nd ed.). St. Louis: Elsevier Sa...

Wilson, B. A., Shannon, M. T., & Shields, K. N. (2009). *Prentice Hall nurse's drug guide 20...* Upper Saddle River, NJ: Pearson Educati...

World Health Organization. (1999). Care of umbilical cord: A review of the evidence line]. Retrieved June 21, 2008 from www... int/rht/documents/MSM98-4

World Health Orgnaization (2008). Male circumcision information package. [On-... Retrieved June 20, 2008 from www.who.i... pub/malecircumcision/infopack/en/inde...

▶ **Key Facts to Remember** summarize important information to recall for student review and for test or clinical preparation.

KEY FACTS TO REMEMBER

Signs of Postpartal Hemorrhage

Excessive or bright-red bleeding (saturation of more than one pad per hour)
A boggy fundus that does not respond to massage
Abnormal clots
High temperature
Any unusual pelvic discomfort or backache
Persistent bleeding in the presence of a firmly contracted uterus
Rise in the level of the fundus of the uterus
Increased pulse or decreased BP
Hematoma formation or bulging/shiny skin in the perineal area
Decreased level of consciousness

Acknowledgments

We are especially grateful to Janet Houser, PhD, RN, for contributing content and boxes on evidence-based practice to this edition, and to Barbara Cheuvront, MS, RN, for developing the Evidence-in-Action boxes. Both have wide, varied backgrounds in nursing and are born teachers.

A project of this scope is not possible without the skill and expertise of many. And so we extend special thanks to the following people.

First and foremost, we are grateful to our editor, Pamela Lappies, for her support and encouragement throughout this process. She remained strong, supportive, and unfailingly optimistic as we dealt with many changes and personal challenges. We appreciate her more than we can say.

As always, we are grateful to Editor-in-Chief Maura Connor, for her support of this book and us as authors. She is committed to providing a wide range of tools to enrich nursing education and we look forward to many years of collaboration.

Julie Alexander, our publisher, has delineated a vision for the future and a commitment to excellence for Pearson Health Science. Her energy, responsiveness, and forward thinking are awe-inspiring and challenge us to give our best. We anticipate a long and exciting relationship with this very special woman.

Special thanks to Marion Waldman and Jill Rembetski, who handled the developmental editing of this edition.

Their organizational skills and eye for detail have helped us produce a strong, readable edition. They make a great team!

We also extend our deep appreciation to Lynn Steines of S4Carlisle Publishing Services. She assumed the Herculean task of steering the book through all phases of production. She was effective in her role, patient and gracious in her interactions, and responsive to our needs when scheduling problems arose.

We are also grateful to Chris Feldman for his skillful copy editing. His work improved our manuscript and helped ensure consistency.

This is a time of possibilities for nursing. The need for skilled nurses has never been higher, nor have the opportunities to make a real difference in the lives of childbearing families ever been greater. Time and again we have seen the difference a skilled nurse can make in the lives of people in need. We, like you, are committed to helping all nurses recognize and take pride in that fact. Thank you for your letters, your comments, and your suggestions. We feel embraced by your support.

PWL
MLL
MRD

Contents

GUIDE TO SPECIAL FEATURES

Key Facts to Remember

Nursing Care Plan

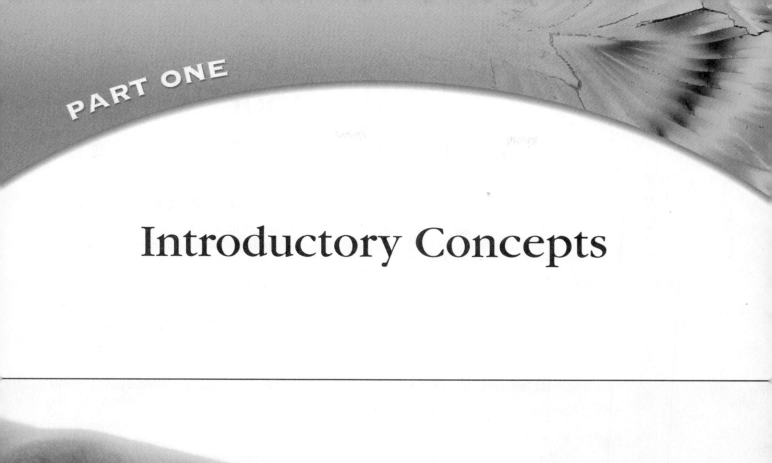

PART ONE

Introductory Concepts

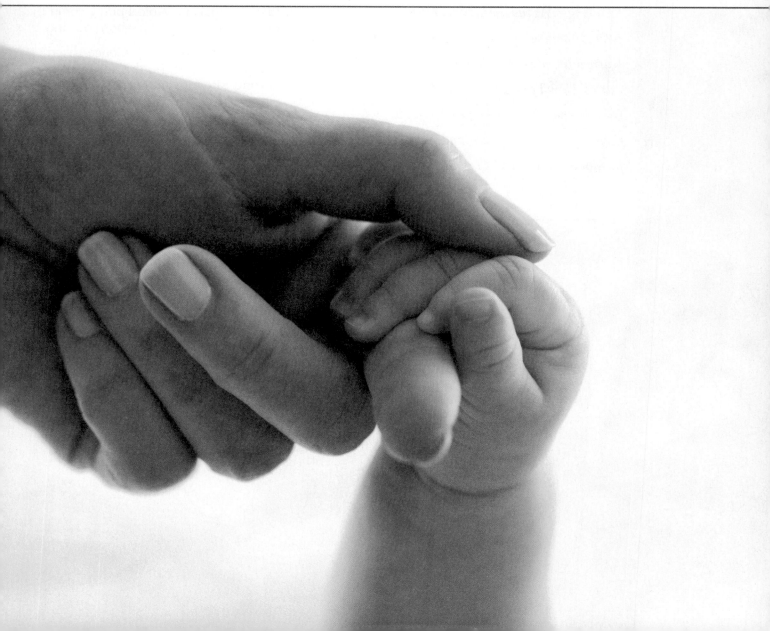

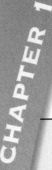

CHAPTER 1

Contemporary Maternal-Newborn Care

The opportunities I've had as a nurse are amazing. I've been an Air Force nurse and a hospital staff nurse. I thought I could never love any type of nursing more than I loved the mother-baby unit, but then I became a nurse practitioner and found wonderful new challenges. At the same time, I became a faculty member at a local university and learned the joy of helping to shape future nurses. Now I am the dean of the program. Do you know how lucky I am? I am 57, I've been a nurse for 36 years, and I am still passionate about what I do!

LEARNING OUTCOMES

1-1. Distinguish between the education, qualifications, and scope of practice in nurses caring for childbearing families.

1-2. Describe the use of community-based nursing care in meeting the needs of childbearing families.

1-3. Identify the nursing roles available to the maternal-newborn nurse.

1-4. Identify legal and ethical principles in the practice of maternal-newborn nursing.

1-5. Identify the impact of evidence-based practice in improving the quality of nursing care for childbearing families.

1-6. Explain how nurses can use descriptive and inferential statistics in clinical practice in maternal-child health nursing.

1-7. Discuss how available statistical data can be used to formulate further research questions.

KEY TERMS

Assisted reproductive technology (ART) **9**
Birth rate **13**
Certified nurse-midwife (CNM) **3**
Certified registered nurse (RNC) **3**
Clinical nurse specialist (CNS) **3**
Evidence-based practice **11**
Infant mortality rate **14**
Informed consent **7**
Intrauterine fetal surgery **9**
Maternal mortality rate **14**
Nurse practitioner (NP) **3**
Nurse researcher **3**
Professional nurse **3**
Therapeutic insemination (TI) **9**

The practice of most nurses is filled with special moments, shared experiences, times in which they know they have practiced the essence of nursing and, in so doing, touched a life. What is the essence of nursing? Simply stated, nurses care *for* people, care *about* people, and use their expertise to help people help themselves. Skilled nurses view clients and families holistically, with a clear realization that a myriad of factors have shaped each individual's perceptions. Such nurses recognize and respect the influence of a host of factors such as upbringing, religious beliefs, culture, socioeconomic status, and life experiences.

The following situation demonstrates the impact a skilled nurse can have by practicing from a framework that considers a client holistically.

Years ago, when I had only been teaching nursing for a few years, before I had even begun working on this text, I had an experience that shaped my view of nursing practice forever. My first pregnancy had ended in a miscarriage at 8 weeks' gestation, so when I became pregnant again we decided to wait until I was a full 3 months along to tell our families. We had had a dinner for both sets of parents to share our news. Everyone was so excited, especially my folks, because this would be their first grandchild. Scarcely 24 hours later, as I was putting away some laundry, I felt a trickle of blood down my leg and knew what it might mean. We rushed to the hospital and, a short time later, I passed a small fetus in the Johnny cap the nurse had placed in the commode. My poor baby was so tiny, only about 3 inches long. We called the nurse, who came and took my baby away.

I sat on the side of the bed and sobbed as my husband sought to console me. The nurse returned a few minutes later and said, "I saw on your record that you are Catholic. Would you like me to baptize your baby?" I was amazed and humbled by her suggestion. She had thought of something that I had not yet even considered. Filled with gratitude, I said, "Oh, yes, please." And she left. Even in my grief, I recognized the meaningfulness of her act.

Later as I relived that day and considered the significance of the care I received, I realized that I had been incredibly fortunate to have a nurse who showed me so very clearly that I was a person, an individual in need of personalized care. I vowed that I would practice nursing in the same holistic way. I also began sharing my story with the students I taught so that they could recognize the difference an expert, caring nurse can make.

We believe that many nurses who work with childbearing families are experts: They are sensitive, intuitive, and technically skilled. They are empowered professionals who can collaborate effectively with others and advocate for those individuals and families who need their support. They view clients holistically and can support the efforts of childbearing families to make decisions about their needs and desires. They can foster independence and self-reliance. Such nurses do make a difference in the quality of care that childbearing families receive.

Nursing Roles

The depth of care provided by nurses caring for women and for childbearing families depends on the nurses' education, qualifications, and scope of practice. A **professional nurse** has graduated from an accredited basic program in nursing, has successfully completed the nursing licensure examination (NCLEX), and is currently licensed as a registered nurse (RN). RNs may be found working as labor nurses, mother-baby nurses, lactation consultants, clinic nurses, newborn nursery nurses, home health nurses, adult or newborn intensive care nurses, gynecology unit nurses, and the like. A **certified registered nurse (RNC)** has shown expertise in a field by taking a national certification exam. A **nurse practitioner (NP)** has received specialized education in a doctor of nursing practice (DNP) program, a master's degree program, or a certificate program and thus can function in an advanced practice role. Nurse practitioners often provide ambulatory care services to expectant families, and, in the case of neonatal nurse practitioners (NNPs), they care for newborns. Some NPs function in acute care, high-risk settings. They focus on physical and psychosocial assessments, including history, physical examination, and certain diagnostic tests and procedures. Nurse practitioners make clinical judgments and begin appropriate treatments, seeking physician consultation when necessary. The emerging emphasis on community-based care has greatly increased opportunities for NPs.

The **clinical nurse specialist (CNS)** has a master's degree and specialized knowledge and competence in a specific clinical area. CNSs are often found on mother-baby units or in the intensive care nursery assisting staff to provide excellent, evidence-based care.

The **certified nurse-midwife (CNM)** is educated in the two disciplines of nursing and midwifery and is certified by the American College of Nurse-Midwives (ACNM). The CNM is prepared to manage independently the care of women at low risk for complications during pregnancy and birth and the care of healthy newborns (Figure 1–1 ■).

The **nurse researcher** has an advanced doctoral degree, typically a PhD, and assumes a leadership role in generating new research. Nurse researchers are generally found in university settings although more and more hospitals are employing them to conduct research relevant to health care, administrative issues, and the like.

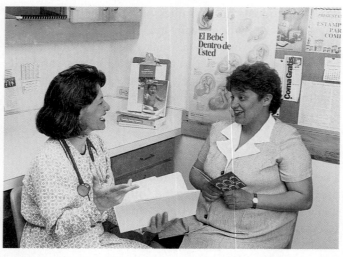

FIGURE 1-1 A certified nurse-midwife confers with her client.

Contemporary Childbirth

Contemporary childbirth is characterized by an emphasis on the family. Today the concept of family-centered childbirth is accepted and encouraged. Fathers are active participants, not simply bystanders; siblings are encouraged to visit and meet the newest family member, and they may even attend the birth. In addition, new definitions of family are evolving. For example, the family of a single mother may include her mother, her sister, another relative, a close friend, the father of the child, or a same-sex partner. Many cultures also recognize the importance of extended families, in which the expectant woman's mother, sister, or other family member may provide care and support (see Chapter 2 ∞).

Contemporary childbirth is also characterized by an increasing number of choices about the birth experience. The family can make choices about the primary caregiver (physician, certified nurse-midwife, or lay midwife), the place of birth (hospital, birthing center, or home), the approaches to childbirth (Lamaze, Bradley, and so forth), birth-related experiences (position for birth and use of analgesia and anesthesia, for example), as well as breast-feeding and childcare choices.

Many women elect to have their pregnancy and birth managed by a certified nurse-midwife (CNM) (see previous discussion). Some women choose to receive care from a direct-entry certified midwife or even a lay midwife (an unlicensed or uncertified midwife who is trained through an informal route such as apprenticeship or self-study rather than a formal educational program (Midwives Alliance of North America [MANA], 2006). Midwives who complete a direct-entry midwifery education program that meets the standards established by ACNM may take a certification exam to become a *certified midwife (CM)*. ACNM has mandated that, by 2010, a master's or doctoral degree will be required for entry into clinical practice as either a CNM or CM (ACNM, 2005).

The North American Registry of Midwives (NARM) is also a certification agency. Midwives certified through NARM may become midwives through a formal educational program at a college, university, or midwifery school, or through apprenticeship or self-study. They are eligible to use the credential *certified professional midwife (CPM)*.

The place of birth is an important decision. As discussed in Chapter 8 ∞, birthing centers and special homelike labor–delivery–recovery–postpartum (LDRP) rooms in hospitals have become increasingly popular. Some women choose to give birth at home, although healthcare professionals do not generally recommend this approach. Most professionals are concerned that, in the event of an unanticipated complication, delay in receiving emergency care might jeopardize the well-being—or even the life—of the mother or her infant. Consequently, the majority of home births are attended by CMs, CPMs, or lay midwives.

In many areas of the United States there is a movement from normal to high-tech birthing. This movement is influenced in part by childbearing families, sometimes called generation Y or the iGeneration, who have grown up with technology and know no other way. They may view elective induction and mother-requested caesarean birth as accepted options, for example. This movement is often reinforced by caregivers who, aware of legal liability issues, practice defensive medicine. Furthermore, many hospitals now support a high-tech model of maternity care because it is "easier" to manage more labouring women if their pain is controlled by epidurals and their contractions are monitored by electronic fetal monitors (Zwelling, 2008). We are troubled by this trend away from family-focused care and encourage nurses to take action to counteract the trend, beginning by analyzing personal attitudes and beliefs about childbirth.

Zwelling (2008) has identified several actions that nurses can take to promote normal childbirth including:

- Advocating vigorously within the community for normal childbirth
- Working to ensure that childbirth preparation classes are readily available
- Increasing personal labor support skills as well as technical skills
- Accepting doulas as part of the labor team
- Promoting changes in the birth environment where they work
- Participating in interdisciplinary committees to develop and implement standardized practices for care

The Healthcare Environment

In 1960, healthcare costs in the United States accounted for approximately 5% of the gross domestic product (GDP). In 2004 the healthcare share of the GDP was 16%, a staggering percentage. Despite this increase in spending, however, not all pregnant women and children in the United States have access to health care. In 2005, 16% of people under age 65 (41 million) were without health insurance (Cohen & Martinez, 2006).

For women who become pregnant, early prenatal care is one of the most important approaches available to reduce adverse pregnancy outcomes. In 2004, 84% of pregnant women in the United States began prenatal care in the first trimester. However, these percentages vary significantly among groups, from 89% for non-Hispanic white women to 70% for American Indian women (National Center for Health Statistics [NCHS], 2006).

Changes in the healthcare environment are influencing women's health and maternal-newborn nursing. Several factors, including demographic changes, the nationally recognized need to improve access to care, public demand for more effective healthcare options, new research findings, and women's preferences for health care, are contributing to changes in the field. Changes are predicted in clinical procedures, provider roles, care settings, and financing of care. As access to health care and the need to control costs increase, so will the need for, and use of, nurses in many roles—especially in advanced practice.

Culturally Competent Care

The U.S. population becomes more diverse every day. Currently more than one-third of all children less than 20 years of age are from families of minority populations. Thus, it is vitally important that nurses who care for women and for childbearing families recognize the importance of a family's cultural values and beliefs, which may be quite different from those of the nurse.

Specific elements that contribute to a family's value system include the following:

- Religion and social beliefs
- Presence and influence of the extended family, as well as socialization within the ethnic group
- Communication patterns
- Beliefs and understanding about the concepts of health and illness
- Beliefs about propriety of physical contact with strangers
- Education

When the family's cultural and social values are incorporated into the plan of care, the family is more likely to cooperate with the plan, especially in the home setting. By learning about the values, religious beliefs, traditions, and practices of local ethnic groups, nurses can develop an individualized nursing care plan for each childbearing woman and her family.

Because of the importance of culturally competent care, this topic is discussed in more depth in Chapter 2 ∞ and throughout the book as well.

CULTURAL PERSPECTIVES

Conflicts can occur with a childbearing woman and her family when traditional rituals and practices of the family's elders do not conform with current healthcare practices. Nurses need to be sensitive to the potential implications for the woman's health and that of her newborn, especially after they are discharged home. When cultural values are not part of the nursing care plan, a woman and her family may be forced to decide whether the family's beliefs should take priority over the healthcare professional's guidance.

Complementary Therapies

Interest in complementary and alternative therapies, sometimes called complementary and alternative medicine (CAM), continues to grow nationwide and affects the care of childbearing families. CAM includes a wide array of therapies including, for example, acupuncture, acupressure, aromatherapy, therapeutic touch, biofeedback, massage therapy, meditation, yoga, herbal therapies, and homeopathic remedies. Concepts related to the use of CAM by childbearing families are addressed in more detail in Chapter 2 ∞ and in special boxed features found throughout the text.

Community-Based Nursing Care

Primary care is the focus of much attention as caregivers search for a new, more effective direction for health care. Primary care includes a focus on health promotion, illness prevention, and individual responsibility for one's own health. These services are best provided in community-based settings. Community-based healthcare systems providing primary care and some secondary care are becoming available in schools, workplaces, homes, churches, clinics, transitional care programs, and other ambulatory settings.

Response to Managed Care

Community-based care has increased in part as a response to third-party payers and managed care organizations, which are beginning to recognize the importance of primary care in containing costs and maintaining health. The growth and diversity of managed care plans offer both opportunities and challenges for women's health care. The potential exists for managed care organizations to work with consumers to provide a model for coordinated and comprehensive well-woman care that includes improved delivery of screening and preventive services. At the same time, managed care organizations face the challenge of integrating essential community providers of care, such as family-planning clinics or women's health centers, which offer a unique service or serve groups of women with special needs (adolescents, women with disabilities, and ethnic or racial minorities). In addition, community-based care remains an essential element of health care for individuals who benefit from public programs such as Medicare or state-sponsored health-related programs.

Response to Consumer Demand

Community-based care is also part of a trend initiated by consumers, who are asking for a "seamless" system of family-centered, comprehensive, coordinated health care, health education, and social services. This seamless system requires coordination as clients move from primary care services to acute care facilities and then back into the community. Nurses can assume this care-management role and perform an important service for individuals and families.

Community-based care is especially important in maternal-child nursing because the vast majority of health care provided to childbearing women and their families takes place outside of hospitals—in clinics, offices, community-based organizations, and private homes. In addition, maternal-child nurses offer specialized services such as childbirth preparation classes and postpartal exercise classes that typically take place outside of hospitals. In essence, we are already expert at providing community-based nursing care; however, it is important that we remain knowledgeable about current practices and trends and open to new ways of meeting the needs of women and children.

Home Care

Providing health care in the home is an especially important dimension of community-based nursing care. Shorter hospital stays end in the discharge of individuals who still require support, assistance, and teaching. Home care helps fill this gap. Conversely, home care enables some individuals to remain at home with conditions such as pregnancy-related complications that formerly would have required hospitalization.

Nurses are the major providers of home care services. Home care nurses perform direct nursing care and also supervise unlicensed assistive personnel who provide less-skilled levels of service. In a home setting, nurses use their skills in assessment, therapeutics, communication, teaching, problem solving, and organization to meet the needs of childbearing women and their families. They also play a major role in coordinating services from other providers, such as physical therapists and lactation consultants.

Postpartum and newborn home visits help ensure a satisfactory transition from the birthing center to the home. We see this trend as positive and hope that this method of meeting the needs of childbearing families will become standard practice. Chapter 32 ∞ discusses home care and provides guidance about making a home visit. Throughout the text we have also provided informa-

tion on the use of home care to meet the needs of pregnant women with health problems, such as diabetes or preterm labor. We believe that home care offers nurses the opportunity to function in an autonomous role and make a significant difference for individuals and families.

Client Teaching in Contemporary Care

The physical and psychologic changes of pregnancy are dramatic and occasionally disconcerting, even for women who have planned their pregnancy. Effective, thoughtful, and carefully timed teaching can help prepare women for the changes they will encounter throughout the trimesters of pregnancy. In addition, anticipatory guidance can help women and their loved ones plan for the birth of the baby and beyond.

In the early 1990s, women who gave birth vaginally remained in the hospital for about 3 days. This provided time for nurses to assess the family's knowledge and skill and to complete essential teaching. In an effort to control costs, discharge within 12 to 24 hours after birth became the norm. This practice did not necessarily cause problems for women with supportive families, thorough prenatal preparation, and adequate resources for necessary follow-up care. However, because early discharge severely limits the time available for client teaching, women with little knowledge, experience, or support were often inadequately prepared to care for themselves and their newborns. Fortunately, the

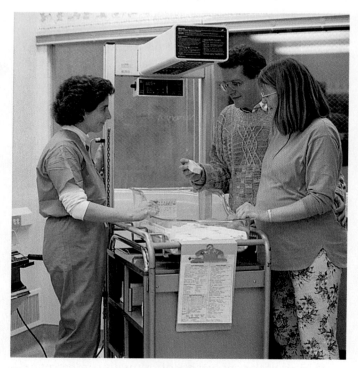

FIGURE 1–2 Individualized education for childbearing couples is one of the prime responsibilities of the maternal-newborn nurse.

negative impact of this practice gained recognition nationwide and resulted in legislation that provides for a postpartum stay of up to 48 hours following a vaginal birth and up to 96 hours following a cesarean birth at the discretion of the mother and her healthcare provider. Nevertheless, nurses are challenged to prepare parents adequately—especially first-time parents—for postpartum and infant care. For this reason, the ability to provide concise and effective teaching is especially important (see Figure 1–2 ■). Nurses can also supplement the teaching they complete with informational handouts and referral to community agencies when indicated.

Legal Considerations

Scope of Practice

The *scope of practice* is defined as the limits of nursing practice set forth in state statutes. Although some state practice acts continue to limit nursing practice to the traditional responsibilities of providing client care related to health maintenance and disease prevention, most state practice acts cover expanded practice roles that include collaboration with other health professionals in planning and providing care, physician-delegated diagnosis and prescriptive privilege, and the delegation of client care tasks to other specified licensed and unlicensed personnel. Specified care activities for certified nurse-midwives and women's health, perinatal, and neonatal nurse practitioners may include diagnosis and prenatal management of uncomplicated pregnancies (CNMs may also manage births) and prescribing and dispensing medications under protocols in specified circumstances. A nurse must function within the scope of practice or risk being accused of practicing medicine without a license.

Standards of Nursing Care

Standards of care establish minimum criteria for competent, proficient delivery of nursing care. Such standards are designed to protect the public and are used to judge the quality of care provided. Legal interpretation of actions within standards of care is based on what a reasonably prudent nurse with similar education and experience would do in similar circumstances.

A number of different sources publish written standards of care. The American Nurses' Association (ANA) has published standards of professional practice written by the ANA Congress for Nursing Practice. The ANA Divisions of Practice have also published standards, including the standards of practice for maternal-child health. Organizations such as the Association of Women's Health, Obstetric, and Neonatal Nurses (AWHONN), the National Association of Neonatal Nurses (NANN), and the

Association of Operating Room Nurses (AORN) have developed standards for specialty practice. Agency policies, procedures, and protocols also provide appropriate guidelines for care standards. The Joint Commission (previously called JCAHO, which is an acronym for the Joint Commission on the Accreditation of Healthcare Organizations), a nongovernmental agency that audits the operation of hospitals and healthcare facilities, has also contributed to the development of nursing standards.

Some standards carry the force of law; others, although not legally binding, carry important legal significance. Any nurse who fails to meet appropriate standards of care may be subject to allegations of negligence or malpractice. However, any nurse who practices within the guidelines established by an agency, or follows local or national standards, is assured that clients are provided with competent nursing care, which, in turn, decreases the potential for litigation.

Clients' Rights

Clients' rights encompass such topics as safety, informed consent, and the right to privacy.

Client/Patient Safety

The Joint Commission has identified patient safety as an important responsibility of healthcare providers, and established the patient safety goals as requirements for accreditation. These goals and requirements, which are updated regularly, can be found on the Joint Commission website.

Informed Consent

Informed consent is a legal concept that protects a client's right to autonomy and self-determination by specifying that no action may be taken without that person's prior understanding and freely given consent. Although this policy is usually enforced for such major procedures as surgery or regional anesthesia, it pertains to any nursing, medical, or surgical intervention. To touch a person without consent (except in an emergency) constitutes battery. Consent is not informed unless the woman understands the recommended procedures or treatments, their rationales, the benefits of each, and any associated risks. To be a truly active participant in decision making about her care, the client should also understand other possible alternatives. When possible, it is important to have translators available for non-English-speaking women. If no translator is available it may be necessary to rely on a family member.

The person who is ultimately responsible for the treatment or procedure should provide the information necessary to obtain informed consent. In most instances, this is the physician. In such cases, the nurse's role is to witness the client's signature giving consent. If the nurse determines that the client does not understand the procedure or risks, the nurse must notify the physician, who must then provide additional information to ensure that the consent is informed. Anxiety, fear, pain, and medications that alter consciousness may influence an individual's ability to give informed consent. An oral consent is legal, but written consent is easier to defend in a court of law.

Society grants parents the responsibility and authority to give consent for their minor children (generally under age 18). Special problems can occur in maternal-newborn nursing when a very young minor gives birth. It is possible that, depending on state law, the very young mother may consent to treatment for her newborn but not for herself. In most states, however, a pregnant teenager is considered an emancipated minor and may therefore give consent for herself as well.

Refusal of a treatment, medication, or procedure after appropriate information is provided also requires that a client sign a form releasing the doctor and clinical facility from liability resulting from the effects of such a refusal. The refusal of blood transfusions or Rh immune globulin by Jehovah's Witnesses is an example of such refusal.

Nurses are responsible for educating clients about any nursing care provided. Before each nursing intervention, the maternal-newborn nurse lets the woman know what to expect, thus ensuring her cooperation and obtaining her consent. Afterward, the nurse documents the teaching and the learning outcomes in the woman's record. The importance of clear, concise, and complete nursing records cannot be overemphasized. These records are evidence that the nurse obtained consent, performed prescribed treatments, reported important observations to the appropriate staff, and adhered to acceptable standards of care.

Right to Privacy

The *right to privacy* is the right of a person to keep her or his person and property free from public scrutiny. Maternity nurses must remember that this includes avoiding unnecessary exposure of the childbearing woman's body. To protect the woman, only those responsible for her care should examine her or discuss her case.

Most states have recognized the right to privacy through statutory or common law, and some states have written that right into their constitution. The ANA, the National League for Nursing (NLN), and the Joint Commission have adopted professional standards protecting clients' privacy. Healthcare agencies should also have written policies dealing with client privacy. The Health Insurance Portability and Accountability Act (HIPAA) of 1996, which was fully implemented in 2002, also has a provision to guarantee the security and privacy of health information.

Laws, standards, and policies about privacy specify that information about clients' treatment, condition, and prognosis can be shared only by health professionals responsible for their care. Information considered as vital statistics (name, age, occupation, and so on) may be revealed legally but is often withheld because of ethical considerations. The client should be consulted regarding what information may be released and to whom. When the client is a celebrity or is considered newsworthy, inquiries by the media are best handled by the agency's public relations department.

Special Ethical Issues in Maternity Care

Although ethical dilemmas confront nurses in all areas of practice, those related to pregnancy, birth, and the newborn seem especially difficult to resolve.

Maternal-Fetal Conflict

Until fairly recently, the fetus was viewed legally as a nonperson. Mother and fetus were viewed as one complex client—the pregnant woman—of which the fetus was an essential part. However, advances in technology have permitted the physician to treat the fetus and monitor fetal development. The fetus is increasingly viewed as a client separate from the mother. This focus on the fetus intensified in 2002 when President George W. Bush announced that "unborn children" would qualify for government healthcare benefits. This move was designed to promote prenatal care but it represented the first time that any U.S. federal policy had defined childhood as starting at conception.

Most women are strongly motivated to protect the health and well-being of their fetus. In some instances, however, women have refused interventions on behalf of the fetus, and forced interventions have occurred. These include forced cesarean birth; coercion of mothers who practice high-risk behaviors such as substance abuse to enter treatment; and, perhaps most controversial, mandating experimental *in utero* therapy or surgery in an attempt to correct a specific birth defect. These interventions infringe on the mother's autonomy. They may also be detrimental to the baby if, as a result, maternal bonding is hindered, the mother is afraid to seek prenatal care, or the mother is herself harmed by the actions taken.

Attempts have also been made to criminalize the behavior of women who fail to follow a physician's advice or who engage in behaviors (such as substance abuse) that are considered harmful to the fetus. This raises two thorny questions: (1) What practices should be monitored? and (2) Who will determine when the behaviors pose such a risk to the fetus that the courts should intervene?

TABLE 1–1	Rationale for Avoiding Coercive and Punitive Approaches to the Maternal-Fetal Relationship

1. Coercive and punitive legal approaches to pregnant women who refuse medical advice fail to recognize that all competent adults are entitled to informed consent and bodily integrity.

2. Court-ordered interventions in cases of informed refusal, as well as punishment of pregnant women for their behavior that may put a fetus at risk, neglect the fact that medical knowledge and predictions of outcomes in obstetrics have limitations.

3. Coercive and punitive policies treat medical problems such as addiction and psychiatric illness as if they were moral failings.

4. Coercive and punitive policies are potentially counter-productive in that they are likely to discourage prenatal care and successful treatment, adversely affect infant mortality rates, and undermine the physician–patient relationship.

5. Coercive and punitive policies directed toward pregnant women unjustly single out the most vulnerable women.

6. Coercive and punitive policies create the potential for criminalization of many types of otherwise legal maternal behavior.

(ACOG, 2005, pp. 6–9)

The American College of Obstetricians and Gynecologists (ACOG) (2004) and the American Academy of Pediatrics (AAP) Committee on Bioethics (1999) both affirm the fundamental right of pregnant women to make informed, uncoerced decisions about medical interventions. Moreover, in 2005 ACOG's Committee on Ethics took a direct stand against coercive and punitive approaches to the maternal-fetal relationship. See Table 1–1, which provides ACOG's rationale for the position.

ACOG and AAP recognize that cases of maternal-fetal conflict involve two clients, both of whom deserve respect and treatment. Such cases are best resolved using internal hospital mechanisms including counseling, the intervention of specialists, and consultation with an institutional ethics committee. Court intervention should be considered a last resort, appropriate only in extraordinary circumstances.

Abortion

Since the 1973 Supreme Court decision in *Roe v. Wade*, abortion has been legal in the United States. Abortion can be performed until the period of viability. After that time, abortion is permissible only when the life or health of the mother is threatened. Before viability, the rights of the mother are paramount; after viability, the rights of the fetus take precedence.

Personal beliefs, cultural norms, life experiences, and religious convictions shape people's attitudes about abortion. Ethicists have thoughtfully and thoroughly argued positions supporting both sides of the question. However, few issues spark the intensity of response seen when the issue of abortion is raised.

At present the decision about abortion is to be made by the woman and her physician. Nurses (and other caregivers) have the right to refuse to assist with the procedure if abortion is contrary to their moral and ethical beliefs. However, if a nurse works in an institution where abortions may be performed, the nurse may be dismissed for refusing to assist. To avoid being placed in a situation contrary to their ethical values and beliefs, nurses should determine the philosophy and practices of an institution before going to work there. A nurse who refuses to participate in an abortion because of moral or ethical beliefs has a responsibility to ensure that someone with similar qualifications is available to provide appropriate care for the client. Clients must never be abandoned, regardless of a nurse's beliefs.

Intrauterine Fetal Surgery

Intrauterine fetal surgery, generally considered experimental, is a therapy for anatomic lesions that can be corrected surgically and are incompatible with life if not treated. The procedure involves opening the uterus during the second trimester (before viability), performing the planned surgery, and replacing the fetus in the uterus. The risks to the fetus are substantial, and the mother is committed to cesarean births for this and subsequent pregnancies (because the upper, active segment of the uterus is entered). The parents must be informed of the experimental nature of the treatment, the risks of the surgery, the commitment to cesarean birth, and alternatives to the treatment.

As in other aspects of maternity care, caregivers must respect the pregnant woman's autonomy. The procedure involves health risks to the woman, and she retains the right to refuse any surgical procedure. Healthcare providers must be careful that their zeal for new technology does not lead them to focus unilaterally on the fetus at the expense of the mother.

Reproductive Assistance

Therapeutic insemination (TI) is accomplished by depositing into a woman sperm obtained from her husband, partner, or other donor. No states prohibit TI using a husband's sperm but legal problems may arise if donor sperm is used. Typically the donor signs a form waiving parental rights. The donor is also required to furnish a complete health history and his sperm is tested for HIV before it is used. If the woman receiving the donor sperm is married, her husband may be asked to sign a form to agree to the insemination and to assume parental responsibility for the child.

Assisted reproductive technology (ART) is the term used to describe highly technologic approaches used to produce pregnancy. *In vitro fertilization and embryo transfer (IVF-ET)*, a therapy offered to selected infertile couples, is perhaps the best-known ART technique. (See the discussion in Chapter 7 ∞.)

Some legislative efforts have been made to address consumer concerns about ART. In the United States, the Federal Fertility Clinic Success Rate and Certification Act (FCSRCA) of 1992 requires standardized reporting of pregnancy success rates associated with ART programs and addresses issues related to laboratory quality. To help ensure data accuracy, a validation process, which includes site visits to a portion of reporting clinics, is completed.

More than one-third of pregnancies that result from ART are multifetal pregnancies (March of Dimes, 2006). Multifetal pregnancy occurs because the use of ovulation-inducing medications typically triggers the release of multiple eggs. When fertilized, they produce multiple embryos, which are then implanted. Multifetal pregnancy increases the risk of miscarriage, preterm birth, and neonatal morbidity and mortality. It also increases the mother's risk of complications including cesarean birth. To help prevent a high-level multifetal pregnancy, the American Society for Reproductive Medicine (ASRM) has issued guidelines to limit the number of embryos transferred. These guidelines are designed to decrease risk while also allowing for individualized care (ASRM, 2006). This practice raises ethical considerations about the handling of the unused embryos. However, when a multifetal pregnancy does occur, the physician may suggest that the woman consider fetal reduction, in which some fetuses are aborted to give the remaining ones a better chance for survival. This procedure raises ethical concerns about the sacrifice of some so that the remainder can survive.

Prevention should be the first approach to the problem of multifetal pregnancy. Prevention begins with careful counselling about the risks of multiple gestation and the ethical issues that relate to fetal reduction. No physician who is morally opposed to fetal reduction should be expected to perform the procedure; however, physicians should be aware of the ethical and medical issues involved and be prepared to respond to families in a professional and ethical manner (ACOG, 2007).

Surrogate childbearing is another approach to infertility. Surrogate childbearing occurs when a woman agrees to become pregnant for a childless couple. She may be artificially inseminated with the male partner's sperm or a donor's sperm or may receive a gamete transfer, depending on the infertile couple's needs. If fertilization occurs, the woman carries the fetus to term and releases the infant to the couple after birth.

These methods of resolving infertility raise ethical issues about candidate selection, responsibility for a child born with a congenital defect, and religious objections to artificial conception. Other ethical questions include the following: What should be done with surplus fertilized oocytes? To whom do frozen embryos belong? Who is liable if a woman or her offspring contracts HIV from donated sperm? Should children be told about their conception?

Embryonic Stem Cell Research

Human stem cells can be found in embryonic tissue and in the primordial germ cells of a fetus. Research has demonstrated that in tissue cultures these cells can be made to differentiate into other types of cells such as blood, nerve, or heart cells, which might then be used to treat problems such as diabetes, Parkinson and Alzheimer diseases, spinal cord injury, or metabolic disorders. The availability of specialized tissue or even organs grown from stem cells might also decrease society's dependence on donated organs for organ transplants.

Positions about embryonic stem cell research vary dramatically, from the view that any use of human embryos for research is wrong to the view that any form of embryonic stem cell research is acceptable, with a variety of other positions that fall somewhere in between these extremes. Other questions also arise: What sources of embryonic tissue are acceptable for research? Is it ever ethical to clone embryos solely for stem cell research? Is there justification for using embryos remaining after fertility treatments?

The question of how an embryo should be viewed—with status in some way as a person or in some sense as property (and, if property, whose?)—is a key question in the debate. Ethicists recognize that it is not necessary to advocate full moral status or personhood for an embryo to have significant moral qualms about the instrumental use of a human embryo in the "interests" of society. The issue of consent, which links directly to an embryo's status, also merits consideration. In truth, the ethical questions and dilemmas associated with embryonic stem cell research are staggeringly complex and require careful analysis and thoughtful dialogue.

Cord Blood Banking

Cord blood, taken from a newborn's umbilical cord at birth, may play a role in combating leukemia, certain other cancers, and immune and blood system disorders. This is possible because cord blood, like bone marrow and embryonic tissue, contains hematopoietic stem cells, which can replace diseased cells in the affected individual. The value of bone marrow transplants is recognized, and a national registry of potential bone marrow donors exists. The process of collecting bone marrow is expensive and uncomfortable, however, and the National Marrow Donor Registry often has difficulty finding a matching bone marrow donor.

Cord blood has numerous advantages over bone marrow: (1) Collecting it involves no risk to the mother or newborn. (2) Large-scale cord blood banking would promote better availability of stem cells for racial and minority groups, who are seriously underrepresented in bone marrow registries. (3) Cord blood is less likely than bone marrow to trigger a potentially fatal rejection response. (4) Cord blood works with a less-than-perfect match. (5) Cord blood is available for use more rapidly than bone marrow.

Cord blood banks that process and store cord blood have now been established in the United States. Cord

MyNursingKit | National Marrow Donor Program

blood banks may be public or private. Public banks receive cord blood units given on a volunteer basis and are designed to support unrelated-donor transplant programs. Private banks are for-profit entities designed primarily for families who plan to use the cord blood for the infant who provided the blood (autologous donation) or for another family member who might need transplantation therapy in the future because of a genetic blood condition, cancer, bone marrow failure, or inborn error of metabolism, for example. Estimates suggest that over 7,000 cord blood transplants have been performed to correct blood-related cancers, inborn errors of metabolism, and certain genetic disorders (ACOG, 2008). This number increases daily.

Ethical concerns vary and focus, for example, on the issue of confidentiality for the mother and family throughout the process; the question of ownership of the blood (donor, parents, the blood bank, or society); the concern about fair distribution of the harvested blood; and obligations to the family that may arise if testing of the blood reveals genetic disorders or infectious diseases.

Both ACOG and the American Academy of Pediatrics (AAP) have issued statements about umbilical cord blood banking. ACOG (2008) stresses the importance of providing balanced information about the advantages and disadvantages of public vs. private banking and stressed the need for healthcare professionals to disclose any financial interests they have in private cord blood banks.

AAP (Lubin & Shearer, 2007) recommendations support the ACOG opinion and address several other clinical considerations as well. Key recommendations include the following:

- Parents are encouraged to bank their newborn's cord blood privately if they have an older child who has a condition that could benefit from a cord blood transfusion.
- In general, parents are encouraged to donate their newborn's cord blood to a public bank because it might help treat someone in need.
- Private cord blood banking as "insurance" against possible future personal or family need is discouraged because often the genetic traits associated with the condition that develops are present in the cord blood.
- Collection centers should test all donated cord blood for infectious and genetic disorders and should have a protocol developed for notifying families of abnormal results.
- Written consent for cord blood donation should be obtained before the onset of labor.

Implications for Nursing Practice

The complex ethical issues facing maternal-newborn nurses have many social, cultural, legal, and professional ramifications. Ethical decisions in maternal-child nursing are often complicated by moral obligations to more than one client. Straightforward solutions to the ethical dilemmas encountered in caring for childbearing families are often, quite simply, not available.

Nurses must learn to anticipate ethical dilemmas, clarify their own positions related to the issues, understand the legal implications of the issues, and develop appropriate strategies for ethical decision making. To accomplish these tasks, they can read about bioethical issues, participate in discussion groups, and attend courses and workshops on ethical topics pertinent to their areas of practice. Nurses also need to refine their skills in logical thinking and critical analysis.

Critical Thinking in Contemporary Care

The abilities to think critically and problem-solve effectively have always been important aspects of skilled nursing care. Today's maternal-newborn and women's healthcare nurses face the need to hone these skills even more as they find themselves dealing with a variety of challenges ranging from less desirable staffing patterns because of the nursing shortage to the availability of ever-evolving technologic tools, which they need to learn to use and interpret. With more clients to care for and less time available in which to do so, nurses need to be constantly assessing, evaluating, integrating information, and acting effectively.

The ability to think critically is an important skill, and nurses have several tools available to help them develop it. As part of their education, nurses learn to use the nursing process, a form of scientific reasoning. *Nursing care plans* are a useful tool in applying the nursing process. Thus, throughout this text we have provided examples of nursing care plans, focusing on one or two key nursing diagnoses, to assist students.

Nurses who use evidence to guide their practice are incorporating a vital critical-thinking tool. Evidence-based practice has emerged as one of the driving forces in health care today. Other tools available to assist nurses to think critically include nursing research, clinical pathways, nursing care plans, and statistical data. These tools are discussed briefly in the following sections and then incorporated throughout the text.

Evidence-Based Practice in Maternal-Newborn Nursing

Evidence-based practice—that is, nursing care in which all interventions are supported by current, valid research evidence—is emerging as a force in health care. It provides a useful approach to problem solving and decision making and to self-directed, client-centered, lifelong learning. Evidence-based practice builds on the actions necessary to transform research findings into clinical practice by also considering other forms of evidence that can be useful in making clinical practice decisions. These other forms of evidence may include, for example, statistical data, quality measurements, risk management measures, and information from support services such as infection control.

As clinicians, nurses need to meet three basic competencies related to evidence-based practice:

1. To recognize which clinical practices are supported by sound evidence, which practices have conflicting findings as to their effect on client outcomes, and which practices have no evidence to support their use.
2. To use data in their clinical work to evaluate outcomes of care.
3. To appraise and integrate scientific bases into practice.

Unfortunately, some agencies and clinical units where nurses practice still operate in the old style, which often generates conflict for nurses who recognize the need for more responsible clinical practice. In truth, market pressures are forcing nurses and other healthcare providers to evaluate routines to improve efficiencies and provide better outcomes for clients.

Nurses need to know what data are being tracked where they work and how care practices and outcomes are improved as a result of quality improvement initiatives. However, there is more to evidence-based practice than simply knowing what is being tracked and how the results are being used. Competent, effective nurses learn to question the very basis of their clinical work.

Throughout this text we have provided *snapshots* of evidence-based practice related to childbearing women and families, such as the one below. We believe that these snapshots will help you understand the concept more clearly. We also expect that these examples may challenge you to question the usefulness of some of the routine care you observe in clinical practice. That is the impact of evidence-based practice—it moves clinicians beyond practices of habit and opinion to practices based on high-quality, current science.

Nursing Research

Research is vital to expanding the science of nursing, fostering evidence-based practice, and improving client care. Research also plays an important role in advancing the profession of nursing. For example, nursing research can help determine the psychosocial and physical risks and benefits of both nursing and medical interventions.

EVIDENCE-BASED PRACTICE

Non-Pharmacologic Nursing Interventions for Dysmenorrhea

Clinical Question
What non-pharmacologic nursing interventions help women control dysmenorrhea?

The Evidence
Dysmenorrhea, or painful menstruation, is a common condition among women. Some reports estimate that up to 10% of women have such difficult periods that they cannot work. Common treatments include medications such as anti-inflammatory drugs. Many women want more natural, non-drug therapies. The scope of practice for nurses encompasses teaching women non-drug interventions such as pain management, relaxation, and guided imagery. Two expert clinicians reviewed research studies focused on the effectiveness of behavioral interventions for dysmenorrhea. Five studies met the quality criteria and were randomized trials. There was evidence that behavioral interventions—specifically pain management techniques and relaxation—ease the symptoms associated with dysmenorrhea. Teaching women relaxation techniques is particularly effective for women whose primary symptom is cramps. Pain management and relaxation techniques helped women maintain a normal level of activity, and these women missed less work. This evidence is a systematic review of multiple studies, but the studies all had limitations in either their methods or their sample. This evidence is considered moderately strong.

What Is Inconclusive?
You can be confident that helping women learn non-drug pain management and relaxation will have an effect on painful menstruation, but it is not clear how completely or consistently the effect is achieved. It is unclear whether different approaches for teaching pain management and relaxation might result in better outcomes. The studies that were reported were so different in terms of samples, interventions, and quality that no one group of interventions emerged as more effective than others. Some women may still need drug therapy to obtain complete relief from severe symptoms.

Best Practice
Understanding a woman's individual needs for relief of dysmenorrhea helps you determine the most appropriate nursing interventions. A variety of approaches may be effective. Teaching women non-drug pain management techniques and relaxation reduces the effects of dysmenorrhea, with or without drug therapy.

References
Proctor, M. I., Murphy, P. A., Pattison, H., Suckling, J., & Farquhar, C. (2007). Behavioral interventions for primary and secondary dysmenorrhea. *Cochrane Database of Systematic Reviews 2007, 3* (CD002248).

The gap between research and practice is being narrowed by the publication of research findings in popular nursing journals, the establishment of departments of nursing research in hospitals, and collaborative research efforts by nurse researchers and clinical practitioners. Interdisciplinary research between nurses and other healthcare professionals is also becoming more common. This ever-increasing recognition of the value of nursing research is important because well-done research supports the goals of evidence-based practice.

Clinical Pathways and Nursing Care Plans

Clinical pathways identify essential nursing activities and provide basic guidelines about expected outcomes at specified time intervals. These guidelines are research based and enable the nurse to determine whether a client's responses meet expected norms at any given time. In the text, we have provided sample clinical pathways.

Nursing care plans, which use the nursing process as an organizing framework, are also invaluable in planning and organizing care. Care plans are especially useful for nursing students and novice nurses. To help organize care, this text also provides several examples of nursing care plans such as the one found on page 320.

Statistical Data and Maternal-Infant Care

Increasingly nurses are recognizing the value and usefulness of statistics. Health-related statistics provide an objective basis for projecting client needs, planning the use of resources, and determining the effectiveness of specific treatments.

The two major types of statistics are descriptive and inferential. *Descriptive statistics* describe or summarize a set of data. They report the facts—what is—in a concise and easily retrievable way. An example of a descriptive statistic is the birth rate in the United States. Although these statistics support no conclusions about why some phenomenon has occurred, they identify certain trends and high-risk target groups and generate possible research questions. *Inferential statistics* allow the investigator to draw conclusions or inferences about what is happening between two or more variables in a population and to suggest or refute causal relationships between them.

Descriptive statistics are the starting point for the formation of research questions. Inferential statistics answer specific questions and generate theories to explain relationships between variables. Theory applied in nursing practice can help to change the specific variables that may be causing or at least contributing to certain health problems.

The following sections discuss descriptive statistics that are particularly important to maternal-newborn health care.

Inferential considerations are addressed as possible research questions that may assist in identifying relevant variables.

Birth Rate

Birth rate refers to the number of live births per 1000 people. In the United States in 2006, the preliminary birth rate rose 1% to 14.2 per 1000. Increases in birth rate were seen in all age groups except the youngest (ages 10 to 14), which dropped slightly, and the oldest (ages 45 to 49), which was unchanged. The birth rate for teenagers ages 15 to 19 increased 3% to 41.9 births per 1000, the first increase since 1991 (Hamilton, Martin, & Ventura, 2007). This increase and its implications for teenage pregnancy prevention efforts have sparked considerable discussion among healthcare professionals (see Chapter 13 ∞).

Preliminary estimates indicate that the number of babies born in 2006 was 4,265,996, which is the largest number of births since 1961 and the largest single-year increase since 1989. In addition, childbearing by unmarried women reached record high levels. Specifically in every age group and for every race, increases in nonmarital births dramatically outpaced increases in total births (Hamilton et al., 2007).

Statistics also indicate that the cesarean birth rate reached a record high at 31.1% of all births. Over the last decade this rate has increased 50% from 20.7 in 1996 (Hamilton et al., 2007).

Table 1–2 compares the birth for selected countries.

TABLE 1–2	Live Birth Rates and Infant Mortality Rates for Selected Countries (2007)	
Country	Birth Rate	Infant Mortality Rate
Afghanistan	46.2	157.4
Argentina	16.5	14.3
Australia	12.0	4.6
Cambodia	25.5	58.5
Canada	10.8	4.6
China	13.5	22.1
Egypt	22.5	29.5
Germany	8.2	4.1
Ghana	29.9	53.6
India	22.7	34.6
Iraq	31.4	47.0
Japan	8.1	2.8
Mexico	20.4	19.6
Russia	10.9	11.1
United Kingdom	10.7	5.0
United States	14.2	6.4

Source: Data from *The World Fact Book 2008*. Washington, DC: The Central Intelligence Agency.

MyNursingKit | Federal Interagency Forum on Child and Family Statistics

Research questions that can be posed about birth rates include the following:

- Is there an association between birth rates and changing social values?
- Do the differences in birth rates among various countries reflect cultural differences, availability of contraceptive information, or other factors?

Infant Mortality

The **infant mortality rate** is the number of deaths of infants under 1 year of age per 1000 live births in a given population. *Neonatal mortality* is the number of deaths of infants less than 28 days of age per 1000 live births, *perinatal mortality* includes both neonatal deaths and fetal deaths per 1000 live births, and *fetal death* is death in utero at 20 weeks or more gestation.

In 2004, the infant mortality rate in the United States was 6.78 per 1000 live births. This rate, although not significantly lower than the 2003 rate of 6.84, is, nevertheless, the lowest rate ever reported in the United States. However, the infant mortality rate varied widely by the race of the mother. Infant mortality rates were highest among non-Hispanic black women (13.6 per 1000 live births). This compares with 5.66 among non-Hispanic white women. Not surprisingly, infant mortality rates are higher among infants born in multiple births, infants born prematurely, and those born to unmarried mothers (Mathews & MacDorman, 2007).

In 2004, 36.5% of all infant deaths were related to preterm birth. Disturbingly the preterm-related infant mortality rate for non-Hispanic black mothers (6.29) was 3.5 times higher than for non-Hispanic white mothers (1.82) (MacDorman, Callaghan, Mathews et al., 2007). Overall, the five leading causes of infant death were congenital malformations and chromosomal abnormalities, disorders related to prematurity and low birth weight, sudden infant death syndrome (SIDS), maternal complications of pregnancy, and accidents (Miniño, Heron, Murphy, & Kochanek, 2007).

The U.S. infant mortality rate continues to be an area of concern because the United States has fallen to 22nd place in infant mortality rankings among industrialized nations. Healthcare professionals, policy makers, and the public continue to stress the need for better prenatal care, coordination of health services, and provision of comprehensive maternal-child services in the United States.

Table 1–2 identifies infant mortality rates for selected countries. As the data indicate, the range is dramatic among the countries listed. Information about birth rates and mortality rates is limited for some countries because of a lack of organized reporting mechanisms.

The information raises questions about access to health care during pregnancy and after birth and about standards of living, nutrition, and sociocultural factors. Additional factors affecting the infant mortality rate may be identified by considering the following research questions:

- What are the leading causes of infant mortality in each country?
- Why do mortality rates differ among racial groups?

Maternal Mortality

Maternal mortality rate is the number of deaths from any cause related to or aggravated by pregnancy or pregnancy management during the pregnancy cycle (including the 42-day postpartal period) per 100,000 live births. It does not include deaths of pregnant women because of external causes such as accidents, homicides, and suicides (Hoyert, 2007). The maternal mortality rate in the United States in 2004 was 13.1 deaths per 100,000 live births. Specifically 540 women died, an increase of 45 deaths over the 2003 total. However, black women have a significantly higher risk of maternal death than white women have. The maternal mortality rate for black women was 34.7 deaths per 100,000 live births as compared with 9.3 deaths for white women. The maternal mortality rate for Hispanic women is cited as 8.5, but inconsistencies in reporting Hispanic origin on death certificates and on censuses and surveys make this number less precise (Miniño et al., 2007).

Factors influencing the long-term decrease in maternal mortality include the increased use of hospitals and specialized healthcare personnel by maternity clients, the establishment of care centers for high-risk mothers and infants, the prevention and control of infection with antibiotics and improved techniques, the availability of blood products for transfusions, and the lowered rates of anesthesia-related deaths.

Additional factors may be identified by asking the following research questions:

- Is there a correlation between maternal mortality and age?
- Is there a correlation between maternal mortality and availability of health care? Economic status?

Implications for Nursing Practice

Nurses can use statistics in a number of ways. For example, they can use statistical data to:

- Determine populations at risk
- Assess the relationship between specific factors
- Help establish databases for specific client populations
- Determine the levels of care needed by particular client populations
- Evaluate the success of specific nursing interventions
- Determine priorities in case loads
- Estimate staffing and equipment needs of hospital units and clinics

Statistical information is available through many sources, including professional literature; state and city health departments; vital statistics sections of private, county, state, and federal agencies; special programs or agencies (such as family planning); and demographic profiles of specific geographic areas. Often the information can be found using the Internet. Many accurate and reliable websites such as the following are available as references for statistical information:

- Centers for Disease Control and Prevention (CDC) www.cdc.gov
- National Center for Health Statistics www.cdc.gov/nchs
- Statistics Canada www.statcan.ca
- March of Dimes www.modimes.org

Nurses who use this information are better prepared to promote the health needs of maternal-newborn clients and their families.

CHAPTER HIGHLIGHTS

- Contemporary childbirth is family-centered, recognizing the needs and roles of the woman and her partner, any siblings, grandparents, and other family members.
- The nurse who provides culturally competent care recognizes the importance of the childbearing family's value system, acknowledges that differences occur among people, and seeks to respect and respond to ethnic diversity in a way that leads to mutually desirable outcomes.
- Interest in complementary and alternative therapies continues to grow nationwide and affects the care of childbearing families.
- Community-based care is especially important in maternal-child nursing because the vast majority of care provided to childbearing women and their families takes place outside of hospitals—in clinics, offices, community-based organizations, and private homes.
- A nurse must perform within the scope of practice or be subject to the accusation of practicing medicine without a license. The standard of care of individual nursing practice is based on a comparison with the care provided by a reasonably prudent nurse.
- Nursing standards provide information and guidelines for nurses in their own practice, in developing policies and protocols in healthcare settings, and in directing the development of quality nursing care.
- Informed consent—based on knowledge of a procedure and its benefits, risks, and alternatives—must be secured before providing treatment.

- Maternal-fetal conflict may arise when the fetus is viewed as a person of equal rights to those of the mother's and external agents attempt to restrict a mother's actions to support the well-being of the fetus.
- Abortion can legally be performed until the fetus reaches the age of viability. The decision to have an abortion is made by a woman in consultation with her physician.
- A variety of procedures are available to help infertile couples achieve a pregnancy. However, some of these procedures provoke serious ethical dilemmas.
- Cord blood banking provides the opportunity to have stem cells available to treat a variety of cancers and blood disorders. Its growing popularity has revealed several ethical issues.
- Evidence-based practice refers to clinical practice based on research findings and other available data. It increases nurses' accountability and results in better client outcomes.
- Nursing research plays a vital role in adding to the nursing knowledge base, expanding clinical practice, and further developing nursing theory.
- Descriptive statistics describe a set of data. Inferential statistics allow the investigator to draw conclusions about what is happening between two or more variables in a population.

PEARSON
EXPLORE **mynursingkit**™

MyNursingKit is your one stop for online chapter review materials and resources. Prepare for success with additional NCLEX®-style practice questions, interactive assignments and activities, web links, animations and videos, and more!

Register your access code from the front of your book at
www.mynursingkit.com

CHAPTER REFERENCES

American Academy of Pediatrics (AAP), Committee on Bioethics. (1999). Fetal therapy—Ethical considerations. *Pediatrics, 103*(5), 1061–1063.

American College of Nurse–Midwives (ACNM). (2005). *Mandatory degree requirements for midwives.* Retrieved March 13, 2006, from http://www.midwife.org

American College of Obstetricians and Gynecologists (ACOG). (2004). *Parent choice: Maternal-fetal* (Committee Opinion No. 214). Washington, DC: Author.

American College of Obstetricians and Gynecologists (ACOG). (2005). *Maternal decision making, ethics, and the law* (Committee Opinion No. 321). Washington, DC: Author.

American College of Obstetricians and Gynecologists (ACOG). (2007). *Multifetal pregnancy reduction* (Committee Opinion No. 369). Washington, DC: Author.

American College of Obstetricians and Gynecologists (ACOG). (2008). *Umbilical cord blood banking* (Committee Opinion No. 399). Washington, DC: Author.

American Society for Reproductive Medicine and the Society for Assisted Reproductive Technology. (2006). Guidelines on number of embryos transferred. *Fertility and Sterility, 86* (suppl. 5), S51–52.

Cohen, R. A., & Martinez, M. E. (2006). Health insurance coverage: Estimates from the National Health Interview Survey, 2005. Retrieved July 25, 2006, from www.cdc.gov/nchs

Hamilton, B. E., Martin, J. A., & Ventura, S. J. (2007). Births: Preliminary data for 2006. *National Vital Statistics Reports, 56*(7), 1–18.

Hoyert, D. L. (2007). Maternal mortality and related concepts. National Center for Health Statistics. *Vital Health Stat, 3*(33), 1–9.

Lubin, B. H., & Shearer, W. T. (2007). Policy statement: Cord blood banking for potential future transplantation. *Pediatrics, 119*(1), 165–171.

MacDorman, M. F., Callaghan, W. M., Mathews, T. J., Hoyert, D. L., & Kochanek, K. D. (2007). Trends in preterm-related infant mortality by race and ethnicity: United States, 1999–2004.

NCHS Health & Stats. Retrieved March 15, 2008, from www.cdc.gov/nchs

March of Dimes. (2006). Multiple pregnancy and birth: Considering fertility options. Retrieved July 17, 2007, from www.modimes.com

Mathews, T. J., & MacDorman, M. F. (2007). Infant mortality statistics from the 2004 period linked birth/infant death data set. *National Vital Statistics Reports, 55*(14), 1–33.

Midwives Alliance of North America (MANA). (2006). *Definitions.* Retrieved March 13, 2006, from www.mana.org/definitions.html

Miniño, A. M., Heron, M. P., Murphy, S. L., & Kochanek, K. D. (2007). Deaths: Final data for 2004. *National Vital Statistics Reports, 55*(19), 1–18.

National Center for Health Statistics. (2006). Health, United States, 2006. With Chartbook on Trends in the Health of Americans. Hyattsville, MD.

Zwelling, E. (2008). The emergence of high-tech birthing. *Journal of Obstetric, Gynecologic, and Neonatal Nursing, 37*(1), 85–93.

CHAPTER 2

Culture and the Childbearing Family

When I first began working at this prenatal clinic I was not very tuned in to the nuances of families. Now I am much better at picking up cues about a family's functioning—who makes decisions, who controls the finances, how power is distributed. I have also come to realize that, unless the family trusts me, they tell me only what they think I need to know. It's not that they mean to be devious, but they may not tell me about the complementary therapies they use or the cultural practices that are important to them if they think I will be judgmental. As I have become more open and accepting, I have become a far better nurse.

LEARNING OUTCOMES

2-1. Describe how family type may influence nursing care of the childbearing family.

2-2. Explain the changes that a childbearing family will undergo based on the developmental tasks to be completed.

2-3. Identify information that would be useful to collect when performing a family assessment.

2-4. Integrate the prevalent cultural norms that affect childbearing and childrearing when providing care to that family.

2-5. Explain the importance of cultural competency in providing nursing care to the childbearing family.

2-6. Interpret the information collected from a cultural assessment to provide culturally sensitive care.

2-7. Identify ways a nurse might accommodate the religious rituals and practices of the childbearing family.

2-8. Distinguish between complementary and alternative therapies.

2-9. Describe the benefits and risks of the various complementary and alternative therapies to the childbearing family.

2-10. Formulate nursing care within the nurse practice act and with the informed consent of the client when using appropriate complementary therapies with childbearing families.

KEY TERMS

Alternative therapy **23**
Complementary therapy **23**
Culture **20**
Ethnicity **20**
Ethnocentrism **22**
Family **18**
Taboo **21**

Individuals do not live in isolation. Their values, beliefs, behaviors, decisions, attitudes, and biases are shaped by many factors including their families, their culture, and their religious beliefs. Nurses who provide effective, holistic care recognize this reality and seek to learn about and care for the entire childbearing family.

This chapter begins with a discussion of family types, functioning, and assessment. It then addresses the impact of culture on the childbearing family, and concludes with a brief examination of complementary and alternative therapies a family might use.

The Family

The U.S. Census Bureau (2006) defines a **family** as individuals who are joined together by marriage, blood, adoption, or residence in the same household. More broadly, however, families are generally characterized by bonds of emotional closeness, sharing, and support.

Within families, members are guided by a common set of values that bind them together. These family values are greatly influenced by external factors including cultural background, social norms, education, environmental influences, socioeconomic status, and beliefs held by peers, coworkers, political and community leaders, and other individuals outside the family unit. Because of the influence of these external factors, a family's values may change considerably over the years.

Types of Families

Various types of families exist in contemporary American society. The following list identifies common types of family structure.

- The *nuclear family* consists of a husband provider, a wife who stays home, and children. Although the nuclear family was once the norm in the United States, it is no longer the most common type of family.
- In the *dual-career/dual-earner family*, both parents work, either by choice or necessity. Today, two-thirds of all two-parent families are this type. Dual-career families have to address issues related to child care, household chores, and spending time together.
- The *childless family* is a growing trend. In some cases a family is childless by choice; in other cases, a family is childless because of issues related to infertility.
- In an *extended family*, a couple shares household and childrearing responsibilities with parents, siblings, or other relatives. Multigenerational arrangements of this sort are more common in non-U.S. cultures and in working class families.
- An *extended kin network family* is a specific form of an extended family in which two nuclear families of primary or unmarried kin live in close proximity to each

other. The family shares a social support network, chores, goods, and services. This type of family model is common in the Latino community.
- Although rare in the past, the *single-parent family* is becoming increasingly common. In some cases, the head of the household is widowed, divorced, abandoned, or separated. In other cases, the head of the household, most often the mother, was never married. Single-parent families often face difficulties because the sole parent may lack social and emotional support, need assistance with child-rearing issues, and face financial strain (Figure 2–1 ■).
- A *stepfamily* consists of a biologic parent with children and a new spouse who may or may not have children. This family structure has become increasingly common because of high rates of divorce and remarriage. These families are also known as *remarried, reconstituted,* or *blended families.* Stepfamily models have both strengths and challenges. Stepfamilies may have fewer financial issues and may offer a child a new support person and role model. Remarriage also provides a new opportunity for a successful relationship for the parents; however, the relationship between stepparents and stepchildren can be strained. Stresses can include discipline issues, adjustment problems, role ambiguity, strain with the other biologic parent, and communication issues.
- A *binuclear family* is a post-divorce family in which the biologic children are members of two nuclear households, both that of the father and that of the mother. The children alternate between the two homes. This is also called co-parenting and involves joint custody. In joint custody, both parents have equal responsibility and legal rights, regardless of where the children live. The binuclear family model enables both parents to be involved

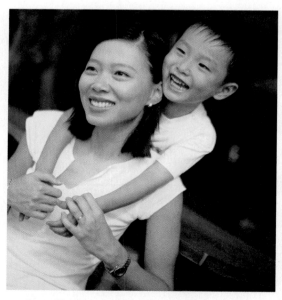

FIGURE 2–1 Single-parent families account for nearly one-third of all U.S. families.
Source: Joyce Choo/CORBIS.

in a child's upbringing and provides additional support and role models from extended family members. However, it often requires negotiation and compromise between the parents about childrearing decisions.

- A *nonmarital heterosexual cohabitating family* describes a heterosexual couple who may or may not have children and who live together outside of marriage. This may include never-married individuals as well as divorced or widowed persons. Although some individuals choose this model for personal reasons, others do so for financial reasons or to seek companionship.
- *Gay and lesbian families* include those in which two or more people who share a same-sex orientation live together (with or without children), and those in which a gay or lesbian single parent rears a child. Small studies that have evaluated children reared by gay and lesbian couples found that the children show no significant differences from children reared in other types of families. Children raised in gay and lesbian families may face unique issues in interacting with peers and in revealing their parents' sexual orientation.

HINTS FOR PRACTICE

It is important to establish which parent has legal custody, current visitation policies, and other variables (restraining orders, supervised visitation, etc.) when communicating information to parents about their children. Certain legal issues may prohibit the nurse from sharing some information with the noncustodial parent.

Family Development Frameworks

Family development refers to the dynamics or changes that a family experiences over time, including changes in relationships, communication patterns, roles, and interactions. Although each family is unique, the members go through a set of fairly predictable changes. For example, Duvall (1977) developed an eight-stage family life cycle that describes the developmental process that each family encounters. This model is based on the nuclear family (Table 2–1). The oldest child serves as a marker for the family's developmental stages except in the last two stages when children are no longer present. Couples with more than one child may find themselves in overlapping stages with developmental advances occurring simultaneously.

Other family development models have been developed to address the stages and developmental tasks facing the unattached young adult, the gay and lesbian family, those who divorce, and those who remarry. For further information on this topic, readers are referred to textbooks on families and on developmental psychology.

Family Assessment

The nurse's understanding of a family's structure helps provide insight into the family's support system and needs. A *family assessment* is a collection of data about the family's type and structure, current level of functioning, support system, sociocultural background, environment, and needs.

To obtain an accurate and concise family assessment, the nurse needs to establish a trusting relationship with the woman and her family. Data are best collected in a comfortable, private environment, free from interruptions.

Basic information should include the following:

- Name, age, sex, and family relationship of all people residing in the household
- Family type, structure, roles, and values

TABLE 2–1	The Eight-Stage Family Life Cycle	
Stage I	Beginning families	Marriage between partners, identification as partners, establishing goals for future, interaction and building relationships with kin.
Stage II	Childbearing families	Birth of first child, new role as parents, integrating new family member into existing family.
Stage III	Families with preschool children	Establishing family network, socialization of children, reinforcing independence in children when separating from parents.
Stage IV	Families with school-age children	Facilitating peer relationships while maintaining family dynamics, adjusting to outside influences.
Stage V	Families with teenagers	Increase in children's independence and autonomy; parents' concerns shift to aging parents, careers, and marital relationship.
Stage VI	Families launching young adults	Readjustment of marital relationship; parents and children establish separate identities outside the family unit.
Stage VII	Middle-aged parents	Renewed marital relationship, new outside interests, fewer family responsibilities, new roles as grandparents and as in-laws, increased concern for aging parents, death, and disability of older generation.
Stage VIII	Retirement and old age	End of career, shift to retirement, maintain functioning during the aging process, maintain marital relationship, adjust to potential loss of spouse, friends, and siblings, prepare for eventual death.

Source: Adapted from Duvall, Elizabeth M. *Marriage and family development* (5th ed.). Published by Allyn and Bacon, Boston, MA. Copyright © 1977 by Pearson Education. Adapted by permission of the publisher; and Friedman, M. M. (1998). *Family nursing: Research, theory, and practice* (4th ed., p. 113). Reprinted by permission of Pearson Education, Upper Saddle River, NJ.

- Cultural associations, including cultural norms and customs related to childbearing, childrearing, and infant feeding (This might include expected activities, forbidden activities, the role of the father, the role of the maternal grandmother, and the like.)
- Religious affiliations, including specific religious beliefs and practices related to childbearing
- Support network, including extended family, friends, and religious and community associations
- Communication patterns, including verbal and written language barriers

In addition, the nurse gathers information about the health of individual family members because their health status can have a major impact on family functioning. When possible it is helpful to have information about the family's home environment as well. In many cases this information is gathered during client interviews. However, a home visit provides far more data about family relationships, roles, needs, and preparation for a new baby.

Cultural Influences Affecting the Family

When caring for families it is critical to consider the influence of culture, which may affect how a family responds to health-related issues. **Culture** can be defined as the beliefs, values, attitudes, and practices that are accepted by a population, a community, or an individual. Culture is learned and not ingrained in our genetic material, yet it can be passed on from generation to generation by means of *enculturation.* When a group is isolated, either geographically or economically, culture is often reinforced.

Ethnicity is a social identity that is associated with shared behaviors and patterns. These include family structure, religious affiliation, language, dress, eating habits, and health behaviors. Many Americans define ethnicity by physical characteristics such as skin color. However, many people consider themselves "biracial" or identify themselves with a specific group not because of skin color but because of a shared ideology or attitudes. More and more, individuals are blends of ethnic backgrounds and it is often difficult to assign a specific ethnic identity to someone. Although some beliefs and practices are common among certain ethnic groups, one must be careful to avoid stereotyping individuals. It is important not to assume that because individuals identify themselves as a specific ethnicity they must practice certain customs.

Acculturation is the process by which people adapt to a new cultural norm. When a group completely changes its cultural identity to become part of the majority culture, *assimilation* occurs.

Acculturation frequently occurs when people leave their country of origin and immigrate to a new country. Often acculturation is associated with improved health status and health behaviors, especially if the immigration is associated with improved socioeconomic status, which leads to better nutrition and access to health care. This is frequently true, for example, for people who immigrate from a developing country. However, health sometimes declines with acculturation. For example, obesity is a problem that is growing rapidly within the United States and particularly among immigrant populations. It may also present problems if a person immigrates from a country with universal health care to a country in which he or she is not eligible for health care or cannot afford it.

Cultural Influences on Childbearing and Childrearing

A family's culture may influence its beliefs about and practices surrounding many aspects of childbearing and childrearing.

Beliefs and Attitudes About Pregnancy

Children are generally valued all over the world, not only for the joy they bring but also because they ensure continuation of the family and cultural values. This valuing of children may manifest itself in different ways, however. Families in the United States and many Western countries commonly have only one or two children out of a desire to provide the children with the best home and education they can afford and to spend as much free time with them as possible. In contrast, in many cultures throughout the world, it is common to have as many children as possible.

In some cultures, a woman who gives birth achieves a higher status, especially if the child is male (Safadi, 2005). This is especially true in the traditional Chinese culture and in some Middle Eastern cultures (Do, 2005). Similarly, in the western United States, people of the Mormon faith view motherhood as the most important aspect of a woman's life, comparable with the male role of priesthood (Faust, 2005). In Mexican American society and among many other Latino groups, having children is evidence of the male's virility and is a sign of manliness or *machismo*, a desired trait.

Culture may also influence attitudes and beliefs about contraception. For example, many Muslims from the Middle East may use birth control but do not believe in sterilization because it is a permanent method (Hammond, White, & Fetters, 2005). Other Muslims might not practice contraception because children are highly valued and it is believed that the traditional role of women is to bear children. In Chinese society, in contrast, where state policy limits the number of children a couple can have, contraception is common.

Health values and beliefs are also important in understanding reactions and behavior. Certain behaviors can be expected if a culture views pregnancy as a sickness, whereas other behaviors can be expected if the culture views pregnancy as a natural occurrence. For example, because Native Americans, African Americans, and Mexican Americans generally view pregnancy as a natural and desirable condition, prenatal care may not be a priority. In other cultures, pregnancy may be seen as a time of increased vulnerability. In Orthodox Judaism, for example, it is a man's responsibility to procreate, but it is a woman's right, not her obligation, to do so. This is because, according to Orthodox Jewish law, the health of the mother, both physically and mentally, is of primary concern, and she should never be obliged to do something that threatens her life (Semenic, Callister, & Feldman, 2004).

Individuals of many cultures take certain protective precautions based on their beliefs. For example, many Southeast Asian women fear that they will have a complicated labor and birth if they sit in a doorway or on a step. Thus they tend to avoid areas near doors in waiting rooms and examining rooms. In the Mexican American culture, the belief is common that *mal aire*, or bad air, may enter the body and cause harm. Preventive measures such as keeping the windows closed or covering the head are used. Some Latinos place a raisin on the cord stump of newborns to prevent drafts from entering their bodies. A **taboo** is a behavior or thing that is to be avoided. Many cultures, including those found in the United States, have taboos centered on the unborn baby and/or newborn that are meant to ensure that the baby will survive. For example, it is common among Muslims to avoid naming the baby until after birth; similarly many Orthodox Jewish women wait to set up the nursery until after the baby is born.

In developing countries, mortality rates among infants and young children are extremely high; thus certain traditions focus on protecting the baby from evil spirits. For example, many Muslim parents will pin an amulet to the newborn's clothes as protection. This may be a palm, an eye, a blue stone, or a verse from the Quaran. Following birth, it is common for a male family member to whisper prayers in the newborn baby's ear to declare faith and protect the baby (Cassar, 2006).

The *equilibrium model of health* is based on the concept of balance between light and dark, heat and cold. Some Eastern philosophies focus on the notion of *yin* and *yang*. Yin represents the female, passive principle—darkness, cold, wetness; yang is the masculine, active principle—light, heat, and dryness. When the two are combined, they are all that can be. The hot–cold classification is seen in cultures in Latin America, the Near East, and Asia.

Some Mexican Americans may consider illness to be an excess of either hot or cold. To restore health, imbalances are often corrected by the proper use of foods, medications, or herbs. These substances are also classified as hot or cold. For example, an illness attributed to an excess of cold will be treated only with hot foods or medications. The classification of foods is not always consistent, but it conforms to a general structure of traditional knowledge. Certain foods, spices, herbs, and medications are perceived to cool or heat the body. These perceptions do not necessarily correspond to the actual temperature; some hot dishes are said to have a cooling quality.

Southeast Asians believe it is important to keep the woman "warm" after birth, because blood, which is considered "hot," has been lost, and the woman is at risk of becoming "cold." Therefore they avoid cold drinks and foods following birth. In contrast, many women in India consider pregnancy a "hot" period and eat "cool" foods to balance the hot state (Holroyd, Twinn, & Yim, 2004).

The concepts of hot and cold are not as important in Native American or African American beliefs. Similarities exist in all of these groups, however, because of their emphasis on a balance in nature.

HINTS FOR PRACTICE

When offering your clients fluids, ask if they would prefer them hot, warm, or iced. This can help ensure both proper hydration and support cultural beliefs.

Health Practices During Pregnancy and Postpartum

Healthcare practices during pregnancy are influenced by numerous factors, such as the prevalence of traditional home remedies and folk beliefs, the importance of indigenous healers, and the influence of professional healthcare workers. In an urban setting, the age, length of time in the city, marital status, and strength of the family may affect these patterns. Socioeconomic status is also important, because modern medical services are more accessible to those who can afford them.

An awareness of alternative health sources is crucial for health professionals, because these practices affect health outcomes. For example, in the traditional Mexican American culture, mothers are often influenced by *familism*, a close-knit, interdependent network of nuclear and extended family members who are connected for the good of the family. Close intergenerational networks exist and young mothers often seek the advice of their mothers or older women about childbirth. In many cases, decisions about health care are made by the family (Eggenberger, Grassley, & Restrepo, 2006).

Indigenous healers are also important to specific cultures. In the Mexican American culture, the healer is called a *curandero* or *curandera* whereas the *partera* is a lay midwife, who gives advice and treats illnesses during pregnancy and also attends labor and birth. In some Native American tribes, the medicine man or woman may fulfill the healing role. Herbalists are often found in Asian cultures, and faith healers, root doctors, and spiritualists are sometimes consulted by members of some African cultures.

Among many people there is a period of isolation post-partally. Chinese women, for example, observe *zuoyuezzi*, often referred to as "doing the month," after childbirth. During this time the mother is typically supported by the baby's grandmother or a close family member. She is encouraged to rest and avoid domestic chores and outside activities. She also avoids bathing, brushing her teeth, and washing her hair. She strives to maintain a balance of hot and cold foods (Callister, 2006). Similarly many Muslim women stay in the house for 40 days following the birth, cared for by female relatives (Cassar, 2006).

Cultural Factors and Nursing Care

Healthcare providers are often unaware of the cultural characteristics they themselves demonstrate. Without cultural awareness, caregivers tend to project their own cultural responses onto foreign-born clients; clients from different socioeconomic, religious, or educational groups; or clients from different regions of the country. This projection leads caregivers to assume that the clients are demonstrating a specific behavior for the same reason that they themselves would. Moreover, healthcare providers often fail to realize that medicine has its own culture, which has been dominated historically by traditional middle class values and beliefs.

Ethnocentrism is the conviction that the values and beliefs of one's own cultural group are the best or only acceptable ones. It is characterized by an inability to understand the beliefs and worldview of another culture. To a certain extent, all of us are guilty of ethnocentrism, at least some of the time. Thus, the nurse who values stoicism during labor may be uncomfortable with the more vocal response of some Latin American women. Another nurse may be disconcerted by a Southeast Asian woman who believes that pain is something to be endured rather than alleviated and who is intent on maintaining self-control in labor (Andrews & Boyle, 2007).

Healthcare providers sometimes believe that if members of other cultures do not share Western values and beliefs, they should adopt them. For example, a nurse who believes strongly in equality of the sexes may find it difficult to remain silent if a woman from a Middle Eastern culture defers to her husband in decision making. It is important to remember that pressure to defy cultural values and beliefs can be stressful and anxiety provoking for these women.

To address issues of cultural diversity in the provision of health care, emphasis is being placed on developing *cultural competence*, that is, the skills and knowledge necessary to appreciate, respect, and work with individuals from different cultures. It requires self-awareness, awareness and understanding of cultural differences, and the ability to adapt clinical skills and practices as needed.

The nurse can begin developing cultural competence by becoming knowledgeable about the cultural practices of local groups. For example, is it considered courteous to avoid eye contact? Should last names be used in conversations as a sign of respect? Is a female healthcare provider necessary? Do communication and language barriers exist? If so, how can they be addressed?

Giger and Davidhizar (2008) suggest that care providers conduct a cultural assessment to glean information about health practices based on the client's beliefs, values, and customs. This kind of assessment might include questions such as the following:

- Who in the family must be consulted before decisions are made about a person's care?
- Does the client see primarily in the present or does he or she have a futuristic time orientation?
- What type of healthcare provider is most appropriate for the client?
- Does the client have beliefs or traditions that may affect the plan of care?

TEACHING TIP

When you care for a family in which the grandparents play a key role in decision making, be sure that they are present if you are teaching something it is important for the family to understand. This might include, for example, signs of illness in the newborn that need immediate follow-up.

Several cultural assessment tools are available to assist the nurse in gathering this information. These tools are becoming increasingly common at healthcare agencies as providers act in response to the expectation of culturally competent care. The nurse who respects cultural diversity is an asset to childbearing families as they adjust to new roles. Establishing a trusting relationship enables the nurse to assist families in meeting educational needs.

Impact of Religion and Spirituality

The terms *religion* and *spirituality* mean different things to different people. Many people consider *religion* to be an institutionalized system that shares a common set of beliefs and practices; others define it more simply as a belief in a transcendent power. The latter definition, however, approaches most people's understanding of *spirituality* as a concern with the spirit or soul.

A childbearing family's religious beliefs, affiliation, and practices can influence deeply their experiences and attitudes toward health care, childbearing, and childrearing. Members of certain religious groups such as Christian Scientists may attempt to avoid all medical interventions whereas others such as Jehovah's Witnesses may refuse specific interventions such as blood transfusions. Roman Catholics may refuse contraception. In most cases, the woman and her family gain comfort from acknowledgment of and respect for their religious beliefs and practices in the healthcare setting. However, the agnostic (one who has doubts about the existence of a transcendent being) or the atheist (one who believes that there is no higher power) may be offended if care providers assume references to God or to a higher power will be comforting.

A religious or spiritual history is often completed when a woman is admitted to a clinic or labor setting. The assessment can include questions about current spiritual beliefs and practices that will affect the mother and baby during the hospital stay or preferences for religious rituals during labor and birth. When possible, the nurse should attempt to accommodate religious rituals and practices requested by the childbearing family.

Considering the diversity of religious beliefs, it is not unusual for nurses to encounter childbearing families whose beliefs conflict with their own. This is not problematic as long as the nurse avoids attempts to influence the client's decision making. For example, a nurse who does not believe in baptism should avoid revealing this to a Catholic mother seeking baptism for her stillborn infant. Nurses should also examine their religious beliefs related to genetic screening procedures, use of assisted reproductive technology to achieve pregnancy, use of technology to support life in a severely compromised newborn, abortion, and even less dramatic issues such as methods of contraception, circumcision, and infant feeding. In many institutions nurses can ask to be reassigned to a different client if their religious beliefs are in conflict; however, if other personnel are not available, it is the nurse's responsibility to provide sensitive, appropriate, and nonjudgmental care to that client.

Complementary and Alternative Therapies and the Childbearing Family

Throughout most of the twentieth century in the United States, it was rare for European American childbearing families to consult anyone except their obstetrician for advice about their pregnancy, birth, and postpartum. Though such clients are still encountered today, perinatal nurses are more likely to care for childbearing families who integrate other types of practitioners and therapies with traditional Western medicine.

A **complementary therapy** may be defined as any procedure or product that is used as an adjunct to conventional medical treatment (National Center for Complementary and Alternative Medicine (NCCAM), 2007c). Although complementary therapies were entirely absent from clinics and hospitals until the last few decades, therapies such as acupuncture, acupressure, and massage therapy are now often used together with conventional medical care, and many health insurance plans cover at least a portion of the cost of such therapies.

In contrast, an **alternative therapy** is usually considered a substance or procedure that is used in place of conventional medicine (NCCAM, 2007c). Thus, alternative therapies are not usually available in conventional clinics and hospitals, and their costs are not typically covered under most health insurance policies. Consequently, a client may be reluctant to discuss them with a conventional physician or nurse.

The dramatic increase in complementary and alternative therapies that began in the 1990s has probably resulted from a combination of several factors.

- Increased consumer awareness of the limitations of conventional Western medicine
- Increased international travel
- Increased media attention
- Advent of the Internet

In this new century, it seems clear that the future of American health care will reveal an ever-increasing integration between conventional medicine and complementary therapies. Some obvious examples of this new integration in perinatal settings include the acceptance of certain herbal teas for antepartal discomforts; the use of massage, reiki, or therapeutic touch during the first stage of labor; music during childbirth; and the increased emphasis on skin-to-skin mother-to-baby bonding in the immediate postpartum period.

Further evidence of this increased integration is the establishment in 1992 of the Office of Alternative Medicine (OAM) at the National Institutes of Health. The OAM was mandated by Congress to promote research into complementary and alternative therapies and dissemination of information to consumers. In 1998, the OAM was incorporated into a new National Center for Complementary and Alternative Medicine (NCCAM) with an expanded mission and increased funding. Recently, NCCAM recognized a new domain of *integrative medicine*, an approach that combines mainstream medical therapies with complementary therapies for which there is some high-quality scientific evidence of safety and effectiveness (NCCAM, 2007c). Many studies of complementary and alternative therapies are currently underway at the NCCAM, which can be accessed via the Internet.

Benefits and Risks

Complementary and alternative therapies undisputedly have many benefits for the childbearing family and other

MyNursingKit | Focus on the Family

MyNursingKit | Religion, Culture and the Family

healthcare consumers. Many complementary and alternative therapies emphasize prevention and wellness, and place a higher value on holistic healing than on physical cure. In addition, many are noninvasive, have few side effects, and are more affordable and available than conventional therapies.

However, many of these remedies have associated risks that must be considered thoughtfully before a decision is made to use them. These risks include lack of standardization, lack of regulation and research substantiating safety and effectiveness, inadequate training and certification of some healers, and financial and health risks of unproven methods.

Types of Complementary and Alternative Therapies

Numerous forms of complementary and alternative therapies are available. Only a few of the most commonly used approaches are presented here.

Homeopathy

Homeopathy is best understood in contrast to conventional Western medicine, which is also called *allopathic medicine.* The term *allopathy* is derived from the Greek words *allos* meaning "different" and *pathos* meaning "suffering." Thus, allopathic medicine uses remedies that produce effects differing from—or in opposition to—those of the disease being treated. For example, conventional healthcare practitioners may prescribe an anti-inflammatory to reduce swelling or a sedative to relieve insomnia.

In contrast, the term *homeopathy* is derived from the Greek word *homos* meaning "the same." It is based on the "law of similars," which says that a substance that can cause symptoms when taken by healthy people can help treat those who are experiencing similar symptoms (Royal College of Midwives, 2006). Thus, it is often described as a healing system that uses like to cure like; specifically, homeopathic remedies are minute dilutions of substances that, if ingested in larger amounts, would produce effects *similar* to the symptoms of the disorder being treated. For example, *Cantharis vesicatoria* is a species of beetle (commonly called Spanish fly) whose poison causes, among other symptoms, burning pains and a frantic urge to urinate. Homeopathic *Cantharis* is a minute dilution of this toxin, and is thus a remedy of choice for women suffering from cystitis.

Naturopathy

Naturopathy is commonly referred to as *natural medicine.* It is more precisely defined as a healing system that combines safe and effective traditional means of preventing and treating human disease with the most current advances in modern medicine (American Association of Naturopathic Physicians, 2005). Many naturopathic physicians are eclectic, employing a variety of therapies in their practice. These might include clinical nutrition, botanical medicine, homeopathy, natural childbirth, traditional Chinese medicine, hydrotherapy, naturopathic manipulative therapy, pharmacology, minor surgery, and counseling for lifestyle modification (American Association of Naturopathic Physicians, 2005).

Traditional Chinese Medicine

Traditional Chinese medicine (TCM) developed more than 3,000 years ago in the Chinese culture and then gradually spread with modifications to other Asian countries. The underlying focus of TCM is prevention, although diagnosis and treatment of disease also play important roles.

TCM seeks to ensure the balance of energy, which is called *chi* or *qi* (pronounced "chee"). Chi is the invisible flow of energy in the body that maintains health and vitality and enables the body to carry out its physiologic functions. Chi flows along certain pathways or meridians.

Another important concept in TCM (mentioned earlier) is that of *yin* and *yang*, opposing internal and external forces that, together, represent the whole.

TCM includes the following therapeutic techniques.

- *Acupuncture* uses very fine (hairlike) stainless steel needles to stimulate specific acupuncture points depending on the client's medical assessment and condition.
- *Acupressure* (Chinese massage) uses pressure from the fingers and thumbs to stimulate pressure points.
- *Herbal therapy* is an important part of TCM but it is sometimes difficult to locate a skilled herbalist because there are relatively few in the United States.
- *Qigong* (pronounced "chee-goong") is a self-discipline that involves the use of breathing, meditation, self-massage, and movement. Typically practiced daily, the movements are nontiring and are designed to stimulate the flow of chi (Figure 2–2 ■).
- *T'ai chi* (pronounced "ty chee") is a form of martial art. It originally focused on physical fitness and self-defense, but is currently used to improve overall health as well (Fontaine, 2005).
- *Moxibustion* involves the application of heat from a small piece of burning herb called *moxa (Artemesia vulgaris)*. The moxa stick is typically burned at the lateral side of the little toe. In TCM moxibustion has many uses. For example, studies from China demonstrate good success when moxibustion is used to help turn a fetus who is breech to a vertex presentation. Controlled research on this use for moxibustion is underway (Grabowska, 2006).

Mind-Based Therapies

Biofeedback is a method used to help individuals learn to control their physiologic responses based on the concept

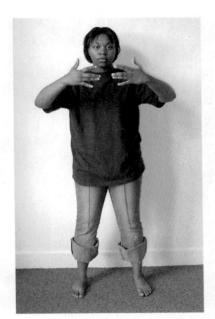

FIGURE 2–2 Pregnant woman practices the movements of Qigong.

that the mind controls the body. An individual is hooked up to a system of highly sensitive instruments that relay information about the body back to that person. Currently biofeedback has more than 150 applications for disease prevention and the restoration of health. The effectiveness of biofeedback has been proven in countless studies and it is now considered a conventional therapy more than a complementary one.

Hypnosis, whether guided by a trained hypnotherapist or induced through self-hypnosis, is a state of great mental and physical relaxation during which a person is very open to suggestions. In this state, the individual is able to modify body responses. Pregnant women who receive hypnosis before childbirth have reported shorter, less painful labors and births. *Visualization* is a complementary therapy in which a person goes into a relaxed state and focuses on or "visualizes" soothing or positive scenes such as a beach or a mountain glade. Visualization helps reduce stress and encourage relaxation. For example, a therapist may work with a woman before childbirth to help the woman create positive images of labor.

Guided imagery is a state of intense, focused concentration used to create compelling mental images. It is sometimes considered a form of hypnosis. Guided imagery is useful in imagining a desired effect such as weight loss or in mentally rehearsing a new procedure or activity.

Chiropractic Therapy

Chiropractic, the third largest independent health profession in the United States (behind medicine and dentistry), is based on concepts of manipulation to address health problems that are thought to be the result of abnormal nerve transmissions (subluxation) caused by misalignment of the spine. In the United States doctors of chiropractic perform more than 90% of all spinal manipulations (NC-CAM, 2007b). Chiropractors also stress the importance of proper nutrition and regular exercise to good health. Chiropractic is widely available and popular demand has earned it a higher level of insurance coverage than most other alternative therapies.

Massage Therapy

Massage has been used for centuries as a form of therapy. *Massage therapy* involves the manipulation of the soft tissues of the body to reduce stress and tension, increase circulation, diminish pain, and promote a sense of well-being. Different techniques have been developed; for example, Swedish massage, shiatsu massage, Rolfing, and trigger point massage. Most forms use techniques such as pressing, kneading, gliding, circular motion, tapping, and vibrational strokes.

Certain massage therapists specialize in massage for women during pregnancy. Massage is often helpful as women adapt to the discomforts of their changing bodies. In addition, certified nurse–midwives often use perineal massage before labor to stretch the muscles of the perineum around the vaginal opening and thereby prevent tearing of the tissues during childbirth. During labor, massage of the back and buttocks by the nurse, labor coach, or *doula* can help the woman relax and may help decrease her discomfort. Infant massage is also growing in popularity in the United States (Figure 2–3 ■).

Herbal Therapies

Herbal therapy or herbal medicine has been used since ancient times to treat illnesses and ailments. Like vitamins and minerals, herbs are a form of dietary supplement, but

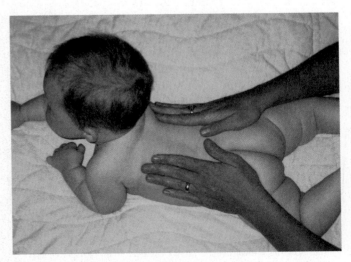

FIGURE 2–3 The calm soothing strokes of infant massage can help sooth an infant and minimize crying.

they are often used to treat the symptoms of specific ailments rather than simply to enhance overall health. Well-known herbal remedies include ginger, rosemary, ginseng, ginkgo, chamomile, oil of evening primrose, echinacea, garlic, lemon balm, and black cohosh.

Currently about 1500 botanical substances are sold in the United States as dietary supplements or as part of traditional ethnic medications. Herbal formulations, however, are not subject to Food and Drug Administration (FDA) premarket testing for safety and effectiveness (National Toxicology Program, 2006). Thus, these products can be sold over the counter with only little control. (The FDA does have the authority to pull a product off the market if it is proven to be dangerous.) Consequently most of what is known about herbs comes from Europe, where they have been studied for some time. Herbal products from Germany, France, England, and Australia are reasonably safe because in these countries herbs are regulated as if they were drugs.

The use of herbs during pregnancy is an especially important consideration for nurses working with childbearing families. Pregnant and lactating women interested in using herbs are best advised to consult with their healthcare provider before taking any herbs, even as teas. Lists identifying common herbs that women are advised to avoid or use with caution during pregnancy and lactation are available.

Therapeutic Touch

Therapeutic touch is a complementary therapy meant to be used with conventional medical care. It was developed in the early 1970s by Dr. Delores Krieger, a nursing professor at New York University, and Dora Kunz, a clairvoyant healer. Therapeutic touch is grounded in the belief that people are a system of energy with a self-healing potential. The therapeutic touch practitioner, often a nurse, can unite his or her energy field with that of the client's, directing it in a specific way to promote well-being and healing. Proponents of therapeutic touch believe that a strong desire to help the recipient is essential as is a conscious use of self to act as a link between the universal life energy and the other person (Fontaine, 2005). Impressive anecdotal evidence and many small studies suggest that therapeutic touch is effective in a variety of conditions. However, as

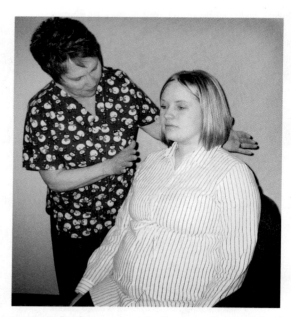

FIGURE 2–4 During pregnancy, therapeutic touch is often helpful in easing pain and reducing anxiety.
Source: Nurse Healers—Professional Associates International, the official organization for Therapeutic Touch. www.therapeutic_touch.org

yet, its effectiveness has not been scientifically proven in large, controlled studies (NCCAM, 2007a).

Like many other conventional and complementary therapies, therapeutic touch should be applied cautiously to pregnant women and newborns by trained providers (Figure 2–4 ■).

Other Types of Complementary and Alternative Therapies

This discussion only touched on some of the most common forms of complementary and alternative therapies. Other examples include ayurveda (the traditional medicine of India), meditation, craniosacral therapy, reflexology, hydrotherapy, Hatha yoga, regular physical exercise, aromatherapy, color and light therapy, music and sound therapies, magnetic therapy, and Reiki, to name a few. Readers interested in these therapies are referred to specialty texts.

Nursing Care of the Childbearing Family Using Complementary Therapies

Some form of complementary and alternative medicine (CAM) is currently being used by 36% of adults in the United States. When prayer for health reasons and megavitamin therapy are added to the definition, that number increases to 62%. Women use CAM more often than men do, as do people with higher educational levels and people who have been hospitalized within the past year. By race,

CULTURAL PERSPECTIVES

The World Health Organization estimates that 80% of Earth's population depends on plants to treat common ailments. Herbalism is an essential part of traditional Indian, Asian, Native American, and naturopathic medicines. Many homeopathic remedies are also developed from herbs.

when megavitamin therapy and prayer are included in the definition, Blacks are the greatest users of CAM. When those elements are excluded, Asians are the greatest users followed by Whites (NCCAM, 2007c).

The reality that women may use CAM and not reveal it raises some concern. Certain CAM modalities such as biofeedback, acupuncture, aromatherapy, and massage are not likely to cause adverse effects during pregnancy. The possibility exists, however, that interactions may occur between herbal therapies and other medications prescribed by the caregiver. Complications may also develop from the use of vitamin supplements.

Nurses who create a climate of respect and openness tend to be more effective in gathering information about a woman's use of complementary or alternative therapies. The following recommendations may be useful to nurses in taking a history (Cady, 2002).

- Ask questions that are direct and nonjudgmental in seeking information about the client's use of CAM.
- Ask questions about specific therapies including the use of herbal therapy and homeopathy. Because many people consider herbs to be natural substances and because they are often sold as dietary supplements, clients may not think to mention them.
- Avoid making negative or disparaging comments about CAM. Such comments send the message that CAM is not desirable and may discourage people from disclosing their use of CAM therapies.

In working with childbearing families, or indeed with any clients, nurses who use CAM therapies should choose those methods that are within the scope of nursing practice in their state and not limited by the licensure of other providers (such as massage therapists). Nurses are also best advised to use CAM therapies that are considered somewhat mainstream and that are supported by evidence about their safety and effectiveness. For example, a nurse working with a pregnant woman might suggest acupressure wristbands for the treatment of nausea. Other therapies that nurses often employ include progressive relaxation, exercise and movement, therapeutic touch, visualization and guided imagery, prayer, meditation, music therapy, massage, storytelling, aromatherapy, and journaling.

Nurses who use complementary modalities should document their use within the context of nursing practice. This is most effective when the modality is identified as an intervention to address a specific nursing diagnosis or identified client need. Thus, music therapy might be used for a laboring woman to address the identified nursing diagnosis of acute pain.

Nurses have a role in conducting and supporting research on CAM. Because of the variety of CAM therapies in use, research is needed in a host of areas. The results of research on CAM can be found in professional journals and at the NIH website. As the evidence supporting the use of certain interventions grows, nurses and other healthcare providers are incorporating the results as part of their evidence-based practice.

CHAPTER HIGHLIGHTS

- Family values, roles, and power are important to consider when attempting to provide holistic health care to childbearing families.
- Nuclear families consist of a mother, father, and children.
- Dual-career/dual-earner families comprise the majority of contemporary families in the United States.
- Childless families are a growing trend in American culture.
- Extended family members can play an active role in family life, decision making, and family roles.
- Single-parent families account for almost one-third of all U.S. families, and stepparent and binuclear families are increasingly common.
- The developmental framework looks at a family over time as it progresses through predictable stages within the life cycle.
- A family assessment provides an in-depth tool to collect pertinent family life information that can assist the nurse in planning care.
- Culture plays a significant part in a family's development, assignment of roles, and observance of traditions, customs, and taboos.

- Cultural norms influence a family's beliefs about the importance of children, pregnancy, health practices, and infant feeding.
- A cultural assessment can assist the nurse in identifying cultural norms and in providing culturally appropriate nursing care.
- A religious history is included when assessing contemporary families. When possible, the nurse accommodates the family's religious-based preferences for care.
- A complementary therapy is an adjunct to conventional medical treatment whereas an alternative therapy is used in place of prescribed medical therapy.
- The National Center for Complementary and Alternative Medicine (NCCAM) promotes research into complementary and alternative therapies and disseminates the information to consumers.
- CAM therapies have several benefits. Many of them emphasize prevention and wellness, place a higher value on holistic healing than on physical cure, are noninvasive, and have few side effects. In addition, many are more affordable and available than conventional therapies.

- Risks include lack of standardization, lack of regulation and research substantiating safety and effectiveness, inadequate training and certification of some healers, and financial and health risks of unproven methods.
- The term *homeopathy* is derived from the Greek word *homos* meaning "the same." It is a healing system that uses like to cure like; that is, homeopathic remedies are minute dilutions of substances that, if ingested in larger amounts, would produce effects *similar* to the symptoms of the disorder being treated.
- Traditional Chinese medicine (TCM) seeks to ensure the balance of energy, called *chi* or *qi*. Techniques of TCM include acupuncture, herbal therapy, nutrition, acupressure, moxibustion, qigong, and t'ai chi.
- Biofeedback is a method used to help individuals learn to control their physiologic responses based on the concept that the mind controls the body.
- Hypnosis, whether guided by a trained hypnotherapist or induced through self-hypnosis, is a state of great mental and physical relaxation during which a person is very open to suggestions.
- Guided imagery is a state of intense, focused concentration used to create compelling mental images.
- Chiropractic, a profession practiced by licensed chiropractors, is based on concepts of manipulation, especially spinal manipulation.
- Therapeutic touch is based on the belief that people are a system of energy with a self-healing potential. The therapeutic touch practitioner, often a nurse, can unite his or her energy field with that of the client's, directing it in a specific way to promote well-being and healing.
- Many nurses are open to and supportive of complementary and alternative therapies. Nurses who incorporate such therapies into their practice must be certain that they are practicing within the framework of their nurse practice act and with the informed consent of their clients.

EXPLORE PEARSON **mynursingkit**™

MyNursingKit is your one stop for online chapter review materials and resources. Prepare for success with additional NCLEX®-style practice questions, interactive assignments and activities, web links, animations and videos, and more!

Register your access code from the front of your book at
www.mynursingkit.com

CHAPTER REFERENCES

American Association of Naturopathic Physicians. (2005). *What is naturopathic medicine?* Retrieved December 7, 2005, from http://www.naturopathic.org/naturopathic_medicine/whatis.aspx

Andrews, M. M., & Boyle, J. S. (2007). *Transcultural concepts in nursing care* (5th ed.). Philadelphia: Wolter/Kluber/Lippincott Williams & Wilkins.

Cady, R. (2002). Are there legal issues of concern for nurses when patients use complimentary (sic) and alternative medicine? *MCN, 27*(2), 119.

Callister, L. C. (2006). Doing the month: Chinese postpartum practices. *MCN: American Journal of Maternal–Child Nursing, 31*(6), 390.

Cassar, L. (2006). Cultural expectations of Muslims and Orthodox Jews in regard to pregnancy and the postpartum period: A study in comparison and contrast. *International Journal of Childbirth Education, 21*(2), 27–30.

Do, H. (2005). Chinese culture. *Ethnomed.* Retrieved November 29, 2005, from http://ethnomed.org

Duvall, E. M. (1977). *Marriage and family development* (5th ed.). New York: Harper Row.

Eggenberger, S. K., Grassley, J., & Restrepo, E. (2006). Culturally competent nursing care for families: Listening to the voices of Mexican-American women. *OJIN: The Online Journal of Issues in Nursing, 11*(3), 1–16.

Faust, J. E. (2005). Instruments in the hands of God. *Liahona Archives.* Retrieved January 4, 2008, from www.lds.org

Fontaine, K. L. (2005). *Complementary and alternative therapies for nursing practice* (2nd ed.). Upper Saddle River, NJ: Prentice Hall Health.

Giger, J. N., & Davidhizar, R. E. (2008). *Transcultural nursing: Assessment and interventions* (5th ed.). St. Louis, MO: Elsevier Mosby.

Grabowska, C. (2006). Turning the breech using moxibustion. *Midwives: The Official Journal of the Royal College of Midwives, 9*(12), 484–485.

Hammond, M. M., White, C. B., & Fetters, M. D. (2005). Opening cultural doors: Providing culturally sensitive healthcare to Arab American and American Muslim patients. *American Journal of Obstetrics & Gynecology, 193*(4), 1307–1311.

Holroyd, E., Twinn, S., & Yim, I. W. (2004). Exploring Chinese women's cultural beliefs and behaviors regarding the practice of "doing the month." *Women's Health, 40*(3), 109–123.

National Center for Complementary and Alternative Medicine. (2007a). *Backgrounder: Energy medicine: An overview.* Retrieved January 4, 2008, from http://nccam.nih.gov

National Center for Complementary and Alternative Medicine. (2007b). *Backgrounder:*

Manipulative and body-based practices: An overview. Retrieved January 4, 2008, from http://nccam.nih.gov

National Center for Complementary and Alternative Medicine. (2007c). *The Use of CAM in the United States.* Retrieved January 4, 2008, from http://nccam.nih.gov

National Toxicology Program. (2006). Herbal medicines. Retrieved May 21, 2008 from http://ntp.niehs.nih.gov/

Royal College of Midwives. (2006). Homeopathy for childbirth: Remedies and research. *Midwives: The Official Journal of the Royal College of Midwives, 9*(11), 438–440.

Safadi, R. (2005). Jordanian women: Perceptions and practices of first-time pregnancy. *International Journal of Nursing Practice, 11*(6), 269–276.

Semenic, S. E., Callister, L. C., & Feldman, P. (2004). Giving birth: The voices of Orthodox Jewish women living in Canada. *Journal of obstetric, gynecologic, and neonatal nursing, 33*(1), 80–87.

US Census Bureau. (2006). American Fact Finder: Glossary. Retrieved September 2, 2006 from http://factfinder.census.gov/home/en/epss/glossary-2.html

CHAPTER 3

Reproductive Anatomy and Physiology

I am amazed by how little many of our students know about anatomy, physiology, and reproduction. As nurses, we must use every opportunity we have to teach young people about their bodies and those of their partners. Information is the key to helping keep them safe and well!
—University Health Clinic Nurse

LEARNING OUTCOMES

3-1. Identify the structures and functions of the female reproductive system.

3-2. Identify the structures and functions of the male reproductive system.

3-3. Explain the significance of specific female reproductive structures during childbirth.

3-4. Describe the actions of the hormones that affect reproductive functioning.

3-5. Identify the two phases of the ovarian cycle and the changes that occur in each phase.

3-6. Describe the phases of the menstrual cycle, their dominant hormones, and the changes that occur in each phase.

KEY TERMS

Understanding childbearing requires more than understanding sexual intercourse or the process by which the female and male sex cells unite. The nurse must also become familiar with the structures and functions that make childbearing possible and the phenomena that initiate it. This chapter presents the anatomic, physiologic, and sexual aspects of the female and male reproductive systems.

The female and male reproductive organs are *homologous;* that is, they are fundamentally similar in structure and function. The primary functions of both female and male reproductive systems are to produce sex cells and transport them to locations where their union can occur. The sex cells, called *gametes*, are produced by specialized organs called *gonads*. A series of ducts and glands within both male and female reproductive systems contributes to the production and transport of the gametes.

Female Reproductive System

The female reproductive system consists of the external and internal genitals and the accessory organs of the breasts. Because of its importance to childbearing, the bony pelvis is also discussed in this chapter.

External Genitals

All the external reproductive organs except the glandular structures can be directly inspected. The appearance of the external genitalia varies greatly among women. Heredity, age, race, and the number of children a woman has borne influence the size, color, and shape of her external organs. The female external genitals, also referred to as the **vulva**, include the following structures (Figure 3–1 ■).

- Mons pubis
- Labia majora
- Labia minora
- Clitoris
- Urethral meatus and opening of the paraurethral (Skene's) glands
- Vaginal vestibule (vaginal orifice, vulvovaginal glands, hymen, and fossa navicularis)
- Perineal body

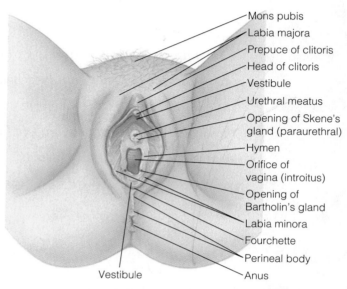

Mons pubis
Labia majora
Prepuce of clitoris
Head of clitoris
Vestibule
Urethral meatus
Opening of Skene's gland (paraurethral)
Hymen
Orifice of vagina (introitus)
Opening of Bartholin's gland
Labia minora
Fourchette
Perineal body
Vestibule
Anus

FIGURE 3–1 Female external genitals, longitudinal view.

Although they are not true parts of the female reproductive system, the urethral meatus and perineal body are considered here because of their proximity and relationship to the vulva.

The vulva has a generous supply of blood and nerves. As a woman ages estrogen secretions decrease, causing the vulvar organs to atrophy.

Mons Pubis

The *mons pubis* is a softly rounded mound of subcutaneous fatty tissue beginning at the lowest portion of the anterior abdominal wall (see Figure 3–1). Also known as the *mons veneris*, this structure covers the front portion of the symphysis pubis. The mons pubis is covered with pubic hair, typically with the hairline forming a transverse line across the lower abdomen. The hair is short and varies from sparse and fine in Asian women to heavy, coarse, and curly in women of African descent. The mons pubis protects the pelvic bones, especially during coitus.

Labia Majora

The *labia majora* are longitudinal, raised folds of pigmented skin, one on either side of the vulvar cleft. As the pair descend, they narrow and merge to form the posterior junction of the perineal skin. Their chief function is to protect the structures lying between them. The labia majora are covered by hair follicles and sebaceous glands, with underlying adipose and muscle tissue.

The inner surface of the labia majora in women who have not had children is moist and looks like mucous membrane, whereas after many births it is more skinlike. With each pregnancy, the labia majora become less prominent.

Because of the extensive venous network in the labia majora, varicosities may occur during pregnancy, and obstetric or sexual trauma may cause hematomas. The labia majora share an extensive lymphatic supply with the other structures of the vulva, which can facilitate the spread of cancer in the female reproductive organs. Because of the nerves supplying the labia majora (from the first lumbar and third sacral segment of the spinal cord), certain regional anesthesia blocks will affect them and cause numbness.

Labia Minora

The *labia minora* are soft folds of skin within the labia majora that converge near the anus, forming the *fourchette*. Each labium minus has the appearance of shiny mucous membrane, moist and devoid of hair follicles. The labia minora are rich in sebaceous glands, which lubricate and waterproof the vulvar skin and provide bactericidal secretions. Because the sebaceous glands do not open into hair follicles but open directly onto the surface of the skin, sebaceous cysts commonly occur in this area. Vulvovaginitis in this area is irritating because the labia minora have many tactile nerve endings. The labia minora increase in size at puberty and decrease after menopause because of changes in estrogen levels.

Clitoris

The *clitoris*, located between the labia minora, is about 5 to 6 mm long and 6 to 8 mm across. Its tissue is essentially erectile. The glans of the clitoris is partly covered by a fold of skin called the *prepuce*, or clitoral hood. This area resembles an opening to an orifice and may be confused with the urethral meatus. Accidental attempts to insert a catheter in this area produce extreme discomfort. The clitoris has rich blood and nerve supplies and is the primary erogenous organ of women. In addition, it secretes *smegma*, which along with other vulval secretions has a unique odor that may be sexually stimulating to the male. In some cultures, the clitoris is removed (see discussion in Chapter 5 ∞).

Urethral Meatus and Paraurethral Glands

The *urethral meatus* is located 1 to 2.5 cm beneath the clitoris in the midline of the vestibule; it often appears as a puckered, slitlike opening. At times the meatus is difficult to visualize because of the presence of blind dimples, small mucosal folds, or wide variations in location.

The paraurethral glands, or *Skene's glands*, open into the posterior wall of the urethra close to its opening (see Figure 3–1). Their secretions lubricate the vaginal opening, facilitating sexual intercourse.

Vaginal Vestibule

The vaginal vestibule is a boat-shaped depression enclosed by the labia majora which is visible when they are separated. The vestibule contains the vaginal opening, or *introitus*, which is the border between the external and internal genitals.

The *hymen* is a thin, elastic collar or semicollar of tissue that surrounds the vaginal opening. The appearance changes during the woman's lifetime. At birth, the hymen is essentially avascular. For thousands of years, some societies have perpetuated the belief that the hymen covers the vaginal opening and thus an intact hymen is a sign of virginity. However, modern studies of female genital anatomy have revealed that the hymen surrounds rather than entirely covers the vaginal opening, and can be torn not only through sexual intercourse but also through strenuous physical activity, masturbation, menstruation, or the use of tampons, thus dispelling old beliefs. For discussion of the nurse's role in discussing these topics see Chapter 5 ∞.

External to the hymen at the base of the vestibule are two small papular elevations containing the openings of the ducts of the *vulvovaginal (Bartholin's) glands*. They lie under the constrictor muscle of the vagina. These glands secrete a clear, thick, alkaline mucus that enhances the viability and motility of the sperm deposited in the vaginal vestibule. These gland ducts can harbor *Neisseria gonorrhea* and other bacteria, which can cause pus formation and abscesses in the Bartholin's glands.

The vestibular area is innervated mainly by the perineal nerve from the sacral plexus. The area is not sensitive to touch generally; however, the hymen contains numerous free nerve endings as receptors to pain.

Perineal Body

The **perineal body** is a wedge-shaped mass of fibromuscular tissue found between the lower part of the vagina and the anus (Figure 3–1). The superficial area between the anus and the vagina is referred to as the *perineum*.

The muscles that meet at the perineal body are the external sphincter ani, both levator ani (the superficial and deep transverse perineal), and the bulbocavernosus. These muscles mingle with elastic fibers and connective tissue in an arrangement that allows a remarkable amount of stretching. During the last part of labor, the perineal body thins out until it is just a few centimeters thick. This tissue is often the site of an episiotomy or lacerations during childbirth (see Chapter 22 ∞).

Female Internal Reproductive Organs

The female internal reproductive organs—the vagina, uterus, fallopian tubes, and ovaries—are target organs for estrogenic hormones and they play a unique part in the reproductive cycle (Figure 3–2 ■). Certain internal reproductive organs can be palpated during vaginal examination and assessed with various instruments.

Vagina

The **vagina** is a muscular and membranous tube that connects the external genitals with the uterus. It extends from the vulva to the uterus in a position nearly parallel to the plane of the pelvic brim. The vagina is often called the *birth canal* because it forms the lower part of the pelvis through which the fetus must pass during birth.

Because the cervix of the uterus projects into the upper part of the anterior wall of the vagina, the anterior wall is approximately 2.5 cm shorter than the posterior wall. Measurements range from 6 to 8 cm for the anterior wall and from 7 to 10 cm for the posterior wall.

In the upper part of the vagina, which is called the vaginal vault, there is a recess or hollow around the cervix.

This area is called the *vaginal fornix*. Since the walls of the vaginal vault are very thin, various structures can be palpated through the walls, including the uterus, a distended bladder, the ovaries, the appendix, the cecum, the colon, and the ureters. The upper fourth of the vagina is separated from the rectum by the pouch of Douglas (sometimes referred to as the cul-de-sac of Douglas). This deep pouch or recess is posterior to the cervix.

When a woman lies on her back after intercourse, the space in the fornix permits the pooling of semen. The collection of a large number of sperm near the cervix at or near the time of ovulation increases the chances of pregnancy.

The walls of the vagina are covered with ridges, or rugae, crisscrossing each other. These rugae allow the vaginal tissues to stretch enough for the fetus to pass through during childbirth.

During a woman's reproductive life, an acidic vaginal environment is normal (pH 4–5). Secretion from the vaginal epithelium provides a moist environment. The acidic environment is maintained by a symbiotic relationship between lactic acid-producing bacilli (Döderlein bacillus or lactobacillus) and the vaginal epithelial cells. These cells contain glycogen, which is broken down by the bacilli into lactic acid. The amount of glycogen is regulated by the

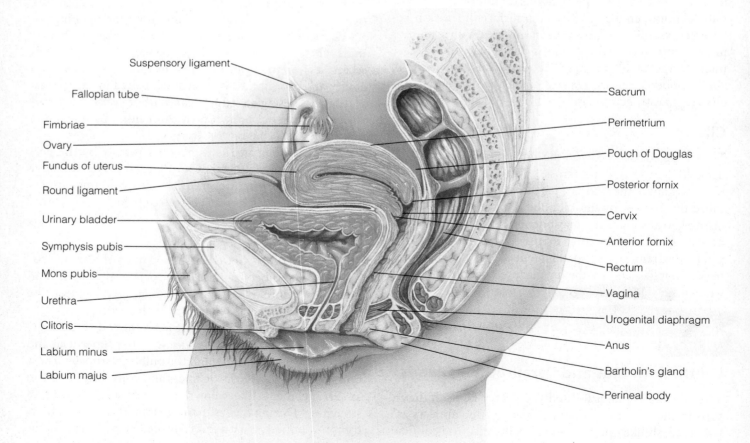

FIGURE 3–2 Female internal reproductive organs.

ovarian hormones. Any interruption of this process can destroy the normal self-cleaning action of the vagina. Such interruption may be caused by antibiotic therapy, douching, or use of perineal sprays or deodorants. (For further discussion, see Chapter 5 ∞.)

The acidic vaginal environment is normal only during the mature reproductive years and in the first days of life, when maternal hormones are operating in the infant. A relatively neutral pH of 7.5 is normal from infancy until puberty and after menopause.

Each third of the vagina is supplied by a distinct vascular and lymphatic pattern (Figure 3–3 ■). In addition to venous drainage going to the heart and lungs, anastomoses of the veins are present and make it possible for a pelvic embolism or carcinoma to bypass the heart and lungs and lodge in the brain, spine, or other remote part of the body.

Vaginal lymphatics drain into the external and internal iliac nodes, the hypogastric nodes, and the inguinal glands. The posterior wall drains into nodes lying in the rectovaginal septum. Any vaginal infection follows these routes.

The pudendal nerve supplies what relatively little somatic innervation there is to the lower third of the vagina. Thus sensation during sexual excitement and coitus is reduced in this area, as is vaginal pain during the second stage of labor.

The vagina has three functions:

- To serve as the passage for sperm and for the fetus during birth
- To provide passage for the menstrual products from the uterine endometrium to the outside of the body
- To protect against trauma from sexual intercourse and infection from pathogenic organisms

Uterus

As the core of reproduction and hence continuation of the human race, the uterus, or womb, has been endowed with a mystical aura. Numerous customs, taboos, mores, and values have evolved about women and their reproductive function. Although scientific knowledge has replaced much of this folklore, remnants of old ideas and superstitions persist. To provide effective care, nurses must be cognizant of their own attitudes and beliefs, as well as those of their clients.

The **uterus** is a hollow, muscular, thick-walled organ shaped like an upside-down pear (Figure 3–4 ■). It lies in the center of the pelvic cavity between the base of the bladder and the rectum and above the vagina. It is level with or slightly below the brim of the pelvis, with the external opening of the cervix (external os) about the level of the ischial spines. The uterus of the mature woman weighs about 40 to 70 g and is 6 to 8 cm long (Cunningham et al., 2005; Krantz, 2007).

The body of the uterus can move freely forward or backward. Only the cervix is anchored laterally. Thus the

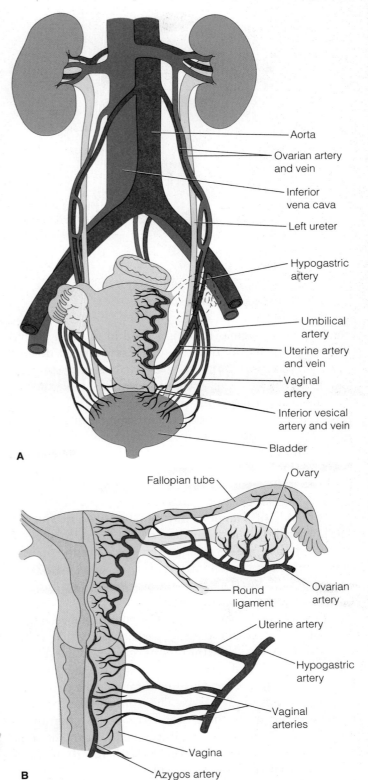

FIGURE 3–3 Blood supply to internal reproductive organs. *A,* Pelvic blood supply. *B,* Blood supply to vagina, ovaries, uterus, and fallopian tube.

position of the uterus can vary, depending on a woman's posture and musculature, number of children borne, bladder and rectal fullness, and even normal respiratory patterns. Generally, the uterus bends forward, forming a sharp

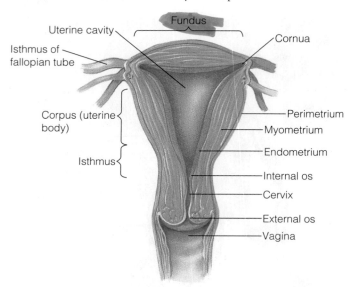

FIGURE 3–4 Structures of the uterus.

angle with the vagina. There is a bend in the area of the isthmus of the uterus; from there the cervix points downward. The uterus is said to be anteverted when it is in this position. The anteverted position is considered normal.

Four pairs of ligaments (i.e., the cardinal, uterosacral, round, and broad) support the uterus. Single anterior and posterior ligaments also support the uterus.

The uterus is divided into two major parts: the upper triangular portion called the **corpus** or uterine body; and the lower cylindric portion called the **cervix**. The corpus comprises the upper two-thirds of the uterus and is composed mainly of a smooth muscle layer (myometrium). The lower third is the cervix or neck. The rounded uppermost portion of the corpus that extends above the points of attachment of the fallopian tubes is called the **fundus**. The elongated portion of the uterus where the fallopian tubes enter is called the **cornua**.

The **isthmus** is that portion of the uterus between the internal cervical os and the endometrial cavity. The isthmus is about 6 mm above the uterine opening of the cervix (the internal os), and it is in this area that the uterine lining changes into the mucous membrane of the cervix; it joins the corpus to the cervix. The isthmus takes on importance in pregnancy because it becomes the lower uterine segment. With the cervix, it is a passive segment and not part of the contractile uterus. At birth, this thin lower segment, situated behind the bladder, is the site for lower-segment cesarean births (see Chapter 23 ∞).

The blood and lymphatic supplies to the uterus are extensive. Innervation of the uterus is entirely by the autonomic nervous system. Even without an intact nerve supply, the uterus can contract adequately for birth; for example, hemiplegic women have adequate uterine contractions.

Pain of uterine contractions is carried to the central nervous system by the 11th and 12th thoracic nerve roots.

Pain from the cervix and upper vagina passes through the ilioinguinal and pudendal nerves. The motor fibers to the uterus arise from the 7th and 8th thoracic vertebrae. Because the sensory and motor levels are separate, epidural anesthesia can be used during labor and birth.

The function of the uterus is to provide a safe environment for fetal development. The uterine lining is cyclically prepared by steroid hormones for implantation of the embryo, a process known as **nidation**. Once the embryo is implanted, the developing fetus is protected until it is expelled.

Both the body of the uterus and the cervix are changed permanently by pregnancy. The body never returns to its prepregnant size, and the external os changes from a circular opening of about 3 mm to a transverse slit with irregular edges.

UTERINE CORPUS The uterine corpus is made up of three layers. The outermost layer is the *serosal layer*, or **perimetrium**, which is composed of peritoneum. The middle layer is the *muscular uterine layer*, or **myometrium**. This muscular uterine layer is continuous with the muscle layers of the fallopian tubes and the vagina. This characteristic helps these organs present a unified reaction to various stimuli—ovulation, orgasm, or the deposit of sperm in the vagina. These muscle fibers also extend into the ovarian, round, and cardinal ligaments and minimally into the uterosacral ligaments, which helps explain the vague but disturbing pelvic "aches and pains" reported by many pregnant women.

The myometrium has three distinct layers of uterine (smooth) involuntary muscles (Figure 3–5 ■). The outer layer, found mainly over the fundus, is made up of longitudinal muscles that cause cervical effacement and expel the fetus during birth. The thick middle layer is made up of interlacing muscle fibers in figure-eight patterns. These muscle fibers surround large blood vessels, and their contraction produces a hemostatic action (a tourniquet-like action on blood vessels to stop bleeding after birth). The inner muscle layer consists of circular fibers that form sphincters at the fallopian tube attachment sites and at the internal os. The internal os sphincter inhibits the expulsion of the uterine contents during pregnancy but stretches in labor as cervical dilatation occurs. An incompetent cervical os can be caused by a torn, weak, or absent sphincter at the internal os. The sphincters at the fallopian tubes prevent menstrual blood from flowing backward into the fallopian tubes from the uterus.

Although each layer of muscle has been discussed as having a unique function, it must be remembered that the uterine musculature works as a whole. The uterine contractions of labor are responsible for the dilatation of the cervix and provide the major force for the passage of the fetus through the pelvis and vaginal canal at birth.

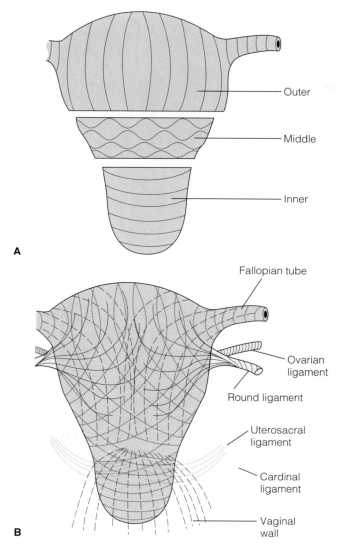

A

B

FIGURE 3–5 Uterine muscle layers. *A,* Muscle fiber placement. *B,* Interlacing of uterine muscle layers.

Outer

Middle

Inner

Fallopian tube

Ovarian ligament

Round ligament

Uterosacral ligament

Cardinal ligament

Vaginal wall

The *mucosal layer,* or **endometrium**, of the uterine corpus is the innermost layer. This single layer consists of columnar epithelium, glands, and stroma. From menarche to menopause, the endometrium undergoes monthly degeneration and renewal in the absence of pregnancy. As it responds to the governing hormonal cycle and prostaglandin influence, the endometrium varies in thickness from 0.5 to 5 mm.

The glands of the endometrium produce a thin, watery, alkaline secretion that keeps the uterine cavity moist. This endometrial milk not only helps sperm travel to the fallopian tubes but also nourishes the developing embryo before it implants in the endometrium (Chapter 4 ∞).

The blood supply to the endometrium is unique. In the myometrium, the radial arteries branch off from the arcuate arteries at right angles. Once inside the endometrium, they become the basal arteries supplying the zona basalis (a layer of the endometrium) and ultimately become the coiled arteries supplying the zona functionalis (also part of the endometrium). The basal arteries are not sensitive to cyclic hormonal control; hence, the zona basalis portion remains intact and is the site of new endometrial tissue generation. The coiled arteries are extremely sensitive to hormonal control. Their response is alternate relaxation and constriction during the ischemic, or terminal, phase of the menstrual cycle. These differing responses allow part of the endometrium to remain intact while other endometrial tissue is shed during menstruation.

When pregnancy occurs and the endometrium is not shed, the reticular stromal cells surrounding the endometrial glands become the decidual cells of pregnancy. The stromal cells are highly vascular, channeling a rich blood supply to the endometrial surface.

THE CERVIX The narrow neck of the uterus is the **cervix**. It meets the body of the uterus at the internal os and descends about 2.5 cm to connect with the vagina at the external os (see Figure 3–4). Thus it provides a protective entrance for the body of the uterus. The cervix is divided by its line of attachment into the vaginal and supravaginal areas. The vaginal cervix projects into the vagina at an angle of from 45 to 90 degrees. The *supravaginal* cervix is surrounded by the attachments that give the uterus its main support: the uterosacral ligaments, the transverse ligaments of the cervix (Mackenrodt's ligaments), and the pubocervical ligaments.

The vaginal cervix appears pink and ends at the external os. The cervical canal appears rosy red and is lined with columnar ciliated epithelium, which contains mucus-secreting glands. Most cervical cancer begins at this *squamocolumnar* junction. The specific location of the junction varies with age and number of pregnancies.

Elasticity is the chief characteristic of the cervix. Its ability to stretch is because of the high fibrous and collagenous content of the supportive tissues and also to the vast number of folds in the cervical lining.

The cervical mucus has three functions:

- To lubricate the vaginal canal
- To act as a bacteriostatic agent
- To provide an alkaline environment to shelter deposited sperm from the acidic vagina

At ovulation, cervical mucus is clearer, thinner, more profuse, and more alkaline than at other times.

Uterine Ligaments

The uterine ligaments support and stabilize the various reproductive organs. The ligaments shown in Figure 3–6 ■ are described as follows:

1. The **broad ligament** keeps the uterus centrally placed and provides stability within the pelvic cavity. It is a double layer that is continuous with the abdominal peritoneum. The broad ligament covers the uterus

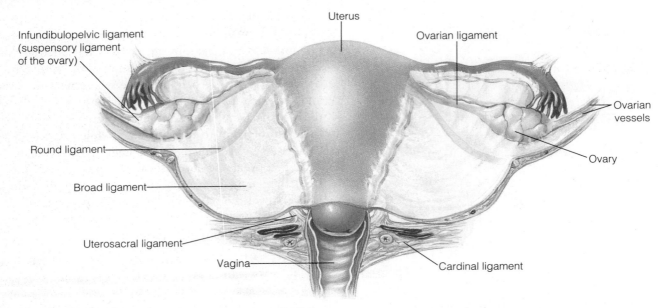

FIGURE 3–6 Uterine ligaments.

anteriorly and posteriorly and extends outward from the uterus to enfold the fallopian tubes. The round and ovarian ligaments are at the upper border of the broad ligament. At its lower border, it forms the cardinal ligaments. Between the folds of the broad ligament are connective tissue, involuntary muscle, blood and lymph vessels, and nerves.

2. The **round ligaments** help the broad ligament keep the uterus in place. The round ligaments arise from the sides of the uterus near the fallopian tube insertions. They extend outward between the folds of the broad ligament, passing through the inguinal ring and canals and eventually fusing with the connective tissue of the labia majora. Made up of longitudinal muscle, the round ligaments enlarge during pregnancy. During labor the round ligaments steady the uterus, pulling downward and forward so that the presenting part of the fetus is moved into the cervix.

3. The **ovarian ligaments** anchor the lower pole of the ovary to the cornua of the uterus. They are composed of muscle fibers that allow the ligaments to contract. This contractile ability influences the position of the ovary to some extent, thus helping the fimbriae of the fallopian tubes to "catch" the ovum as it is released each month.

4. The **cardinal ligaments** are the chief uterine supports and suspend the uterus from the side walls of the true pelvis. These ligaments, also known as Mackenrodt's or transverse cervical ligaments, arise from the sides of the pelvic walls and attach to the cervix in the upper vagina. These ligaments prevent uterine prolapse and also support the upper vagina.

5. The **infundibulopelvic ligament** suspends and supports the ovaries. Arising from the outer third of the broad ligament, the infundibulopelvic ligament contains the ovarian vessels and nerves.

6. The **uterosacral ligaments** provide support for the uterus and cervix at the level of the ischial spines. Arising on each side of the pelvis from the posterior wall of the uterus, the uterosacral ligaments sweep back around the rectum and insert on the sides of the first and second sacral vertebrae. The uterosacral ligaments contain smooth muscle fibers, connective tissue, blood and lymph vessels, and nerves. They also contain sensory nerve fibers that contribute to dysmenorrhea (painful menstruation) (see Chapter 5 ∞).

Fallopian Tubes

The two **fallopian tubes**, also known as the *oviducts* or *uterine tubes*, arise from each side of the uterus and reach almost to the sides of the pelvis, where they turn toward the ovaries (Figure 3–7 ■). Each tube is approximately 8 to 13.5 cm long. A short section of each fallopian tube is inside the uterus; its opening into the uterus is only 1 mm in diameter. The fallopian tubes link the peritoneal cavity with the uterus and vagina. This linkage increases a woman's biologic vulnerability to disease processes.

Each fallopian tube may be divided into three parts: the *isthmus*, the *ampulla*, and the infundibulum or *fimbria*. The fallopian tube isthmus is straight and narrow, with a thick muscular wall and an opening (lumen) 2 to 3 mm in diameter. It is the site of tubal ligation, a surgical procedure to prevent pregnancy (see Chapter 5 ∞).

Next to the isthmus is the curved **ampulla**, which comprises the outer third of the tube. Fertilization of the secondary oocyte by a spermatozoon usually occurs here. The ampulla ends at the **fimbria**, which is a funnel-like en-

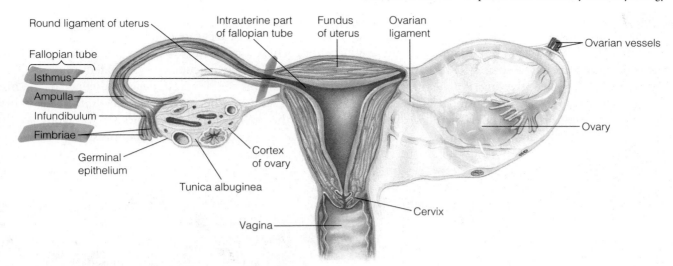

FIGURE 3–7 Fallopian tubes and ovaries.

largement with many fingerlike projections (fimbriae) reaching out to the ovary. The longest of these, the fimbria ovarica, is attached to the ovary to increase the chances of intercepting the ovum as it is released.

The wall of the fallopian tube consists of four layers: peritoneal (serous), subserous (adventitial), muscular, and mucous tissues. The peritoneum covers the tubes. The subserous layer contains the blood and nerve supply, and the muscular layer is responsible for the peristaltic movement of the tube. The mucosal layer, immediately next to the muscular layer, is composed of ciliated and nonciliated cells, with the number of ciliated cells more abundant at the fimbria. Nonciliated cells secrete a protein-rich, serous fluid that nourishes the ovum. The constantly moving tubal cilia propel the ovum toward the uterus. Because the ovum is a large cell, this ciliary action is needed to assist the tube's muscular layer peristalsis. Any malformation or malfunction of the tubes can result in infertility, ectopic pregnancy, or even sterility.

A well-functioning tubal transport system involves active fimbriae close to the ovary, peristalsis of the tube created by the muscular layer, ciliated currents beating toward the uterus, and the proximal contraction and distal relaxation of the tube caused by different types of prostaglandins.

A rich blood and lymphatic supply serves each fallopian tube. Thus the tubes have an unusual ability to recover from an inflammatory process (see Figure 3–3). The fallopian tubes have three functions:

- To provide transport for the ovum from the ovary to the uterus (transport time through the fallopian tubes varies from 3 to 4 days)
- To provide a site for fertilization
- To serve as a warm, moist, nourishing environment for the ovum or zygote (fertilized egg) (See Chapter 4 ∞ for further discussion.)

Ovaries

The **ovaries** are two almond-shaped structures just below the pelvic brim. One ovary is located on each side of the pelvic cavity. Their size varies among women and with the stage of the menstrual cycle. Each ovary weighs approximately 6 to 10 g and is 1.5 to 3 cm wide, 2 to 5 cm long, and 1 to 1.5 cm thick. The ovaries of girls are small, but they become larger after puberty and then decrease in size following menopause. They also change in appearance from a dull white, smooth-surfaced organ to a pitted gray organ as the woman ages. The pitting is caused by scarring due to ovulation. The ovaries are held in place by the broad, ovarian, and infundibulopelvic ligaments. It is rare for both ovaries to be at the same level in the pelvic cavity.

There is no peritoneal covering for the ovaries. Although this lack of covering assists the mature ovum to erupt, it also allows easier spread of malignant cells from cancer of the ovaries. A single layer of cuboidal epithelial cells, called the germinal epithelium, covers the ovaries. The ovaries are composed of three layers: the tunica albuginea, the cortex, and the medulla. The *tunica albuginea* is dense and dull white and serves as a protective layer. The *cortex* is the main functional part because it contains ova, graafian follicles, corpora lutea, the degenerated corpora lutea (corpora albicantia), and degenerated follicles. The *medulla* is completely surrounded by the cortex and contains the nerves and the blood and lymphatic vessels.

The ovaries are the primary source of two important hormones: the estrogens and progesterone. *Estrogens* are associated with those characteristics contributing to femaleness, including breast alveolar lobule growth and duct development. The ovaries secrete large amounts of estrogen, while the adrenal cortex (extraglandular sites) produces minute amounts of estrogen in nonpregnant women. *Progesterone* is often called the *hormone of pregnancy* because its effects on the uterus allow pregnancy to be maintained. The placenta is the primary source of progesterone during pregnancy. This hormone also inhibits the action of prolactin in alpha-lactalbumin synthesis, thereby preventing lactation during pregnancy (Riordan, 2005).

The interplay between the ovarian hormones and other hormones such as follicle-stimulating hormone (FSH) and luteinizing hormone (LH) is responsible for the cyclic changes that allow pregnancy to occur. The hormonal and physical changes that occur during the female reproductive cycle are discussed in depth later in this chapter. Between the ages of 45 and 55, a woman's ovaries secrete decreasing amounts of estrogen. Eventually, ovulatory activity ceases and menopause occurs.

Bony Pelvis

The female bony pelvis has two unique functions:

- To support and protect the pelvic contents
- To form the relatively fixed axis of the birth passage

Because the pelvis is so important to childbearing, its structure must be understood clearly.

Bony Structure

The pelvis is made up of four bones: two innominate bones, the sacrum, and the coccyx. The pelvis resembles a bowl or basin; its sides are the innominate bones, and its back is the sacrum and coccyx. Lined with fibrocartilage and held tightly together by ligaments (Figure 3–8 ■), the four bones join at the symphysis pubis, the two sacroiliac joints, and the sacrococcygeal joints.

The *innominate bones*, also known as the hip bones, are made up of three separate bones: the ilium, ischium, and pubis. These bones fuse to form a circular cavity, the *acetabulum*, which articulates with the femur.

The *ilium* is the broad, upper prominence of the hip. The iliac crest is the margin of the ilium. The ischial spines, the foremost projections nearest the groin, are the site of attachment for ligaments and muscles.

The *ischium*, the strongest bone, is under the ilium and below the acetabulum. The L-shaped ischium ends in a marked protuberance, the ischial tuberosity, on which the weight of a seated body rests. The **ischial spines** arise near the junction of the ilium and ischium and jut into the pelvic cavity. The shortest diameter of the pelvic cavity is between the ischial spines. The ischial spines serve as reference points during labor to evaluate the descent of the fetal head into the birth canal (see Chapter 17 and Figure 17–7 ∞).

The **pubis** forms the slightly bowed front portion of the innominate bone. Extending medially from the acetabulum to the midpoint of the bony pelvis, each pubis meets the other to form a joint called the **symphysis pubis**. The triangular space below this junction is known as the pubic arch. The fetal head passes under this arch during birth. The symphysis pubis is formed by heavy fibrocartilage and the superior and inferior pubic ligaments. The mobility of the inferior ligament increases during a first pregnancy and to a greater extent in subsequent pregnancies.

The sacroiliac joints also have a degree of mobility that increases near the end of pregnancy as the result of an upward, gliding movement. The pelvic outlet may be in-

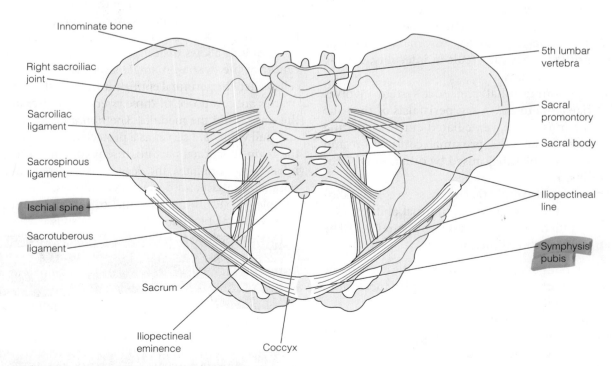

FIGURE 3–8 Pelvic bones with supporting ligaments.

creased by 1.5 to 2 cm in the squatting, sitting, and dorsal lithotomy positions. These relaxations of the joints are induced by the hormones of pregnancy.

The *sacrum* is a wedge-shaped bone formed by the fusion of five vertebrae. The anterior upper portion of the sacrum has a projection into the pelvic cavity known as the **sacral promontory**. This projection is another obstetric guide in determining pelvic measurements. (For a discussion of pelvic measurements, see Chapter 10 ∞.)

The small triangular bone last on the vertebral column is the coccyx. It articulates with the sacrum at the sacrococcygeal joint. The coccyx usually moves backward during labor to provide more room for the fetus.

Pelvic Floor

The muscular floor of the bony pelvis is designed to overcome the force of gravity exerted on the pelvic organs. It acts as a buttress to the irregularly shaped pelvic outlet, thereby providing stability and support for surrounding structures.

Deep fascia, the levator ani, and coccygeal muscles form the part of the pelvic floor known as the **pelvic diaphragm**. The components of the pelvic diaphragm function as a whole, yet they are able to move over one another. This feature provides an exceptional capacity for dilatation during birth and return to pre-pregnancy condition following birth. Above the pelvic diaphragm is the pelvic cavity; below and behind it is the perineum. The sacrum is located posteriorly.

The levator ani muscle makes up the major portion of the pelvic diaphragm and consists of four muscles: the iliococcygeus, pubococcygeus, puborectalis, and pubovaginalis. The iliococcygeal muscle, a thin muscular sheet underlying the sacrospinous ligament, helps the levator ani support the pelvic organs. Muscles of the pelvic floor are shown in Figure 3–9 ■ and discussed in Table 3–1.

Pelvic Division

The **pelvic cavity** is divided into the false pelvis and the true pelvis (Figure 3–10A ■). The **false pelvis**, the portion above the pelvic brim, or linea terminalis, serves to support the weight of the enlarged pregnant uterus and direct the presenting fetal part into the true pelvis below.

The **true pelvis** is the portion that lies below the linea terminalis. The bony circumference of the true pelvis is made up of the sacrum, coccyx, and innominate bones and represents the bony limits of the birth canal. The relationship between the true pelvis and the fetal head is of paramount importance: The size and shape of the true pelvis must be adequate for normal fetal passage during labor and at birth. The true pelvis consists of three parts: the inlet, the pelvic cavity, and the outlet (Figure 3–10B). Each part has distinct measurements that aid in evaluating the adequacy of the pelvis for childbirth. Measurement techniques are discussed in Chapter 10 ∞. The effects of inadequate or abnormal pelvic diameters on labor and birth are considered in Chapter 18 ∞.

The **pelvic inlet** is the upper border of the true pelvis and is typically rounded. Its size and shape are determined by assessing three anteroposterior diameters. The **diagonal conjugate** extends from the subpubic angle to the middle of the sacral promontory and is typically 11.5 cm. The diagonal conjugate can be measured manually during a pelvic examination. The **obstetric conjugate** extends from

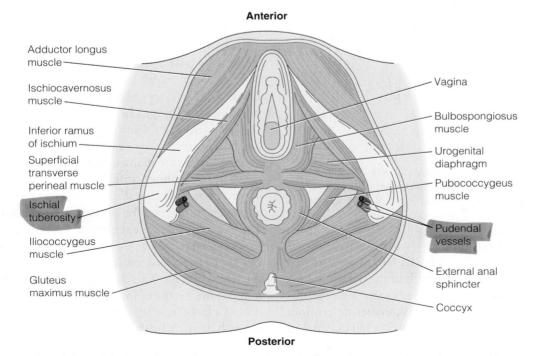

Anterior

Adductor longus muscle

Ischiocavernosus muscle

Inferior ramus of ischium

Superficial transverse perineal muscle

Ischial tuberosity

Iliococcygeus muscle

Gluteus maximus muscle

Vagina

Bulbospongiosus muscle

Urogenital diaphragm

Pubococcygeus muscle

Pudendal vessels

External anal sphincter

Coccyx

Posterior

FIGURE 3–9 Muscles of the pelvic floor. (The puborectalis, pubovaginalis, and coccygeal muscles cannot be seen from this view.)

TABLE 3–1	Muscles of the Pelvic Floor			
Muscle	Origin	Insertion	Innervation	Action
Levator ani	Pubis, lateral pelvic wall, and ischial spine	Blends with organs in pelvic cavity	Inferior rectal, second, and third sacral nerves, plus anterior rami of third and fourth sacral nerves	Supports pelvic viscera; helps form pelvic diaphragm
Iliococcygeus	Pelvic surface of ischial spine and pelvic fascia	Central point of perineum, coccygeal raphe, and coccyx		Assists in supporting abdominal and pelvic viscera
Pubococcygeus	Pubis and pelvic fascia	Coccyx		
Puborectalis	Pubis	Blends with rectum; meets similar fibers from opposite side		Forms sling for rectum, just posterior to it; raises anus
Pubovaginalis	Pubis	Blends into vagina		Supports vagina
Coccygeus	Ischial spine and sacrospinous ligament	Lateral border of lower sacrum and upper coccyx	Third and fourth sacral nerves	Supports pelvic viscera; helps form pelvic diaphragm; flexes and abducts coccyx

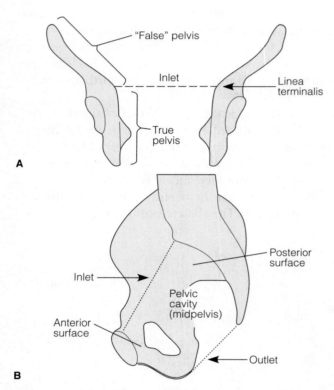

FIGURE 3–10 Female pelvis. *A,* False pelvis is a shallow cavity above the inlet; true pelvis is the deeper portion of the cavity below the inlet. *B,* True pelvis consists of inlet, cavity (midpelvis), and outlet.

the middle of the sacral promontory to an area approximately 1 cm below the pubic crest. Its length is estimated by subtracting 1.5 cm from the length of the diagonal conjugate (Figure 3–11 ■). The fetus passes through the obstetric conjugate, and the size of this diameter determines whether the fetus can move down into the birth canal in order for engagement to occur. The true (anatomic) conjugate, or **conjugate vera**, extends from the middle of the

sacral promontory to the middle of the pubic crest (superior surface of the symphysis). One additional measurement, the transverse diameter, helps determine the shape of the inlet. The **transverse diameter** is the largest diameter of the inlet and is measured by using the linea terminalis as the point of reference.

The *pelvic cavity* (canal) is a curved canal with a longer posterior than anterior wall. A change in the lumbar curve can increase or decrease the tilt of the pelvis and can influence the progress of labor because the fetus has to adjust itself to this curved path as well as to the different diameters of the true pelvis (see Figure 3–10B).

The **pelvic outlet** is at the lower border of the true pelvis. The size of the pelvic outlet can be determined by assessing the *transverse diameter*. The anteroposterior diameter of the pelvic outlet increases during birth as the presenting part pushes the coccyx posteriorly at the mobile sacrococcygeal joint. Decreased mobility, a large head, and/or a forceful birth can cause the coccyx to break. As the infant's head emerges, the long diameter of the head (occipital frontal) parallels the long diameter of the outlet (anteroposterior).

The transverse diameter *(bi-ischial* or *intertuberous)* extends from the inner surface of one ischial tuberosity to the other. It is the shortest diameter of the pelvic outlet and becomes even shorter if the woman has a narrowed pubic arch. The pubic arch is of great importance because the fetus must pass under it during birth. If it is narrow, the baby's head may be pushed backward toward the coccyx, making extension of the head difficult. This situation, known as outlet dystocia, may require the use of forceps or a cesarean birth. The shoulders of a large baby may also become wedged under the pubic arch, making birth more difficult (see Chapter 23 ∞). The clinical assessment of each of these obstetrical diameters is discussed further in Chapter 10 ∞.

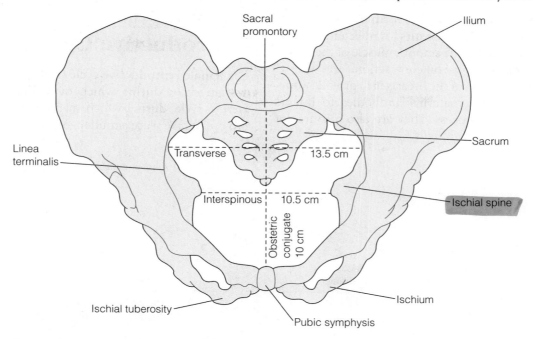

FIGURE 3–11 Pelvic planes: coronal section and diameters of the bony pelvis.

Pelvic Types

The Caldwell–Moloy classification of pelves is widely used to differentiate bony pelvic types (Caldwell & Moloy, 1933). The four basic types are *gynecoid, android, anthropoid,* and *platypelloid* (see Figure 17–1 ∞). However, variations in the female pelvis are so great that classic types are not usual. Each type has a characteristic shape, and each shape has implications for labor and birth which are discussed in detail in Chapter 22 ∞.

Breasts

The **breasts,** or *mammary glands,* considered accessories of the reproductive system, are specialized sebaceous glands (Figure 3–12 ■). They are conical and symmetrically placed on the sides of the chest. The greater pectoral and anterior serratus muscles underlie each breast. Suspending the breasts are fibrous tissues, called *Cooper's ligaments,* which extend from the deep fascia in the chest outward to just under the skin covering the breast. Frequently, the left breast is larger than the right. In different racial groups breasts develop at slightly different levels in the pectoral region of the chest.

In the center of each mature breast is the **nipple,** a protrusion about 0.5 to 1.3 cm in diameter. The nipple is composed mainly of erectile tissue, which becomes more rigid and prominent during the menstrual cycle, sexual excitement, pregnancy, and lactation. The nipple is surrounded by the heavily pigmented **areola,** which is 2.5 to 10 cm in diameter. Both the nipple and the areola are roughened by small papillae called *tubercles of Montgomery.* As an infant suckles, these tubercles secrete a fatty substance that helps lubricate and protect the breasts.

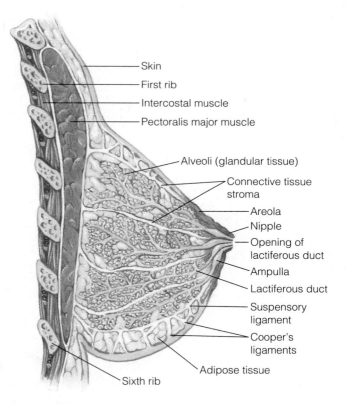

FIGURE 3–12 Anatomy of the breast: sagittal view of left breast.

The breasts are composed of glandular, fibrous, and adipose tissue. The glandular tissue is arranged in a series of 15 to 24 lobes separated by fibrous and adipose tissue.

Each lobe is made up of several lobules composed of many alveoli clustered around tiny ducts. The lining of these ducts secretes the various components of milk. The ducts from several lobules merge to form the larger lactiferous ducts which serve as reservoirs for milk and open on the surface of the nipple. The smooth muscle of the nipple causes erection of the nipple on contraction.

The biologic function of the breasts is to provide nourishment and protective maternal antibodies to infants through the lactation process. They are also a source of pleasurable sexual sensation.

The Female Reproductive Cycle

The **female reproductive cycle (FRC)** is composed of the ovarian cycle, during which ovulation occurs, and the uterine cycle, during which menstruation occurs. These two cycles take place simultaneously (Figure 3–13 ■).

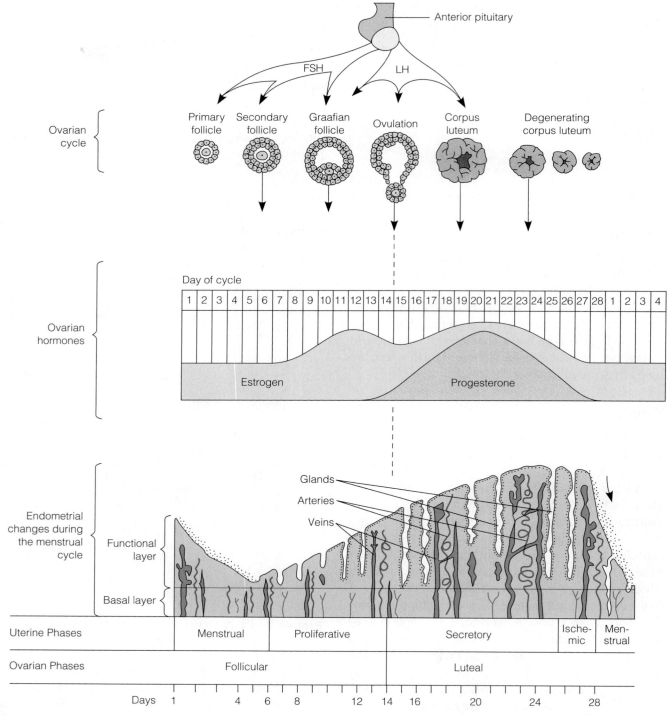

FIGURE 3–13 Female reproductive cycle: interrelationships of hormones with the four phases of the uterine cycle and the two phases of the ovarian cycle in an ideal 28-day cycle.

Effects of Female Hormones

After menarche, a female undergoes a cyclic pattern of ovulation and menstruation, which is disrupted only by pregnancy for a period of 30 to 40 years. This cycle is an orderly process under neurohormonal control. Each month one oocyte matures, ruptures from the ovary, and enters the fallopian tube. The ovary, vagina, uterus, and fallopian tubes are major target organs for female hormones.

The ovaries produce mature gametes and secrete hormones. Ovarian hormones include the estrogens, progesterone, and testosterone. The ovary is sensitive to follicle-stimulating hormone (FSH) and luteinizing hormone (LH). The uterus is sensitive to estrogen and progesterone. The relative proportion of these hormones to each other controls the events of both ovarian and menstrual cycles.

Estrogens

Estrogens are hormones that are associated with characteristics contributing to "femaleness." The major estrogenic effects are due primarily to three classical estrogens: estrone, β-estradiol, and estriol. The major estrogen is β-estradiol.

Estrogens control the development of the female secondary sex characteristics: breast development, growth of body hair, widening of the hips, and deposits of tissue (fat) in the buttocks and mons pubis. Estrogens also assist in the maturation of the ovarian follicles and cause the endometrial mucosa to proliferate following menstruation. The amount of estrogens is greatest during the proliferative (follicular or estrogenic) phase of the menstrual cycle. Estrogens also cause the uterus to increase in size and weight because of increased glycogen, amino acids, electrolytes, and water. Blood supply is expanded as well. Under the influence of estrogens, myometrial contractility increases in both the uterus and the fallopian tubes, and uterine sensitivity to oxytocin increases. Estrogens inhibit FSH production and stimulate LH production.

Estrogens have effects on many hormones and other carrier proteins, such as contributing to the increased amount of protein-bound iodine in pregnant women and women who use oral contraceptives containing estrogen. Estrogens may also increase libidinal feelings in humans. They decrease the excitability of the hypothalamus, which may cause an increase in sexual desire.

Progesterone

Progesterone is secreted by the corpus luteum and is found in greatest amounts during the secretory (luteal or progestational) phase of the menstrual cycle. It decreases uterine motility and contractility caused by estrogens, thereby preparing the uterus for implantation after the ovum is fertilized. The endometrial mucosa is in a ready state as a result of estrogenic influence. Progesterone causes the uterine endometrium to further increase its supply of glycogen, arterial blood, secretory glands, amino acids, and water.

This hormone is often called the *hormone of pregnancy* because its effects on the uterus allow pregnancy to be maintained. Under the influence of progesterone, the vaginal epithelium proliferates and the cervix secretes thick, viscous mucus. Breast glandular tissue increases in size and complexity. Progesterone also prepares the breasts for lactation.

The temperature rise of about 0.3°C to 0.6°C (0.5°F to 1.0°F) that accompanies ovulation and persists throughout the secretory phase of the menstrual cycle is due to progesterone.

Prostaglandins

Prostaglandins (PGs) are oxygenated fatty acids that are produced by the cells of the endometrium and are also classified as hormones. Prostaglandins have varied action in the body. The two primary types of prostaglandins are group E and F. Generally PGE relaxes smooth muscles and is a potent vasodilator; PGF is a potent vasoconstrictor and increases the contractility of muscles and arteries. Although the primary actions of PGE and PGF seem antagonistic, their basic regulatory functions in cells are achieved through an intricate pattern of reciprocal events.

Prostaglandin production increases during follicular maturation, is dependent on gonadotropins, and seems to be critical to follicular rupture (Cunningham et al., 2005). Extrusion of the ovum, resulting from follicular swelling and increased contractility of the smooth muscle in the theca externa layer of the mature follicle, is thought to be caused in part by $PGF_{2\alpha}$. Significant amounts of PGs are found in and around the follicle at the time of ovulation.

Neurohumoral Basis of the Female Reproductive Cycle

The female reproductive cycle is controlled by complex interactions between the nervous and endocrine systems and their target tissues. These interactions involve the hypothalamus, anterior pituitary, and ovaries.

The hypothalamus secretes **gonadotropin-releasing hormone (GnRH)** to the pituitary gland in response to signals received from the central nervous system. This releasing hormone is often called both luteinizing hormone-releasing

MyNursingKit | Progesterone: The Forgotten Hormone

hormone (LHRH) and follicle-stimulating hormone-releasing hormone (FSHRH) (Blackburn, 2007).

In response to GnRH, the anterior pituitary secretes the gonadotropic hormones **follicle-stimulating hormone (FSH)** and **luteinizing hormone (LH)**. FSH is primarily responsible for the maturation of the ovarian follicle. As the follicle matures, it secretes increasing amounts of estrogen, which enhance the development of the follicle (Cunningham et al., 2005). (This estrogen is also responsible for the building or proliferation phase of the endometrium after it is shed during menstruation.)

Final maturation of the follicle cannot come about without the action of LH. The anterior pituitary's production of LH increases six- to tenfold as the follicle matures. The peak production of LH can precede ovulation by as much as 12 hours (Cunningham et al., 2005). The LH is also responsible for the "luteinizing" of the theca and granulosa cells of the ruptured follicle. As a result, estrogen production is reduced and progesterone secretion continues. Thus estrogen levels fall a day before ovulation; tiny amounts of progesterone are in evidence. **Ovulation** takes place following the very rapid growth of the follicle, as the sustained high level of estrogen diminishes and progesterone secretion begins.

The ruptured follicle undergoes rapid change, complete luteinization is accomplished, and the mass of cells becomes the **corpus luteum**. The lutein cells secrete large amounts of progesterone with smaller amounts of estradiol. (Concurrently, the excessive amounts of progesterone are responsible for the secretory phase of the uterine cycle.) On day 7 or 8 following ovulation, the corpus luteum begins to involute, losing its secretory function. The production of both progesterone and estrogen is severely diminished. The anterior pituitary responds with increasingly large amounts of FSH; a few days later LH production begins. As a result, new follicles become responsive to another ovarian cycle and begin maturing.

Ovarian Cycle

The ovarian cycle has two phases: the *follicular phase* (days 1–14) and the *luteal phase* (days 15–28 in a 28-day cycle). Figure 3–14 ■ depicts the changes that the follicle undergoes during the ovarian cycle. In women whose menstrual cycles vary, usually only the length of the follicular phase varies, because the luteal phase is of fixed length. During the follicular phase, the immature follicle matures as a result of FSH. Within the follicle, the oocyte grows.

A mature graafian follicle appears on about the 14th day under dual control of FSH and LH. It is a large structure, measuring about 5 to 10 mm. The mature follicle produces increasing amounts of estrogen. In the mature

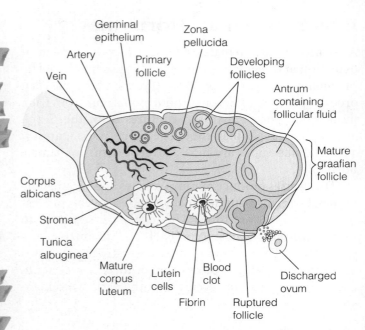

FIGURE 3–14 Various stages of development of the ovarian follicles.

graafian follicle, the cells surrounding the fluid-filled antral cavity are granulosa cells. The mass of granulosa cells surrounding the oocyte and follicular fluid is called the *cumulus oophorus*. In the fully mature graafian follicle, the zona pellucida, a thick elastic capsule, develops around the oocyte. Just before ovulation, the mature oocyte completes its first meiotic division (see Chapter 4 ∞ for a description of meiosis). As a result of this division, two cells are formed: a small cell, called a *polar body,* and a larger cell, called the *secondary oocyte.* The secondary oocyte matures into the ovum (see Figure 4–2 ∞).

As the graafian follicle matures and enlarges, it comes close to the surface of the ovary. The ovary surface forms a blisterlike protrusion 10 to 15 mm in diameter, and the follicle walls become thin. The secondary oocyte, polar body, and follicular fluid are pushed out. The ovum is discharged near the fimbria of the fallopian tube and is pulled into the tube to begin its journey toward the uterus.

In some women, ovulation is accompanied by midcycle pain known as *mittelschmerz*. This pain may be caused by a thick tunica albuginea or by a local peritoneal reaction to the expelling of the follicular contents. Vaginal discharge may increase during ovulation, and a small amount of blood (midcycle spotting) may be discharged as well.

The body temperature increases about 0.3°C to 0.6°C (0.5°F to 1.0°F) 24 to 48 hours after the time of ovulation. It remains elevated until the day before menstruation begins. There may be an accompanying sharp basal body temperature drop before the increase. These temperature changes are useful clinically to determine the approximate time ovulation occurs (Blackburn, 2007).

Generally the ovum takes several minutes to travel through the ruptured follicle to the fallopian tube opening. The contractions of the tube's smooth muscle and its ciliary action propel the ovum through the tube. The ovum remains in the ampulla, where, if it is fertilized, cleavage can begin. The ovum is thought to be fertile for only 6 to 24 hours. It reaches the uterus 72 to 96 hours after its release from the ovary.

The luteal phase begins when the ovum leaves its follicle. Under the influence of LH, the corpus luteum develops from the ruptured follicle. Within 2 or 3 days, the corpus luteum becomes yellowish and spherical and increases in vascularity. If the ovum is fertilized and implants in the endometrium, the fertilized egg begins to secrete **human chorionic gonadotropin (hCG)**, which is needed to maintain the corpus luteum. If fertilization does not occur, within about a week after ovulation the corpus luteum begins to degenerate, eventually becoming a connective tissue scar called the *corpus albicans*. With degeneration comes a decrease in estrogen and progesterone. This allows for an increase in LH and FSH, which trigger the hypothalamus.

Menstrual Cycle

Menstruation is cyclic uterine bleeding in response to cyclic hormonal changes. Menstruation occurs when the ovum is not fertilized and begins about 14 days after ovulation in an ideal 28-day cycle. The menstrual discharge, also referred to as the *menses*, or *menstrual flow*, is composed of blood mixed with fluid, cervical and vaginal secretions, bacteria, mucus, leukocytes, and other cellular debris. The menstrual discharge is dark red and has a distinctive odor.

Menstrual parameters vary greatly among individuals. Generally, menstruation occurs every 29 days, but varies from 21 to 35 days. Some women normally have longer cycles, which can skew standard calculations of the estimated date of birth (EDB). Emotional and physical factors such as illness, excessive fatigue, stress or anxiety, and vigorous exercise programs can alter the cycle interval. Certain environmental factors such as temperature and altitude may also affect the cycle.

The duration of menses is from 2 to 8 days, with the blood loss averaging 25 to 60 mL, and the loss of iron averaging 0.5 to 1 mg daily.

The uterine (menstrual) cycle has four phases: menstrual, proliferative, secretory, and ischemic. Menstruation occurs during the *menstrual phase*. Some endometrial areas are shed, although others remain. Some of the remaining tips of the endometrial glands begin to regener-ate. The endometrium is in a resting state following menstruation. Estrogen levels are low, and the endometrium is 1 to 2 mm deep. During this part of the cycle, the cervical mucosa is scanty, viscous, and opaque.

The *proliferative phase* begins when the endometrial glands enlarge, becoming twisted and longer in response to increasing amounts of estrogen. The blood vessels become prominent and dilated, and the endometrium increases in thickness six- to eightfold. This gradual process reaches its peak just before ovulation. The cervical mucosa becomes thin, clear, watery, and more alkaline, making the mucosa more favorable to spermatozoa. As ovulation nears, the cervical mucosa shows increased elasticity, called *spinnbarkeit*. At ovulation, the mucus will stretch more than 5 cm. The cervical mucosa pH increases from below 7.0 to 7.5 at the time of ovulation. On microscopic examination, the mucosa shows a characteristic ferning pattern (see Figure 7–3 ∞). This fern pattern is a useful aid in assessing ovulation time.

The *secretory phase* follows ovulation. The endometrium, under estrogenic influence, undergoes slight cellular growth. Progesterone, however, causes such marked swelling and growth that the epithelium is warped into folds. The amount of tissue glycogen increases. The glandular epithelial cells begin to fill with cellular debris, become twisted, and dilate. The glands secrete small quantities of endometrial fluid in preparation for a fertilized ovum. The vascularity of the entire uterus increases greatly, providing a nourishing bed for implantation. If implantation occurs, the endometrium, under the influence of progesterone, continues to develop and become even thicker (see Chapter 4 ∞ for a discussion of implantation).

If fertilization does not occur, the *ischemic phase* begins. The corpus luteum begins to degenerate, and as a result both estrogen and progesterone levels fall. Areas of necrosis appear under the epithelial lining. Extensive vascular changes also occur. Small blood vessels rupture, and the spiral arteries constrict and retract, causing a deficiency of blood in the endometrium, which becomes pale. This ischemic phase is characterized by the escape of blood into the stromal cells of the uterus. The menstrual flow begins, thus beginning the menstrual cycle again. After menstruation the basal layer remains, so that the tips of the glands can regenerate the new functional endometrial layer. For further discussion, see Key Facts to Remember: Summary of Female Reproductive Cycle.

Male Reproductive System

The primary reproductive functions of the male genitals are to produce and transport sex cells (sperm) through and eventually out of the male genital tract and into the

KEY FACTS TO REMEMBER

Summary of Female Reproductive Cycle

Ovarian Cycle

Follicular phase (days 1–14): Primordial follicle matures under influence of FSH and LH up to the time of ovulation.

Luteal phase (days 15–28): Ovum leaves follicle; corpus luteum develops under LH influence and produces high levels of progesterone and low levels of estrogen.

Menstrual Cycle

Menstrual phase (days 1–6): Estrogen levels are low. Cervical mucus is scant, viscous, and opaque. Endometrium is shed.

Proliferative phase (days 7–14): Endometrium and myometrium thickness increases. Estrogen peaks just before ovulation. Cervical mucus at ovulation:
   Is clear, thin, watery, alkaline
   Is more favorable to sperm; shows ferning pattern on microscopic exam
   Has spinnbarkeit greater than 5 cm
Just before ovulation, body temperature may drop slightly, then at ovulation basal body temperature increases 0.3°C to 0.6°C (0.5°F to 1.0°F), and mittelschmerz and/or midcycle spotting may occur.

Secretory phase (days 15–26): Estrogen drops sharply, and progesterone dominates. Vascularity of entire uterus increases. Tissue glycogen increases, and the uterus is made ready for implantation.

Ischemic phase (days 27–28): Both estrogen and progesterone levels drop. Endometrium becomes pale, blood vessels rupture. Blood escapes into uterine stromal cells, gets ready to be shed.

female genital tract. The external and internal genitals of the male reproductive system are shown in Figure 3–15 ■

External Genitals

The two external reproductive organs are the penis and scrotum.

Penis

The *penis* is an elongated, cylindrical structure consisting of a body, called the *shaft*, and a cone-shaped end, called the *glans*. The penis lies in front of the scrotum. The shaft of the penis is made up of three longitudinal columns of erectile tissue: the paired *corpora cavernosa* and the *corpus spongiosum*. These columns are covered by dense fibrous connective tissue and then enclosed by elastic tissue. The penis is covered by a thin outer layer of skin.

The corpus spongiosum contains the urethra and becomes the glans at the distal end of the penis. The urethra widens within the glans and ends in a slitlike opening, located in the tip of the glans, called the *urethral meatus*. A circular fold of skin arises just behind the glans and covers it. Known as the *prepuce*, or *foreskin*, it may be removed by the surgical procedure of circumcision (see Chapter 26 ∞). If the corpus spongiosum does not surround the urethra completely, the urethral meatus may occur on the ventral aspect of the penile shaft (hypospadias) or on the dorsal aspect (epispadias).

The penis is innervated by the pudendal nerve. Sexual stimulation causes the penis to elongate, thicken, and stiffen, a process called *erection*. The penis becomes erect when its blood vessels become engorged, a consequence of parasympathetic nerve stimulation. If sexual stimulation is intense enough, the forceful and sudden expulsion of semen occurs through the rhythmic contractions of the penile muscles. This phenomenon is called *ejaculation*.

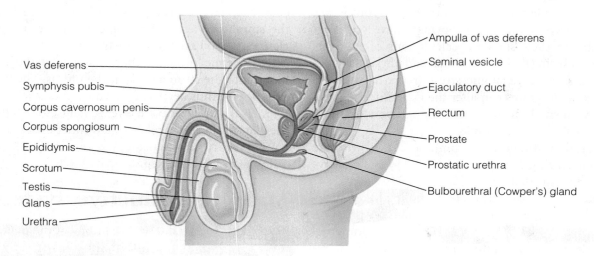

Vas deferens
Symphysis pubis
Corpus cavernosum penis
Corpus spongiosum
Epididymis
Scrotum
Testis
Glans
Urethra

Ampulla of vas deferens
Seminal vesicle
Ejaculatory duct
Rectum
Prostate
Prostatic urethra
Bulbourethral (Cowper's) gland

FIGURE 3–15 Male reproductive system, sagittal view.

The penis serves both the urinary and the reproductive systems. Urine is expelled through the urethral meatus. The reproductive function of the penis is to deposit sperm in the vagina so that fertilization of the ovum can occur.

Scrotum

The *scrotum* is a pouchlike structure that hangs in front of the anus and behind the penis. Composed of skin and the *dartos* muscle, the scrotum shows increased pigmentation and scattered hairs. The sebaceous glands open directly onto the scrotal surface; their secretion has a distinctive odor. Contraction of the dartos and cremasteric muscles shortens the scrotum and draws it closer to the body, thus wrinkling its outer surface. The degree of wrinkling is greatest in young men and at cold temperatures and is least in older men and at warm temperatures.

Inside the scrotum are two lateral compartments. Each compartment contains a testis with its related structures. Because the left spermatic cord grows longer, the left testis and its scrotal sac hang lower than the right. A ridge (raphe) on the external scrotal surface marks the position of the medial septum and continues anteriorly on the urethral surface of the penis, disappearing in the perineal area.

The function of the scrotum is to protect the testes and the sperm by maintaining a temperature lower than that of the body. Spermatogenesis cannot occur if the testes fail to descend and thus remain at body temperature. Because it is sensitive to touch, pressure, temperature, and pain, the scrotum defends against potential harm to the testes.

Male Internal Reproductive Organs

The male internal reproductive organs include the gonads (testes or testicles), a system of ducts (epididymides, vas deferens, ejaculatory duct, and urethra), and accessory glands (seminal vesicles, prostate gland, bulbourethral glands, and urethral glands). See Key Facts to Remember: Summary of Male Reproductive Organ Functions.

Testes

The *testes* are a pair of oval, compound glandular organs contained in the scrotum. In the sexually mature male, they are the site of spermatozoa production and the secretion of several male sex hormones.

Each testis is 4 to 6 cm long, 2 to 3 cm wide, and 3 to 4 cm thick and weighs about 10 to 15 g. Each is covered by an outer serous membrane and an inner capsule that is tough, white, and fibrous. The connective tissue sends projections inward to form septa, dividing the testis into 250 to 400 lobules. Each lobule contains one to three

---

KEY FACTS TO REMEMBER

Summary of Male Reproductive Organ Functions

The testes house seminiferous tubules and gonads.

- Seminiferous tubules contain sperm cells in various stages of development and undergoing meiosis.
- Sertoli's cells nourish and protect spermatocytes (phase between spermatids and spermatozoa—see Chapter 4 ∞).
- Leydig's cells are the main source of testosterone.
- Epididymides provide an area for maturation of sperm and a reservoir for mature spermatozoa.
- The vas deferens connects the epididymis with the prostate gland, then connects with ducts from the seminal vesicle to become an ejaculatory duct.
- Ejaculatory ducts provide a passageway for semen and seminal fluid into the urethra.
- Seminal vesicles secrete yellowish fluid rich in fructose, prostaglandins, and fibrinogen. This provides nutrition that increases motility and fertilizing ability of sperm. Prostaglandins also aid fertilization by making the cervical mucus more receptive to sperm.
- The prostate gland secretes thin, alkaline fluid containing calcium, citric acid, and other substances. Alkalinity counteracts acidity of ductus and seminal vesicle secretions.
- Bulbourethral (Cowper's) glands secrete alkaline, viscous fluid into semen, aiding in neutralization of acidic vaginal secretions.

---

tightly packed, convoluted *seminiferous tubules* containing sperm cells in all stages of development.

The seminiferous tubules are surrounded by loose connective tissue that houses abundant blood and lymph vessels and *interstitial (Leydig's) cells*. The interstitial cells produce testosterone, the primary male sex hormone. The tubules also contain Sertoli's cells, which nourish and protect the spermatocytes. The seminiferous tubules come together to form 20 to 30 straight tubules, which in turn form an anastomotic network of thin-walled spaces, the *rete testis*. The rete testis forms 10 to 15 efferent ducts that empty into the duct of the epididymis.

Most of the cells lining the seminiferous tubules undergo **spermatogenesis**, a process of maturation in which spermatocytes become spermatozoa. (Chapter 4 ∞ further discusses the process of spermatogenesis.) Sperm production varies among and within the tubules, with cells in different areas of the same tubule undergoing different stages of spermatogenesis. The sperm are eventually released from the tubules into the epididymis, where they mature further.

Like the female reproductive cycle, the process of spermatogenesis and other functions of the testes are the result of complex neural and hormonal controls. The hypothalamus secretes releasing factors that stimulate the anterior pituitary to release the gonadotropins—FSH and LH. These hormones cause the testes to produce testosterone, which maintains spermatogenesis, increases sperm production by the seminiferous tubules, and stimulates production of seminal fluid.

Testosterone is the most prevalent and potent of the testicular hormones. It is also responsible for the development of secondary male characteristics and certain behavioral patterns. The effects of testosterone include structural and functional development of the male genital tract, emission and ejaculation of seminal fluid, distribution of body hair, promotion of growth and strength of long bones, increased muscle mass, and enlargement of the vocal cords. The action of testosterone on the central nervous system is thought to produce aggressiveness and sexual drive. The action of testosterone is constant, not cyclic like that of the female hormones. Its production is not limited to a certain number of years, but it is thought to decrease with age.

The testes have two primary functions:

- To serve as the site of spermatogenesis
- To produce testosterone

Epididymis

The *epididymis* (plural, *epididymides*) is a duct about 5.6 m long, although it is convoluted into a compact structure about 3.75 cm long. An epididymis lies behind each testis. It arises from the top of the testis, courses downward, and then passes upward, where it becomes the vas deferens.

The epididymis provides a reservoir for maturing spermatozoa. When discharged from the seminiferous tubules into the epididymis, the sperm are immotile and incapable of fertilizing an ovum. The spermatozoa usually remain in the epididymis for 2 to 10 days but can be stored in the body for up to 42 days. As the sperm move along the tortuous course of the epididymis they become both motile and fertile.

Vas Deferens and Ejaculatory Ducts

The *vas deferens*, also known as the *ductus deferens*, is about 40 cm long and connects the epididymis with the prostate. One vas deferens arises from the posterior border of each testis. It joins the spermatic cord and weaves over and between several pelvic structures until it meets the vas deferens from the opposite side. Each vas deferens terminus expands to form the *terminal ampulla*. It then unites with the seminal vesicle duct (a gland) to form the ejaculatory duct, which enters the prostate gland and ends in the prostatic urethra. The ejaculatory ducts serve as passageways for semen and fluid secreted by the seminal vesi-

cles. The main function of the vas deferens is to rapidly squeeze the sperm from their storage sites (the epididymis and distal part of the vas deferens) into the urethra.

Men who choose to take total responsibility for birth control may elect to have a vasectomy. In this procedure, the scrotal portion of the vas deferens is surgically incised or cauterized. Although sperm continues to be produced for the next several years, they can no longer reach the outside of the body. Eventually, the sperm deteriorate and are reabsorbed.

Urethra

The *male urethra* is the passageway for both urine and semen. The urethra begins in the bladder and passes through the prostate gland, where it is called the *prostatic urethra*.

The urethra emerges from the prostate gland to become the *membranous urethra*. It terminates in the penis, where it is called the *penile urethra*. In the penile urethra, goblet secretory cells are present, and smooth muscle is replaced by erectile tissue.

Accessory Glands

The male accessory glands secrete a unique and essential component of the total seminal fluid in an ordered sequence.

The *seminal vesicles* are two glands composed of many lobes. Each vesicle is about 7.5 cm long. They are situated between the bladder and the rectum, immediately above the base of the prostate. The epithelium lining the seminal vesicles secretes an alkaline, viscous, clear fluid rich in high-energy fructose, prostaglandins, fibrinogen, and amino acids. During ejaculation, this fluid mixes with the sperm in the ejaculatory ducts. This fluid helps provide an environment favorable to sperm motility and metabolism.

The *prostate gland* encircles the upper part of the urethra and lies below the neck of the bladder. Made up of several lobes, it measures about 4 cm in diameter and weighs 20 to 30 g. The prostate is made up of both glandular and muscular tissue. It secretes a thin, milky, alkaline fluid containing high levels of zinc, calcium, citric acid, and acid phosphatase. This fluid protects the sperm from the acidic environment of the vagina and the male urethra, which would otherwise be spermicidal.

The *bulbourethral (Cowper's) glands* are a pair of small, round structures on either side of the membranous urethra. The glands secrete a clear, thick, alkaline fluid rich in mucoproteins that becomes part of the semen. This secretion also lubricates the penile urethra during sexual excitement and neutralizes the acid in the male urethra and the vagina, thereby enhancing sperm motility.

The *urethral (Littré's) glands* are tiny mucus-secreting glands found throughout the membranous lining of the penile urethra. Their secretions add to those of the bulbourethral glands.

Semen

The male ejaculate, *semen* or *seminal fluid,* is made up of spermatozoa and the secretions of all the accessory glands. The seminal fluid transports viable and motile sperm to the female reproductive tract. Effective transportation of sperm requires adequate nutrients, an adequate pH (about 7.5), a specific concentration of sperm to fluid, and an optimal osmolarity.

A spermatozoon is made up of a head and a tail (Figure 3–16 ■). The head's main components are the acrosome and nucleus. The head carries the male's haploid number of chromosomes (23), and it is the part that enters the ovum at fertilization (see Chapter 4 ∞). The tail, or *flagellum,* is divided into the middle and end piece and is specialized for motility.

Sperm may be stored in the epididymis and distal vas deferens for up to 42 days, depending primarily on the frequency of ejaculations. The average volume of ejaculate following abstinence for several days is 2 to 5 mL but may vary from 1 to 10 mL. Repeated ejaculation results in decreased volume. Once ejaculated, sperm can live only 2 or 3 days in the female genital tract.

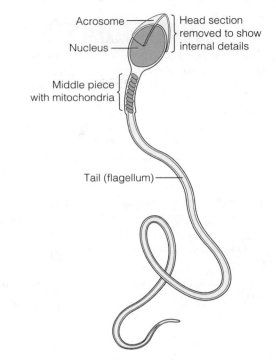

FIGURE 3–16 Schematic representation of a mature spermatozoon.

CHAPTER HIGHLIGHTS

- Reproductive activities require a complex interaction between the reproductive structures, the central nervous system, and such endocrine glands as the pituitary, hypothalamus, testes, and ovaries.
- The female reproductive system consists of the ovaries, where female germ cells and female sex hormones are formed; the fallopian tubes, which capture the ovum and allow transport to the uterus; the uterus, which is the implantation site for the fertilized ovum; the cervix, which is a protective portal for the body of the uterus and the connection between the vagina and the uterus; and the vagina, which is the passageway from the external genitals to the uterus and provides for discharge of menstrual products out of the body.
- The female reproductive cycle may be described in terms of the ovarian cycle, during which ovulation occurs, and the menstrual cycle, during which menstruation occurs. These two cycles take place simultaneously and are under neuro-humoral control.
- The ovarian cycle has two phases: the follicular phase and the luteal phase. During the follicular phase, the primordial follicle matures under the influence of FSH and LH until ovulation occurs. The luteal phase begins when the ovum leaves the follicle and the corpus luteum develops under the influence of LH. The corpus luteum produces high levels of progesterone and low levels of estrogen.
- The menstrual cycle has four phases: menstrual, proliferative, secretory, and ischemic. Menstruation is the actual shedding of the endometrial lining, when estrogen levels are low. The proliferative phase begins when the endometrial glands begin to enlarge under the influence of estrogen and cervical mucosal changes occur; the changes peak at ovulation. The secretory phase follows ovulation, and, influenced primarily by progesterone, the uterus increases its vascularity to make ready for possible implantation. The ischemic phase is characterized by degeneration of the corpus luteum, decreases in both estrogen and progesterone levels, constriction of the spiral arteries, and escape of blood into the stromal cells of the endometrium.
- The male reproductive system consists of the testes, where male germ cells and male sex hormones are formed; a series of continuous ducts through which spermatozoa are transported outside the body; accessory glands that produce secretions important to sperm nutrition, survival, and transport; and the penis, which serves as the reproductive organ of intercourse.

CHAPTER REFERENCES

Blackburn, S. T. (2007). *Maternal, fetal, & neonatal physiology: A clinical perspective* (2nd ed.). St. Louis, MO: Saunders.

Caldwell, W. E., & Moloy, H. C. (1933). Anatomical variations in the female pelvis and their effect on labor with a suggested classification [Historical article]. *American Journal of Obstetrics and Gynecology, 26*, 479–505.

Cunningham, F. G., Leveno, K. J., Bloom, S. L., Hauth, J. C., & Wenstrom, K. D. (2005). *William's obstetrics* (22nd ed.). New York: McGraw Hill.

Krantz, K. E. (2007). Anatomy of the female reproductive system. In A. H. Decherney, L. Nathan, T. M. Goodwin, & N. Laufer (Eds.), *Current diagnosis and treatment: Obstetrics & gynecology* (10th ed.). Boston: McGraw Hill.

Riordan, J. (2005). Anatomy and physiology of lactation. In J. Riordan, *Breastfeeding and human lactation* (3rd ed.). Boston: Jones and Bartlett Publishers.

CHAPTER 4

Conception and Fetal Development

I love teaching the course content on conception and fetal development. Each time, I am struck anew by the absolute magic of human reproduction.

—Department of Nursing Faculty Member

LEARNING OUTCOMES

4-1. Differentiate between meiotic cellular division and mitotic cellular division.

4-2. Compare the processes by which ova and sperm are produced.

4-3. Analyze the components of the process of fertilization as to how each may impact fertilization.

4-4. Compare the factors and processes by which fraternal (dizygotic) and identical (monozygotic) twins are formed.

4-5. Analyze the processes that occur during the cellular multiplication and differentiation stages of intrauterine development and their effect on the structures that form.

4-6. Describe the development, structure, and functions of the placenta and umbilical cord during intrauterine life (embryonic and fetal development).

4-7. Contrast the significant changes in growth and development of the fetus at 4, 6, 12, 16, 20, 24, 28, 36, and 40 weeks' gestation.

4-8. Compare the vulnerable periods during which malformations of the various organ systems may occur to the resulting congenital malformations.

KEY TERMS

Acrosomal reaction 54
Amnion 57
Amniotic fluid 57
Bag of waters (BOW) 57
Blastocyst 56
Capacitation 54
Chorion 57
Cleavage 56
Cotyledons 61
Decidua basalis 56
Decidua capsularis 56
Decidua vera (parietalis) 56

The human genome contains *genes*, which are units of genetic information. Genes are encoded in the DNA that makes up the chromosomes in the nucleus of each cell. These chromosomes, which determine the structure and function of organ systems and traits, are of the same biochemical substances. How then does each person become unique? The answer lies in the physiologic mechanisms of heredity, the processes of cellular division, and the environmental factors that influence our development from the moment we are conceived. This chapter explores the processes involved in conception and fetal development—the basis of human uniqueness.

Cellular Division

Each human begins life as a single cell called a fertilized ovum or zygote. This single cell reproduces itself, and in turn each resulting cell also reproduces itself in a continuing process. The new cells are similar to the cells from which they came. Cells are reproduced by either mitosis or meiosis, two different but related processes.

Mitosis results in the production of diploid body (somatic) cells, which are exact copies of the original cell. Mitosis makes growth and development possible, and in mature individuals it is the process by which our body cells continue to divide and replace themselves. **Meiosis** is a process of cell division leading to the development of eggs and sperm needed to produce a new organism. Unlike cells produced during mitosis, the cells produced during meiosis contain only half the genetic material or number of chromsomes (the haploid number).

Mitosis

During mitosis, the cell undergoes several changes ending in cell division. As the last phase of cell division nears completion, a furrow develops in the cell cytoplasm, which divides it into two daughter cells, each with its own nucleus. Daughter cells have the same **diploid number of chromosomes** (46) and same genetic makeup as the cell from which they came. After a cell with 46 chromosomes goes through mitosis, the result is two identical cells, each with 46 chromosomes.

Meiosis

Meiosis is a special type of cell division by which diploid cells in the testes and ovaries give rise to gametes (sperm and ova) with the **haploid number of chromosomes**, which is 23.

Meiosis consists of two successive cell divisions. In the first division, the chromosomes replicate. Next, a pairing takes place between homologous chromosomes (Sadler, 2006). Instead of separating immediately, as in mitosis, the chromosomes become closely intertwined. At each point of contact, there is a physical exchange of genetic material between the chromatids (the arms of the chromosomes). New combinations are provided by the newly formed chromosomes; these combinations account for the wide variation of traits in people (e.g., hair or eye color). The chromosome pairs then separate, and the members of the pair move to opposite sides of the cell. (In contrast, during mitosis the chromatids of each chromosome separate and move to opposite poles.) The cell divides, forming two daughter cells, each with 23 double-structured chromosomes—the same amount of deoxyribonucleic acid (DNA) as a normal somatic cell. In the second division, the chromatids of each chromosome separate and move to opposite poles of each of the daughter cells. Cell division occurs, resulting in the formation of four cells, each containing 23 single chromosomes (the haploid number of chromosomes). These daughter cells contain only half the DNA of a normal somatic cell (Sadler, 2006). See Key Facts to Remember: Comparison of Meiosis and Mitosis.

Mutations may occur during the second meiotic division, if two of the chromatids do not move apart rapidly enough when the cell divides. The still-paired chromatids are carried into one of the daughter cells and eventually form an extra chromosome. This condition, *autosomal nondisjunction* (chromosomal mutation), is harmful to the offspring that may result should fertilization occur. Another type of chromosomal mutation can occur if chromosomes break during meiosis. If the broken segment is lost, the result is a shorter chromosome; this situation is known as *deletion*. If the broken segment becomes attached to another chromosome, a harmful mutation called a *translocation* is the result. The implications of

MyNursingKit | Animation: Cell Division

◆

KEY FACTS TO REMEMBER

Comparison of Meiosis and Mitosis

MEIOSIS
Purpose
Produce reproductive cells (gametes). Reduction of chromosome number by half (from diploid [46] to haploid [23]), so that when fertilization occurs the normal diploid number is restored. Introduces genetic variability.

Cell Division
Two-stage reduction.

Number of Daughter Cells
Four daughter cells, each containing one-half the number of chromosomes as the mother cell, or 23 chromosomes. Nonidentical to original cell.

MITOSIS
Purpose
Produce cells for growth and tissue repair. Cell division characteristic of all somatic cells.

Cell Division
One-stage cell division.

Number of Daughter Cells
Two daughter cells identical to the mother cell, each with the diploid number (46 chromosomes).

---

nondisjunction and the effects of translocation are described in Chapter 7 ∞.

Gametogenesis

Meiosis occurs during **gametogenesis**, the process by which germ cells, or **gametes** *(ovum and sperm)*, are produced. These cells contain only half the genetic material of a typical body cell. The gametes must have a haploid number (23) of chromosomes so that when the female gamete (egg or ovum) and the male gamete (sperm or spermatozoon) unite to form the **zygote** (fertilized ovum), the normal human diploid number of chromosomes (46) is reestablished.

Oogenesis

Oogenesis is the process that produces the female gamete, called an ovum (egg). As discussed in Chapter 3 ∞, the ovaries begin to develop early in the fetal life of the female. All the ova that the female will produce in her lifetime are present at birth. The ovary gives rise to oogonial cells, which develop into oocytes. Meiosis begins in all oocytes before the female fetus is born but stops before the first division is complete and remains in this arrested phase until puberty. During puberty, the mature primary oocyte proceeds (by oogenesis) through the first meiotic division in the graafian follicle of the ovary.

The first meiotic division produces two cells of unequal size with different amounts of cytoplasm but with the same number of chromosomes. These two cells are the *secondary oocyte* and a minute *polar body*. Both the secondary oocyte and the polar body contain 22 double-structured autosomal chromosomes and one double-structured sex chromosome (X).

At the time of ovulation, a second meiotic division begins immediately and proceeds as the oocyte moves down the fallopian tube. Division is again not equal, and the secondary oocyte moves into the metaphase stage of cell division, where its meiotic division is arrested until and unless the oocyte is fertilized.

When the secondary oocyte completes the second meiotic division after fertilization, the result is a mature ovum with the haploid number of chromosomes and virtually all the cytoplasm. In addition, the second polar body (also haploid) forms at this time. The first polar body has now also divided, producing two additional polar bodies. Thus, at the completion of meiosis, four haploid cells have been produced: the three polar bodies, which eventually disintegrate, and one ovum (Sadler, 2006) (Figure 4–1 ■).

Spermatogenesis

During puberty, the germinal epithelium in the seminiferous tubules of the testes begins the process of spermatogenesis, which produces the male gamete (sperm). The diploid spermatogonium replicates before it enters the first meiotic division, during which it is called the *primary spermatocyte*. During this first meiotic division, the spermatogonium replicates and forms two cells called *secondary spermatocytes*, each of which contains 22 double-structured autosomal chromosomes and either a double-structured X sex chromosome or a double-structured Y sex chromosome. During the second meiotic division, they divide to form four spermatids, each with the haploid number of chromosomes. The spermatids undergo a series of changes during which they lose most of their cytoplasm and become sperm (spermatozoa) (Figure 4–1). The nucleus becomes compacted into the head of the sperm, which is covered by a cap called an *acrosome* that is, in turn, covered by a plasma membrane. A long tail is produced from one of the centrioles.

The Process of Fertilization

Fertilization is the process by which a sperm fuses with an ovum to form a new diploid cell, or zygote. The zygote begins life as a single cell with a complete set of genetic material, 23 chromosomes from the mother's ovum and 23 chromosomes from the father's sperm for a total of 46 chromosomes. The following events lead to fertilization.

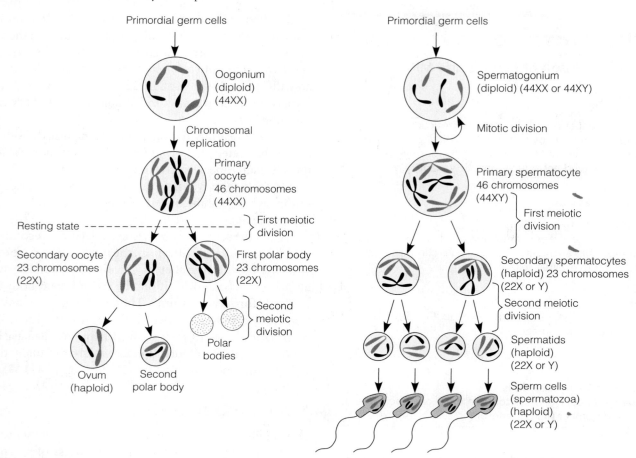

FIGURE 4–1 Gametogenesis involves meiosis within the ovary and testis. *A,* During meiosis each oogonium produces a single haploid ovum once some cytoplasm moves into the polar bodies. *B,* Each spermatogonium produces four haploid spermatozoa.

Preparation for Fertilization

The mature ovum and spermatozoa have only a brief time to unite. Ova are considered fertile for about 12 to 24 hours after ovulation. Sperm can survive in the female reproductive tract for 48 to 72 hours, but are believed to be healthy and highly fertile for only about 24 hours.

The ovum's cell membrane is surrounded by two layers of tissue. The layer closest to the cell membrane is called the *zona pellucida.* It is a clear, noncellular layer whose thickness influences the fertilization rate. Surrounding the zona pellucida is a ring of elongated cells, called the *corona radiata* because they radiate from the ovum like the gaseous corona around the sun. These cells are held together by hyaluronic acid. The ovum has no inherent power of movement. During ovulation, high estrogen levels increase peristalsis within the fallopian tubes, which helps move the ovum through the tube toward the uterus. The high estrogen levels also cause a thinning of the cervical mucus, facilitating movement of the sperm through the cervix, into the uterus, and up the fallopian tube.

The process of fertilization takes place in the ampulla (outer third) of the fallopian tube. In a single ejaculation, the male deposits approximately 200 to 300 million spermatozoa into the vagina, of which only hundreds of sperm actually reach the ampulla (Sadler, 2006). Fructose in the semen, secreted by the seminal vesicles, is the energy source for the sperm. The spermatozoa propel themselves up the female tract by the flagellar movement of their tails. Transit time from the cervix into the fallopian tube can be as short as 5 minutes but usually takes an average of 2 to 7 hours after ejaculation (Sadler, 2006). Prostaglandins in the semen may increase uterine smooth muscle contractions, which help transport the sperm. The fallopian tubes have a dual ciliary action that facilitates movement of the ovum toward the uterus and movement of the sperm from the uterus toward the ovary.

The sperm must undergo two processes before fertilization can occur: capacitation and the acrosomal reaction. **Capacitation** is the removal of the plasma membrane overlying the spermatozoa's acrosomal area and the loss of seminal plasma proteins. If the glycoprotein coat is not removed, the sperm will not be able to fertilize the ovum (Sadler, 2006). Capacitation occurs in the female reproductive tract (aided by uterine enzymes) and is thought to take about 7 hours. Sperm that undergo capacitation now take on three characteristics: (1) the ability to undergo the acrosomal reaction, (2) the ability to bind to the zona pellucida, and (3) the acquisition of hypermotility.

The **acrosomal reaction** follows capacitation, whereby the acrosomes of the sperms surrounding the

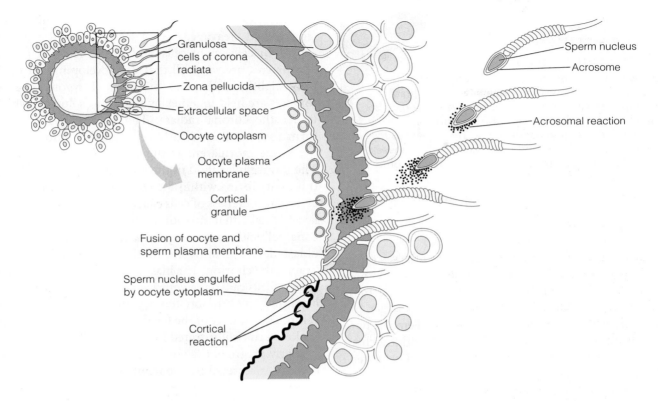

Granulosa cells of corona radiata

Zona pellucida

Extracellular space

Oocyte cytoplasm

Oocyte plasma membrane

Cortical granule

Fusion of oocyte and sperm plasma membrane

Sperm nucleus engulfed by oocyte cytoplasm

Cortical reaction

Sperm nucleus

Acrosome

Acrosomal reaction

A

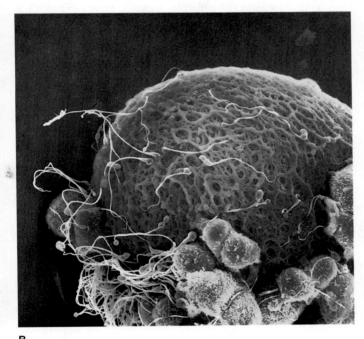

B

FIGURE 4–2 Sperm penetration of an ovum. *A*, The sequential steps of oocyte penetration by a sperm are depicted moving from top to bottom. *B*, Scanning electron micrograph of a human sperm surrounding a human ovum (750X). The smaller spherical cells are granulosa cells of the corona radiata. *Source: B*, Scanning electron micrograph from Nilsson, L. (1990). *A child is born.* New York: Dell Publishing.

ovum release their enzymes (hyaluronidase, a protease called acrosin, and trypsinlike substances) and thus break down the hyaluronic acid in the ovum's corona radiata (Sadler, 2006). Hundreds of acrosomes must rupture before enough hyaluronic acid is cleared for a single sperm to penetrate the ovum's zona pellucida successfully.

At the moment of penetration by a fertilizing sperm, the zona pellucida undergoes a reaction that prevents additional sperm from entering a single ovum. This is known as the *block to polyspermy*. This cellular change is mediated by release of materials from the cortical granules, organelles found just below the ovum's surface, and is called the *cortical reaction* (Figure 4–2 ■).

The Moment of Fertilization

After the sperm enters the ovum, a chemical signal prompts the secondary oocyte to complete the second meiotic division, forming the nucleus of the ovum and ejecting the second polar body. Then the nuclei of the ovum and sperm swell and approach each other. The true moment of fertilization occurs as the nuclei unite. Their individual nuclear membranes disappear, and their chromosomes pair up to produce the diploid zygote. Because each nucleus contains a haploid number of chromosomes (23), this union restores the diploid number (46). The zygote contains a new combination of genetic material that results in an individual different from either parent and from anyone else.

The moment of fertilization is also when the sex of the zygote is determined. The two chromosomes (the sex chromosomes) of the 23rd pair—either XX or XY—determine the sex of an individual. The X chromosome is larger and bears more genes than the Y chromosome. Females have two X chromosomes, and males have an X and a Y chromosome. Whereas the mature ovum produced by oogenesis can have only one type of sex chromosome—an X—spermatogenesis produces two sperm with an X chromosome and two sperm with a Y chromosome. When each gamete contributes an X chromosome, the resulting zygote is female. When the ovum contributes an X and the sperm contributes a Y chromosome, the resulting zygote is male. Certain traits are termed *sex linked* because they are controlled by the genes on the X sex chromosome. Two examples of sex-linked traits are color blindness and hemophilia.

Preembryonic Development

The first 14 days of development, starting the day the ovum is fertilized (conception), are called the *preembryonic stage*, or the *stage of the ovum*. Development after fertilization can be divided into two phases: cellular multiplication and cellular differentiation. These phases are characterized by rapid cellular multiplication, and differentiation and establishment of the primary germ layers and embryonic membranes. Synchronized development of both the endometrium and embryo is a prerequisite for implantation to succeed (Moore & Persaud, 2008). These phases and the process of implantation (nidation), which occurs between them, are discussed next.

Cellular Multiplication

Cellular multiplication begins as the zygote moves through the fallopian tube toward the cavity of the uterus. This transport takes 3 days or more and is accomplished mainly by a very weak fluid current in the fallopian tube resulting from the beating action of the ciliated epithelium that lines the tube.

The zygote now enters a period of rapid mitotic divisions called **cleavage**, during which it divides into two cells, four cells, eight cells, and so on. These cells, called *blastomeres*, are so small that the developing cell mass is only slightly larger than the original zygote. The blastomeres are held together by the zona pellucida, which is under the corona radiata. The blastomeres eventually form a solid ball of 12 to 16 cells called the **morula**.

As the morula enters the uterus, two things happen: The intracellular fluid in the morula increases, and a central cavity forms within the cell mass. Inside this cavity is an inner solid mass of cells called the **blastocyst**. The outer layer of cells that surrounds the cavity and replaces the zona pellucida is the **trophoblast**. Eventually, the trophoblast develops into one of the two embryonic membranes, the chorion. The blastocyst develops into a double layer of cells called the *embryonic disc*, from which the embryo and the amnion (embryonic membrane) will develop. The journey of the fertilized ovum to its destination in the uterus is illustrated in Figure 4–3 ■.

Early pregnancy factor (EPF), an immunosuppressant protein, is secreted by the trophoblastic cells. This factor appears in the maternal serum within 24 to 48 hours after fertilization and forms the basis of a pregnancy test during the first 10 days of development (Moore & Persaud, 2008).

Implantation (Nidation)

While floating in the uterine cavity, the blastocyst is nourished by the uterine glands, which secrete a mixture of lipids, mucopolysaccharides, and glycogen. The trophoblast attaches itself to the surface of the endometrium for further nourishment. The most frequent site of attachment is the upper part of the posterior uterine wall. Between days 7 and 10 after fertilization, the zona pellucida disappears and the blastocyst implants itself by burrowing into the uterine lining and penetrating down toward the maternal capillaries until it is completely covered (Moore & Persaud, 2008). The lining of the uterus thickens below the implanted blastocyst, and the cells of the trophoblast grow down into the thickened lining, forming processes that will be called chorionic villi.

Under the influence of progesterone, the endometrium increases in thickness and vascularity in preparation for implantation and nutrition of the ovum. After implantation, the endometrium is called the decidua. The portion of the decidua that covers the blastocyst is called the **decidua capsularis**, the portion directly under the implanted blastocyst is the **decidua basalis**, and the portion that lines the rest of the uterine cavity is the **decidua vera (parietalis)**. The maternal part of the placenta develops from the decidua basalis, which contains large numbers of blood vessels (see magnified inset in Figure 4–3) (Moore & Persaud, 2008). The chorionic villi (discussed shortly) in contact with the decidua basalis will form the fetal portion of the placenta.

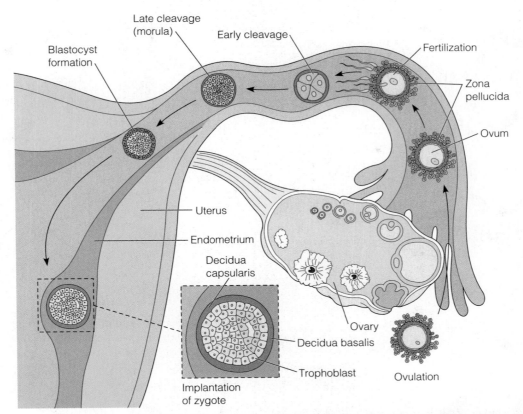

FIGURE 4–3 During ovulation, the ovum leaves the ovary and enters the fallopian tube. Fertilization generally occurs in the outer third of the fallopian tube. The figure depicts subsequent changes in the fertilized ovum from conception to implantation.

Cellular Differentiation

Primary Germ Layers

About the 10th to 14th day after conception, the homogeneous mass of blastocyst cells differentiates into the primary germ layers (Figure 4–4 ■). These three layers, the **ectoderm**, **mesoderm**, and **endoderm**, are formed at the same time as the embryonic membranes. All tissues, organs, and organ systems will develop from these primary germ cell layers (see Table 4–1). For example, differentiation of the endoderm results in the formation of epithelium lining the respiratory and digestive tracts (Figure 4–5 ■).

Embryonic Membranes

The **embryonic membranes** begin to form at the time of implantation (Figure 4–6 ■). These membranes protect and support the embryo as it grows and develops inside the uterus. The first and outermost membrane to form is the **chorion**. This thick membrane develops from the trophoblast, and has many fingerlike projections called *chorionic villi* on its surface. These chorionic villi can be used for early genetic testing of the embryo at 8 to 11 weeks' gestation by chorionic villi sampling (see Chapter 14 ∞). As the pregnancy progresses, the chorionic villi begin to degenerate, except for those just under the embryo, which grow and branch into depressions in the uterine wall, form-

ing the fetal portion of the placenta. By the fourth month of pregnancy, the surface of the chorion is smooth except at the place of attachment to the uterine wall.

The second membrane to form, the amnion, originates from the ectoderm, a primary germ layer, during the early stages of embryonic development. The **amnion** is a thin protective membrane that contains amniotic fluid. The space between the membrane and the embryo is the *amniotic cavity*. This cavity surrounds the embryo and yolk sac, except where the developing embryo (germ-layer disc) attaches to the trophoblast via the umbilical cord. As the embryo grows, the amnion expands until it comes into contact with the chorion. These two slightly adherent membranes form the fluid-filled amniotic sac, also called the **bag of waters** (**BOW**), which protects the floating embryo.

Amniotic Fluid

The *primary functions* of **amniotic fluid** are to:

- Act as a cushion to protect the embryo against mechanical injury
- Help control the embryo's temperature (relies on the mother to release heat)
- Permit symmetrical external growth and development of the embryo
- Prevent adherence of the embryo–fetus to the amnion (decreases chance of amniotic band syndrome) to allow

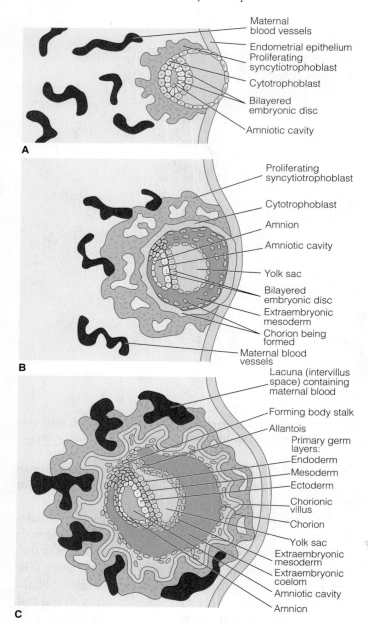

FIGURE 4–4 Formation of primary germ layers. *A,* Implantation of a 7½-day blastocyst in which the cells of the embryonic disc are separated from the amnion by a fluid-filled space. The erosion of the endometrium by the syncytiotrophoblast is ongoing. *B,* Implantation is completed by day 9, and extraembryonic mesoderm is beginning to form a discrete layer beneath the cytotrophoblast. *C,* By day 16 the embryo shows all three germ layers, a yolk sac, and an allantois (an outpouching of the yolk sac that forms the structural basis of the body stalk, or umbilical cord). The cytotrophoblast and associated mesoderm have become the chorion, and chorionic villi are developing.

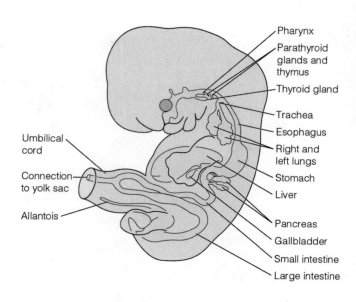

5-week embryo

FIGURE 4–5 Endoderm differentiates to form the epithelial lining of the digestive and respiratory tracts and associated glands.

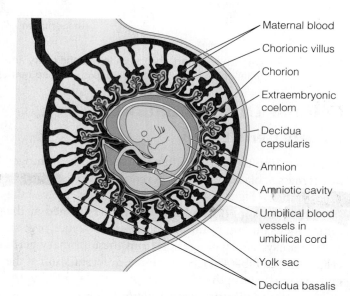

FIGURE 4–6 Early development of primary embryonic membranes. At 4½ weeks, the decidua capsularis (placental portion enclosing the embryo on the uterine surface) and decidua basalis (placental portion encompassing the elaborate chorionic villi and maternal endometrium) are well formed. The chorionic villi lie in blood-filled intervillous spaces within the endometrium. The amnion and yolk sac are well developed.

freedom of movement so that the embryo–fetus can change position (flexion and extension), thus aiding in musculoskeletal development
- Allow the umbilical cord to be relatively free of compression

- Act as an extension of fetal extracellular space (hydropic infants have increased amniotic fluid)
- Act as a wedge during labor
- Provide fluid for analysis to determine fetal health and maturity

TABLE 4–1	Derivation of Body Structures from Primary Cell Layers	
Ectoderm	**Mesoderm**	**Endoderm**
Epidermis	Dermis	Respiratory tract epithelium
Sweat glands	Wall of digestive tract	Epithelium (except nasal), including pharynx, tongue, tonsils, thyroid, parathyroid, thymus, tympanic cavity
Sebaceous glands	Kidneys and ureter (suprarenal cortex)	
Nails	Reproductive organs (gonads, genital ducts)	Lining of digestive tract
Hair follicles		Primary tissue of liver and pancreas
Lens of eye	Connective tissue (cartilage, bone, joint cavities)	Urethra and associated glands
Sensory epithelium of internal and external ear, nasal cavity, sinuses, mouth, anal canal	Skeleton	Urinary bladder (except trigone)
	Muscles (all types)	Vagina (parts)
Central and peripheral nervous systems	Cardiovascular system (heart, arteries, veins, blood, bone marrow)	
Nasal cavity		
Oral glands and tooth enamel	Pleura	
Pituitary gland	Lymphatic tissue and cells	
Mammary glands	Spleen	

Amniotic fluid is slightly alkaline and contains albumin, uric acid, creatinine, lecithin, sphingomyelin, bilirubin, vernix, leukocytes, epithelial cells, enzymes, and fine hair called **lanugo**. The amount of amniotic fluid at 10 weeks is about 30 mL, and it increases to 350 mL at 20 weeks. After 20 weeks, the volume ranges from 700 to 1000 mL. The amniotic fluid volume is constantly changing as the fluid moves back and forth across the placental membrane. Water and solutes must pass between the amniotic fluid and fetus. As the pregnancy continues, the fetus contributes to the volume of amniotic fluid by excreting urine. The fetus also swallows up to 262 mL/kg/day. About 400 mL of lung fluid flows out of the fetal lungs each day (Gilbert, 2007). Abnormal variations in amniotic fluid volume are *oligohydramnios* (less than 400 mL of amniotic fluid) and *hydramnios* (more than 2000 mL or amniotic fluid index greater than 97.5 percentile for the corresponding gestational age). Hydramnios is also called *polyhydramnios*. See Chapter 22 ∞ for an in-depth discussion of alterations in amniotic fluid volume.

Yolk Sac

In humans, the yolk sac is small and functions early in embryonic life. It develops as a second cavity in the blastocyst on about day 8 or 9 after conception. It forms primitive red blood cells during the first 6 weeks of development, until the embryo's liver takes over the process. As the embryo develops, the yolk sac is incorporated into the umbilical cord, where it can be seen as a degenerated structure after birth.

Umbilical Cord

As the placenta is developing, the **umbilical cord** is also being formed from the amnion. The *body stalk*, which at-

taches the embryo to the yolk sac, contains blood vessels that extend into the chorionic villi. The body stalk fuses with the embryonic portion of the placenta to provide a circulatory pathway from the chorionic villi to the embryo. As the body stalk elongates to become the umbilical cord, the vessels in the cord decrease to one large vein and two smaller arteries. About 1% of umbilical cords have only two vessels, an artery and a vein; this condition may be associated with congenital malformations primarily of the renal, gastrointestinal, and cardiovascular systems. A specialized connective tissue known as **Wharton's jelly** surrounds the blood vessels in the umbilical cord. This tissue, plus the high blood volume pulsating through the vessels, prevents compression of the umbilical cord in utero. The umbilical cord has no sensory or motor innervation, so cutting the cord after birth is not painful. At term (38 to 42 weeks' gestation), the average cord is 2 cm (0.8 in.) across and about 55 cm (22 in.) long. The cord can attach itself to the placenta in various sites. Central insertion into the placenta is considered normal. (See Chapter 22 ∞ for a discussion of the various attachment sites.)

Umbilical cords appear twisted or spiraled, which is most likely caused by fetal movement. A true knot in the umbilical cord rarely occurs; if it does, the cord is longer than usual. More common are so-called false knots, caused by the folding of cord vessels. A *nuchal cord* is said to exist when the umbilical cord encircles the fetal neck.

Twins

Twins normally occur in approximately 1 in 80 pregnancies, and triplets occur in 1 in 8,000 pregnancies. Fraternal (nonidentical or dizygotic) twins have been reported to occur more often among black than among white women and more often among white women than among women of Asian origin (Moore & Persaud, 2008). Among all groups, as parity (having given birth to a viable infant) increases, so does the chance for multiple births.

Twins may be either fraternal or identical (Figure 4–7 ■). If twins are fraternal, they are dizygotic, which means they arise from two separate ova fertilized by two separate spermatozoa. There are two placentas, two chorions, and two amnions; however, the placentas sometimes fuse and look as if they are one. Despite their birth relationship, fraternal twins are no more similar to each other than they would be to siblings born singly. They may be of the same or different sex.

Dizygotic twinning increases with maternal age up to about age 35 and then decreases abruptly. The chance of dizygotic twins increases with parity, in conceptions that occur in the first 3 months of marriage, and also with coital frequency. The chance of dizygotic twinning decreases during periods of malnutrition and during winter and spring for women living in the Northern Hemisphere. Studies indicate that dizygotic twins occur in certain families, perhaps because of genotype (genetic constitution) of the mother that results in elevated serum gonadotropin levels leading to double ovulation

(Moore & Persaud, 2008). The incidence of dizygotic twinning varies greatly from approximately 1 in 500 in Asians, 1 in 125 in whites, and as high as 1 in 20 in some African populations, whereas the incidence of monozygotic twins is approximately the same in all populations (Moore & Persaud, 2008).

Identical, or monozygotic, twins develop from a single fertilized ovum. They are of the same sex and have the same phenotype (appearance). Identical twins usually have a common placenta. Monozygosity is not affected by environment, race, physical characteristics, or fertility.

Monozygotic twins originate from division of the fertilized ovum at different stages of early development, after the zygote consists of thousands of cells. Complete separation of the cellular mass into two parts is necessary for twin formation. The number of amnions and chorions present depends on the timing of the division.

1. If division occurs within 3 days of fertilization (before the inner cell mass and chorion are formed), two embryos, two amnions, and two chorions will develop. This dichorionic–diamniotic situation occurs about 20% to 30% of the time, and there may be two distinct placentas or a single fused placenta.

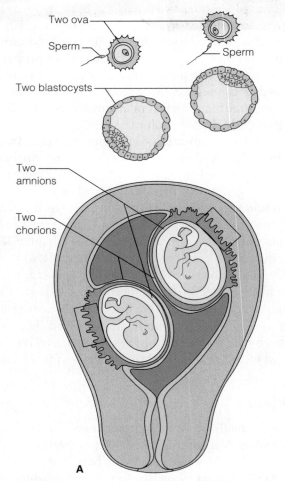

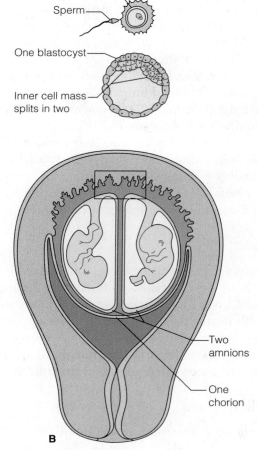

FIGURE 4–7 *A,* Formation of fraternal twins. (Note separate placentas.) *B,* Formation of identical twins.

2. If division occurs about 5 days after fertilization (when the inner cell mass is formed and the chorion cells have differentiated but those of the amnion have not), two embryos develop with separate amnion sacs. These sacs will eventually be covered by a common chorion; thus there will be a monochorionic–diamniotic placenta (see Figure 4–7B).

3. If the amnion has already developed, approximately 7 to 13 days after fertilization, division results in two embryos with a common amnion sac and a common chorion (a monochorionic–monoamniotic placenta). This type rarely occurs.

Monozygotic twinning is considered a random event and occurs in approximately 3 to 4 per 1,000 live births (Sadler, 2006). The survival rate of monozygotic twins is lower than that of dizygotic twins, and congenital anomalies are more prevalent. Both twins may have the same malformation.

Development and Functions of the Placenta

The **placenta** is the means of metabolic and nutrient exchange between the embryonic and maternal circulations. Placental development and circulation do not begin until the third week of embryonic development. The placenta develops at the site where the embryo attaches to the uterine wall. Expansion of the placenta continues until about 20 weeks, when it covers approximately one-half of the internal surface of the uterus. After 20 weeks' gestation, the placenta becomes thicker but not wider. At 40 weeks' gestation, the placenta is about 15 to 20 cm (5.9 to 7.9 in.) in diameter and 2.5 to 3.0 cm (1.0 to 1.2 in.) in thickness. At that time, it weighs about 400 to 600 g (14 to 21 oz).

The placenta has two parts: the maternal and fetal portions. The maternal portion consists of the decidua basalis and its circulation. Its surface is red and fleshlike. The fetal portion consists of the chorionic villi and their circulation. The fetal surface of the placenta is covered by the amnion, which gives it a shiny, gray appearance (Figures 4–8 and 4–9 ■).

Development of the placenta begins with the chorionic villi. The trophoblastic cells of the chorionic villi form spaces in the tissue of the decidua basalis. These spaces fill with maternal blood, and the chorionic villi grow into them. As the chorionic villi differentiate, two trophoblastic layers appear: an outer layer, called the *syncytium* (consisting of syncytiotrophoblasts), and an inner layer, known as the *cytotrophoblast* (see Figure 4–4). The cytotrophoblast thins out and disappears about the fifth month, leaving only a single layer of syncytium covering the chorionic villi. The syncytium is in direct contact with the maternal blood in the intervillous spaces. It is the functional layer of the placenta and secretes the placental hormones of pregnancy.

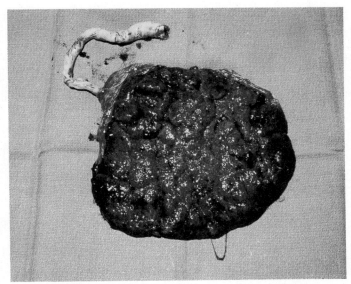

FIGURE 4–8 Maternal side of placenta. *Dirty Duncan* (Photo courtesy of Marcia London.)

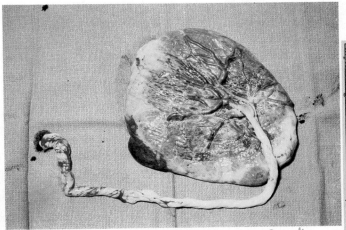

FIGURE 4–9 Fetal side of placenta. *Shiny Shutz comes out this way.* (Photo courtesy of Marcia London.)

MyNursingKit | Animation: Development of the Placenta

A third, inner layer of connective mesoderm develops in the chorionic villi, forming *anchoring villi*. These anchoring villi eventually form the *septa* (partitions) of the placenta. The septa divide the mature placenta into 15 to 20 segments called **cotyledons** (subdivisions of the placenta made up of anchoring villi and decidual tissue). In each cotyledon, the *branching villi* form a highly complex vascular system that allows compartmentalization of the uteroplacental circulation. The exchange of gases and nutrients takes place across these vascular systems.

Exchange of substances across the placenta is minimal during the first 3 to 5 months of development because the villous membrane is initially too thick, which limits its permeability. As the villous membrane thins, placental permeability increases until about the last month of pregnancy, when permeability begins to decrease as the placenta ages. In the fully developed placenta, fetal blood in the villi and maternal blood in the intervillous spaces are separated by three to four thin layers of tissue.

Placental Circulation

After implantation of the blastocyst, the cells distinguish themselves into fetal cells and trophoblastic cells. The proliferating trophoblast successfully invades the decidua basalis of the endometrium, first opening the uterine capillaries and later opening the larger uterine vessels. The chorionic villi are an outgrowth of the blastocystic tissue. As these villi continue to grow and divide, the fetal vessels begin to form. The intervillous spaces in the decidua basalis develop as the endometrial spiral arteries are opened.

By the end of the fourth week, the placenta has begun to function as a means of metabolic exchange between embryo and mother. The completion of the maternal–placental–fetal circulation occurs about 17 days after conception, when the embryonic heart begins functioning (Moore & Persaud, 2008). By 14 weeks, the placenta is a discrete organ. It has grown in thickness as a result of growth in the length and size of the chorionic villi and accompanying expansion of the intervillous space.

In the fully developed placenta's umbilical cord, fetal blood flows through the two umbilical arteries to the capillaries of the villi, becomes oxygen enriched, and then flows back through the umbilical vein into the fetus (Figure 4–10 ■). Late in pregnancy, a soft blowing sound (*funic souffle*) can be heard over the area of the umbilical cord. The sound is synchronous with the fetal heartbeat and fetal blood flow through the umbilical arteries.

Maternal blood, rich in oxygen and nutrients, spurts from the spiral uterine arteries into the intervillous spaces. These spurts are produced by the maternal blood pressure. The spurt of blood is directed toward the chorionic plate, and as the blood loses pressure, it becomes lateral (spreads out). Fresh blood enters continuously and exerts pressure on the contents of the intervillous spaces, pushing blood toward the exits in the basal plate. The blood then drains through the uterine and other pelvic veins. A *uterine souffle*, timed precisely with the mother's pulse, is also heard just above the mother's symphysis pubis during the last months of pregnancy. This souffle is caused by the augmented blood flow entering the dilated uterine arteries.

Braxton Hicks contractions are intermittent painless uterine contractions that may occur every 10 to 20 minutes and occur more frequently near the end of pregnancy (see Chapter 17 ∞). These contractions are believed to facilitate placental circulation by enhancing the movement of blood from the center of the cotyledon through the intervillous space. Placental blood flow is enhanced when the woman is lying on her side because venous return from the lower extremities is not compromised (Blackburn, 2007).

Placental Functions

Placental exchange functions occur only in those fetal vessels that are in intimate contact with the covering syncytial

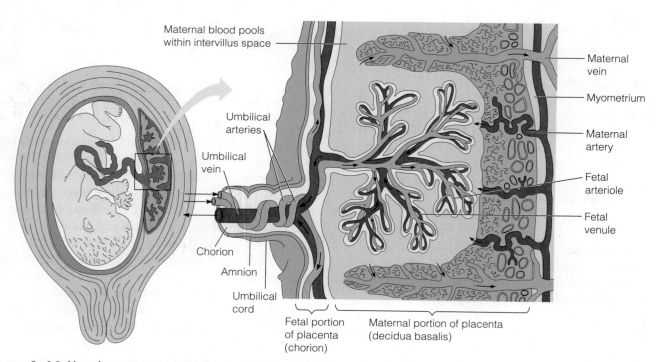

FIGURE 4–10 Vascular arrangement of the placenta. Arrows indicate the direction of blood flow. Maternal blood flows through the uterine arteries to the intervillous spaces of the placenta and returns through the uterine veins to maternal circulation. Fetal blood flows through the umbilical arteries into the villous capillaries of the placenta and returns through the umbilical vein to the fetal circulation.

membrane. The syncytium villi have brush borders containing many microvilli, which greatly increase the exchange rate between maternal and fetal circulation (Sadler, 2006).

The placental functions, many of which begin soon after implantation, include fetal respiration, nutrition, and excretion. To carry out these functions, the placenta is involved in metabolic and transfer activities. In addition, it has endocrine functions and special immunologic properties; see discussion later in this section.

Metabolic Activities

The placenta continuously produces glycogen, cholesterol, and fatty acids for fetal use and hormone production. The placenta also produces numerous enzymes (such as sulfatase [enhances excretion of fetal estrogen precursors] and insulinase [which increases the barrier to insulin]) required for fetoplacental transfer, and breaks down certain substances such as epinephrine and histamine (Blackburn, 2007). In addition, it stores glycogen and iron.

Transport Function

The placental membranes actively control the transfer of a wide range of substances by a variety of transport mechanisms.

Simple diffusion moves substances from an area of higher concentration to an area of lower concentration. Substances that move across the placenta by simple diffusion include water, oxygen, carbon dioxide, electrolytes (sodium and chloride), anesthetic gases, and drugs. Insulin and steroid hormones originating from the adrenals, as well as thyroid hormones, also cross the placenta. However, this happens at a very slow rate. The rate of oxygen transfer across the placental membrane is greater than that allowed by simple diffusion, indicating that oxygen is also transferred by some type of facilitated diffusion transport. Unfortunately many substances of abuse, such as cocaine and heroin, cross the placenta via simple diffusion.

Facilitated transport involves a carrier system to move molecules from an area of greater concentration to an area of lower concentration. Molecules such as glucose, galactose, and some oxygen are transported by this method. The glucose level in the fetal blood ordinarily is approximately 20% to 30% lower than the glucose level in the maternal blood, because the fetus is metabolizing glucose rapidly. This in turn causes rapid transport of additional glucose from the maternal blood into the fetal blood.

Active transport can work against a concentration gradient and allows molecules to move from areas of lower concentration to areas of higher concentration. Amino acids, calcium, iron, iodine, water-soluble vitamins, and glucose are transferred across the placenta in this way. The measured amino acid content of fetal blood is greater than that of maternal blood, and calcium and inorganic phosphate occur in greater concentration in fetal blood than in maternal blood (Blackburn, 2007).

Other modes of transfer also exist. *Pinocytosis* is important for transferring large molecules such as albumin and gamma globulin. Materials are engulfed by amoeba-like cells, forming plasma droplets. *Hydrostatic* and *osmotic pressures* allow the bulk flow of water and some solutes. Also fetal red blood cells can pass into the maternal circulation through breaks in the capillaries and placental membrane, particularly during labor and birth. Certain cells, such as maternal leukocytes, and microorganisms, such as viruses (e.g., the human immunodeficiency virus [HIV], which causes acquired immunodeficiency syndrome [AIDS]), rubella, cytomegalovirus, polio, and the bacterium *Treponema pallidum* (which causes syphilis), can also cross the placental membrane under their own power (Moore & Persaud, 2008). Some bacteria and protozoa infect the placenta by causing lesions and then entering the fetal blood system.

Reduction of the placental surface area, as with abruptio placentae (partial or complete premature separation of an abnormally implanted placenta), lessens the area that is functional for exchange. Placental diffusion distance also affects exchange. In conditions such as diabetes and placental infection, edema of the villi increases the diffusion distance, thus increasing the distance the substance has to be transferred.

Blood flow alteration changes the transfer rate of substances. Decreased blood flow in the intervillous space is seen in labor and with certain maternal diseases such as hypertension. Mild fetal hypoxia increases the umbilical blood flow, but severe hypoxia results in decreased blood flow.

As the maternal blood picks up fetal waste products and carbon dioxide, it drains back into the maternal circulation through the veins in the basal plate. Fetal blood is hypoxic by comparison; it therefore attracts oxygen from the mother's blood. Affinity for oxygen increases as the fetal blood gives up its carbon dioxide, which also decreases its acidity.

Endocrine Functions

The placenta produces hormones that are vital to the survival of the fetus. These include human chorionic gonadotropin (hCG); human placental lactogen (hPL); and two steroid hormones, estrogen and progesterone.

The hormone hCG is similar to luteinizing hormone (LH) and prevents the normal involution of the corpus luteum at the end of the menstrual cycle (see Chapter 3 ∞). If the corpus luteum stops functioning before the 11th week of pregnancy, spontaneous abortion occurs. The hCG also causes the corpus luteum to secrete increased amounts of estrogen and progesterone.

After the 11th week, the placenta produces enough progesterone and estrogen to maintain pregnancy. In the male fetus, hCG also exerts an interstitial cell-stimulating effect on the testes, resulting in the production of testosterone. This small secretion of testosterone during embryonic development is the factor that causes male sex organs to grow. Human chorionic gonadotropin may play a role in the trophoblast's immunologic capabilities (ability to exempt the placenta and embryo from rejection by the mother's system). This hormone is used as a basis for pregnancy tests (see Chapter 9 ∞).

Human chorionic gonadotropin is present in maternal blood serum 8 to 10 days after fertilization, just as soon as implantation has occurred, and is detectable in maternal urine at the time of missed menses. After reaching its maximum level at 50 to 70 days' gestation, hCG begins to decrease as placental hormone production increases.

Progesterone is an essential hormone for pregnancy. It increases the secretions of the fallopian tubes and uterus to provide appropriate nutritive matter for the developing morula and blastocyst. It also appears to aid in ovum transport through the fallopian tube. Progesterone causes decidual cells to develop in the uterine endometrium, and it must be present in high levels for implantation to occur. Progesterone also decreases the contractility of the uterus, thus preventing uterine contractions from causing spontaneous abortion.

Before stimulation by hCG, the production of progesterone by the corpus luteum reaches a peak about 7 to 10 days after ovulation. Implantation occurs at about the same time as this peak. At 16 days after ovulation, progesterone reaches a level between 25 and 50 mg per day and continues to rise slowly in subsequent weeks. After 11 weeks, the placenta (specifically, the syncytiotrophoblast) takes over the production of progesterone and secretes it in tremendous quantities, reaching levels of more than 250 mg per day late in pregnancy.

By 7 weeks, the placenta produces more than 50% of the estrogens in the maternal circulation. *Estrogens* serve mainly a proliferative function, causing enlargement of the uterus, breasts, and breast glandular tissue. Estrogens also have a significant role in increasing vascularity and vasodilation, particularly in the villous capillaries toward the end of pregnancy. Placental estrogens increase markedly toward the end of pregnancy, to as much as 30 times the daily production in the middle of a normal monthly menstrual cycle. The primary estrogen secreted by the placenta is different from that secreted by the ovaries. The placenta secretes mainly *estriol*, whereas the ovaries secrete primarily estradiol. The placenta cannot synthesize estriol by itself. Essential precursors such as dehydroepiandrosterone sulfate (DHEA-S) is provided by the fetal adrenal glands, is processed by fetal liver, and is transported to the placenta for the final conversion to estrone, estradiol, and estriol (Blackburn, 2007; Knuppel, 2007).

The hormone human placental lactogen (hPL), also referred to as human chorionic somatomammotropin (hCS), is similar to human pituitary growth hormone; hPL stimulates certain changes in the mother's metabolic processes. These changes ensure that more protein, glucose, and minerals are available for the fetus. Secretion of hPL can be detected by about 4 weeks after conception.

Immunologic Properties

The placenta and embryo are transplants of living tissue within the same species and are therefore considered *homografts*. Unlike other homografts, the placenta and embryo appear exempt from immunologic reaction by the host. Most recent data suggest that there is a suppression of cellular immunity by the placental hormones (progesterone and hCG) during pregnancy (Knuppel, 2007). One theory suggests that chorionic villi syncytiotrophoblastic tissue is immunologically inert. The chorionic villi may lack major histocompatibility (MHC) antigens and thus do not evoke rejection responses. It does, however, protect against antibody formation. Extravillous trophoblast (EVT) cells, which invade the uterine deciduas, have HLA-G which is not readily recognized by sensitized t lymphocytes and natural killer cells (Moore & Persaud, 2008).

Development of the Fetal Circulatory System

The circulatory system of the fetus has several unique features that, by maintaining the blood flow to the placenta, provide the fetus with oxygen and nutrients while removing carbon dioxide and other waste products.

Most of the blood supply bypasses the fetal lungs because they do not carry out respiratory gas exchange. The placenta assumes the function of the fetal lungs by supplying oxygen and allowing the fetus to excrete carbon dioxide into the maternal bloodstream. Figure 4–11 ■ shows the fetal circulatory system. The blood from the placenta flows through the umbilical vein, which enters the abdominal wall of the fetus at the site that, after birth, is the umbilicus (belly button). As umbilical venous blood approaches the liver, a small portion of the blood enters the liver sinusoids, mixes with blood from the portal circulation, and then enters the inferior vena cava via hepatic veins. Most of the umbilical vein's blood flows through the **ductus venosus** directly into the fetal inferior vena cava, bypassing the liver. This blood then enters the right atrium, passes through the **foramen ovale** into the left atrium, and pours into the left ventricle, which pumps blood into the aorta. Some blood returning from the head and upper extremities by way of the superior vena cava is emptied into the right atrium and passes through the tricuspid valve into the right ventricle. This blood is pumped into the pulmonary artery, and a small amount passes to the lungs for nourishment only. The larger portion of blood passes from the pulmonary artery through

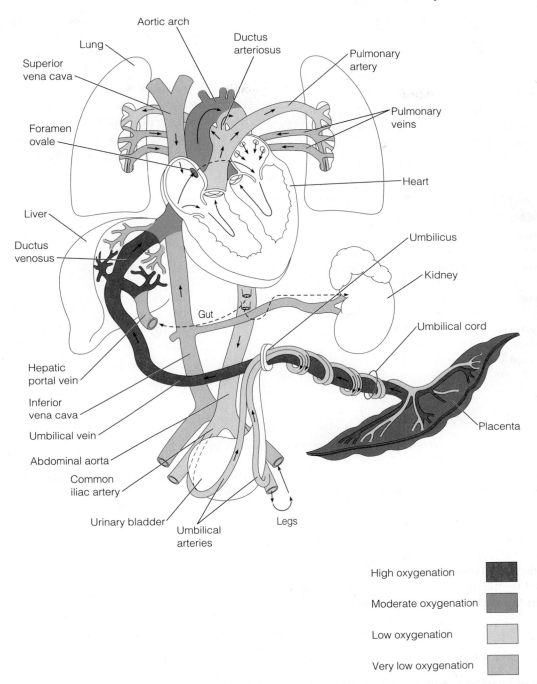

FIGURE 4–11 Fetal circulation. Blood leaves the placenta and enters the fetus through the umbilical vein. After circulating through the fetus, the blood returns to the placenta through the umbilical arteries. The ductus venosus, the foramen ovale, and the ductus arteriosus allow the blood to bypass the fetal liver and lungs.

the **ductus arteriosus** into the descending aorta, bypassing the lungs. Finally, blood returns to the placenta through the two umbilical arteries, and the process is repeated.

The fetus obtains oxygen via diffusion from the maternal circulation because of the gradient difference of PO_2 of 50 mmHg in maternal blood in the placenta to 30 mm Hg PO_2 in the fetus. At term the fetus receives oxygen from the mother's circulation at a rate of 20 to 30 mL per minute (Sadler, 2006). Fetal hemoglobin facilitates obtaining oxy-

gen from the maternal circulation, because it carries as much as 20% to 30% more oxygen than adult hemoglobin. For further discussion, see Chapter 24 ∞.

Fetal circulation delivers the highest available oxygen concentration to the head, neck, brain, and heart (coronary circulation) and a lesser amount of oxygenated blood to the abdominal organs and the lower body. This circulatory pattern leads to cephalocaudal (head-to-tail) development in the fetus.

Embryonic and Fetal Development

Pregnancy is calculated to last an *average* of 10 lunar months: 40 weeks, or 280 days. This period of 280 days is calculated from the onset of the last normal menstrual period to the time of birth. Estimated date of birth (EDB), sometimes referred to as the *estimated date of delivery (EDD)*, is usually calculated by this method. Most fetuses are born within 10 to 14 days of the calculated date of birth. The fertilization age (or postconception age) of the fetus is calculated to be *about* 2 weeks less, or 266 days (38 weeks) or 9.5 calendar months. The latter measurement is more accurate because it measures time from the fertilization of the ovum, or conception.

The basic events of organ development in the embryo and fetus are outlined in Table 4–2. The time periods in the table are **postconception age periods**. During the

---

TABLE 4–2	Summary of Organ System Development

Age: 2 to 3 Weeks
Length: 2 mm C–R (crown to rump)
Nervous system: Groove forms along middle back as cells thicken; neural tube forms from closure of neural groove.
Cardiovascular system: Beginning of blood circulation; tubular heart begins to form during third week.
Gastrointestinal system: Liver begins to function.
Genitourinary system: Formation of kidneys beginning.
Respiratory system: Nasal pits forming.
Endocrine system: Thyroid tissue appears.
Eyes: Optic cup and lens pit have formed; pigment in eyes.
Ears: Auditory pit is now enclosed structure.

Age: 4 Weeks
Length: 4 to 6 mm C–R
Weight: 0.4 g.
Nervous system: Anterior portion of neural tube closes to form brain; closure of posterior end forms spinal cord.
Musculoskeletal system: Noticeable limb buds.
Cardiovascular system: Tubular heart beats at 28 days, and primitive red blood cells circulate through fetus and chorionic villi.
Gastrointestinal system: Mouth: formation of oral cavity; primitive jaws present; esophagotracheal septum begins division of esophagus and trachea. Digestive tract: stomach forms; esophagus and intestine become tubular; ducts of pancreas and liver forming.

Age: 5 Weeks
Length: 8 mm C–R
Weight: Only 0.5% of total body weight is fat (to 20 weeks).
Nervous system: Brain has differentiated and cranial nerves are present.
Musculoskeletal system: Developing muscles have innervation.
Cardiovascular system: Atrial division has occurred.

Age: 6 Weeks
Length: 12 mm C–R
Musculoskeletal system: Bone rudiments present; primitive skeletal shape forming; muscle mass begins to develop; ossification of skull and jaws begins.
Cardiovascular system: Chambers present in heart; groups of blood cells can be identified.
Gastrointestinal system: Oral and nasal cavities and upper lip formed; liver begins to form red blood cells.
Respiratory system: Trachea, bronchi, and lung buds present.
Ears: Formation of external, middle, and inner ear continues.
Sexual development: Embryonic sex glands appear.

Age: 7 Weeks
Length: 18 mm C–R
Cardiovascular system: Fetal heartbeats can be detected.
Gastrointestinal system: Mouth: tongue separates; palate folds. Digestive tract: stomach attains final form.
Genitourinary system: Separation of bladder and urethra from rectum.
Respiratory system: Diaphragm separates abdominal and thoracic cavities.
Eyes: Optic nerve formed; eyelids appear, thickening of lens.
Sexual development: Differentiation of sex glands into ovaries and testes begins.

TABLE 4–2	Summary of Organ System Development *(Continued)*

Age: 8 Weeks

Length: 2.5 to 3 cm C–R

Weight: 2 g.

Musculoskeletal system: Digits formed; further differentiation of cells in primitive skeleton; cartilaginous bones show first signs of ossification; development of muscles in trunk, limbs, and head; some movement of fetus now possible.

Cardiovascular system: Development of heart essentially complete; fetal circulation follows two circuits—four extraembryonic and two intraembryonic. Heartbeat can be heard with Doppler at 8 to 12 weeks.

Gastrointestinal system: Mouth: completion of lip fusion. Digestive tract: rotation in midgut; anal membrane has perforated.

Ears: External, middle, and inner ear assuming final forms.

Sexual development: Male and female external genitals appear similar until end of ninth week.

Age: 10 Weeks

Length: 5 to 6 cm C–H (crown to heel)

Weight: 14 g.

Nervous system: Neurons appear at caudal end of spinal cord; basic divisions of brain present.

Musculoskeletal system: Fingers and toes begin nail growth.

Gastrointestinal system: Mouth: separation of lips from jaw; fusion of palate folds. Digestive tract: developing intestines enclosed in abdomen.

Genitourinary system: Bladder sac formed.

Endocrine system: Islets of Langerhans differentiated.

Eyes: Eyelids fused closed; development of lacrimal duct.

Sexual development: Males: production of testosterone and physical characteristics between 8 and 12 weeks.

Age: 12 Weeks

Length: 8 cm C–R; 11.5 cm C–H

Weight: 45 g.

Musculoskeletal system: Clear outlining of miniature bones (12 to 20 weeks); process of ossification is established throughout fetal body; appearance of involuntary muscles in viscera.

Gastrointestinal system: Mouth: completion of palate. Digestive tract: appearance of muscles in gut; bile secretion begins; liver is major producer of red blood cells.

Respiratory system: Lungs acquire definitive shape.

Skin: Pink and delicate.

Endocrine system: Hormonal secretion from thyroid; insulin present in pancreas.

Immunologic system: Appearance of lymphoid tissue in fetal thymus gland.

Age: 16 Weeks

Length: 13.5 cm C–R; 15 cm C–H

Weight: 200 g.

Musculoskeletal system: Teeth beginning to form hard tissue that will become central incisors.

Gastrointestinal system: Mouth: differentiation of hard and soft palate. Digestive tract: development of gastric and intestinal glands; intestines begin to collect meconium.

Genitourinary system: Kidneys assume typical shape and organization.

Skin: Appearance of scalp hair; lanugo present on body; transparent skin with visible blood vessels; sweat glands developing.

Eyes, ears, and nose: Formed.

Sexual development: Sex determination possible.

Age: 18 Weeks

Musculoskeletal system: Teeth beginning to form hard tissue (enamel and dentine) that will become lateral incisors.

Cardiovascular system: Fetal heart tones audible with fetoscope at 16 to 20 weeks.

Age: 20 Weeks

Length: 19 cm C–R; 25 cm C–H

Weight: 435 g (6% of total body weight is fat).

Nervous system: Myelination of spinal cord begins.

Musculoskeletal system: Teeth beginning to form hard tissue that will become canine and first molar. Lower limbs are of final relative proportions.

Gastrointestinal system: Fetus actively sucks and swallows amniotic fluid; peristaltic movements begin.

Skin: Lanugo covers entire body; brown fat begins to form; vernix caseosa begins to form.

Immunologic system: Detectable levels of fetal antibodies (IgG type).

Blood formation: Iron is stored and bone marrow is increasingly important.

(Continued)

TABLE 4–2 Summary of Organ System Development *(Continued)*

Age: 24 Weeks

Length: 23 cm C–R; 28 cm C–H

Weight: 780 g.

Nervous system: Brain looks like mature brain.

Musculoskeletal system: Teeth are beginning to form hard tissue that will become the second molars.

Respiratory system: Respiratory movements may occur (24 to 40 weeks). Nostrils reopen. Alveoli appear in lungs and begin production of surfactant; gas exchange possible.

Skin: Reddish and wrinkled, vernix caseosa present.

Immunologic system: IgG levels reach maternal levels.

Age: 28 Weeks

Length: 27 cm C–R; 35 cm C–H

Weight: 1,200 to 1,250 g.

Nervous system: Begins regulation of some body functions.

Skin: Adipose tissue accumulates rapidly; nails appear; eyebrows and eyelashes present.

Eyes: Eyelids open (26 to 29 weeks).

Sexual development: Males: testes descend into inguinal canal and upper scrotum.

Age: 32 Weeks

Length: 31 cm C–R; 38–43 cm C–H

Weight: 2,000 g.

Nervous system: More reflexes present.

Age: 36 Weeks

Length: 35 cm C–R; 42 to 48 cm C–H

Weight: 2,500 to 2,750 g.

Musculoskeletal system: Distal femoral ossification centers present.

Skin: Pale; body rounded, lanugo disappearing, hair fuzzy or woolly; few sole creases; sebaceous glands active and helping to produce vernix caseosa (36 to 40 weeks).

Ears: Earlobes soft with little cartilage.

Sexual development: Males: scrotum small and few rugae present; descent of testes into upper scrotum to stay (36 to 40 weeks). Females: labia majora and minora equally prominent.

Age: 38 to 40 Weeks

Length: 40 cm C–R; 48 to 52 cm C–H

Weight: 3,200+ g (16% of total body weight is fat).

Respiratory system: At 38 weeks, lecithin–sphingomyelin (L/S) ratio approaches 2:1 (indicates decreased risk of respiratory distress from inadequate surfactant production if born now).

Skin: Smooth and pink; vernix present in skin folds; moderate to profuse silky hair; lanugo on shoulders and upper back; nails extend over tips or digits; creases cover sole.

Ears: Earlobes firmer because of increased cartilage.

Sexual development: Males: rugous scrotum. Females: labia majora well developed and minora small or completely covered.

Source: Data from Sadler, T. W. (2006). *Langman's medical embryology* (10th ed.). Baltimore: Lippincott Williams & Wilkins.

Note: Age refers to postfertilization or postconception age.

period from fertilization to the end of the embryonic period (8 weeks), age is often expressed in days but can be given in weeks. During the fetal period (ninth week until birth) age is given in weeks (Moore & Persaud, 2008). The foldout poster in the middle of the book also summarizes fetal development.

In review, human development follows three stages. The preembryonic stage, as discussed earlier in the chapter, consists of the first 14 days of development after the ovum is fertilized; then the embryonic stage covers the period from day 15 until approximately the end of the eighth week, and the fetal stage extends from the end of the eighth week until birth. (See the detailed discussion of the embryonic and fetal stages next.)

Embryonic Stage

The stage of the **embryo** starts on day 15 (the beginning of the third week after conception) and continues until approximately the eighth week, or until the embryo reaches a crown-to-rump (C–R) length of 3 cm (1.2 in.). This length is usually reached about 56 days after fertilization (the end of the eighth gestational week). During the embryonic stage, tissues differentiate into essential organs and the main external features develop (see Figure 4–12 ■). The embryo is the most vulnerable to *teratogens* during this period. These are discussed in more depth later in the chapter.

Three Weeks

In the third week, the embryonic disk becomes elongated and pear shaped, with a broad cephalic end and a narrow caudal end. The ectoderm has formed a long cylindrical tube for brain and spinal cord development. The gastrointestinal tract, created from the endoderm, appears as another tube-like structure communicating with the yolk sac. The most advanced organ is the heart. At 3 weeks, a single tubular heart forms just outside the body cavity of the embryo.

Four to Five Weeks

During days 21 to 32, *somites* (a series of mesodermal blocks) form on either side of the embryo's midline. The vertebrae that form the spinal column will develop from these somites. Before 28 days, arm and leg buds are not visible, but the tail bud is present. The pharyngeal arches—which will form the lower jaw, hyoid bone, and larynx—develop at this time. The pharyngeal pouches appear now; these pouches will form the eustachian tube and cavity of the middle ear, the tonsils, and the parathy-roid and thymus glands. The primordia of the ear and eye are also present. By the end of 28 days, the tubular heart is beating at a regular rhythm and pushing its own primitive blood cells through the main blood vessels.

During the fifth week, the optic cups and lens vessels of the eye form and the nasal pits develop. Partitioning in the heart occurs with the dividing of the atrium. The embryo has a marked C-shaped body, accentuated by the rudimentary tail and the large head folded over a protuberant trunk (Figure 4–13 ■). By day 35, the arm and leg buds are well developed, with paddle-shaped hand and foot plates. The heart, circulatory system, and brain show the most advanced development. The brain has differentiated into five areas, and 10 pairs of cranial nerves are recognizable.

Six Weeks

At 6 weeks the head structures are more highly developed and the trunk is straighter than in earlier stages. The upper and lower jaws are recognizable, and the external nares are well formed. The trachea has developed, and its caudal end is bifurcated for beginning lung formation. The upper lip has formed, and the palate is developing. The ears are developing rapidly. The arms have begun to extend ventrally across the chest, and both arms and legs have digits, although they may still be webbed. There is a slight elbow

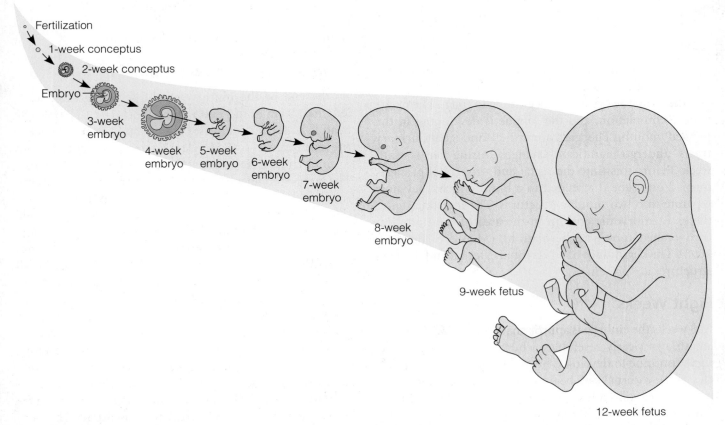

FIGURE 4–12 The actual size of a human conceptus from fertilization to the early fetal stage. The embryonic stage begins in the third week after fertilization; the fetal stage begins in the ninth week.

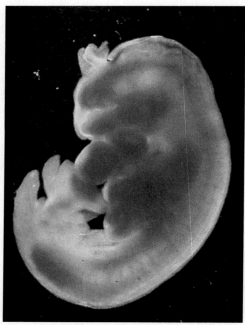

FIGURE 4–13 The embryo at 5 weeks. The embryo has a marked C-shaped body and a rudimentary tail.
Source: © Petit Format/Nestle/Science Source/Photo Researchers Inc.

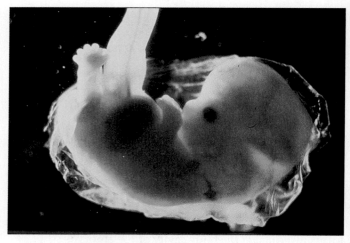

FIGURE 4–14 The embryo at 7 weeks. The head is rounded and nearly erect. The eyes have shifted forward and closer together, and the eyelids begin to form.
Source: © Petit Format/Nestle/Science Source/Photo Researchers Inc.

bend in the arms, which are more advanced in development than the legs. Beginning at this stage, the prominent tail will recede. The heart now has most of its definitive characteristics, and fetal circulation begins to be established. The liver starts to produce blood cells.

Seven Weeks

At 7 weeks the head of the embryo is rounded and nearly erect (Figure 4–14 ■). The eyes have shifted and are closer together, and the eyelids are beginning to form. The palate is near completion, and the tongue is developing in the formed mouth. The gastrointestinal and genitourinary tracts undergo significant changes during the seventh week. Before this time the rectal and urogenital passages formed one tube that ended in a blind pouch; they now separate into two tubular structures. The intestines enter the extraembryonic coelom in the area of the umbilical cord (called umbilical herniation) (Moore & Persaud, 2008). The beginnings of all essential external and internal structures are present.

Eight Weeks

At 8 weeks the embryo is approximately 3 cm (1.2 in.) C–R length and clearly resembles a human being. Facial features continue to develop. The eyelids begin to fuse. Auricles of the external ears begin to assume their final shape, but they are still set low (Moore & Persaud, 2008). External genitals appear, but the embryo's sex is not clearly identifiable. The rectal passage opens with the perforation of the anal membrane. The circulatory system through the umbilical cord is well established. Long bones are beginning to form, and the large muscles are now capable of contracting.

Fetal Stage

By the end of the eighth week, the embryo is sufficiently developed to be called a **fetus**. Every organ system and external structure that will be found in the full-term newborn is present. The remainder of gestation is devoted to refining structures and perfecting function.

Nine to Twelve Weeks

By the end of the ninth week the fetus reaches a C–R length of 5 cm (2 in.) and weighs about 14 g (0.5 oz). The head is large and comprises almost half of the fetus's entire size (Figure 4–15 ■). At 12 weeks, the fetus reaches 8 cm (3.2 in.) C–R length and weighs about 45 g (1.6 oz). The face is well formed, with the nose protruding, the chin small and receding, and the ear acquirng a more adult shape. The eyelids close at about the 10th week and will not reopen until about the 26 to 29 week period. Some movement of the lips suggestive of the sucking reflex has been observed at 3 months. Tooth buds now appear for all 20 of the child's first teeth (baby teeth). The limbs are long and slender, with well-formed digits. The fetus can curl the fingers toward the palm and begins to make a tiny fist. The legs are still shorter and less developed than the arms. The urogenital tract completes its development, well-differentiated genitals appear, and the kidneys begin to produce urine. Red blood cells are produced primarily by the liver. Spontaneous movements of the fetus now occur. Fetal heart rates can be ascertained by electronic devices between 8 and 12 weeks. The rate is 120 to 160 beats per minute.

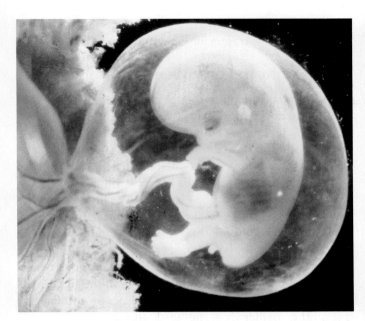

FIGURE 4–15 The fetus at 9 weeks. Every organ system and external structure is present.
Source: Nilsson, L. (1990). *A child is born.* New York: Dell Publishing.

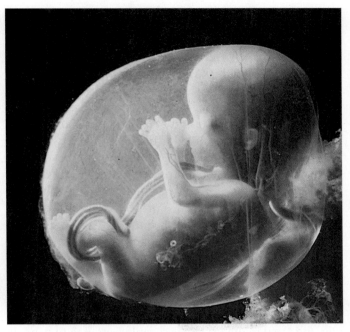

FIGURE 4–16 The fetus at 14 weeks. During this period of rapid growth the skin is so transparent that blood vessels are visible beneath it. More muscle tissue and body skeleton have developed, and they hold the fetus more erect.
Source: Nilsson, L. (1990). *A child is born.* New York: Dell Publishing.

Thirteen to Sixteen Weeks

This is a period of rapid growth. At 13 weeks, the fetus weighs 55 to 60 g (1.9 to 2.1 oz) and is about 9 cm (3.6 in.) in C–R length. Lanugo, or fine hair, begins to develop, especially on the head. The skin is so transparent that blood vessels are clearly visible beneath it. More muscle tissue and body skeleton have developed and hold the fetus more erect (Figure 4–16 ■). Active movements are present; the fetus stretches and exercises its arms and legs. It makes sucking motions, swallows amniotic fluid, and produces meconium in the intestinal tract. Bronchial tubes are branching out in the primitive lungs, and sweat glands are developing. The liver and pancreas now begin production of their appropriate secretions. By the beginning of week 16, skeletal ossification is clearly identifiable.

Twenty Weeks

The fetus doubles its C–R length and now measures 19 cm (8 in.) long. Fetal weight is between 435 and 465 g (15.2 and 16.3 oz). Lanugo covers the entire body and is especially prominent on the shoulders. Subcutaneous deposits of brown fat, which has a rich blood supply, make the skin less transparent. Nipples now appear over the mammary glands. The head is covered with fine, "woolly" hair, and the eyebrows and eyelashes are beginning to form. Nails are present on both fingers and toes. Muscles are well developed, and the fetus is active (Figure 4–17 ■). The mother feels fetal movement, known as *quickening.* The fetal heartbeat is audible through a fetoscope. Quickening and fetal heartbeat can help in validating the EDB.

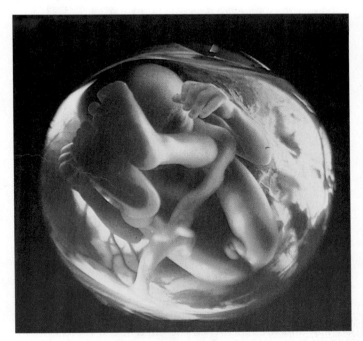

FIGURE 4–17 The fetus at 20 weeks. The fetus now weighs 435 to 465 g (15.2 to 16.3 oz) and measures about 19 cm (7.5 in.). Subcutaneous deposits of brown fat make the skin a little less transparent. "Woolly" hair covers the head, and nails have developed on the fingers and toes.
Source: Nilsson, L. (1990). *A child is born.* New York: Dell Publishing.

Twenty-Four Weeks

The fetus at 24 weeks reaches a crown-to-heel (C–H) length of 28 cm (11.2 in.). It weighs about 780 g (1 lb, 10 oz). The hair on the head is growing long, and eyebrows and eyelashes have formed. The eye is structurally complete and will soon open. The fetus has a reflex hand grip (grasp reflex) and, by the end of 6 months, a startle reflex. Skin covering the body is reddish and wrinkled, with little subcutaneous fat. Skin on the hands and feet have thickened, with skin ridges on palms and soles forming distinct foot- and fingerprints. The skin over the entire body is covered with **vernix caseosa**, a protective cheeselike, fatty substance secreted by the sebaceous glands. The alveoli in the lungs are just beginning to form.

Twenty-Five to Twenty-Eight Weeks

At 6 calendar months, the fetal skin is still red, wrinkled, and covered with vernix caseosa. The brain is developing rapidly, and the nervous system is complete enough to provide some degree of regulation of body functions. The eyelids, under neural control, open and close. The fetus has nails on both fingers and toes. In the male fetus, the testes begin to descend into the scrotal sac. Even though the lungs are still physiologically immature, they are sufficiently developed to provide gas exchange. A fetus born at this time will require immediate and prolonged intensive care to survive and then to decrease the risk of major handicap. The fetus at 28 weeks is about 35 to 38 cm (14 to 15 in.) long C–H and weighs 1200 to 1250 g (2 lb, 10.5 oz to 2 lb, 12 oz).

Twenty-Nine to Thirty-Two Weeks

At 30 weeks the pupillary light reflex is present (Moore & Persaud, 2008). The fetus is gaining weight from an increase in body muscle and fat and weighs about 2000 g (4 lb, 6.5 oz), with a C–H length of about 38 to 43 cm (15 to 17 in.), by 32 weeks of age. The CNS has matured enough to direct rhythmic breathing movements and partially control body temperature; however, the lungs are not yet fully mature. Bones are fully developed but soft and flexible. The fetus begins storing iron, calcium, and phosphorus. In males the testicles may be located in the scrotal sac but are often still high in the inguinal canals.

Thirty-Five to Thirty-Six Weeks

The fetus begins to get plump, and less wrinkled skin covers the deposits of subcutaneous fat. Lanugo begins to disappear, and the nails reach the edge of the fingertips. By 35 weeks of age the fetus has a firm grasp and exhibits spontaneous orientation to light. By 36 weeks of age the weight is usually 2500 to 2750 g (5 lb, 12 oz to 6 lb, 11.5 oz), and the C–H length of the fetus is about 42 to 48 cm (16 to 19 in.). An infant born at this time has a good chance of surviving but may require special care, especially if there is intrauterine growth restriction.

Thirty-Eight to Forty Weeks

The fetus is considered full term at 38 weeks and up to 40 weeks after conception. The C–H length varies from 48 to 52 cm (19 to 21 in.), with males usually longer than females. Males also usually weigh more than females. The weight at term is about 3000 to 3600 g (6 lb, 10 oz to 7 lb, 15 oz) and varies in different ethnic groups. The skin is pink and has a smooth, polished look. The only lanugo left is on the upper arms and shoulders. The hair on the head is no longer woolly but is coarse and about 1 in. long. Vernix caseosa is present, with heavier deposits remaining in the creases and folds of the skin. The body and extremities are plump, with good skin turgor, and the fingernails extend beyond the fingertips. The chest is prominent but still a little smaller than the head, and mammary glands protrude in both sexes. In males, the testes are in the scrotum or palpable in the inguinal canals.

As the fetus enlarges, amniotic fluid diminishes to about 500 mL or less, and the fetal body mass fills the uterine cavity. The fetus assumes what is called its *position of comfort*, or lie. The head is generally pointed downward, following the shape of the uterus (and possibly because the head is heavier than the feet). The extremities, and often the head, are well flexed. After 5 months, patterns in feeding, sleeping, and activity become established, so at term the fetus has its own body rhythms and individual style of response. See Key Facts to Remember: Fetal Development: What Parents Want to Know for important developmental milestones. For a detailed discussion of each body system's transition to and functioning in the newborn see Chapter 24 ∞.

Factors Influencing Embryonic and Fetal Development

Factors that may affect embryonic development include the quality of the sperm or ovum from which the zygote was formed, the genetic code established at fertilization, and the adequacy of the intrauterine environment. If the environment is unsuitable before cellular differentiation occurs, all the cells of the zygote are affected. The cells may die, which causes spontaneous abortion, or growth may be slowed, depending on the severity of the situation. When differentiation is complete and the fetal membranes have formed, an injurious agent has the greatest effect on those cells undergoing the most rapid growth. Thus the time of injury is critical in the development of anomalies.

Because organs are formed primarily during embryonic development, the growing organism is considered

KEY FACTS TO REMEMBER

Fetal Development: What Parents Want to Know

4 weeks:	The fetal heart begins to beat.
8 weeks:	All body organs are formed.
8 to 12 weeks:	Fetal heart rate can be heard by ultrasound Doppler device.
16 weeks:	Baby's sex can be seen.
	Although thin, the fetus looks like a baby.
20 weeks:	Heartbeat can be heard with fetoscope.
	Mother feels movement (quickening).
	Baby develops a regular schedule of sleeping, sucking, and kicking.
	Hands can grasp.
	Baby assumes a favorite position in utero.
	Vernix (lanolinlike covering) protects the body, and lanugo (fine hair) keeps oil on skin.
	Head hair, eyebrows, and eyelashes present.
24 weeks:	Weighs 780 g (1 lb, 10 oz).
	Activity is increasing.
	Fetal respiratory movements begin.
28 weeks:	Eyes open and close.
	Baby can breathe at this time.
	Surfactant needed for breathing at birth is formed.
	Baby is two-thirds its final length.
32 weeks:	Baby has fingernails and toenails.
	Subcutaneous fat is being laid down.
	Baby appears less red and wrinkled.
38+ weeks:	Baby fills total uterus.
	Baby gets antibodies from mother.

most vulnerable to hazardous agents during the first months of pregnancy. Any agent (e.g., drug, virus, or radiation) that can cause development of abnormal structures in an embryo is called a **teratogen**. It is important to remember that the effects of teratogens depend on the (1) maternal and fetal genotype, (2) stage of development when exposure occurs, and (3) dose and duration of exposure of the agent. Chapter 9 ∞ discusses the effects of specific teratogenic agents on the developing fetus.

Adequacy of the maternal environment is also important during the periods of rapid embryonic and fetal development. Maternal nutrition can affect brain and neural tube development. The period of maximum brain growth and myelination begins with the fifth lunar month before birth and continues during the first 6 months after birth, when there is a twofold increase in myelination (Volpe, 2008). Amino acids, glucose, and fatty acids are considered to be the primary dietary factors in brain growth. A subtle type of damage that affects the associative capacity of the brain, possibly leading to learning dis-

CRITICAL THINKING

Melodie Chong, in her third week of pregnancy, develops a fever of 104°F (40°C) but refuses to take any medication because she is afraid that drugs will harm her baby. Is she correct?

See Appendix F ∞ for possible responses.

abilities, may be caused by nutritional deficiency at this stage. Vitamins and folic acid supplements taken before conception can reduce the incidence of neural tube defects (Volpe, 2008). Maternal nutrition may also predispose offspring to the development of adult coronary heart disease, hypertension, and diabetes in babies who were small or disproportionate at birth. Maternal nutrition is discussed in depth in Chapter 12 ∞.

Another prenatal influence on the intrauterine environment is maternal hyperthermia associated with sauna or hot tub use. Studies of the effects of maternal hyperthermia during the first trimester have raised concern about possible CNS defects and failure of neural tube closure (Table 4–3). Maternal substance abuse also affects the intrauterine environment and is discussed in Chapters 15 and 28 ∞.

TABLE 4–3	Developmental Vulnerability Timetable
Weeks Since Conception	**Potential Teratogen-Induced Malformation**
3	Ectromelia (congenital absence of one or more limbs)
	Ectopia cordis (heart lies outside thoracic cavity)
4	Omphalocele (herniation of abdominal viscera into the umbilical cord)
	Tracheoesophageal fistula (abnormal connection between trachea and esophagus) (4 to 5 weeks)
	Hemivertebra (4 to 5* weeks)
5	Nuclear cataract
	Microphthalmia (abnormally small eyeballs) (5 to 6* weeks)
	Facial clefts
	Carpal or pedal ablation (5 to 6* weeks)
6	Gross septal or aortic abnormalities
	Cleft lip, agnathia (absence of the lower jaw)
7	Interventricular septal defects
	Pulmonary stenosis
	Cleft palate, micrognathia (smallness of the jaw)
	Epicanthus
	Brachycephalism (shortness of the head) (7 to 8* weeks)
	Mixed sexual characteristics
8	Persistent ostium primum (persistent opening in atrial septum)
	Digital stunting (shortening of fingers and toes)

*May occur in several time periods after conception.

Source: Modified from Danforth, D. N., & Scott, J. R. (1986). *Obstetrics and gynecology* (5th ed., p. 319). Philadelphia: Lippincott.

- Humans have 46 chromosomes, which are divided into 23 pairs—22 pairs of autosomes and 1 pair of sex chromosomes.
- Mitosis is the process by which additional somatic (body) cells are formed. It provides growth and development of the organisms and replacement of body cells.
- Meiosis is the process by which gametes (ova and sperm) are formed. It occurs during gametogenesis (oogenesis and spermatogenesis) and consists of two successive cell divisions (reduction division), which produce a gamete with 23 chromosomes (22 autosomal chromosomes and 1 sex chromosome), the haploid number of chromosomes.
- Gametes must have a haploid number of chromosomes (23) so that when the female gamete (ovum) and the male gamete (spermatozoon) unite (fertilization) to form the zygote, the normal human diploid number of chromosomes (46) is reestablished.
- An ovum is considered fertile for about 12 to 24 hours after ovulation, and the sperm is capable of fertilizing the ovum for only about 24 hours after it is deposited in the female reproductive tract.
- Fertilization usually takes place in the ampulla (outer third) of the fallopian tube. Both capacitation and acrosomal reaction must occur for the sperm to fertilize the ovum. Capacitation is the removal of the plasma membrane, which exposes the acrosomal covering of the sperm head. Acrosomal reaction is the deposit of hyaluronidase in the corona radiata, which allows the sperm head to penetrate the ovum.
- Sex chromosomes are referred to as X and Y. Females have two X chromosomes, and males have an X and a Y chromosome. Y chromosomes are carried only by the sperm. To produce a female child, both the mother and the father contribute an X chromosome. To produce a male child, the mother contributes an X chromosome and the father contributes a Y chromosome.
- Intrauterine development first proceeds via cellular multiplication in which the zygote undergoes rapid mitotic division called cleavage. As a result of cleavage, the zygote divides and multiplies into cell groupings called blastomeres, which are held together by the zona pellucida. The blastomeres eventually become a solid ball of cells called the morula. When a cavity forms in the morula cell mass, the inner solid cell mass is called the blastocyst.
- Implantation usually occurs in the upper part of the posterior uterine wall when the blastocyst burrows into the uterine lining.
- After implantation, the endometrium is called the decidua. Decidua capsularis is the portion that covers the blastocyst. Decidua basalis is the portion that is directly under the blastocyst. Decidua vera is the portion that lines the rest of the uterine cavity.
- Primary germ layers will give rise to all tissues, organs, and organ systems. The three primary germ cell layers are ectoderm, endoderm, and mesoderm.

- Embryonic membranes are called the amnion and the chorion. The amnion is formed from the ectoderm and is a thin protective membrane that contains the amniotic fluid and the embryo. The chorion is a thick membrane that develops from the trophoblast and encloses the amnion, embryo, and yolk sac.
- Amniotic fluid cushions the fetus against mechanical injury, controls the embryo's temperature, allows symmetrical external growth, prevents adherence to the amnion, and permits freedom of movement.
- The umbilical cord contains two umbilical arteries, which carry deoxygenated blood from the fetus to the placenta, and one umbilical vein, which carries oxygenated blood from the placenta to the fetus. The umbilical cord normally has a central insertion into the placenta. Wharton's jelly, a specialized connective tissue, helps prevent compression of the umbilical cord in utero.
- Twins are either monozygotic (identical) or dizygotic (fraternal). Dizygotic twins arise from two separate ova fertilized by two separate spermatozoa. Monozygotic twins develop from a single ovum fertilized by a single spermatozoon.
- The placenta develops from the chorionic villi and decidua basalis and has two parts: The maternal portion, consisting of the decidua basalis, is red and fresh looking; the fetal portion, consisting of chorionic villi, is covered by the amnion and appears shiny and gray. The placenta is made up of 15 to 20 segments called cotyledons.
- The placenta serves endocrine (production of hPL, hCG, estrogen, and progesterone), metabolic, and immunologic functions. It acts as the fetus's respiratory organ, is an organ of excretion, and aids in the exchange of nutrients.
- Fetal circulation is a specially designed circulatory system that provides for oxygenation of the fetus while bypassing the fetal lungs.
- Stages of fetal development include the preembryonic stage (the first 14 days of human development starting at the time of fertilization), the embryonic stage (from day 15 after fertilization, or the beginning of the third week, until approximately 8 weeks), and the fetal stage (from 8 weeks until birth, at approximately 38+ weeks after the last normal menstrual period).
- Significant events that occur during the embryonic stage include the fetal heart beginning to beat at 4 weeks and the establishment of fetal circulation at 6 weeks.
- The fetal stage is devoted to refining structures and perfecting function. Significant developments during the fetal stage are discussed in Key Facts to Remember: Fetal Development: What Parents Want to Know.
- The embryo is particularly vulnerable to teratogenesis during the first 8 weeks of cell differentiation and organ system development.

CHAPTER REFERENCES

Blackburn, S. T. (2007). *Maternal, fetal, & neonatal physiology: A clinical perspective* (3rd ed.). St. Louis: Saunders.

Gilbert, W. M. (2007). Amniotic fluid disorders. In S. G. Gabbe, J. R. Niebyl, & J. L. Simpson (Eds.), *Obstetrics: Normal and problem pregnancies.* (5th ed., pp. 834–845). Philadelphia: Churchill Livingstone Elsevier

Knuppel, R. A. (2007). Maternal–placental–fetal unit: Fetal & early neonatal physiology. In A. H. Decherney, L. Nathan, T. M Goodwin, & N. Laufer (Eds.), *Current diagnosis and treatment: Obstetrics & gynecology* (10th ed.). Boston: McGraw-Hill.

Moore, K. L., & Persaud, T. V. N. (2008). *The developing human: Clinical oriented embryology* (8th ed.). Philadelphia: Saunders.

Sadler, T. W. (2006). *Langman's medical embryology* (10th ed.). Philadelphia: Lippincott Williams & Wilkins.

Volpe, J. J. (2008). *Neurology of the newborn* (5th ed.). Philadelphia: Saunders.

PART TWO

Women's Health: The Reproductive Years

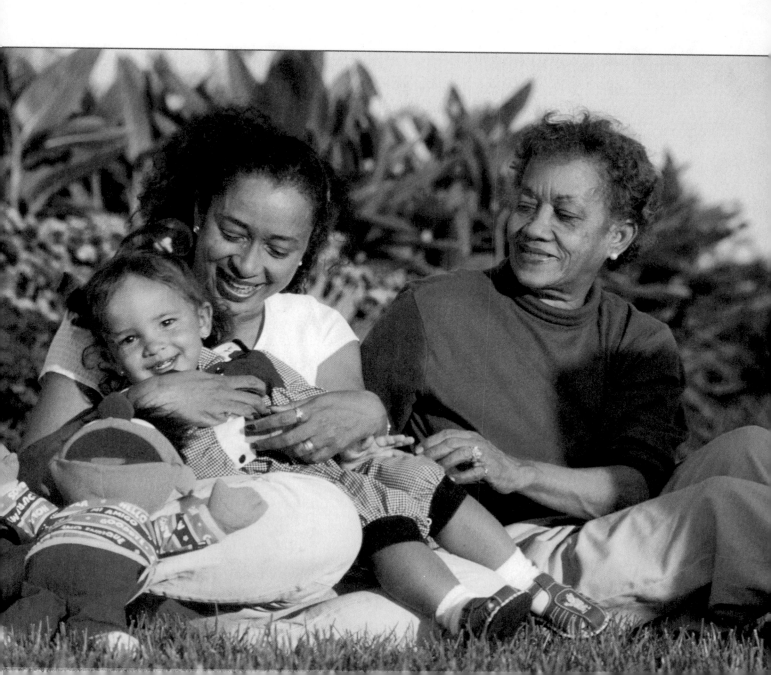

CHAPTER 5

Health Promotion for Women

I have started caring for the teenage daughters of many of my longtime clients. Making each teen's first pelvic exam a positive experience has become something of a mission for me. Yesterday I completed a young woman's first GYN exam and as I finished she said, "That was easy. Why do women make such a fuss about a pelvic?" I wanted to jump up and shout, "Yes!" Attitudes are changed one person at a time.

—A Women's Health Nurse Practitioner

LEARNING OUTCOMES

5-1. Identify appropriate nursing care based on the results of the client's sexual history.

5-2. Describe accurate information to be provided to girls and women so that they can implement effective self-care measures for dealing with menstruation.

5-3. Discriminate between the signs, symptoms, and nursing management of women with dysmenorrhea and premenstrual syndrome.

5-4. Compare the advantages, disadvantages, and effectiveness of the various methods of contraception available today.

5-5. Delineate basic gynecologic screening procedures indicated for well women.

5-6. Explain the physical and psychologic aspects and clinical treatment options of menopause when caring for menopausal women.

5-7. Examine the nurse's role in screening and caring for women who have experienced domestic violence or rape.

KEY TERMS

A woman's healthcare needs change throughout her life-time. As a young girl she needs health teaching about menstruation, sexuality, and personal responsibility. As a teen she needs information about reproductive choices and safe sexual activity. During this time she should also be introduced to the importance of healthcare practices such as breast self-examination and regular Pap smears. The mature woman may need to be reminded of these self-care issues and prepared for physical changes that accompany childbirth and aging. By educating women about their bodies, their healthcare choices, and their right to be knowledgeable consumers, nurses can help women assume responsibility for the health care they receive.

This chapter provides information about selected aspects of women's health care with an emphasis on conditions typically addressed in a community-based setting.

Community-Based Nursing Care

Women's health refers to a holistic view of women and their health-related needs within the context of their everyday lives. It is based on the awareness that a woman's physical, mental, and spiritual status are interdependent and affect her state of health or illness. The woman's view of her situation, her assessment of her needs, her values, and her beliefs are valid and important factors to be incorporated into any healthcare intervention.

Nurses can work with women to provide health teaching and information about self-care practices in schools, during routine examinations in a clinic or office, at senior centers, at meetings of volunteer organizations, through classes offered by local agencies or schools, or in the home. This community-based focus is the key to providing effective nursing care to women of all ages.

In reality, the vast majority of women's health care is provided outside of acute care settings. Nurses oriented to community-based care are especially effective in recognizing the autonomy of each individual and in dealing with clients holistically. This holistic approach is important in addressing not only physical problems but also major health issues such as violence against women, which may go undetected unless care providers are alert for signs of it.

The Nurse's Role in Addressing Issues of Sexuality

Because sexuality and its reproductive implications are such an intrinsic and emotion-laden part of life, people have many concerns, problems, and questions about sex roles, behaviors, education, inhibitions, morality, and related areas such as family planning. Health factors are another consideration. The increase in the incidence of sexually transmitted infections, especially human immunodeficiency virus/acquired immunodeficiency syndrome (HIV/AIDS) and genital herpes, has caused many people to modify their sexual practices and activities. Women frequently ask questions or voice concerns about these issues to the nurse in a clinic or ambulatory setting. Thus the nurse may need to assume the role of counselor on sexual and reproductive matters.

Nurses who assume this role must be secure about their own sexuality. They must also recognize their own feelings, values, and attitudes about sexuality so they can be more sensitive and objective when they encounter the values and beliefs of others. Nurses need to have accurate, up-to-date information about topics related to sexuality, sexual practices, and common gynecologic problems. They also need to know about the structures and functions of the female and male reproductive systems. In addition, when a woman is accompanied by her partner, it is important that the nurse be sensitive to the dynamics of the relationship between the partners.

Continuing education for the practicing nurse and appropriate courses in undergraduate and graduate nursing education programs can help nurses achieve the requisite knowledge about aspects of sexuality. These courses can help nurses learn about sexual values, attitudes, alternative lifestyles, cultural factors, and misconceptions and myths about sex and reproduction.

Taking a Sexual History

Nurses are often responsible for taking a woman's initial history, including her gynecologic and sexual history. To be effective, the nurse must have good communication skills and should conduct the interview in a quiet, private place free of distractions.

Opening the discussion with a brief explanation of the purpose of such questions is often helpful. For example, the nurse might say, "As your nurse I'm interested in all aspects of your well-being. Often women have concerns or questions about sexual matters, especially as their life situations change. I will be asking you some questions about your sexual history as part of your general health history." This explanation will help women understand the nature of this part of the history and allow for more open, honest answers.

It may be helpful to use direct eye contact as much as possible unless the nurse knows it is culturally unacceptable to the woman. The nurse should do little, if any, writing during the interview, especially if the woman seems ill at ease or is discussing very personal issues. Open-ended questions are often useful in eliciting information. For example, "What, if anything, would you change about your sex life?" will elicit more information than "Are you happy with your sex life now?" The nurse needs to clarify terminology and proceed from easier topics to those that are more difficult to discuss. Throughout the interview the nurse should be alert to body language and nonverbal cues. It is important that the nurse not assume that the client is heterosexual. Some women are open about lesbian relationships; others are more reserved until they develop a sense of trust in their caregivers.

After completing the sexual history, the nurse assesses the information obtained. If there is a problem that requires further medical tests and assessments, the nurse refers the woman to a nurse practitioner, certified nurse–midwife, physician, or counselor as necessary. In many instances the nurse alone will be able to develop a nursing diagnosis and then plan and implement therapy. For example, if the nurse determines that a woman who is interested in conceiving a child does not have a clear understanding of when she ovulates, the nurse may formulate the following nursing diagnosis: Health-Seeking Behaviors: Information About Ovulation related to an expressed desire to time intercourse to enhance the possibility of conception. The nurse can then evaluate the woman's knowledge through discussion and review and work with the woman to provide necessary information. The nurse might also suggest that the woman keep a menstrual calendar and monitor basal body temperatures to identify the time of ovulation.

The nurse must be realistic in making assessments and planning interventions. It requires insight and skill to recognize when a woman's problem requires interventions that are beyond a nurse's preparation and ability. In such situations, the nurse must make appropriate referrals.

Menstruation

Girls today begin to learn about puberty and menstruation at a surprisingly young age. Unfortunately the source of their "education" is sometimes their peers or the media;

thus the information is often incomplete, inaccurate, and sensationalized. Nurses who work with young girls and adolescents recognize this and are working hard to provide accurate health teaching and to correct misinformation about menarche (the onset of menses) and the menstrual cycle.

Cultural, religious, and personal attitudes about menstruation are part of the menstrual experience and often reflect negative attitudes toward women. In the past, many misconceptions surrounded menstruation. Women were often isolated or restricted to the company of other women during their monthly flow because they were considered "unclean." Currently in the Western world there are few restrictions associated with menstruation, although some women remain uncomfortable about discussing it. Sexual intercourse during menses is a common practice and is not generally contraindicated. For most couples, the decision is one of personal preference. (The physiology of menstruation is discussed in Chapter 3 ∞.)

Counseling the Premenstrual Girl About Menarche

Many young women find it embarrassing or stressful to discuss the menstrual experience, both because of the many taboos associated with the subject and because of their immaturity. However, the most critical factor in successful adaptation to menarche is the adolescent's level of preparedness. Information should be given to premenstrual girls over time rather than all at once. This allows them to absorb information and develop questions.

The following basic information is helpful for young clients.

- *Cycle length.* Cycle length is determined from the first day of one menses to the first day of the next menses. Initially, cycle length may be irregular. Once established, a female's cycle length is about 29 days, but the normal length may vary from 21 to 35 days. Cycle length often varies by a day or two from one cycle to the next, although greater normal variations may also occur.
- *Amount of flow.* The average flow is approximately 25 to 60 mL per period. Usually women characterize the amount of flow in terms of the number of pads or tampons used. Flow is often heavier at first and lighter toward the end of the period.
- *Length of menses.* Menses usually lasts from 2 to 8 days, although this may vary.

The nurse should make it clear that variations in age at menarche, length of cycle, and duration of menses are normal because girls may worry if their experience varies from that of their peers. It also is helpful to acknowledge the negative aspects of menstruation (messiness and embarrassment) while stressing its positive role as a symbol of maturity and womanhood.

Educational Topics

The nurse's primary role is to provide accurate information and assist in clarifying misconceptions, so that girls will develop positive self-images and progress smoothly through this phase of maturation.

Pads and Tampons

Since early times women have made pads and tampons from cloth or rags, which required washing but were reusable. Commercial tampons were introduced in the 1930s.

Today adhesive-stripped minipads and maxipads and flushable tampons are readily available. However, the deodorants and increased absorbency that manufacturers have added to both sanitary napkins and tampons may prove harmful. The chemical used to deodorize can create irritation of the vulva and inner aspects of the vagina. Excessive or inappropriate use of tampons can produce dryness or even small sores or ulcers in the vagina.

The use of super-absorbent tampons has been linked to the development of toxic shock syndrome (TSS) (see Chapter 6 ∞). Women may prevent problems by using tampons with the minimum absorbency necessary to control menstrual flow, changing them every 3 to 6 hours, and avoiding using them for vaginal discharge or very light bleeding. Because *Staphylococcus aureus*, the causative organism of TSS, is frequently found on the hands, a woman should wash her hands before inserting a fresh tampon and should avoid touching the tip of the tampon when unwrapping it or before insertion.

In the absence of a heavy menstrual flow, tampons absorb moisture, leaving the vaginal walls dry and subject to injury. The absorbency of regular tampons varies. If the tampon is hard to pull out or shreds when removed, or if the vagina becomes dry, the tampon is probably too absorbent. If a woman is worried about accidental spotting, she can check the diagrams on the packages of regular tampons; those that expand in width are better able to prevent leakage without being too absorbent.

A woman may want to use tampons only during the day and switch to napkins at night to avoid vaginal irritation. If a woman experiences vaginal irritation, itching, or soreness or notices an unusual odor while using tampons, she should stop using them and be evaluated for infection. The choice of sanitary protection—whether napkins or tampons—must meet the individual's needs and feel comfortable. Cultural factors may play a role in this decision (see Cultural Perspectives). Young women should be taught to track their periods and to carry feminine hygiene products when their menses is due so that they are prepared for its onset.

CULTURAL PERSPECTIVES

In certain religious or cultural groups unmarried women are expected to avoid the use of tampons. This is more common among those groups that highly value a girl's virginity, for fear of breaking the hymen. Thus it is wise to ask the girl (or her mother if the girl is uncertain) about the issue.

TEACHING TIP

If you work with teens and preteens, keep a variety of pads and tampons on hand so that you can help these young girls become familiar with the options available for dealing with menstruation. You can also put colored water in a small glass and insert a tampon to show a girl how much fluid a tampon absorbs. Girls often think that they lose far more blood with a period than they actually do.

Vaginal Spray, Douching, and Cleansing

Vaginal sprays are unnecessary and can cause infections, itching, burning, rashes, and other problems. Generally healthcare providers do not recommend them. If a woman chooses to use a spray, she needs to know that these sprays are for external use only, should be used infrequently, and should never be applied to irritated or itching skin.

Douching as a hygiene practice is unnecessary because the vagina cleanses itself. Douching washes away the natural mucus and upsets the vaginal ecology, which can make the vagina more susceptible to infection. Douching with perfumed douches can cause allergic reactions. Propelling water up the vagina may force bacteria and germs from the vagina into the uterus. Women should avoid douching during menstruation because the cervix is dilated to permit the downward flow of menstrual fluids from the uterine lining. Douching is also contraindicated during pregnancy.

The mucous secretions that continually bathe the vagina are odorless while they are in the vagina; odor develops only when they mingle with perspiration and are exposed to the air. Keeping one's skin clean and free of bacteria with plain soap and water is the most effective method of controlling odor. A soapy finger or soft washcloth should be used to wash gently between the vulvar folds. Bathing is as important during menses as at any other time. A long, leisurely soak in a warm tub promotes menstrual blood flow and relieves cramps by relaxing the muscles.

Keeping the vulva fresh throughout the day means keeping it dry and clean. A woman can ensure adequate ventilation by wearing cotton panties and clothes loose enough to permit the vaginal area to breathe. After using the toilet, a woman should always wipe herself from front to back and, if necessary, follow up with a moistened paper towel or premoistened wipe. If an unusual odor persists despite these efforts, a visit to one's healthcare provider is indicated. Certain conditions such as vaginitis produce a foul-smelling discharge.

Associated Menstrual Conditions

A variety of menstrual irregularities have been identified. An abnormally short duration of menstrual flow is termed *hypomenorrhea;* an abnormally long one is called *hypermenorrhea.* Excessive, profuse flow is called *menorrhagia,* and bleeding between periods is known as *metrorrhagia.* Infrequent and too frequent menses are termed *oligomenorrhea* and *polymenorrhea,* respectively. An *anovulatory cycle* is one in which ovulation does not occur. Such irregularities should be investigated to rule out any disease process.

Amenorrhea

Primary **amenorrhea** necessitates a thorough assessment of the young woman to determine its cause. Possible causes include genetic disorders such as Turner syndrome; congenital obstructions; congenital absence of the uterus, ovaries, or vagina; testicular feminization (external genitals appear female but uterus and ovaries are absent and testes are present); chronic anovulation related to polycystic ovarian syndrome, or thyroid or adrenal disorders; or absence or imbalance of hormones. Success of treatment depends on the causative factors. Many causes are not correctable.

Secondary amenorrhea is caused most frequently by pregnancy. Additional causes include lactation, hormonal imbalances, poor nutrition (anorexia nervosa, obesity, and fad dieting), ovarian lesions, strenuous exercise (associated with long-distance runners, dancers, and other athletes with low body fat ratios), debilitating systemic diseases, stress of high intensity and/or long duration, stressful life events, a change in season or climate, use of oral contraceptives, use of the phenothiazine and chlorpromazine group of tranquilizers, exposure to radiation or chemotherapy, viral infection, and syndromes such as Cushing and Sheehan.

Treatment is dictated by the causative factors. The nurse can explain that once the underlying condition has been corrected—for example, when sufficient body weight is gained—menses will resume. Female athletes and women who participate in strenuous exercise routines may be advised to increase their caloric intake or reduce their exercise levels for a month or two to see whether a normal cycle ensues. If it does not, medical referral is indicated.

Dysmenorrhea

Dysmenorrhea, or painful menstruation, occurs at, or a day before, the onset of menstruation and disappears by the end of menses. Dysmenorrhea is classified as primary or secondary. Primary dysmenorrhea is defined as cramps without underlying disease. Prostaglandins E_2 and F_{2a}, which are produced by the uterus in higher concentrations during menses, are the primary cause. They increase uterine contractility and decrease uterine artery blood flow, causing ischemia. The end result is the painful sensation of cramps. Dysmenorrhea typically disappears after a first pregnancy and does not occur if cycles are anovulatory.

Treatment of primary dysmenorrhea includes oral contraceptives (which inhibit ovulation); nonsteroidal anti-inflammatory drugs (NSAIDs) such as ibuprofen, aspirin, and naproxen, which act as prostaglandin inhibitors; and self-care measures such as regular exercise, rest, application of heat, and good nutrition. Some nutritionists suggest that vitamins B and E help relieve the discomforts associated with menstruation. Vitamin B_6 may help relieve the premenstrual bloating and irritability some women experience. Vitamin E, a mild prostaglandin inhibitor, may help decrease menstrual discomfort. Avoiding salt can decrease discomfort from fluid retention.

Biofeedback has been used with some success. Hysterectomy may be the treatment of choice if there are anatomic disorders and childbearing is not desired.

Secondary dysmenorrhea is associated with pathology of the reproductive tract and usually appears after menstruation has been established. Conditions that most frequently cause secondary dysmenorrhea include endometriosis, residual pelvic inflammatory disease (PID), cervical stenosis, uterine fibroids, ovarian cysts, benign or malignant tumors of the pelvis or abdomen, and the presence of an intrauterine device. Because primary and secondary dysmenorrhea may coexist, accurate differential diagnosis is essential for appropriate treatment.

Premenstrual Syndrome

Premenstrual syndrome (PMS) refers to a symptom complex associated with the luteal phase of the menstrual cycle (2 weeks before the onset of menses). The symptoms must, by definition, occur between ovulation and the onset of menses. They repeat at the same stage of each menstrual cycle and include some or all of the following:

- *Psychologic:* irritability, lethargy, depression, low morale, anxiety, sleep disorders, crying spells, and hostility
- *Neurologic:* classic migraine, vertigo, and syncope
- *Respiratory:* rhinitis, hoarseness, and occasionally asthma
- *Gastrointestinal:* nausea, vomiting, constipation, abdominal bloating, and craving for sweets
- *Urinary:* retention and oliguria
- *Dermatologic:* acne
- *Mammary:* swelling and tenderness

Most women experience only some of these symptoms. The symptoms usually are most pronounced 2 or 3 days before the onset of menstruation and subside as menstrual flow begins, with or without treatment.

Premenstrual dysphoric disorder (PMDD) is a diagnosis that may be applied to a small subgroup of women with PMS whose symptoms are primarily mood related and severe. Women with PMDD must experience five or more symptoms in the given time frame, which are relieved with menstruation. PMDD markedly interferes with work, school, and relationships, and must not merely be worsened symptoms of another disorder such as major depressive disorder, panic disorder, or personality disorder (Shulman, 2005).

The exact cause of PMS is unknown, although a variety of theories have been put forth to explain it. These include, for example, hormone imbalance, nutritional deficiency, prostaglandin excess, and endorphin deficiency. Currently researchers speculate that PMS may be related to decreased serotonin levels (Shulman, 2005).

Nursing Care Management

The focus of management, at least initially, involves lifestyle changes and natural approaches. After assessment, counseling for PMS may include advising the woman to restrict her intake of foods containing methylxanthines such as chocolate, cola, and coffee; restrict her intake of alcohol, nicotine, red meat, and foods containing salt and sugar; increase her intake of complex carbohydrates and protein; and increase the frequency of meals. For women whose primary symptoms are psychologic, supplementation with B complex vitamins, especially B$_6$, may decrease anxiety and depression. Vitamin E supplements may help reduce breast tenderness. Supplementation with 1,200 mg calcium carbonate may help relieve certain physical and psychologic symptoms. Magnesium supplements may help reduce fluid retention and breast tenderness including negative mood, food cravings, water retention, and pain.

A program of aerobic exercise such as fast walking, jogging, and aerobic dancing is generally beneficial. In addition to vitamin supplements, pharmacologic treatments for PMS include diuretics and prostaglandin inhibitors.

Women with PMDD may benefit from selective serotonin reuptake inhibitors (SSRI) such as fluoxetine hydrochloride (Prozac), sertraline hydrochloride (Zoloft), and paroxeline CR (Paxil CR) taken during the entire cycle or intermittently (half the cycle) (Endicott, 2007). The FDA has also approved the use of an oral contraceptive called YAZ for PMDD. YAZ may be a good choice for women who choose an oral contraceptive as their method of contraception and who experience side effects from SSRIs or dislike the idea of taking them (Endicott, 2007).

An empathic relationship with a healthcare professional to whom the woman feels free to voice concerns is highly beneficial. The nurse can encourage the woman to keep a diary to help track activities, diet, exercise, stressful events, and symptoms associated with PMS. Self-care groups and self-help literature can help women feel they have control over their bodies. Some women elect to use complementary therapies such as homeopathic remedies or herbs. It is important that women using such alternatives seek advice from knowledgeable, experienced homeopaths or herbalists.

Contraception

The decision to use a method of contraception may be made individually by a woman (or, in the case of vasectomy, by a man) or jointly by a couple. The decision may be motivated by a desire to avoid pregnancy, to gain control over the number of children conceived, or to determine the spacing of future children. In choosing a specific method, consistency of use outweighs the absolute reliability of the given method.

Decisions about contraception should be made voluntarily, with full knowledge of advantages, disadvantages, effectiveness, side effects, contraindications, and long-term effects. Many outside factors influence this choice, including cultural practices, religious beliefs, attitudes and personal preferences, cost, effectiveness, misinformation, practicality of method, and self-esteem. Different methods of contraception may be appropriate at different times for couples.

MyNursingKit | Contraception Online

CULTURAL PERSPECTIVES

- Maternal morbidity and mortality remain a major health challenge in developing countries. In 2005 approximately 536,000 women died from pregnancy-related causes. Less than 1% of maternal deaths occur in developed countries (World Health Organization [WHO], 2007).
- Up to 100,000 maternal deaths per year could be avoided if contraception was available and used by women who did not desire children (WHO, 2005).
- In the developing world, 137 million women have an unmet need for contraception, and an additional 64 million have an unmet need for a modern contraceptive method. This is especially apparent in Sub-Saharan Africa where maternal mortality rates are very high (Sonfield, 2006).
- Most of the causes of maternal mortality are treatable or preventable with adequate health care including contraceptive services. Thus, maternal healthcare services must improve if maternal mortality and morbidity are to be reduced.

Fertility Awareness Methods

Fertility awareness-based methods (FAB), also known as *natural family planning*, are based on an understanding of the changes that occur throughout a woman's ovulatory cycle. FAB takes into account the lifespan of sperm (2 to 7 days) and the ovum (1 to 3 days) in the female reproductive tract. Maximum fertility for the woman occurs approximately 5 days before ovulation and decreases rapidly the day after (Speroff & Darney, 2005). All these methods require periods of abstinence and recording of certain events throughout the cycle; cooperation of the partners is important.

Fertility awareness methods are free, safe, and acceptable to many whose religious beliefs prohibit other methods. They provide an increased awareness of the body, involve no artificial substances or devices, encourage a couple to communicate about sexual activity and family planning, and are useful in helping a couple plan a pregnancy.

However, these methods require extensive initial counseling to be used effectively. They may interfere with sexual spontaneity; they require careful maintenance of records for several cycles before beginning to use them; they may be difficult or impossible for women with irregular cycles to use; and, although theoretically they should be very reliable, in practice they may not be as reliable in preventing pregnancy as other methods.

The *basal body temperature (BBT) method* to detect ovulation requires that a woman take her BBT every morning upon awakening (before any activity) and record the readings on a temperature graph. To do this, she uses a basal body temperature thermometer, which shows tenths of a degree rather than the two-tenths shown on standard thermometers. She may also use tympanic thermometry (an "ear thermometer"). After 3 to 4 months of recording temperatures, a woman with regular cycles should be able to predict when ovulation will occur. The method is based on the fact that the temperature sometimes drops just be-

fore ovulation and almost always rises and remains elevated for several days after. The temperature rise occurs in response to the increased progesterone levels that occur in the second half of the cycle. Figure 5–1 ■ shows a sample BBT chart. To avoid conception, the couple abstains from intercourse on the day of the temperature rise and for 3 days after. Because the temperature rise does not occur until after ovulation, a woman who had intercourse just before the rise is at risk of pregnancy. To decrease this risk, some couples abstain from intercourse for several days before the anticipated time of ovulation and then for 3 days after.

The *calendar rhythm method* is based on the assumptions that ovulation tends to occur about 14 days before the start of the next menstrual period, sperm are viable for up to 7 days, and the ovum is viable for up to 3 days. To use this method, the woman must record her menstrual cycles for 6 months to identify the shortest and longest cycles. The first day of menstruation is the first day of the cycle. The fertile phase is calculated from 18 days before the end of the shortest recorded cycle through 11 days from the end of the longest recorded cycle. For example, if a woman's cycle lasts from 24 to 28 days, the fertile phase would be calculated as day 6 through day 17. Once this information is obtained, the woman can identify the fertile and infertile phases of her cycle. For effective use of this method, she must abstain from intercourse during the fertile phase. The calendar method is the least reliable of the fertility awareness methods and has largely been replaced by other, more scientific approaches.

The *ovulation method*, sometimes called the *cervical mucus method* or the *Billings method*, involves the assessment of cervical mucus changes that occur during the menstrual cycle. The amount and character of cervical mucus change because of the influence of estrogen and progesterone. At the time of ovulation the mucus (estrogen-dominant mucus) is clearer, more stretchable (a quality called *spinnbarkeit*), and more permeable to sperm. It also shows a characteristic fern pattern when placed on a glass slide and allowed to dry (see Figure 7–3 ∞). During the luteal phase, the cervical mu-

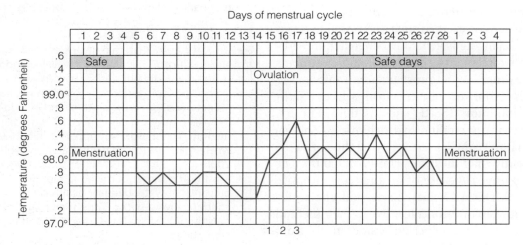

Figure 5–1 Sample basal body temperature chart.

cus is thick and sticky (progesterone-dominant mucus) and forms a network that traps sperm, making their passage more difficult.

To use the cervical mucus method, the woman abstains from intercourse for the first menstrual cycle. Each day she assesses her cervical mucus for amount, feeling of slipperiness or wetness, color, clearness, and spinnbarkeit, as she becomes familiar with varying characteristics.

The peak day of wetness and clear, stretchable mucus is assumed to be the time of ovulation. To use this method correctly, the woman should abstain from intercourse from the time she *first* notices that the mucus is becoming clear, more elastic, and slippery until 4 days *after* the last wet mucus (ovulation) day. Because this method evaluates the effects of hormonal changes, it can be used by women with irregular cycles.

The *symptothermal method* consists of various assessments made and recorded by the couple. These include information regarding cycle days, coitus, cervical mucus changes, and secondary signs such as increased libido, abdominal bloating, *mittelschmerz* (midcycle abdominal pain), and basal body temperature. Through the various assessments, the couple learns to recognize signs that indicate ovulation. This combined approach tends to improve the effectiveness of fertility awareness as a method of birth control.

Situational Contraceptives

Abstinence can be considered a method of contraception, and, partly because of changing values and the increased risk of infection with intercourse, it is gaining increased acceptance.

Coitus interruptus, or withdrawal, is one of the oldest and least reliable methods of contraception. This method requires that the male withdraw from the female's vagina when he feels that ejaculation is impending. He then ejaculates away from the external genitalia of the woman. Failure tends to occur for two reasons: (1) This method demands great self-control on the part of the man, who must withdraw just as he feels the urge for deeper penetration with impending orgasm, and (2) some preejaculatory fluid, which can contain sperm, may escape from the penis during the excitement phase before ejaculation. The fact that the quantity of sperm in this preejaculatory fluid is increased after a recent ejaculation is especially significant for couples who engage in repeated episodes of intercourse within a short period of time. Couples who use this method should be aware of postcoital contraceptive options in case the man fails to withdraw in time.

Douching after intercourse is an ineffective method of contraception and is not recommended. It may actually facilitate conception by pushing sperm farther up the birth canal.

Spermicides

The **spermicide** approved for use in the United States, nonoxynol-9 (N-9), is available as a cream, jelly, foam, vaginal film, and suppository. A spermicide is inserted into the vagina before intercourse. It destroys sperm by disrupting the cell membrane. A spermicide that effervesces in a moist environment offers more rapid protection, and coitus may take place immediately after it is inserted. A suppository may require up to 30 minutes to dissolve and will not offer protection until it has done so. The nurse instructs the woman to insert any of these spermicide preparations high in the vagina and maintain a supine position.

N-9 is minimally effective when used alone, but its effectiveness increases in conjunction with a diaphragm or condom. The major advantages of spermicides are their wide availability and low toxicity. Skin irritation and allergic reactions to spermicides are the primary disadvantages. In 2007 the Food and Drug Administration (FDA) issued a ruling requiring that a warning and label information be added for all over-the-counter vaginal contraceptives containing N-9. The ruling states that N-9 does not offer protection against infection from the human immunodeficiency virus, which causes HIV/AIDS, or against any other sexually transmitted infection. Moreover, N-9 may actually increase a woman's risk of HIV infection because it irritates vaginal tissue, making them more susceptible to invasion by organisms such as HIV (FDA, 2007).

Barrier Methods of Contraception

Barrier methods of contraception prevent the transport of sperm to the ovum, immobilize sperm, or are lethal against sperm.

Male and Female Condoms

The male **condom** offers a viable means of contraception when used consistently and properly (Figure 5–2 ■). Acceptance has been increasing as a growing number of men are assuming responsibility for regulation of fertility. The condom is applied to the erect penis, rolled from the tip to the end of the shaft, before vulvar or vaginal contact. A small space must be left at the end of the condom to allow for collection of the ejaculate, so that the condom will not break at the time of ejaculation. If the condom or vagina is dry, water-soluble lubricants such as K-Y jelly should be used to prevent irritation and possible condom breakage.

Care must be taken in removing the condom after intercourse. For optimal effectiveness, the man should withdraw his penis from the vagina while it is still erect and hold the condom rim to prevent spillage. If after ejaculation the penis becomes flaccid while still in the vagina, the male should hold on to the edge of the condom while

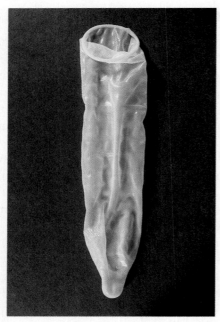

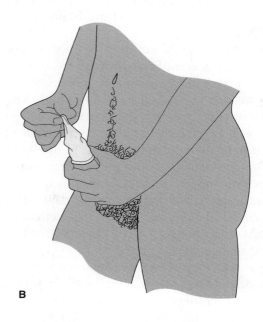

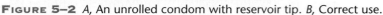

FIGURE 5–2 *A,* An unrolled condom with reservoir tip. *B,* Correct use.

withdrawing to avoid spilling the semen and to prevent the condom from slipping off.

The effectiveness of male condoms is largely determined by their use. The condom is small, disposable, and inexpensive; it has no side effects (if not allergic to latex), requires no medical examination or supervision, and offers visual evidence of effectiveness. Most condoms are made of latex, although polyurethane and silicone rubber condoms are available for individuals allergic to latex. All condoms except natural "skin" condoms, made from lamb's intestines, offer protection against both pregnancy and sexually transmitted infections (STIs). Breakage, displacement, perineal or vaginal irritation, and dulled sensation are possible disadvantages. Condoms should not be stored in hot conditions because heat accelerates their deterioration making them more susceptible to breaking. Thus, men should avoid placing them in their car glove box or in their wallets in a rear pant's pocket.

The male condom is becoming increasingly popular because of the protection it offers from infections. For women, sexually transmitted infection increases the risk of PID and resultant infertility. Many women are beginning to insist that their sexual partners use condoms, and many women carry condoms with them.

The *Reality female condom* (Figure 5–3 ■) is a thin polyurethane sheath with a flexible ring at each end. The

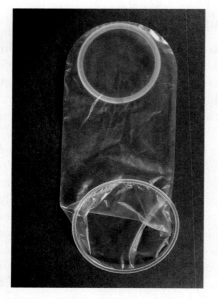

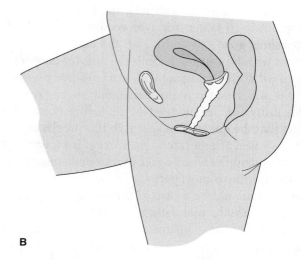

FIGURE 5–3 *A,* The female condom. *B,* When properly inserted, the outer ring should rest on the folds of skin around the vaginal opening, and the inner ring (closed end) should fit loosely against the cervix.

inner ring, at the closed end of the condom, serves as the means of insertion and fits over the cervix like a diaphragm. The second ring remains outside the vagina and covers a portion of the woman's perineum. It also covers the base of the man's penis during intercourse. Available over the counter and designed for one-time use, the condom may be inserted up to 8 hours before intercourse. The inner sheath is prelubricated but does not contain spermicide and is not designed to be used with a male condom. Because it also covers a portion of the vulva, it probably provides better protection than other contraceptive methods against some pathogens. High cost, noisiness during intercourse, and the cumbersome feel of the device make acceptability a problem for some couples.

Diaphragm and Cervical Cap

The **diaphragm** (Figure 5–4 ■) is used with spermicidal cream or jelly and offers a good level of protection from conception. The woman must be fitted with a diaphragm and instructed in its use by trained personnel. The di-

aphragm should be rechecked for correct size after each childbirth and whenever a woman has gained or lost 10 to 15 pounds or more.

The diaphragm must be inserted before intercourse, with approximately 1 teaspoonful (or 1.5 inches from the tube) of spermicidal jelly placed around its rim and in the cup. This chemical barrier supplements the mechanical barrier of the diaphragm. The diaphragm is inserted through the vagina and covers the cervix. The last step in insertion is to push the edge of the diaphragm under the symphysis pubis, which may result in a "popping" sensation. When fitted properly and correctly in place, the diaphragm should not cause discomfort to the woman or her partner. Correct placement of the diaphragm can be checked by touching the cervix with a fingertip through the cup. The cervix feels like a small, firm, rounded structure and has a consistency similar to that of the tip of the nose. The center of the diaphragm should be over the cervix. If more than 6 hours elapse between insertion of the diaphragm and intercourse, additional spermicidal cream should be used. It is necessary to leave the

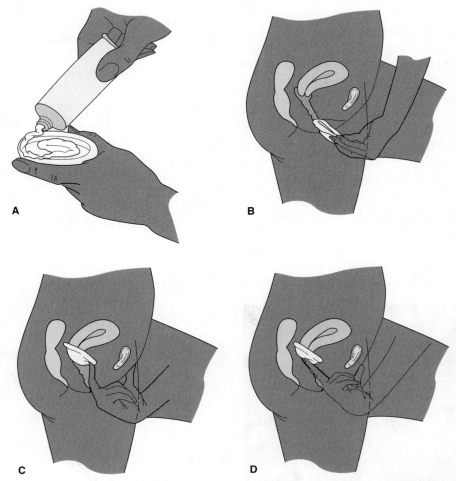

FIGURE 5–4 Inserting the diaphragm. *A*, Apply jelly to the rim and center of the diaphragm. *B*, Insert the diaphragm. *C*, Push the rim of the diaphragm under the pubic symphysis. *D*, Check placement of the diaphragm. The cervix should be felt through the diaphragm.

diaphragm in place for at least 6 hours after coitus. If intercourse is desired again within the 6 hours, another type of contraception must be used or additional spermicidal jelly placed in the vagina with an applicator, taking care not to disturb the placement of the diaphragm. The diaphragm should not remain in the vagina for more than 24 hours. Periodically the diaphragm should be held up to the light and inspected for tears or holes.

Some couples feel that the use of a diaphragm interferes with the spontaneity of intercourse. The nurse can suggest that the partner insert the diaphragm as part of foreplay. The woman can then easily verify the placement herself.

Diaphragms are an excellent contraceptive method for women who are lactating, who cannot or do not wish to use the pill (oral contraceptives), who are smokers over age 35, or who wish to avoid the increased risk of PID associated with intrauterine devices. A silicone diaphragm is available for women with a latex allergy.

Women who object to touching their genitals to insert the diaphragm, check its placement, and remove it may find this method unsatisfactory. Women who are very obese or who have short fingers may find the diaphragm difficult to insert. It is not recommended for women with a history of urinary tract infection (UTI), because pressure from the diaphragm on the urethra may interfere with complete bladder emptying and lead to recurrent UTIs. Women with a history of toxic shock syndrome should not use diaphragms or any of the barrier methods because they are left in place for prolonged periods. For the same reason, the diaphragm should not be used during a menstrual period or if a woman has abnormal vaginal discharge.

The Prentiff Cavity Rim **cervical cap** (Figure 5–5 ■) is a latex cup-shaped device, used with spermicidal cream or jelly, that fits snugly over the cervix and is held in place by suction. Effectiveness rates and method of insertion are similar to those for the diaphragm. The cap may be left in place for up to 48 hours, and repeated acts of intercourse do not require additional spermicide. Advantages, disadvantages, and contraindications are similar to those associated with the diaphragm. The cervical cap may be more

difficult to fit because of limited size options. It also tends to be more difficult for women to insert and remove. A newer form of cervical cap—the FemCap—is also available. It looks like a small sailor's cap and has a strap placed over the dome that allows easier removal.

A systematic research review indicates that the Prentiff cervical cap is comparable to the diaphragm in preventing pregnancy; however, the FemCap is not as effective as a diaphragm. Both forms of cap are medically safe to use (Gallo, Grimes, & Schulz, 2006).

Lea's shield is a reusable silicone vaginal barrier method that completely covers the cervix. It is similar to the cervical cap but contains a centrally located valve that permits the passage of cervical secretions and air. A spermicide should be used with it, and it should not be worn for more than 48 hours with a single application of spermicide. The device has been available over the counter in several European countries for over a decade because one size fits virtually all women. In the United States, a woman must see her practitioner to obtain one.

Vaginal Sponge

The *Today vaginal sponge*, available without a perscription, is a pillow-shaped, soft, absorbent synthetic sponge containing spermicide. It is made with a concave or cupped area on one side that fits over the cervix, and has a loop for easy removal. The sponge is moistened thoroughly with water before insertion to activate the spermicide, and then inserted into the vagina with the cupped side against the cervix (Figure 5–6 ■). It should be left in place for 6 hours following intercourse and may be worn for up to 24 hours, then removed and discarded.

The sponge has the following advantages: professional fitting is not required, it may be used for multiple acts of coitus for up to 24 hours, one size fits all, and it acts as both a barrier and a spermicide. Problems associated with the

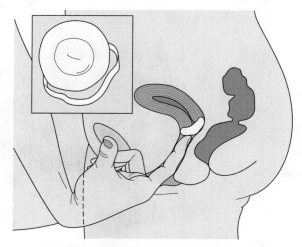

FIGURE 5–6 The contraceptive sponge is moistened well with water and inserted into the vagina with the concave portion positioned over the cervix.

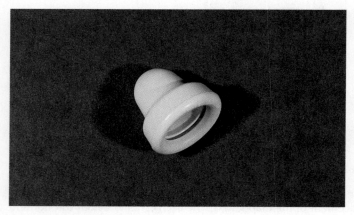

FIGURE 5–5 A cervical cap.

sponge include difficulty removing it and irritation or allergic reactions. Some women report a problem because the sponge absorbs vaginal secretions, contributing to vaginal dryness. For women without children the failure rate is comparable to that of the diaphragm and cervical cap. It is higher for women who have borne children, possibly because of changes in the shape of the cervix.

Intrauterine Devices

The **intrauterine device (IUD)** is a safe, effective method of reversible contraception that is designed to be inserted into the uterus by a qualified healthcare provider and left in place for an extended period, providing continuous contraceptive protection. Traditionally the IUD was believed to act by preventing the implantation of a fertilized ovum. Thus the IUD was considered an abortifacient (abortion-causing) method. This belief is not accurate. IUDs truly are contraceptives; they trigger a spermicidal type reaction in the body, thereby preventing fertilization. The IUD is also known to have local inflammatory effects on the endometrium.

Advantages of the IUD include high rate of effectiveness, continuous contraceptive protection, no coitus-related activity, and relative inexpensiveness over time. Possible adverse reactions to the IUD include discomfort to the wearer, increased bleeding during menses, increased risk of pelvic infection for about 3 weeks following insertion, perforation of the uterus during insertion, intermenstrual bleeding, dysmenorrhea, and expulsion of the device.

Two IUDs are currently available in the United States. The copper T380A (ParaGard) is nonhormonal, highly effective, and can be left in place for up to 10 years. The levonorgestrel-releasing intrauterine system (LNG-IUS) (Mirena) is a small, T-shaped frame with a reservoir that releases levonorgestrel gradually (Figure 5–7 ■). It is com-

parable in effectiveness to the Copper T, and may be left in place for up to 5 years. After 3 months of use of the LNG-IUS, bleeding and length of menstrual cycles are reduced, and some women experience amenorrhea, which they welcome once they are advised that the absence of menses is safe and not an indication of pregnancy.

Formerly the IUD was recommended only for women who have at least one child and were in a stable, mutually monogamous relationship, because these women have the lowest risk of developing a pelvic infection. At the request of the company that manufactures the Copper T380A, the FDA removed a "patient or partner with multiple sexual partners" as a contraindication for its use. This change can apply as well to the LNG-IUS (Ogburn & Espey, 2007). Research indicates that, contrary to common belief, the IUD is reliable and effective for women who have never been pregnant; it is effective against ectopic pregnancy because of their overall effectiveness in preventing any pregnancy. Moreover the copper IUD is a good choice for women who cannot use hormonal forms of contraception (Jacobstein, 2007).

The IUD is inserted into the uterus with its string or tail protruding through the cervix into the vagina. It may be inserted at any time during a woman's cycle, providing she is not pregnant, or during the 4- to 6-week postpartum check. The Copper IUD may be inserted up to 5 days after unprotected intercourse as a method of emergency contraception. After insertion, the clinician instructs the woman to check for the presence of the string once a week for the first month and then after each menses. She is told that she may have some cramping or bleeding intermittently for 2 to 6 weeks and that her first few menses may be irregular. Follow-up examination is suggested 4 to 8 weeks after insertion.

Women with IUDs should contact their healthcare providers if they are exposed to an STI or if they develop the following warning signs: late period, abnormal spotting or bleeding, pain with intercourse, abdominal pain, abnormal discharge, signs of infection (fever, chills, and malaise), or missing string. If the woman becomes pregnant with an IUD in place, the device should be removed as soon as possible to prevent infection.

Hormonal Contraceptives

Hormonal contraceptives are available in a variety of forms. They may be progestin-only hormones, most often using a synthetic form of progesterone called progestin, or a combination of estrogen and a progestin.

Combined Estrogen–Progestin Approaches

Combined hormonal approaches work by inhibiting the release of an ovum, by creating an atrophic endometrium, and by maintaining a thick cervical mucus that slows

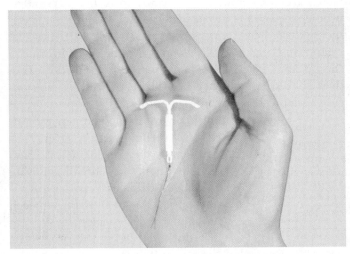

FIGURE 5–7 The Mirena Intrauterine Contraceptive, which releases levonorgestrel gradually, may be left in place for up to 5 years.
Source: Courtesy of Berlex, Inc.

sperm transport and inhibits the process that allows sperm to penetrate the ovum.

COMBINED ORAL CONTRACEPTIVES Combined oral contraceptives (COCs), also called *birth control pills*, are a combination of estrogen and progestin. COCs are safe, highly effective, and rapidly reversible. COCs are generally taken daily for 21 days, typically beginning on the Sunday after the first day of the menstrual cycle although the woman can also start on day 1 of her menstrual cycle. In most cases menses occurs 1 to 4 days after the last pill is taken. Seven days after taking her last pill, the woman restarts the pill. Thus the woman always begins the pill on the same day. Some companies offer a 28-day pack with seven "blank" pills so that the woman never stops taking a pill. The pill should be taken at approximately the same time each day—usually upon arising or before retiring in the evening.

Research suggests that traditional 21/7 approaches may need to be modified. With today's low-dose COCs, the 7 hormone-free days may result in failure to completely suppress ovarian function, resulting in the development of an ovarian follicle and possible ovulation (Sulak, 2008). Consequently there is growing interest in extended oral contraceptives. Seasonale and Seasonique are the first FDA-approved extended cycle COCs. They both are 91-day regimens in which a woman takes an active pill daily for 84 consecutive days followed by 7 days of inactive tablets during which the woman has a period. Thus a woman has only four periods a year. Extended use reduces the side effects of COCs such as bloating, headache, breast tenderness, and cramping (Abboud, 2006). Another COC, Lybrel, has been approved by the FDA for continuous 365-day use with no scheduled hormone-free periods.

Although they are highly effective when taken correctly, COCs may produce a variety of side effects, which may be either progesterone or estrogen related (Table 5–1). The use of low-dose (35 mcg or less estrogen) preparations has reduced many of the side effects. The newer 20 or 25 mcg pills have even fewer side effects but they may result in less contraceptive effectiveness and in weaker cycle control.

Absolute contraindications to the use of oral contraceptives include pregnancy, previous history of thrombophlebitis or thromboembolic disease, acute or chronic liver disease of cholestatic type with abnormal function, presence of estrogen-dependent carcinomas, undiagnosed uterine bleeding, heavy smoking, gallbladder disease, hypertension, diabetes, and hyperlipidemia. In addition, women with the following relative contraindications need to be monitored frequently: migraine headaches, epilepsy, depression, oligomenorrhea,

TABLE 5–1	Side Effects Associated with Oral Contraceptives
Estrogen Effects	**Progestin Effects**
Alterations in lipid metabolism	Acne, oily skin
Breast tenderness; engorgement; increased breast size	Breast tenderness; increased breast size
Cerebrovascular accident	Decreased libido
Changes in carbohydrate metabolism	Decreased high-density lipoprotein (HDL) cholesterol levels
Chloasma	
Fluid retention; cyclic weight gain	Depression
Headache	Fatigue
Hepatic adenomas	Hirsutism
Hypertension	Increased appetite; weight gain
Leukorrhea, cervical erosion, ectopia	Increased low-density lipoprotein (LDL) cholesterol levels
Nausea	Oligomenorrhea, amenorrhea
Nervousness, irritability	Pruritus
Telangiectasia	Sebaceous cysts
Thromboembolic complications—thrombophlebitis, pulmonary embolism	

and amenorrhea. Women who choose this method of contraception should be fully advised of its potential side effects.

COCs also have some important noncontraceptive benefits. Many women experience relief of uncomfortable menstrual symptoms. Cramps are lessened, flow is decreased, and cycle regularity is increased. Mittelschmerz is eliminated, and the incidence of functional ovarian cysts is decreased. There is also a substantial reduction in the incidence of ectopic pregnancy, ovarian cancer, endometrial cancer, iron deficiency anemia, and benign breast disease. COCs are considered a good solution to the physiologic problems some women experience during the perimenopause. Because of the increased risk of myocardial infarction (heart attack), women over age 35 who smoke should not take COCs. The woman using oral contraceptives should contact her healthcare provider if she becomes depressed, becomes jaundiced, develops a breast lump, or experiences any of the following warning signs: severe abdominal pain, severe chest pain or shortness of breath, severe headaches, dizziness, changes in vision (vision loss or blurring), speech problems, or severe leg pain.

Another COC is the progestin-only pill, also called the *minipill*. It is used primarily by nursing mothers because it does not interfere with breast milk production. It is also used by women who have a contraindication to the estrogen component of

---

EVIDENCE IN ACTION

Oral contraceptives increase the risk of premenopausal breast cancer, especially if used before a first full-term pregnancy.
(Meta-analysis) (Kahlenborn, Modugno, Potter, & Severs, 2006)

the combination preparation, such as history of thrombophlebitis, but are strongly motivated to use this form of contraception. The major problems with this preparation are amenorrhea or irregular spotting and bleeding patterns.

OTHER COMBINED HORMONAL METHODS

Hormones can now be administered transdermally using a *contraceptive skin patch* called Ortho Evra. Roughly the size of a silver dollar, but square, the woman applies the patch weekly for 3 weeks to one of four sites: her abdomen, buttocks, upper outer arm, or trunk (excluding the breasts). During the fourth week, no patch is worn and menses occurs. The patch is highly effective in women who weigh less than 198 pounds. The patch is as safe and reliable as COCs and has a better rate of compliance.

Because skin absorption of transdermal estrogen is 60% greater than oral absorption of a 35 mcg COC, questions have arisen as to whether this increases a woman's risk of serious side effects or complications. It has been noted that women using the patch still have about a 25% lower peak blood level of estrogen than women taking typical COCs (U.S. Food and Drug Administration, 2006). Preliminary research suggests that the incidence of stroke and acute MI is no higher in women using the patch than in women using 35 mcg COCs (Jick & Jick, 2007). Research is ongoing. In the meantime, this method is considered a safe birth control option.

NuvaRing vaginal contraceptive ring (manufactured by Orgonon), another form of low-dose, sustained release hormonal contraceptive, is a flexible soft ring that the woman inserts into her vagina (Figure 5–8 ■). The ring is left in place for 3 weeks and then removed for 1 week to allow for withdrawal bleeding. One size fits virtually all women. The ring is highly effective and has minimal side effects. The ring can be worn during intercourse and is comfortable for both the woman and her partner. Replacement rings should be kept in the refrigerator to maintain integrity.

Lunelle, an injectable combination of medroxyprogesterone acetate (MPA) and estradiol cypionate (E_2C), is now off the market in the United States and Canada but is available in many countries worldwide under the name Cyclofem. Administered every 28 to 30 days (not to exceed 33 days) intramuscularly, it is a highly effective contraceptive that has a side effect pattern similar to that of COCs.

Long-Acting Progestin Contraceptives

Norplant, a system consisting of six silastic capsules containing levonorgestrel (a progestin), which are implanted in a woman's arm, was the original **subdermal implant**. It is now off the market in the United States. Norplant II, which consists of a two-rod system that is effective for up to 5 years, was never introduced in the United States, although it is marketed elsewhere as Jadelle.

Implanon, a single-capsule implant also inserted under the skin of the arm, is effective for up to 3 years. It is impregnated with etonogestrel, another progestin. Its release in the United States has been postponed, but remains anticipated.

Subdermal implants prevent ovulation in most women. They also stimulate the production of thick cervical mucus, which inhibits sperm penetration. Norplant provides effective continuous contraception removed from the act of coitus. Possible side effects include spotting, irregular bleeding or amenorrhea, an increased incidence of ovarian cysts, weight gain, headaches, fluid retention, acne, mood changes, and depression.

Implants are mentioned in this chapter because some women may not have had their six Norplant rods removed or the nurse may care for women from foreign countries who use Jadelle or Implanon. A minor surgical procedure is required to insert and remove the implants.

Depot-medroxyprogesterone acetate (DMPA) (**Depo-Provera**), another long-acting progesterone, provides highly effective birth control for 3 months when given as a single injection of 150 mg. DMPA, which acts primarily by suppressing ovulation, is safe, convenient, private, and relatively inexpensive. It also separates birth control from the act of coitus. It can safely be given to nursing mothers because it contains no estrogen. DMPA provides levels of progesterone high enough to block the LH surge, thereby suppressing ovulation. It also thickens the cervical mucus to block sperm penetration. Side effects include menstrual irregularities, headache, weight gain, breast tenderness, and depression. Return of fertility may be delayed for an average of 9 months.

Depo-Provera is not recommended for use longer than 2 years without specific informed consent by the woman. It has been associated with calcium loss from the bones that may not resolve after discontinuing use. Women who remain on DMPA longer than 2 years must be educated

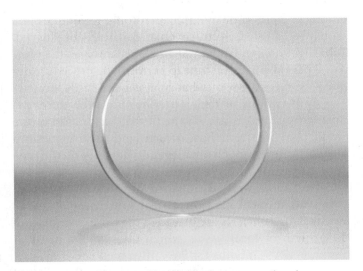

FIGURE 5–8 The NuvaRing vaginal contraceptive ring.
Source: Courtesy of Orgonon, Inc.

CRITICAL THINKING

Monique Hermann, age 37, was divorced 3 years ago. Her only son, now 19, is away at college. Recently, with some trepidation, Monique began dating, and she is now enjoying an active social life. She is being seen today for advice about contraception, which had not been an issue during her marriage because her husband had had a vasectomy. She reports that she is a little nervous about becoming sexually active because until this point her husband had been her only sexual partner. She is very attracted to two different men but does not prefer one over the other at this point. She states that she wants a reliable method that would permit her to have intercourse at any time without having to take action beforehand because she thinks that would be embarrassing for her. Similarly she is not interested in the patch, which is visible. She is not willing to consider a tubal ligation. She is a nonsmoker who drinks occasionally. She has no known contraindications to any available methods. Which methods of contraception might be appropriate for Monique?

Answer found in Appendix F ∞.

about this serious side effect and need to exercise and take 1200 mg of calcium daily.

Depo-Provera 104 mg subcutaneously is an alternative to Depo-Provera 150 mg. Originally approved by the FDA for the treatment of endometriosis, it subsequently was approved as a contraceptive. Because there is 30% less drug available compared with the 150 mg preparation, it may result in less bone density loss for long-term users. It is administered subcutaneously every 10–13 weeks.

Emergency Postcoital Contraception

Emergency **postcoital contraception** (EC) is indicated when a woman is worried about pregnancy because of unprotected intercourse, rape, or possible contraceptive failure (e.g., broken condom, slipped diaphragm, missed COCs, or too long a time between DMPA injections). Plan B, a progestin-only (levonorgestrel) approach, is the only emergency contraceptive currently available in the United States.

The phrase "morning after pill" is misleading. The woman actually takes her first dose as soon after intercourse as possible (but not longer than 72 hours) and a second dose 12 hours later. Emergency contraception taken within 72 hours can reduce the risk of pregnancy after a single act of intercourse by 89% (Office of Population Research & Association of Reproductive Health Professionals, 2007). In 2006 Plan B was approved by the FDA for over-the-counter sale to women 18 years and older. A prescription for this pill is still required for teens under age 18.

A combined hormonal approach (levonorgestrel and ethinyl estradiol) called Preven is no longer available in the United States. However, a woman can use COCs for emergency contraception if necessary. She is advised to consult her healthcare provider about specifics. Placement of the Copper IUD within 5 days of unprotected intercourse may reduce pregnancy risk by as much as 99% (Hatcher et al., 2004).

Operative Sterilization

Operative **sterilization** is an inclusive term that refers to surgical procedures that permanently prevent pregnancy. Before sterilization is performed on either partner, the physician provides a thorough explanation of the procedure to both. Each needs to understand that sterilization is not a decision to be taken lightly or entered into when psychologic stresses, such as separation or divorce, exist. Even though both male and female procedures are theoretically reversible, the permanency of the procedure should be stressed and understood.

Male sterilization is achieved through a relatively minor procedure called a **vasectomy**. This procedure involves surgically severing the vas deferens in both sides of the scrotum. It takes about 4 to 6 weeks and 6 to 36 ejaculations to clear the remaining sperm from the vas deferens. During that period, the couple is advised to use another method of birth control and to bring in two or three semen samples for a sperm count. The man is rechecked at 6 and 12 months to ensure that fertility has not been restored by recanalization. Side effects of a vasectomy include pain, infection, hematoma, sperm granulomas, and spontaneous reanastomosis (reconnecting).

Vasectomies can sometimes be reversed by using microsurgery techniques. Restored fertility, as measured by subsequent pregnancy, ranges from 38% to 82% (Hatcher et al., 2004).

Female sterilization is most frequently accomplished by **tubal ligation**. The tubes are located through a small subumbilical incision or by minilaparotomy techniques and are clipped, ligated, electrocoagulated, banded, or plugged. Tubal ligation may be done at any time; however, the postpartal period is an ideal time to perform the procedure because the tubes are somewhat enlarged and easily located.

Complications of female sterilization procedures include coagulation burns on the bowel, perforation of the bowel, pain, infection, hemorrhage, and adverse anesthesia effects. Reversal of a tubal ligation depends on the type of procedure performed.

The *Essure* method of permanent sterilization requires no surgical incision. Under hysteroscopy, stainless steel microinserts are placed in the tubes stimulating the growth of local tissue, which then results in tubal blockage—by 3 months for 96% of women and 6 months postprocedure for 100% (Memmel & Gilliam, 2008). Essure eliminates the need for transabdominal surgery but it does require some specialized training and a hysterosalpingogram (HSG) 3 months following the procedure to confirm that the tubes are occluded. The woman should use a backup contraceptive method until the HSG confirms that the tubes are occluded.

Male Contraception

The vasectomy and the condom, discussed previously, are currently the only forms of male contraception available in the United States. Hormonal contraception for men has yet to be developed, although studies are underway. Developing safe, effective, and reversible male contraceptives is challenging: It is easier to interrupt a woman's cyclic process than to interrupt a man's continuous fertility.

Nursing Care Management

In most cases, the nurse who provides information and guidance about contraceptive methods works with the female partner, because most contraceptive methods are for women. Because a man can purchase condoms without seeing a healthcare provider, only with vasectomy does a man require counseling and interaction with a nurse. The nurse can play an important role in helping a woman choose a method of contraception that is acceptable to her and to her partner.

In addition to completing a history and assessing for any contraindications to specific methods, the nurse can spend time with a woman learning about her lifestyle, personal attitudes about particular contraceptive methods, religious beliefs, personal biases, and plans for future childbearing, before helping the woman select a particular contraceptive method. Once the method is chosen, the nurse can help the woman learn to use it effectively. Table 5–2 summarizes factors to consider in choosing an appropriate method of contraception.

TABLE 5–2	Factors to Consider in Choosing a Method of Contraception
Effectiveness of method in preventing pregnancy	Personal preferences, biases
Safety of the method:	Lifestyle:
Are there inherent risks?	How frequently does client have intercourse?
Does it offer protection against STIs or other conditions?	Does she have multiple partners?
	Does she have ready access to medical care in the event of complications?
Client's age and future childbearing plans	Is cost a factor?
Any contraindications in client's health history	Partner's support and willingness to cooperate
Religious or moral factors influencing choice	Personal motivation to use method

The nurse also reviews any possible side effects and warning signs related to the method chosen and counsels the woman about what action to take if she suspects she is pregnant. In many cases the nurse is involved in telephone counseling of women who call with questions and concerns about contraception. Thus it is vital that the nurse be knowledgeable about this topic and have resources available to find answers to less common questions.

Client Teaching: Using a Method of Contraception provides guidelines for helping women use a method of contraception effectively. It is summarized on the teaching card: Teaching About Methods of Contraception inserted in the center of this text.

Clinical Interruption of Pregnancy

Although abortion was legalized in the United States in 1973, the associated controversy over moral and legal issues continues. This controversy is as readily apparent in the medical and nursing professions as in other groups.

Many women are strongly opposed to abortion for religious, ethical, or personal reasons. Other women feel that access to a safe, legal abortion is every woman's right. A number of physical and psychosocial factors influence a woman's decision to seek an abortion. The presence of a disease or health state that jeopardizes the mother's life and serious, life-threatening fetal problems are frequently suggested as indications for abortion. In other instances, the timing or circumstance of the pregnancy creates an inordinate stress on the woman and she chooses an abortion. Some of these situations may involve contraceptive failure, sexual assault, or incest.

Medical abortion, now available in the United States, provides an effective alternative to surgical abortion for many women with unintended pregnancy. *Mifepristone* (Mifeprex), originally called RU 486, may be used to induce abortion medically during the first 7 weeks of pregnancy (up to 49 days following conception). (*Note:* Some clinicians support the use of a slightly modified dosage regimen through 63 days' gestation [Creinin, Blumenthal, & Shulman, 2006].)

Mifepristone blocks the action of progesterone, thereby altering the endometrium. After the length of the woman's gestation is confirmed, she takes a dose of mifepristone. Between 1 to 3 days later (depending upon gestation) she returns to her caregiver and takes a dose of the prostaglandin misoprostol, which induces contractions that expel the embryo/fetus. About 14 days after taking the misoprostol, the woman is seen a third time to confirm that the abortion was successful.

Client Teaching USING A METHOD OF CONTRACEPTION

Content	Teaching Method
Discuss the factors that a woman should consider in choosing a method of contraception (Table 5–2). Stress that the different methods may be appropriate at different times in the woman's life. Review the woman's reasons for selecting a particular method and confirm any contraindications to specific methods.	Contraception is a personal decision, so the discussion should take place in a private area free of interruptions. Create a supportive, warm, and comfortable atmosphere by attitude and communication style—both verbal and nonverbal. Provide accurate information in an open, nonjudgmental way.
Discuss the advantages, disadvantages, and risks of the chosen method.	Focus on open discussion. It may help to have written information about the method chosen. If a signed permit is required (as with sterilization or IUD insertion), the physician should also discuss the advantages, disadvantages, and risks.
Describe the correct procedure for using a method. Go through step by step. Periodically stop and have the woman review the information. If a technique is to be learned (as with inserting a diaphragm or charting basal body temperature), demonstrate and then have the woman do a return demonstration as appropriate. (*Note:* If certain aspects are beyond the nurse's level of expertise, the nurse can review the content and confirm that the woman has the opportunity to do a return demonstration. For example, an office nurse who does not do cervical cap fittings may cover information on its use, have the woman try inserting the cap herself, and then have the placement checked by the nurse practitioner or physician.)	Learning is best accomplished when material is broken down into smaller steps. Have a model or chart available to enable the woman to visualize what is being described. Have a sample of the chosen method available: a package of oral contraceptives, an open IUD, or a symptothermal chart.
Provide information on what the woman should do if unusual circumstances arise (she forgets a pill or misses a morning temperature). Stress warning signs that require immediate action on the part of the woman and explain why these signs indicate a risk. Carefully delineate the actions the woman should take.	Provide a written handout identifying the warning signs of her chosen method and listing the actions a woman should take. The handout should also cover actions the woman should take if an unusual situation develops. For example, what should she do if she vomits or has diarrhea while taking oral contraceptives? Arrange to talk with the woman again soon, either on the phone or at a return visit, to determine if she has any questions about the method and to ensure that no problems have arisen.

Since 2001, seven deaths that may possibly have been related to the oral mifepristone/vaginal misoprostol regimen have been reported. Four of these deaths were related to an infection caused by a rare organism, *Clostridium sordelli* (Creinin et al., 2006). Therefore, *any* woman who has taken the oral mifepristone/vaginal misoprostol regimen within the last 24 hours who develops stomach pain, weakness, nausea, vomiting or diarrhea, with or without fever, should contact her healthcare provider *immediately* (U.S. FDA, 2007). Currently, mifepristone is still considered safe and use of routine prophylactic antibiotics is not recommended.

In the first trimester, surgical abortion may be performed by dilatation and curettage (D&C), minisuction, or vacuum curettage. The major risks include perforation of the uterus, laceration of the cervix, systemic reaction to the anesthetic agent, hemorrhage, and infection. Second trimester abortion may be done using dilatation and extraction (D&E), hypertonic saline, systemic prostaglandins, and intrauterine prostaglandins. Surgical abortion in the first trimester is technically easier and safer than abortion in the second trimester.

Nursing Care Management

Important aspects of nursing care for a woman who chooses to have an abortion include providing information about the methods of abortion and associated risks; counseling regarding available alternatives to abortion and their implications; encouraging verbalization by the woman; providing support before, during, and after the procedure; monitoring vital signs, intake, and output; providing for physical comfort and privacy throughout the procedure; and health teaching about self-care, the importance of the postabortion checkup, and contraception review.

Health Promotion for Women

Healthcare providers and consumers alike are becoming increasingly aware of the importance of activities that promote health and prevent illness, and the value of regular screenings to detect any health problems early.

Lifestyle Choices

Women can make lifestyle choices that promote health and well-being. These choices involve a variety of factors, including:

- Eating a nutritious, balanced diet
- Maintaining normal weight for height (no fad dieting)
- Performing regular aerobic exercise and weight training several times a week
- Getting adequate sleep
- Refraining from smoking and/or stopping smoking
- Consuming alcohol in moderation, if at all
- Managing stress effectively
- Developing enjoyable hobbies and leisure activities
- Developing an inner life in some form through religion, spirituality, personal reflection, yoga, and so forth
- Fostering bonds of support and affection with family and friends
- Ensuring that immunizations are up to date
- Obtaining regular health screenings and assessments

Health screening recommendations vary by age. General screening and immunization guidelines for women can be found on MyNursingKit.

EVIDENCE IN ACTION
The risk of CVD is increased in women who are obese and don't exercise.
(Organization Guidelines) (American Heart Association, 2007)

Body Piercing, Tattoos, and Branding

Body piercing and tattooing, often called *body art*, are becoming commonplace in today's culture among people of all ages. *Tattooing* is the application of minute amounts of pigments into the skin with indelible inks. Body piercing sites include ear lobes and ear cartilage, lips, nose, tongue, eyebrow, nipples, umbilicus, and the external genitalia for the purpose of displaying some form of adornment or jewelry. Estimates suggest that, in the United States, as many as 50% of undergraduates have had some form of body piercing (Donohoe, 2006).

These forms of body art carry an element of health risk. For tattooing and body piercing, risks include infections such as HIV and hepatitis B and C because of the use of inadequately sterilized equipment as well as allergic reactions, local swelling and burns, granulomas, and keloid formation (more common in people of African descent). Oral piercing has been associated with tooth and gum damage. Among pregnant or breastfeeding women, nipple piercing has been associated with mastitis, damaged milk ducts, difficulty with breastfeeding, and galactorrhea (Camann, 2006).

Educating clients about the risks associated with these practices should include information about infection, permanent scarring, keloid formation, and care afterward. It is important for the nurse to avoid passing judgment or making generalizations about clients who have these types of body alterations.

Recommended Gynecologic Screening Procedures

The accepted standard of care for women today involves the regular completion of a variety of screening procedures designed to detect potential problems early to permit the most effective treatment. This section focuses on some of the most commonly used screening procedures: breast self-examination and breast examination by a trained healthcare provider, mammography, Pap smear, and pelvic examination.

Breast Examination

Like the uterus, the breast undergoes regular cyclical changes in response to hormonal stimulation. Each month, in rhythm with the cycle of ovulation, the breasts become engorged with fluid in anticipation of pregnancy, and the woman may ex-perience sensations of tenderness, lumpiness, or pain. If conception does not occur, the accumulated fluid drains away via the lymphatic network. *Mastodynia* (premenstrual swelling and tenderness of the breasts) is common. It usually lasts for 3 to 4 days before the onset of menses, but the symptoms may persist throughout the month.

After menopause, adipose breast tissue atrophies and is replaced by connective tissue. Elasticity is lost, and the breasts may droop and become pendulous. The recurring breast engorgement associated with ovulation ceases. If estrogen replacement therapy is used to counteract other symptoms of menopause, breast engorgement may resume.

Monthly **breast self-examination (BSE)** is the best method for detecting breast masses early. A woman who knows the texture and feel of her own breasts is far more likely to detect changes that develop. Thus it is important for a woman to develop the habit of doing routine BSE as early as possible, preferably as an adolescent. Women at high risk for breast cancer are especially encouraged to be attentive to the importance of early detection through routine BSE.

In the course of a routine physical examination or during an initial visit to the caregiver, the woman should be taught BSE technique and its importance as a monthly practice. The effectiveness of BSE is determined by the woman's ability to perform the procedure correctly.

Breast self-examination should be performed on a regular monthly basis about 1 week after each menstrual period, when the breasts are typically not tender or swollen. After menopause, BSE should be performed on the same day each month (chosen by the woman for ease of remembrance).

Breast self-examination is most effective when it uses a dual approach incorporating both inspection and palpation. See Client Teaching: Breast Self-Examination.

Clinical breast examination by a trained healthcare provider, such as a physician, nurse–practitioner, or nurse–midwife, is an essential element of a routine gynecologic examination. Experience in differentiating among benign, suspicious, and worrisome breast changes enables the caregiver to reassure the woman if the findings are normal or move forward with additional diagnostic procedures or referral if the findings are suspicious or worrisome.

Mammography

A **mammogram** is a soft tissue X-ray of the breast without the injection of a contrast medium. It can detect lesions in the breast before they can be felt and has gained wide acceptance as an effective screening tool for breast cancer. Currently the American Cancer Society (2006) recommends that all women age 40 and over have an annual mammogram. The National Cancer Institute (2006) recommends mammograms every 1 to 2 years for women ages 40 to 49 and annually for all women ages 50 and older.

Pap Smear and Pelvic Examination

The *Papanicolaou smear* (**Pap smear**) is a form of cervical cytology testing used to screen for cellular abnormalities by obtaining a sample containing cells from the cervix and the endocervical canal. Precancerous and cancerous conditions, as well as atypical findings and inflammatory changes, can be identified by microscopic examination.

Traditionally the test has been performed by preparing a Pap smear slide. More recently, another test—the liquid-based medium Pap smear—was approved by the Food and Drug Administration (FDA). In this test, no slide is prepared; instead, the cervical cells are transferred directly to a vial of preservative fluid, thereby preserving the entire specimen. The specimen is sent to a laboratory where a special processor prepares a slide.

Liquid-based Pap smear preparations have become the method of choice for cervical cancer screening. These types of preparations allow for removal of debris from the sample, such as blood and mucus, thereby increasing accuracy. Additionally, these preparations allow for human papillomavirus (HPV) screening and for some STI infection screening. Pap smear findings are reported using the Bethesda System (see Chapter 6 ∞). A definitive diagnosis of cervical cancer is made by studying tissue samples obtained by biopsies.

Currently, both the American Cancer Society (ACS) and the American College of Obstetricians and Gynecologists (ACOG) recommend that all women begin having Pap smears when they reach the age of 18 or when they become sexually active, whichever comes first. ACOG recommends annual Pap smears thereafter. Alternatively, the ACS states that, following three consecutive negative Pap smears, the Pap smear may sometimes be done less frequently at the discretion of the caregiver. Less frequent Pap smears might be suggested, for example, for a woman with no history of STI or gynecologic cancer who is in a stable, monogamous relationship with a partner who is also monogamous and infection free. Some caregivers are reluctant to extend the time between Pap smears, however, because they worry that women may delay the test beyond the recommended time frames.

Women should be advised to avoid douching, intercourse, female hygiene products, and spermicidal agents immediately before a specimen is obtained for screening. Specimens should not be obtained during menstruation or when visible cervicitis exists.

HINTS FOR PRACTICE

When you teach about pelvic examination and cervical cytology testing, be certain that the woman understands that she should not douche for at least 24 hours beforehand. Douching can interfere with the accuracy of the test. Occasionally a caregiver will specifically request that a woman use a douche before cervical cytology testing; douching should only be done in this circumstance.

The *pelvic examination* enables the healthcare provider to assess a variety of factors about the woman's vagina, uterus, ovaries, and lower abdominal area. It is often performed after cervical cytology testing but may also be performed without it for diagnostic purposes. Women sometimes perceive the pelvic exam as uncomfortable and embarrassing. The negative feelings may cause women to delay having yearly gynecologic examinations, and this avoidance may pose a threat to life and health.

Client Teaching BREAST SELF-EXAMINATION

MyNursingKit | Video: Nursing in Action: Breast Self-Exam

Content

Discuss the risk factors associated with breast cancer.

Stress the unique risk factors associated with the woman's personal history and lifestyle.

Discuss the use of BSE in breast cancer detection.

Describe and Demonstrate the Correct Procedure for BSE

A. Instruct the woman to inspect her breasts by standing or sitting in front of a mirror. She needs to inspect her breasts in three positions: with both arms relaxed down at her sides, both arms stretched straight over her head, and both hands placed on her hips while leaning forward (Figure 5–9 ■).

Teaching Method

Breast cancer should be discussed in a private area free of interruptions. The room needs to have a mirror; bed, couch, or examining table; pillows; a patient gown; and private area for the woman to disrobe.

Create a supportive, warm, and comfortable atmosphere by attitude and communication style—both verbal and nonverbal. A discussion of breast cancer may bring forth many emotions in the woman, including grief for previous breast cancer-related losses.

Focus on open discussion. A brochure with statistics and illustrations may be useful. Stress the positive outcomes of early detection to counterbalance fears.

Learning is best accomplished when material is broken down into smaller steps and presented with multiple approaches. Before asking the woman to perform BSE, use a model or a chart to demonstrate the procedure. Then have the woman perform BSE. Be very supportive and give a lot of positive feedback because some women may be embarrassed. Demonstrate a nonjudgmental, accepting attitude.

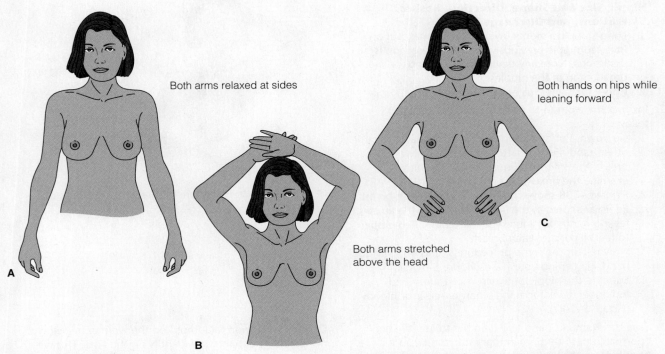

Both arms relaxed at sides

Both hands on hips while leaning forward

Both arms stretched above the head

A

B

C

FIGURE 5–9 Positions for inspection of the breasts. *A,* Both arms relaxed at sides. *B,* Both arms stretched above the head. *C,* Both hands on hips while leaning forward.

(Continued on next page)

Client Teaching BREAST SELF-EXAMINATION (*Continued*)

B. Advise the woman to look at her breasts individually and in comparison with one another. Note and record the following characteristics for each position:

Size and Symmetry of the Breasts
1. Breasts may vary, but the variations should remain constant during rest or movement—note abnormal contours.
2. Some size difference between the breasts is normal.

Shape and Direction of the Breasts
1. The shape of the breasts can be rounded or pendulous with some variation between breasts.
2. The breasts should be pointing slightly laterally.

Color, Thickening, Edema, and Venous Patterns
1. Check for redness or inflammation.
2. A blue hue with a marked venous pattern that is focal or unilateral may indicate an area of increased blood supply because of tumor. Symmetric venous patterns are normal.
3. Skin edema observed as thickened skin with enlarged pores ("orange peel") may indicate blocked lymphatic drainage because of tumor.

Surface of the Breasts
1. Skin dimpling, puckering, or retraction (pulling) when the woman presses her hands together or against her hips suggests malignancy.
2. Striae (stretch marks) red at onset and whitish with age are normal.

Nipple Size and Shape, Direction, Rashes, Ulcerations, and Discharge
1. Long-standing nipple inversion is normal, but an inverted nipple previously capable of erection is suspicious. Note any deviation, flattening, or broadening of the nipples.
2. Check for rashes, ulcerations, or discharge.

C. Instruct the woman to palpate (feel) her breasts as follows:
1. Lie down. Put one hand behind your head. With the other hand, fingers flattened, gently feel your breast. Press lightly (Figure 5–10A ■). Now examine the breast.
2. Figure 5–10B shows you how to check each breast. Begin as shown in the figure and follow the arrows, feeling gently for a lump or thickening. Remember to feel all parts of each breast.
3. Now repeat the same procedure sitting up, with the hand still behind your head (Figure 5–10C).
4. Squeeze the nipple between your thumb and forefinger. Look for any discharge—clear or bloody (Figure 5–10D).

D. Take the woman's hand and help her to identify her "normal lumps" (e.g., mammary ridge, ribs, and nodularity in the upper outer quadrants).

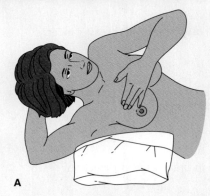

With one hand behind your head, flatten your fingers and press lightly on your breast, feeling gently for a lump or thickening.

A

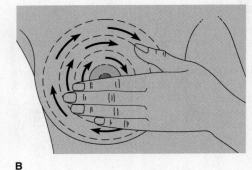

Check each breast in a circular manner, feeling all parts of the breast.

B

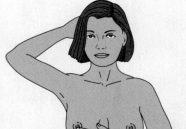

Repeat the same procedure sitting up with your hand still behind your head.

C

FIGURE 5–10 Procedure for breast self-examination.

Demonstrate "normal lumps" on the woman herself while guiding her hand and identifying the area. This will increase confidence that she will recognize an abnormal finding. Checking her immediately afterward will positively reinforce her and diminish the fear associated with BSE.

Client Teaching BREAST SELF-EXAMINATION (Continued)

E. After she examines her breasts and identifies her normal lumps, instruct her to palpate her breasts once more to identify any areas that she may have questions about. If questions arise, the nurse should palpate the area and attempt to identify whether it is normal.

F. If a breast model is available, instruct the woman to palpate it and identify the lumps.

G. Provide information on the warning signs of breast cancer and what she should do if she identifies any of these signs during BSE.

Explain When and How to Perform BSE

Instruct the woman to perform BSE on a monthly basis. Be specific based on whether she is premenopausal, pregnant, postmenopausal, or postmenopausal receiving hormone replacement therapy.

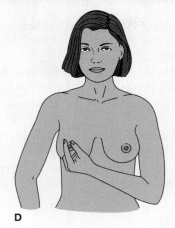

Squeeze your nipple between your thumb and forefinger; look for any clear or bloody discharge.

D

FIGURE 5–10 Procedure for breast self-examination. *Source:* American Cancer Society. (1973). *Breast self-examination and the nurse* (No. 3408 PB). New York: Author.

To make the pelvic examination less threatening, and hopefully improve the woman's health-seeking behavior, it is important to create an atmosphere of trust and incorporate practices that help the woman maintain a sense of control. Some healthcare providers are performing what is called an educational pelvic exam. During this type of exam the woman becomes an active participant. She is positioned and draped so that she can maintain eye contact with the practitioner. She is encouraged to participate by asking questions and giving feedback. The nurse can assist the woman by encouraging her to relax with specific suggestions such as, "Wiggle your toes if you find yourself beginning to tense your muscles."

TEACHING TIP

With the examiner's consent obtained beforehand, offer the woman a hand mirror so that she can watch all or part of the examination. This practice removes the "mystery" from the procedure and enables the woman to become familiar with the appearance of her body and the procedure. The nurse points out anatomic parts and positions and drapes her to allow eye-to-eye contact with the practitioner. The woman is encouraged to participate by asking questions and giving feedback.

Nurse practitioners, certified nurse–midwives, and physicians all perform pelvic examinations. Nurses assist the practitioner and the woman during the examination. See Clinical Skill: Assisting with a Pelvic Examination.

Menopause

Menopause, defined as the absence of menstruation for 1 full year, is a time of transition for a woman, marking the end of her reproductive abilities. *Climacteric*, or change of life (often used synonymously with menopause), refers to the host of psychologic and physical alterations that occur around the time of menopause.

Although menopause usually occurs between 45 and 52 years of age, the current median age at menopause is 51.3 years. A woman's psychologic adaptation to menopause and the climacteric is multifactorial. She is influenced by her own expectations and knowledge, physical well-being, family views, marital stability, and sociocultural expectations. As the number of women reaching menopause increases, the negative emotional connotations society once attached to menopause are diminishing, enabling menopausal women to cope more effectively and even encouraging them to view menopause as a time of personal growth.

Perimenopause refers to the period of time before menopause during which a woman moves from normal ovulatory cycles to cessation of menses. Typically lasting from 2 to 8 years, perimenopause is characterized by decreasing ovarian function, unstable endocrine physiology, and highly variable hormone profiles. Symptoms of perimenopause may be nonexistent or bothersome. They may include PMS, hot flashes, irregular periods, insomnia, and mood changes.

Contraception remains a concern during perimenopause. Combined oral contraceptives (the pill, patches, and vaginal rings) are becoming increasingly popular among healthy nonsmokers because many women also benefit from the noncontraceptive effects including regulation of menses, relief of symptoms of estrogen deficiency, and a decreased risk of endometrial and ovarian cancers. Other contraceptive options for perimenopausal women

MyNursingKit | Menopause Online

Clinical Skill Assisting with a Pelvic Examination

NURSING ACTION	RATIONALE

Preparation

1. Ensure that the room is sufficiently warm by checking room temperature and adjusting the thermostat if necessary. If overhead heat lamps are available, turn them on.

2. Explain the procedure to the woman. If she has never had a pelvic examination, show her the equipment to be used as part of the explanation.

   Explaining the procedure helps reduce anxiety and increase cooperation.

3. Ask the woman to empty her bladder and to remove clothing below the waist.

   An empty bladder promotes comfort during the internal examination.

4. Have padding on the stirrups. If stirrups are not padded, the woman may prefer to leave her shoes on during the procedure.

   Stirrups are usually padded to ease the pressure of the feet against the metal and to decrease the discomfort associated with the touch of the cold stirrups. If they are not padded, however, wearing shoes accomplishes the same purpose.

5. Give the woman a disposable drape or sheet to use during the exam. Ask her to sit at the end of the examining table with the drape opened across her lap.

6. Position the woman in the lithotomy position with her thighs flexed and abducted. Place her feet in the stirrups. Her buttocks should extend slightly beyond the edge of the examining table.

   This position provides the exposure necessary to conduct the examination effectively. The drape helps preserve the woman's sense of dignity and privacy.

7. Drape the woman with the sheet, leaving a flap so that the perineum can be exposed.

Equipment and Supplies

- Vaginal specula of various sizes, warmed with water or on the heating pad before insertion
- Sterile gloves
- Water-soluble lubricant

  Lubricant may alter the results of tests and cultures and is not used during the speculum examination. Its use is reserved for the bimanual examination.

- Materials for Pap smear or ThinPrep Pap test and cultures
- Good light source

Procedure

1. The examiner dons gloves for the procedure. Explain each part of the procedure as the certified nurse–midwife, nurse practitioner, or physician performs it. Let the woman know that the examiner begins with an inspection of the external genitalia. The speculum is then inserted to allow visualization of the cervix and vaginal walls and to obtain specimens for testing. After the speculum is withdrawn the examiner performs a bimanual examination of the internal organs using the fingers of one hand inserted in the woman's vagina while the other hand presses over the woman's uterus and ovaries. The final step of the procedure is generally a rectal examination.

2. Ask the woman to breathe slowly and regularly and to use any method she finds effective in helping her to remain relaxed.

   Relaxation helps decrease muscle tension.

3. Let her know when the examiner is ready to insert the speculum and ask her to bear down.

   Bearing down helps open the vaginal orifice and relaxes the perineal muscles.

4. After the speculum is withdrawn, lubricate the examiner's fingers before the bimanual examination.

   Lubrication decreases friction and eases insertion of the examiner's fingers.

5. After the examiner has completed the bimanual and rectal examination and moved away from the woman, move to the end of the examination table and face the woman. Cover her with the drape. Apply gentle pressure to her knees and encourage her to move toward the head of the table. Assist her to remove her feet from the stirrups, then offer your hand and assist her to sit up.

   Assistance is important because the lithotomy position is an awkward one and many women, but especially those women who are pregnant, obese, or older, may find it difficult to get out of the stirrups.

6. Provide her with tissues to wipe the lubricant from her perineum.

   Vaginal secretions and lubricant may be discharged from the vagina when the woman sits upright.

7. Provide the woman with privacy while she dresses. Be sure that she is not dizzy and that she is standing or sitting safely before leaving the room.

   Lying supine may cause postural hypotension.

include sterilization, IUDs, progestin-only methods, and barrier methods such as condoms, diaphragm, cervical cap, and spermicides.

Physical Aspects

The physical characteristics of menopause are linked to the shift from a cyclic to a noncyclic hormonal pattern. Generally ovulation ceases 1 to 2 years before menopause, but individual variations exist. Atrophy of the ovaries occurs gradually. FSH levels rise, and less estrogen is produced. Menopausal symptoms include atrophic changes in the vagina, vulva, and urethra and in the trigonal area of the bladder.

Many menopausal women experience a vasomotor disturbance commonly known as a *hot flash*, a feeling of heat arising from the chest and spreading to the neck and face. Hot flashes are often accompanied by sweating and sleep disturbances. These episodes may occur as often as 20 to 30 times a day and generally last 3 to 5 minutes. Some women also experience dizzy spells, palpitations, and weakness. Many women find their own most effective ways to deal with the hot flashes. Some report that using a fan or drinking a cool liquid helps relieve distress; others seek relief through hormone replacement therapy or complementary therapies (see later discussion).

The uterine endometrium and myometrium atrophy, as do the cervical glands. The uterine cavity constricts. The fallopian tubes and ovaries atrophy extensively. The vaginal mucosa becomes smooth and thin, and the rugae disappear, leading to loss of elasticity. As a result, intercourse can be painful, but this problem may be overcome by using lubricating gel. Dryness of the mucous membrane can lead to burning and itching. The vaginal pH level increases as the number of Döderlein's bacilli decreases.

Postmenopausal women can still be multiorgasmic. Some women find that their sexual interest and activity improve as the need for contraception disappears and personal growth and awareness increase. Other women experience a decrease in libido at this time. Vulvar atrophy occurs late, and the pubic hair thins, turns gray or white, and may ultimately disappear. The labia shrivel and lose their heightened pigmentation. Pelvic fascia and muscles atrophy, resulting in decreased pelvic support. The breasts become pendulous and decrease in size and firmness.

Long-range physical changes may include **osteoporosis**, a decrease in the bony skeletal mass. This change is thought to be associated with lowered estrogen and androgen levels, lack of physical exercise, inadequate vitamin D, and a chronic low intake of calcium. Moreover, the estrogen deprivation that occurs in menopausal women may significantly increase their risk of coronary heart disease. Loss of protein from the skin and supportive tissues causes wrinkling. Postmenopausal women frequently gain weight, which may be because of excessive caloric intake or to lower caloric need with the same level of intake.

Psychologic Aspects

A woman's psychologic adaptation to menopause and the climacteric is multifactorial. It is often complicated because women of this age may be dealing with other life circumstances such as adjustment to an "empty nest" or caring for aging parents. Numerous personal factors influence a woman's ability to deal with these changes, such as self-concept, physical health, marital stability, relationships with others, and cultural values. Some women express disappointment in approaching this time of their lives, whereas many others may see it as a positive transition that offers freedom from menses or concern about contraception. Often night sweats and insomnia affect a woman's ability to cope because of increased fatigue.

In reality the average woman in the United States will live one-third of her life after menopause. The changing perceptions of menopause and the years beyond are enabling menopausal women to cope more effectively and to view menopause as a time of personal growth.

Clinical Therapy

Hormone Replacement Therapy

Hormone replacement therapy (HRT), often simply called *hormone therapy (HT)*, refers to the administration of specific hormones, usually estrogen alone (ET) or combined estrogen–progestogen (EPT), to alleviate menopausal symptoms, especially hot flashes, night sweats, and urogenital symptoms. ET is used for women who have had a hysterectomy whereas EPT is used for women with an intact uterus. When estrogen is given alone, it can produce endometrial hyperplasia and increase the risk of endometrial cancer. Thus, in women who still have a uterus, estrogen is opposed by giving a progestin.

In 2002 the advisability of HRT, specifically EPT, was called into question because of the results of the Women's Health Initiative study, which suggested that the risks of HRT outweigh the benefits, especially for long-term use because of the slightly increased risk of breast cancer, thromboembolic disease, and stroke (Writing Group for the Women's Health Initiative Investigators, 2002). At present, the treatment of severe vasomotor symptoms (hot flashes and night sweats) is the primary indication for HT. It is also indicated for the treatment of moderate to severe symptoms of vulvar and vaginal atrophy (dyspareunia, vaginal dryness, and atrophic vaginitis). It is not recommended for the prevention of coronary heart disease (North American Menopause Society [NAMS], 2007). Generally short-term therapy (1 to 4 years) is advised. Women considering HRT should clearly understand the associated risks so that they can make an informed decision about using it.

HT may be prescribed in a number of ways including orally; transdermally (patch); topically as a gel, lotion, or vaginal cream; and through a vaginal ring. It is given in a continuous manner, daily administration of both estrogen and progestogen, or as a cyclic or sequential therapy, with estrogen use daily and a progestogen added on a set sequence. Combination estrogen–progestogen preparations are also available.

Postmenopausal women experiencing decreased libido may experience improved sexual desire, responsiveness, and frequency when testosterone is added to their HT. Options for providing testosterone in doses low enough for women are still limited. Estratest, a combined estrogen–androgen pill, is used by some women. Custom-compounded testosterone preparations are available by prescription and work is underway on low-dose testosterone patches (Shifren, 2006).

Before starting HT a woman should undergo a thorough history; physical examination, including Pap smear; measurement of cholesterol, lipids, and liver enzyme levels; and baseline mammogram. An initial endometrial biopsy is indicated for women with an increased risk of endometrial cancer; biopsy is also indicated if excessive, unexpected, or prolonged vaginal bleeding occurs. Women taking estrogen should be advised to stop immediately if they develop headaches, visual changes, signs of thrombophlebitis, or chest pain.

Complementary and Alternative Therapies

For women who do not wish to take HRT or who have medical contraindications to it, a variety of approaches have been proposed as complementary or alternative treatment or preventive measures for the discomforts of the perimenopausal and postmenopausal years. These include diet and nutrition, specifically a high-fiber, low-fat diet with supplements of calcium and vitamins D, E, and B complex. *Phytoestrogens* (plant products with estrogen properties), found in a number of plant foods, especially soy products, may be helpful. See Complementary and Alternative Therapies for a discussion of the use of botanicals.

Weight-bearing exercises such as walking, jogging, tennis, and low-impact aerobics help increase bone mass and decrease the risk of osteoporosis. Exercise also improves cholesterol profiles and contributes to overall health. Stress management and relaxation techniques such as biofeedback, meditation, yoga, visualization, and massage may provide a sense of well-being.

Prevention and Treatment of Osteoporosis

Osteoporosis is becoming a significant health risk for older adults, especially women. In fact, in the United States

---

COMPLEMENTARY AND ALTERNATIVE THERAPIES

Use of Botanicals for Menopausal Symptoms

The following botanicals were reviewed during a 2005 National Institutes of Health (NIH) State-of-the-Science conference on the management of menopausal symptoms. The panel found the following:

- *Black cohosh.* This substance has received the most attention of all the botanicals. It does not act as an estrogen, as was once believed. Studies of its effectiveness in relieving hot flashes have had mixed results but it has a good safety record over many years.
- *Red clover.* Five controlled studies found no conclusive or consistent evidence that hot flashes were reduced in women using red clover leaf extract. Few side effects have been reported and no serious health problems have been cited in the literature. Animal studies have raised a concern as to whether red clover might be harmful to estrogen-sensitive tissue such as the uterus and breasts.
- *Dong quai.* In the only randomized controlled study reported, dong quai was not found to be effective in reducing hot flashes. Because dong quai is known to interact with and increase the activity of warfarin (coumadin), its use by women on warfarin can lead to bleeding problems.
- *Ginseng.* Although it has not been found to be effective in relieving hot flashes, ginseng may help with other menopausal symptoms such as sleep disturbances and mood swings.
- *Kava.* No evidence supports its effectiveness in relieving hot flashes although it may decrease anxiety. The FDA has issued a warning about kava because it has been associated with liver disease.
- *Soy.* Results about the use of soy to relieve hot flashes (see discussion of phytoestrogens) are mixed. Its use as a dietary supplement for short periods of time is not associated with any serious side effects although long-term use has been associated with a thickening of the uterine lining.

Source: National Center for Complementary and Alternative Medicine (NCCAM). (2006). Do CAM therapies help menopausal symptoms? Retrieved March 8, 2006, from http://nccam.nih.gov/health/menopauseandcam/

13% to 18% of women age 50 and older have osteoporosis (ACOG, 2004). Table 5–3 identifies risk factors associated with osteoporosis.

Bone mineral density (BMD) testing is useful in identifying individuals who are at risk for osteoporosis. The National Osteoporosis Foundation (NOF) (2008) recommends BMD testing for the following:

- All postmenopausal women ages 65 or older and men 70 years and older
- Postmenopausal women under age 65 and men ages 50 to 70 with one or more risk factors
- Postmenopausal women and men who have had a fracture to determine the severity of the disease

TABLE 5–3	Risk Factors for Osteoporosis

- Middle-age and elderly women
- European American or Asian ethnic origin
- Small-boned and thin body type
- Low body weight (less than 127 pounds)
- Family history of osteoporosis
- Lack of regular weight-bearing exercise
- Nulliparity
- Early onset of menopause
- Consistently low intake of calcium
- Cigarette smoking
- Moderate to heavy alcohol intake
- Use of certain medications such as anticonvulsants, corticosteroids, or lithium

In addition to the changes in bone density often found following menopause, a variety of conditions such as malabsorption syndromes, inflammatory bowel disease, AIDS, chronic obstructive pulmonary disease, certain cancers, eating disorders and inadequate diet, multiple sclerosis, and insulin-dependent diabetes mellitus may be associated with an increased risk of osteoporosis in adults. In addition, certain medications such as some anticonvulsants, lithium, long-term heparin use, glucocortico-steroids, and tamoxifen may also lead to osteoporosis.

Prevention of osteoporosis is a primary goal of care. Peri- and postmenopausal women are advised to have a calcium intake of at least 1200 mg/day (NAMS, 2006). Most women require supplements to achieve this level. Vitamin D supplements (800 to 1000 international units per day) may also be indicated for those at risk of deficiency (NOF, 2008). In addition, women are advised to participate regularly in weight-bearing exercise, to consume only modest quantities of alcohol and caffeine, and to stop smoking. Alcohol and smoking have a negative effect on the rate of bone resorption. In caring for women at menopause and beyond, it is important to ensure that the woman's height is measured at each visit, because a loss of height is often an early sign that vertebrae are being compressed because of reduced bone mass. The effectiveness of estrogen in preventing osteoporosis is well documented. However, because of the increased risks associated with long-term use of hormone replacement therapy, other pharmacologic agents are being used more frequently to prevent and treat osteoporosis. These include the following:

- *Bisphosphonates* are calcium regulators that act by inhibiting bone resorption and increasing bone mass. Alendronate (Fosamax) and risedronate (Actonel) are the two most commonly prescribed.

- *Selective estrogen receptor modulators (SERMs)* such as raloxifene (Evista) preserve the beneficial effects of estrogen, including its protection against osteoporosis, but do not stimulate uterine or breast tissue.
- *Salmon calcitonin* is a calcium regulator that may inhibit bone loss. Generally administered as a nasal spray, although it is also available as an injection, its value is less clear than that of the other medications listed.
- *Parathyroid hormone,* taken daily as a subcutaneous injection, activates bone formation, which results in substantial increases in bone density.
- Ultra-low-dose estrogen patches (Menostar) can be used without a progestogen. These small doses can provide effective prevention of fracture without the increased side effects or risks of endometrial stimulation found in larger dose estrogen patches (Ettinger, 2004).

EVIDENCE IN ACTION

Soy isoflavone intake has been shown to increase the bone mineral density in the spine of menopausal women.
(Meta-analysis) (Ma, Qin, Wang, & Katoh, 2008)

Women who are taking medication for osteoporosis should have BMD testing 2 years after beginning therapy and every 2 years thereafter (NOF, 2008).

Nursing Care Management

Most menopausal women deal well with this developmental phase of life, although some women may need counseling to adjust successfully. Reaction to menopause is determined to a large extent by the life the woman has lived, by the security she has in her feminine identity, and by her feelings of self-worth and self-esteem.

Nurses and other healthcare professionals can help the menopausal woman achieve high-level functioning at this time in her life. Of paramount importance is the nurse's ability to understand and provide support for the woman's views and feelings. Whether the woman expresses relief and delight or tearfulness and fear, the nurse needs to use an empathic approach in counseling, health teaching, and providing physical care.

Nurses should explore the question of the woman's comfort during sexual intercourse. In counseling, the nurse may say, "After menopause many women notice that their vagina seems dryer and intercourse can be uncomfortable. Have you noticed any changes?" This gives the woman information and may open discussion. The nurse can then go on to explain that dryness and shrinking of the vagina can be addressed by use of a water-soluble jelly. Use of estrogen, orally or in vaginal creams, may also be indicated. Increased frequency of intercourse will maintain some elasticity in the vagina. When assessing the menopausal woman, the nurse should address the question of sexual activity openly but tactfully, because the woman may have been socialized to be reticent in discussing sex.

The crucial need of women in the perimenopausal period of life is for adequate information about the changes taking place in their bodies and their lives. Supplying that information provides both a challenge and an opportunity for nurses.

HINTS FOR PRACTICE

Women respond differently to the experience of menopause, so it is important to avoid generalizations. However, in working with menopausal women—and indeed, any women—touch, listening, and caring, as nursing measures, may enhance your self-actualization and that of your client.

Violence Against Women

Violence against women has become endemic in society today. Violence affects women of all ages, races, ethnic backgrounds, socioeconomic levels, educational levels, and walks of life. Two of the most common forms of violence are domestic violence and rape. Often people not only accept these forms of violence but also shift the blame for the violence to the women themselves by asking questions such as, "How did she make him so mad?" "Why does she stay?" "What was she doing out so late?" and "Why did she dress that way?"

Violence against women is also a major health concern: In addition to causing injuries, associated physical and mental health outcomes, and fatalities, violence costs the healthcare system millions of dollars annually. In response to this epidemic, healthcare providers are becoming more knowledgeable about actions they should take to identify women at risk, implement preventive measures, and provide effective care.

Domestic Violence

Domestic violence is defined as a pattern of coercive behaviors and methods used to exert power and control by one individual over another in an adult domestic or intimate relationship. It is also termed **intimate partner violence (IPV)**. This section focuses on domestic violence experienced by women in heterosexual relationships. Among heterosexual couples estimates indicate that in at least 95% of the cases, the perpetrators are men. It is important to note, however, that heterosexual men, as well as gays and lesbians, experience domestic violence in their relationships as well.

Although the incidence has decreased significantly in the last decade, domestic violence is still staggeringly common in the United States where one in four women will experience domestice violence (National Coalition Against Domestic Violence [NCADV], 2007a). Worldwide, as many as one in three women will be the victim of violence or sexual coercion at some point in her life (NCADV, 2007c).

The woman may be married to her abuser, or she may be living with, dating, or divorced from him. Domestic violence takes many forms, including verbal attacks, insults, intimidation, threats, emotional abuse, social isolation, economic deprivation, intellectual derision, ridicule, stalking, and physical attacks and injury. Physical battering includes slapping, kicking, shoving, punching, forms of torture, attacks with objects or weapons, and sexual assault. Women who are physically abused can also suffer psychologic and emotional abuse.

Cycle of Violence

In an effort to explain the experience of battered women, Walker (1984) developed the theory of the cycle of violence. Battering takes place in a cyclic fashion through three phases:

1. In the *tension-building phase*, the batterer demonstrates power and control. This phase is characterized by anger, arguing, blaming the woman for external problems, and possibly minor battering incidents. The woman may blame herself and believe she can prevent the escalation of the batterer's anger by her own actions.

2. The *acute battering incident* is typically triggered by some external event or internal state of the batterer. It is an episode of acute violence distinguished by lack of control, lack of predictability, and major destructiveness. The cycle of violence can be interrupted before the acute battering incident if proper interventions take place.

3. The *tranquil phase* is sometimes termed the honeymoon period. This phase may be characterized by extremely kind and loving behavior on the part of the batterer as he tries to make up with the woman, or it may simply be manifested as an absence of tension and violence. Without intervention, this phase will end and the cycle of violence will continue. Over time the violence increases in severity and frequency.

Characteristics of Battered Women

Battered women often hold traditional views of sex roles. Many were raised to be submissive, passive, and dependent and to seek approval from male figures. Some battered women were exposed to violence between their parents, whereas others first experienced it from their partners. Many battered women do not work outside the home. As part of the manipulation of batterers, they are isolated from family and friends and totally dependent on their partners for their financial and emotional needs.

Women with physically abusive partners nearly always experience psychologic abuse as well and have been told repeatedly by their batterers that the family's problems are all their fault. Many believe their batterers' insults and accusations. As these women become more isolated, they find it harder to judge who is right. Eventually they fully believe in their inadequacy, and their low self-esteem reinforces their belief that they deserve to be beaten. Battered women often feel a pervasive sense of guilt, fear, and depression. Their sense of hopelessness and helplessness reduces their problem-solving ability. Battered women may also experience a lack of support from family, friends, and their religious community.

Characteristics of Batterers

Batterers come from all backgrounds, professions, religious groups, and socioeconomic levels. Batterers often have feelings of insecurity, socioeconomic inferiority, powerlessness, and helplessness that conflict with their assumptions of male supremacy. Emotionally immature and aggressive men have a tendency to express these overwhelming feelings of inadequacy through violence. Many batterers feel undeserving of their partners, yet they blame and punish the very women they value.

Battered women often describe their husbands or partners as lacking respect toward women in general, having come from homes where they witnessed abuse of their mothers or were themselves abused as children, and having a hidden rage that erupts occasionally. Batterers accept traditional macho values, yet when they are not angry or aggressive, they appear childlike, dependent, seductive, manipulative, and in need of nurturing. They may be well respected in the community. This dual personality of batterers reflects the conflict between their belief that they must live up to their macho image and their feelings of inadequacy in the role of husband or provider. Combined with low frustration tolerance and poor impulse control, their pervasive sense of powerlessness leads them to strike out at life's inequities by abusing women.

Nursing Care Management

Nurses in various healthcare settings often come in contact with abused women but fail to recognize them, especially if their bruises are not visible. Women who are at high risk of battering often have a history of alcohol or drug abuse, child abuse, or abuse in the previous or present relationship. Other possible signs of abuse include expressions of helplessness and powerlessness; low self-esteem revealed by the woman's dress, appearance, and the way she relates to healthcare providers; signs of depression evidenced by fatigue, hopelessness, and somatic problems such as headache, insomnia, chest pain, back pain, or pelvic pain; and possible suicide attempts. In addition, the abused woman may have a history of missed or frequently changed appointments, perhaps because she had signs of abuse that kept her from coming in or her partner prevented it.

Because domestic violence is so prevalent, many caregivers now advocate *universal screening of all female clients at every healthcare encounter*. Screening should be done privately, with only the caregiver and client present, in a safe and quiet place. Specific language leads to higher disclosure rates. Possible screening questions include the following:

1. During the past year, have you been slapped, kicked, hit, choked, or hurt physically by someone?
2. Has your partner or anyone else ever forced you to have sex?
3. Are you afraid of an ex-partner or of anyone at home?

During the screening the nurse should assure the woman that her privacy will be respected (see Figure 5–11 ■). It is essential that the nurse remain nonjudgmental; create a warm, caring climate conducive to sharing; and demonstrate a willingness to talk about violence. A battered woman often interprets the nurse's willingness to discuss violence as permission for her to discuss it as well.

When a woman seeks care for an injury, the nurse should be alert to the following cues of abuse:

- Hesitation in providing detailed information about the injury and how it occurred
- Inappropriate affect for the situation
- Delayed reporting of symptoms
- Pattern of injury consistent with abuse, including multiple injury sites involving bruises, abrasions, and contusions to the head (eyes and back of the neck), throat, chest, abdomen, or genitals
- Inappropriate explanation for the injuries
- Lack of eye contact
- Signs of increased anxiety in the presence of the possible batterer, who frequently does much of the talking

When a woman who has been battered comes in for treatment, she needs to feel safe physically and secure in

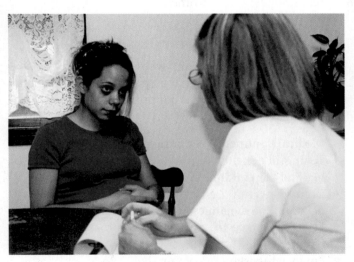

FIGURE 5–11 Screening for domestic violence should be done privately.
Source: Courtesy of Al Dodge.

talking about her injuries and problems. If a man is with her, the nurse should ask or tell him to remain in the waiting room while the woman is examined. A battered woman also needs to reestablish a feeling of control over her world. She needs to regain a sense of predictability by knowing what to expect and how she can interact. The nurse should provide sufficient information about what to expect in terms the woman can understand.

In providing care the nurse needs to let the woman work through her story, problems, and situation at her own pace. The nurse should reassure the woman that she is believed and that her feelings are reasonable and normal. The nurse should anticipate the woman's ambivalence (because of her fear and possible love–hate relationship with her batterer) but also respect the woman's capacity to change and grow when she is ready. Thus any assessment should include information about a woman's strengths and support system. The woman may require assistance in identifying specific problems and in developing realistic ideas for reducing or eliminating those problems. In all interactions the nurse should stress that no one should be abused and that the abuse is not the woman's fault.

Nurses need to be aware that immigrant women who experience domestic violence may face barriers to seeking help including the following (NCADV, 2007b):

- *Language barriers* if English is not the primary language
- *Fear of law enforcment or the legal system* if they have had negative experiences in their country of origin or if their abuser has given them misinformation
- *Fear of deportation* if they are in the country illegally or if the abuser has led them to believe that it is possible if they complain or call the police
- *Cultural or religious factors* if they were raised with strict guidelines about gender roles and the subservient position of women

Community-Based Nursing Care

The nurse should inform any woman suspected of being in an abusive situation of the services available in the healthcare agency and the community. Specifically the woman may need the following:

- Medical treatment for injuries
- Temporary shelter to provide a safe environment for her and her children
- Counseling to raise her self-esteem and help her understand the dynamics of family violence
- Legal assistance for protection or prosecution of the batterer
- Financial assistance to obtain shelter, food, and clothing
- Job training or employment counseling
- An ongoing support group with counseling

If the woman returns to an abusive situation, the nurse should encourage her to develop an exit plan for herself and her children, if any. As part of the plan, she should pack a change of clothing for herself and her children, including toiletries and an extra set of car and house keys. She should store these items away from the house with a friend or relative and ask a neighbor to call the police if violence begins. In planning she should be aware that her abuser may monitor mail, telephone, and Internet communications. If possible she should have money, identification papers (driver's license, social security card, and birth certificates for herself and her children), checkbook, bank account information, other financial information (such as mortgage papers, automobile papers, and pay stubs), court papers or orders, and information about the children to help her enroll them in school. She should also plan where she will go, regardless of the time of day. The nurse should ensure that the woman has a planned escape route and emergency telephone numbers she can call, including local police, a phone hotline, and a women's shelter if one is available in the community.

Working with battered women is challenging, and many healthcare providers feel frustrated and impotent when women repeatedly return to their abusive situations. Nurses must realize that they cannot rescue battered women; battered women must decide on their own how to handle their situations. Effective nurses provide battered women with information that empowers them in decision making and supports their decisions, knowing that incremental assistance over the years may be the only alternative until the woman is ready to explore other options.

Sexual Assault and Rape

In its broadest sense, **sexual assault** is involuntary sexual contact with another person. The National Crime Victimization Survey defines **rape** as follows: "Rape is forced sexual intercourse and includes both psychological coercion as well as physical force. Forced sexual intercourse means vaginal, anal, or oral penetration by the offender(s)." The person who commits a sexual assault may be an acquaintance, spouse, other relative, employer, or stranger. Sexual assault is an act of violence expressed sexually—most commonly, a man's aggression and rage acted out against a woman.

Research indicates that one in six American women over age 12 has been the victim of an attempted or completed sexual assault or rape. However, the incidence of sexual assault is still down by 69% since 1993 (Rape, Abuse, and Incest National Network [RAINN], 2008a). Experts attribute this dramatic decline to two trends (Rape, Abuse, and Incest National Network [RAINN], 2003):

1. *Tough-on-crime policies with longer sentences and three strike laws.* All types of criminals commit rapes and rapists often commit other forms of crime.

2. *Generational changes.* Over 75% of rape victims are under 30 years of age. Women now in this age group have grown up knowing that "no means no." These young women are more cautious about potentially risky situations and more willing to express their wishes forcefully.

No woman of any age or ethnicity is immune. However, statistics indicate that young, unmarried women, women who are unemployed or have a low family income, and students have the highest incidence of sexual assault or attempted assault. In fact, over half (54%) of rape victims are under age 18, whereas 22% are younger than 12 (National Center for Injury Prevention and Control, 2006). Like their victims, the assailants come from all ethnic backgrounds and walks of life. The majority are white (52%) with an average age of 31 years. Almost two-thirds know their victim. Of those imprisoned for rape, 22% are married (RAINN, 2008b).

Why do men rape? Of the many theories put forth, none provides a completely satisfactory explanation. So few assailants are actually caught and convicted that a clear characteristic of the assailant has not been developed. However, rapists tend to be emotionally weak and insecure and may have difficulty maintaining interpersonal relationships. Many assailants also have trouble dealing with the stresses of daily life. Such men may become angry and overcome by feelings of powerlessness. They then commit a sexual assault as an expression of power or anger.

Acquaintance rape, which occurs when the assailant is someone with whom the victim has had previous nonviolent interaction, is the most common form of rape. In fact, 67% of female rape victims know their assailant as an acquaintance, friend, relative, or intimate (Catalano, 2005). One type of acquaintance rape, **date rape**, which occurs between a dating couple, is an increasing problem on high school and college campuses. In some cases an assailant uses alcohol or other drugs to sedate his intended victim (*drug-facilitated sexual assault*). One drug, flunitrazepam (Rohypnol), has gained notoriety as a date rape drug because it frequently produces amnesia in its victims. In date rape situations, the male is usually determined to have sex and will do whatever he feels necessary if denied.

Responses to Sexual Assault

Sexual assault is a situational crisis. It is a traumatic event that the victim cannot be prepared to handle because it is unforeseen. Following the assault, the victim generally experiences a cluster of symptoms, described by Burgess and Holmstrom (1979) as the *rape trauma syndrome*, that last far beyond the rape itself. These phases are described in Table 5–4. Although the phases of response are listed individually, they often overlap, and individual responses and their duration may vary. Recently a fourth phase—integration and recovery—has been suggested (Holmes, 1998).

Research also suggests that survivors of sexual assault may exhibit high levels of posttraumatic stress disorder (PTSD), the same disorder that develops in many combat veterans. PTSD is marked by varying degrees of intensity. Assault victims with this disorder often require lengthy, intensive therapy to regain a sense of trust and feeling of personal control.

Nursing Care Management

Survivors of sexual assault often enter the healthcare system by way of the emergency room. Thus the emergency room nurse is often the first person to counsel them. Because the values, attitudes, and beliefs of the caregiver will necessarily affect the competence and focus of the care, it is essential that nurses clearly understand their feelings about sexual assault and assault survivors and resolve any conflicts that may exist. In many communities, specially trained sexual assault nurse examiner (SANE) nurses coordinate the care of survivors of sexual assault, gather necessary forensic evidence, and are then available as expert witnesses when assailants are tried for the crime.

TABLE 5–4	Phases of Recovery Following Sexual Assault
Phase	Response
Acute Phase (Disorganization)	Fear, shock, disbelief, desire for revenge, anger, anxiety, guilt, denial, embarrassment, humiliation, helplessness, dependence, self-blame, wide variety of physical reactions, lost or distorted coping mechanisms
Outward Adjustment (Denial) Phase	Survivor appears outwardly composed, denying and repressing feelings (e.g., she returns to work, buys a weapon); refuses to discuss the assault; denies need for counseling
Reorganization	Survivor makes many life adjustments, such as moving to a new residence or changing her phone number; uses emotional distancing; may engage in risky sexual behaviors; may experience sexual dysfunction, phobias, flashbacks, sleep disorders, nightmares, anxiety; has a strong urge to talk about or resolve feelings; may seek counseling or remain silent
Integration and Recovery	Time of resolution; survivor begins to feel safe and be comfortable trusting others; places blame on assailant; may become an advocate for others

The first priority in caring for a survivor of a sexual assault is to create a safe, secure milieu. Admission information is gathered in a quiet, private room. The woman should be reassured that she is safe and not alone. The nurse assesses the survivor's appearance, demeanor, and ways of communicating for the purpose of planning care. Initially, the woman is evaluated to determine the need for emergency care. Obtaining a careful, detailed history is essential. After the woman has received any necessary emergency care, a forensic chart and kit are completed.

HINTS FOR PRACTICE

Strive to listen nonjudgmentally. Impartial listening can often make the difference in a survivor's readiness to disclose the full details of the assault and can also assist her in the recovery process.

The woman is given a thorough explanation of the procedures to be carried out and signs a consent form for the forensic examination and collection of materials. Sexual assault kits contain all the necessary supplies for collecting and labeling evidence. The woman's clothing is collected and bagged, swabs of stains and secretions are taken, hair samples and any fingernail scrapings are collected, blood samples are drawn, tissue swabs are obtained, and photographs are taken. Vaginal and rectal examinations are performed, along with a complete physical examination for trauma. If possible photographs are taken of any injuries. The woman is offered prophylactic treatment for sexually transmitted infections. If the assailant's HIV status is not known, consideration should be given to offering postexposure prophylaxis with HIV antiviral medications. In such cases, consultation with an HIV specialist is advised. The woman is also questioned about her menstrual cycle and contraceptive practices. If she could become pregnant as a result of the rape, she is offered postcoital contraceptive therapy.

Throughout the experience the nurse acts as the sexual assault survivor's advocate, providing support without usurping decision making. The nurse need not agree with all the survivor's decisions but should respect and defend her right to make them.

The family members and friends on whom the survivor calls will also need nursing care. Like those of the survivor, the reactions of the family will depend on the values to which they ascribe. Many families or partners blame the survivor for the assault and feel angry with her for not having been more careful. They may also incorrectly view the assault as a sexual act rather than an act of violence. They may feel personally wronged and see the survivor as devalued or unclean. Their reactions may compound the survivor's crisis. By spending some time with family members before their first interaction with the survivor, the nurse may be able to reduce their anxiety and absorb some of their frustrations, sparing the woman further trauma.

Sexual assault counseling, provided by qualified nurses or other counselors, is a valuable tool in helping the survivor come to terms with her assault and its impact on her life. In counseling, the woman is encouraged to explore and identify her feelings and determine appropriate actions to resolve her problems and concerns. It is important for the counselor to avoid reinforcing the prevalent myth that the assault was somehow the woman's fault. The fault lies with the assailant. The counselor also plays an important role in emphasizing that the loss of control the woman experienced during the rape was temporary and that the woman can regain a feeling of control over life.

Prosecution of the Assailant

Legally, sexual assault is considered a crime against the state, and prosecution of the assailant is a community responsibility. The survivor, however, must begin the process by reporting the assault and pressing charges against her assailant. In the past, the police and the judicial system were notoriously insensitive in dealing with survivors. However, many communities now have classes designed to help officers work effectively with sexual assault survivors or have special teams to carry out this important task.

Many women who have sought to use the judicial process have had such a traumatic experience that they refer to it as a second assault. The woman may be asked repeatedly to describe the experience in intimate detail, and her reputation and testimony will be attacked by the defense attorney. In addition, publicity may intensify her feelings of humiliation, and, if her assailant is released on bail or found not guilty, she may fear retaliation.

The nurse acting as a counselor needs to be aware of the judicial sequence to anticipate rising tension and frustration in the survivor and her support system. She will need consistent, effective support at this crucial time.

CHAPTER HIGHLIGHTS

- Nurses should provide girls and women with clear information about menstrual issues, such as use of tampons (deodorant and absorbency); vaginal spray and douching practices; and self-care comfort measures during menstruation, such as maintaining good nutrition, exercising, and using heat and massage.

- Dysmenorrhea usually begins at, or a day before, onset of menses and disappears by the end of menstruation. Hormone therapy (e.g., combined oral contraceptives), nonsteroidal anti-inflammatory drugs, or prostaglandin inhibitors can ease symptoms. Self-care measures include improved nutrition, exercise, applications of heat, and extra rest.
- Premenstrual syndrome occurs most often in women over age 30. Symptoms occur 2 to 3 days before onset of menstruation and subside as menstruation starts, with or without treatment. Medical management usually includes prostaglandin inhibitors and calcium supplementation. Self-care measures include improving nutrition (vitamins B complex and E supplementation and avoiding methylxanthines, which are found in chocolate and caffeine), a program of aerobic exercise, and participation in self-care support groups. In some cases medications such as selective serotonin reuptake inhibitors may be indicated.
- Fertility awareness methods are natural, noninvasive methods of contraception often used by people whose religious beliefs prevent their using other methods.
- Barrier contraceptives such as the diaphragm, cervical cap, and condom act as barriers to prevent the transport of sperm. These methods are used in conjunction with a spermicide.
- Spermicides are far less effective in preventing pregnancy when they are not used with a barrier method.
- The intrauterine device (IUD) is a mechanical contraceptive. Although its exact method of action is not clearly understood, research suggests it acts by immobilizing sperm or by impeding the progress of sperm from the cervix to the fallopian tubes. In addition, the IUD has a local inflammatory effect.
- Combined oral contraceptives (the pill) are combinations of estrogen and progesterone. When taken correctly, they are one of the most effective reversible methods of fertility control.
- Combined hormonal options (estrogen and progestin) now available worldwide include the patch (Ortho Evra) and the vaginal ring (NuvaRing). The combined injection, Lunelle, and progestin-only implants such as Norplant are not available in the United States although they can be obtained in other parts of the world.

- Permanent sterilization is accomplished by tubal ligation for women and vasectomy for men. Although theoretically reversible, clients are advised that the method should be considered irreversible.
- Recommendations about the frequency of screening mammograms vary somewhat. Currently the American Cancer Society recommends annual mammography in women beginning at age 40. The National Cancer Institute recommends mammograms every 1 to 2 years for women ages 40 to 49 and annually for all women ages 50 and older.
- Menopause is a physiologic, maturational change in a woman's life. Physiologic changes include the cessation of menses and decrease in circulating hormones. Hormonal changes sometimes bring unsettling emotional responses. The most common physiologic symptoms are hot flashes, palpitations, dizziness, and increased perspiration at night. The woman's anatomy also undergoes changes, such as atrophy of the vagina, reduction in size and pigmentation of the labia, and myometrial atrophy. Osteoporosis becomes an increasing concern.
- Current management of menopause centers around hormone replacement therapy, complementary therapies, and client healthcare education. Decisions about the use of HRT should be made individually based on each woman's symptoms and risks, and the woman should be advised about the known risks.
- Batterers use physical, psychologic, and sexual abuse to maintain power and control in a sexual relationship. Battering occurs in a cyclic pattern called the "cycle of violence" and increases in frequency and severity over time.
- Nurses are in an excellent position to intervene and assist battered women by recognizing their cues, diagnosing their problems appropriately, and understanding the complex dynamics of the battering family. Nurses provide information about available community resources, medical attention, and community support.
- Rape is a form of violence acted out sexually. Most sexual assaults are expressions of anger or power.
- Following sexual assault, the survivor will usually experience an assortment of symptoms known as the rape trauma syndrome. Research also links the effects of rape to the posttraumatic stress disorder.

CHAPTER REFERENCES

Abboud, R. L. (2006). Delaying your period through oral contraceptives. Retrieved March 17, 2008, from www.mayoclinic.com/health/womens-health/WO00069/METHOD=print

American Cancer Society. (2006). *Breast cancer facts and figures 2005–2006.* Retrieved July 6, 2006, from www.cancer.org

American College of Obstetricians and Gynecologists (ACOG). (2003). *Benefits and risks of sterilization* (ACOG Practice Bulletin No. 46). Washington, DC: Author.

American College of Obstetricians and Gynecologists (ACOG). (2004). *Osteoporosis.* (ACOG Practice Bulletin No. 50). Washington, DC: Author.

Burgess, A. W., & Holmstrom, L. L. (1979). *Rape: Crisis and recovery.* Englewood Cliffs, NJ: Prentice Hall.

Catalano, S. M. (2005). *Criminal victimization 2004.* Bureau of Justice Statistics National Crime Victimization Survey. Retrieved July 1, 2006 from www.ojp.usdoj.gov/bjs

Camann, W. (2006). Obstetric and anesthetic implications of "body art" (piercing and tattooing). *Medscape OB/GYN & Women's Health, 11,* 1–3. Retrieved April 17, 2006, from www.medscape.com/viewarticle/527920_print

Creinin, M., Blumenthal, P., & Shulman, L. (2006). Mifepristone–misoprostol medical abortion mortality. *Medscape General Medicine, 8*(2), 26. Retrieved May 6, 2006, from http://www.medscape.com/viewarticle/529318_print

Donohoe, M. (2006). Beauty and body modification. *Medscape OB/GYN & Women's Health, 11,* 1–6. Retrieved on April 26, 2006, from www.medscape.com/viewarticle/529442_print

Endicott, J. (2007). PMDD spotlight: Redefined expectations: Improving quality of life in women with PMDD. *Medscape OB/GYN & Women's Health.* Retrieved January 11, 2008, from www.medscape.com/viewarticle.567290_print

Ettinger, B. (2004). Unopposed ultra-low-dose estradiol: A new approach to osteoporosis prevention. *OBG Management* (suppl), 17–19.

Food and Drug Administration (FDA). (2007). Over-the-counter vaginal contraceptive and spermicide drug products containing nonoxynol 9; required labeling. Final rule. *Federal Register, 72*(243), 71769–71785.

Gallo, M. F., Grimes, D. A., & Schulz, K. F. (2006). Cervical cap versus diaphragm for contraception (Accession No. 2009134249). Cochrane Library, 2008(1).

Hatcher, R. A., Trussell, J., Stewart, F., Nelson, A., Cates, W., Guest, F., & Kowal, D. (2004). *Contraceptive technology* (18th ed.). New York: Ardent Media, Inc.

Holmes, M. M. (1998). The clinical management of rape in adolescents. *Contemporary OB/GYN, 43*(5), 62–78.

Jacobstein, R. (2007). Long-acting and permanent sterilization: An international development, service delivery perspective. *Journal of Midwifery & Women's Health, 52*(4), 361–367.

Jick, S. S., & Jick, H. (2007). The *contraceptive patch* in relation to ischemic stroke and acute myocardial infarction. *Pharmacotherapy, 27*(2), 218–220.

Kahlenborn, C., Modugno, F., Potter, D. M., & Severs, W. B. (2006). Oral contraceptive use as a risk factor for premenopausal breast cancer: A meta-analysis. *Mayo Clinic Proceedings, 81*(10), 1290–1302.

Ma, D., Qin, L., Wang, P., & Katoh, R. (2008). Soy isoflavone intake increases bone mineral density in the spine of menopausal women: Meta-analysis of randomized controlled trials. *Clinical Nutrition, 27,* 57–64.

Memmel, L., & Gilliam, M. (2008). Contraception. In *Danforth's Obstetrics and Gynecology* (10th ed.). Gibbs, R. S., Karlan, B.Y., Haney, A.F., & Nygaard, I.E. (Eds.). Philadelphia: Wolters Kluwer/Lippincott Williams & Wilkins.

National Cancer Institute. (2006). *Screening mammograms: Questions and answers.* Fact sheet retrieved July 6, 2006, from http://www.cancer.gov

National Center for Injury Prevention and Control (NCIPC). (2006). *Sexual violence: Fact sheet.* Centers for disease control and prevention. Retrieved July 1, 2006, from www.cdc.gov/ncipc/factsheets/svfacts.htm

National Coalition Against Domestic Violence (NCADV). (2007a). Domestic violence facts. Retrieved June 2, 2008, from www.ncadv.org

National Coalition Against Domestic Violence (NCADV). (2007b). Immigrant victims of domestic violence. Retrieved March 17, 2008, from www.ncadv.org

National Coalition Against Domestic Violence (NCADV). (2007c). International violence against women. Retrieved March 17, 2008, from www.ncadv.org

National Osteoporosis Foundation (NOF). (2008). *Clinician's guide to prevention and treatment of osteoporosis.* Retrieved March 17, 2008, from www.nof.org

North American Menopause Society (NAMS). (2006). The role of calcium in peri- and postmenopausal women: 2006 position statement of The North American Menopause Society. *Menopause, 13*(6), 862–877.

North American Menopause Society (NAMS). (2007). Estrogen and progestogen use in peri- and postmenopausal women: March 2007 position statement of The North American Menopause Society. *Menopause, 14*(2), 168–182.

Ogburn, T., & Espey, E. (2007). Encouraging more patients to choose an IUD. *Contemporary OB/GYN, 52*(6), 72–77.

Office of Population Research & Association of Reproductive Health Professionals. (2007). Emergency contraception pills ("Morning after pills"). Retrieved September 9, 2007, from http://ec.princeton.edu/info/ecp.html

Rape, Abuse, & Incest National Network (RAINN). (2003). RAINN News: New report shows dramatic increase in willingness to report rape to the police. Retrieved December 6, 2003, from www.rainn.org/news/ncvs2002.html

Rape, Abuse, & Incest National Network (RAINN). (2008a). Sexual assault statistics. Retrieved March 17, 2008, from www.rainn.org/print/81

Rape, Abuse, & Incest National Network (RAINN). (2008b). The offenders. Retrieved March 17, 2008, from www.rainn.org/print/289

Shifren, J. L. (2006). Testosterone therapy in postmenopausal women. *The Female Patient, 21*(4), 29–31.

Shulman, L. P. (2005). Unique progestational impact on PMS/PMDD. Innovative options for patient care, a new way of thinking. CE Monograph. Released February 2005.

Sonfield, A. (2006). Working to eliminate the world's unmet need for contraception. *Guttmacher Policy Review, 9*(1), 10–13.

Speroff, L., & Darney, P. (2005). *A clinical guide for contraception* (4th ed.). Philadelphia: Lippincott Williams & Wilkins.

Sulak, P. J. (2008). Continuous oral contraception: changing times. *Best Practice & Research in Clinical Obstetrics and Gynaecology, 22*(2), 355–374.

U.S. Food and Drug Administration (FDA). (2006). Patient information sheet: Norlegstromin/ethinyl estradiol (marketed as Ortho Evra). Retrieved September 9, 2007, from www.fda.gov

U.S. Food and Drug Administration (FDA). (2007). Mifeprex (mifepristone) information. Retrieved March 17, 2008, from www.fda.gov

Walker, L. (1984). *The battered woman syndrome.* New York: Springer.

World Health Organization (WHO). (2005). Facts and figures from the world health report, 2005. Retrieved January 6, 2006, from www.who.org

World Health Organization (WHO). (2007). Maternal mortality in 2005: Estimates developed by WHO, UNICEF, UNFPA, and the World Bank. Retrieved June 2, 2008, from www.who.org

Writing Group for the Women's Health Initiative Investigators. (2002). Risks and benefits of estrogen plus progestin in healthy postmenopausal women: Principal results from the Women's Health Initiative randomized controlled trial. *Journal of the American Medical Association, 288,* 321–333.

CHAPTER 6

Common Gynecologic Problems

When I first started working here I was stunned by how little young women knew about sexually transmitted infections. They would come to the clinic devastated to have an infection or worried about AIDS without being aware of the long-term implications of infections such as herpes or genital warts. I decided that I had to do something to try to prevent infection, not just treat it, so now I am working with three of our local high schools offering classes on prevention. Judging from what several of the students have told me, I am making a difference. I'm proud of that.

—Nurse Working at a Sexually Transmitted Infection Clinic in a Major Urban Area

LEARNING OUTCOMES

6-1. Contrast the contributing factors, signs and symptoms, treatment options, and nursing care management of women with common benign breast disorders.

6-2. Explain the signs and symptoms, medical therapy, and implications for fertility in determining the nursing care management of women with endometriosis.

6-3. Identify the risk factors, treatment options, and nursing interventions for a woman with toxic shock syndrome.

6-4. Compare the causes, signs and symptoms, treatment options, and nursing care for women with vulvovaginal candidiasis versus bacterial vaginosis.

6-5. Compare the prevention, causes, treatment, signs and symptoms, treatment options, and nursing care of women for the common sexually transmitted infections.

6-6. Relate the implications of pelvic inflammatory disease (PID) for future fertility to its pathology, signs and symptoms, treatment, and nursing care.

6-7. Compare the cause and implications of an abnormal finding during a pelvic examination in the provision of nursing care.

6-8. Contrast the causes, signs and symptoms, treatment options, and nursing care for women with cystitis versus pyelonephritis.

6-9. Describe the nursing care management of a woman requiring a hysterectomy.

Throughout her lifetime, a woman is likely to face a variety of gynecologic or urinary tract problems. Some may be minor and easily treated, whereas others may be more serious. This chapter provides information about a variety of gynecologic conditions with an emphasis on problems commonly addressed in community-based settings.

Care of the Woman with a Benign Disorder of the Breast

This section discusses the most common benign breast disorders women encounter. For information on breast cancer, readers should refer to a medical–surgical nursing textbook.

Fibrocystic Breast Changes

Fibrocystic breast changes, the most common of the benign breast disorders, are most prevalent in women 30 to 50 years of age. *Fibrosis* is a thickening of the normal breast tissue. Cyst formation that may accompany fibrosis is considered a later change in the condition. The exact etiology of fibrocystic breast changes is unclear, but they are probably caused by an imbalance in estrogen and progesterone that distorts the normal changes of the menstrual cycle. The symptoms often increase as the woman approaches menopause and generally decrease after menopause. However, if a postmenopausal woman is treated with hormone replacement therapy, the cyclic breast changes may resume. Only women with fibrocystic breast changes who show certain histologic changes (usually found incidentally when a biopsy is done) have an increased risk of developing cancer.

The woman often reports pain, tenderness, and swelling that occur cyclically. These symptoms are most pronounced just before menses and improve about 1 to 2 days into the menstrual cycle. Physical examination may reveal only mild signs of irregularity, or the breasts may feel dense, with areas of irregularity and nodularity. Women often refer to this irregularity as "lumpiness." Some women may also have expressible nipple discharge. Unilateral discharge and serosanguineous discharge are the most worrisome findings because they may indicate conditions such as intraductal papilloma or, if a mass is also present, breast cancer. Consequently, all significant nipple discharge should be investigated further.

If the woman has a large, fluid-filled cyst, she may experience a localized painful area as the capsule containing the accumulated fluid distends coincident with her cycle. If small cysts form, however, the woman may experience not a solitary tender lump but a diffuse tenderness. A cyst may often be differentiated from a malignancy because a cyst is more mobile (easily moved with palpation) and tender, whereas a cancer may be fixed (not movable) and may be associated with skin retraction (pulling) in the surrounding tissue.

Mammography, sonography, magnetic resonance imaging, palpation, and fine-needle aspiration may be used to confirm fibrocystic breast changes. Often, fine-needle aspiration is the treatment as well, affording relief from the tenderness or pain. Treatment of palpable cysts is conservative; invasive procedures such as biopsy are used only if the diagnosis is questionable.

Women with mild symptoms may benefit from restricting sodium intake and taking a mild diuretic during the week before the onset of menses. This counteracts fluid retention, relieves pressure in the breast, and helps decrease the pain. In other cases, a mild analgesic is necessary. In severe cases, the hormone inhibitor danazol is often helpful because it suppresses FSH and LH, resulting in anovulation. However, it can cause undesirable side effects including masculinization.

Some researchers suggest that methylxanthines (found in caffeine products, such as coffee, tea, colas, and chocolate, and in some medications) may contribute to the development of fibrocystic breast changes and that limiting intake of these substances will help decrease fibrocystic changes. Other research fails to demonstrate a clear association between methylxanthines and fibrocystic breast changes. Additional medical therapies that are helpful in varying degrees include oral contraceptives, progestins, bromocriptine, and the antiestrogen medication tamoxifen (although this is an "off-label" use for it). All work on the principle of estrogen suppression and progesterone stimulation or augmentation.

Other Benign Breast Disorders

Fibroadenoma is a common benign tumor seen in women in their teens and early twenties. It has not been significantly associated with breast cancer. Fibroadenomas are freely movable, solid tumors that are well defined, sharply delineated, and rounded, with a rubbery texture. Asymptomatic and nontender, they are often found by the woman or her partner.

If there are any disquieting features to the appearance of a lump, fine-needle biopsy or excision of the mass may be indicated. Caution is exercised when deciding on biopsy because excision of the mass in a young girl may interfere with normal breast development. Watchful observation and possible surgical excision are the only treatments for fibroadenomas. Surgery is often deferred. When advisable, surgical removal of the fibroadenoma concludes its treatment.

Intraductal papillomas, most often occurring during the menopausal years, are tumors growing in the terminal portion of a duct or, sometimes, throughout the duct system within a section of the breast. They are typically benign but have the potential to become malignant. Although relatively uncommon, they are the most frequent cause of nipple discharge in women who are not pregnant or lactating.

The majority of papillomas are present as solitary nodules. These small, ball-like lesions may be detected on mammography but often are nonpalpable. The presence of a papilloma is often frightening to the woman, because her primary symptom is a discharge from the nipple that may be serosanguineous or brownish green because of old blood. The location of the papilloma within the duct system and its pattern of growth determine whether nipple discharge will be present.

If the woman reports a nipple discharge, the breast should be milked to obtain fluid, which is sent for a Pap smear. The diagnosis is confirmed if papilloma cells are present. The lesion must be excised and histologically examined because of the difficulty in differentiating between a benign papilloma and a papillary carcinoma. Treatment for benign intraductal papilloma is excision with followup care.

Duct ectasia (comedomastitis), an inflammation of the ducts behind the nipple, commonly occurs during or near the onset of menopause and is not associated with malignancy. The condition typically occurs in women who have borne and nursed children. It results because of an increase in maternal glandular secretions with the resulting production of an irritating lipid fluid that can produce nipple discharge. Duct ectasia is characterized by a thick, sticky nipple discharge and by burning pain, pruritus, and inflammation. Nipple retraction may also be noted, especially in postmenopausal women. Treatment is conservative, with drug therapy aimed at symptomatic relief. The major central ducts of the breast occasionally have to be excised.

Nursing Care Management

Nursing Assessment and Diagnosis

During the period of diagnosis of any breast disorder, the woman may be anxious about a possible change in body image or a diagnosis of cancer. The nurse can use therapeutic communication to assess the significance the woman places on her breasts; her current emotional status, coping mechanisms used during periods of stress, and knowledge and beliefs about cancer; and other variables that may influence her coping and adjustment.

Nursing diagnoses that may apply to a woman with a benign disorder of the breast include the following:

- *Health-Seeking Behavior: Information About Diagnostic Procedures for Breast Disorders* related to an expressed desire for further information
- *Anxiety* related to threat to body image

Nursing Plan and Implementation

During the prediagnosis period the nurse should clarify misconceptions and encourage the woman to express her anxiety. Once a diagnosis is made, the nurse should ensure that the woman clearly understands her condition, its association to breast malignancy, and the treatment options.

The nurse can also point out that frequent professional breast examinations and regular mammograms are tools that help detect any abnormalities. Although recommendations about the importance of monthly breast self-examination (BSE) have modified since research has failed to demonstrate that survival rates were improved in women who did regular BSE (Ruhl, 2007), most professionals agree that women should be familiar with their own breasts so that they are able to note changes should they occur.

Evaluation

Expected outcomes of nursing care include the following:

- The woman is able to discuss her fears, concerns, and questions during the period of diagnosis.
- The diagnosis is made quickly and accurately, and treatment is initiated if indicated.

Care of the Woman with Endometriosis

Endometriosis, a condition characterized by the presence of endometrial tissue outside the uterine cavity, occurs in about 12% to 32% of women of childbearing age who undergo laparoscopy to determine the cause of pelvic pain

(Schenken, 2003). Endometriosis has been found almost everywhere in the body, including the vagina, lungs, cervix, central nervous system, and gastrointestinal tract. The most common location, however, is the pelvic cavity. Endometrial tissue bleeds cyclically in response to the hormonal changes of the menstrual cycle. The bleeding results in inflammation, scarring of the peritoneum, and formation of adhesions.

Endometriosis may occur at any age after puberty, although it is most common in women between ages 20 and 45. The exact cause is unknown. Leading theories include retrograde menstrual flow and inflammation of the endometrium, hereditary tendency, and a possible immunologic defect.

The most common symptom of endometriosis is pelvic pain, which is often dull or cramping. Because the pain is usually related to menstruation, the woman typically assumes it is dysmenorrhea. **Dyspareunia** (painful intercourse) and abnormal uterine bleeding are other common signs. The condition is often diagnosed when the woman seeks evaluation for infertility. Bimanual examination may reveal a fixed, tender, retroverted uterus and palpable nodules in the cul-de-sac. Diagnosis is confirmed by laparoscopy.

Treatment may be medical, surgical, or a combination of the two. During the laparoscopic examination, the physician may surgically remove any visible implants of endometrial tissue by excision, endocoagulation, electrocautery, or laser vaporization. Surgery is effective in relieving pain symptoms, at least for a period of time. In women with minimal disease and symptoms, treatment includes observation, analgesics, and nonsteroidal anti-inflammatory drugs (NSAIDs). If the woman does not currently desire pregnancy, she may be started on a combined oral contraceptive (COC) often in combination with NSAIDs. The COC creates a pseudopregnancy state with decreased menstrual bleeding. If the COC does not relieve symptoms, therapy with medroxyprogesterone acetate (MPA), danazol, or a gonadotropin-releasing hormone (GnRH) agonist may be indicated.

MPA causes endometrial tissue to atrophy, thereby decreasing symptoms. It is administered intramuscularly every 3 months and the effectiveness of treatment is evaluated every 3 to 6 months. Side effects include weight gain, bloating, acne, headaches, emotional lability, and irregular bleeding.

Danazol is a testosterone derivative that suppresses GnRH and has high-androgen and low-estrogen effects that inhibit the growth of the endometrium. It suppresses ovulation and causes amenorrhea. Danazol has some significant side effects, however, including hirsutism, vaginal bleeding, acne, oily skin, weight gain, reduced libido, voice changes and hoarseness, clitoral enlargement, and decreased breast size.

GnRH agonists such as nafarelin acetate (given as a metered nasal spray twice daily) and leuprolide acetate (Lupron) (given once a month as an intramuscular injection) are gaining popularity because many women tolerate them better than danazol and their results in treating endometriosis are comparable. GnRH agonists suppress the menstrual cycle through estrogen antagonism. This may result in the hypoestrogen side effects of hot flashes, vaginal dryness, decreased libido, pain in muscles and joints, and loss of bone density. These side effects can be reduced by adding an oral progestin or a combination of low-dose estrogen and progestin. In more advanced cases, surgery may be done to remove implants and break up adhesions. If severe dyspareunia or dysmenorrhea are symptoms, the surgeon may perform a presacral neurectomy. In advanced cases in which childbearing is not an issue, treatment may be a hysterectomy with bilateral salpingo-oophorectomy (removal of fallopian tubes and ovaries).

Nursing Care Management

Nursing Assessment and Diagnosis

The nurse should be aware of the common symptoms of endometriosis and elicit an accurate history if a woman mentions these symptoms. If a woman is being treated for endometriosis, the nurse should assess the woman's understanding of the condition, its implications, and the treatment alternatives.

Nursing diagnoses that may apply to a woman with endometriosis include the following:

- *Acute Pain* related to peritoneal irritation secondary to endometriosis
- *Compromised Family Coping* related to depression secondary to infertility

Nursing Plan and Implementation

The nurse can be available to explain the condition, its symptoms, treatment alternatives, and prognosis. The nurse can help the woman evaluate treatment options and make appropriate choices. If the woman begins taking medication, the nurse can review the dosage, schedule, possible side effects, and any warning signs. A woman with endometriosis is often advised not to delay pregnancy because of the increased risk of infertility that women with endometriosis face. The woman may wish to discuss the implications of this decision on her life choices, relationship with her partner, and personal preferences. The nurse acts as a nonjudgmental listener and helps the woman consider her options.

Evaluation

Expected outcomes of nursing care include the following:

- The woman is able to discuss her condition, its implications for fertility, and her treatment options.
- After considering the alternatives, the woman chooses appropriate treatment options.

Care of the Woman with Polycystic Ovarian Syndrome

Polycystic ovarian syndrome (PCOS) is a complex endocrine disorder of ovarian dysfunction that is evidenced by amenorrhea or oligomenorrhea and clinical signs of androgen excess (typically hirsutism, acne) in the absence of other conditions that might have these same signs and symptoms (King, 2007).

The most common clinical signs and symptoms of PCOS include:

- *Menstrual dysfunction.* Irregular menses, ranging from total absence of periods (amenorrhea) to intermittent or infrequent periods (oligomenorrhea), to heavy periods (menorrhagia), are the hallmark of PCOS (Jackson, 2004/2005).
- *Hyperandrogenism.* Women with PCOS consistently have elevated serum androgen levels, specifically testosterone and androsterone. These elevated androgen levels often lead to clinical manifestations such as acne, alopecia (male-patterned hair loss), hirsutism, deepening voice, increased muscle mass, and menstrual irregularities. Estimates suggest that 70% of women with PCOS have hirsutism (King, 2007).
- *Obesity.* About half the women who have PCOS are clinically obese. The obesity is generally of the android type, with an increased hip-to-waist ratio.
- *Hyperinsulinemia.* Women with PCOS are insulin resistant. This insulin resistance, characterized by the failure of insulin to enter the cells appropriately, places these women at increased risk for impaired glucose tolerance and type 2 diabetes mellitus (King, 2007).
- *Infertility.* Nearly 75% of women who have been diagnosed with PCOS struggle with some degree of infertility related to anovulation, and obese women with PCOS have even higher rates of infertility (Hill, 2003). The diagnosis of PCOS is one of exclusion of other conditions. The diagnostic process is fourfold: history, physical examination, laboratory studies, and endovaginal ultrasound to evaluate the uterus and ovaries.

Clinical Therapy

The goals for treatment include decreasing the effects of hyperandrogenism (hirsutism, acne, etc.), restoring reproductive functioning for women desiring pregnancy, protecting the endometrium (increased risk for uterine cancer), and reducing long-term risks, specifically type 2 diabetes and cardiovascular disease.

If pregnancy is not an immediate goal, menstrual irregularities can be treated with a combined oral contraceptive or cyclic progesterone. Combined oral contraceptives (COCs) help to regulate menstrual cycles; provide a balance between estrogen and progesterone, thereby protecting the endometrium and decreasing the risk of uterine cancer; and may improve acne by inhibiting ovarian androgen production (Jackson, 2004/2005). If pregnancy is an immediate goal then another option is the use of medications that improve insulin sensitivity and utilization.

Antiandrogens such as spironolactone (Aldactone) may be used to decrease symptoms of androgen excess. Metformin (Glucophage) inhibits glucose production in the liver and improves glucose uptake by fat and muscle cells. It improves ovarian function, reduces the degree of hyperandrogenism, restores normal ovulation in women with PCOS, and is associated with an improved ability to lose weight. Women desiring pregnancy may be given low doses of clomiphene citrate (Clomid) (see Chapter 7 ∞). In addition, lifestyle changes should also be a major component in the treatment of PCOS. Modifications should include weight loss, regular exercise, balanced diet, and smoking cessation.

Long-term, PCOS may increase a woman's risk for developing type 2 diabetes, hypertension, cardiovascular disease, endometrial cancer, breast cancer, and ovarian cancer. Additionally, the woman with PCOS may struggle with significant emotional responses to this chronic disorder. She will likely face issues related to body image, infertility, problematic menses, and depression.

Nursing Care Management

The nurse plays a vital role in the identification, evaluation, management, and follow-up when caring for a woman with PCOS. Sometimes it is the nurse who puts the bigger picture together, especially in a community-health setting where knowledge of PCOS may be lacking. The signs of PCOS, especially hirsutism, negatively impact women's feelings of femininity and lead them to invest considerable time and effort in hair removal treatments. Women with PCOS also feel a strong desire to "be normal," with regular menstrual cycles and a more feminine appearance, and struggle with a sense of guilt over their difficulty losing weight (Snyder, 2006). Nurses can help women recognize these feelings and find ways to develop a more positive body image. The nurse also has an important role in providing accurate information, education, and counseling for a woman diagnosed with PCOS. Finally, because the woman with PCOS is at risk for developing long-term complications, the nurse can play a key role in follow-up and continuity of care throughout the life of a woman facing this challenging disorder.

Care of the Woman with Toxic Shock Syndrome

Although **toxic shock syndrome (TSS)** has been reported in children, postmenopausal women, and men, it is primarily a disease of women in their reproductive years, especially women at or near menses or during the postpartum period. The causative organism is a toxin released by a strain of *Staphylococcus aureus*. The use of superabsorbent tampons has been widely related to the incidence of TSS. However, occluding the cervical os with a contraceptive device such as a diaphragm or cervical cap during menses may also increase the risk of TSS.

Early diagnosis and treatment are important in preventing a fatal outcome. The most common signs of TSS include fever (often greater than 38.9°C [102°F]); rash on the trunk initially followed by desquamation of the skin, especially the palms and soles, which usually occurs 1 to 2 weeks after the onset of symptoms; hypotension; and dizziness. Systemic symptoms often include vomiting, diarrhea, severe myalgia, and inflamed mucous membranes (oropharyngeal, conjunctival, or vaginal). Disorders of the central nervous system, including alterations in consciousness, disorientation, and coma, may also occur. Laboratory findings reveal elevated blood urea nitrogen (BUN), creatinine, aspartate aminotransferase (AST), alanine aminotransferase (ALT), and total bilirubin levels, whereas platelets are often less than 100,000/mm³.

Women with TSS are generally hospitalized and given supportive therapy, including intravenous fluids to maintain blood pressure. Severe cases may require renal dialysis, administration of vasopressors, and intubation. Broad-spectrum antibiotic therapy (including antistaphylococcal agents) is initiated immediately until septicemia is excluded as a diagnosis; antibiotic therapy also reduces the risk of recurrence.

Nursing Care Management

Nurses play a major role in helping educate women about ways to prevent the development of TSS. Women should understand the importance of avoiding prolonged use of tampons. They should change tampons every 3 to 6 hours and avoid using superabsorbent tampons. Some women may choose to use other products, such as sanitary napkins or minipads. Women who choose to continue using tampons may reduce their risk of TSS by alternating them with napkins and avoiding overnight use of tampons.

Postpartal women should avoid the use of tampons for 6 to 8 weeks after childbirth. Women with a history of TSS should never use tampons. Women who use diaphragms or cervical caps should not leave them in place for prolonged periods and should not use them during the postpartum period or when they are menstruating. Nurses can also help make women aware of the signs and symptoms of TSS so that they will seek treatment promptly if symptoms occur.

Care of the Woman with a Vaginal Infection

Vaginitis is the most common reason women seek gynecologic care. Symptoms of vaginitis or vulvovaginitis may include increased vaginal discharge, vulvar irritation and pruritis, foul odor, and pain when urine touches irritated vulvar tissue. It may be caused directly by an infection or it may result when normal flora is altered making the vagina vulnerable to organisms, as in the case of bacterial vaginosis or *Candida albicans*.

Bacterial Vaginosis

Bacterial vaginosis (BV), the most prevalent form of vaginal infection worldwide, is an alteration of normal vaginal bacterial flora that results in the loss of hydrogen peroxide-producing lactobacilli, which are normally the main vaginal flora. With the loss of this natural defense, bacteria such as *Gardnerella*, mycoplasmas, and anaerobes overgrow in large numbers, causing vaginitis. The cause of this overgrowth is not clear, although trauma from douching, frequent sexual intercourse without condom use, and an upset in normal vaginal flora are predisposing factors.

The infected woman often notices an excessive amount of thin, watery, white or gray vaginal discharge with a foul odor described as "fishy." The characteristic "clue" cell is seen on a wet-mount preparation (Figure 6–1 ■). The addition of 10% potassium hydroxide (KOH) solution to the vaginal secretions, called a "whiff" test, releases a strong, fishy odor. The vaginal pH is usually greater than 4.5.

The nonpregnant, symptomatic woman is generally treated with metronidazole (Flagyl) orally or as a vaginal cream (see Drug Guide: Metronidazole). If metronidazole is prescribed, the woman and her partner should be cautioned to avoid alcohol while taking it; the combination has an effect similar to that of alcohol and Antabuse—abdominal pain, flushing, and tremors. Alternately clindamycin (Cleocin) vaginal cream may be used, although it is slightly less effective (CDC, 2006).

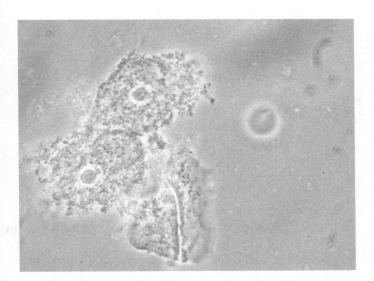

Figure 6–1 The characteristic "clue cells" seen in bacterial vaginosis. Unlike normal epithelial cells, which appear translucent and have a clear border, clue cells are desquamated epithelial cells with bacteria adhering to them. The presence of the bacteria makes the cell appear to be speckled with black dots. The borders are also obscured because of the bacteria.
Source: Centers for Disease Control and Prevention (CDC).

Until recently, metronidazole was avoided during pregnancy because of its potential teratogenic effects. However, the CDC (2006) now reports that multiple studies failed to document a relationship between metronidazole use in pregnancy and teratogenesis in the newborn. Thus the recommended treatment for pregnant women with BV is currently either oral metronidazole or oral

Drug Guide Metronidazole (Flagyl)

Overview of Action Metronidazole is an antiprotozoal and antibacterial agent. It possesses direct trichomonacidal and amebicidal activity against *T vaginalis* and *E histolytica*. Metronidazole is active in vitro against most obligate anaerobes but does not appear to possess any clinically relevant activity against facultative anaerobes or obligate aerobes. It is used in the treatment of various infections caused by organisms that are sensitive to this drug. It is used predominantly to treat the following infections in women: *T vaginalis*, bacterial vaginosis, endometritis, endomyometritis, tubo-ovarian abscess, and postsurgical vaginal cuff infection.

Route, Dosage, Frequency
Trichomoniasis—nonpregnant woman: 1 day treatment 2 g orally in a single dose, 7-day treatment: 500 mg orally twice a day for 7 consecutive days (CDC, 2006).

Amebiasis—Adults: 750 mg orally three times a day for 5–10 days; children: 35–50 mg/kg/24 hours orally divided into three doses for 10 days.

Bacterial vaginosis—nonpregnant woman: 500 mg orally twice a day for 7 consecutive days or one full applicator of metronidazole gel 0.75% intravaginally, once daily for 5 days (CDC, 2006).

Contraindications
Blood dyscrasias
Breastfeeding women (drug secreted in breast milk)
Impaired kidney or liver function
Active CNS disease

Side Effects
Convulsive seizures	Weakness
Peripheral neuropathy	Insomnia
Nausea/Vomiting	Cystitis
Headache	Dysuria

Anorexia	Reversible neutropenia and thrombocytopenia
Diarrhea	Flattening of the T wave on ECG
Epigastric distress	Polyuria
Abdominal cramping	Incontinence
Constipation	Pelvic pressure
Metallic taste in mouth	Proliferation of *Candida* in the vagina and mouth
Dizziness	Joint pains
Vertigo	Decreased libido
Uncoordination	Dryness in the mouth, vulva, and vagina
Ataxia	Dyspareunia
Confusion	Depression
Irritability	

Nursing Considerations
- Inform woman about potential side effects.
- Stress the importance of contraceptive compliance during course of treatment.
- Obtain baseline renal and liver function tests as ordered.
- Teach woman about the signs, symptoms, and treatment of vulvovaginal candidiasis.
- Counsel the woman to avoid alcoholic beverages while taking the medication.
- If the woman is taking oral contraceptives, a backup nonhormonal contraceptive method is recommended during treatment.
- Take thorough history to rule out the woman's exposure to this medication within the last 6 weeks.
- Teach woman to monitor the signs and symptoms of her infection.
- Encourage cooperation with the entire course of treatment.

clindamycin. BV during pregnancy may be a factor in premature rupture of the membranes and preterm birth.

Vulvovaginal Candidiasis

Vulvovaginal candidiasis (VVC), also called moniliasis or yeast infection, is one of the most common forms of vaginitis that women experience. Estimates suggest that, in their lifetime, 75% of women will have at least one episode of VVC (CDC, 2006). Recurrences are frequent for some women. *Candida albicans* is the fungal species responsible for most vaginal yeast infections. Factors that contribute to the occurrence of this infection are the use of oral contraceptives, immunosuppressants, and antibiotics, which destroy populations of normal bacteria that usually keep the yeast cells in check. Other factors are frequent douching, pregnancy, and diabetes mellitus.

The woman with VVC often complains of thick, curdy vaginal discharge, severe itching, dysuria, and dyspareunia. A male sexual partner may experience a rash or excoriation of the skin of the penis and possibly pruritus. The male may be symptomatic and the female asymptomatic.

On physical examination, the woman's labia may be swollen and excoriated if pruritus has been severe. A speculum examination reveals thick, white, tenacious cheeselike patches adhering to the vaginal mucosa. Diagnosis is confirmed by microscopic examination of the vaginal discharge; hyphae and spores are usually seen on a wet-mount preparation (Figure 6–2 ■).

Medical treatment of VVC includes intravaginal butoconazole, miconazole, tioconazole, terconazole, clotrimazole, or nystatin suppositories, cream, or tablets. Single-dose and short-course (3 days) approaches are effective for 80% to 90% of women with uncomplicated VVC. Oral fluconazole, 150 mg in a single dose, is also effective for mild VVC (CDC, 2006). If the vulva is also infected, the cream is applied topically. Some of the topical medications indicated for women with a history of yeast infections who clearly recognize the symptoms are available over the counter.

Treatment of the male partner is generally not necessary unless candidal balanitis (inflammation of the glans penis) is present or if the man's partner has recurrent infection. Then treatment with a topical antifungal medication is indicated (CDC, 2006).

If a woman experiences recurrent VVC (four or more symptomatic episodes in a year), she should be tested for an elevated blood glucose level to determine whether a diabetic or prediabetic condition is present. Women at high risk for sexually transmitted infections should also be tested for HIV. Recurrent infection is then treated with an intensive regimen of oral and local agents for 7 to 14 days followed by maintenance antifungal therapy. Pregnant women with VVC are treated only with topical azole preparations applied for 7 days (CDC, 2006). Infection at the time of birth may cause thrush (a mouth infection) in the newborn.

Nursing Care Management

Nursing Assessment and Diagnosis

The nurse should suspect VVC if a woman complains of intense vulvar itching and a curdy, white discharge. Because pregnant women with diabetes mellitus are especially susceptible to this infection, the nurse should be alert for symptoms in these women. In some areas nurses are trained to do speculum examinations and wet-mount preparations and can confirm the diagnosis themselves. In most cases, however, the nurse who suspects a vaginal infection reports it to the woman's healthcare provider (see Key Facts to Remember: Vaginitis).

Nursing diagnoses that might apply to the woman with VVC include the following:

- *Risk for Impaired Skin Integrity* related to scratching secondary to discomfort of the infection
- *Health-Seeking Behaviors: Information About Yeast Infection* related to an expressed desire to learn about ways of preventing the development of VVC

Nursing Plan and Implementation

If the woman is experiencing discomfort because of pruritus, the nurse can recommend gentle bathing of the vulva with a weak sodium bicarbonate solution. If a topical treatment is being used, the woman will need to bathe the area before applying the medication.

The nurse also discusses with the woman the factors that contribute to the development of VVC and suggests ways to prevent recurrences, such as wearing cotton underwear and avoiding vaginal powders or sprays that may irritate the vulva. Some women report that the addition

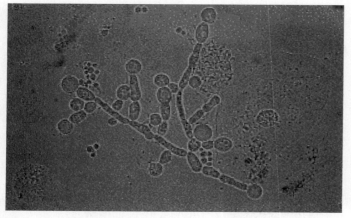

Figure 6–2 Hyphae and spores of *Candida albicans*, the fungus responsible for vulvovaginal candidiasis.
Source: Centers for Disease Control and Prevention (CDC).

KEY FACTS TO REMEMBER

Vaginitis

To distinguish among the common types of vaginitis and their treatments, it is useful to remember the following:

Vulvovaginal Candidiasis (Moniliasis)

Cause: Candida albicans
Appearance of discharge: Thick, curdy, like cottage cheese
Diagnostic test: Slide of vaginal discharge (treated with potassium hydroxide [KOH]) shows characteristic hyphae and spores
Treatment: Clotrimazole vaginal cream or suppositories

Bacterial Vaginosis (*Gardnerella Vaginalis* Vaginitis)

Cause: Gardnerella vaginalis
Appearance of discharge: Gray, milky
Diagnostic test: Slide of vaginal discharge shows characteristic "clue" cells
Treatment: Metronidazole

Trichomoniasis

Cause: Trichomonas vaginalis
Appearance of discharge: Greenish white and frothy
Diagnostic test: Saline slide of vaginal discharge shows motile flagellated organisms
Treatment: Metronidazole

of yogurt to the diet or the use of activated culture of plain yogurt as a vaginal douche helps prevent recurrence by maintaining high levels of lactobacilli. For the same reason, some clinicians recommend that women who are taking antibiotics consume "probiotics" supplements (containing acidophilus and other helpful bacteria) simultaneously.

Evaluation

Expected outcomes of nursing care include the following:

- The woman's symptoms are relieved and the infection is cured.
- The woman is able to identify self-care measures to prevent further episodes of VVC.

Care of the Woman with a Sexually Transmitted Infection

The occurrence of **sexually transmitted infection (STI)**, or *sexually transmitted disease (STD)*, has increased over the past few decades. In fact, vaginitis and STIs are the most common reasons for outpatient, community-based treatment of women.

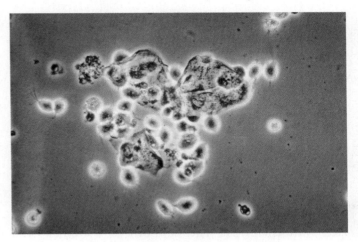

FIGURE 6–3 Microscopic appearance of *Trichomonas vaginalis*.
Source: Courtesy of Centers for Disease Control and Prevention (CDC).

Trichomoniasis

Trichomoniasis is an infection caused by *Trichomonas vaginalis*, a microscopic motile protozoan that thrives in an alkaline environment. Almost all infections are acquired through sexual intimacy. Transmission by shared bath facilities, wet towels, or wet swimsuits—though possible—is unlikely.

Symptoms of trichomoniasis include a yellow-green, frothy, odorous discharge frequently accompanied by inflammation of the vagina and cervix, vulvar itching, dysuria, and dyspareunia. Visualization of *T. vaginalis* under the microscope on a wet-mount preparation of vaginal discharge confirms the diagnosis (Figure 6–3 ■).

Treatment for trichomoniasis is metronidazole (Flagyl) administered in a single 2-g dose for both male and female sexual partners; a 7-day regimen is also available (CDC, 2006). Partners should avoid intercourse until both are cured (see Key Facts to Remember: Vaginitis). Pregnant women with trichomoniasis may be at increased risk for premature rupture of the membranes, preterm birth, and low birth weight. Pregnant women who are symptomatic should be treated with a single 2-g dose of metronidazole (CDC, 2006).

CRITICAL THINKING

Ella Matlosz is a 21-year-old, single woman, never pregnant, who comes to the office today complaining of excessive, odorous vaginal discharge. She uses an IUD for contraception and has several sex partners. She states that she douches with a medicated douche after intercourse. What should you tell Ella about feminine hygiene? What would you tell Ella about the relationship between contraceptives and sexually transmitted infections?

Answers can be found in Appendix F ∞.

Chlamydial Infection

Chlamydial infection, caused by *Chlamydia trachomatis*, is the most common bacterial STI in the United States. The organism is an intracellular bacterium with several different immunotypes. Strains of chlamydia are responsible for lymphogranuloma venereum and trachoma, which is the world's leading cause of preventable blindness.

Chlamydia is a major cause of nongonococcal urethritis (NGU) in men. In women it can cause infections similar to those that occur with gonorrhea. It can infect the fallopian tubes, cervix, urethra, and Bartholin's glands. Pelvic inflammatory disease, infertility, and ectopic pregnancy are associated with chlamydia. The newborn of a woman with untreated chlamydia is at risk of developing ophthalmia neonatorum, which responds to erythromycin ophthalmic ointment but not to silver nitrate eye prophylaxis at birth. The newborn may also develop chlamydia pneumonia.

Symptoms of chlamydia include a thin or purulent discharge, burning and frequency of urination, and lower abdominal pain. Women, however, are often asymptomatic. Diagnosis is often made after treatment of a male partner for NGU or in a symptomatic woman with a negative gonorrhea culture. Of the laboratory tests available to diagnose chlamydia, nucleic acid amplification testing (NAAT) is the most sensitive. Other tests for diagnosis include culture, direct immunofluorescence, EIA, and nucleic acid hybridization tests (CDC, 2006). The recommended treatment is a single 1-g dose of azithromycin orally or doxycycline orally twice daily for 7 days. Sexual partners should be treated, and couples should abstain from intercourse for 7 days (CDC, 2006). Doxycycline is contraindicated in pregnancy. The CDC (2006) recommends that pregnant women be treated with azithromycin or amoxacillin.

Gonorrhea

Gonorrhea is an infection caused by the bacteria *Neisseria gonorrhoeae*. If a nonpregnant woman contracts the disease, she is at risk of developing pelvic inflammatory disease. If a woman becomes infected after the third month of pregnancy, the mucous plug in the cervix will prevent the infection from ascending, and it will remain localized in the urethra, cervix, and Bartholin's glands until the membranes rupture. Then it can spread upward.

Because the majority of women with gonorrhea are asymptomatic, it is accepted practice to screen for this infection by doing a cervical culture during the initial prenatal examination. For women at high risk, the culture may be repeated during the last month of pregnancy. Cultures of the urethra, throat, and rectum may also be required for diagnosis, depending on the body orifices used for intercourse.

The most common symptoms of gonorrheal infection include a purulent, greenish yellow vaginal discharge, dysuria, and urinary frequency. Some women also develop inflammation and swelling of the vulva. The cervix may appear swollen and eroded and may secrete a foul-smelling discharge in which gonococci are present.

Treatment for nonpregnant women consists of antibiotic therapy with ceftriaxone or cefixime plus treatment for chlamydia if chlamydia has not been ruled out (CDC, 2007b). This combined approach is used because gonorrhea and chlamydia often occur together. Additional treatment may be required if the cultures remain positive 7 to 14 days after completion of treatment. All sexual partners must also be treated or the woman may become reinfected. Pregnant women should be treated with ceftriaxone intramuscularly or cefixime orally. This treatment is combined with azithromycin or amoxicillin to address the risk of co-infection with chlamydia (CDC, 2006).

Women should be informed of the need for reculture to verify cure and the need for abstinence or condom use until a cure is confirmed. Both sexual partners should be treated if either has a positive test for gonorrhea.

Herpes Genitalis

Herpes infections are caused by the herpes simplex virus (HSV). Two types of herpes infections can occur: HSV-1 (the cold sore), which can cause genital herpes through oral–genital contact, and HSV-2, which is usually associated with genital infections. The clinical symptoms and treatment of both types are the same. At least 50 million people in the United States have been diagnosed with genital HSV-2 infection—**herpes genitalis** (Hill-Brusselle, 2008).

The primary episode of herpes genitalis is characterized by the development of single or multiple blisterlike vesicles, which usually occur in the genital area and sometimes affect the vaginal walls, cervix, urethra, and anus. The vesicles may appear within a few hours to 20 days after exposure and rupture spontaneously to form very painful, open, ulcerated lesions. Inflammation and pain secondary to the presence of herpes lesions can cause difficult urination and urinary retention. Inguinal lymph node enlargement may be present. Flulike symptoms and genital pruritus or tingling also may be noticed. Primary episodes usually last the longest and are the most severe. Lesions heal spontaneously in 2 to 4 weeks.

After the lesions heal, the virus enters a dormant phase, residing in the nerve ganglia of the affected area. Some individuals never have a recurrence, whereas others have regular recurrences. Such recurrences are usually less severe than the initial episode and seem to be triggered by emotional stress, menstruation, ovulation, pregnancy, frequent or vigorous intercourse, poor health status or a generally run-down physical condition, tight clothing, or overheating. Diagnosis is made on the basis of the clinical appearance of the lesions, culture of the lesions, polymerase chain reaction (PCR) identification, and glycoprotein G-based Type-specific assays (Herpe Select™, Biokit HSV-2, and Sure Vue HSV-2) (CDC, 2006).

No known cure for herpes exists. Medications are available to provide relief from pain and prevent complications from secondary infection. The recommended treatment of the first clinical episode of genital herpes is oral acyclovir, valacyclovir, or famciclovir. These same medications, in somewhat different dosages, are also recommended for recurrent herpes infection and for daily suppression therapy for people who have frequent recurrences. Therapy should be started during the prodromal period for the greatest benefit. Because there is more documented information on use of acyclovir during pregnancy it may be administered orally to pregnant women with first-episode genital herpes or severe recurrent herpes. Its use in the third trimester may reduce the incidence of cesarean births by decreasing the incidence of recurrences at term (CDC, 2006).

Self-help suggestions include cleansing with povidone-iodine (Betadine) solution to prevent secondary infection and with Burow's solution to relieve discomfort. Use of vitamin C or lysine is frequently suggested to prevent recurrence, although studies have not documented the effectiveness of these supplements. Keeping the genital area clean and dry, wearing loose clothing, and wearing cotton underwear or none at all will promote healing. Primary and recurrent lesions will heal without prescriptive therapies.

If herpes is present in the genital tract of a woman during childbirth, it can have a devastating, even fatal, effect on the newborn. For further discussion, see Chapter 16 ∞.

Syphilis

Syphilis is a chronic infection caused by the spirochete *Treponema pallidum*. Syphilis can be acquired congenitally through transplacental inoculation and can result from maternal exposure to infected exudate during sexual contact or from contact with open wounds or infected blood. The incubation period varies from 10 to 90 days, and even though no symptoms or lesions are noted during this time, the woman's blood contains spirochetes and is infectious.

Syphilis is divided into early and late stages. During the early stage (primary), a chancre appears at the site where the *T. pallidum* organism entered the body. Symptoms include slight fever, weight loss, and malaise. The chancre persists for about 4 weeks and then disappears. In 6 weeks to 6 months, secondary symptoms appear. Skin eruptions called condylomata lata, which resemble wartlike plaques and are highly infectious, may appear on the vulva. Other secondary symptoms are acute arthritis, enlargement of the liver and spleen, nontender enlarged lymph nodes, iritis, and a chronic sore throat with hoarseness. When infected in utero, the newborn exhibits secondary-stage symptoms of

syphilis. Transplacentally transmitted syphilis may cause intrauterine growth restriction, preterm birth, and stillbirth.

As a result of the disease's impact on the fetus in utero, serologic testing of every pregnant woman is recommended; some state laws require it. Testing is done at the initial prenatal screening and repeated in the third trimester. Blood studies in early pregnancy may be negative if the woman has only recently contracted the infection. Diagnosis is made by dark-field examination for spirochetes. Blood tests such as the venereal disease research laboratory (VDRL) test, rapid plasma reagin (RPR) test, or the more specific fluorescent treponemal antibody-absorption (FTA-ABS) test are commonly done.

For pregnant and nonpregnant women with syphilis of less than a year's duration, the CDC (2006) recommends 2.4 million units of benzathine penicillin G administered intramuscularly in a single dose. If syphilis is of long (more than a year) or unknown duration, 2.4 million units of benzathine penicillin G is given intramuscularly once a week for 3 weeks. If a woman is allergic to penicillin and nonpregnant, doxycycline or tetracycline can be given. The pregnant woman who is allergic to penicillin should be desensitized to penicillin and then treated with it (CDC, 2006). Maternal serologic testing may remain positive for 8 months, and the newborn may have a positive test for 3 months.

Human Papillomavirus/ Condylomata Acuminata

Condylomata acuminata, also called genital or *venereal warts*, is a common sexually transmitted condition caused by the human papillomavirus (HPV). Transmission can occur through vaginal, oral, or anal sex. The infection has received considerable attention because HPV is almost always the cause of cervical cancer (Schmidt, 2007).

Over 120 HPV subtypes have been identified. Of these about 30 can infect the genital tract (Scheinfeld & Lehman, 2006). HPV types 6 and 11 account for 90% of visible genital warts whereas HPV types 16 and 18 cause about 70% of cervical cancer (Schmidt, 2007).

Often a woman seeks medical care after noticing single or multiple soft, grayish pink, cauliflowerlike lesions in her genital area (Figure 6–4 ■). The moist, warm environment of the genital area is conducive to the growth of the warts, which may be present on the vulva, vagina, cervix, and anus. The incubation period following exposure is 3 weeks to 3 years, with the average being about 3 months.

Because condylomata sometimes resemble other lesions and malignant transformation is possible, all atypical, pigmented, and persistent warts should be biopsied and treatment should be instituted promptly. The CDC (2006) does not specify a treatment of choice for genital warts but recommends that treatment be determined

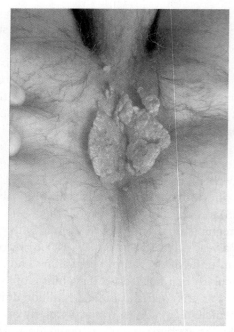

FIGURE 6–4 Condylomata acuminata on the vulva.
Source: Biophoto Associates/Photo Researchers, Inc.

based on client preference, available resources, and experience of the healthcare provider. Client-applied therapies include podofilox solution or gel or imiquimod cream. Provider-administered therapies include cryotherapy with liquid nitrogen or cryoprobe; topical podophyllin; trichloroacetic acid (TCA); bichloroacetic acid (BCA); intralesional interferon; surgical removal by tangential scissor excision, shave excision, curettage, or electrosurgery; or laser surgery (CDC, 2006). Imiquimod, podophyllin, and podofilox are not used during pregnancy because they are thought to be teratogenic and in large doses have been associated with fetal death.

In 2006 the U.S. Food and Drug Administration approved the first vaccine designed to protect against four types of HPV—types 6, 11, 16, and 18. The vaccine—Gardasil®—given in three doses, is recommended for females ages 11 to 26 (preferably before they are sexually active). The vaccine does not treat existing infections. However, if a woman in this age group has already been diagnosed with one of the vaccine virus strains, she can still receive the vaccine. Clinical trials have shown the vaccine offers protection against the other strains covered by the vaccine (CDC, 2007a). (See Evidence-Based Practice.)

Women who have received Gardasil® should still receive regular Pap smears because the vaccine does not protect against all HPV types. Women with diagnosed HPV infections should have frequent Pap smears to monitor cervical cellular changes. Sex partners are probably infected but do not require treatment unless large lesions are present. The use of male or female condoms may reduce the risk of transmitting the virus to an uninfected partner.

Acquired Immunodeficiency Syndrome

Acquired immunodeficiency syndrome (AIDS) is a fatal disorder caused by the human immunodeficiency virus (HIV). Medical–surgical texts more fully describe care of individuals with HIV and AIDS. However, because the diagnosis of HIV/AIDS or the presence of the HIV antibody has profound implications for a fetus if the woman is pregnant, AIDS is discussed in more detail in Chapter 15 ∞.

Nursing Care Management

Nursing Assessment and Diagnosis

Nurses working with women must become adept at taking a thorough history and identifying women at risk for STIs. Risk factors include multiple sexual partners, a partner's involvement with other partners, high-risk sexual behaviors such as intercourse without barrier contraception or anal intercourse, partners with high-risk behaviors, treatment with antibiotics while taking oral contraceptives, and young age at onset of sexual activity. Nurses should be alert for signs and symptoms of STIs and be familiar with diagnostic procedures if an STI is suspected.

Although each STI has certain distinctive characteristics, the following complaints suggest the possibility of infection and warrant further investigation:

- Presence of a sore or lesion on the vulva
- Increased vaginal discharge or malodorous vaginal discharge
- Burning with urination
- Vulvar/vaginal itching or irritation
- Dyspareunia
- Bleeding after intercourse
- Pelvic pain

In many instances the woman is asymptomatic but may report symptoms in her partner, especially painful urination or urethral discharge. It is often helpful to ask the woman whether her partner is experiencing any symptoms.

Nursing diagnoses that may apply when a woman has an STI include the following:

- *Interrupted Family Processes* related to the effects of a diagnosis of STI on the couple's relationship
- *Health-Seeking Behavior: Information on Preventing STIs* related to an expressed desire to prevent infection

Nursing Plan and Implementation

In a supportive, nonjudgmental way the nurse provides the woman who has an STI with information about the infec-

EVIDENCE-BASED PRACTICE

Recommendations for Administering the Human Papillomavirus Vaccines

Clinical Question
Who needs the human papillomavirus vaccine? When should it be administered?

The Evidence
Human papillomavirus (HPV) infection is a highly prevalent sexually transmitted infection. Prevalence rates as high as 82% have been found in some sexually active adolescent populations. The danger of this infection is its identification as a causal factor in cervical cancer. Two vaccines have been developed that prevent HPV types associated with more than 70% of cervical cancers. The Centers for Disease Control and Prevention convened an expert workgroup to review published and unpublished randomized trials of the HPV vaccine, including data on safety, efficacy, acceptability, and cost-effectiveness. The resulting recommendations represent the highest level of evidence resulting from the systematic review of multiple studies.

What Is Effective?
Clinical trials have demonstrated that the HPV vaccines are safe, effective, and well-tolerated without serious side effects. The CDC's Advisory Committee on Immunization Practices (ACIP) recommends routine vaccination with the quadrivalent HPV vaccine for all 11- to 12-year-old girls and catch-up vaccination for women 13 to 26 years old who have not been previously vaccinated. The vaccine is targeted at younger girls because it is most effective when initiated before sexual activity. Pap testing is not required before administration of the vaccine. Administer the vaccines at baseline, 2, and 6 months. When this schedule cannot be followed, separate the first and second doses by at least 4 weeks, and the second and third doses by at least 12 weeks. If the schedule is interrupted at any point, do not restart it, but administer the required dose as soon as possible. No therapeutic effects have been demonstrated in women with existing HPV infection, and so administration of the vaccines as a treatment option is not supported.

What Is Inconclusive?
The benefit for girls younger than 11 has not been determined. The ACIP recommendations leave the decision to vaccinate 9- or 10-year-old girls for the provider or parent to make. The vaccination is not harmful at this younger age, but it is unclear as to whether it provides adequate protection against subsequent infection with HPV. The vaccine is most effective when given before a girl becomes sexually active, but it may still provide protection among sexually active young women. Having initiated sexual activity is not identified as an exclusion criterion by the Committee. Sustained immunity has been measured at 5 years; protection beyond that time period is not confirmed. Vaccine efficacy in men has not yet been demonstrated.

Best Practice
Administration of the HPV vaccine to young girls before the initiation of sexual activity can prevent HPV safely. Given the association of HPV with cervical cancer, encourage routine administration of the vaccine for young women 11 to 12 years of age, and older women who have not previously been vaccinated. Vaccination provides an opportunity to discuss sexual health with both young women and their parents.

References
Brown, D., Shew, M., Quadadri, B., et al. (2005). A longitudinal study of genital human papillomavirus infection in a cohort of closely followed adolescent women. *Journal of Infectious Disease, 191,* 182–192.

Centers for Disease Control and Prevention. (2007). Quadrivalent human papillomavirus vaccine: recommendations of the Advisory Committee on Immunization Practices (ACIP). *MMWF, 56*(No. RR-2), 1–26.

Kahn, J., Lan, D., & Kahn, R. (2007). Sociodemographic factors associated with high-risk HPV infection in a national sample of U.S. women. *Obstetrics and Gynecology, 110,* 87–95.

tion, methods of transmission, implications for pregnancy or future fertility, and the importance of thorough treatment. If treatment of her partner is indicated, the woman must understand that it is necessary to prevent a cycle of reinfection. She should also understand the need to abstain from sexual activity, if necessary, during treatment.

Some STIs such as trichomoniasis or chlamydia may cause a woman concern but, once diagnosed, are rather simply treated. Other STIs may also be fairly simple to treat medically but may carry a stigma and be emotionally devastating for the woman. Thus the nurse should stress prevention with all women and encourage them to require partners, especially new partners, to use condoms.

The nurse can be especially helpful in encouraging the woman to explore her feelings about the diagnosis. She may experience anger or feel betrayed by a partner, she may feel guilt or see her diagnosis as a form of punishment, or she may feel concern about the long-term implications for future childbearing or ongoing intimate relationships. She may experience a myriad of emotions that she never expected. Opportunities to discuss her feelings in a nonjudgmental environment can be very helpful. The nurse can offer suggestions about support groups, if indicated.

More subtly, the nurse's attitude of acceptance and matter-of-factness conveys to the woman that she is still an acceptable person who happens to have an infection. Table 6–1 provides basic information the nurse should share with women who have an STI or who are at risk for infection.

TABLE 6–1	Preventing STIs and Their Consequences

The risk of contracting an STI increases with the number of sexual partners. Because of the extended time between infection with HIV and evidence of infection, intercourse with an individual exposes a female or male to all the other sexual partners of that individual for the past 5 or more years. In light of this risk, it is important to take the following actions:

- Plan ahead and develop strategies to refuse sex (especially important for adolescents who may be less confident about saying "no" to casual sexual encounters), because abstinence is the best method of preventing STIs.

- Limit the number of sexual contacts and practice mutual monogamy.

- The condom is the best contraceptive method currently available (other than abstinence) for protection from STIs. Use one for every act of vaginal and anal intercourse. Other contraceptives such as the diaphragm, cervical cap, and spermicides also offer some protection against STIs.

- Plan strategies for negotiating condom use with a partner.

- Reduce high-risk behaviors. Use of recreational drugs and alcohol can increase sexual risk taking.

- Refrain from oral sex if your partner has active sores in mouth, vagina, or anus or on penis.

- Seek care as soon as you notice symptoms and make sure your partner gets treatment if indicated. Absence of symptoms or disappearance of symptoms does not mean that treatment is unnecessary if you suspect an STI. Take all prescribed medications completely.

- The presence of a genital infection may lead to an abnormal Pap smear. Women with certain infections should have more frequent Pap tests according to a schedule recommended by their caregiver. Ask your healthcare provider if you need more frequent Paps.

Evaluation

Expected outcomes of nursing care include the following:

- The infection is identified and cured, if possible. If not, supportive therapy is provided.
- The woman and her partner can describe the infection, its method of transmission, its implications, and the therapy.
- The woman copes successfully with the impact of the diagnosis on her self-concept.

Care of the Woman with Pelvic Inflammatory Disease

Pelvic inflammatory disease (PID) is a clinical syndrome of inflammatory disorders of the upper female genital tract that includes any combination of endometritis, salpingitis (tubal infection), tubo-ovarian abscess, pelvic abscess, and pelvic peritonitis (CDC, 2006). In the United States an estimated 1 million cases of PID are diagnosed annually and more than 100,000 women become infertile as a result of it (CDC, 2004). The disease is more common in women who have had multiple sexual partners, a history of PID, early onset of sexual activity, or recent insertion of an intrauterine device and in women who douche regularly (Mayo Clinic, 2005). Perhaps the greatest problem of PID is postinfection tubal damage, which is closely associated with infertility.

The organisms most frequently identified with PID include *Chlamydia trachomatis* and *Neisseria gonorrhoeae*. Bacterial vaginosis may facilitate the ascending spread of pathogens.

Symptoms of PID include bilateral sharp, cramping pain in the lower quadrants, fever, chills, purulent vaginal discharge, irregular bleeding, malaise, nausea, and vomiting. However, it is also possible to be asymptomatic and have normal laboratory values.

Diagnosis consists of a clinical examination to define symptoms, plus cultures for gonorrhea and chlamydia, a complete blood count (CBC) with differential, and an RPR or VDRL to test for syphilis. Often the woman with PID has an elevated C-reactive protein and elevated sedimentation rate. Physical examination usually reveals direct abdominal tenderness with palpation, adnexal tenderness, and cervical and uterine tenderness with movement (chandelier sign). A palpable mass is evaluated with ultrasound. Laparoscopy may be used to confirm the diagnosis and to enable the examiner to obtain cultures from the fimbriated ends of the fallopian tubes.

The decision to hospitalize is based on clinical judgment. Inpatient treatment includes intravenous (IV) fluids, pain medications, and IV antibiotics—often either cefotetan or cefoxitin, plus doxycycline or clindamycin plus gentamicin. Outpatient oral therapy usually includes ceftriaxone plus doxycycline with or without metronidazole (CDC, 2004). Other antibiotic combinations may also be used. In addition, supportive therapy is often indicated for severe symptoms. The sexual partner should be treated. If the woman has an IUD, it is generally removed 24 to 48 hours after antibiotic therapy is started.

Nursing Care Management

Nursing Assessment and Diagnosis

The nurse is alert to factors in a woman's history that put her at risk for PID. Even though fewer types of IUDs are available, many women still have them, and the nurse should question the woman about possible symptoms, such as aching pain in the lower abdomen, foul-smelling discharge, malaise, and the like. The woman who is acutely ill will have obvious symptoms, but a low-grade infection is more difficult to detect.

Nursing diagnoses that may apply to a woman with PID include the following:

- *Acute Pain* related to peritoneal irritation
- *Deficient Knowledge* related to a lack of information about the possible effects of PID on fertility

Nursing Plan and Implementation

The nurse plays a vital role in helping to prevent or detect PID. Accordingly, the nurse spends time discussing risk factors related to this infection. The woman who uses an IUD for contraception and has multiple sexual partners needs to understand clearly the risk she faces. The nurse discusses signs and symptoms of PID and stresses the importance of early detection.

The woman who develops PID should be counseled on the importance of completing her antibiotic treatment and of returning for follow-up evaluation. She should also understand the possibility of decreased fertility following the infection.

Evaluation

Expected outcomes of nursing care include the following:

- The woman describes her condition, her therapy, and the possible long-term implications of PID on her fertility.
- The woman completes her course of therapy and the PID is cured.

Care of the Woman with an Abnormal Finding During Pelvic Examination

Except in the most benign situations, an abnormal finding resulting from a pelvic examination typically sparks concern and even fear. It requires careful follow-up, appropriate interventions, and good psychologic support for the woman and her family.

Abnormal Pap Smear Results

As discussed in Chapter 5 ∞, a Papanicolaou (Pap) smear is a cervical cytology test done to screen for the presence of cellular abnormalities by obtaining a sample containing cells from the cervix and the endocervical canal. Although the Pap smear is useful in detecting a variety of abnormalities, it has had its greatest impact on *cervical cancer*, once the leading type of cancer in women in the United States. Cervical cancer is now considered a preventable disease because it is slow growing, has a lengthy preinvasive state, has inexpensive and readily available screening programs, and has effective treatment approaches for preinvasive lesions.

The *Bethesda system* (Table 6–2) has become the most widely used system in the United States for reporting Pap smear results. The system provides a uniform format and classification of terminology based on current understanding of cervical disease.

The Pap smear is a screening tool; consequently, an abnormal finding requires further assessment. Notification of an abnormal Pap smear usually causes anxiety for a woman, so it is important that she be told in a caring way. The woman needs accurate, complete information about the meaning of the results and the next steps to be taken. She should also be given time to ask questions and express her concerns.

Diagnostic or therapeutic procedures employed in cases of abnormalities include repetition of the Pap smear using the liquid-based medium Pap smear, Pap tests at shorter intervals, colposcopy and endocervical biopsy, cryotherapy, laser conization, or loop electrosurgical excision procedure (LEEP). Management is based on the specific report.

Colposcopy, the direct, detailed visualization and examination of the cervix, is done in most gynecologic offices and clinics. It has evolved as an appropriate second step in many cases of abnormal Pap. The examination permits more detailed visualization of the cervix in bright light, using a microscope with 6 to 40 times magnification. The cervix can be visualized directly and again following application of 3% acetic acid. The acetic acid causes abnormal epithelium to assume a characteristic white appearance. The colposcope can be used to localize and obtain a directed biopsy.

Women who had first coitus at an early age or have a history of (or a sex partner with a history of) multiple sexual partners, exposure to sexually transmitted infections, immunosuppressive therapy, or antenatal exposure to diethylstilbestrol (DES) have an increased risk of abnormal cell changes and cervical cancer.

Ovarian Masses

Ovarian masses may be palpated during the pelvic exam. Between 70% and 80% of ovarian masses are benign. More than 50% are functional cysts (cysts that develop from ovarian follicles, from the corpus luteum, or from the theca luteum), occurring most commonly in women 20 to 40 years of age. Functional cysts are associated with abnormal hormone production and are rare in women who take oral contraceptives.

Ovarian cysts usually represent physiologic variations in the menstrual cycle. Dermoid cysts (cystic teratomas) comprise 10% of all benign ovarian masses. Cartilage, bone, teeth, skin, or hair can be observed in these cysts. Endometriomas, or "chocolate cysts," are another common type of ovarian mass.

No relationship exists between the presence of benign ovarian masses and the subsequent development of ovarian cancer. However, ovarian cancer is the most fatal of all cancers in women because it is difficult to diagnose and often has spread throughout the pelvis before it is detected. Although ovarian cancer is occasionally diagnosed by a palpable mass, the most common initial symptoms include

MyNursingKit | Common Gynecological Cancers

TABLE 6–2	The Bethesda System for Classifying Pap Smears

Specimen Type

Indicate conventional smear (Pap smear) vs. liquid based vs. other

Specimen Adequacy

Satisfactory for evaluation *(describe presence or absence of endocervical/transformation zone component and any other quality indicators, e.g., partially obscuring blood inflammation, etc.)*

Unsatisfactory for evaluation… *(specify reason)*

Specimen rejected/not processed *(specify reason)*

Specimen processed and examined, but unsatisfactory for evaluation of epithelial abnormality because of *(specify reason)*

General Categorization (optional)

Negative for intraepithelial lesion or malignancy.

Epithelial cell abnormality. See Interpretation/Result *(specify 'squamous' or 'glandular' as appropriate).*

Other: See Interpretation/Result *(e.g., endometrial cells in a woman 40 years of age).*

Automated Review

If case examined by automated device, specify device and result.

Ancillary Testing

Provide a brief description of the test methods and report the result so that it is easily understood by the clinician.

Interpretation/Result

Negative for intraepithelial lesion or malignancy

(when there is no cellular evidence of neoplasia, state this in the General Categorization above and/or in the Interpretation/Result section of the report, whether or not there are organisms or other nonneoplastic findings)

ORGANISMS
   Trichomonas vaginalis

Fungal organisms morphologically consistent with *Candida* spp.

Shift in flora suggestive of bacterial vaginosis.

Bacteria morphologically consistent with *Actinomyces* spp.

Cellular changes associated with herpes simplex virus.

Other Nonneoplastic Findings *(Optional to report list not inclusive):* Reactive cellular changes associated with

- Inflammation (includes typical repair)
- Radiation
- Intrauterine contraceptive device (IUD)

Glandular cells status posthysterectomy

Atrophy

Other

Endometrial cells (in a woman 40 years of age) (Specify if negative for squamous intraepithelial lesion.)

Epithelial cell abnormalities

SQUAMOUS CELL

Atypical squamous cells

- Of undetermined significance (ASC-US)
- Cannot exclude HSIL (ASC-H)

Low-grade squamous intraepithelial lesion (LSIL)

- Encompassing HPV/mild dysplasia/CIN-1

High-grade squamous intraepithelial lesion (HSIL)

- Encompassing: moderate and severe dysplasia CIS/CIN-2 and CIN-3
- With features suspicious for invasion *(if invasion is suspected)*

Squamous cell carcinoma

GLANDULAR CELL

Atypical

- Endocervical cells *(NOS or specify in comments)*
- Endometrial cells *(NOS or specify in comments)*
- Glandular cells *(NOS or specify in comments)*

Atypical

- Endocervical cells, favor neoplastic
- Glandular cells, favor neoplastic

Endocervical adenocarcinoma in situ

Adenocarcinoma

- Endocervical
- Endometrial
- Extrauterine
- Not otherwise specified (NOS)

Other malignant neoplasms (specify)

Educational Notes and Suggestions (optional)

Suggestions should be concise and consistent with clinical follow-up guidelines published by professional organizations (references to relevant publications may be included).

Source: Courtesy of National Cancer Institute.

feelings of abdominal bloating, distention, pain, and weight loss. Gastrointestinal symptoms such as nausea, dyspepsia, diarrhea, or constipation also occur.

Many women with a benign ovarian mass are asymptomatic; the mass may be noted on a routine pelvic examination. Others experience a sensation of fullness or cramping in the lower abdomen (often unilateral), dyspareunia, irregular bleeding, or delayed menstruation.

Diagnosis is made on the basis of a palpable mass with or without tenderness and other related symptoms. Radi-

ography or ultrasonography may be used to assist in the diagnosis.

The woman is frequently kept under observation for a month or two because most cysts will resolve on their own and are harmless. Oral contraceptives may be prescribed for 1 to 2 months to suppress ovarian function. If this regimen is effective, a repeat pelvic examination should be normal. If the mass is still present after 60 days of observation and oral contraceptive therapy, a diagnostic laparoscopy or laparotomy may be considered. Tubal or ovarian lesions, ectopic pregnancy, cancer, infection, or appendicitis also must be ruled out before a diagnosis can be confirmed.

Surgery is not always necessary but will be considered if the mass is larger than 6 to 7 cm in circumference; if the woman is over 40 years of age with an adnexal mass, a persistent mass, or continuous pain; or if the woman is taking oral contraceptives. Surgical exploration is also indicated when a palpable mass is found in an infant, a young girl, or a postmenopausal woman.

Women who are taking oral contraceptives should be informed of their preventive effect against ovarian masses. Women may need clear explanations about why the initial therapy is observation. A discussion of the origin and resolution of ovarian cysts may clarify this treatment plan. If a surgical treatment removes or impairs the function of one ovary, the woman needs to be assured that the remaining ovary can be expected to take over ovarian functioning and that pregnancy is still possible.

Uterine Abnormalities

Fibroid tumors, or *leiomyomas*, are among the most common benign disease entities in women and are the most common reason for gynecologic surgery. Between 25% and 44% of premenopausal women over age 30 develop leiomyomas (Hutchins, 2008). The potential for cancer is minimal. Leiomyomas are more common in women of African heritage.

Fibroid tumors develop when smooth muscle cells are present in whorls and arise from uterine muscles and connective tissue. The size varies from 1 to 2 cm to the size of a 10-week fetus. Frequently the woman is asymptomatic. Lower abdominal pain, fullness or pressure, menorrhagia, metrorrhagia, or increased dysmenorrhea may occur, particularly with large leiomyomas. Ultrasonography revealing masses or nodules can assist and confirm the diagnosis. Leiomyoma is also considered when masses or nodules involving the uterus are palpated on a pelvic examination.

During pregnancy, if a leiomyoma is present in the lower uterine segment or cervix, it may prevent the normal vertex (head-first) presentation of the infant, leading to a breech presentation or transverse lie (see Chapter 17 ∞). If a section of the placenta implants over a leiomyoma, it increases the risk that the placenta will separate too soon (abruptio placentae), which is a serious complication. Often this problem can be detected on ultrasound and an early elective birth can be scheduled.

The majority of these masses require no treatment and will shrink after menopause. Close observation for symptoms or an increase in size of the uterus or the masses is the only management most women will require. Routine pelvic examinations every 3 to 6 months are recommended unless new symptoms appear.

If a woman is troubled by symptoms, or pelvic examination reveals that the mass is increasing in size, interventions are recommended. *Myomectomy* (surgical removal of the fibroid) is used most often if the woman wishes to maintain her ability to have a child. However, fibroids may re-grow after myomectomy. *Hysterectomy* is often used to treat fibroids when the primary symptom is heavy menstrual bleeding. It is a definitive treatment but does have potential complications. *Uterine artery embolization (UAE)* is gaining popularity as a viable alternative for women who wish to avoid hysterectomy (Hehenkamp, Volkers, Birnie et al., 2008). Small particles are injected through a catheter placed in the umbilical artery. These particles block the blood supply to the fibroid, leading to shrinkage and symptom relief. If symptoms recur, hysterectomy may be necessary.

Endometrial cancer is the most common female genital tract malignancy, occurring in about 1 of every 45 women. Fortunately it has a high rate of cure if detected early. The hallmark sign is vaginal bleeding in postmenopausal women not treated with hormone replacement therapy. Diagnosis is made by endometrial biopsy, by transvaginal ultrasound, or by posthysterectomy pathology examination of the uterus. The treatment is total abdominal hysterectomy (TAH) and bilateral salpingo-oophorectomy (BSO). Radiation therapy may also be indicated, depending on the stage of the cancer.

> **EVIDENCE IN ACTION**
> There is a strong association with lower pregnancy rates in women with submucosal fibroids.
> (Systematic literature review) (Klatsky, Tran, Caughey, & Fujimoto, 2008)

Nursing Care Management

Pelvic examinations and Pap smears are not done by nurses unless they have special training. In most cases, nursing assessment is directed toward an evaluation of the woman's understanding of the findings and their implications and her psychosocial response.

The woman needs accurate information on etiology, symptomatology, and treatment options. She should be encouraged to report symptoms and keep appointments for follow-up examination and evaluation. The woman needs realistic reassurance if her condition is benign; she may require counseling and effective emotional support if a malignancy is likely. If the management plan includes surgery, she may need the nurse's support in obtaining a second opinion and making her decision.

Care of the Woman with a Urinary Tract Infection

A **urinary tract infection (UTI)** is defined as significant bacteriuria in the presence of symptoms. Estimates indicate that about 11% of women have at least one diagnosed UTI per year, and approximately 60% of women will experience a UTI in their lifetime (American College of Obstetricians and Gynecologists [ACOG], 2008). Bacteria usually enter the urinary tract by way of the urethra. The organisms are capable of migrating against the downward flow of urine. The shortness of the female urethra facilitates the passage of bacteria into the bladder. Other conditions that are associated with bacterial entry are relative incompetence of the urinary sphincter, frequent enuresis (bedwetting) before adolescence, and urinary catheterization. Wiping from back to front after urination may transfer bacteria from the anorectal area to the urethra.

Voluntarily suppressing the desire to urinate is a predisposing factor. Retention overdistends the bladder and can lead to an infection. Sexual activity is a strong risk factor for UTI, especially in younger women. General poor health or lowered resistance to infection can increase a woman's susceptibility to UTI.

Asymptomatic bacteriuria (ASB) (bacteria in the urine actively multiplying without accompanying clinical symptoms) is a condition that becomes significant if a woman is pregnant because about 30% of pregnant women with untreated ASB will develop symptomatic UTIs (Smail, 2007). ASB is almost always caused by a single organism, typically *Escherichia coli*. If more than one type of bacteria is cultured, the possibility of urine-culture contamination must be considered.

A woman who has had a UTI is susceptible to recurrent infection. If a pregnant woman develops an acute UTI, especially with a high temperature, amniotic fluid infection may develop and retard the growth of the placenta.

Lower Urinary Tract Infection (Cystitis)

Because urinary tract infections are ascending, it is important to recognize and diagnose a lower UTI early to avoid the sequelae associated with upper UTI. *E. coli* is present in about 72% of women with UTIs. *Klebsiella pneumonia*, *Proteus mirabilis*, and *Enterococcus* species are the next most common causative organisms, especially in women over 50. *Staphylococcus* saprophyticus is more common in younger women (Czaja & Hooton, 2006).

When cystitis develops the initial symptom is often dysuria, specifically at the end of urination. Urgency and frequency also occur. Cystitis is usually accompanied by a low-grade fever (38.3°C [101°F] or lower), and hematuria is occasionally seen. Urine specimens usually contain an abnormal number of leukocytes and bacteria. Diagnosis is made with a urine culture.

Treatment depends on the causative organism. A 3-day course of an oral trimethoprim-sulfamethoxazole (TMP-SMZ) is recommended as first-line treatment. However TMP-SMZ resistant strains of organisms have developed.

In areas of high resistance, alternative treatments such as trimethoprim alone or a fluoroquinolone such as ciprofloxacin, levofloxacin, gatifloxacin, or noefloxacin is recommended (ACOG, 2008). (For treatment options during pregnancy, see Table 15–3 ∞.)

Upper Urinary Tract Infection (Pyelonephritis)

Pyelonephritis (inflammatory disease of the kidneys) is less common but more serious than cystitis and is often preceded by lower UTI. It is more common during the latter part of pregnancy or early postpartum and poses a serious threat to maternal and fetal well-being. Women with symptoms of pyelonephritis during pregnancy have an increased risk of preterm birth and of intrauterine growth restriction.

Acute pyelonephritis has a sudden onset, with chills, high temperature of 39.6°C to 40.6°C (103°F to 105°F), and flank pain (either unilateral or bilateral). The right side is almost always involved if the woman is pregnant because the large bulk of intestines to the left pushes the uterus to the right, putting pressure on the right ureter and kidney. Nausea, vomiting, and general malaise may ensue. With accompanying cystitis, the woman may experience frequency, urgency, and burning with urination.

Edema of the renal parenchyma or ureteritis with blockage and swelling of the ureter may lead to temporary suppression of urinary output. This is accompanied by severe colicky (spastic, intense) pain, vomiting, dehydration, and ileus of the large bowel. Women with acute pyelonephritis generally have increased diastolic blood pressure, positive fluorescent antibody titer (FA test), low creatinine clearance, significant bacteremia in urine culture, pyuria, and presence of white blood cell casts.

Women with acute pyelonephritis should have a urine culture and sensitivity done to determine the appropriate antibiotic. A woman who is severely ill or has complications may require hospitalization. She should be started on broad-spectrum intravenous (IV) antibiotics until the results of the culture and sensitivity are obtained. This treatment should be followed with an appropriate antibiotic. Therapy also includes IV hydration, urinary analgesics such as Pyridium, pain management, and medication to manage fever.

Many women can be treated as outpatients or given IV fluids and one IV dose of antibiotics, then discharged on oral medications. A 14-day regimen using a fluoroquinolone is first-line therapy although TMP-SMZ may be used in areas of low resistance (ACOG, 2008).

In the case of obstructive pyelonephritis, a blood culture is necessary. The woman is kept on bed rest. After the sensitivity report is received, the antibiotic is changed as necessary. If signs of urinary obstruction occur or continue, the ureter may be catheterized to establish adequate drainage.

With appropriate drug therapy, the woman's temperature should return to normal. The pain subsides and the urine shows no bacteria within 2 to 3 days. Follow-up urinary cultures are needed to determine that the infection has been eliminated completely.

Nursing Care Management

Nursing Assessment and Diagnosis

During a woman's visit, the nurse obtains a sexual and medical history to identify whether the client is at risk for UTI. A clean-catch urine specimen is evaluated for evidence of ASB.

Nursing diagnoses that may apply to a woman with an upper UTI include the following:

- *Acute Pain* related to dysuria, systemic discomforts, or renal pain secondary to upper UTI
- *Fear* related to the possible long-term effects of the disease

Nursing Plan and Implementation

The nurse provides the woman with information to help her recognize the signs of UTI, so she can contact her caregiver as soon as possible. The nurse also discusses hygiene practices, the advantages of wearing cotton underwear, and the need to void frequently to prevent urinary stasis. See Key Facts to Remember: Information for Women About Ways to Avoid Cystitis.

◈

KEY FACTS TO REMEMBER

Information for Women About Ways to Avoid Cystitis

- If you use a diaphragm for contraception, try changing methods or using another size of diaphragm.
- Avoid bladder irritants such as alcohol, caffeine products, and carbonated beverages.
- Increase fluid intake, especially water, to a minimum of six to eight glasses per day.
- Make regular urination a habit; avoid long waits.
- Practice good genital hygiene, including wiping from front to back after urination and bowel movements.
- Be aware that vigorous or frequent sexual activity may contribute to urinary tract infection.
- Urinate before and after intercourse to empty the bladder and cleanse the urethra.
- Complete medication regimens even if symptoms decrease.
- Do not use medication left over from previous infections.
- Drink cranberry juice to acidify the urine. This has been found to relieve symptoms in some cases.

The nurse stresses the importance of maintaining a good fluid intake. The nurse should also reinforce instructions and answer any questions the woman may have. UTIs usually respond quickly to treatment, but follow-up clinical evaluation and urine cultures are important.

Evaluation

Expected outcomes of nursing care include the following:

- The woman completes her prescribed course of antibiotic therapy.
- The woman's infection is cured.
- The woman incorporates preventive self-care measures into her daily regimen.

Care of the Woman with Pelvic Relaxation

A **cystocele** is the downward displacement of the bladder, which appears as a bulge in the anterior vaginal wall. Arbitrary classifications of mild to severe are frequently given. Genetic predisposition, childbearing, obesity, and increased age are factors that may contribute to cystocele.

Symptoms of stress urinary incontinence are most common, including loss of urine with coughing, sneezing, laughing, or sudden exertion. Vaginal fullness, a bulging out of the vaginal wall, or a dragging sensation may also be noticeable.

If pelvic relaxation is mild, Kegel exercises are helpful in restoring tone. The exercises involve contraction and relaxation of the pubococcygeal muscle (see Chapter 11 ∞). Women have found these exercises helpful before and after childbirth in maintaining vaginal muscle tone. Estrogen may improve the condition of vaginal mucous membranes, especially in menopausal women. Vaginal pessaries or rings may be used if surgery is undesirable or impossible or until surgery can be scheduled. Surgery may be considered for cystoceles considered moderate to severe.

The nurse can instruct the woman in the use of Kegel exercises. Information on causes and contributing factors and discussion of possible alternative therapies will greatly assist the woman.

A **rectocele** may develop when the posterior vaginal wall is weakened. The anterior wall of the rectum can then sag forward, ballooning into the vagina, pushing the weakened posterior wall of the vagina in front of it. When the woman strains to have a bowel movement, a pocket of rectum develops that traps stool, and constipation results. To defecate, a woman with a rectocele may find it necessary to press the tissue between the vagina and rectum, which elevates the rectocele.

Diagnosis is based on history and physical examination. Decisions about treatment are based on the size of the rectocele, the presence and severity of symptoms, and the woman's individual situation, including her overall health. Surgery is often indicated.

Uterine prolapse occurs when the uterus protrudes downward (drops) into the upper vagina, pulling the vagina with it. The extent of the prolapse is determined by the location of the cervix in the vagina. In severe cases the uterus may prolapse below the vaginal introitus. The woman may report a "dragging" sensation in her groin and a backache over the sacrum, which is caused by pulling on the uterosacral ligaments. Typically these symptoms are relieved when the woman lies down. As with cystocele, conservative treatment includes the use of topical or systemic estrogen and vaginal pessaries. Surgery for uterine prolapse often involves hysterectomy and repair of the prolapsed vaginal walls.

Care of the Woman Requiring a Hysterectomy

Hysterectomy is the surgical removal of the uterus. In the United States it is the most common nonpregnancy-related surgical procedure that women undergo. Removal of the uterus through a surgical incision is called a *total abdominal hysterectomy (TAH)* and removal of both fallopian tubes and ovaries is called a *bilateral salpingo-oophorectomy (BSO)*. When both procedures are performed at the same time it is called a TAH-BSO. When the uterus is removed through the vagina it is termed a *total vaginal hysterectomy (TVH)*.

Abdominal hysterectomy is the usual treatment for several conditions including cancer of the cervix, endometrium, or ovary; large fibroids; severe endometriosis; chronic pelvic inflammatory disease (PID); and adenomyosis. TAH is preferred when cancer is expected because it permits easier exploration of the abdomen. It is also helpful when large uterine masses are present.

Vaginal hysterectomy is generally done for pelvic relaxation, abnormal uterine bleeding, or small fibroids. Advantages of vaginal hysterectomy include earlier ambulation, less postoperative pain, less anesthesia and operative time, less blood loss, no visible scar, and a shorter hospital stay. The major disadvantage is the increased risk of trauma to the bladder.

Nursing Care Management

Nursing Assessment and Diagnosis

Preoperatively the nurse needs to identify the woman's physiologic and psychologic needs as she approaches surgery. Additionally it is important to evaluate her learning needs in relation to the surgery and its implications postoperatively. In assessing the woman, it is important to consider her age, her culture and educational level, the attitudes of her partner and family, her preoperative status, and whether the hysterectomy is being performed because of a cancer diagnosis. The significance of her reproductive health to her self-image is also a consideration.

Nursing diagnoses that may apply to a woman having a hysterectomy include the following:

- *Deficient Knowledge* related to a lack of information about preoperative routines, postoperative activities, and expected postoperative changes
- *Fear* related to the risk of possible surgical complications

Nursing Plan and Implementation

Preoperative teaching should include information about the procedure, expected preparation, effects of the anesthesia to be used, possible risks and complications, postoperative care routines, and expected recovery time. See Figure 6–5.

Routine postoperative care includes monitoring of physiologic and emotional responses and implementation of nursing interventions to ensure physical well-being and comfort. The woman should be aware of possible complications and when to follow up with her surgeon. Additionally it is important to follow up with the woman regarding any psychosocial implications discussed preoperatively, such as support at home and potential for sadness or depression related to perception of changed sexuality or self-image.

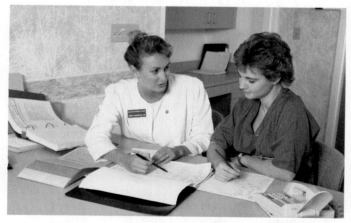

FIGURE 6–5 The nurse provides information for the woman during preoperative teaching.

Evaluation

Expected outcomes of nursing care include the following:

- The woman can discuss the reasons for her hysterectomy and the type of procedure performed, the alternatives, and aspects of self-care following surgery.
- The woman has an uneventful recovery without complications.
- The woman participates in decision making about her care.
- The woman can identify available resources if she has physical or emotional concerns in the postoperative period.

CHAPTER HIGHLIGHTS

- In fibrocystic breast changes, the cysts tend to be round, mobile, and well-delineated. The woman generally experiences increased discomfort premenstrually.
- Because of the increased risk of breast cancer, women with fibrocystic breast changes should understand the importance of monthly breast self-examination.
- Endometriosis is a condition in which endometrial tissue occurs outside the endometrial cavity. This tissue bleeds in a cyclic fashion in response to the menstrual cycle. The bleeding leads to inflammation, scarring, and adhesions. The primary symptoms include dysmenorrhea, dyspareunia, and infertility.
- Treatment of endometriosis may be medical, surgical, or a combination. For the woman not desiring pregnancy at present, oral contraceptives are used. Women desiring pregnancy are treated with danazol or GnRH analogs.
- Toxic shock syndrome, caused by a toxin of *Staphylococcus aureus*, is most common in women of childbearing age. There is an increased incidence in women who use tampons or barrier methods of contraception, such as the diaphragm and cervical cap.
- Bacterial vaginosis, a common vaginal infection, is diagnosed by its characteristic fishy odor and by the presence of "clue" cells on a vaginal smear. It is treated with metronidazole.
- Vulvovaginal candidiasis (moniliasis), a vaginal infection caused by *Candida albicans*, is most common in women who use oral contraceptives, are on antibiotics, are currently pregnant, or have diabetes mellitus. It is generally treated with intravaginal miconazole or clotrimazole suppositories or fluconazole orally.
- Chlamydial infection is difficult to detect in a woman but may result in pelvic inflammatory disease (PID) and infertility. It is treated with antibiotic therapy.
- Gonorrhea, a common sexually transmitted infection, may be asymptomatic in women initially but may cause PID if not diagnosed early. The treatment of choice is ceftriaxone and doxycycline or azithromycin.
- Herpes genitalis, caused by the herpes simplex virus, is a recurrent infection with no known cure. Acyclovir (Zovirax),

valacyclovir, or famciclovir may reduce the symptoms and decrease the length of viral shedding.
- Syphilis, caused by *Treponema pallidum*, is a sexually transmitted infection that is treatable if diagnosed. The characteristic lesion is the chancre. Syphilis can also be transmitted in utero to the fetus of an infected woman. The treatment of choice is penicillin.
- Condylomata acuminata (venereal or genital warts) are transmitted by the human papillomavirus (HPV). Treatment is indicated, because research suggests a link between certain strains of HPV and the development of cervical cancer. The treatment chosen depends on the size and location of the warts.
- Pelvic inflammatory disease may be life threatening and may lead to infertility. *C. trachomatis* and *N. gonorrhoeae* are the organisms that cause PID most frequently.
- Women with an abnormal finding on a pelvic examination need a careful explanation of the finding and techniques of diagnosis and emotional support during the diagnostic period.
- The classic symptoms of a lower urinary tract infection (UTI) are dysuria, urgency, frequency, and sometimes hematuria.
- An upper UTI is a serious infection that can permanently damage the kidneys if untreated. Generally the woman is acutely ill and requires supportive therapy as well as antibiotics.
- Three common forms of pelvic relaxation exist: A cystocele is a downward displacement of the bladder into the vagina. Often it is accompanied by stress incontinence. Kegel exercises may help restore tone in mild cases. A rectocele is displacement of the rectum into the vagina. Prolapse of the uterus is downward displacement of the cervix into the vagina.
- Hysterectomy is the most common nonpregnancy-related surgery performed in the United States. It may be done vaginally or abdominally and is sometimes accompanied by removal of the ovaries and fallopian tubes.

CHAPTER REFERENCES

American College of Obstetricians and Gynecologists (ACOG). (2008). Treatment of urinary tract infections in nonpregnant women (ACOG Practice Bulletin, No. 91). Washington, DC: Author.

Centers for Disease Control and Prevention (CDC). (2004). *Fact sheet: Pelvic inflammatory disease.* Retrieved October 24, 2007, from www.cdc.gov/std/PID/STDFact-PID.htm

Centers for Disease Control and Prevention (CDC). (2006). Sexually transmitted diseases treatment guidelines, 2006. *Mortality and Morbidity Weekly Report, 55*(RR-11), 1–94.

Centers for Disease Control and Prevention (CDC). (2007a). CDC questions and answers concerning the safety and efficacy of Gardasil®. Retrieved March 22, 2008, from www.CDC.gov

Centers for Disease Control and Prevention (CDC). (2007b). Update to CDC's sexually transmitted diseases treatment guidelines, 2006: Fluoroquinolones no longer recommended for treatment of gonococcal infection. *Mortality and Morbidity Weekly Report, 56*(14), 332–336.

Czaja, C. A., & Hooton, T. M. (2006). Update on acute uncomplicated urinary tract infection in women. *Postgraduate Medicine, 119*(1), 39–45.

Hehenkamp, W. J., Volkers, N. A., Birnie, E., Reekers, J. A., & Ankum, W. M. (2008).

Symptomatic uterine fibroids: Treatment with uterine artery embolization or hysterectomy–results from the randomized clinical Embolisation (sic) versus Hysterectomy (EMMY) Trial. *Radiology, 246*(3), 823–832.

Hill, K. (2003). Update: The pathogenesis and treatment of PCOS. *The Nurse Practitioner, 28,* 8–23.

Hill-Brusselle, D. L. (2008). Genital herpes: Diagnosis and counseling. *The Female Patient, 33*(3), 14–22.

Hutchins, F. L. (2008). New developments in uterine fibroid ablation. *The Female Patient, 33*(2), 47–52.

Jackson, M. L. (2004/2005). Ovarian syndrome: What nurses need to know about this misunderstood disorder. *AWHONN Lifelines, 8*(6), 512–518.

King, J. (2007). Polycystic ovary syndrome. *Journal of Midwifery and Women's Health, 51*(6), 415–422.

Klatsky, P. C., Tran, N. D., Caughey, A. B., & Fujimoto, V. Y. (2008). Fibroids and reproductive outcomes: A systematic literature review from conception to delivery. *American Journal of Obstetrics & Gynecology, April,* 357–366.

Mayo Clinic. (2005). *Pelvic inflammatory disease.* Retrieved February 20, 2006, from www.mayoclinic.com/health/pelvic-inflammatory-disease/DS00402/DSECTION-4

Ruhl, C. (2007). Breast health screening: What all women should know. *Nursing for Women's Health, 11*(3), 326–330.

Scheinfeld, N., & Lehman, D. S. (2006). An evidence-based review of medical and surgical treatments of genital warts. *Dermatology Online Journal, 12*(3), 1–19.

Schenken, R. S. (2003). Endometriosis. In J. R. Scott, R. S. Gibbs, B. Y. Karlan, & A. F. Haney (Eds.), *Danforth's obstetrics and gynecology* (9th ed., pp. 713–720). Philadelphia: Lippincott Williams & Wilkins.

Schmidt, J. V. (2007). HPV vaccine: Implications for nurses and patients. *Nursing for Women's Health, 11*(1), 83–87.

Snyder, B. S. (2006). The lived experience of women diagnosed with polycystic ovary syndrome. *Journal of Obstetric, Gynecologic and Neonatal Nursing, 35*(3), 385–392.

Smail, F. (2007). Asymptomatic bacteriuria in pregnancy. *Best Practice & Research Clinical Obstetrics and Gynaecology, 21*(3), 439–450.

CHAPTER 7

Families with Special Reproductive Concerns

When I first began working in genetics I focused primarily on the science of it, on the odds, on the disorders. Now I recognize the courage of those with known genetic disorders who must decide whether to risk childbirth, the commitment of those who care for and love children with profound disabilities, and the constant sorrow of those who lose a child because of a previously undetected genetic problem. This work is about people—not genes, not DNA, but people.

—A Nurse Genetic Counselor

LEARNING OUTCOMES

7-1. Compare the essential components of fertility with the possible causes of infertility.

7-2. Describe the elements of the preliminary investigation of infertility and the nurse's role in supporting/teaching clients during this phase.

7-3. Compare the indications for the tests and associated treatments, including assisted reproductive technologies, that are done in an infertility workup.

7-4. Explain the physiologic and psychologic effects of infertility on a couple to the nursing care management of the couple.

7-5. Describe the nurse's role as counselor, educator, and advocate for couples during infertility evaluation and treatment.

7-6. Distinguish couples who may benefit from preconceptual chromosomal analysis and prenatal testing when providing care to couples with special reproductive concerns.

7-7. Identify the characteristics of autosomal dominant, autosomal recessive, and X-linked (sex-linked) recessive disorders.

7-8. Compare prenatal and postnatal diagnostic procedures used to determine the presence of genetic disorders and the nursing considerations for each.

7-9. Examine the emotional impact on a couple undergoing genetic testing or coping with the birth of a baby with a genetic disorder, and explain the nurse's role in supporting the family undergoing genetic counseling.

Most couples who want children are able to conceive them with little difficulty. Pregnancy and childbirth usually take their normal course, and a healthy baby is born without problems. But some less fortunate couples are unable to fulfill their dream of having the desired baby because of infertility or genetic problems.

This chapter explores two particularly troubling reproductive problems facing some couples: the inability to conceive and the risk of bearing babies with genetic abnormalities.

Infertility

Infertility, a lack of conception despite unprotected sexual intercourse for at least 12 months (Kumar, Ghadir, Eskandari, & DeCherney, 2007), has a profound emotional, psychologic, and economic impact on affected couples and society. The term *sterility* is applied when there is an absolute factor preventing reproduction. **Subfertility** is used to describe a couple who has difficulty conceiving because both partners have reduced fertility. The term *secondary infertility* is applied to couples who have been unable to conceive after one or more successful pregnancies or who cannot sustain a pregnancy.

Approximately 10–15% of couples in their reproductive years are infertile in the United States (Wright & Johnson, 2008). Public perception is that the incidence of infertility is increasing, but in fact there has been no significant change in the proportion of infertile couples in the United States. What has changed is the composition of the infertile population; the infertility diagnosis has increased in the age group 25 to 44 because of delayed childbearing and the entry of the baby boom cohort into this age range in Western society.

The perception that infertility is on the rise may be related to the following factors:

- The deferring of marriage and then the desire to have a family shortly after marriage
- The increase in assisted reproductive techniques
- The increase in availability and use of infertility services
- The increase in insurance coverage of some ethnic groups for diagnosis of and treatment for infertility

- The increased number of childless women over age 35 seeking medical attention for infertility

Essential Components of Fertility

Understanding the elements essential for normal fertility can help the nurse identify the many factors that may cause infertility. The following components must be present for normal fertility.

Female partner

- The cervical mucus must be favorable to ensure survival of spermatozoa and facilitate passage to the upper genital tract.
- The fallopian tubes must be patent and have normal fimbriae with peristaltic movements toward the uterus to facilitate transport and interaction of ovum and sperm.
- The ovaries must produce and release normal ova in a regular, cyclic fashion.
- There must be no obstruction between the ovaries and the uterus.
- The endometrium must be in a physiologic state to allow implantation of the blastocyst and to sustain normal growth.
- Adequate reproductive hormones must be present.

Male partner

- The testes must produce spermatozoa of normal quality, quantity, and motility.
- The male genital tract must not be obstructed.
- The male genital tract secretions must be normal.
- Ejaculated spermatozoa must be deposited in the female vaginal tract in such a manner that they reach the cervix.

These normal findings are correlated with possible causes of deviation in Table 7–1. With timing and environment playing such a crucial role, it is an impressive natural phenomenon that the majority of couples in the United States are able to conceive. The remaining couples suffer infertility because of a male factor (40%), a female factor (40%), or either an unknown cause (unexplained infertility) or a problem with both partners (20%) (American Society of Reproductive Medicine, 2006b). Profes-

TABLE 7-1 Possible Causes of Infertility

Necessary Norms	Deviations from Normal
Female	
Favorable cervical mucus	Cervicitis, cervical stenosis, use of coital lubricants, antisperm antibodies (immunologic response)
Clear passage between cervix and tubes	Myomas, adhesions, adenomyosis, polyps, endometritis, cervical stenosis, endometriosis, congenital anomalies (e.g., septate uterus, diethylstilbestrol [DES] exposure)
Patent tubes with normal motility	Pelvic inflammatory disease, peritubal adhesions, endometriosis, intrauterine device (IUD), salpingitis (e.g., chlamydia, recurrent sexually transmitted infections [STIs]), neoplasm, ectopic pregnancy, tubal ligation
Ovulation and release of ova	Primary ovarian failure, polycystic ovarian disease, hypothyroidism, pituitary tumor, lactation, periovarian adhesions, endometriosis, premature ovarian failure, hyperprolactinemia, Turner syndrome
No obstruction between ovary and tubes	Adhesions, endometriosis, pelvic inflammatory disease
Endometrial preparation	Anovulation, luteal phase defect, malformation, uterine infection, Asherman syndrome
Male	
Normal semen analysis	Abnormalities of sperm or semen, polyspermia, congenital defect in testicular development, mumps after adolescence, cryptorchidism, infections, gonadal exposure to X-rays, chemotherapy, smoking, alcohol abuse, malnutrition, chronic or acute metabolic disease, medications (e.g., morphine, aspirin [ASA], ibuprofen), cocaine, marijuana use, constrictive underclothing, heat
Unobstructed genital tract	Infections, tumors, congenital anomalies, vasectomy, strictures, trauma, varicocele
Normal genital tract secretions	Infections, autoimmunity to semen, tumors
Ejaculate deposited at the cervix	Premature ejaculation, impotence, hypospadias, retrograde ejaculation (e.g., diabetic), neurologic cord lesions, obesity (inhibiting adequate penetration)

sional intervention can help approximately 65% of infertile couples achieve pregnancy.

Young couples with no history that is suggestive of reproductive disorders should be referred for infertility evaluation if they have been unable to conceive after at least 1 year of attempting to achieve pregnancy. An earlier workup is indicated in couples with positive history for fertility-lowering disease or advancing maternal age (Wright & Johnson, 2008). If the woman is over age 35, it may be appropriate to refer the couple after only 6 to 9 months of unprotected intercourse without conception. At age 25, when couples are the most fertile, in about 25% of cases, conception occurs within the first month of unprotected intercourse (Wright & Johnson, 2008).

Initial Investigation: Physical and Psychosocial Issues

The easiest and least intrusive infertility testing approach is used first. Extensive testing for infertility is avoided until data confirm that the timing of intercourse and length of coital exposure have been adequate. The nurse provides information about the most fertile times to have intercourse during the menstrual cycle. Teaching the couple the signs and timing of ovulation, the most effective times for intercourse within the cycle, and other fertility awareness behaviors may solve the problem (see Table 7–2). Primary assessment, including a comprehensive history (with a discussion of genetic conditions) and physical examination for any obvious causes of infertility, is done before a costly, time-consuming, and emotionally trying investigation is initiated.

During the first visit for the preliminary investigation, the nurse explains the basic infertility workup. The basic investigation depends on the couple's history and usually

TABLE 7-2 Suggestions for Improving Fertility

Avoid douching and artificial lubricants (gels, oils, saliva) that can alter sperm mobility. Prevent alteration of pH of vagina and introduction of spermicidal agents.

Promote retention of sperm. The male superior position with female remaining recumbent for at least 20 to 30 minutes after intercourse maximizes the number of sperm reaching the cervix.

Avoid leakage of sperm. Elevate the woman's hips with a pillow after intercourse for 20 to 30 minutes to allow liquefaction of seminal fluid and motility of the sperm toward the egg. Avoid getting up to urinate or shower for 1 hour after intercourse.

Maximize the potential for fertilization. Instruct the couple that it is optimal if sexual intercourse occurs every other day during the fertile period. Because each woman's menstrual cycle varies in length, the fertile period can extend from cycle day [CD] 7 through CD 17. Note CD 1 is considered the first day of actual menstrual flow.

Avoid emphasizing conception during sexual encounters to decrease anxiety and potential sexual dysfunction.

Maintain adequate nutrition and reduce stress. Stress-reduction techniques and good nutritional habits increase sperm production.

Explore other methods to increase fertility awareness, such as home assessment of cervical mucus and basal body temperature (BBT) recordings, and use of a home ovulation predictor kit (tests LH surge to time intercourse).

Consider incorporating culturally appropriate methods to enhance fertility.

includes assessment of ovarian function, cervical mucus adequacy and receptivity to sperm, sperm adequacy, tubal patency, and the general condition of the pelvic organs. Because about 40% of infertility is related to a male factor, a semen analysis should be one of the first diagnostic tests done before moving on to more invasive diagnostic procedures involving the woman.

The mutual desire to have children is a cornerstone of many marriages. A fertility problem is a deeply personal, emotion-laden area in a couple's life. The self-esteem of one or both partners may be threatened if the inability to conceive is perceived as a lack of virility or femininity (Klock, 2004). It is never easy to discuss one's sexual activ-

ity, especially when potentially irreversible problems with fertility exist. The nurse can provide comfort to couples by offering a sympathetic ear, a nonjudgmental approach, and appropriate information and instructions throughout the diagnostic and therapeutic process. Because counseling includes discussion of very personal matters, nurses who are comfortable with their own sexuality are able to establish rapport and elicit relevant information from couples with fertility problems.

The first interview should involve both partners and include a comprehensive history and physical examination. Table 7–3 lists the items in a complete infertility physical workup and laboratory evaluation for both part-

---

TABLE 7–3 Initial Infertility Physical Workup and Laboratory Evaluations

Female

Physical examination
Assessment of height, weight, blood pressure, temperature, and general health status
Endocrine evaluation of thyroid for exophthalmos, lid lag, tremor, or palpable gland
Optic fundi evaluation for presence of increased intracranial pressure, especially in oligomenorrheal or amenorrheal women (possible pituitary tumor)
Reproductive features (including breast and external genital area)
Physical ability to tolerate pregnancy

Pelvic examination
Papanicolaou (PAP) smear
Culture for gonorrhea if indicated and possibly chlamydia or mycoplasma culture (opinions vary)
Signs of vaginal infections (Chapter 6 ∞)
Shape of escutcheon (e.g., does pubic hair distribution resemble that of a male?)
Size of clitoris (enlargement caused by endocrine disorders)
Evaluation of cervix: old lacerations, tears, erosion, polyps, condition and shape of os, signs of infections, cervical mucus (evaluate for estrogen effect of spinnbarkeit and cervical ferning)

Bimanual examination
Size, shape, position, and motility of uterus
Presence of congenital anomalies
Evaluation for endometriosis
Evaluation of adnexa: ovarian size, cysts, fixations, or tumors

Rectovaginal examination
Presence of retroflexed or retroverted uterus
Presence of rectouterine pouch masses
Presence of possible endometriosis

Laboratory examination
Complete blood count
Sedimentation rate, if indicated
Serology
Urinalysis
Rh factor and blood grouping
Rubella IgG
Follicle-stimulating hormone (FSH) level regardless of age and regularity of menstrual cycles
If indicated depending on age and regularity of menstrual cycles: thyroid-stimulating hormone (TSH), prolactin levels (PRL), glucose tolerance test, hormonal assays including estradiol (E$_2$), luteinizing hormone (LH), mid-luteal progesterone (MLP), dehydroepiandrosterone (DHEA), androstenedione, testosterone, 17 alpha-hydroxy progesterone (17–OHP).

Male

Physical examination
General health (assessment of height, weight, blood pressure)
Endocrine evaluation (e.g., presence of gynecomastia)
Visual fields evaluation for bitemporal hemianopia (blindness in one-half of the visual field)
Abnormal hair patterns

Urologic examination
Presence or absence of phimosis (narrowing of the preputial orifice)
Location of urethral meatus
Size and consistency of each testis, vas deferens, and epididymis
Presence of varicocele (enlargement of spermatic cord veins above testicles)

Rectal examination
Size and consistency of prostate, with microscopic evaluation of prostate fluid for signs of infection
Size and consistency of seminal vesicles

Laboratory examination
Complete blood count
Sedimentation rate, if indicated
Serology
Urinalysis
Rh factor and blood grouping
Semen analysis
If indicated, testicular biopsy, buccal smear (to determine number of Barr bodies)
Hormonal assays, FSH, LH, prolactin

ners. Figure 7–1 ■ outlines the historical database, diagnostic tests usually performed, and healthcare interventions used in cases of infertility.

Assessment of the Woman's Fertility

After a thorough history and physical examination, both partners may undergo tests to identify causes of infertility. A thorough female evaluation includes assessment of the hypothalamic–pituitary axis in terms of ovulatory function, as well as structure and function of the cervix, uterus, fallopian tubes, and ovaries. See Chapter 3 ∞ for an in-depth discussion of the fertility cycle.

Evaluation of Ovulatory Factors

Ovulation problems account for approximately 15% of couples' infertility. For a review of female reproductive cycle characteristics, see Chapter 3 ∞.

BASAL BODY TEMPERATURE RECORDING One basic test of ovulatory function is the **basal body temperature (BBT)** recording, which aids in identifying follicular and luteal phase abnormalities. At the initial visit, the nurse instructs the woman in the technique of recording BBT on a special form. The woman is instructed to begin a new chart on the first day of every monthly cycle. The temperature can be taken with an oral or rectal thermometer that is calibrated by tenths of a degree, making slight temperature changes readily apparent. A special kind of thermometer (BBT) may be used to measure temperatures only between 35.6°C and 37.8°C (96°F and 100°F). In addition to the traditional or digital thermometers, tympanic thermometry, which provides a reading in only a few seconds, may also be a valid method.

The woman records daily variations on the temperature graph. The temperature graph shows a typical biphasic pattern during ovulatory cycles, whereas in anovulatory cycles it remains monophasic. The woman uses the readings on

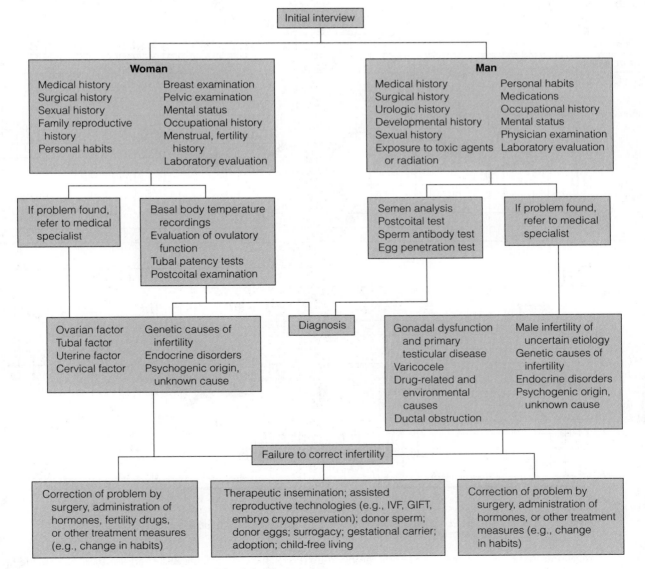

FIGURE 7–1 Flow chart for management of the infertile couple.

the temperature graph to detect ovulation and timing of intercourse (see Figure 7–2 ■).

Basal temperature for females in the preovulatory (follicular) phase is usually below 36.7°C (98°F). As ovulation approaches, production of estrogen increases and at its peak may cause a slight drop, then a rise, in the basal temperature. The slight drop in temperature before ovulation is often difficult to capture on the BBT chart. After ovulation, there is a surge of luteinizing hormone (LH), which stimulates production of progesterone. Because progesterone is thermogenic (produces heat), it causes a 0.3°C to 0.6°C (0.5°F to 1.0°F) sustained rise in basal temperature during the second half of the menstrual cycle (luteal phase). Immediately before or coincident with the onset of menses, the temperature falls below 36.7 °C (98°F). These changes in the basal temperature create the typical biphasic pattern. Figure 7–2B shows a biphasic ovulatory BBT chart. Temperature elevation does not predict the day of ovulation, but it does provide supportive evidence of ovulation about a day after it has occurred.

Although there are other, more reliable methods to detect ovulatory function, BBT offers couples a low-tech, noninvasive, and inexpensive option. Based on serial BBT charts, the clinician might recommend sexual intercourse *every other day* beginning 3 to 4 days before and continuing for 2 to 3 days after the expected time of ovulation. See Client Teaching: Methods of Determining Ovulation.

HORMONAL ASSESSMENTS OF OVULATORY FUNCTION Hormonal assessments of ovulatory function fall into the following categories.

1. *Gonadotropin levels (FSH, LH)*. Baseline hormonal assessment of FSH and LH provides valuable information about normal ovulatory function. Measured on cycle day (CD) 3, FSH is the single most valuable test of ovarian reserve (number of remaining oocytes or follicles in the ovary) and function. FSH should always be measured, particularly in women over age 30, to predict the potential for successful treatment with ovulation–induction treatment cycles (Wright & Johnson, 2008). LH levels

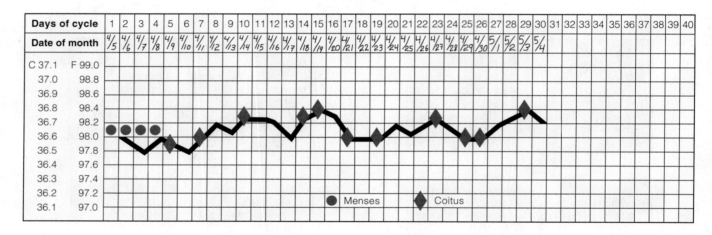

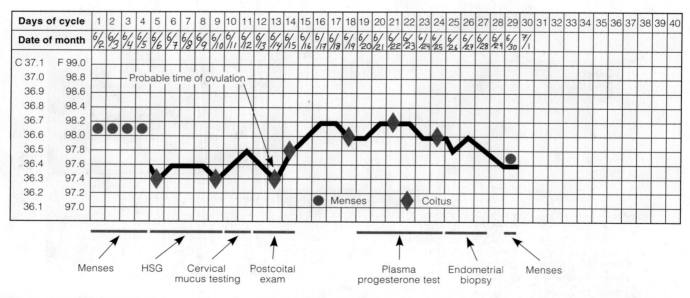

FIGURE 7–2 *A*, Monophasic, anovulatory basal body temperature (BBT) chart. *B*, Biphasic BBT chart illustrating probable time of ovulation, the different types of testing, and the time in the cycle that each would be performed.

Client Teaching METHODS OF DETERMINING OVULATION

Content

Basal Body Temperature (BBT) Method

The basal body temperature (BBT) method relies on assessing the woman's temperature pattern.

Describe the expected findings with an ovulatory (biphasic) cycle and stress the need to monitor BBT for 3 to 4 months to establish a pattern. BBT can be used to time intercourse if pregnancy is desired or as a method of natural family planning. Describe the timing of intercourse to achieve or avoid pregnancy.

Describe the procedure for measuring BBT:

- Using a BBT thermometer, the woman chooses one site (oral, vaginal, or rectal), which she uses consistently.
- The woman takes her temperature every day before arising and before starting any activity, including smoking. Any activity can produce an increase in body temperature.
  Note: Read and follow manufacturers' instructions for each type of BBT thermometer in regard to the amount of time needed for an accurate reading.
- The result is then recorded immediately on a BBT chart, and the temperature dots for each day are connected to form a graph.
- The woman then shakes the thermometer down and cleans it in preparation for use the next day.

Explain that certain situations can disturb body temperature such as large alcohol intake, sleeplessness, fever, warm climate, jet lag, shift work, the use of an electric blanket, or use of heated waterbed.

Cervical Mucus Method

Explain that cervical mucus changes throughout a woman's menstrual cycle and that the quality of the mucus can be used to predict ovulation. Describe the various characteristics of the cervical mucus throughout the menstrual cycle.

Describe the procedure for assessing cervical mucus changes:

- Every day when she uses the bathroom the woman checks her vagina, either by dabbing the vaginal opening with toilet paper or by putting a finger in the opening.
- She notes the wetness (presence of mucus), collects some mucus, determines its color and consistency, and records her findings on a chart. For discussion of mucus characteristics, see page 140.
- She washes her hands before and after the procedure.

Stress that it may take several cycles for the woman to become familiar with the pattern.

Teaching Method

Choose a private location, free of distractions, for the discussion.

Create a supportive, comfortable atmosphere by attitude and communication style.

Briefly explain why BBT can predict ovulation.

Use pictures or graphs to demonstrate the BBT changes that indicate ovulatory and anovulatory cycles.

Learning is best accomplished when content is broken down into smaller steps.

Show the woman the BBT thermometer and demonstrate its use.
  Note: A tympanic (ear) electric thermometer may also be used. Remind the women to use the same type of thermometer throughout the menstrual cycle.

Provide a blank chart. Ask the woman to chart 3 days' findings using temperature results you identify.

Remind the woman that BBT charts are not a prediction of ovulation and that the temperature rise is a response to ovulation that has already occurred.

Provide the woman with an example of LH testing results for comparison

Provide a handout summarizing the procedure.

Provide frequent opportunities for questions and discussion.

Discuss the characteristics of the mucus and the rationale for the changes.

Explore the woman's feelings about using the procedure.

Show pictures of the mucus changes including spinnbarkeit of different degrees of elasticity (see Figure 7–3A).

Encourage the woman to ask questions.

Stress that the presence and consistency of the mucus are altered by vaginal infection, vaginal medications, spermicides, lubricants, douching, sexual arousal, and semen.

Provide a written handout describing the process and findings so that the woman has information readily available.

---

may be measured early in the cycle to rule out androgen excess disorders, which disrupt normal follicular development and oocyte maturation. Daily sampling of LH at midcycle can detect the LH surge. The day of the LH surge is believed to be the day of maximum fertility. Ovulation occurs 24 to 36 hours after the onset of the LH surge and 10 to 12 hours after the peak of the LH surge.

Urine LH ovulation prediction and serum LH assay kits are available for home use to better time postcoital testing, insemination, and intercourse (Kumar, Ghadir, Eskandari et al., 2007).

2. *Progesterone assays.* Progesterone levels furnish the best evidence of ovulation and corpus luteum function. Serum levels begin to rise with the LH surge and

peak about 8 days later. A level of 3 ng/ml 3 days after the LH surge confirms ovulation (Wright & Johnson, 2008). On day 21 (7 days postovulation) a level of 10 ng/ml or higher indicates an adequate luteal phase.

Hormonal assessment may also be conducted for prolactin, thyroid-stimulating hormone, and androgen (testosterone, dehydroepiandrosterone [DHEAS], and androstenedione) levels.

ENDOMETRIAL BIOPSY (EMB) Endometrial biopsy provides information about the effects of progesterone produced by the corpus luteum after ovulation and endometrial receptivity. The biopsy is performed not earlier than 10 to 12 days after ovulation (usually day 22 or 23 of a 28-day menstrual cycle), preferably 2 to 3 days before the expected onset of menses and involves removing a sample of endometrium with a small pipette attached to suction (Kumar, Ghadir, Eskandari et al., 2007; Varney, Kriebs, & Gegor, 2004). The woman should be informed that some pelvic discomfort, cramping, and vaginal spotting are normal during and following the procedure. The woman should be pretreated with NSAIDs to help reduce the pain or cramping associated with procedure (Speroff & Fritz, 2005). The onset of menses following biopsy should be disclosed for accurate interpretation of the biopsy report.

A dysfunction may exist if the endometrial lining does not show the expected amount of secretory tissue for that day of the woman's menstrual cycle. Histological evidence of a secretory endometrium detected by endometrial biopsy shows ovulation and corpus luteum formation. EMB is reliable for determining the presence of ovulation. However it is not effective for diagnosing luteal phase deficiency (Wright & Johnson, 2008).

TRANSVAGINAL ULTRASOUND Transvaginal ultrasound is the method of choice for follicular monitoring of women undergoing induction cycles, for timing ovulation for insemination and intercourse, for retrieving oocytes for in vitro fertilization (IVF), and for monitoring early pregnancy.

The use of a transvaginal color flow Doppler to investigate uterine blood flow may in the future help the endocrinologist evaluate the adequacy of the developing follicle, further assess oocyte maturity and endometrial development and patterns, and improve the diagnosis of luteal phase defects. For the procedure, the woman doesn't need to have a full bladder. In addition, if the woman is more comfortable she can insert the lubricated transvaginal probe herself (Storment, 2006).

Evaluation of Cervical Factors

The mucous cells of the endocervix consist predominantly of water. As ovulation approaches, the ovary increases its secretion of estrogen and produces changes in the cervical mucus. The amount of mucus increases tenfold, and the water content rises significantly. At ovulation, mucus elasticity (**spinnbarkeit**) increases to at least 5 cm in length and viscosity decreases. Excellent spinnbarkeit exists when the mucus can be stretched 8 to 10 cm or longer. Mucous elasticity is determined by using two glass slides (Figure 7–3A ■) or by grasping some mucus at the external os and stretching it through the vagina toward the introitus (see Client Teaching: Methods of Determining Ovulation).

The **ferning capacity** (crystallization) (Figures 7–3B and 7–3C) of the cervical mucus also increases as ovulation approaches. Ferning is caused by decreased levels of salt and water interacting with the glycoproteins in the mucus during the ovulatory period and is thus an indirect indication of estrogen production. To test for ferning, mucus is obtained from the cervical os, spread on a glass slide, allowed to air dry, and examined under the microscope. Within 24 to 48 hours postovulation, rising levels of progesterone markedly decrease the quantity of cervical mucus and increase its viscosity and cellularity. The resulting absence of spinnbarkeit and ferning capacity decreases sperm survival.

To be receptive to sperm, cervical mucus must be thin, clear, watery, profuse, alkaline, and acellular. As shown in Figure 7–4 ■, the mazelike microscopic mucoid strands align in a parallel manner to allow for easy sperm passage. The mucus is termed *inhospitable* if these changes do not occur.

Cervical mucus inhospitable to sperm survival can have several causes, some of which are treatable. For example, estrogen secretion may be inadequate for development of receptive mucus. Cone biopsy, electrocautery, or cryosurgery of the cervix may remove large numbers of mucus-producing glands, creating a "dry cervix" that decreases sperm survival. Treatment with clomiphene citrate may have harmful effects on cervical mucus because of its antiestrogenic properties. Therapy with supplemental estrogen for approximately 6 days before expected ovulation encourages the formation of suitable spinnbarkeit. However, intrauterine insemination (IUI) is more often the most appropriate therapy to overcome these obstacles. When mucosal hostility to sperm is because of cervical infection, antimicrobial therapy may be effective.

The cervix can also be the site of secretory immunologic reactions in which antisperm antibodies are produced, causing agglutination or immobilization of sperm. The most widely used serum–sperm bioassay to detect specific classes of antibodies in serum and seminal fluid is immunobead testing (IBT) (Lu, Huang & Lu, 2008; Kumar et al., 2007). The IBT is considered clinically significant when 50% of the sperm are coated with immunobeads. The treatment for antisperm antibodies may include IUI of the man's washed sperm to bypass the cervical factor.

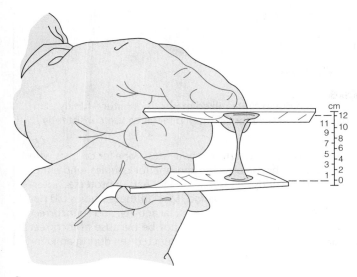

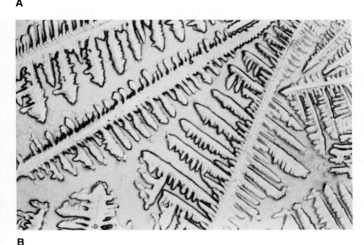

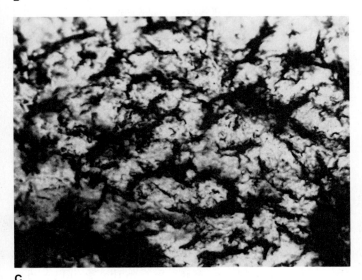

FIGURE 7–3 *A*, Spinnbarkeit (elasticity). *B*, Ferning pattern. *C*, Lack of ferning.
Source: (B) Courtesy of Lavena Porter OB/GYN NP *(C)* From *Clinical gynecologic endocrinology and infertility*, 5e, by L. Speroff, et al., p. 818. Copyright 1994 Lippincott, Williams and Wilkins. Reprinted with permission. (http://www.com)

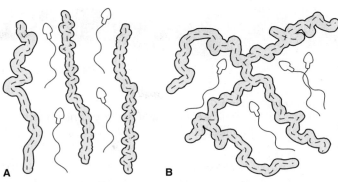

FIGURE 7–4 Sperm passage through cervical mucus. *A*, Appearance at the time of ovulation with channels favoring efficient sperm penetration and migration upward. *B*, Unfavorable mazelike configuration found at other times during the menstrual cycle.
Source: Corson, S. (1998). Conquering infertility, in *A guide for couples* (4th ed., p. 16). Vancouver, BC: EMIS-Canada.

The **postcoital test (PCT)**, also called the **Huhner test**, is performed 1 or 2 days before the expected date of ovulation as determined by previous BBT charts, the length of prior cycles, or a urinary LH kit. This examination evaluates the cervical mucus, the number of active sperm in the cervical mucus, and the length of sperm survival (in hours) after intercourse.

The couple can have intercourse 2 to 8 hours before the examination. If the results are abnormal, the test should be repeated at the optimal time of 2 to 3 hours after intercourse. A small plastic catheter attached to a 10 ml syringe is placed in the cervix. Mucus is aspirated from the endocervical canal, measured, and examined microscopically for signs of infection, spinnbarkeit, ferning, number and motility of active spermatozoa per high-power field (HPF), and number of sperm with poor or no motility. The focus of the postcoital exam on the timing of intercourse may promote sexual difficulties in some infertile couples. Its use is controversial and has limited use in infertility workups because its value in assessing cervical hostility to sperm has never been proven (Kumar et al., 2007). Tests that can potentially predict the fertilizing ability of sperm include the zona-free hamster egg penetration assay and the hemizona test.

Evaluation of Uterine Structures and Tubal Patency

Uterine abnormalities are a relatively uncommon cause of infertility, but should be considered. A few tests offer the ability to evaluate the uterine cavity and tubal patency simultaneously. These tests are usually done after BBT evaluation, semen analysis, and other less invasive tests. Tubal patency and uterine structure are usually evaluated by hysterosalpingography or laparoscopy. Other invasive tests used to evaluate only the uterine cavity are hysteroscopy and sonohysterography. Hysteroscopy may be performed

EVIDENCE-BASED PRACTICE

Natural Family Planning

Clinical Question
What is the effectiveness of natural family planning methods for determining times of fertility?

The Evidence
The most common natural methods for estimating the fertile phase of the menstrual cycle are calendar-based formulas, daily measurement of basal body temperature (BBT) and observation of the characteristics of cervical mucus. A technology-based approach to fertility monitoring is a handheld, home-use device that measures urinary luteinizing hormones. Data about the effectiveness of each method when used singly or in combination has been generated through meta-analysis, a multisite prospective clinical efficacy trial, and a longitudinal study of more than 900 women. The data from these sources is the strongest evidence for practice.

What Is Effective?
Identifying the peak fertility period and avoiding unprotected sex during this time is essential for natural family planning methods to work. Calendar-based methods are the least accurate and require the longest periods of abstinence; when used alone, 15% to 18% of women became pregnant in 1 year. Two methods—BBT and urine hormone detection—identify ovulation at its peak. Because fertilization is most common in the 2 days before ovulation, these methods do not present a long enough warning period. Cervical mucus observation alone had a much lower pregnancy rate (1% to 3.4%) but women often found it confusing to use correctly. When used incorrectly, the cervical mucus method resulted in 15.2 to 22.5 pregnancies per 100 women. The best results were achieved when two methods were used in tandem. The cervical mucus method combined with BBT detection had an associated pregnancy rate of 1.8%. Combining urine hormone detection with cervical mucus had a correct use pregnancy rate of 2.1%. One of the studies found that nearly 10% of women discontinue mixed methods of natural family planning because they found them difficult to use consistently.

What Is Inconclusive?
Efficacy is usually reported as two rates—one for couples who used the methods correctly, and one for couples who either used the methods incorrectly or who had unprotected intercourse during the fertile period. Most of these studies did not require the subjects to report sexual activity, and so incorrect application of the method may not be because of incorrect usage but rather because of unprotected sex during an identified fertile period.

Best Practice
Professional nurses are often in a position to recommend natural family planning methods to women who desire nonpharmacologic methods of protection against unintended pregnancy. Teaching focused on the correct use of any natural family planning method is essential. Focus on both the use of the method and the need to avoid unprotected intercourse during times of peak fertility. Encourage women to use multiple methods, specifically cervical mucus observation along with BBT monitoring or a home urine hormone detection device, to get maximum effectiveness from these methods.

References
Colombo, B., Mion, A., Passarin, K., & Scarpa, B. (2006). Cervical mucus symptom and daily fecundability: First results from a new database. *Statistical Methods in Medical Research, 15*, 161–180.

Fehring, R., Schneider, M., Raviele, K., & Barron, K. (2007). Efficacy of cervical mucus observations plus electronic hormonal fertility monitoring as a method of natural family planning. *JOGNN: The Journal of Obstetric, Gynecological & Neonatal Nursing, 36*, 152–160.

Frank-Herrmann, P., et al. (2007). The effectiveness of a fertility awareness based method to avoid pregnancy in relation to a couple's sexual behaviour during the fertile time: A prospective longitudinal study. *Human Reproduction, 22*(5), 1310–1319.

---

earlier in the evaluation if the woman's history suggests potential for adhesive disease or uterine abnormalities.

HYSTEROSALPINGOGRAPHY Hysterosalpingography (HSG) or *hysterogram* involves an instillation of a radiopaque substance into the uterine cavity. In addition the oil-based dye and injection pressure used in HSG may have a therapeutic effect. This effect may be caused by the flushing of debris, breaking of adhesions, or induction of peristalsis by the instillation.

The HSG should be performed in the follicular phase of the cycle to avoid interrupting an early pregnancy. This timing also avoids the lush secretory changes in the endometrium that occur after ovulation, which may prevent the passage of the dye through the tubes and present a false picture of obstruction of the entry point of the fallopian tube into the uterus. HSG causes moderate discomfort.

The pain is referred from the peritoneum (which is irritated by the subdiaphragmatic collection of gas) to the shoulder. The cramping may be decreased if the radiopaque dye is warmed to body temperature before instillation. Women can take an over-the-counter (OTC) prostaglandin synthesis inhibitor (such as ibuprofen) 30 minutes before the procedure to decrease the pain, cramping, and discomfort. HSG can also cause recurrence of pelvic inflammatory disease, so prophylactic antibiotics are recommended to prevent infection that could be triggered by the procedure (Wright & Johnson, 2008).

HYSTEROSCOPY *Hysteroscopy* is the definitive method for both diagnosis and treatment of intrauterine pathology (Speroff & Fritz, 2005). Hysteroscopy allows the physician to further evaluate any areas of suspicion within the uterine cavity or fallopian tubes revealed by the HSG. It can be done in conjunction with a laparoscopy or independently in the office and does not require general anesthesia. A fiberoptic instrument called a hysteroscope is placed into the uterus for further evaluation of polyps, fibroids, or structural variations (Goldstein, 2008).

LAPAROSCOPY Laparoscopy enables direct visualization of the pelvic organs and is not routinely advised after a normal HSG unless symptoms suggest the need for earlier evaluation (Wright & Johnson, 2008). Diagnostic laparoscopy is an outpatient procedure requiring the use of general anesthesia. Generally, a three-puncture approach is used, entry is made through the umbilical area, and supporting instruments are inserted in two suprapubic incisions. The peritoneal cavity is distended with carbon dioxide gas so that the pelvic organs can be directly visualized with a fiberoptic instrument. Tube patency can be assessed by instillation of dye into the uterine cavity through the cervix. The pelvis is evaluated for endometriosis, adhesions, organ fixations, pelvic inflammatory disease, tumors, and cysts. The intraperitoneal gas is usually manually expressed at the end of the procedure. In routine preanesthesia instructions, the woman is told that she may have some discomfort from organ displacement and shoulder and chest pain caused by gas in the abdomen. She should be informed that she can resume normal activities as tolerated after 24 hours. Using postoperative pain medication and assuming a supine position may help relieve discomfort caused by any remaining gas.

Assessment of the Man's Fertility

Male infertility can be caused by numerous factors and categorized as ductal obstruction or abnormalities of sperm production or sperm function (Speroff & Fritz, 2005). Sperm function abnormalities may be because of problems with sperm binding or penetration of the egg, prostatitis, or varocele. Varocele accounts for approximately 40% of male infertility (Speroff & Fritz, 2005). If the man's history indicates the need, he may be referred to a urologist for testing. A semen analysis of sperm quality, quantity, and motility is the single most important initial diagnostic study of the man. It should be done early in the couple's evaluation, before invasive testing of the woman.

To obtain accurate results, the specimen is collected after 2 to 3 days of abstinence, usually by masturbation to avoid contamination or loss of any ejaculate. If the man has difficulty producing sperm by masturbation, special medical-grade condoms are available to collect the sperm during intercourse. Regular latex and nonlatex condoms should not be used because they contain agents that impair the mobility of sperm, which can result in sperm loss in the condom. Most lubricants also are spermicidal and should not be used unless approved by the andrology laboratory. If the specimen is obtained at home, it needs to be

brought to the lab within 1 hour and kept at body temperature so as not to impair motility.

Both seasonal and incidental variability may be seen in count and motility in successive semen analyses from the same individual. Thus a repeat semen analysis may be required to assess the man's fertility potential adequately; a minimum of two separate analyses is recommended for confirmation. In cases in which a known testicular insult has occurred (infection, high fevers, or surgery), a repeat analysis may not be done for at least 2.5 months to allow for new sperm maturation.

Sperm analysis provides information about sperm motility and morphology and a determination of the absolute number of spermatozoa present (Table 7–4). Although low numbers and motility may indicate compromised fertility, other parameters, such as morphology, motion patterns, and progression, are important prognostic indicators. Values previously thought to indicate subfertility may in fact be compatible with normal fertility when morphology, motion patterns, and progression factors are considered. An infertile specimen is one that has fewer than 20 million sperm per milliliter, less than 50% motility at 6 hours, or less than 30% normal sperm forms (Kumar et al., 2007). The quality of sperm decreases with increasing paternal age and may result in chromosomal damage. For example, fathers older than 50 years have infants at increased risk for trisomies.

A variety of environmental factors can affect male fertility. Causes of increased scrotal heat, such as jockey shorts, hot tubs, or occupations requiring long hours of sitting, are thought to decrease fertility potential, but there are no clinical studies to substantiate this belief (Honig, 2005). Heavy use of marijuana, alcohol, or cocaine within 2 years of testing can depress sperm count and testosterone levels; cigarette smoking may depress sperm motility (Quallich, 2006). The use of anabolic steroids lowers the body's ability to make endogenous testosterone, causing low sperm counts, which may not be reversible (Honig,

TABLE 7–4	Normal Semen Analysis
Factor	Value
Volume	Greater than 2 ml
pH	7.0 to 8.0
Total sperm count	Greater than 20 million/ml
Liquefaction	Complete in 1 hour
Motility	50% or greater forward progression
Normal forms	30% or greater
Round cells	Less than 5 million/ml
White cells	Less than 1 million/ml

Source: World Health Organization. (1993). *The WHO laboratory manual for the examination of human semen and sperm-cervical mucus interaction* (3rd ed.). Geneva: Author.

2005). Neurologic ejaculatory dysfunction can be associated with the use of drugs such as alpha blockers; for example, phentolamine, methyldopa, guanethidine, and reserpine. Sperm quality may be affected by medicines such as calcium channel blockers, propranolol, cimetidine, nitrofurantoin, or allopurinol/colchicines (Honig, 2005). Heavy metals (lead) and pesticide exposure can also reduce sperm count (Denson, 2006). A low sperm count of at least 10 million/ml may benefit from IUI because an increased concentrated amount of sperm can be deposited directly into the uterine cavity. For a sperm count of less than 5% normal forms, IVF with intracytoplasmic sperm injection (ICSI) is recommended (Speroff & Fritz, 2005).

Spermatozoa have been shown to possess intrinsic antigens that can provoke male immunologic infertility. Immunologic infertility is especially apparent following vasectomy reversals or genital trauma, such as testicular torsion, in which autoimmunity to sperm (the man produces antibodies to his own sperm) develops. Research indicates that it is the actual presence of antibodies on the spermatozoal surface (not just the presence of antibodies in the serum) that affects sperm function and thus leads to subfertility. Antisperm antibodies can be screened for by an immunobead binding test (Kumar et al., 2007). Treatment for antisperm antibodies is directed toward preventing the formation of antibodies or arresting the underlying mechanism that compromises sperm function. Therapies such as immunosuppression with corticosteriods and IUI have not proved effective. The treatment of choice for clinically significant antisperm antibodies is intracytoplasmic sperm injection (ICSI) in conjunction with IVF.

Methods of Infertility Management

Methods of managing infertility include pharmacologic agents, therapeutic insemination, in vitro fertilization, and other assisted reproductive techniques.

Pharmacological Agents

This section provides a brief overview of the drugs commonly used for ovarian stimulation in the follicular phase, control of midcycle release, and support of the luteal phase. The pharmacologic treatment chosen depends on the specific cause of infertility. Table 7–5 lists some of the drugs commonly used and indications for use.

CLOMIPHENE CITRATE If a woman has normal ovaries, a normal prolactin level, and an intact pituitary gland, *clomiphene citrate* (Clomid or Serophene) is often used. This medication induces ovulation in 70% of women by actions at both the hypothalamic and ovarian levels; 30% to 40% of these women will become pregnant.

Approximately 10% of women develop multiple-gestation pregnancies, almost exclusively twins (Stormont, 2006). Clomiphene citrate works by stimulating the hypothalamus to secrete more gonadotropin-releasing hormone (GnRH). This increases the secretion of LH and FSH, which stimulates follicle growth and facilitates the release of ova (Speroff & Fritz, 2005).

For the first course the woman usually takes 50 mg/day orally for 5 days from cycle day (CD) 3 to day 7 or CD 5 to day 9. In nonresponders, the dose may be increased to 100 mg/day to a maximum of 250 mg/day, although doses in excess of 100 mg/day are not approved by the FDA (Wilson, Shannon, Shields et al., 2009). The woman may need to take estrogen simultaneously if a decrease in cervical mucus occurs.

The woman is informed that if ovulation occurs, it is expected 5 to 9 days after the last dose. The nurse determines if the couple has been advised to have sexual intercourse every other day for 1 week, beginning 5 days after the last day of medication. Upon a negative pregnancy test, another trial of clomiphene can be initiated. After the first treatment cycle, a pelvic ultrasound should be done to rule out ovarian enlargement, ovarian cysts, or hyperstimulation. Ovarian enlargement and abdominal discomfort (bloating) may result from follicular growth and formation of multiple corpora lutea. Persistence of ovarian cysts is a contraindication for further treatment regimens. Other side effects include hot flashes, abdominal distention, bloating, breast discomfort, nausea and vomiting, vision problems (such as visual spots), headache, and dryness or loss of hair (Wright & Johnson, 2008). Supplemental low-dose estrogen may be given to ensure appropriate quality and quantity of cervical mucus, or IUI may be employed to overcome this obstacle. Women can assess the presence of ovulation and possible response to clomiphene therapy by doing BBT and urinary LH tests. The woman should be knowledgeable about side effects and call her healthcare provider if they occur. When visual disturbances (flashes, blurring, or spots) occur, bright lighting should be avoided. This side effect disappears within a few days or weeks after discontinuation of therapy. The occurrence of hot flashes may be because of the antiestrogenic properties of clomiphene citrate. The woman can obtain some relief by increasing intake of fluids and using fans.

GONADOTROPINS Therapy using *human menopausal gonadotropins (hMGs)*, which include menotropins (Repronex and Menopur) and urofollitropin (Bravelle), is indicated as a first line of therapy for anovulatory infertile women with low to normal levels of gonadotropins (FSH and LH). It is a second line of therapy in women who fail to ovulate or conceive with clomiphene citrate therapy and in women undergoing controlled ovarian stimulation with assisted reproduction. Menotropin is a combination of FSH

TABLE 7–5	Drugs Commonly Used to Treat Infertility	
	Indications	
Drugs	**Women**	**Men**
Clomiphene citrate (Clomid, Serophene)	• PCOS • Hyper-androgenemia • Premature follicle rupture	• Low levels of gonadotrophins • Hypothalamic hypogonadism
Human menopausal gonadotropin (hMG), (Repronex, Bravelle)	• Hypothalamic ovulatory dysfunction (after failure of clomiphene) • Hypopituitarism • PCOS (rarely) • Luteinized unruptured follicle syndrome (after failure of hCG alone) • Inadequate cervical mucus • In vitro fertilization, GIFT, ZIFT • Controlled super-ovulation	• Hypothalamic pituitary failure due to Kallmann syndrome or delayed puberty • Hypo-gonadotrophic hypogonadism (deficiency of FSH and LH)
Recombinant follicle-stimulating hormone (rFSH) (Follistim, Gonal-F)	• PCOS • Too long cycles • In vitro fertilization, GIFT, ZIFT	
Human chorionic gonadotropin (hCG) (Pregnyl, Novarel, A.P.L)	• Induces dominant follicle to release egg • Luteinized unruptured follicle syndrome	
Bromocriptine (Parlodel) Cabergoline (Dostinex)	• Pituitary adenoma • Hyper-pituitarism	• Hyper-prolactinemia (functional or pituitary adenoma)
Gonadotropin releasing hormone (GnRh) (Factral, Lutre-pulse) **GnRh analogs** • Leuprolide acetate (Lupron) • Nafarelin acetate (Synarel) • Goserelin acetate (Zoladex) **GnRH antagonists** • Ganirelix acetate (Antagon)	• Hypothalamic ovulatory dysfunction—to ensure a pulsatile release of GnRH by a small pump • Premature follicular rupture • In vitro fertilization, GIFT, ZIFT • Endometriosis • Same as GnRH analogs	• Hypothalmic pituitary failure due to Kallmann syndrome or delayed puberty (pulsed infusion) • Hypo-gonadotrophic hypogonadism
Progesterone (Crinone, Prometrium, progesterone in oil)	• Luteal phase dysfunction • Luteal phase support	

Source: Adapted from American Society for Reproductive Medicine Booklet. (2006). *Medications for inducing ovulation—A guide for patients.* http://www.org/patientbooklets/ovulation_drugs.pdf; Shane. J. (1993). Evaluation and treatment of infertility. *Clinical Symposia, 45,2*; Wilson, B. A., Shannon, M. T., Shields, K. M., & Stang, C. L. (2009). *Prentice Hall nurse's drug guide 2009.* Upper Saddle River, NJ: Pearson Education.

and LH, and urofollitropin is a further purified form and contains mainly FSH with trace amounts of LH. Immediately before injection, the powder is reconstituted with diluent and injected subcutaneously.

More recently, however, recombinant gonadotropins (rFSH and rLH) have been produced, giving rise to more consistent preparations. Recombinant FSH is homogenous and free of contaminants by proteins. Luveris, a recombinant form of LH, is used concomitantly with recombinant FSH in women with profound LH deficiency. It is thought that the use of recombinant gonadotropins will eventually become the preferred preparation and that the use of urinary preparations will be phased out.

Gonadotropin therapy requires close observation by use of serum estradiol levels and ultrasound. Monitoring of follicle development is necessary to minimize the risk of multiple fetuses and to avoid ovarian hyperstimulation syndrome. The daily dose of medication given is titrated

based on serum estradiol and ultrasound findings. Then once follicle maturation has occurred, hCG may be administered by intramuscular or subcutaneous injection to induce final follicular maturation and stimulate ovulation. The couple is advised to have intercourse 24 to 36 hours after hCG administration and for the next 2 days. Women who elect to undergo ovarian stimulation with gonadotropins have usually passed through all other forms of management without conceiving. Strong emotional support and thorough education are needed because of the numerous office visits and injections. Often the male partner is instructed, with return demonstration, to administer the daily injections.

BROMOCRIPTINE   High prolactin levels may impair the glandular production of FSH and LH or block their action on the ovaries. When hyperprolactinemia accompanies anovulation, the infertility may be treated with bromocriptine (Parlodel). This medication acts directly on the prolactin-secreting cells in the anterior pituitary. It inhibits the pituitary's secretion of prolactin, thus preventing suppression of the pulsatile secretion of FSH and LH. This restores normal menstrual cycles and induces ovulation by allowing FSH and LH production. If treatment is successful, the tests of ovulatory function will indicate that ovulation is occurring with a normal luteal phase. Bromocriptine should be discontinued if pregnancy is suspected or at the anticipated time of ovulation because of its possible teratogenic effects. Other side effects include nausea, diarrhea, dizziness, headache, and fatigue, which can be attributed to the dopaminergic action of bromocriptine. To minimize side effects for women who are extremely sensitive, treatment may be initiated with a dose of 1.25 mg, slowly building tolerance toward the usual dose of 2.5 mg bid. An intravaginal preparation may also be used to decrease the occurrence of side effects (Wright & Johnson, 2008).

AROMATASE INHIBITORS   Aromatase inhibitors (letrozole [Femara] and anastrozole [Arimidex]) are medications that reduce estrogen levels and have been successfully used for ovulation induction. They are currently FDA approved for postmenopausal breast cancer. Pregnancy rates have been reported to be comparable to clomiphene citrate (American Society of Reproductive Medicine, 2006c). Recent data has raised concern that letrozole may be associated with an increased risk of congenital abnormalities.

PROGESTERONE   Treatment of luteal phase defects may include the use of progesterone to augment luteal phase progesterone levels. Ovulation–induction agents, such as clomiphene citrate or menotropins, may be used to augment proliferative phase FSH production in the developing follicle, as women with luteal phase defects have been found to have decreased FSH production in the proliferative phase. This is associated with a decline in luteal phase progesterone and estrogen production and is manifested by an out-of-phase endometrial biopsy. It is also common to use progesterone supplementation in conjunction with these ovulation–induction agents for luteal phase support, thereby increasing endometrial receptivity for embryonic implantation. Occasionally hCG therapy may be used in the luteal phase to stimulate corpus luteum production of progesterone.

Other Pharmacologic Agents

Pharmacologic treatments for endometriosis-related infertility involve use of danazol (Danocrine), oral contraceptives or oral medroxyprogesterone acetate, and gonadotropin-releasing hormone (GnRH) agonists. The management and care of endometriosis is further discussed in Chapter 6 ∞.

COMPLEMENTARY AND ALTERNATIVE THERAPIES
Common Treatments for Infertility

Couples experiencing infertility may seek out alternative treatments. Some common treatments include acupuncture and herbs.

Acupuncture: Acupuncture is a therapy used in traditional Chinese medicine (TCM), and has become a popular complementary treatment. Acupuncture involves inserting sterile needles into specific points on the body to control the flow of chi, or life energy. Acupuncture treatment would focus on balancing the flow of chi in the kidneys and adrenal glands. Several clinical studies have shown acupuncture to be effective in treating infertility in both men and women (Gurfinkel, Cedenho, Yamamura et al., 2003; White, 2003).

Herbal Treatments: Herbs frequently recommended to treat infertility include ginseng and astragalus. Herbalists cite the healing and hormone-balancing effects of these herbs. Ginseng has historically been used in TCM to enhance male virility and fertility. Several studies also cite ginseng, as well as astragalus, in enhancing in vitro sperm motility (Skidmore-Roth, 2006).

The nurse should be alert for signs that the couple is pursuing complementary therapies out of desperation. A sensitive, nonjudgmental approach will go a long way toward comforting a couple and assuring them that many complementary therapies used are helpful and not harmful.

Therapeutic Insemination

Therapeutic insemination has replaced the previously used term *artificial insemination* and involves the depositing of semen at the cervical os or in the uterus by mechanical means. *Therapeutic donor insemination (TDI)* is the current term for use of donor semen, and *therapeutic husband insemination (THI)* is the current term for use of the husband's semen.

THI is generally indicated for such seminal deficiencies as oligospermia (low sperm count), asthenospermia (decreased motility), and teratospermia (low percentage, abnormal morphology); for anatomic defects accompanied by inadequate deposition of semen such as hypospadia (a congenital abnormal male urethral opening on the underside of the penis); and for ejaculatory dysfunction (such as retrograde ejaculation). THI is also indicated in cases of unexplained infertility and some cases of female factor infertility, such as scant or inhospitable mucus, persistent cervicitis, or cervical stenosis. In some cases, IUI would be indicated to bypass the cervical factor. Seminal fluid contains high levels of prostaglandins, which can cause nausea, severe cramps, abdominal pain, and diarrhea when absorbed by the uterine lining. Therefore, sperm preparation for IUI involves washing sperm from the seminal plasma. IUI, with or without ovulation induction therapy, is an option for many couples before more aggressive treatments such as in vitro fertilization are employed.

TDI is considered in cases of azoospermia (absence of sperm), severe oligospermia or asthenospermia, inherited male sex-linked disorders, and autosomal dominant disorders. In the past several years, indications for donor insemination have expanded to include single women or lesbians desirous of pregnancy. Some states have specified the parental rights of single women and donors, but most are silent on this issue.

Therapeutic donor insemination has become more complicated and expensive in the past decade because of the need for strict screening and processing procedures to prevent transmission of a genetic defect or sexually transmitted infection to the offspring or recipient. Guidelines have been established that include mandatory medical (genetic) and infectious disease screening of both donor and recipient, the need for informed consent from all parties, the need to limit the number of pregnancies per donor, and the need for accurate means of record keeping. Finally, because of the risk of transmitting infectious diseases, donated sperm must be frozen and quarantined for 6 months from the time of acquisition, and the donor must be retested before sperm can be released for use.

Numerous factors need to be evaluated before TDI is performed. Has every possible effort been made to diagnose and treat the cause of the male infertility? Do tests indicate normal fertility and sperm–ovum transport in the woman? Has the couple had an opportunity to discuss this option with an infertility counselor to explore the issues of secrecy, disclosure, and potential feelings of loss the couple (particularly the male partner) may feel about not having a genetic child? Are there any religious constraints? After making the decision, the couple should allow themselves time to further assess their concerns and explore their feelings individually and together to ensure that this option is acceptable to both.

In Vitro Fertilization

In vitro fertilization (IVF) is selectively used in cases when infertility has resulted from tubal factors, mucous abnormalities, male infertility, unexplained infertility, male and female immunologic infertility, and cervical factors. In IVF a woman's eggs are collected from her ovaries, fertilized in the laboratory, and placed into her uterus after normal embryo development has begun. If the procedure is successful, the embryo continues to develop in the uterus, and pregnancy proceeds naturally.

The potential for a successful pregnancy with IVF is maximized when three to four embryos (rather than one) are placed into the uterus. For this reason, fertility drugs

CULTURAL PERSPECTIVES

Infertility Treatments

The acceptance of infertility treatments varies widely around the world. Some belief systems do not allow various treatments, because using a treatment is considered interfering with God's design or because the treatment itself is seen as tainted or sinful. For example, fertility practices in Arab cultures are influenced by traditional Arab Bedouin values that support tribal dominance and beliefs that "God decides family sizes." In Arab cultures, procreation is the purpose of marriage.

If a couple is infertile, the approved methods for treating infertility are limited to use of therapeutic insemination using the husband's sperm and *in vitro* fertilization involving the fertilization of the wife's ovum by the husband's sperm because of lineage concerns (Purnell & Paulanka, 2008).

Sterility in a woman can lead to rejection and divorce. Also with the use of ICSI, male-initiated divorce is becoming more common for aging wives of infertile husbands (Inhorn, 2002). Contemporary Islamic religious opinion forbids any kind of egg, embryo, or semen donation, as well as surrogacy (Inhorn, 2002).

In Jewish cultures, infertile couples are to try all possible means to have children including egg and sperm donation. However, Orthodox Jewish opinion is virtually unanimous in prohibiting therapeutic insemination when the semen donor is a Jewish man other than the woman's husband, because it may constitute adultery (Purnell & Paulanka, 2008). If the infertility is because of a male factor, therapeutic insemination with sperm from a non-Jewish sperm donor is acceptable because "Jewishness" is conferred through the matrilineal. IVF and embryo transfer (ET) are also acceptable artificial insemination methods because they do not involve putting sperm into another's wife (Kahn, 2002).

are used to induce ovulation before the process. Follicular development and oocyte maturity are monitored frequently with ultrasound and hormonal assays. Monitoring usually begins around cycle day 5, and medications are titrated according to individual response. When follicles appear mature, hCG is given to stimulate final egg maturation and control the induction of ovulation. Egg retrieval is performed approximately 35 hours later, before ovulation occurs.

In the majority of cases, egg retrieval is performed by a transvaginal approach under ultrasound guidance (Figure 7–5 ■). It is an outpatient procedure performed with intravenous sedation and a cervical block for anesthesia. Many follicles can be aspirated with only one puncture, and the procedure generally lasts no more than 30 minutes. Once the eggs are fertilized and progress to the embryo stage, the embryos are placed in the uterus. This occurs 1 to 2 days after conception. After the procedure, the woman is advised to engage in only minimal activity

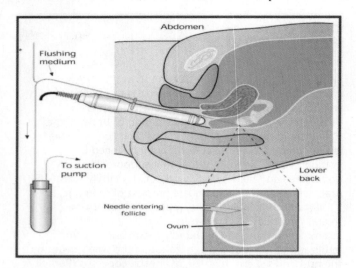

FIGURE 7–5 Transvaginal ultrasound-guided oocyte retrieval.
Source: Courtesy of Serono, Inc., Rockland, MA.

for 12 to 24 hours, and progesterone supplementation is prescribed. The progesterone supplementation is given to promote implantation and support the early pregnancy; therefore, she will not have a period even if she is not pregnant (the pregnancy is usually determined by transvaginal ultrasound).

Sperm used to fertilize the eggs in vitro can be obtained naturally or via microsurgical epididymal sperm aspiration (MESA) or testicular sperm aspiration (TESA). These are procedures that address severe male factor infertility. MESA and TESA involve the retrieval of sperm from the gonadal tissue of men who have azoospermia or an ejaculatory disorder (Figure 7–6 ■). Percutaneous epididymal sperm aspiration (PESA) and TESA are replacing MESA as the preferred techniques for retrieval of sperm because they are not surgical procedures. ICSI is a microscopic procedure to inject a single sperm into the outer layer of an ovum so that fertilization will occur (Devine, 2008).

Success with IVF depends on many factors, but especially the woman's age and the specific indication. Women have a good chance of achieving pregnancy with an average of three cycles of IVF. Many couples find the emotional, physical, and financial costs of going beyond three cycles too great. Costs vary by treatment and by region of the country: one cycle of IVF-ET averages $12,400 (American Society of Reproductive Medicine, 2006a). Clinical birth rates reported by the Society of Assisted Reproductive Technology (SART) were 40% to 45% per egg donation for women regardless of age or indication in the United States (American Society of Reproductive Medicine, 2007). The increase in

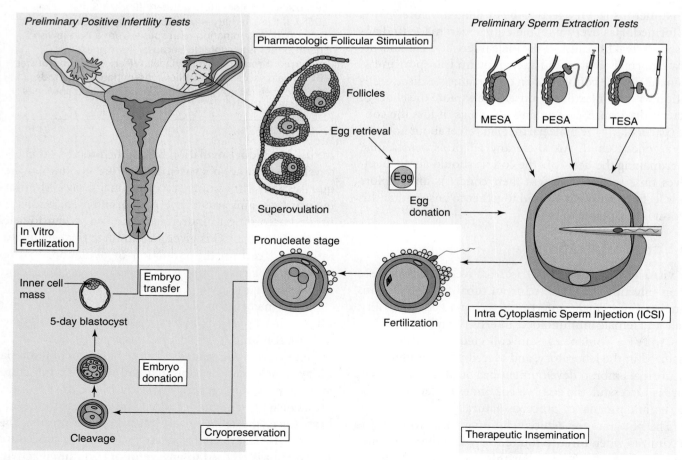

FIGURE 7–6 Assisted reproductive techniques.

maternal and neonatal morbidity associated with IVF because of the rates of multiple fetuses remains an issue

Other Assisted Reproductive Techniques

Other assisted reproductive techniques include procedures for transfer of gametes, zygotes, or embryos; cryopreservation of embryos; IVF using donor oocytes; micromanipulation techniques; and use of a gestational carrier.

GAMETE INTRAFALLOPIAN TRANSFER Gamete **intrafallopian transfer (GIFT)** involves the retrieval of oocytes by laparoscopy; immediate placement of the oocytes in a catheter with washed, motile sperm; and placement of the gametes into the fimbriated end of the fallopian tube. Fertilization occurs in the fallopian tube as with normal conception (in vivo) rather than in the laboratory (in vitro). The fertilized egg then travels through the fallopian tube to the uterus for implantation as in normal reproduction. This practice is acceptable to the Roman Catholic Church.

From the GIFT technology evolved procedures such as **zygote intrafallopian transfer (ZIFT)** and **tubal embryo transfer (TET)**. In these procedures eggs are retrieved and incubated with the man's sperm. However, the eggs are transferred back to the woman's body at a much earlier stage of cell division than in IVF and, as in GIFT, are placed in the fallopian tube or tubes and not the uterus. In TET the placement is done at the embryo stage. These procedures allow fertilization to be documented, which is not possible with GIFT, and the pregnancy rate is theoretically increased when the fertilized ovum is placed in the fallopian tube.

When considering IVF and the transfer procedures, several factors must be weighed. IVF success rates approximate those that have been achieved with the transfer procedures, and IVF is a much less invasive and costly procedure. For these reasons, GIFT and other tubal procedures have lost some acceptance and IVF techniques are more often employed. However, GIFT may be more acceptable to adherents of some religions, because fertilization does not occur outside the woman's body.

PREIMPLANTATION GENETIC DIAGNOSIS (PGD) Other recent advances in micromanipulation allow a single cell to be removed from the embryo for genetic study. Couples at risk for having a detectable single gene or chromosomal anomaly may wish to undergo such preimplantation genetic testing, called *blastomere analysis* or, more recently, *preimplantation genetic diagnosis (PGD)*. The single cell is obtained from a six- to eight-cell embryo by a process known as blastomere biopsy. The genetic content of the cell is examined using polymerase chain reaction (PCR) technique or fluorescence in situ (FISH). Results of genetic testing on the preimplantation embryos are available in 4 to 24 hours, so unaffected embryos may still be transferred during the required biologic window of time without the need for cryopreservation.

The diagnosis of genetic disorders before implantation provides couples with the option of forgoing the attempt to establish a pregnancy and thereby avoiding a difficult decision about terminating an affected pregnancy (Simpson & Holzgreve, 2007). This technology also raises several ethical issues, including the following:

- Identification of couples at risk. There is a need for criteria that identify couples at risk for diseases that constitute significant hardship and suffering so that "wrongful birth" cases can be avoided.
- Availability of and access to centers providing PGD. Should society provide access for those at risk for genetic transfer of disease but without the financial resources to pay for the services?
- Analysis of blastomeres for sex chromosome testing when a genetic disorder carried on the sex chromosomes is suspected. In X-linked diseases, the only way to prevent the disorder is to select against the blastomere with the Y chromosome.
- Identification of late-onset diseases. The Human Genome Project has aided in the identification of genetic markers for late-onset disease. Couples may wish to choose to implant blastomeres that do not carry these markers.
- Effect on the offspring as a result of removing cells from the embryo
- Selection for nonmedical reasons and potential concern of eugenics "designer babies"

A micromanipulation procedure called *assisted embryo hatching* has proved to be an effective adjunct therapy in IVF. In vitro fertilization using a *gestational carrier* allows infertile women who are genetically sound but unable to carry a pregnancy to exercise the option of having their own biologic child. Other technologies involve oocyte donation and cryopreservation of the embryo.

Adoption

Infertile couples consider various alternatives for resolving their infertility; adoption is one option that will be considered at several points during the treatment process. As couples begin to consider adoption, an important aspect of this exploration is the gathering of information from magazines, books, informational websites, and organizations such as the National Adoption Information Clearinghouse; attending adoption support groups and conferences; and meeting with adoptive parents to discuss their experiences with adoption.

The adoption of a healthy American infant can be difficult and frustrating, often involving long waiting periods, continual setbacks, and high costs. Thus many couples seek international adoption or consider adopting older children,

children with handicaps, or children of mixed parentage because the adoption process in such cases is quicker and more children are available. Nurses in the community can assist couples considering adoption by providing information on community resources for adoption and support through the adoption process. Couples need support if they remain childless, either by choice or circumstance. Informational books, websites such as Childless by Choice, and support groups such as San Francisco RESOLVE's "living without children" are available for couples who remain childless by choice or circumstance at www.resolve.org.

Pregnancy After Infertility

The feeling of being infertile does not necessarily disappear with pregnancy. Although there may be initial ecstasy, couples may face a whole new arena of fear and anxiety, and the parents-to-be often do not know where they "fit in." They may feel a great sense of isolation because those who have had no trouble conceiving cannot relate to the physical and emotional pain they endured to achieve the pregnancy. Contact with their past support system of other infertile couples may vanish when peers learn the couple has resolved their infertility. Although the desperation to become pregnant may have superseded the couple's ability to acknowledge their concerns about undergoing various treatments or procedures, questions about the repeated cycle of fertility drugs or the achievement of pregnancy through IVF technology or cryopreservation may now arise. The expectant couple may be very concerned about the potential of these treatments to adversely affect the fetus (Wright & Johnson, 2008). Couples may need reassurance throughout the pregnancy to allay these anxieties. The nurse can assist couples who conceive after infertility by acknowledging their past experiences of infertility treatment; validating their fears and anxieties as they face childbirth classes, birth, and parenting issues; and providing support and education about what to anticipate physically and emotionally throughout the pregnancy. The nurse can also counsel couples that infertility because of nonstructural causes may correct itself following a successful pregnancy and birth; therefore, post-childbirth contraception counseling may be warranted. These interventions will go a long way toward normalizing the experience for the couple.

Nursing Care Management

Infertility therapy taxes a couple's financial, physical, and emotional resources. Treatment can be costly, and insurance coverage is limited. Years of effort and numerous evaluations and examinations may take place before conception occurs, if it occurs at all. In a society that values children and considers them to be the natural result of marriage, infertile couples face a myriad of tensions and discrimination.

Clinic nurses need to be constantly aware of the emotional needs of the couple confronting infertility evaluation and treatment. Often an intact marriage will become stressed with intrusive infertility procedures and treatments. Constant attention to temperature charts and instructions about their sex life from a person outside the relationship naturally affects the spontaneity of a couple's interactions. Tests and treatments may heighten feelings of frustration or anger between partners. The need to share this intimate area of a relationship, especially when one or the other is identified as "the cause" of infertility, may precipitate feelings of guilt or shame. Infertility often becomes a central focus for role identity, especially for women (Devine, 2008).

The couple may experience feelings of loss of control, feelings of reduced competency and defectiveness, loss of status and ambiguity as a couple, a sense of social stigma, stress on the marital and sexual relationship, and a strained relationship with healthcare providers. The nurse's roles can be summarized as those of counselor, educator, and advocate.

Tasks of the infertile couple and appropriate nursing interventions are summarized in Table 7–6. Throughout the evaluation process nurses play a key role in lessening the stress these couples must endure by providing resources and accurate information about what is entailed in treatment and what physical, emotional, and financial demands they can anticipate throughout the process (Klock, 2004).

The nurse's ability to assess and respond to emotional and educational needs is essential to give infertile couples a sense of control and help them negotiate the treatment process. An assessment tool such as an infertility questionnaire (Table 7–7) may be helpful. Extensive and repeated explanations and written instruction may be necessary because the couple's anxiety often overwhelms their ability to retain all the information given. It is important to use a

TABLE 7–6	Tasks of the Infertile Couple
Tasks	Nursing Interventions
Recognize how infertility affects their lives and express feelings (may be negative toward self or mate)	Supportive: help to understand and facilitate free expression of feelings
Grieve the loss of potential offspring	Help to recognize feelings
Evaluate reasons for wanting a child	Help to understand motives
Decide about management	Identify alternatives; facilitate partner communication

Source: Sawatzky, M. (1981). Tasks of the infertile couple. *Journal of Obstetric, Gynecologic, and Neonatal Nursing, 10,* 132.

TABLE 7–7	Infertility Questionnaire

Self-Image

1. I feel bad about my body because of our inability to have a child.
2. Since our infertility, I feel I can do anything as well as I used to.
3. I feel as attractive as before our infertility.
4. I feel less masculine/feminine because of our inability to have a child.
5. Compared with others, I feel I am a worthwhile person.
6. Lately, I feel I am sexually attractive to my wife/husband.
7. I feel I will be incomplete as a man/woman if we cannot have a child.
8. Having an infertility problem makes me feel physically incompetent.

Guilt/Blame

1. I feel guilty about somehow causing our infertility.
2. I wonder if our infertility problem is because of something I did in the past.
3. My spouse makes me feel guilty about our problem.
4. There are times when I blame my spouse for our infertility.
5. I feel I am being punished because of our infertility.

Sexuality

1. Lately I feel I am able to respond to my spouse sexually.
2. I feel sex is a duty, not a pleasure.
3. Since our infertility problem, I enjoy sexual relations with my spouse.
4. We have sexual relations for the purpose of trying to conceive.
5. Sometimes I feel like a "sex machine," programmed to have sex during the fertile period.
6. Impaired fertility has helped our sexual relationship.
7. Our inability to have a child has increased my desire for sexual relations.
8. Our inability to have a child has decreased my desire for sexual relations.

Note: The questionnaire is scored on a Likert scale, with responses ranging from "strongly agree" to "strongly disagree." Each question is scored separately, and the mean score is determined for each section (Self-Image, Guilt/Blame, and Sexuality). The total mean score is then divided by 3. A final mean score of greater than 3 indicates distress.

Source: From Bernstein, J., Potts, N., & Mattox, J. H. (1985). Assessment of psychological dysfunction association with infertility. *Journal of Obstetric, Gynecologic, and Neonatal Nursing,* 14 (Suppl.), 64S, Table 1. Washington DC: Author. © 1985 by the Association of Women's Health, Obstetric and Neonatal Nurses. All rights reserved.

resolution, if ever, may depend on the cause and on the duration of treatment. Each partner may progress through the stages at different rates (Kumar et al., 2007). Nonjudgmental acceptance and a professional, caring attitude on the nurse's part can go far in dissipating the negative emotions the couple may experience while going through these stages. Recognition of these stages can assist the nurse in providing appropriate support and counseling or referral for additional therapy.

This is also a time when the nurse may assess the couple's relationship: Are both partners able and willing to communicate verbally and share feelings? Are the partners mutually supportive? The answers to such questions may help the nurse to identify areas of strength and weakness and to construct an appropriate plan of care.

Referral to mental health professionals is helpful when the emotional issues become too disruptive in the couple's relationship or life. The couple should be aware of infertility support and education organizations such as RESOLVE (National Infertility Association) which may help meet some of their needs and validate their feelings. Finally, individual or group counseling with other infertile couples can help the couple resolve feelings brought about by their own difficult situation.

Genetic Disorders

Even when conception has been achieved, families can have special reproductive concerns. The desired and expected outcome of any pregnancy is the birth of a healthy, "perfect" baby. Parents experience grief, fear, and anger when they discover that their baby has been born with a defect or a genetic disease. Such an abnormality may be evident at birth or may not appear for some time. The baby may have inherited a disorder from one parent or both, creating guilt and strife within the family.

Regardless of the type or scope of the problem, parents will have many questions: "What did I do?" "What caused it?" "How do I cope with it?" "Will it happen again?" The nurse must anticipate the couple's questions and concerns and guide, direct, and support the family. To do so, the nurse must have a basic knowledge of genetics and genetic counseling. Professional nurses can help expedite this process if they understand the principles involved and can direct the family to the appropriate resources.

Chromosomes and Chromosomal Analysis

All hereditary material is carried on tightly coiled strands of DNA known as **chromosomes**. The chromosomes carry the *genes*, the smallest units of inheritance, as discussed in greater detail in Chapter 4 ∞. The Human

nursing framework that recognizes the multidimensional needs of the infertile individual or couple within physical, social, psychologic, spiritual, and environmental contexts.

Infertility may be perceived as a loss by one or both partners. Affected individuals have described this as a loss of their relationship with spouse, family, or friends; their health; their status or prestige; their self-esteem and self-confidence; their security; and the potential child. Any one of these losses may lead to depression, but in many cases the crisis of infertility evokes feelings similar to those associated with all these losses (Klock, 2004). Each couple passes through several stages of feelings: surprise, denial, anger, isolation, guilt, grief, and resolution. The impact of these feelings on the couple and how fast they move into

Genome Project has made remarkable advances toward determining the exact DNA sequence of human genes and the precise genes that are associated with certain abnormalities such as fragile X syndrome and cystic fibrosis, as discussed in greater detail later in the chapter (Ward, 2008).

All *somatic (body) cells* contain 46 chromosomes, which is the *diploid* number; the sperm and egg contain half as many (23) chromosomes, or *the haploid* number (see Chapter 4 ∞). There are 23 pairs of homologous chromosomes (a matched pair of chromosomes, one inherited from each parent). Twenty-two of the pairs are **autosomes** (nonsex chromosomes), and one pair is made up of the sex chromosomes, X and Y. A normal female has a 46, XX chromosome constitution, the normal male, 46, XY (Figures 7–7 ■ and 7–8 ■).

The **karyotype**, or pictorial analysis of these chromosomes, is usually obtained from specially treated and stained peripheral blood lymphocytes. Placental tissue taken from a site near the insertion of the cord and deep enough to include chorion can also be sent for karyotyping of the fetus.

Chromosome abnormalities can occur in either the autosomes or the sex chromosomes and can be divided into two categories: abnormalities of number and abnormalities of structure. Even small alterations in chromosomes can cause problems, especially those associated with delayed growth and development. Some of these abnormalities can be passed on to other offspring. Thus in some cases chromosomal analysis is appropriate even if clinical manifestations are mild.

Abnormalities of Chromosomal Number

Abnormalities of chromosomal number are most commonly seen as trisomies, monosomies, and mosaicism. In all three

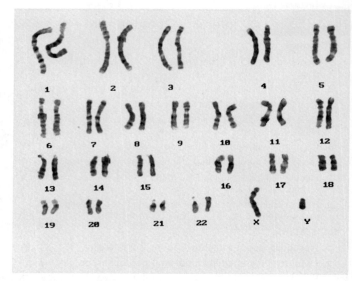

FIGURE 7–8 Normal male karyotype.
Source: Courtesy of David Peakman, Reproductive Genetics Center, Denver, CO.

cases, the abnormality is most often caused by *nondisjunction*, a failure of paired chromosomes to separate during cell division. If nondisjunction occurs in either the sperm or the egg before fertilization, the resulting zygote (fertilized egg) will have an abnormal chromosome makeup in all of the cells (trisomy or monosomy). If nondisjunction occurs after fertilization, the developing zygote will have cells with two or more different chromosome makeups, evolving into two or more different cell lines (mosaicism).

Trisomies are the product of the union of a normal gamete (egg or sperm) with a gamete that contains an extra chromosome. The individual will have 47 chromosomes and be trisomic (has three copies of the same chromosome) for whichever chromosome is extra (Table 7–8). Down syndrome (formerly called mongolism) is the most common trisomy abnormality seen in children (see Figure 7–9 ■).

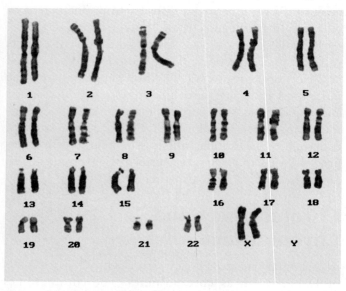

FIGURE 7–7 Normal female karyotype.
Source: Courtesy of David Peakman, Reproductive Genetics Center, Denver, CO.

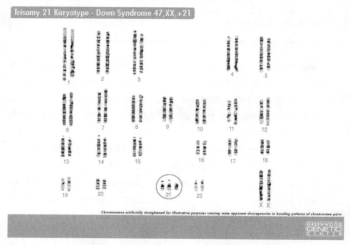

FIGURE 7–9 Karyotype of a female who has trisomy 21, Down syndrome. Note the extra 21 chromosome.
Source: Courtesy of Greenwood Genetics Center. (2007). *Genetic counseling aids,* 5th ed.

TABLE 7-8	Chromosomal Syndromes

Altered Chromosome: 21

Genetic defect: trisomy 21 (Down syndrome) (secondary nondisjunction or 14/21 unbalanced translocation)

Incidence: average 1 in 700 live births, incidence variable with age of woman (Figures 7–9 and 7–10)

Characteristics

CNS: mental retardation; hypotonia at birth

Head: flattened occiput; depressed nasal bridge; mongoloid slant of eyes; epicanthal folds; white specking of the iris (Brushfield spots); protrusion of the tongue; high, arched palate; low-set ears

Hands: broad, short fingers; abnormalities of finger and foot; dermal ridge patterns (dermatoglyphics); transverse palmar crease

Other: congenital heart disease

Altered Chromosome: 18

Genetic defect: trisomy 18

Incidence: 1 in 3000 live births

Characteristics

CNS: mental retardation; severe hypotonia

Head: prominent occiput; low-set ears; corneal opacities; ptosis (drooping eyelids)

Hands: third and fourth fingers overlapped by second and fifth fingers; abnormal dermatoglyphics; syndactyly (webbing of fingers)

Other: congenital heart defects; renal abnormalities; single umbilical artery; gastrointestinal tract abnormalities; rocker-bottom feet; cryptorchidism; various malformations of other organs

Altered Chromosome: 13

Genetic defect: trisomy 13

Incidence: 1 in 5000 live births

Characteristics

CNS: mental retardation; severe hypotonia; seizures

Head: microcephaly; microphthalmia, and/or coloboma (keyhole-shaped pupil); malformed ears; aplasia of external auditory canal; micrognathia (abnormally small lower jaw); cleft lip and palate

Hands: polydactyly (extra digits); abnormal posturing of fingers; abnormal dermatoglyphics

Other: congenital heart defects; hemangiomas; gastrointestinal tract defects; various malformations of other organs

Altered Chromosome: 5P

Genetic defect: deletion of short arm of chromosome 5 (cri du chat, or cat-cry syndrome)

Incidence: 1 in 20,000 live births

Characteristics

CNS: severe mental retardation; a catlike cry in infancy

Head: microcephaly; hypertelorism (widely spaced eyes); epicanthal folds; low-set ears

Other: failure to thrive; various organ malformations

Altered Chromosome: XO (Sex Chromosome)

Genetic defect: only one X chromosome or partially missing second X chromosome in female (Turner syndrome)

Incidence: 1 in 300 to 7000 live female births (Figure 7–13)

Characteristics

CNS: no intellectual impairment; some perceptual difficulties

Head: low hairline; webbed neck

Trunk: short stature; cubitus valgus (increased carrying angle of arm); excessive nevi (congenital discoloration of skin because of pigmentation); broad, shieldlike chest with widely spaced nipples; puffy feet; no toenails

Other: fibrous streaks in ovaries; underdeveloped secondary sex characteristics; primary amenorrhea; usually infertile; renal anomalies; coarctation of the aorta

Altered Chromosome: XXY (Sex Chromosome)

Genetic defect: extra X chromosome in male (Klinefelter syndrome)

Incidence: 1 in 1000 live male births, approximately 1% to 2% of institutionalized males

Characteristics

CNS: mild mental retardation

Trunk: occasional gynecomastia (abnormally large male breasts); eunuchoid body proportions (lack of male muscular and sexual development)

Other: small, soft testes; underdeveloped secondary sex characteristics; usually sterile

The presence of the extra chromosome 21 produces distinctive clinical features (see Table 7–7 and Figure 7–10 ■). Although children born with Down syndrome have a variety of physical ailments, advances in medical science have extended their life expectancy.

Two other common trisomies are trisomy 18 and trisomy 13 (refer to Table 7–8 and Figures 7–11 and 7–12 ■). The prognosis for both trisomies 13 and 18 is extremely poor. Most children (70%) die within the first 3 months of life sec-

ondary to complications related to respiratory and cardiac abnormalities. However, 10% survive the first year of life; therefore, the family needs to plan for the possibility of long-term care of a severely affected infant and for family support.

Monosomies occur when a normal gamete unites with a gamete that is missing a chromosome. In this case, the individual has only 45 chromosomes and is said to be monosomic. Monosomy of an entire autosomal chromosome is incompatible with life.

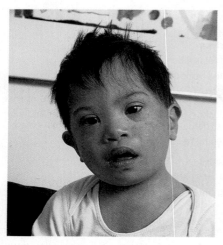

FIGURE 7–10 A boy with Down syndrome.

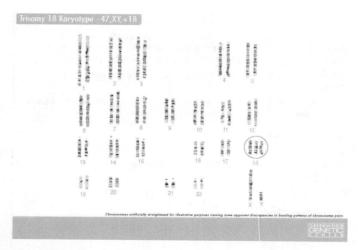

FIGURE 7–11 Karyotype of a male who has trisomy 18.
Source: Courtesy of Greenwood Center. (2007). *Genetic counseling aids,* 5th ed.

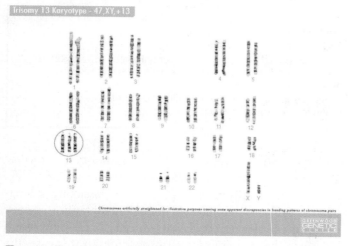

FIGURE 7–12 Karyotype of male with trisomy 13.
Source: Courtesy of Greenwood Center. (2007). *Genetic counseling aids,* 5th ed.

Mosaicism occurs after fertilization and results in an individual who has two different cell lines, each with a different chromosomal number. Mosaicism tends to be more common in the sex chromosomes than in the autosomes; when it occurs in the autosomes, it is most common in Down syndrome. An individual with many classic signs of Down syndrome but with normal or near-normal intelligence should be investigated for the possibility of mosaicism.

Abnormalities of Chromosome Structure

Abnormalities of chromosome structure involve only parts of the chromosome and occur in two forms: translocation and deletions or additions. Some children born with Down syndrome have an abnormal rearrangement of chromosomal material known as a *translocation.* Clinically the two types of Down syndrome are indistinguishable; the only way to distinguish them is to do a chromosome analysis.

The translocation occurs when the carrier parent has 45 chromosomes, usually with one chromosome fused to another. For example, a common translocation is one in which a particle of chromosome 14 breaks and fuses to chromosome 21. The parent has one normal 14, one normal 21, and one 14/21 chromosome. Because all the chromosomal material is present and functioning normally, the parent is clinically normal. This individual is known as a *balanced translocation carrier.* When a person who is a balanced translocation carrier has a child with a partner who has a structurally normal chromosome constitution, the child can have a normal number of chromosomes, be a carrier, or have an extra chromosome 21. Such a child has an *unbalanced translocation* and has Down syndrome.

Structure abnormality is also caused by *additions* or *deletions* of chromosomal material. Any portion of a chromosome may be lost or added, generally leading to some adverse effect. Depending on how much chromosomal material is involved, the clinical effects may be mild or severe. Many types of additions and deletions have been described, such as the deletion of the short arm of chromosome 5 (*cri du chat,* or cat-cry syndrome) or the deletion of the long arm of chromosome 18 (Edwards syndrome). Table 7–8 lists other chromosomal syndromes.

Sex Chromosome Abnormalities

To better understand abnormalities of the sex chromosomes, the nurse should know that in a female, at an early embryonic stage, one of the two normal X chromosomes becomes inactive. The inactive X chromosome forms a dark staining area known as the *Barr body.* The normal female has one Barr body, because one of her two X chromosomes has been inactivated. The normal male has no Barr bodies because he has only one X chromosome.

The most common sex chromosome abnormalities are Turner syndrome in females (45, XO with no Barr bodies present; see Figure 7–13 ■) and Klinefelter syndrome in males (47, XXY with one Barr body present). See Table 7–8 for clinical descriptions of these abnormalities.

The mosaic form of the XO chromosome is associated with daughters of women who took the drug diethylstilbestrol (DES) during pregnancy. The fertility of women with the mosaic form of the XO chromosome may not be impaired; however, there is a higher percentage of uterine malformation and hormonal difficulty associated with it and therefore a high degree of miscarriage.

There is a concern that children born as a result of ICSI might be at increased risk for chromosomal and other major congenital anomalies, cancer, or infertility, because ICSI may override natural safeguards that serve to prevent fertilization. Therefore it is strongly recommended that karyotyping and Y chromosome deletion analysis be offered to all men with severe male factor infertility who are candidates for IVF and ICSI (Speroff & Fritz, 2005).

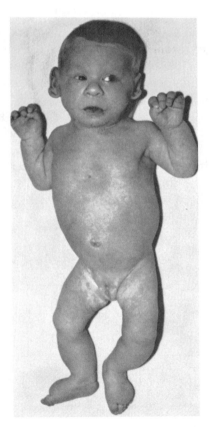

FIGURE 7–13 Infant with Turner syndrome at 1 month of age. Note prominent ears.
Source: Lemli, L., & Smith, D. W. (1963). The XO syndrome: A study of the differentiated phenotype in 25 patients. *Journal of Pediatrics, 63,* 577, with permission from Elsevier Science.

Modes of Inheritance

Many inherited diseases are produced by an abnormality in a single gene or pair of genes. In such instances, the chromosomes are grossly normal. The defect is at the gene level. Some of these gene defects can be detected by technologies such as DNA and other biochemical assays.

The two major categories of inheritance are **Mendelian (single-gene) inheritance** and **non-Mendelian (multifactorial) inheritance**. Each single-gene trait is determined by a pair of genes working together. These genes are responsible for the observable expression of the traits (e.g., brown eyes, dark skin), referred to as the **phenotype**. The total genetic makeup of an individual is referred to as the **genotype** (pattern of the genes on the chromosomes).

One of the genes for a trait is inherited from the mother, the other from the father. An individual who has two identical genes at a given locus is considered to be *homozygous* for that trait. Individuals are considered to be *heterozygous* for a particular trait when they have two different alleles (alternate forms of the same gene) at a given locus on a pair of homologous chromosomes.

The best known modes of single-gene inheritance are autosomal dominant, autosomal recessive, and X-linked (sex-linked) recessive. There is also an X-linked dominant mode of inheritance, which is less common, and the new identified mode of inheritance, fragile X syndrome.

Autosomal Dominant Inheritance

A person is said to have an autosomal dominant inherited disorder if the disease trait is heterozygous—that is, the abnormal gene overshadows the normal gene of the pair to produce the trait. It is essential to remember that in autosomal dominant inheritance the following occurs:

- An affected individual generally has an affected parent. Thus the family **pedigree** (graphic representation of a family tree) usually shows multiple generations with the disorder.
- Affected individuals have a 50% chance of passing on the abnormal gene to each of their children (Figure 7–14 ■).
- Males and females are equally affected, and a father can pass the abnormal gene on to his son. This is an important principle when distinguishing autosomal dominant disorders from X-linked disorders.
- Autosomal dominant inherited disorders have varying degrees of presentation. This is an important factor when counseling families concerning autosomal dominant disorders. Although a parent may have a mild form of the disease, the child may have a more severe form.

Autosomal dominant conditions such as phocomelia (a developmental anomaly characterized by the absence of the upper portion of the limbs) can have minimal expression in

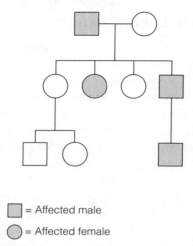

= Affected male

= Affected female

FIGURE 7–14 Autosomal dominant pedigree. One parent is affected. Statistically 50% of offspring will be affected regardless of sex.

a parent but severe effects in a child. Other common autosomal dominant inherited disorders are Huntington disease, polycystic kidney disease, neurofibromatosis (von Recklinghausen disease), and achondroplastic dwarfism.

Autosomal Recessive Inheritance

In an autosomal recessive inherited disorder, the individual must have two abnormal genes to be affected. The notion of a carrier state is appropriate here. A *carrier* is an individual who is heterozygous for the abnormal gene and clinically normal. It is not until two individuals mate and pass on the same abnormal gene that affected children may appear. It is essential to remember that in autosomal recessive inheritance the following occurs:

- An affected individual may have clinically normal parents, but both parents are carriers of the abnormal gene (Figure 7–15 ■).

- In the case where both parents are carriers, there is a 25% chance that the abnormal gene will be passed on to any of their offspring. Each pregnancy has a 25% chance of resulting in an affected child.
- If a child of two carrier parents is clinically normal, there is a 50% chance that the child is a carrier of the gene.
- Both males and females are equally affected.
- There is an increased history of consanguineous matings (mating of close relatives).

Some common autosomal recessive inherited disorders are cystic fibrosis, phenylketonuria (PKU), galactosemia, sickle cell anemia, Tay–Sachs disease, and most metabolic disorders.

X-Linked Recessive Inheritance

X-linked, or sex-linked, disorders are those for which the abnormal gene is carried on the X chromosome. Thus an X-linked disorder is manifested in a male who carries the abnormal gene on his X chromosome. His mother is considered to be a carrier when the normal gene on one X chromosome overshadows the abnormal gene on the other X chromosome. It is essential to remember that in X-linked recessive inheritance the following occurs:

- There is no male-to-male transmission. Affected males are related through the female line (see Figure 7–16 ■).
- There is a 50% chance that a carrier mother will pass the abnormal gene to each of her sons, who will thus be affected.
  - There is a 50% chance that a carrier mother will pass the normal gene to each of her sons, who will thus be unaffected.
  - There is a 50% chance that a carrier mother will pass the abnormal gene to each of her daughters, who become carriers.

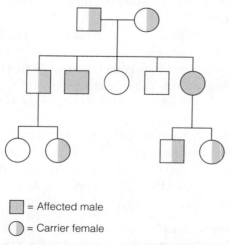

= Affected male

= Carrier female

FIGURE 7–15 Autosomal recessive pedigree. Both parents are carriers. Statistically 25% of offspring are affected regardless of sex.

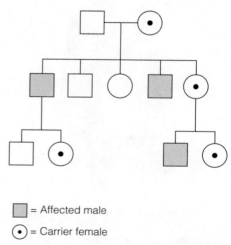

= Affected male

= Carrier female

FIGURE 7–16 X-linked recessive pedigree. The mother is the carrier. Statistically 50% of male offspring are affected, and 50% of female offspring are carriers.

• Fathers affected with an X-linked disorder cannot pass the disorder to their sons, but all their daughters become carriers of the disorder.

Common X-linked recessive disorders are hemophilia, Duchenne muscular dystrophy, and color blindness.

X-Linked Dominant Inheritance

X-linked dominant disorders are extremely rare, the most common being vitamin D-resistant rickets and fragile X syndrome. When X-linked dominance does occur, the pattern is similar to that of X-linked recessive inheritance except that heterozygous females are affected. It is essential to remember that in X-linked dominant inheritance there is no male-to-male transmission. Affected fathers will have affected daughters; however, because they pass only the Y chromosome to male offspring, any sons will not be affected.

Fragile X Syndrome

Fragile X syndrome is a common inherited form of mental retardation second only to Down syndrome among all causes of moderate mental retardation in males. Fragile X syndrome is a central nervous system disorder linked to a "fragile" site on the X chromosome. It is characterized by moderate mental retardation, large protuberant ears, and large testes after puberty. The carrier females do not have the abnormal features, but about one-third are mildly retarded.

Multifactorial Inheritance

Many common congenital malformations such as cleft palate, heart defects, spina bifida, dislocated hips, clubfoot, and pyloric stenosis are caused by an interaction of many genes and environmental factors. They are, therefore, multifactorial in origin. It is essential to remember that in multifactorial inheritance the following occurs:

• The malformations may vary from mild to severe. For example, spina bifida may range in severity from mild (spina bifida occulta) to more severe (myelomeningocele). It is believed that the more severe the defect, the greater the number of genes present for that defect.
• There is often a sex bias. For example, pyloric stenosis is more common in males, whereas cleft palate is more common in females. When a member of the less commonly affected sex shows the condition, a greater number of genes must usually be present to cause the defect.
• In the presence of environmental influences (such as seasonal changes, altitude, radiation exposure, chemicals in the environment, or exposure to toxic substances), fewer genes are needed to manifest the disease in the offspring.

• In contrast to single-gene disorders, there is an additive effect in multifactorial inheritance. The more family members who have the defect, the greater the risk that the next pregnancy will also be affected (Ward, 2008).

Although most congenital malformations are multifactorial, a careful family history should always be taken, because cleft lip and palate, certain congenital heart defects, and other malformations occasionally can be inherited as autosomal dominant or recessive traits. Other disorders thought to be within the multifactorial inheritance group are diabetes, hypertension, some heart diseases, and mental illness.

Prenatal Diagnostic Tests

Parent–child and family-planning counseling have become a major responsibility of professional nurses. To be effective counselors, nurses must have the most up-to-date information about prenatal diagnosis. Appropriate counseling should occur before prenatal screening is done. It is essential that couples be completely informed about the known and potential risks of each of the genetic diagnostic procedures. The prescreening counseling should include the conditions detectable by the screen, diagnostic test available if the screen is positive, risk to the mother and child of the test performed, accuracy of the test, and limitations of the test (Lashley, 2007). The nurse needs to recognize the emotional impact on the family of a decision to undergo or not to undergo a genetic diagnostic procedure.

The ability to diagnose certain genetic diseases has enormous implications for the practice of preventive health care. Several methods are available for prenatal diagnosis, although some are still experimental.

Genetic Ultrasound

Ultrasound may be used to assess the fetus for genetic or congenital problems. With ultrasound, one can visualize the fetal head for fetal abnormalities in size, shape, and structure. (For a detailed discussion of ultrasound technology, see Chapter 14 ∞.) Craniospinal defects (anencephalus, microcephaly, hydrocephalus), thoracic malformations (diaphragmatic hernia), gastrointestinal malformations (omphalocele, gastroschisis), renal malformations (dysplasia or obstruction), and skeletal malformations (caudal regression, conjoined twins) are only some of the disorders that have been diagnosed in utero by ultrasound. Screening by ultrasound for congenital anomalies is best done at 18 to 20 weeks, when fetal structures have developed completely. With the addition of fetal nuchal translucency measurement at 10 to 13 weeks, there is high correlation with fetal chromosome abnormalities (Lashley, 2007). There is no information documenting harm to the fetus or long-term effects with exposure to ultrasound. However, there is no guarantee of complete safety; therefore, the practitioner and the parents must evaluate the risks against the benefits on an individual basis.

Genetic Amniocentesis

A major method of prenatal diagnosis is genetic amniocentesis (Figure 7–17 ■). The procedure is described in Chapter 14 ∞. The indications for genetic amniocentesis include the following:

1. *Maternal age 35 or older.* Women age 35 or older are at greater risk for having children with chromosomal abnormalities (see Chapter 9 ∞ for further discussion). Chromosomal abnormalities because of maternal age include trisomy 21, trisomy 13, trisomy 18, XXX, or XXY. The risk of having a live-born infant with a chromosome problem is 1 in 192 for a 35-year-old woman; the risk for trisomy 21 is 1 in 386. At age 44, the risks are 1 in 26 and 1 in 40, respectively (Ward, 2008).
2. *Previous child born with a chromosomal abnormality.* Young couples who have had a child with a trisomy 21, 18, or 13 have an approximately 1% to 2% risk of a future child having a chromosomal abnormality.
3. *Parent carrying a chromosomal abnormality (balanced translocation).* A woman who carries a balanced 14/21 translocation has a risk of approximately 10% to 15% that her children will be affected with the unbalanced translocation of Down syndrome; if the father is the carrier, there is a 2% to 5% risk.
4. *Mother carrying an X-linked disease.* In families in which the woman is a known or possible carrier of an X-linked disorder such as hemophilia A or B or Duchenne muscular dystrophy, options may include genetic amniocentesis, chorionic villus sampling (CVS), or percutaneous umbilical blood sampling (PUBS). For a known female carrier, the risk of an affected male fetus is 50%. Now DNA testing may make it possible to identify affected males from nonaffected males in some disorders. In disorders in which female carriers can be distinguished from noncarriers, only the carrier females would be offered prenatal diagnosis.
5. *Parents carrying an inborn error of metabolism that can be diagnosed in utero.* Inborn error of metabolism disorders detectable in utero include argininosuccinic-

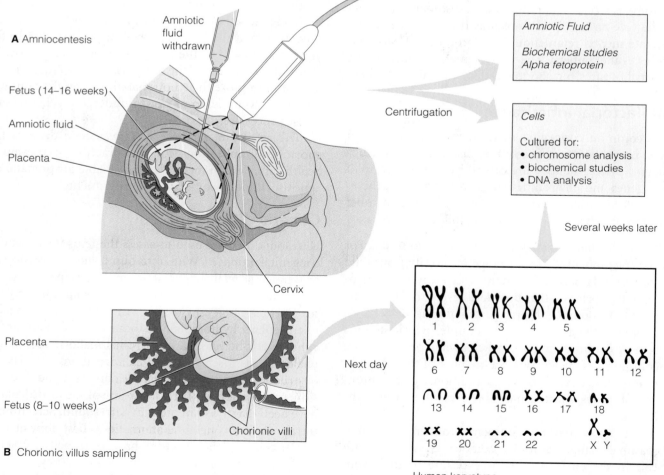

FIGURE 7–17 *A,* Genetic amniocentesis for prenatal diagnosis is done at 14 to 16 weeks' gestation. *B,* Chorionic villus sampling is done at 8 to 10 weeks, and the cells are karyotyped within 48 to 72 hours.

aciduria, cystinosis, Fabry disease, galactosemia, Gaucher disease, homocystinuria, Hunter syndrome, Hurler disease, Krabbe disease, Lesch–Nyhan syndrome, maple syrup urine disease, metachromatic leukodystrophy, methylmalonic aciduria, Niemann–Pick disease, Pompe disease, Sanfilippo syndrome, and Tay–Sachs disease.

6. *Both parents carrying an autosomal recessive disease.* When both parents are carriers of an autosomal recessive disease, there is a 25% risk for *each pregnancy* that the fetus will be affected. Diagnosis is made by testing the cultured amniotic fluid cells (enzyme level, substrate level, product level, or DNA) or the fluid itself. Autosomal recessive diseases identified by amniocentesis are hemoglobinopathies such as sickle cell anemia, thalassemia, and cystic fibrosis (Dugoff, 2008).

7. *Family history of neural tube defects.* Genetic amniocentesis is available to couples who have had a child with neural tube defects or who have a family history of these conditions, which include anencephaly, spina bifida, and myelomeningocele. Neural tube defects are usually multifactorial traits.

Percutaneous Umbilical Blood Sampling and Chorionic Villus Sampling

Percutaneous umbilical blood sampling (PUBS) is a technique used for obtaining blood that allows for rapid chromosome diagnosis, genetic studies, or transfusion for Rh isoimmunization or hydrops fetalis. *Chorionic villus sampling (CVS)* is used in selected regional centers, and its diagnostic capability is similar to that of amniocentesis. Its advantage is that diagnostic information is available at 8 to 10 weeks' gestation and that products of conception are tested directly. Some potential risks include loss of pregnancy or limb-reduction defects especially if performed before 10 weeks gestation. For further discussion, see Chapter 14 ∞.

Alpha-Fetoprotein

The maternal circulation or amniotic fluid is tested for alpha-fetoprotein (AFP). The maternal serum AFP (MSAFP) level is elevated in cases of infants with open neural tube defects, anencephaly, omphalocele, or gastroschisis, and in multiple gestations (Lashley, 2007). Low MSAFP level has been associated with Down syndrome. MSAFP testing is done at 15 to 22 weeks' gestation (Lashley, 2007). In addition other screening labs may include maternal serum free beta human chorionic gonadotropin (hCG) and maternal serum-pregnancy-associated plasma protein (PAPP-A) to detect Down syndrome. Ultrasound and amniocentesis are offered to clients with low or high MSAFP levels. Inaccurate dating is the most common cause for abnormal AFP; therefore, ultrasound dating is very important. With high MSAFP levels, normal amniotic fluid AFP, and normal ultrasound, there is an increased risk for preterm labor, perinatal death, and intrauterine growth restriction.

Implications of Prenatal Diagnostic Testing

It is imperative that counseling precede any procedure for prenatal diagnosis. Many questions and points must be considered if the family is to reach a satisfactory decision. See Key Facts to Remember: Couples Who May Benefit from Prenatal Diagnosis and Cultural Perspectives: Genetic Screening Recommendations for Various Ethnic and Age Groups.

With the advent of diagnostic techniques such as amniocentesis, at-risk couples who would not otherwise have a first child or additional children can decide to conceive. Following prenatal diagnosis, a couple can decide not to have a child with a genetic disease. For many couples, prenatal diagnosis is not a solution because they choose not to prevent the genetic disease by aborting the fetus. The decision about whether to use prenatal diagnosis can only be made by the family. Even when termination is not an option, prenatal diagnosis can give parents an opportunity to prepare for the birth of a child with special needs, contact the families of children with similar problems, or access support services before the birth.

❖

KEY FACTS TO REMEMBER

Couples Who May Benefit from Prenatal Diagnosis

- Women age 35 or over at time of birth
- Couples with a balanced translocation (chromosomal abnormality)
- Family history of known or suspected Mendelian genetic disorder (e.g., cystic fibrosis, hemophilia A and B, Duchenne muscular dystrophy)
- Couples with a previous child with chromosomal abnormality
- Couples in which either partner or a previous child is affected with, or in which both partners are carriers for, a diagnosable metabolic disorder
- Family history of birth defects and/or mental retardation (e.g., neural tube defects, congenital heart disease, cleft lip and/or palate)
- Ethnic groups at increased risk for specific disorders (see Cultural Perspectives: Genetic Screening Recommendations for Various Ethnic and Age Groups)
- Couples with history of two or more first trimester spontaneous abortions
- Women with an abnormal maternal serum alpha-fetoprotein (MSAFP or AFP) test
- Women with a teratogenic risk secondary to an exposure or maternal health condition (e.g., diabetes)

Every pregnancy has a 3% to 4% risk of resulting in an infant with a birth defect. When an abnormality is detected or suspected before birth, an attempt is made to determine the diagnosis by assessing the family health history (via the pedigree) and the pregnancy history and by evaluating the fetal anomaly or anomalies via ultrasound. Once experts on a specific disorder are consulted, healthcare professionals can then present the parents with options.

Treatment of prenatally diagnosed disorders may begin during the pregnancy, thus possibly preventing irreversible damage. For example, a mother carrying a fetus with galactosemia may follow a galactose-free diet. In light of the philosophy of preventive health care, information that can be obtained prenatally should be made available to all couples who are expecting a baby or who are contemplating pregnancy.

Postnatal Diagnosis

Questions concerning genetic disorders (cause, treatment, and prognosis) are most often first discussed in the new-born nursery or during the infant's first few months of life. When a child is born with anomalies, has a stormy newborn period, or does not progress as expected, a genetic evaluation may be warranted. An accurate diagnosis and an optimal treatment plan incorporate the following:

- Complete detailed history to determine whether the problem is prenatal (congenital), postnatal, or familial in origin
- Complete physical examination that includes a dermatoglyphics analysis (Figure 7–18 ■)
- Laboratory analysis, which includes chromosome analysis; enzyme assay for inborn errors of metabolism (see Chapter 28 ∞ for further discussion of these tests); DNA studies (both direct and by linkage); and antibody titers for infectious teratogens, such as toxoplasmosis, rubella, cytomegalovirus, and herpes virus (TORCH syndrome) (see Chapter 16 ∞).

To make an accurate diagnosis, the geneticist consults with other specialists and reviews the current literature.

CULTURAL PERSPECTIVES
Genetic Screening Recommendations for Various Ethnic and Age Groups

Background of Population at Risk	Disorder	Screening Test	Definitive Test
Ashkenazic Jewish, French-Canadians, Cajuns	Tay–Sachs disease	Decreased serum hexosaminidase-A	CVS* or amniocentesis for hexosaminidase-A assay
African; Hispanic from Caribbean, Central America, or South America; Arabs; Egyptians; Asian Indians	Sickle cell anemia	Presence of sickle-cell hemoglobin; confirmatory hemoglobin electrophoresis	CVS or amniocentesis for genotype determination; direct molecular studies
Greek, Italian	Beta-thalassemia	Mean corpuscular volume less than 80%; confirmatory hemoglobin electrophoresis	CVS or amniocentesis for genotype determination (direct molecular studies or indirect RFLP†l analysis)
Southeast Asian (Vietnamese, Laotian, Cambodian), Filipino	Alpha-thalassemia	Mean corpuscular volume less than 80%; confirmatory hemoglobin electrophoresis	CVS or amniocentesis for genotype determination (direct molecular studies)
Women over age 35 (all ethnic groups)	Chromosomal trisomies	None	CVS or amniocentesis for cytogenetic analysis
Women of any age (all ethnic groups; particularly suggested for women from British Isles, Ireland)	Neural tube defects and selected other anomalies	Maternal serum alpha-fetoprotein (MSAFP)	Amniocentesis for amniotic fluid, alpha-fetoprotein, and acetylcholinesterase assays
Ashkenazic Jewish	Gaucher disease	Decrease glucocerebrosidase	CVS
Caucasians (Northern Europeans, Celtic population), Ashkenazic Jewish	Cystic fibrosis	Transmembrane regulation (CFTR) gene	CVS or amniocentesis for genotype determination; definitive diagnosis for all fetuses not possible

*Chorionic villus sampling.

†lRestriction fragment length polymorphism.

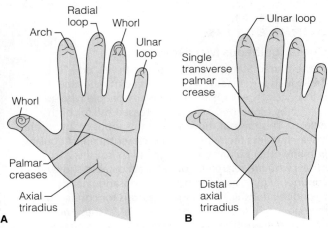

FIGURE 7–18 Dermatoglyphic patterns of the hands in *A,* a normal individual, and *B,* a child with Down syndrome. Note the single transverse palmar crease, distally placed axial triradius, and increased number of ulnar loops.

This lets the geneticist evaluate all the available information before arriving at a diagnosis and plan of action.

The Human Genome Project has significant implications for the identification and management of inherited disorders. Once genes are identified, it will be possible to detect their presence in carriers and lead to better genetic counseling. New genetic material might be inserted into cells to provide important missing information (gene transfer) as may be possible in cystic fibrosis, or medications can be specifically designed to target the disease on a molecular level (Simpson & Holzgreve, 2007).

However, concerns have been voiced about ethical considerations with genetic research. What guidelines are needed to protect children and families so that genetic testing does not lead to discrimination in future employment or health insurance? Who should be tested for genetic diseases, and who should have access to the results? Because children cannot yet give informed consent for genetic testing (see Chapter 1 ∞ for discussion of informed consent), it is recommended that children and adolescents should have genetic testing only when medical treatment could help if the disease is identified, or when another family member might benefit from the knowledge for their own health and the child will not be harmed by testing (Simpson & Holzgreve, 2007). Whenever genetic testing is performed, counseling about the results must be available.

Perinatal and neonatal nurses must keep abreast of new genomic knowledge and prenatal/neonatal screening and testing that can be done to impact long-term health (Williams et al., 2004). Because of nursing's frontline position in healthcare systems and their emphasis on providing holistic, family-centered care, nurses are likely the first healthcare professionals individuals and families will turn to with questions about genetic risk and susceptibility, as well as to seek guidance regarding the complex-

ities of genetic testing and interpretation. All health professionals at every level of education must have knowledge of genomics. In 2001 the National Coalition of Health Professional Education in Genetics (NCHPEG) published a list of core competencies for all health professionals in all disciplines (Jenkins, 2001). Currently a nursing group led by Dr. Jean Jenkins and colleagues are adapting these to reflect the nursing profession and care. Some nurses with a subspecialty in genomics enable them to work in the growing field of genetics and health care. They can act as a genetic counselor, informing families of their genetic risks, providing information, and giving support during the initial diagnosis and thorough follow-up.

Genetic Counseling

Genetic counseling is a communication process in which a genetic counselor, physician, or specially trained and certified nurse tries to provide a family with the most complete and accurate information about the occurrence or the risk of recurrence of a genetic disease in that family. Genetic counseling is thus an appropriate course of action for any family wondering, "Will it happen again?"

Referral

Genetic counseling referral is advised for any of the following categories:

- *Congenital abnormalities, including mental retardation.* Any couple who has a child or a relative with a congenital malformation may be at increased risk and should be so informed. If mental retardation of unidentified cause has occurred in a family, there may be an increased risk of recurrence. In some cases, the genetic counselor will identify the cause of a malformation as a teratogen (see Chapter 11 ∞). The family should be aware of teratogenic substances so they can avoid exposure during any subsequent pregnancy.
- *Familial disorders.* Families should be told that certain diseases may have a genetic component and that the risk of their occurrence in a particular family may be higher than that in the general population. Such disorders as diabetes, heart disease, cancer, and mental illness fall into this category.
- *Known inherited diseases.* Families may know that a disease is inherited but not know the mechanism or the specific risk for them. An important point to remember is that family members who are not at risk for passing on a disorder should be as well informed as family members who are at risk.
- *Metabolic disorders.* Any families at risk for having a child with a metabolic disorder or biochemical defect should be referred for genetic counseling. Because

most inborn errors of metabolism are autosomal recessively inherited, a family may not be identified as being at risk until the birth of an affected child; for example, a child with cystic fibrosis or sickle cell anemia. Carriers of the sickle cell trait and cystic fibrosis can be identified before conception or a pregnancy has occurred, and the risk of having an affected child can be determined. Prenatal diagnosis of an affected fetus is available on an experimental basis only.

• *Chromosomal abnormalities.* As discussed previously, any couple who has had a child with a chromosomal abnormality may be at increased risk of having another child similarly affected. This group includes families in which there is concern about a possible translocation.

After a couple has been referred to the genetics clinic, they are sent a form requesting information on the health status of various family members. This information assists the genetic counselor in creating the family's pedigree.

Together, the pedigree and history facilitate identification of other family members who might also be at risk for the same disorder (Figure 7–19 ■). The family being

CULTURAL PERSPECTIVES

Consanguineous Marriages

In the United States, marriage between related individuals is generally taboo. In Western medicine, there is a concern that a child conceived by people who are related by blood may have an increased risk for birth defects. This has not, however, been supported by recent research unless the relationship is closer than first cousins. In many other cultures, marriage of first cousins and others who are related by blood is acceptable and even common. Egypt has a high rate of consanguineous (blood relationship) marriages. Reasons for consanguineous marriage include: "increase family links," "they knew each other and everything would be clear before marriage," "customs and traditions," and "less cost." The most common type of consanguineous marriage in Egypt is between first cousins.

counseled may wish to notify relatives at risk so that they, too, can begin genetic counseling. When done correctly, the family history and pedigree can be powerful tools for determining a family's risk.

Initial Session

During the initial session, the counselor gathers additional information about the pregnancy, the affected child's growth and development, and the family's understanding of the problem. The counselor also elicits information concerning ethnic background and family origin. Many genetic disorders are more common among certain ethnic groups or in particular geographic areas.

Generally the child undergoes a physical examination. Other family members may also be examined. If laboratory tests such as chromosomal analyses, metabolic studies, or viral titers are indicated, they are performed at this time. The genetic counselor may then give the parents some preliminary information based on the data at hand.

Follow-Up Counseling

When all the data have been carefully examined and analyzed, the couple returns for a follow-up visit. At this time, the genetic counselor gives the parents all the information available, including the medical facts, diagnosis, probable course of the disorder, and any available management; the inheritance pattern for this particular family and the risk of recurrence; and the options or alternatives for dealing with the risk of recurrence. The remainder of the counseling session is spent discussing the course of action that seems appropriate to the family in view of the risk and family goals. For couples who desire to become parents or who want a subsequent child, options include prenatal diagnosis, early detection and treatment, and, in some cases, adoption, therapeutic insemination, and delayed childbearing.

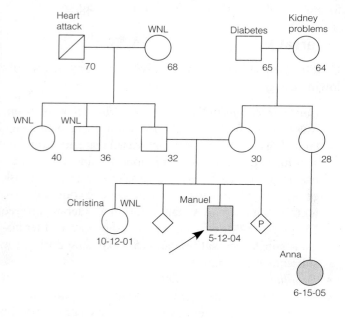

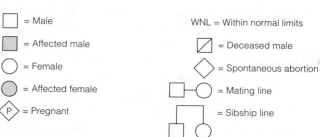

FIGURE 7–19 Screening pedigree. Arrow indicates the nearest family member affected with the disorder being investigated. Basic data have been recorded. Numbers refer to the ages of the family members.

The couple may consider therapeutic donor insemination (TDI), discussed earlier in the chapter. This alternative is appropriate, for example, if the male partner has an autosomal dominant disease; TDI would decrease to zero the risk of having an affected child (if the sperm donor is not at risk) because the child would not inherit any genes from the affected parent. If the man has an X-linked disorder and does not wish to continue the gene in the family (all his daughters would be carriers), TDI is an alternative to terminating all pregnancies with a female fetus. If the man is a carrier for a balanced translocation and if termination of pregnancy is against family ethics, TDI is the most appropriate alternative. If both parents are carriers of an autosomal recessive disorder, TDI lowers the risk to a very low level or to zero if a carrier test is available. TDI also may be appropriate if the couple is at high risk for a multifactorial disorder.

Couples who are young and at risk may decide to delay childbearing. These couples may find in a few years that prenatal diagnosis is available or that a disease can be detected and treated early to prevent irreversible damage.

When the parents have completed the counseling sessions, the counselor sends them and their certified nurse–midwife or physician a letter detailing the contents of the sessions. The parents keep this document for reference. See Key Facts to Remember: Nursing Responsibilities in Genetic Counseling.

Nursing Care Management

In both prospective and retrospective genetic counseling, timely nursing intervention is a crucial factor. During annual exam and other clinical appointments, the nurse should interview all women of childbearing age to determine any family history or other risk factors for genetic disorders. If the woman is planning to conceive, genetic counseling should be encouraged before discontinuation of contraception.

The nurse has a key role in preventing recurrence. One cannot expect a couple who has just learned that their child has a birth defect or Down syndrome to take in any information concerning future risks. However, the couple should never be "put off" from genetic counseling for so long that they conceive another affected child because of lack of information. The perinatal nursing team frequently has the first contact with the family who has a newborn with a congenital abnormality. At the birth of an affected child, the nurse can inform the parents that genetic counseling is available.

After genetic counseling, the nurse with the appropriate knowledge of genetics is in an ideal position to help couples review what has been discussed during the counseling sessions and to answer any additional questions they might have. As families return to daily living, the nurse can provide helpful information on the day-to-day aspects of caring for a child, answer questions as they arise, support parents in their decisions, and refer families to other health and community agencies.

The family may return to the genetic counselor a number of times to ask questions and express concerns, especially if the couple is considering having more children, or if siblings want information about their affected brother or sister. It is most desirable for the nurse working with the family to attend many or all of these counseling sessions. Because the nurse has already established a rapport with the couple, she or he can act as a liaison between the family and the genetic counselor. Hearing directly what the genetic counselor says helps the nurse clarify the issues for the family, which in turn helps them formulate questions. Many genetic centers have found the public health nurse to be the ideal health professional to provide such follow-up care. Nurses must be careful not to assume a diagnosis, determine carrier status or recurrence risks, or provide genetic counseling without adequate information and training. Inadequate, inappropriate, or inaccurate information may be misleading or harmful. Healthcare professionals need to learn the appropriate referral systems and options for care in their region.

CHAPTER HIGHLIGHTS

- Couples are considered infertile when they do not conceive after 1 year of unprotected coitus.
- Around 8% of couples in the United States are infertile.
- A thorough history and physical exam of both partners are essential as a basis for infertility investigation.
- General fertility investigations include evaluation of ovarian function, cervical mucus adequacy and receptivity to sperm, sperm number and function, tubal patency, general condition of the pelvic organs, and certain laboratory tests.
- Among cases of infertility, 40% involve male factors, 40% involve female factors, and 20% have either no identifiable cause or have multifactorial causes.
- Medications may be prescribed to induce ovulation, facilitate cervical mucus formation, reduce antibody concentration, increase sperm count and motility, and suppress endometriosis.
- The emotional aspects of infertility may be even more difficult for the couple than the testing and therapy.
- The nurse needs to be prepared to dispel myths and provide accurate information about infertility.
- The nurse assesses coping responses and initiates counseling referrals as indicated.
- In autosomal dominant inherited disorders, an affected parent has a 50% chance of having an affected child. Such disorders equally affect males and females. The characteristic presentation varies in each individual with the gene. Some of the common autosomal dominant inherited disorders are Huntington disease, polycystic kidney disease, and neurofibromatosis (von Recklinghausen disease).
- Autosomal recessive inherited disorders are characterized by both parents being carriers; each offspring having a 25% chance of having the disease, a 25% chance of not being affected, and a 50% chance of being a carrier; and males and females being equally affected. Some common autosomal recessive inherited disorders are cystic fibrosis, phenylketonuria, galactosemia, sickle cell anemia, Tay–Sachs disease, and most metabolic disorders.
- X-linked recessive disorders are characterized by no male-to-male transmission, effects limited to males, a 50% chance that a carrier mother will pass the abnormal gene to her son, a 50% chance that a carrier mother will not transmit the abnormal gene to her son; a 50% chance that the daughter of a carrier mother will be a carrier; and a 100% chance that daughters of affected fathers will be carriers. Common X-linked recessive disorders are hemophilia, some forms of color blindness, and Duchenne muscular dystrophy.
- Multifactorial inheritance disorders include cleft lip and palate, spina bifida, developmental dysplasia of the hips, clubfoot, and pyloric stenosis.
- Some genetic conditions that can currently be diagnosed prenatally are neural tube and craniospinal defects, renal malformations, hemophilia, fragile X syndrome, thalassemia, cystic fibrosis, and many inborn errors of metabolism such as Tay–Sachs disease. This list expands daily as new technology allows for the detection of more conditions.
- The chief tools of prenatal diagnosis are ultrasound, serum alpha-fetoprotein testing, amniocentesis, chorionic villus sampling, and percutaneous umbilical blood sampling.
- Based on sound knowledge about common genetic problems, the nurse should prepare the family for counseling and act as a resource person during and after the counseling sessions. Many nurses with advanced training are entering the field of genetic counseling.

EXPLORE PEARSON **mynursingkit**™

MyNursingKit is your one stop for online chapter review materials and resources. Prepare for success with additional NCLEX®-style practice questions, interactive assignments and activities, web links, animations and videos, and more!

Register your access code from the front of your book at
www.mynursingkit.com

CHAPTER REFERENCES

American Society of Reproductive Medicine (ASRM). (2006a). *Frequently asked questions about infertility*. Retrieved March 24, 2008, from www.asrm.org/patients/faqs.htm

American Society of Reproductive Medicine (ASRM). (2006b). *Frequently asked questions. The psychological component of infertility.* Retrieved March 24, 2008, from www.asrm.org/patients/faqs.htm

American Society of Reproductive Medicine (ASRM). (2006c). *Medications for inducing ovulation: A guide for patients.* Retrieved March 24, 2008, from www.asrm.org/patientbooklets/ovulation_drugs.pdf

American Society of Reproductive Medicine (ASRM). (2007). *Assisted reproductive technologies: A guide for parents.* Retrieved March 24, 2008, from www.asrm.org/patientbooklets/assisted

Denson, V. (2006). Diagnosis and management of infertility. *Journal for Nurse Practitioners, 2(6),* 380–386.

Devine, K. S. (2008). *Challenges and management of infertility, including assisted reproductive technologies.* White Plains, NY: March of Dimes Foundation.

Dugoff, L. (2008). Prenatal diagnosis. In R. S. Gibbs, B. Y. Karlan, A. F. Haney, & I. Nygaard (Eds.), *Danforth's obstetrics and gynecology* (10th ed., pp. 111–121). Philadelphia, PA: Lippincott Williams & Wilkins.

Goldstein, S. R. (2008). Abnormal uterine bleeding. In R. S. Gibbs, B. Y. Karlan, A. F. Haney, & I. Nygaard (Eds.), *Danforth's obstetrics and gynecology* (10th ed., pp. 664–681). Philadelphia, PA: Lippincott Williams & Wilkins.

Gurfinkel, E., Cedenho, A. P., Yamamura, Y., & Srougi, M. (2003). Effects of acupuncture and moxa treatment in patients with semen abnormalities. *Asian Journal of Andrology, 5,* 345–348.

Honig, S. (2005). Preventive medicine and male factor infertility: Facts & fiction. Retrieved December 17, 2005, from www.resolve.org/site/PageServer?pagename=lrn _jfm_pm

Inhorn, M. C. (2002). "Local" confronts the "Global": Infertile bodies and the new reproductive technology in Egypt. In M. C. Inhorn & F. Van Balen (Eds.), *Infertility around the globe: New thinking on childness, gender, and reproductive technologies.* Berkeley and Los Angeles: University of California Press.

Jenkins, J. (2001). *Core competencies in genetics essential for all health care professionals.* Rockville, MD: National Coalition for Health Professional Education in Genetics (NCHPEG).

Kahn, S. M. (2002). Rabbis and reproduction: The uses of new reproductive technologies among Ultraorthodox Jews in Israel. In M. C. Inhorn & F. Van Balen (Eds.), *Infertility around the globe: New thinking on childness, gender, and reproductive technologies.* Berkeley and Los Angeles: University of California Press.

Klock, S. C. (2004). Psychological issues related to infertility. In J. J. Sciarri (Ed.), *Gynecology and obstetrics* (Vol. 6, chap. 74, pp. 1–8). Philadelphia: Lippincott Williams & Wilkins.

Kumar, A., Ghadir, S., Eskandari, N., & DeCherney, A. H. (2007). Infertility. In A. H. DeCherney, L. Nathan, T. M. Goodwin, & N. Laufer (Eds.), *Current diagnosis and treatment: Obstetrics & gynecology* (10th ed.). Boston: McGraw Hill.

Lashley, F. R. (2007). *Essentials of clinical genetics in nursing practice.* New York: Springer Publishing Company.

Lu, Jin-Chun, Huang, Yu-Feng, & Lu, Nian-Qing. (2008). Antisperm immunity and infertility. *Expert Review Clinical Immunology, 4*(1), 113–126.

Purnell, L. D., & Paulanka, B. J. (2008). *Transcultural health care: A culturally competent approach.* Philadelphia: F. A. Davis.

Quallich, S. (2006). Examining male infertility. *Urological Nurses, 26*(4), 277–288.

Simpson, J. L., & Holzgreve, W. (2007). Genetic counseling and genetic screening. In S. G. Gabbe, J. R. Niebyl, & J. L. Simpson (Eds.), *Obstetrics: Normal and problem pregnancies* (5th ed., pp. 138–151). Philadelphia, PA: Churchill Livingstone.

Skidmore-Roth, L. (2006). Mosby's handbook of herbs & natural supplements. St. Louis, MO: Elsevier Mosby.

Speroff, L., & Fritz, M. (2005). *Clinical gynecologic endocrinology and infertility.* Philadelphia, PA: Lippincott Williams & Wilkins.

Storment, J. M. (2006). Infertility and recurrent pregnancy loss. In M. G. Curtis, S. Overholt, & M. P. Hopkins, *Glass' office gynecology* (6th ed.). Philadelphia. PA: Lippincott Williams & Wilkins.

Varney, H., Kriebs, J. M., & Gegor, C. L. (2004). *Varney's midwifery* (4th ed.). Boston: Jones and Bartlett Publishers.

Ward, K. (2008). Genetics in obstetrics and gynecology. In R. S. Gibbs, B. Y. Karlan, A. F. Haney, & I. Nygaard (Eds.), *Danforth's obstetrics and gynecology* (10th ed., pp. 88–110). Philadelphia, PA: Lippincott Williams & Wilkins.

White, A. R. (2003). A review of controlled trials of acupuncture for women's reproductive health care. *Journal of Family Planning and Reproductive Health Care, 29*(4), 233–236.

Williams, J. K., et al. (2004). Advancing genetic nursing knowledge. *Nursing Outlook, 52,* 73–79.

Wilson, B. A., Shannon, M. T., Shields, K. M., & Stang, C. L. (2009). *Prentice Hall nurse's drug guide—2009.* Upper Saddle River, NJ: Pearson Education, Inc.

Wright, K. P., & Johnson, J. (2008). Infertility. In R. S. Gibbs, B. Y. Karlan, A. F. Haney, & I. Nygaard (Eds.), *Danforth's obstetrics and gynecology* (10th ed., pp. 705–715). Philadelphia, PA: Lippincott Williams & Wilkins.

CHAPTER 8

Preparation for Parenthood

One of the most important things I can do for couples is to help them expand their awareness—awareness of the inherent "rightness" and naturalness of the birth process, awareness of the multitude of options that are available to them, awareness of the healthcare environment, awareness that control is an illusion, and awareness of the intuitions and strengths that they already possess.

—A Certified Childbirth Educator (CBE) and Nurse

LEARNING OUTCOMES

8-1. Describe the most appropriate nursing care for couples during preconception counseling to help ensure their best possible health state.

8-2. Assist expectant parents in making the best decisions possible in issues related to pregnancy, labor, and birth.

8-3. Explain the basic goals of childbirth education in providing care to expectant couples and their families.

8-4. Explain the goals and content of the various types of antepartal education programs when providing nursing care for expectant couples and their families.

8-5. Describe interventions that can be implemented by the childbirth educator to decrease pregnant women's anxiety.

8-6. Compare methods of childbirth preparation and the nursing interventions for each.

8-7. Examine ways in which the nurse conveys respect for client individuality in preparing for childbirth.

KEY TERMS

Abdominal effleurage **173**
Birth plan **169**
Doula **171**
La Leche League **173**
Prenatal education **171**

As pregnancy progresses, expectant parents begin to look forward to their birth experience and the challenges of parenthood. In addition to gathering information about the pregnancy, they also need to make many decisions and plans. Where will the birth be? Who do they wish to be present? What steps can they take to prepare themselves for this wonderful occasion? How do they approach their new roles as parents?

Today's professional nurse can assist a pregnant woman or expectant couple, if the father or significant other is involved, to make the choices that are part of pregnancy and birth. The nurse can help them select a healthcare provider, find prenatal classes that meet their needs, and make informed choices based on accurate and adequate information. Even more important, as the parents work through these decisions, the nurse is able to affirm their decision-making abilities and prepare them for their roles as parents. For first-time parents, the decisions may seem numerous and complicated, and the nurse has a unique opportunity to help them establish a pattern of decision making that will serve them well in their years as parents.

Preconception Counseling

One of the first questions a couple should ask before conception is whether they wish to have children. This decision involves consideration of each person's goals, expectations of the relationship, and desire to be a parent. Sometimes one individual wishes to have a child, but the other does not. In such situations, an open discussion is essential to reach a mutually acceptable decision.

Couples who wish to have children face a decision about the timing of pregnancy. At what point in their lives do they believe it would be best to become parents? Pregnancy is a life-changing event and comes as a surprise even when the decision about timing is made.

For couples who have religious beliefs that do not support contraception or who feel that fertility planning is unnatural, planning the timing of the pregnancy is unacceptable and irrelevant. These couples can still take steps to ensure that they are in the best possible physical and mental health when pregnancy occurs.

Preconception Health Measures

Most preconception recommendations focus on helping the couple attain their best possible health state so that they do not enter pregnancy with unnecessary risks. The nurse begins by teaching the couple about known or suspected health risks. The nurse advises the woman to cease smoking or at least to limit her cigarette intake as much as possible. Because of the hazards of secondhand smoke, it is helpful for the woman to avoid environments where sec-

ondhand smoke is common and to ask her partner to refrain from smoking around her. Although the effects of caffeine are less clearly understood, the woman is advised to avoid or limit her intake of caffeine. Alcohol, social drugs, and street drugs pose a real threat to the fetus. A woman who uses any prescription or over-the-counter medications needs to discuss the implications of their use with her healthcare provider. Women with chronic health problems, such as thyroid disorders, seizures, hypertension, and diabetes, should have a preconception visit with the appropriate specialist to determine if pregnancy is advised and medication changes or treatment plan changes are warranted. Because of the possible teratogenic effects of environmental hazards, the nurse urges the couple contemplating pregnancy to determine possible exposure to any environmental hazards, such as radiation or chemical exposure, at work or in their community.

Physical Examination

It is advisable for both partners to have a physical examination to identify any health problems so that they can be corrected if possible. These problems might include medical conditions such as high blood pressure, diabetes, or obesity; problems that pose a threat to fertility, such as certain sexually transmitted infections; or conditions that keep the individual from achieving optimal health, such as anemia or colitis. If the family history indicates previous genetic disorders, or if the couple is planning pregnancy when the woman is over age 35, the healthcare provider may suggest that the couple consider genetic counseling. In addition to the history and physical exam, the woman may have a variety of laboratory tests. (See Assessment Guide: Initial Prenatal Assessment, in Chapter 10 ∞.) Before conception the woman is also advised to have a dental examination and any necessary dental work to avoid exposure to X-rays, local anesthetics, and the risk of infection while pregnant.

Nutrition

Before conception it is advisable for the woman to be at an average weight for her body build and height. Women who are underweight should be advised to gain weight, whereas women who are more than ideal weight should try to get their weight down because maternal obesity is a risk factor for multiple pregnancy complications. The woman is advised to follow a nutritious diet that contains ample quantities of all the essential nutrients. Some nutritionists advocate emphasizing the following nutrients: calcium, protein, iron, B complex vitamins, vitamin C, and magnesium. Folic acid supplementation before conception is recommended as these supplements decrease the risk of neural tube defects. Intake of vitamins in greater than the recommended dietary allowance (RDA) can cause severe fetal problems and should be avoided. (See Chapter 13 ∞ for further discussion of nutrition.) An assessment that includes unique dietary practices that can impact nutrition should also be explored. Cultural norms that affect nutritional intake should also be reviewed.

Exercise

A woman is advised to continue her present pattern of exercise or to establish a regular exercise plan beginning at least 3 months before she attempts to become pregnant. An exercise routine that she enjoys and maintains will provide the best results. Exercise that includes some aerobic conditioning and some general muscle toning will improve the woman's circulation and general health. Once an exercise program is well established, the woman is generally encouraged to continue it during pregnancy. During pregnancy at least 30 minutes of moderate exercise daily or at least most days is recommended (Penney, 2008).

Contraception

A woman who uses hormonal contraception—such as combined oral contraceptives, mini-pills, the NuvaRing, Ortho Evra patch, or Depo-Provera—is advised to stop using the hormonal birth control method and have two or three normal menstrual cycles before attempting to conceive. This waiting period allows the natural hormonal cycle to return and facilitates dating the subsequent pregnancy. A woman using an intrauterine device is advised to have it removed and wait 1 month before attempting to conceive. During the waiting period she can use barrier methods of contraception (condoms, diaphragm, or cervical cap with spermicides). Women who have used Depo-Provera should be advised that it could take up to 12 months to conceive after discontinuation.

Conception

Conception is a personal and emotional experience. Even if a couple is prepared, they may feel some ambivalence when it actually occurs. Ambivalence is a normal response, especially if the conception is unintended. Couples may require reassurance that this feeling typically passes. Although couples in the United States have access to more contraceptive choices than those in developing countries, the percentage of unintended pregnancies that occur in the United States is approximately 50% (CDC, 2007). Women or couples with unplanned pregnancies need additional nursing support, such as information on community resources, and encouragement to examine their feelings regarding the unintended pregnancy.

Couples who fervently desire a child may get so caught up in preparation and in their efforts to "do things right" that they lose sight of the pleasure they derive from each other and their lives together. They may even cease to value the joy of spontaneity in their relationship. It is often helpful for the healthcare provider to remind an overly zealous couple to take pleasure in the present moment.

Healthcare providers can assist the couple in achieving conception by identifying the woman's most fertile period. The nurse should identify possible days of ovulation based on the length of her menstrual cycle and educate the woman about possible signs of ovulation (presence of ovulatory mucus, changes in the woman's temperature, and the presence of mittelschmerz (ovulation-related pain)). After a year of attempting to conceive, the couple should be referred for medical evaluation. These factors are discussed in Chapter 3 ∞.

Childbearing Decisions

Once the couple has achieved conception, they should begin exploring options for a healthcare provider and birth setting, as well as labor support and sibling preparation, if appropriate.

Care Provider

One of the first decisions facing expectant parents is the selection of a healthcare provider. The nurse assists them by explaining the various options and outlining what can be expected from each. A thorough understanding of the differences in educational preparation, skill level, practice characteristics, and general philosophy of certified nurse–midwives, obstetricians, family practice physicians, and lay midwives is essential. For instance, research shows that as many as one-third of adults use some form of complementary or alternative medicine (Institute of Medicine, 2005). To determine whether a particular practice is safe during pregnancy, an open avenue for communication must exist between the expectant parent and the primary care provider. In addition to concerns about philosophy, the nurse should encourage expectant parents to investigate the specific care provider's credentials, education and training, fee schedule, availability to new clients, and on-call coverage issues; this information is often obtained by telephoning the provider's office. The nurse can also help the expectant parents develop a list of questions for their first visit to a care provider to help determine compatibility. Questions could include the following:

- Who is in practice with you, or who covers for you when you are unavailable?
- How do your partners' philosophies compare with yours?
- How do you feel about my partner, other support person, or other children coming to the prenatal visits?
- What are your feelings about _____ (fill in special desires for the birth event, such as different positions

assumed during labor, episiotomy, induction of labor, other people present during the birth, breastfeeding immediately after the birth, no separation of infant and parents following birth, and so on)?

- If a cesarean birth is necessary, could my partner be present?
- Are you familiar with _____ (fill in complementary or alternative forms of health care that may be used currently)? How will this practice impact my plan of care?

Choosing a care provider is just one of the decisions pregnant women and couples make. A method that has assisted many couples in making these decisions is called a **birth plan**. By writing down preferences, prospective parents identify aspects of the childbearing experience that are most important to them (Figure 8–1 ■). Used as a tool for communication among the expectant parents, the healthcare provider, and the healthcare professionals at the birth setting, the written plan identifies options that are available as well as those that are not.

The birth plan also helps pregnant women and couples set priorities. Using the plan, they identify areas that they want to incorporate into their own birth experience. They can then discuss the document at a visit with their prospective care provider and use it to compare their wishes with the philosophy and beliefs of the provider. They can also take the birth plan to the birth setting and use it as a basis for communicating their needs during the childbirth experience.

Expectant parents also need to discuss the qualities they want in a care provider for the newborn. They may want to visit several before the birth to select someone who will meet their needs as well as those of their child.

Pregnant women and couples will make many more choices. Some are explored in Table 8–1. Although most birth experiences are very close to the desired experience, at times expectations cannot be met because of the unavailability of some choices in the community, limitations set by insurance providers, or unexpected problems during pregnancy or birth. It is important for nurses to help expectant parents keep sight of what is realistic for their situation while also acting as an advocate for them.

Birth Setting

The nurse can help expectant parents choose a birth setting by suggesting they tour facilities and talk with nurses there and with friends or acquaintances who are recent parents. However, it is important to note that the birth setting may be largely determined by the choice of the care provider. The vast majority of births in the United States occur in the acute care or hospital setting. Other birth settings include a birthing center or birth in the woman's home. Women who opt for these less traditional birth settings should be carefully screened. Women with medical risk factors, including those who have had a previous cesarean birth, are not good candidates for alternative birth settings. Questions that expectant parents may ask of new parents include the following:

- What kind of care and support did you receive during labor?
- If the setting has both labor and birthing rooms, was a birthing room available when you wanted it?
- Were you encouraged to be mobile during labor or to do what you wanted to do (walking, sitting in a rocking chair, sitting in a whirlpool bath, standing in a shower, and so on)? If not, were there reasonable circumstances that prevented you from doing so?
- Were you encouraged to be actively involved in your plan of care and kept well informed of progress or proposed changes?
- Was your labor partner or support person treated well?
- Were your birth preferences respected? Did you share them with the facility before the birth? If something did not work, why do you think there were problems?

Sample Birth Plan	
Choice	*Choice*
Care provider:	Position during birth:
Certified nurse–midwife	On side
Obstetrician	Hands and knees
Family physician	Kneeling
Lay midwife	Squatting
Birth setting	Birthing chair
Hospital:	Birthing bed
Birthing room	Other:
Delivery room	Family present (sibs)
Birth center	Filming of birth (videotaping)
Home	Photography of birth
Support during labor and birth:	Leboyer
Partner present	Episiotomy
Doula present	No sterile drapes
Other support person present	Partner to cut umbilical cord
During labor:	Baby placed on maternal abdomen
Ambulate as desired	immediately after birth
Shower if desired	Hold baby immediately after birth
Wear own clothes	Breastfeed immediately after birth
Use hot tub	No separation after birth
Use of rocking chair	Save the placenta
Have perineal prep	Collect cord blood for banking
Have enema	Newborn care:
Water birth	Eye treatment for the baby
Electronic fetal monitoring	Vitamin K injection
Doppler monitoring	Heptovac injection
Membranes:	Breastfeeding
Rupture naturally	Formula-feeding
Amniotomy if needed	Pacifier use
Labor stimulation if needed	Glucose water
Medication:	Circumcision
Identify type desired	Postpartum care:
Fluids or ice as desired	Short stay
Music during labor and birth	48-hour stay after vaginal birth
Massage	Home visits after discharge
Therapeutic touch	Home doula
Healing touch	Other

FIGURE 8–1 Birth plan listing various choices that the woman or the couple may consider during their childbirth experience. Once the woman or the couple has considered each of the choices, they may circle the items they desire.

TABLE 8-1	Benefits and Risks of Some Consumer Decisions During Pregnancy, Labor, and Birth	
Issue	Benefits	Disadvantages
Breastfeeding	• No additional expense • Contains maternal antibodies to decrease illness • Decreases incidence of infant otitis media, vomiting, and diarrhea, hospitalizations during the first year of life, and allergies • Easier to digest than formula • Immediately after birth, promotes uterine contractions and decreases incidence of postpartum hemorrhage • Promotes maternal–infant bonding	• Transmission of maternal infections to newborn, such as HIV • Irregular ovulation and menses can cause false sense of security and nonuse of hormonal contraceptives • Increased nutritional requirement in mother • Limitation of birth-control options in the postpartal period
Perineal prep	• May decrease risk of infection • Facilitates episiotomy repair	• Nicks can be portal for bacteria • Discomfort as hair grows back
Enema	• May facilitate labor • Increases space for infant in pelvis • May increase strength of contractions • May prevent contamination of sterile field	• Increases discomfort and anxiety

Ambulation during labor	• Comfort for laboring woman
	• May assist in labor progression by: if appropriate
	  • Stimulating contractions
	  • Allowing gravity to help descent of fetus
	  • Giving sense of independence and control
		• Cord prolapse will rupture membranes unless engagement has occurred
		• Birth of infant in undesirable locations (hallways, outdoors, waiting area)
		• Inability to monitor fetal heart rate if telemetry unit is not available

Electronic fetal monitoring	• Helps evaluate fetal well-being • Helps identify nonreassuring fetal status • Useful in diagnostic testing • Helps evaluate labor progress	• Supine postural hypotension • Intrauterine perforation (with internal uterine pressure device) • Infection (with internal monitoring) • Decreases personal interaction with mother because of attention paid to the machine • Mother is unable to ambulate or change her position freely
Whirlpool (jet hydrotherapy)	• Increased relaxation • Decreased anxiety • Stimulation of labor • Provides pain relief • Slight decrease in blood pressure • Increased diuresis • Decreased incidence of vacuum and forceps-assisted births • Increased pain threshold • Higher satisfaction with birth • Decreased use of pain medication	• May slow contractions if used before active labor is established • Possible risk of infection if membranes are ruptured • Slight increase in maternal temperature and pulse in tub • Hypothermia • Increases FHR by 10 to 20 bpm (Teschendorf & Evans, 2000)
Analgesia	• Maternal relaxation facilitates labor	• All drugs reach the fetus in varying degrees and with varying effects
Episiotomy	• Decreases irregular tearing of perineum • Easier to repair for practitioner	• Increased pain after birth and for 1 to 3 months following birth • Dyspareunia • Infection • Increased frequency of third- and fourth-degree lacerations (Low, Seng, Murtland et al., 2000)

• During labor, did the nurse offer or suggest a variety of comfort measures?
• How were medications handled during labor? Were you comfortable with this arrangement?
• Were siblings welcomed in the birth setting? After the birth?
• Was the nursing staff helpful after the baby was born? Did you receive self-care and infant care information?
• Did you have a choice about what information was provided?

Labor Support

Another important choice the expectant family faces is how active a support role the father or other partner wants to take during labor and birth. Although many partners are comfortable acting as the primary physical and emotional support for the laboring woman, some partners are not. Studies have found that the role of fathers has undergone tremendous transformation because today's fathers are more actively involved in providing care to children and childrearing than ever before because of the large numbers of working mothers. Fathers often play a key role in the support of mothers during labor, birth, and the postpartum period (Friedewald, Fletcher, & Fairborn, 2005). One study revealed that the father's motivation in attending childbirth education classes was to feel informed, to listen and share with other parents, to be there for his partner, to help imagine what the future would be like once he was a parent, and to be the second parent in the child's life (Premburg & Lundgren, 2006).

Over the past decade a variety of options for labor support have emerged as families and healthcare providers have come to understand and respect individual needs. Some possible choices include asking a friend or family member to attend the birth and help with comfort needs, or contacting a local childbirth advocate group for a volunteer referral. Advocacy groups offer labor support services to certain groups of women who lack social support during labor. These include teen mothers and military spouses whose husbands are deployed during the time of birth.

Some women or couples hire a specialized childbirth support person, known as a *doula*. The role of the **doula** is to act as an advocate and to attend to the needs of the childbearing family. Doulas do not perform clinical tasks. However, because the doula is specially trained to offer guidance, provide labor support, assist with births and provide encouragement to new parents and family members, the doula is an adjunct to the healthcare team. A knowledgeable doula can be an asset to the nurse by attending to the many comfort needs of the laboring mother and her family.

Sibling Preparation for Birth

Some expectant parents may wish to have their other children present at the birth. Children who will attend a birth can be prepared through books, audiovisual materials, models, discussion, and sibling classes. Nurses can assist parents with sibling preparation by helping them understand the stresses a child may experience. For example, the child may become frightened if the laboring mom is irritable and visibly showing pain, feel left out when there is a new child to love, or feel disappointed if a brother is born when a sister was expected.

It is imperative that a sibling have his or her own support person whose sole responsibility is tending to the child's needs. The support person needs to be familiar to the child; warm, sensitive, and flexible; knowledgeable about the birth process; and comfortable with sexuality and birth. This person must be prepared to interpret what is happening for the child and to intervene when necessary. For example, the support person needs to be prepared to remove the child from the birthing room at the child's request or if the situation warrants that action.

Siblings should be given the option of relating to the birth in whatever manner they choose, as long as it is not disruptive. They should understand that they may stay or leave the room as they choose. The nurse may elicit from the children exactly what they expect from the experience and ensure that they feel free to ask questions and express feelings.

Children should be educated about the normal birth process and what they will be seeing. Information should be straightforward and age appropriate. Most children present in the room during the birth of a sibling cope adequately and are not fearful (Kitzinger, 2005). Being present at the birth appears to increase siblings' acceptance of the new baby. In general, siblings who are present at birth tend to have feelings of interest and the desire to nurture "our" baby, as opposed to jealousy and rivalry directed at "Mom's" baby. The mother does not disappear mysteriously into the hospital and return with a demanding outsider. Instead, the family attending the birth together finds a new opportunity for closeness and growth by sharing in the birth of a new member.

CULTURAL PERSPECTIVES

Women from Hispanic cultures typically want their partner with them during labor. These women like both emotional and physical support, such as verbal reassurance, hand-holding, or assistance with ambulation. The woman may also want female relatives present during the labor and birth to provide additional support.

Classes for Family Members During Pregnancy

Prenatal education programs provide important opportunities to share information about pregnancy and childbirth and to enhance the parents' decision-making skills. The content of each class is generally directed by the overall goals of the program. For example, in classes that aim to provide preconceptual information, preparations for becoming pregnant and optimizing the woman's health status are the major topics. Other classes may be directed toward childbirth choices available today, preparation of the mother and her partner for pregnancy and birth, preparation for a vaginal birth after a (previous) cesarean (VBAC) birth, and preparation for the birth by specific people such as grandparents or siblings. The nurse who knows the types of prenatal programs available in the community can direct expectant parents to programs that meet their special needs and learning goals. See Key Facts to Remember: Possible Content of Classes for Childbirth Preparation.

From the expectant parents' point of view, class content is best presented in chronology with the pregnancy. It is important to begin the classes by finding out what each parent wants to learn and including a discussion of related choices. Whereas both parents may expect to learn breathing and relaxation techniques and infant care, fathers usually expect facts and mothers expect coping strategies. Classes for fathers only provide a forum for expectant fathers to ask questions and interact with other men who are sharing similar circumstances and have the same types of

concerns (Premburg & Lundgren, 2006). Prenatal classes are often divided into early and late classes.

Early Classes: First Trimester

Early prenatal classes often include prepregnant women and couples as well as those in early pregnancy. The classes cover early gestational changes; self-care during pregnancy; fetal development and environmental dangers for the fetus; sexuality in pregnancy; birth settings and types of care providers; nutrition, rest, and exercise suggestions; common discomforts of pregnancy and relief measures; psychologic changes in pregnancy for the woman and man; methods of coping with stress; and the benefits of following a healthful lifestyle. Early classes also provide information about factors that place the woman at risk for preterm labor or other adverse pregnancy-related conditions, as well as how to recognize symptoms and what to do if they occur.

Early classes should also present information about breastfeeding and formula-feeding. The majority of women have made their infant feeding decision before the sixth month of pregnancy. Factors influencing a woman's choice of feeding method include husband's (partner's) preference, ability to breastfeed independently at hospital discharge, influence of family and friends, perceptions of professional support, society's view of breastfeeding, and knowledge about breastfeeding (McFadden, 2006; Scott, 2006).

Later Classes: Second and Third Trimesters

The later classes focus on preparation for the birth, including birth choices (position for birth, episiotomy, medications, fetal monitoring, epidural, and so forth), postpartum self-care, infant care and feeding, and newborn safety issues. Because many expectant parents purchase a car seat before the birth of their child, later classes should also include information about the importance of car seats, how they work, and how to select an approved car seat. Because the majority of car seats installed by parents are installed incorrectly, parents should be encouraged to read the directions thoroughly or have the seat professionally installed or checked by the local police or fire department. Sibling preparation is also an important topic that should be covered if any of the participants have other children.

◇

KEY FACTS TO REMEMBER

Possible Content of Classes for Childbirth Preparation

Early Classes (First Trimester)

Early gestational changes
Self-care during pregnancy
Fetal development and environmental dangers for the fetus
Sexuality in pregnancy
Birth settings and types of care providers
Nutrition, rest, and exercise suggestions
Relief measures for common discomforts of pregnancy
Psychologic changes in pregnancy
Information for getting pregnancy off to a good start
Prenatal and genetic testing available

Later Classes (Second and Third Trimesters)

Preparation for birth process
Postpartum self-care
Birth choices (e.g., episiotomy, medications, fetal monitoring, enema)
Relaxation techniques
Breathing techniques
Infant stimulation or infant massage
Newborn safety issues such as car seats
Sibling preparation and adjustment

Adolescent Preparation Classes

How to be a good parent
Newborn care
Health dangers for the baby
Healthy diet during pregnancy
How to recognize when the baby is ill
Baby care: physical and emotional
Sexuality
Peer relationships

Breastfeeding Programs

Advantages and disadvantages
Techniques of breastfeeding
Methods of breast milk storage
Involvement of fathers in the feeding process
Breastfeeding and returning to work

TEACHING TIP

Advise parents of community resources available for inspecting the installation of car seats. Many police departments and fire stations have car seat inspection clinics that are conducted within the community. Some fire stations have set hours when parents can bring in their car seat and have it installed free of charge. Remind new parents that newborns should be in a rear-facing position until the age of 12 months.

Childbirth preparation classes are an ideal time to incorporate infant stimulation concepts. These concepts aid in the development of parenting skills and enhance prenatal and neonatal bonding. Tactile, vestibular, and auditory stimulation can be explained. Information regarding tactile stimulation can be presented while discussing maternal anatomy and physiology. As the uterine wall thins during the pregnancy, the mother and father are better able to feel the baby, and the fetus can sense the parents' stroking and patting through the abdominal wall. **Abdominal effleurage** (a light stroking movement made over the abdominal wall with the fingertips) can be used to provide tactile stimulation to the fetus.

Vestibular stimulation through movement of the fetus is provided while the expectant woman does the pelvic-tilt exercise. Rocking in a rocking chair is also a comfortable way to provide both relaxation for the expectant woman and vestibular stimulation for the fetus. Prenatal yoga is gaining popularity and is another means of providing vestibular stimulation to the newborn. Auditory stimulation can be provided by playing music. Classical music (such as works by Vivaldi, Bach, Beethoven, and Mozart) is found to stimulate the fetus.

Adolescent Parenting Classes

Adolescents have special learning needs during pregnancy. Areas of concern for teens focus on how to be a good parent, how to care for the new baby, health dangers to the baby, and healthful foods to eat during pregnancy. Teens also have information needs about how to recognize when the baby is sick, protect the baby from accidents, and make the baby feel happy and loved. Expectant teens are often eager to hear more about the birth process (especially ways to cope with pain during the birth process), the personal health of the mother, the discomforts and life changes that accompany pregnancy, body image issues, and sexuality.

Breastfeeding Programs

Programs offering information on breastfeeding are increasing. For many years, a primary source of information has been the **La Leche League**, a nonprofit organization that promotes breastfeeding. Information can also be obtained from certified lactation educators, clinical lactation consultants, peer counselors, birthing centers, hospitals, and health clinics. Online support groups can also be an important resource for new mothers. Expectant parents learn positioning and techniques of breastfeeding, advantages and disadvantages, and methods of breast pumping and milk storage. The father's support and encouragement of the mother is vital, so it is important to include him in the educational programs and decision making. Some fathers may feel ambivalent or resentful about breastfeeding

and need opportunities in the prenatal period for discussion and sharing of feelings and experiences. The nurse can identify ways for including the father in the breastfeeding process. This may include bringing the baby to the mother for feedings, burping the baby between breasts and/or after feeding, or rocking the baby back to sleep.

Sibling Preparation: Adjustment to a Newborn

The birth of a new sibling is a significant event in a child's life. Positive adjustment can be enhanced by attendance at sibling preparation classes (see Figure 8–2 ■). The classes usually focus on reducing anxiety in the child, providing opportunities for the child to express feelings and concerns, and encouraging realistic expectations of the newborn. Many classes teach siblings how to feed and burp the baby, safely hold a newborn, or change diapers. This enables the sibling to be an active participant when the new baby arrives. Parents learn strategies to help prepare the child for the birth and to assist the child in coping with a new family member.

Sibling preparation can be addressed through a formal class or in a less formal way by providing a booklet for parents that addresses issues affecting both parents and children. Many facilities now offer sibling classes. Parents can be referred to the office of childbirth education or family education at their hospital where they will give birth. Many facilities offer family tours so the younger children can see where Mom and baby will stay and where they will come and visit.

Classes for Grandparents

Grandparents are an important source of support and information for prospective and new parents. They are now often included in the birthing process. Prenatal programs

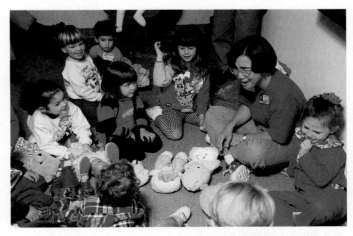

FIGURE 8–2 It is especially important that siblings be well prepared when they are going to be present for the birth. However, all siblings benefit from information about birth and the new baby ahead of time.

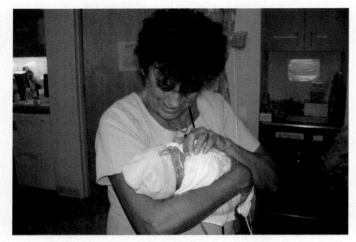

FIGURE 8–3 Grandparents play a key role in many childbearing families' lives by taking an active role with grandchildren.

for grandparents can be an important source of information about current beliefs and practices in childbearing. The most useful content may include changes in birthing and parenting practices and helpful tips for being a supportive grandparent. Grandparents who will be integral members of the labor and birth team need information about that role (see Figure 8–3 ■).

Education of the Family Having Cesarean Birth

Cesarean birth is an alternative method of birth. However, because the need for a cesarean birth is rarely known in advance, specific classes covering this alternative are uncommon. The number of cesarean births has been steadily rising since the warnings about vaginal birth after cesarean were issued. In 2006, 31.1% of women gave birth by cesarean (National Center for Health Statistics [NCHS], 2007). Because the cesarean rate is so high, preparation for this possibility should be an integral part of every childbirth education curriculum.

Preparation for Cesarean Birth

Cesarean birth class content should cover what the parents can expect to happen during a cesarean birth, what they might feel, and what choices are available to them. All pregnant women and couples should be encouraged to discuss with their certified nurse–midwife or physician the progression of events if a cesarean birth becomes necessary. They can also discuss their needs and preferences regarding the following:

- Choice of anesthetic
- Father (or significant other) being present during the birth
- Immediate initial contact with their newborn

Preparation for Repeat Cesarean Birth

When expectant parents are anticipating a repeat cesarean birth, they have time to plan and prepare. The incidence of repeated cesarean births has risen dramatically over the past decade because of concern over possible uterine rupture associated with labor in women who previously gave birth via cesarean. In addition, once a woman has had two previous cesarean births, she is no longer a candidate for a vaginal birth after cesarean (VBAC) (ACOG, 2004). Repeat cesarean births have nonmedical advantages such as allowing the parents to plan for child care and work-related absences, and prearranging assistance at home for the new mother and infant. Many birthing units provide preparation classes for repeat cesarean birth. Parents who have had previous negative experiences need an opportunity to describe what contributed to their feelings. They should be encouraged to identify what they would like to change and to list interventions that would make the experience more positive. Those who have had positive experiences require reassurance that their needs and desires will be met in a similar manner. In addition, all parents are encouraged to air any fears or anxieties.

A specific concern of the woman facing a repeat cesarean is anticipation of pain. She needs reassurance that subsequent cesarean births are often less painful than the first. In addition, planned cesarean births involve less fatigue than unplanned procedures because they are not preceded by a long, strenuous labor. Providing this information will help the woman cope more effectively with stressful stimuli, including pain. The nurse can remind the client that she has already had experience with how to reduce, cope with, and alleviate discomfort during the first few days following surgery.

Preparation for Parents Desiring Vaginal Birth After Cesarean Birth (VBAC)

Parents who have had a cesarean birth and are now anticipating a vaginal birth have unique needs. They may feel disappointed in their previous birthing experience, have unresolved questions and concerns about the last birth, or have fears about the upcoming birth. They may have concern over the risk involved, despite making the choice to attempt a trial of labor. For these reasons, it is helpful to begin the series of classes with an informational session. Couples should be aware that current practice is to await the onset of labor and that induction is not offered in many settings. The use of oxytocin administration has been associated with a higher incidence of uterine rupture in some studies. In addition, the use of prostaglandin agents is contraindicated because it dramatically increases the risk of uterine rupture (ACOG, 2004). During this session, couples can ask questions, share experiences, and begin to form bonds with each other. The nurse can supply information regarding the criteria necessary to attempt a trial of labor, the risks and benefits involved, and the decisions to be made regarding the birth experience. In addition to teaching and empathetic listening, the nurse provides the parents with emotional support and encouragement. At one time, 26% of women who had previously given birth via cesarean opted for a VBAC, whereas in 2006, only 11% did so (Lothian, 2006); therefore, many women look to the nurse to provide objective information on the birthing options available for a woman who has had a previous cesarean birth.

Some childbirth educators suggest that parents prepare two birth preference plans: one for vaginal birth and one for cesarean birth. Preparation of the birth plans seems to give parents some sense of control over the birth experience and tends to increase the positive aspects of the experience.

HINTS FOR PRACTICE

Provide reassurance that the healthcare team's main objective will be to ensure the safety and well-being of both the mother and the baby. Often, pointing out that the most important outcome is not the type of birth, but that the mother and newborn are safe, allows the couple to focus on the most important aspects of birth rather than the way the birth occurred.

After an informational session, the classes may be divided according to the needs of the expectant parents. Those with recent childbirth experiences may need only refresher classes, whereas others may need complete training. Some parents may choose to attend regular classes after participating in the informational session.

Childbirth Preparation Methods

Childbirth preparation classes are usually taught by *certified childbirth educators* (*CBE* or *CCE*). Various types of childbirth preparation are available. Vital to each method is the educational component, which helps alleviate fear. The classes vary in coverage of subjects related to the maternity cycle, but all teach relaxation and coping techniques, as well as what to expect during labor and birth. Most classes also feature exercises to relax and condition muscles and breathing exercises for use in labor. The greatest differences among the methods lie in the theories of why they work and in the specific comfort techniques and breathing patterns they teach. Some classes are tailored to women who receive care from specific healthcare providers or hospitals and include information that is specific to that provider or setting.

Childbirth preparation offers several advantages, including the satisfaction of the parents, for whom childbirth becomes a shared and profound emotional experience. In addition, each method has been shown to shorten labor. All nurses should know how these techniques differ, so that they can effectively support each birth experience.

Programs for Preparation

The evolution of childbirth education began in the 1930s when Grantly Dick-Read published several books on theories focusing on pain and fear in childbirth. This began a movement of childbirth education that has continued to evolve. Some antepartal classes, specifically oriented to preparation for labor and birth, have a name associated with a theory of pain reduction in childbirth. The most common methods of this type are the Lamaze (psychoprophylactic), Kitzinger (sensory–memory), Bradley (partner-coached childbirth), and HypnoBirthing. Each of these programs is designed to provide the woman or couple with self-help measures so that the pregnancy and birth are healthful and happy events. See Table 8–2 for differentiating characteristics of each method.

One of the most important components of childbirth education is instilling confidence in a woman's ability to give birth (Lothian, 2006). The Council of Childbirth Education Specialists encourages education that focuses on the interconnectedness of the body and spirit. After that connection is established and understood by pregnant women, coping strategies, stress reduction, and relaxation techniques can then be taught.

One organization that provides educational resources and certification for educators is the International Childbirth Education Association (ICEA). This organization does not advocate a particular method of childbirth preparation but rather promotes a philosophy of "freedom of choice based on knowledge of alternatives" (ICEA, 2006). Many expectant parents find this approach consistent with their own desires to experience birth as informed healthcare consumers. ICEA educators often teach a combination of techniques designed to meet individual needs.

TEACHING TIP

Remind women using Internet childbirth education resources that some sites may not use health professionals or experts in the childbirth field and may be written by individuals who lack formal education and training. Advise women to look for resources that are supported by licensed professionals or well-known, credible organizations.

As the demands and numbers of dual-career families increase, many women seek alternative childbirth education methods. Examples include videotapes, books, magazines, condensed private education seminars, and Internet-accessed preparation classes and online discussion groups.

MyNursingKit | International Childbirth Education Association

TABLE 8–2	Summary of Selected Childbirth Preparation Methods			
Method	Purpose or Philosophy	Goals	Techniques	Class Content
Bradley	To have the best, safest, and most rewarding birth experience possible.	• Natural childbirth • Active participation of the husband as coach • Excellent nutrition • Breastfeeding, beginning at birth	• Working in harmony with your body using controlled breathing and deep abdominopelvic breathing (American Academy of Husband-Coached Childbirth, 2008) • Promoting general body relaxation (American Academy of Husband-Coached Childbirth, 2008)	• Nutrition • Coach's role • Introduction to stages of labor • Birth planning • Variations and complications of labor • Postpartum preparation • Advanced first- and second-stage techniques • Preparation for the new family • Advocacy for the family unit
Lamaze	Childbirth education empowers women to make informed choices in health care, to assume responsibility for their health, and to trust their inner wisdom.	• Birth is normal, natural, and healthy. • The experience of birth profoundly affects women and their families. • Women's inner wisdom guides them through birth. • Women have the right to give birth free from routine medical interventions.	• Disassociation relaxation • Controlled muscular relaxation • Breathing patterns	• Nutrition • Gestational changes • Labor and birth techniques for easing pain • Breathing techniques • Positioning during labor
Kitzinger	• Sheila Kitzinger campaigns for women to have the information they need to make choices about childbirth. • She is a strong believer in the benefits of home birth for women who are not at high risk.	• Uses sensory memory to help the woman understand and work with her body in preparation for birth.	• Uses chest breathing in conjunction with abdominal relaxation • Incorporates elements of the Stanislavsky method of acting in a way to teach relaxation	• Antenatal care • Birth plans • Therapeutic touch during labor • Posttraumatic stress following childbirth • Breastfeeding
HypnoBirthing	Eliminate fear and experience birth in a stress-free, calm, and gentle environment that most resembles nature's own design.	• With both mind and body relaxed, the muscles of the uterus work in complete neuromuscular harmony. • When in a relaxed state, the body releases endorphins, the body's natural anesthesia.	• Relaxation techniques • Deep breathing • Slow breathing • Breathing your baby down • Maintaining comfort and eliminating pain	• HynoBirthing philosophy • Rapid, progressive relaxation/deepening techniques for transition • Visualizations for labor • Composing a birth plan • Early signs of labor • Birthing companion's integral role in labor • Pushing techniques • Postnatal bonding of parents with baby
Birthworks ©	Promotion of confidence, trust, and faith in a woman's ability to give birth.	• Seeks to facilitate a woman's or a couple's personal process of birth. • Proactive decision making by the couple. • Maintaining an ideal environment. • Promotion of beliefs that increase self-awareness.	• Exercise • Pelvic body positioning • Support • Relaxation	• Beliefs about pregnancy, labor, and birth. • Safety of VBAC. • Physical and emotional aspects. • Risks and benefits of medical procedures. • Personal support and comfort measures. • Nutrition, exercise, and pelvic body work.

Nurses should ensure that women who have used alternative childbirth education methods have an opportunity to address issues that are unclear to them or have not been previously discussed. In a study of 1,500 women who gave birth in a hospital setting, 56% of the women having their first baby attended childbirth classes and only 9% of experienced mothers took some form of classroom education course. Only 4% of these women reported that classes were their most important source of information. Technology has played a key role in childbirth education over the last decade. Many women now turn to the Internet as a resource for childbirth preparation information (Lothian, 2006).

Body-Conditioning Exercises

Some body-conditioning exercises, such as the pelvic tilt, pelvic rock, and Kegel exercises, are taught in childbirth preparation classes. Other exercises strengthen the abdominal muscles for the expulsive phase of labor. (See Chapter 10 ∞ for a description of recommended exercises.)

Relaxation Exercises

Relaxation during labor allows the woman to conserve energy and allows the uterine muscles to work more efficiently. Without practice it is difficult to relax the whole body in the midst of intense uterine contractions. However, *progressive relaxation* exercises such as those taught to induce sleep can be helpful during labor. Instructions for one relaxation exercise is as follows:

- Lie down on your back or side. (Lying on the left side is best for pregnant women.)
- Tighten your muscles in both feet. Hold the tightness for a few seconds and then relax the muscles completely, letting all the tension drain out.
- Tighten your lower legs, hold for a few seconds, and then relax the muscles, letting all the tension drain out.
- Continue tensing and relaxing parts of your body, moving up the body as you do so.

Another relaxation technique, called *touch relaxation*, is based on interaction between the woman and her partner (see an example in Table 8–3).

An additional exercise specific to Lamaze is *disassociation relaxation*. The woman is taught to become familiar with the sensation of contracting and relaxing the voluntary muscle groups throughout her body. She then learns to contract a specific muscle group and relax the rest of her body. The exercise conditions the woman to relax uninvolved muscles while the uterus contracts, creating an active relaxation pattern.

The relaxation techniques described are most effective if the woman practices them regularly both alone and with the participation of her support person. During a practice session, the partner can begin by checking the woman's neck, shoulders, arms, and legs for relaxation. As tense areas are found, the support person encourages the woman to relax those particular body parts. By gentle touch and verbal cues the woman learns to respond to her own perceptions of tense muscles and also to the suggestion from others. The exercises are usually practiced each day so that they become comfortable and easy to do.

Relaxation may also be promoted by cutaneous stimulation. The same abdominal effleurage useful to stimulate the fetus may also be used before the transitional phase of

TABLE 8–3	Touch Relaxation

Touch relaxation technique often combines patterned abdominal breathing with focused relaxation. It may be used to achieve relaxation of specific body parts or for general body relaxation.

Goals: The woman learns to release tension in the areas that her partner touches. The partner learns to watch his or her partner carefully and becomes attuned to tense, tightened muscles.

Technique

- The partner gently touches the woman's brow.
- The woman uses abdominal breathing. As she breathes in through her nose, her abdomen rises, and as she breathes out through her mouth, her abdomen falls. As each breath is released, she lets all tightness and tension flow out with the breath.
- The partner continues to lightly touch her brow until relaxation is felt. The partner may want to provide quiet encouragement such as, "You are doing fine, you are releasing the tension in your forehead." After at least five breaths, the partner may now touch the woman's shoulders and repeat the pattern described earlier.
- The partner moves on to the arms, chest, abdomen, thighs, and calves. The last aspect is to breathe in, let the whole body relax and go limp, and slowly release the breath. It will be helpful at the end of each labor contraction to let the body go limp and release all tension.
- As the couple practices, it is important for the woman to relax each part of her body. When she is in labor it will not be possible to go through the whole body; however, the woman can indicate what would be most helpful (e.g., touch her shoulder during each contraction). The partner can also be alert for signs of muscle tension and tightening. As the partner and woman practice touch relaxation, they may want to make the situation more realistic. They could decide that uterine contractions are occurring every 5 minutes and are lasting for 30 seconds. A clock will help the partner keep track of time. The partner can indicate that a contraction is beginning and suggest the woman begin her breathing. To help her focus, the partner may touch her shoulder or hand. In some instances, it is helpful for the partner to breathe along with the woman. Each couple can determine what works best for them.

labor (Figure 8–4 ■). This light abdominal stroking effectively relieves mild pain. Deep pressure over the sacrum is effective for relieving back pain. In addition to the measures just described, the nurse can promote relaxation by encouraging and supporting the expectant mother's breathing techniques.

HINTS FOR PRACTICE

Call the birthing facilities in your community and inquire about what options and choices are available for childbearing women at each facility.

Breathing Techniques

Breathing techniques are a key element of most childbirth preparation programs. They help keep the mother and her unborn baby adequately oxygenated and help the mother relax and focus her attention appropriately. Breathing techniques are best taught during the final trimester of pregnancy, when the expectant mother's attention is focused on the birth experience. The nurse can

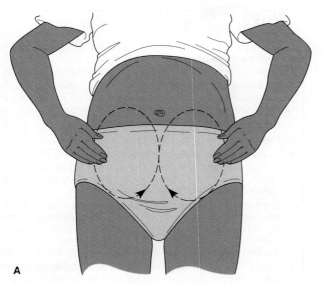
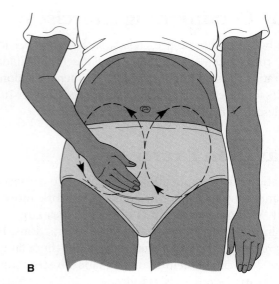

A   B

FIGURE 8-4 Effleurage is light stroking of the abdomen with the fingertips. *A,* Starting at the symphysis, the woman lightly moves her fingertips up and around in a circular pattern. *B,* An alternative approach involves using one hand in a figure-eight pattern. This light stroking can also be done by the support person.

then support the mother's use of breathing techniques during labor. See Key Facts to Remember: Goals of Breathing Techniques. Breathing techniques are described in detail in Chapter 19 ∞.

Preparation for Childbirth That Supports Individuality

Nurses involved in childbirth education need to include the concept of individuality when providing information to expectant parents about the process of childbirth. The current focus in childbirth education is to encourage women to incorporate their own natural responses into coping with the pain of labor and birth. Self-care activities that may be used include the following:

- Vocalization or "sounding" to relieve tension in pregnancy and labor
- Massage (light touch) to facilitate relaxation
- Use of warm water for showers or tub or whirlpool baths during labor

- Visualization (imagery)
- Relaxing music and subdued lighting
- Use of birthing ball, bean bag chair, and so on (Figure 8–5 ■)

Nurses should encourage expectant mothers and couples to make the birth a personal experience. Women

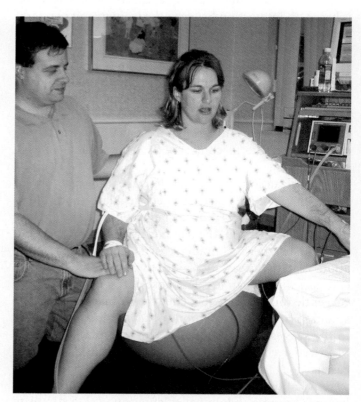

FIGURE 8-5 A birthing ball is just one of many options that a family may choose to promote maternal comfort during labor.

◈

KEY FACTS TO REMEMBER

Goals of Breathing Techniques

- Provide adequate oxygenation of mother and baby, open maternal airways, and avoid inefficient use of muscles.
- Increase physical and mental relaxation.
- Decrease pain and anxiety.
- Provide a means of focusing attention.
- Control inadequate ventilation patterns that are related to pain and stress.

might choose to bring items from home that help them create a more personal birthing space to enhance relaxation and comfort. These items might include warm socks, extra pillows, bath powder, lotion, or a favorite blanket. She may wish to bring photos of special people or places. Many expectant parents enjoy listening to tapes of favorite music or watching favorite home videos. Such personalization of the birth experience may give expectant parents feelings of increased serenity and empowerment.

CHAPTER HIGHLIGHTS

- Preconception counseling may help couples make decisions regarding childbearing.
- Prenatal classes may be offered early and late in the pregnancy. Expectant parents tend to want information in chronological sequence with the pregnancy.
- Adolescents have special learning needs related to pregnancy, the birthing process, and newborn care.
- Breastfeeding programs are offered in the prenatal period.
- Siblings are often included in the whole birthing process, and special classes are available for them.
- Grandparents have unique needs for information.

- Information regarding cesarean birth is beneficial in prenatal classes.
- Prenatal education programs vary in their goals, content, and method of teaching, but all seek to enhance knowledge and decrease anxiety.
- Childbirth education groups, such as the ICEA and the Council of Childbirth Education Specialists, provide consumer health information and certification for teaching prenatal classes.
- Childbirth classes must meet the individual needs of families and their members.

PEARSON
EXPLORE mynursingkit™

MyNursingKit is your one stop for online chapter review materials and resources. Prepare for success with additional NCLEX®-style practice questions, interactive assignments and activities, web links, animations and videos, and more!

Register your access code from the front of your book at
www.mynursingkit.com

CHAPTER REFERENCES

American Academy of Husband-Coached Childbirth. (2008). The Bradley Method. Retrieved on February 11, 2008, from http://www.bradleybirth.com/Main.aspx

American College of Obstetricians & Gynecologists [ACOG]. (2004). Vaginal birth after cesarean. ACOG Practice Bulletin No. 54. ACOG: Washington, DC.

American College of Obstetricians & Gynecologists [ACOG] and American Academy of Pediatricians [AAP]. (2008). *Guidelines for perinatal care* (6th ed.). Washington DC: ACOG & AAP.

Center for Disease Control and Prevention [CDC]. (2007). Unintended pregnancy prevention. Retrieved on February 11, 2008, from http://www.cdc.gov/reproductivehealth/UnintendedPregnancy/index.htm

Friedewald, M., Fletcher, R., & Fairborn, H. (2005). All-male discussion forums for expectant

fathers: Evaluation of a model. *Journal of Perinatal Education, 14*(2), 8–18.

Institute of Medicine [IOM]. (2005). *Complementary and alternative medicine.* Institute of Medicine: Washington, DC.

International Childbirth Education Association. (2006). ICEA philosophy statement. Retrieved on February 11, 2008, from http://www.icea.org

Kitzinger, S. (2005). Home birth: A social process, not a medical crisis. *Practicing Midwife, 8*(4), 26–29.

Lothian, J. A. (2006). Listening to mothers: Take two. *Journal of Perinatal Education, 15*(4).

Low, L. K., Seng, G. S., Murtland, T. L., & Oakley, D. (2000). Clinician-specific episiotomy rates: Impact on perinatal outcomes. *Journal of Nurse-Midwifery and Women's Health, 45*(2), 87–93.

McFadden, A. (2006). Exploring women's views of breastfeeding: A focus group study within an area with high levels of socio-economic

deprivation. *Maternal & Child Nutrition, 2*(3), 156–168.

National Center for Health Statistics [NCHS]. (2007). Teen birth rate rises for the first time in 15 years. Retrieved on February 11, 2008, from http://www.cdc.gov/NCHS/pressroom/07newsreleases/teenbirth.htm

Penney, D. S. (2008). The effects of vigorous exercise during pregnancy. (2008). *Journal of Midwifery and Women's Health, 53*(2), 155–159.

Premburg, A., & Lundgren, I. (2006). Fathers' experiences of childbirth education. *Journal of Perinatal Education, 15*(2), 21–28.

Scott, J. A. (2006). Temporal changes in the determinants of breastfeeding initiation. *Birth, 33*(1), 37–45.

Teschendorf, M., & Evans, C. (2000). Hydrotherapy during labor: An example of a developing practice policy. *American Journal of Maternal-Child Nursing, 25*(4), 198–203.

PART THREE

Pregnancy and Family

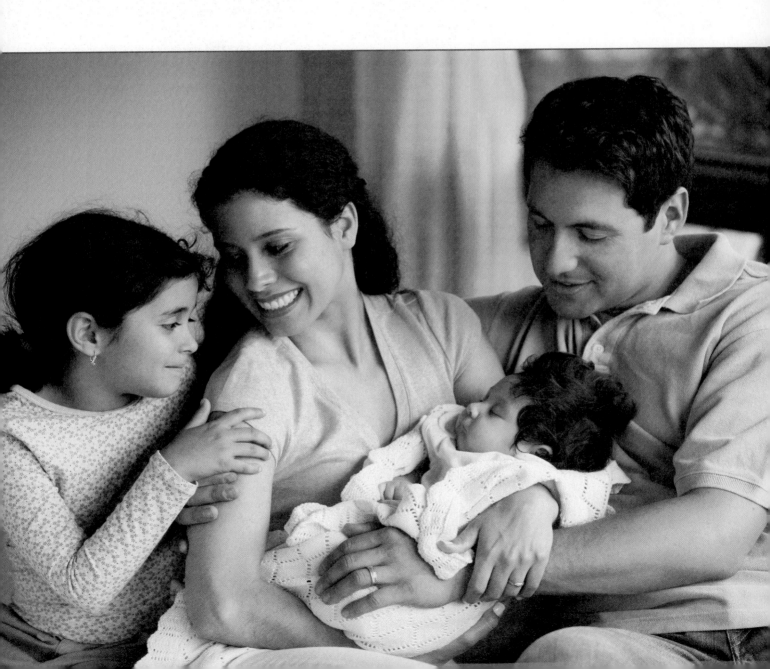

CHAPTER 9

Physical and Psychologic Changes of Pregnancy

In my experience, few women are ever really prepared for all the changes they experience during pregnancy, especially a first pregnancy. That is why early prenatal care is important. Yes, starting care early gives us a better chance to identify risk factors, but it also enables us to do a better job of prenatal education. I am constantly amazed by what a difference it makes for a woman when she has a good idea of what to expect and why.

—A Nurse Working with an Obstetrician in Private Practice

LEARNING OUTCOMES

9-1. Identify the anatomic and physiologic changes that occur during pregnancy in providing nursing care to expectant women.

9-2. Assess the subjective (presumptive), objective (probable), and diagnostic (positive) changes of pregnancy in clients.

9-3. Contrast the various types of pregnancy tests.

9-4. Examine the emotional and psychologic changes that commonly occur in a woman, her partner, and her family during pregnancy when providing nursing care.

9-5. Discuss cultural factors that may influence a family's response to pregnancy in the provision of nursing care.

KEY TERMS

Ballottement **190**
Braxton Hicks contractions **183**
Chadwick's sign **183**
Chloasma (melasma gravidarum) **185**
Couvade **195**
Diastasis recti **186**
Goodell's sign **183**
Hegar's sign **189**
Linea nigra **185**
McDonald's sign **189**
Morning sickness **188**
Mucous plug **183**
Physiologic anemia of pregnancy **184**
Quickening **189**
Striae **184**
Supine hypotensive syndrome (vena caval syndrome, aortocaval compression) **184**

No matter how much we learn about pregnancy and the changes that occur in the woman and the developing fetus, we never cease to be amazed. First, it is nothing short of a miracle that the union of two microscopic entities—an ovum and a sperm—can produce a living being. Second, the woman's body must undergo extraordinary physical changes to maintain a pregnancy.

Pregnancy is divided into three trimesters, each approximately a 3-month period. Each trimester brings predictable changes for both the mother and fetus. This chapter describes these physical and psychologic changes. It also presents the various cultural factors that can affect a pregnant woman's well-being. Subsequent chapters build on this information in describing effective approaches to planning and providing care.

Anatomy and Physiology of Pregnancy

The changes that occur in the pregnant woman's body may result from hormonal influences, the growth of the fetus, or the mother's physiologic adaptation to the pregnancy. Please see the foldout chart in the center of this text for a summary of these changes.

Reproductive System

Some of the most dramatic changes of pregnancy occur in the reproductive organs.

Uterus

The changes in the uterus during pregnancy are amazing. Before pregnancy, the uterus is a small, semisolid, pear-shaped organ measuring approximately $7.5 \times 5 \times 2.5$ cm and weighing about 60 g (2 oz). At the end of pregnancy it measures about $28 \times 24 \times 21$ cm and weighs approximately 1,100 g (2.5 lb); its capacity has also increased from about 10 mL to 5,000 mL (5 L) or more (Cunningham, Leveno, Bloom et al., 2005).

The enlargement of the uterus is primarily because of the enlargement (hypertrophy) of the preexisting myometrial cells as a result of the stimulating influence of estrogen and the distention caused by the growing fetus. Only a limited increase in cell number (hyperplasia) occurs. The fibrous tissue between the muscle bands increases markedly, which adds to the strength and elasticity of the muscle wall. The enlarging uterus, developing placenta, and growing fetus require additional blood flow to the uterus. By the end of pregnancy, one-sixth of the total maternal blood volume is contained within the vascular system of the uterus.

Braxton Hicks contractions, which are irregular, generally painless contractions of the uterus, occur intermittently throughout pregnancy. They may be felt through the abdominal wall beginning about the fourth month of pregnancy. In later months, these contractions become uncomfortable and may be confused with true labor contractions.

HINTS FOR PRACTICE

Beginning early in pregnancy, have the woman feel her uterus periodically so that she becomes familiar with its size and the way it feels. As her pregnancy progresses she then will be more likely to identify Braxton Hicks contractions and preterm labor, if it occurs.

Cervix

Estrogen stimulates the glandular tissue of the cervix, which increases in cell number and becomes hyperactive. The endocervical glands secrete a thick, sticky mucus that accumulates and forms a **mucous plug**, which seals the endocervical canal and prevents the ascent of microorganisms into the uterus. This plug is expelled when cervical dilatation begins. The hyperactivity of the glandular tissue also increases the normal physiologic mucorrhea, at times resulting in profuse discharge. Increased cervical vascularity also causes both the softening of the cervix (**Goodell's sign**) and its bluish discoloration (**Chadwick's sign**).

Ovaries

The ovaries stop producing ova during pregnancy, but the corpus luteum continues to produce hormones until about weeks 6 to 8. It secretes progesterone until about the seventh week of pregnancy to maintain the endometrium until the placenta assumes the task. The corpus luteum then begins to disintegrate slowly.

Vagina

Estrogen causes a thickening of the vaginal mucosa, a loosening of the connective tissue, and an increase in vaginal secretions. These secretions are thick, white, and acidic (pH 3.5 to 6.0). The acid pH helps prevent bacterial infection but favors the growth of yeast organisms. Thus the pregnant woman is more susceptible to *Candida* infection than usual.

The supportive connective tissue of the vagina loosens throughout pregnancy. By the end of pregnancy, the vagina and perineal body are sufficiently relaxed to permit passage of the infant. Because blood flow to the vagina is increased, the vagina may show the same blue–purple color (Chadwick's sign) as the cervix.

Breasts

Estrogen and progesterone cause many changes in the mammary glands. The breasts enlarge and become more nodular as the glands increase in size and number in preparation for lactation. Superficial veins become more prominent, the nipples become more erectile, and the areolas darken. Montgomery's follicles (sebaceous glands) enlarge, and **striae** (reddish stretch marks that slowly turn silver after childbirth) may develop.

Colostrum, an antibody-rich yellow secretion, may leak or be expressed from the breasts during the last trimester. Colostrum gradually converts to mature milk during the first few days after childbirth.

Respiratory System

Many respiratory changes occur to meet the increased oxygen requirements of a pregnant woman. The volume of air breathed each minute increases 30% to 40%. In addition, progesterone decreases airway resistance, permitting a 15% to 20% increase in oxygen consumption, as well as increases in carbon dioxide production and in the respiratory functional reserve.

As the uterus enlarges, it presses upward and elevates the diaphragm. The subcostal angle increases, so that the rib cage flares. The anteroposterior diameter increases, and the chest circumference expands by as much as 6 cm; as a result, there is no significant loss of intrathoracic volume. Breathing changes from abdominal to thoracic as pregnancy progresses, and descent of the diaphragm on inspiration becomes less possible. Some hyperventilation and difficulty in breathing may occur.

Nasal stuffiness and epistaxis (nosebleeds) may also occur because of estrogen-induced edema and vascular congestion of the nasal mucosa.

Cardiovascular System

During pregnancy, blood flow increases to organ systems with an increased workload. Thus blood flow increases to the uterus, placenta, and breasts, whereas hepatic and cerebral flow remains unchanged. Cardiac output begins to increase early in pregnancy and peaks at 25 to 30 weeks' gestation at 30% to 50% above prepregnant levels. In the third trimester cardiac output becomes less predictable; it is likely that any changes are individually determined (Gordon, 2007).

The pulse may increase by as many as 10 to 15 beats per minute at term. The blood pressure decreases slightly, reaching its lowest point during the second trimester. It gradually increases to near prepregnant levels by the end of the third trimester.

The enlarging uterus puts pressure on pelvic and femoral vessels, interfering with returning blood flow and causing stasis of blood in the lower extremities. This condition may lead to dependent edema and varicosity of the veins in the legs, vulva, and rectum (hemorrhoids) in late pregnancy. This increased blood volume in the lower legs may also make the pregnant woman prone to postural hypotension.

When the pregnant woman lies supine, the enlarging uterus may press on the vena cava, thus reducing blood flow to the right atrium, lowering blood pressure, and causing dizziness, pallor, and clamminess. Research indicates that the enlarging uterus may also press on the aorta and its collateral circulation (Cunningham et al., 2005). This condition is called **supine hypotensive syndrome**. It may also be referred to as **vena caval syndrome** or **aortocaval compression** (Figure 9–1 ■). It can be corrected by having the woman lie on her left side or by placing a pillow or wedge under her right hip as she lies in a supine position.

Blood volume progressively increases beginning in the first trimester, increases rapidly until about 30 to 34 weeks, and then plateaus until birth at about 40% to 50% above nonpregnant levels. This increase occurs because of increases in both erythrocytes and plasma (Gordon, 2007).

The total erythrocyte (red blood cell) volume increases by about 30% in women who receive iron supplementation (but only about 18% without iron supplementation). This increase in erythrocytes is necessary to transport the additional oxygen required during pregnancy. However, the increase in plasma volume during pregnancy averages about 50%. Because the plasma volume increase (50%) is greater than the erythrocyte increase (30%), the hematocrit, which measures the concentration of red blood cells in the plasma, decreases slightly (Gordon, 2007). This decrease is referred to as the **physiologic anemia of pregnancy** (pseudoanemia).

Iron is necessary for hemoglobin formation, and hemoglobin is the oxygen-carrying component of erythrocytes. Thus the increase in erythrocyte levels results in an increased need for iron by the pregnant woman. Even though the gastrointestinal absorption of iron is moderately increased during pregnancy, it is usually necessary to add supplemental iron to the diet to meet the expanded red blood cell and fetal needs.

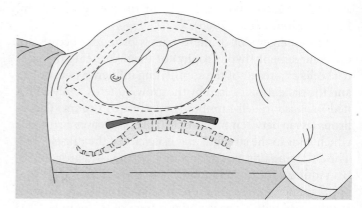

Figure 9–1 Vena caval syndrome. The gravid uterus compresses the vena cava when the woman is supine. This reduces the blood flow returning to the heart and may cause maternal hypotension.

Leukocyte production increases slightly to an average of 8,500 mm³ with a range of 5,600 to 12,200 mm³. During labor and the early postpartum period, these levels may reach 20,000 to 30,000/mm³. Because of this normal increase in WBCs, the result should not be used clinically to diagnose the presence of infection (Gordon, 2007).

Both the fibrin and plasma fibrinogen levels increase during pregnancy. Although the blood-clotting time of the pregnant woman does not differ significantly from that of the nonpregnant woman, clotting factors VII, VIII, IX, and X increase; thus pregnancy is a somewhat hypercoagulable state. These changes, coupled with venous stasis in late pregnancy, increase the pregnant woman's risk of developing venous thrombosis.

Gastrointestinal System

Nausea and vomiting are common during the first trimester because of elevated human chorionic gonadotropin levels and changed carbohydrate metabolism. Gum tissue may soften and bleed easily. The secretion of saliva may increase and even become excessive (ptyalism).

Elevated progesterone levels cause smooth muscle relaxation, resulting in delayed gastric emptying and decreased peristalsis. As a result, the pregnant woman may complain of bloating and constipation. These symptoms are aggravated as the enlarging uterus displaces the stomach upward and the intestines are moved laterally and posteriorly. The cardiac sphincter also relaxes, and heartburn (pyrosis) may occur because of reflux of acidic secretions into the lower esophagus. Hemorrhoids frequently develop in late pregnancy from constipation and from pressure on vessels below the level of the uterus.

Only minor liver changes occur with pregnancy. Plasma albumin concentrations and serum cholinesterase activity decrease with normal pregnancy, as with certain liver diseases.

The emptying time of the gallbladder is prolonged during pregnancy as a result of smooth muscle relaxation from progesterone. This, coupled with the elevated levels of cholesterol in the bile, can predispose the woman to gallstone formation.

Urinary Tract

During the first trimester, the enlarging uterus is still a pelvic organ and presses against the bladder, producing urinary frequency. This symptom decreases during the second trimester, when the uterus becomes an abdominal organ and pressure against the bladder lessens. Frequency reappears during the third trimester, when the presenting part descends into the pelvis and again presses on the bladder, reducing bladder capacity, contributing to hyperemia, and irritating the bladder.

The ureters (especially the right ureter) elongate and dilate above the pelvic brim. The glomerular filtration rate (GFR) rises by as much as 50% beginning in the second trimester and remains elevated until birth. To compensate for this increase, renal tubular reabsorption also increases. However, glycosuria is seen sometimes during pregnancy because of the kidneys' inability to reabsorb all the glucose filtered by the glomeruli. Glycosuria may be normal or may indicate gestational diabetes, so it always warrants further testing.

Skin and Hair

Changes in skin pigmentation commonly occur during pregnancy. They are thought to be stimulated by increased estrogen, progesterone, and α-melanocytic-stimulating hormone levels. Pigmentation of the skin increases primarily in areas that are already hyperpigmented: the areola, the nipples, the vulva, and the perianal area. The skin in the middle of the abdomen may develop a pigmented line, the **linea nigra**, which usually extends from the umbilicus or above to the pubic area (Figure 9–2 ■). Facial **chloasma** or **melasma gravidarum** (also known as the "mask of pregnancy"), a darkening of the skin over the cheeks, nose, and forehead, may develop. Chloasma or melasma is more prominent in dark-haired women and is aggravated by exposure to the sun. Fortunately, the condition fades or becomes less prominent soon after childbirth when the hormonal influence of pregnancy subsides.

In addition, the sweat and sebaceous glands are often hyperactive during pregnancy.

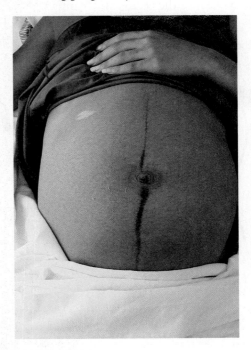

FIGURE 9–2 Linea nigra.

Striae, or stretch marks, are reddish, wavy streaks that may appear on the abdomen, thighs, buttocks, and breasts. They result from reduced connective tissue strength because of elevated adrenal steroid levels.

Vascular spider nevi—small, bright red elevations of the skin radiating from a central body—may develop on the chest, neck, face, arms, and legs. They may be caused by increased subcutaneous blood flow in response to elevated estrogen levels.

The rate of hair growth may decrease during pregnancy; the number of hair follicles in the resting or dormant phase also decreases. After birth, the number of hair follicles in the resting phase increases sharply and the woman may notice increased hair shedding for 1 to 4 months. Practically all hair is replaced within 6 to 12 months, however (Cunningham et al., 2005).

Musculoskeletal System

No demonstrable changes occur in the teeth of pregnant women. The dental caries that sometimes accompany pregnancy are probably caused by inadequate oral hygiene and dental care, especially if the woman has problems with bleeding gums or nausea and vomiting.

The joints of the pelvis relax somewhat because of hormonal influences. The result is often a waddling gait. As the pregnant woman's center of gravity gradually changes, the lumbar spinal curve becomes accentuated, and her posture changes (Figure 9–3 ■). This posture change compensates for the increased weight of the uterus anteriorly and frequently results in low backache.

Pressure of the enlarging uterus on the abdominal muscles may cause the rectus abdominis muscle to sepa-

rate, producing **diastasis recti**. If the separation is severe and muscle tone is not regained postpartally, subsequent pregnancies will not have adequate support and the woman's abdomen may appear pendulous.

Central Nervous System

Pregnant women frequently describe decreased attention, concentration, and memory during and shortly after pregnancy, but few studies have explored this phenomenon. One study did compare a group of pregnant women against a control group, finding a decline in memory that could not be attributed to depression, anxiety, sleep deprivation, or other physical changes of pregnancy. This memory loss disappears soon after childbirth (Cunningham et al., 2005).

Eyes

During pregnancy, intraocular pressure decreases, probably because of increased vitreous outflow, and the cornea thickens slightly because of fluid retention. As a result, some pregnant women experience difficulty wearing previously comfortable contact lenses (Cunningham et al., 2005). These changes usually disappear by 6 weeks postpartum.

Metabolism

Most metabolic functions increase during pregnancy because of the increased demands of the growing fetus and its support system. The expectant mother must meet both her own tissue replacement needs and those of her unborn

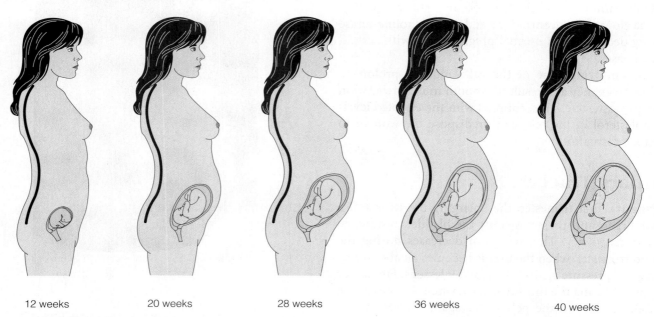

| 12 weeks | 20 weeks | 28 weeks | 36 weeks | 40 weeks |

FIGURE 9–3 Postural changes during pregnancy. Note the increasing lordosis of the lumbosacral spine and the increasing curvature of the thoracic area.

child. Her body must also anticipate the needs of labor and lactation. For a detailed discussion of nutrient, vitamin, and mineral metabolism, see Chapter 13 ∞.

Weight Gain

As discussed in Chapter 13 ∞, adequate nutrition and weight gain are important during pregnancy. The recommended weight gain for women of normal weight before pregnancy is 11.4 to 15.9 kg (25 to 35 lb), whereas women who are overweight should limit their gain to 6.8 kg (15 lb). Underweight women may gain up to 18.1 kg (40 lb) (Johnson, Gregory, & Niebyl, 2007). The average pattern of weight gain is 1.6 to 2.3 kg (3.5 to 5 lb) during the first trimester and 5.5 to 6.8 kg (12 to 15 lb) during each of the last two trimesters.

Water Metabolism

Increased water retention, a basic alteration of pregnancy, is caused by several interrelated factors. The increased level of steroid sex hormones affects sodium and fluid retention. The lowered serum protein also influences fluid balance, as do increased intracapillary pressure and permeability. The extra water is needed for the fetus, placenta, and amniotic fluid and the mother's increased blood volume, interstitial fluids, and enlarged organs.

Nutrient Metabolism

The fetus makes its greatest protein and fat demands during the second half of pregnancy, doubling in weight during the last 6 to 8 weeks. Protein (contributing nitrogen) must be stored during pregnancy to maintain a constant level within the breast milk and to avoid depletion of maternal tissues. Carbohydrate needs also increase, especially during the second and third trimesters.

Fats are more completely absorbed during pregnancy, and the level of free fatty acids increases in response to human placental lactogen. The levels of lipoproteins and cholesterol also increase. Because of these changes, increased levels of dietary fat or reduced carbohydrate production may lead to ketonuria in the pregnant woman. See Chapter 12 ∞ for a complete discussion of the mother's nutritional requirements.

Endocrine System

Thyroid

The thyroid gland often enlarges slightly during pregnancy because of increased vascularity and hyperplasia of glandular tissue. Its capacity to bind thyroxine is greater, resulting in an increase in serum protein-bound iodine. These changes are because of higher blood levels of estrogen during pregnancy.

> ## COMPLEMENTARY AND ALTERNATIVE THERAPIES
>
> ### Herbs During Pregnancy
>
> Pharmaceutical companies have not included pregnant women and children in their studies of drug safety, claiming excessive costs and other research problems. As a result, very few over-the-counter or prescription drugs can claim to be safe for pregnant women and nursing mothers. The same can be said for herbal medicines. Many herbs have been researched extensively in Europe and Asia, although there has been little clinical research done in the United States on the use of herbs in pregnancy. Nurses would do well to learn about many of the commonly used herbs so that they can provide pregnant women with accurate information. Every pregnant or nursing woman must be cautious about everything she ingests—foods, liquids, medications, and herbs. If a problem warrants intervention, she and her primary healthcare provider should discuss the benefits and risks of all treatments, synthetic and natural.

The basal metabolic rate increases by as much as 20% to 25% during pregnancy. The increased oxygen consumption is primarily because of fetal metabolic activity. Within a few weeks after birth all thyroid function returns to normal limits.

Pituitary

Pregnancy is made possible by the hypothalamic stimulation of the anterior pituitary gland. The anterior pituitary produces follicle-stimulating hormone (FSH), which stimulates ovum growth, and luteinizing hormone (LH), which brings about ovulation. Stimulation of the pituitary also prolongs the ovary's corpus luteal phase, which maintains the endometrium in case conception occurs. Prolactin, another anterior pituitary hormone, is responsible for lactation.

The posterior pituitary secretes vasopressin (antidiuretic hormone) and oxytocin. Vasopressin causes vasoconstriction, which results in increased blood pressure; it also helps regulate water balance. Oxytocin promotes uterine contractility and stimulates ejection of milk from the breasts (the letdown reflex) in the postpartum period.

Adrenals

No significant increase in the weight of the adrenal glands occurs during pregnancy. Circulating cortisol, which regulates carbohydrate and protein metabolism, increases in response to increased estrogen levels. Cortisol blood levels return to normal within 1 to 6 weeks postpartum.

The adrenals secrete increased levels of aldosterone by the early part of the second trimester. This increase in aldosterone in a normal pregnancy may be the body's protective response to the increased sodium excretion associated with progesterone (Cunningham et al., 2005).

Pancreas

The pregnant woman has increased insulin needs, and the pancreatic islets of Langerhans, which secrete insulin, are stressed to meet this increased demand. Any marginal pancreatic function quickly becomes apparent, and the woman may show signs of gestational diabetes (see Chapter 15 ∞).

Hormones in Pregnancy

Several hormones are required to maintain pregnancy. Most of them are initially produced by the corpus luteum; then the placenta takes over production.

HUMAN CHORIONIC GONADOTROPIN (hCG) The trophoblast secretes human chorionic gonadotropin (hCG) in early pregnancy. This hormone stimulates progesterone and estrogen production by the corpus luteum to maintain the pregnancy until the placenta is developed sufficiently to assume that function. HCG can be detected in maternal blood and urine as early as 8 days post-fertilization and peaks at 9 to 10 weeks (Burton, Sibley, & Jauniaux, 2007).

HUMAN PLACENTAL LACTOGEN (hPL) Also called human chorionic somatomammotropin, human placental lactogen (hPL) is produced by the syncytiotrophoblast. Human placental lactogen is an antagonist of insulin; it increases the amount of circulating free fatty acids for maternal metabolic needs and decreases maternal metabolism of glucose to favor fetal growth.

Estrogen, secreted originally by the corpus luteum, is produced primarily by the placenta as early as the seventh week of pregnancy. Estrogen stimulates uterine development to provide a suitable environment for the fetus. It also helps develop the ductal system of the breasts in preparation for lactation.

PROGESTERONE Progesterone, also produced initially by the corpus luteum and then by the placenta, plays the greatest role in maintaining pregnancy. It maintains the endometrium and inhibits spontaneous uterine contractility, thus preventing early spontaneous abortion. Progesterone also helps develop the acini and lobules of the breasts in preparation for lactation.

RELAXIN Relaxin is detectable in the serum of a pregnant woman by the time of the first missed menstrual period. Relaxin inhibits uterine activity, diminishes the strength of uterine contractions, aids in the softening of the cervix, and has the long-term effect of remodeling collagen. Its primary source is the corpus luteum, but small amounts are believed to be produced by the placenta and uterine decidua.

Prostaglandins in Pregnancy

Prostaglandins (PGs) are lipid substances that can arise from most body tissues but occur in high concentrations in the female reproductive tract and are present in the decidua during pregnancy. The exact functions of PGs during pregnancy are still unknown, although it has been proposed that they are responsible for maintaining reduced placental vascular resistance. Decreased prostaglandin levels may contribute to hypertension and preeclampsia. Prostaglandins are also believed to play a role in the complex biochemistry that initiates labor.

Signs of Pregnancy

Many of the changes women experience during pregnancy are used to diagnose the pregnancy itself. They are called the subjective, or presumptive, changes; the objective, or probable, changes; and the diagnostic, or positive, changes of pregnancy. The guidelines for differentiating among these three are identified in Key Facts to Remember: Differentiating the Signs of Pregnancy.

Subjective (Presumptive) Changes

The subjective changes of pregnancy are the symptoms the woman experiences and reports. Because they can be caused by other conditions, they cannot be considered proof of pregnancy (Table 9–1). The following subjective signs can be diagnostic clues when other signs and symptoms of pregnancy are also present.

Amenorrhea, or the absence of menses, is the earliest symptom of pregnancy. The missing of more than one menstrual period, especially in a woman whose cycle is ordinarily regular, is an especially useful diagnostic clue.

Nausea and vomiting in pregnancy (NVP) occur frequently during the first trimester and may be the result of elevated hCG levels and changed carbohydrate metabolism. Because these symptoms often occur in the early part of the day, they are commonly referred to as **morning sickness**. In reality, the symptoms may occur at any time

---

◆

KEY FACTS TO REMEMBER
Differentiating the Signs of Pregnancy

These guidelines help differentiate among the presumptive, probable, and positive changes of pregnancy.

Subjective (Presumptive) Changes
- Symptoms the woman experiences and reports
- May have causes other than pregnancy

Objective (Probable) Changes
- Signs perceived by the examiner
- May have causes other than pregnancy

Diagnostic (Positive) Changes
- Signs perceived by the examiner
- Can be caused only by pregnancy

TABLE 9–1	Differential Diagnosis of Pregnancy—Subjective Changes
Subjective Changes	**Possible Alternative Causes**
Amenorrhea	Endocrine factors: early menopause; lactation; thyroid, pituitary, adrenal, ovarian dysfunction
	Metabolic factors: malnutrition, anemia, climatic changes, diabetes mellitus, degenerative disorders, long-distance running
	Psychologic factors: emotional shock, fear of pregnancy or sexually transmitted infection, intense desire for pregnancy (pseudocyesis), stress
	Obliteration of endometrial cavity by infection or curettage
	Systemic disease (acute or chronic), such as tuberculosis or malignancy
Nausea and vomiting	Gastrointestinal disorders
	Acute infections such as encephalitis
	Emotional disorders such as pseudocyesis or anorexia nervosa
Urinary frequency	Urinary tract infection
	Cystocele
	Pelvic tumors
	Urethral diverticula
	Emotional tension
Breast tenderness	Premenstrual tension
	Chronic cystic mastitis
	Pseudocyesis
	Hyperestrogenism
Quickening	Increased peristalsis
	Flatus ("gas")
	Abdominal muscle contractions
	Shifting of abdominal contents

and can range from a mere distaste for food to severe vomiting. Research indicates that women who experience NVP often have a more favorable pregnancy outcome than those who do not (Gordon, 2007).

Excessive fatigue may be noted within a few weeks after the first missed menstrual period and may persist throughout the first trimester.

Urinary frequency is experienced during the first trimester as the enlarging uterus presses on the bladder.

Changes in the breasts are frequently noted in early pregnancy. These changes include tenderness and tingling sensations, increased pigmentation of the areola and nipple, and changes in Montgomery's glands. The veins also become more visible and form a bluish pattern beneath the skin.

Quickening, or the mother's perception of fetal movement, occurs about 18 to 20 weeks after the last menstrual period in a woman pregnant for the first time but may occur as early as 16 weeks in a woman who has been pregnant before. Quickening is a fluttering sensation in the abdomen that gradually increases in intensity and frequency.

HINTS FOR PRACTICE

Some women suggest that it is easiest to imagine the fluttering associated with quickening by letting the outer tips of the eyelashes brush a finger and then imagining that same sensation deep inside the abdomen.

Objective (Probable) Changes

An examiner can perceive the objective changes that occur in pregnancy. Because these changes can also have other causes, they do not confirm pregnancy (Table 9–2).

Changes in the pelvic organs—the only physical changes detectable during the first 3 months of pregnancy—are caused by increased vascular congestion. These changes are noted on pelvic examination. As noted earlier, there is a softening of the cervix called Goodell's sign. Chadwick's sign is a bluish, purple, or deep red discoloration of the mucous membranes of the cervix, vagina, and vulva (some sources consider this a presumptive sign). **Hegar's sign** is a softening of the isthmus of the uterus, the area between the cervix and the body of the uterus (Figure 9–4 ■).

McDonald's sign is an ease in flexing the body of the uterus against the cervix.

General enlargement and softening of the body of the uterus can be noted after the eighth week of pregnancy. The

TABLE 9–2	Differential Diagnosis of Pregnancy—Objective Changes
Objective Changes	**Possible Alternative Causes**
Changes in pelvic organs	Increased vascular congestion
Goodell's sign	Estrogen–progestin oral contraceptives
Chadwick's sign	Vulvar, vaginal, cervical hyperemia
Hegar's sign	Excessively soft walls of nonpregnant uterus
Uterine enlargement	Uterine tumors
Braun von Fernwald's sign	Uterine tumors
Enlargement of abdomen	Obesity, ascites, pelvic tumors
Braxton Hicks contractions	Hematometra, pedunculated, submucous, and soft myomas
Uterine souffle	Large uterine myomas, large ovarian tumors, or any condition with greatly increased uterine blood flow
Pigmentation of skin	Estrogen–progestin oral contraceptives
Chloasma (Melasma)	Melanocyte hormonal stimulation
Linea nigra	
Nipples/areola	
Abdominal striae	Obesity, pelvic tumor
Ballottement	Uterine tumors/polyps, ascites
Pregnancy tests	Increased pituitary gonadotropins at menopause, choriocarcinoma, hydatidiform mole
Palpation for fetal outline	Uterine myomas

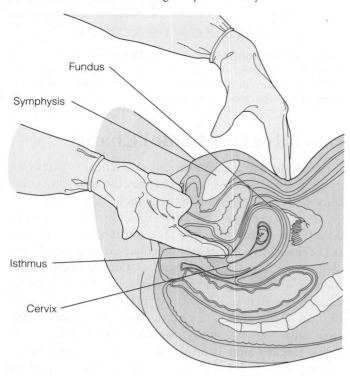

FIGURE 9–4 Hegar's sign, a softening of the isthmus of the uterus, can be determined by the examiner during a vaginal examination.

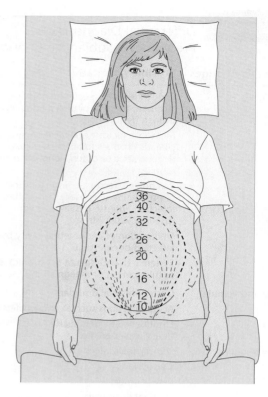

FIGURE 9–5 Approximate height of the fundus at various weeks of pregnancy.

fundus of the uterus is palpable just above the symphysis pubis at about 10 to 12 weeks' gestation and at the level of the umbilicus at 20 to 22 weeks' gestation (Figure 9–5 ■).

Enlargement of the abdomen during the childbearing years is usually regarded as evidence of pregnancy, especially if it is continuous and accompanied by amenorrhea.

Braxton Hicks contractions can be palpated most commonly after 28 weeks. As the woman approaches the end of pregnancy, these contractions may become uncomfortable. They are then often called false labor.

Uterine souffle may be heard when the examiner auscultates the abdomen over the uterus. It is a soft, blowing sound that occurs at the same rate as the maternal pulse and is caused by the increased uterine blood flow and blood pulsating through the placenta. It is sometimes confused with the *funic souffle,* a soft, blowing sound of blood pulsating through the umbilical cord. The funic souffle occurs at the same rate as the fetal heart rate.

Changes in pigmentation of the skin are common in pregnancy. The nipples and areola may darken, and the linea nigra may develop. Facial melasma (chloasma) may become noticeable, and striae may appear.

The *fetal outline* may be identified by palpation in many pregnant women after 24 weeks' gestation. **Ballottement** is the passive fetal movement elicited when the examiner inserts two gloved fingers into the vagina and pushes against the cervix. This action pushes the fetal body up, and, as it falls back, the examiner feels a rebound.

Pregnancy tests detect the presence of hCG in the maternal blood or urine. These are not considered a positive sign of pregnancy because other conditions can cause elevated hCG levels.

Clinical Pregnancy Tests

A variety of assay techniques are available to detect hCG during early pregnancy. Historically, the following two tests were commonly used urine tests done on the first morning urine specimen. These tests become positive within 10 to 14 days after the first missed period.

- *Hemagglutination inhibition test* (Pregnosticon R test), an immunoassay, is based on the fact that no clumping of cells occurs when the urine of a pregnant woman is added to the hCG-sensitized red blood cells of sheep.
- *Latex agglutination test* (Gravindex and Pregnosticon Slide tests), also an immunoassay, is based on the fact that latex particle agglutination is inhibited in the presence of urine containing hCG.

Several newer pregnancy tests are available, including the following:

- β-*subunit radioimmunoassay (RIA)* uses an antiserum with specificity for the β-subunit of hCG in maternal blood. This accurate pregnancy test becomes positive a few days after presumed implantation, thereby permitting early diagnosis of pregnancy. This test is also used in the diagnosis of ectopic pregnancy or trophoblastic disease. However, because it requires several hours to perform and has only limited sensitivity, it is being replaced by other, technically simpler tests such as the immunoradiometric assay.

- *Immunoradiometric assay (IRMA)* (Neocept, Pregnosis) uses a radioactive antibody to identify the presence of hCG in the serum. This test can detect very low concentrations of hCG and requires only about 30 minutes to perform.
- *Enzyme-linked immunosorbent assay (ELISA)* (Model Sensichrome, Quest Confidot) does not use radioisotopes but a substance that results in a color change after binding. The test is sensitive, quick, and can detect hCG levels as early as 7 to 9 days after ovulation and conception, which is 5 days before the first missed period.
- *Fluoroimmunoassay (FIA)* (Opus hCG, Stratus hCG) uses an antibody tagged with a fluorescent label to detect serum hCG. The test, which takes about 2 to 3 hours to perform, is extremely sensitive and is used primarily to identify and follow hCG concentrations.

Over-the-Counter Pregnancy Tests

Home pregnancy tests are available over the counter at a reasonable cost. These enzyme immunoassay tests, performed on urine, are very sensitive and detect even low levels of hCG.

Home pregnancy test instructions are quite explicit and should be followed carefully for optimal results. The false-positive rate of these tests is low, but the false-negative results are higher and so follow-up is indicated if symptoms of pregnancy occur. If the results are negative, the woman should repeat the test in 1 week if she has not started her period.

Diagnostic (Positive) Changes

The positive signs of pregnancy are completely objective, cannot be confused with a pathologic state, and offer conclusive proof of pregnancy.

The *fetal heartbeat* can be detected with an electronic Doppler device as early as weeks 10 to 12. The heartbeat can be detected with a fetoscope by weeks 17 to 20.

Fetal movement is actively palpable by a trained examiner after about week 20 of pregnancy.

Visualization of the fetus by ultrasound examination confirms a pregnancy. The gestational sac can be observed by 4 to 5 weeks' gestation (2 to 3 weeks after conception). Fetal parts and fetal heart movement can be seen as early as 8 weeks' gestation. More recently ultrasound using a vaginal probe has been used to detect a gestational sac as early as 10 days after implantation (Cunningham et al., 2005).

Psychologic Response of the Expectant Family to Pregnancy

Pregnancy is a turning point in a family's life, accompanied by stress and anxiety, whether the pregnancy is desired or not. Especially if this is their first child, the expectant couple may be unaware of the physical, emotional, and cognitive changes of pregnancy and may anticipate no problems from such a normal event. Thus they may be confused and distressed by new feelings and behaviors that are essentially normal.

For beginning families, pregnancy is the transition period from childlessness to parenthood. If the expectant woman is married or has a stable partner, she no longer is only a mate but must also assume the role of mother. Her partner, whether male or female, will become a parent, too. The anticipation of parenthood brings significant role changes for them. Career goals and mobility may be affected, and the couple's relationship takes on a different meaning to them and their families and community. If the pregnancy results in the birth of a child, the couple enters a new, irreversible stage of their life together. With each subsequent pregnancy, routines and family dynamics are again altered, requiring readjustment and realignment.

In most pregnancies, finances are an important consideration. Traditional lore relegates to the father the role of primary breadwinner, and indeed finances are often a very real concern for fathers. In today's society, however, there are many types of families (see Chapter 2 ∞) and even pregnant women with stable partners recognize the financial impact of a child and may feel concern about financial issues. Decisions about financial matters need to be made at this time. Will the woman work during her pregnancy and return to work after her child is born? If so, who will provide child care? Couples may also need to decide about the division of domestic tasks. Any differences of opinion must be discussed openly and resolved so that the family can meet the needs of its members.

If the pregnant woman has no stable partner, she must deal alone with the role changes, fears, and adjustments of pregnancy or seek support from family or friends. She also faces the reality of planning for the future as a single parent. Finances may be a major source of concern. Even if the pregnant woman plans to relinquish her infant, she must still deal with the adjustments of pregnancy. This adjustment can be especially difficult without a good support system.

Developmental Tasks of the Expectant Couple

Pregnancy can be viewed as a developmental stage with its own distinct developmental tasks. For a couple, it can be a time of support or conflict, depending on the amount of adjustment each is willing to make to maintain the family's equilibrium.

During a first pregnancy, the couple plans together for the child's arrival, collecting information on how to be parents. At the same time, each continues to participate in some separate activities with friends or family members. The availability of social support is an important factor in psychosocial well-being during pregnancy. The social network is often a major source of advice for the pregnant woman; however, both sound and unsound information may be conveyed.

During pregnancy, the expectant parents both face significant changes and must deal with major psychosocial adjustments (Table 9–3). Other family members, especially other children of the woman or couple and the grandparents-to-be, must also adjust to the pregnancy.

For some, pregnancy is more than a developmental stage; it is a crisis. *Crisis* can be defined as a disturbance or conflict in which the individual cannot maintain a state of equilibrium. Pregnancy can be considered a *maturational*

crisis, as it is a common event in the normal growth and development of the family. During such a crisis, the individual or family is in disequilibrium. Egos weaken, usual defense mechanisms are not effective, unresolved material from the past reappears, and relationships shift. The period of disequilibrium and disorganization is marked by unsuccessful attempts to solve the perceived problems. If the crisis is not resolved, it will result in maladaptive behaviors in one or more family members and possible disintegration of the family. Families that are able to resolve a maturational crisis will return successfully to normal functioning and can even strengthen the bonds in the family relationship.

The Mother

Pregnancy is a condition that alters body image and necessitates a reordering of social relationships and changes in roles of family members. The way each woman meets the stresses of pregnancy is influenced by her emotional makeup, her sociologic and cultural background, and her acceptance or re-

TABLE 9–3 Parental Reactions to Pregnancy		
First Trimester	**Second Trimester**	**Third Trimester**
Mother's Reactions	**Mother's Reactions**	**Mother's Reactions**
Informs father secretively or openly.	Remains regressive and introspective, projects all problems with authority figures onto partner, may become angry as if lack of interest is sign of weakness in him.	Experiences more anxiety and tension, with physical awkwardness.
Feels ambivalent toward pregnancy, anxious about labor and responsibility of child.		Feels much discomfort and insomnia from physical condition.
Is aware of physical changes, daydreams of possible miscarriage.	Continues to deal with feelings as a mother and looks for furniture as something concrete.	Prepares for birth, assembles layette, picks out names.
Develops special feelings for and renewed interest in her own mother, with formation of a personal identity.	May have other extreme of anxiety and wait until ninth month to look for furniture and clothes for baby.	Dreams often about misplacing baby or not being able to give birth, fears birth of deformed baby.
	Feels movement and is aware of fetus and incorporates it into herself.	Feels ecstasy and excitement, has spurt of energy during last month.
	Dreams that partner will be killed, telephones him often for reassurance.	
	Experiences more distinct physical changes; sexual desires may increase or decrease.	
Father's Reactions	**Father's Reactions**	**Father's Reactions**
Differ according to age, parity, desire for child, economic stability.	If he can cope, will give her extra attention she needs; if he cannot cope, will develop a new time-consuming interest outside of home.	Adapts to alternative methods of sexual contact.
Acceptance of pregnant woman's attitude or complete rejection and lack of communication.	May develop a creative feeling and a "closeness to nature."	Becomes concerned over financial responsibility.
Is aware of his own sexual feelings, may develop more or less sexual arousal.	May become involved in pregnancy and buy or make furniture.	May show new sense of tenderness and concern, treats partner like doll.
Accepts, rejects, or resents mother-in-law.	Feels for movement of baby, listens to heartbeat, or remains aloof, with no physical contact.	Daydreams about child as if older and not newborn, dreams of losing partner.
May develop new hobby outside of family as sign of stress.	May have fears and fantasies about himself being pregnant, may become uneasy with this feminine aspect in himself.	Renewed sexual attraction to partner.
	May react negatively if partner is too demanding, may become jealous of physician and of physician's importance to partner and her pregnancy.	Feels he is ultimately responsible for whatever happens.

jection of the pregnancy. However, many women manifest similar psychologic and emotional responses during pregnancy, including ambivalence, acceptance, introversion, mood swings, and changes in body image.

A woman's attitude toward her pregnancy can be a significant factor in its outcome. Even if the pregnancy is planned, there is an element of surprise at first. Many women commonly experience feelings of ambivalence during early pregnancy. This ambivalence may be related to feelings that the timing is somehow wrong; worries about the need to modify existing relationships or career plans; fears about assuming a new role; unresolved emotional conflicts with the woman's own mother; and fears about pregnancy, labor, and birth. These feelings may be more pronounced if the pregnancy is unplanned or unwanted. Indirect expressions of ambivalence include complaints about considerable physical discomfort, prolonged or frequent depression, significant dissatisfaction with changing body shape, excessive mood swings, and difficulty in accepting the life changes resulting from the pregnancy.

Many pregnancies are unintended, but not all unintended pregnancies are unwanted. A pregnancy can be unintended and wanted at the same time. For some women, an unintended pregnancy has more psychologic and social advantages than disadvantages. It provides purpose and direction to life and allows a woman to test the devotion and love of her partner and family. However, an unintended pregnancy can be a risk factor for depression. Women with an unintended pregnancy may also perceive life events as being more stressful than women with an intended pregnancy—another contributor to depression. Depression, in turn, can negatively impact a woman's health choices and behaviors (Messer, Dole, Kaufman et al., 2005).

Conflicts about adapting to pregnancy are no more pronounced for older pregnant women (age 35 and over) than for younger ones. Moreover, older pregnant women tend to be less concerned about the normal physical changes of pregnancy and are confident about handling issues that arise during pregnancy and parenting. This difference may result because mature pregnant women have more experience with problem solving. However, mature pregnant women may have fewer pregnant peers and thus may have fewer people with whom to share concerns and expectations.

Pregnancy produces marked changes in a woman's body within a relatively short period of time. Pregnant women experience changes in body image because of physical alterations and may feel a loss of control over their bodies during pregnancy and later during childbirth. These perceptions are related to a certain extent to personality factors, social network responses, and attitudes toward pregnancy. Although changes in body image are normal, they can be very stressful for the woman. Expla-

nation and discussion of the changes may help both the woman and her partner deal with the stress associated with this aspect of pregnancy.

Fantasies about the unborn child are common among pregnant women. The themes of the fantasies (baby's appearance, gender, traits, impact on parents, and so forth) vary by trimester and also differ between women who are pregnant for the first time and women who already have children.

First Trimester

During the first trimester, feelings of disbelief and ambivalence are paramount. The woman's baby does not seem real, and she focuses on herself and her pregnancy. She may experience one or more of the early symptoms of pregnancy, such as breast tenderness or morning sickness, which are unsettling and at times unpleasant.

At this time, the expectant mother also begins to exhibit some characteristic behavioral changes. She may become increasingly introspective and passive. She may be emotionally labile, with characteristic mood swings from joy to despair. She may fantasize about a miscarriage and feel guilt because of these fantasies. She may worry that these thoughts will harm the baby in some way.

Second Trimester

During the second trimester, quickening occurs. This perception of fetal movement helps the woman think of her baby as a separate person, and she generally becomes excited about the pregnancy even if earlier she was not. The woman becomes increasingly introspective as she evaluates her life, her plans, and her child's future. This introspection helps the woman prepare for her new mothering role. Emotional lability, which may be unsettling to her partner, persists. In some instances, the partner may react by withdrawing. This withdrawal is especially distressing to the woman, because she needs increased love and affection. Once the couple understands that these behaviors are characteristic of pregnancy, it is easier for the couple to deal with them effectively, although they may be sources of stress to some extent throughout pregnancy.

As pregnancy becomes more noticeable, the woman's body image changes. She may feel great pride, embarrassment, or concern. Generally, women feel best during the second trimester, which is a relatively tranquil time.

Third Trimester

In the third trimester, the woman feels both pride about her pregnancy and anxiety about labor and birth. Physical discomforts increase, and the woman is eager for the pregnancy to end. She experiences increased fatigue, her body movements are more awkward, and her interest in sexual activity may decrease. During this time, the woman tends to be concerned about the health and safety of her unborn child and may worry that she will not cope well during childbirth. Toward the end of this period, there is often a surge of energy as the woman prepares a "nest" for the infant. Many women report bursts of energy, during which they vigorously clean and organize their homes.

Psychologic Tasks of the Mother

Rubin (1984) identified four major tasks that the pregnant woman undertakes to maintain her intactness and that of her family and at the same time incorporate her new child into the family system. These tasks form the foundation for a mutually gratifying relationship with her infant.

1. *Ensuring safe passage through pregnancy, labor, and birth.* The pregnant woman feels concern for both her unborn child and herself. She looks for competent maternity care to provide a sense of control. She may seek information from literature, observation of other pregnant women and new mothers, and discussion with others. She also attempts to ensure safe passage by engaging in self-care activities related to diet, exercise, alcohol consumption, and so forth. In the third trimester she becomes more aware of external threats in the environment—a toy on the stairs, the awkwardness of an escalator—that pose a threat to her well-being. She may worry if her partner is late or if she is home alone. Sleep becomes more difficult and she longs for birth even though it, too, is frightening.

2. *Seeking acceptance of this child by others.* The birth of a child alters a woman's primary support group (her family) and her secondary affiliative groups. The woman slowly and subtly alters her network to meet the needs of her pregnancy. In this adjustment, the woman's partner is the most important figure. The partner's support and acceptance help form a maternal identity. If there are other children in the home, the mother also works to ensure their acceptance of the coming child. Acceptance of the anticipated change is sometimes stressful, and the woman may work to maintain some special time with her partner or older children. The woman without a partner looks to others such as a family member or friend for this support.

3. *Seeking commitment and acceptance of herself as mother to the infant (binding in).* During the first trimester, the child remains a rather abstract concept. With quickening, however, the child begins to become a real person, and the mother begins to develop bonds of attachment. The mother experiences the movement of the child within her in an intimate, exclusive way, and out of this experience bonds of love form. This binding-in process, characterized by its strong emotional component, motivates the pregnant woman to become competent in her role and provides satisfaction for her in the role of mother. This possessive love increases her maternal commitment to protect her fetus now and her child after he or she is born.

4. *Learning to give of oneself on behalf of one's child.* Childbirth involves many acts of giving. The man "gives" a child to the woman; she in turn "gives" a child to him. Life is given to an infant; a sibling is given to older children of the family. The woman begins to develop a capacity for self-denial and learns to delay immediate personal gratification to meet the needs of another. Baby showers and gifts are acts of giving that increase the mother's self-esteem and help her recognize the separateness and needs of the coming baby.

Accomplishment of these tasks helps the expectant woman develop her self-concept as mother. The expectant woman who was well nurtured by her own mother may view her mother as a role model and emulate her; the woman who views her mother as a "poor mother" may worry that she will make similar mistakes. A woman's self-concept as a mother expands with actual experience and continues to grow through subsequent childbearing and childrearing. Occasionally a woman fails to accept the mother role, instead playing the role of baby-sitter or older sister to her child.

The Father

For the expectant father, pregnancy is a psychologically stressful time because he, too, must make the transition from nonparent to parent or from parent of one or more to parent of two or more. Research indicates that most men handle the transition to fatherhood well, and in general, any anxieties they feel resolve over time. However, the anxieties they have are sometimes missed prenatally because most attention is devoted to the expectant mother (Buist, Morse, & Durkin, 2003).

Initially, expectant fathers may feel pride in their virility, which pregnancy confirms, but also have many of the same ambivalent feelings as expectant mothers. The extent of ambivalence depends on many factors, including the father's relationship with his partner, his previous experience with pregnancy, his age, his economic stability, and whether the pregnancy was planned.

In adjusting to his role, the expectant father must first deal with the reality of the pregnancy and then struggle to gain recognition as a parent from his partner, family, friends, coworkers, and society—and from his baby as well. The expectant mother can help her partner be a participant and not merely a helpmate to her if she has a definite sense of the experience as *their* pregnancy and *their* infant and not *her* pregnancy and *her* infant.

The expectant father must establish a fatherhood role, just as the woman develops a motherhood role. Fathers who are most successful at this task generally like children, are excited about the prospect of fatherhood, are eager to nurture a child, and have confidence in their ability to be a parent. They also share the experiences of pregnancy and birth with their partners (see Table 9–3).

First Trimester

After the initial excitement attending the announcement of the pregnancy, an expectant father may begin to feel left out. He may be confused by his partner's mood changes. He might resent the attention she receives and her need to modify their relationship as she experiences fatigue and possibly a decreased interest in sex. In addition, he might be concerned about what kind of father he will be. During this time, his child is a "potential" baby. Fathers often picture interacting with a child of 5 or 6 years, not a newborn. The pregnancy itself may seem unreal until the woman shows more physical signs.

Second Trimester

The father's role in the pregnancy is still vague in the second trimester, but his involvement may increase as he watches and feels fetal movement and listens to the fetal heartbeat during a prenatal visit. For many men, seeing their infant on ultrasound is an important experience in accepting the reality of pregnancy. Like expectant mothers, expectant fathers need to confront and resolve some of their conflicts about the fathering they received. A father needs to sort out which behaviors of his own father he wants to imitate and which he wants to avoid.

Evidence suggests that the father-to-be's anxiety is lessened if both parents agree on the paternal role the man is to assume. For example, if both see his role as that of breadwinner, the man's stress is low. However, if the man views his role as that of breadwinner and the woman expects him to be actively involved in child care, his stress increases. An open, honest discussion about the expectations the parents have about their roles will help the father-to-be in his transition to fatherhood (Goodman, 2005).

As the woman's appearance begins to change, her partner may have several reactions. Her changed appearance may decrease his sexual interest, or it may have the opposite effect. Because of the variety of emotions both partners may feel, continued communication and acceptance are important.

Third Trimester

If the couple's relationship has grown through effective communication of their concerns and feelings, the third trimester is often a rewarding time. They may attend childbirth classes and make concrete preparations for the arrival of the baby. If the father has developed a detached attitude about the pregnancy, however, it is unlikely he will become a willing participant, even though his role becomes more obvious.

Concerns and fears may recur. The father may worry about hurting the unborn baby during intercourse or become concerned about labor and birth. Also, he may wonder what kind of parents he and his partner will be.

Couvade

Couvade has traditionally referred to the observance of certain rituals and taboos by the male to signify the transition to fatherhood. This observance affirms his psychosocial and biophysical relationship to the woman and child. Some taboos restrict his actions. For example, in some cultures the man may be forbidden to eat certain foods or carry certain weapons before and immediately after the birth. More recently, the term has been used to describe the unintentional development of physical symptoms such as fatigue, increased appetite, difficulty sleeping, depression, headache, or backache by the partner of a pregnant woman. Men who demonstrate couvade syndrome tend to have a higher degree of paternal role preparation and be involved in more activities related to this preparation.

Siblings

Bringing a new baby home often marks the beginning of sibling rivalry. The siblings view the baby as a threat to the security of their relationships with their parents. Parents who recognize this potential problem early in pregnancy and begin constructive actions can minimize the problem of sibling rivalry.

Preparation of the young child begins several weeks before the anticipated birth. Because they do not have a clear concept of time, young children should not be told too early about the pregnancy. From the toddler's point of view, several weeks is an extremely long time. The mother may let the child feel the baby moving in her uterus, explaining that the uterus is "a special place where babies grow." The child can help the parents put the baby clothes in drawers or prepare the nursery.

The concept of consistency is important in dealing with young children. They need reassurance that certain people, special things, and familiar places will continue to exist after the new baby arrives. The crib is often an important though transient object in a child's life. If it is to be given to the new baby, the parents should thoughtfully help the older child adjust to this change. Any move from crib to bed or from one room to another should precede the baby's birth by at least several weeks. If the new baby is to share a room with siblings, the parents must also discuss this situation with the older child or children.

Some parents advocate cosleeping (one or both parents sleeping with the baby or young child), and so the crib is less an issue. Cosleeping, common in many non-Western cultures, is on the increase in the United States. Opinion varies sharply about the advantages and risks of the practice, especially in light of an American Academy of Pediatrics policy statement (2005) recommending against cosleeping because of the increased risk of sudden infant death syndrome (SIDS). The AAP stresses that the infant can be brought to the bed to be comforted or for breastfeeding, but should be placed supine in a separate bed ("back to bed") to sleep. (See discussion in Chapter 32 ∞.) Parents who choose to cosleep must make decisions about the sleeping arrangements of other siblings following the birth of the baby.

If the child is ready, toilet training is most effective several months before or after the baby's arrival. It is not unusual for an older, toilet-trained child to regress to wetting or soiling because of the attention the newborn gets for such behavior. The older, weaned child may want to nurse or drink from the bottle again after the baby arrives. If the new mother anticipates these behaviors, they will be less frustrating during her early postpartum days.

Pregnant women may find it helpful to bring their children on a prenatal visit to the certified nurse-midwife or physician to give them an opportunity to listen to the fetal heartbeat. Such a visit helps make the baby more real to the children; they may also become involved in the prenatal care.

If siblings are school-age children, pregnancy should be viewed as a family affair. Teaching should be suitable to the child's level of understanding and may be supplemented with appropriate books. Taking part in family discussions, attending sibling preparation classes, feeling fetal movement, and listening to the fetal heartbeat help the school-age child take part in the experience of pregnancy and not feel like an outsider.

Older children or adolescents may appear to have sophisticated knowledge but may have many misconceptions about pregnancy and birth. The parents should make opportunities to discuss their concerns and involve the children in preparations for the new baby.

Even after birth, siblings need to feel that they are taking part. Having siblings visit their mother and the new baby at the hospital or birthing center will help. After the baby comes home, siblings can share in "showing off" the new baby.

Sibling preparation is essential, but other factors are equally important. These factors include how much parental attention the new arrival receives, how much attention the older child receives after the baby comes home, and how well the parents handle regressive or aggressive behavior.

Grandparents

The first relatives told about a pregnancy are usually the grandparents. Often, the expectant grandparents become increasingly supportive of the couple, even if conflicts previously existed. But it can be difficult for even sensitive grandparents to know how deeply to become involved in the childrearing process.

Because grandparenting can occur over a wide expanse of years, people's response to this role can vary considerably. Younger grandparents leading active lives may not demonstrate as much interest as the young couple would like. In other cases, expectant grandparents may give advice and gifts unsparingly. For grandparents, conflict may be related to the expectant couple's need to feel in control of their lives, or it may stem from events signaling changing roles in the grandparents' own lives (e.g., retirement, financial concerns, menopause, or death of a friend). Some parents of expectant couples may already be grandparents with a developed style of grandparenting. This influences their response to the pregnancy.

Because childbearing and childrearing practices have changed, family cohesiveness is promoted by effective communication and frank discussion between young cou-

---

CULTURAL PERSPECTIVES

Providing Culturally Sensitive Care

Nurses who are interacting with expectant families from a different culture or ethnic group can provide more effective, culturally sensitive nursing care by:

- Critically examining their own cultural beliefs
- Identifying personal biases, attitudes, stereotypes, and prejudices
- Making a conscious commitment to respect and study the values and beliefs of others
- Using sensitive, current language when describing others' cultures
- Learning the rituals, customs, and practices of the major cultural and ethnic groups with whom they have contact
- Including cultural assessment and assessment of the family's expectations of the healthcare system as a routine part of prenatal nursing care
- Incorporating the family's cultural and spiritual practices into prenatal care as much as possible
- Fostering an attitude of respect for and cooperation with alternative healers and caregivers when possible
- Providing for the services of an interpreter if language barriers exist
- Learning the language (or at least several key phrases) of at least one of the cultural groups with whom they interact
- Recognizing that ultimately it is the woman's right to make her own healthcare choices
- Evaluating whether the client's healthcare beliefs have any potential negative consequences for her health

ples and interested grandparents about the changes and the reasons for them. Clarifying the role of the helping grandparent ensures a comfortable situation for all.

Classes for grandparents may provide information about changes in birth and parenting practices. These classes help familiarize grandparents with new parents' needs and may offer suggestions for ways in which the grandparents can support the childbearing couple.

Cultural Values and Pregnancy

A universal tendency exists to create ceremonial rituals or rites around important life events. Thus pregnancy, childbirth, marriage, and death are often tied to ritual. The rituals and customs of a group are a reflection of the group's values. Thus the identification of cultural values is useful in predicting reactions to pregnancy. An understanding of male and female roles, family lifestyles, religious values, or the meaning of children in a culture may explain reactions of joy or shame.

Generalization about cultural characteristics or values is difficult because not every individual in a culture may display these characteristics. Just as variations are seen between cultures, variations are also seen within cultures.

For example, because of their exposure to the American culture, a third-generation Chinese-American family might have very different values and beliefs from those of a Chinese family that has recently immigrated to America. For this reason, the nurse needs to supplement a general knowledge of cultural values and practices with a complete assessment of the individual's values and practices. The accompanying Cultural Perspectives: Providing Culturally Sensitive Care feature summarizes the key actions a nurse can take to become more culturally aware.

Cultural assessment is an important aspect of prenatal care. Healthcare professionals are becoming increasingly aware that they must address cultural needs in the prenatal assessment to provide culturally sensitive health care during pregnancy. The nurse needs to identify the prospective parents' main beliefs, values, and behaviors related to pregnancy and childbearing. This includes information about ethnic background, amount of affiliation with the ethnic group, patterns of decision making, religious preference, language, communication style, and common etiquette practices. The nurse can also explore the woman's (or family's) expectations of the healthcare system. Once this information is gathered, the nurse can then plan and provide care that is appropriate and responsive to family needs. These topics are discussed in more detail in Chapter 2 ∞.

CHAPTER HIGHLIGHTS

- Virtually all systems of a woman's body are altered in some way during pregnancy.
- Blood pressure decreases slightly during pregnancy. It reaches its lowest point in the second trimester and gradually increases to near normal levels in the third trimester.
- The enlarging uterus may cause pressure on the vena cava when the woman lies supine, causing supine hypotensive syndrome.
- A physiologic anemia may occur during pregnancy because the total plasma volume increases more than the total number of erythrocytes. This difference produces a drop in the hematocrit.
- The glomerular filtration rate increases somewhat during pregnancy. Glycosuria may be caused by the body's inability to reabsorb all the glucose filtered by the glomeruli.
- Changes in the skin include the development of chloasma; linea nigra; darkened nipples, areola, and vulva; striae; and spider nevi.
- Insulin needs increase during pregnancy. A woman with a latent deficiency state may respond to the increased stress on the islets of Langerhans by developing gestational diabetes.
- The subjective (presumptive) signs of pregnancy are symptoms experienced and reported by the woman, such as amenorrhea, nausea and vomiting, fatigue, urinary frequency, breast changes, and quickening.

- The objective (probable) signs of pregnancy can be perceived by the examiner but may be caused by conditions other than pregnancy.
- The diagnostic (positive) signs of pregnancy can be perceived by the examiner and can be caused only by pregnancy.
- During pregnancy, the expectant mother may experience ambivalence, acceptance, introversion, emotional lability, and changes in body image.
- Rubin (1984) identified four developmental tasks for the pregnant woman: (1) ensuring safe passage through pregnancy, labor, and birth; (2) seeking acceptance of this child by others; (3) seeking commitment and acceptance of herself as mother to the infant; and (4) learning to give of oneself on behalf of one's child.
- The father faces a series of adjustments as he accepts his new role. The father must deal with the reality of pregnancy, gain recognition as a parent, and confront and resolve any personal conflicts about the fathering he himself received.
- Siblings of all ages require assistance in dealing with the birth of a new baby.
- Cultural values, beliefs, and behaviors influence a family's response to childbearing and the healthcare system.
- A cultural assessment does not have to be exhaustive, but it should focus on factors that will influence the practices of the childbearing family with regard to health needs.

CHAPTER REFERENCES

American Academy of Pediatrics (AAP). (2005). Policy statement: The changing concept of sudden infant death syndrome: Diagnostic coding shifts, controversies regarding the sleeping environment, and new variables to consider in reducing risk. *Pediatrics,116*(5), 1245–1255.

Buist, A., Morse, C. A., & Durkin, S. (2003). Men's adjustment to fatherhood: Implications for obstetric health care. *Journal of Obstetric, Gynecologic, and Neonatal Nursing, 32*(2), 172–180.

Burton, G. J., Sibley, C. P., & Jauniaux, E. R. M. (2007). Placental anatomy and physiology. In S. G. Gabbe, J. R. Niebyl, & J. L. Simpson (Eds.), *Obstetrics: Normal and problem pregnancies* (5th ed.). New York: Churchill-Livingstone.

Cunningham, F. G., Leveno, K. J., Bloom, S. L., Hauth, J. C., Gilstrap III, L. C., & Wenstrom, K. D. (2005.) *Williams obstetrics* (22nd ed.). New York: McGraw-Hill.

Goodman, J. H. (2005). Becoming an involved father of an infant. *Journal of Obstetric, Gynecologic, and Neonatal Nursing, 34*(2), 190–200.

Gordon, M. C. (2007). Maternal physiology. In S. G. Gabbe, J. R. Niebyl, & J. L. Simpson (Eds.), *Obstetrics: Normal and problem pregnancies* (5th ed.). New York: Churchill-Livingstone.

Johnson, T. R. B., Gregory, K. D., & Niebyl, J., R. (2007). Preconception and prenatal care: Part of the continuum. In S. G. Gabbe, J. R. Niebyl, & J. L. Simpson (Eds.), *Obstetrics: Normal and problem pregnancies* (5th ed.). New York: Churchill-Livingstone.

Messer, L. C., Dole, N., Kaufman, J. S., & Savitz, D. A. (2005). Pregnany intendedness, maternal psychosocial factors and preterm birth. *Maternal and Child Health Journal, 9*(4), 403–412.

Rubin, R. (1984). *Maternal identity and the maternal experience.* New York: Springer.

CHAPTER 10

Antepartal Nursing Assessment

When I work the prenatal clinic I constantly remind myself to look past stereotypes about people of different cultures and ethnic groups to see each woman and family as unique. It has helped me tremendously to do some reading about various cultural groups and their common practices—that way I don't make glaring mistakes during my initial contact with a family. However, I have found it most useful simply to ask people about their preferences in a respectful, accepting way. Almost always they tell me gladly because their childbearing experience is important to them and they sense that I am sincere.

—A Nurse Working in a Large County Health Department

LEARNING OUTCOMES

10-1. Use information provided on a prenatal history to identify risk factors for the mother and/or fetus.

10-2. Define common obstetric terminology found in the history of maternity clients.

10-3. Identify factors related to the father's health that are generally recorded on the prenatal record in assessing risk factors for the mother and/or fetus.

10-4. Evaluate those areas of the initial assessment that reflect the psychosocial and cultural factors related to a woman's pregnancy.

10-5. Predict the normal physiologic changes a nurse would expect to find when performing a physical assessment of a pregnant woman.

10-6. Calculate the estimated date of birth using the common methods.

10-7. Describe the essential measurements that can be determined by clinical pelvimetry.

10-8. Describe the results of the major screening tests used during the prenatal period in the assessment of the prenatal client.

10-9. Assess the prenatal client for the danger signs of pregnancy.

10-10. Relate the components of the subsequent prenatal history and assessment to the progress of pregnancy and the nursing care of the prenatal client.

The registered nurse caring for a woman who is pregnant establishes an environment of comfort and open communication with each antepartal visit. The nurse conveys interest in the woman as an individual and discusses the woman's concerns and desires. This nurse can also complete many areas of prenatal assessment. Advanced practice nurses such as certified nurse-midwives (CNMs) and certified women's health nurse practitioners have the education and skill to perform full and complete antepartal assessments.

This chapter focuses on the prenatal assessments completed initially and at subsequent visits to provide optimum care for the childbearing family.

Initial Client History

The course of a pregnancy depends on a number of factors, including the woman's prepregnancy health, presence of disease states, emotional status, and past health care. A thorough history is useful in determining the status of a woman's prepregnancy health.

Definition of Terms

The following terms are used in recording the history of maternity clients:

Gestation: the number of weeks since the first day of the last menstrual period

Abortion: birth that occurs before the end of 20 weeks' gestation or the birth of a fetus–newborn who weighs less than 500 g (Cunningham, Leveno, Bloom et al., 2005)

Term: the normal duration of pregnancy (38 to 42 weeks' gestation)

Antepartum: time between conception and the onset of labor; often used to describe the period during which a woman is pregnant; used interchangeably with *prenatal*

Intrapartum: time from the onset of true labor until the birth of the infant and placenta

Postpartum: time from birth until the woman's body returns to an essentially prepregnant condition

Preterm or premature labor: labor that occurs after 20 weeks' but before completion of 37 weeks' gestation

Postterm labor: labor that occurs after 42 weeks' gestation

Gravida: any pregnancy, regardless of duration, including present pregnancy

Nulligravida: a woman who has never been pregnant

Primigravida: a woman who is pregnant for the first time

Multigravida: a woman who is in her second or any subsequent pregnancy

Para: birth after 20 weeks' gestation regardless of whether the infant is born alive or dead

Nullipara: a woman who has had no births at more than 20 weeks' gestation

Primipara: a woman who has had one birth at more than 20 weeks' gestation, regardless of whether the infant was born alive or dead

Multipara: a woman who has had two or more births at more than 20 weeks' gestation

Stillbirth: an infant born dead after 20 weeks' gestation

The terms *gravida* and *para* are used in relation to pregnancies, not to the number of fetuses. Thus twins, triplets, and so forth count as one pregnancy and one birth.

The following examples illustrate how these terms are applied in clinical situations.

1. Jean Sanchez has one child born at 38 weeks' gestation and is pregnant for the second time. At her initial prenatal visit, the nurse indicates her obstetric history as "gravida 2 para 1 ab 0." Jean Sanchez's present pregnancy terminates at 16 weeks' gestation. She is now "gravida 2 para 1 ab 1."

2. Tracy Hopkins is pregnant for the fourth time. At home she has a child who was born at term. Her second pregnancy ended at 10 weeks' gestation. She then gave birth to twins at 35 weeks. One of the twins died soon after birth. At her antepartal assessment the nurse records her obstetric history as "gravida 4 para 2 ab 1."

This approach is confusing, however, because it fails to identify the number of children that a woman might have. To provide more comprehensive data, a more detailed approach is used in some settings. Using the detailed system, *gravida* keeps the same meaning, but the meaning of *para* changes because the detailed system counts each infant *born* rather than the number of pregnancies carried to viability (Varney, Kriebs, & Gegor, 2004). Thus for example, triplets count as one pregnancy but *three* babies.

A useful acronym for remembering the detailed system is TPAL:

T: number of **t**erm infants born—that is, the number of infants born after 37 weeks' gestation

P: number of **p**reterm infants born—that is, the number of infants born after 20 weeks' but before the completion of 37 weeks' gestation

A: number of pregnancies ending in either spontaneous or therapeutic **a**bortion

L: number of currently **l**iving children

Using this approach, the nurse would have initially described Jean Sanchez (see the first example) as "gravida 2 para 1001." Following Jean's spontaneous abortion, she would be "gravida 2 para 1011." Tracy Hopkins would be described as "gravida 4 para 1212." (Figure 10–1 ■ illustrates this method.)

HINTS FOR PRACTICE

In general, it is best to avoid an initial discussion of a woman's gravida and para in front of her partner. It is possible that the woman had a previous pregnancy that she has not mentioned to her partner, and revealing the information could violate her right to privacy.

Client Profile

The history is essentially a screening tool that identifies factors that may place the mother or fetus at risk during the pregnancy. The following information is obtained for each pregnant woman at the first prenatal assessment.

1. *Current pregnancy*
   - First day of last normal menstrual period (LMP). Is she sure of the date or uncertain? Do her cycles normally occur every 28 days, or do her cycles tend to be longer?
   - Presence of cramping, bleeding, or spotting since LMP
   - Woman's opinion about the time when conception occurred and when infant is due
   - Woman's attitude toward pregnancy (Is this pregnancy planned? Wanted?)
   - Results of pregnancy tests, if completed
   - Any discomforts since LMP such as nausea, vomiting, urinary frequency, fatigue, or breast tenderness

2. *Past pregnancies*
   - Number of pregnancies
   - Number of abortions, spontaneous or induced
   - Number of living children
   - History of previous pregnancies, length of pregnancy, length of labor and birth, type of birth (vaginal, forceps or vacuum-assisted birth, or cesarean), type of anesthesia used (if any), woman's perception of the experience, and complications (antepartal, intrapartal, and postpartal)

   - Neonatal status of previous children: Apgar scores, birth weights, general development, complications, and feeding patterns (breast milk or formula)
   - Loss of a child (miscarriage, elective or medically indicated abortion, stillbirth, neonatal death, relinquishment, or death after the neonatal period). What was the experience like for her? What coping skills helped? How did her partner, if involved, respond?
   - If Rh negative, was medication received after birth to prevent sensitization?
   - Prenatal education classes and resources (books)

3. *Gynecologic history*
   - Date of last Pap smear; any history of abnormal Pap smear; any follow-up therapy completed
   - Previous infections: vaginal, cervical, tubal, sexually transmitted
   - Previous surgery
   - Age at menarche
   - Regularity, frequency, and duration of menstrual flow
   - History of dysmenorrhea
   - Sexual history
   - Contraceptive history (If birth control pills were used, did pregnancy occur immediately following cessation of pills? If not, how long after?)
   - Any issues related to infertility or fertility treatments

4. *Current medical history*
   - Weight
   - Blood type and Rh factor, if known
   - General health including nutrition (dietary practices such as vegetarianism), regular exercise program (type, frequency, and duration)
   - Any medications presently being taken (including nonprescription, homeopathic, or herbal medications) or taken since the onset of pregnancy
   - Previous or present use of alcohol, tobacco, or caffeine (Ask specifically about the amounts of alcohol, cigarettes, and caffeine [specify coffee, tea, colas, or chocolate] consumed each day.)
   - Illicit drug use or abuse (Ask about specific drugs such as cocaine, crack, methamphetamines, and marijuana.)
   - Drug allergies and other allergies (Ask about latex allergies or sensitivies.)
   - Potential teratogenic insults to this pregnancy such as viral infections, medications, x-ray examinations, surgery, or cats in the home (possible source of toxoplasmosis)

Name	Gravida	Term	Preterm	Abortions	Living Children
Jean Sanchez	2	1	0	1	1
Tracy Hopkins	4	1	2	1	2

FIGURE 10–1 The TPAL approach provides more detailed information about a woman's pregnancy history.

- Presence of disease conditions such as diabetes, hypertension, cardiovascular disease, renal problems, or thyroid disorder
- Record of immunizations (especially rubella)
- Presence of any abnormal symptoms

5. *Past medical history*
   - Childhood diseases
   - Past treatment for any disease condition (Any hospitalizations? History of hepatitis? Rheumatic fever? Pyelonephritis? Cancer?)
   - Surgical procedures
   - Presence of bleeding disorders or tendencies (Has she received blood transfusions?)

6. *Family medical history*
   - Presence of diabetes, cardiovascular disease, cancer, hypertension, hematologic disorders, tuberculosis, or preeclampsia–eclampsia
   - Occurrence of multiple births
   - History of congenital diseases or deformities
   - History of mental illness
   - Causes of death of deceased parents or siblings
   - Occurrence of cesarean births and cause, if known

7. *Religious, spiritual, and cultural history*
   - Does the woman wish to specify a religious preference on her chart? Does she have any spiritual beliefs or practices that might influence her health care or that of her child, such as prohibition against receiving blood products, dietary considerations, or circumcision rites?
   - What practices are important to maintain her spiritual well-being?
   - Might practices in her culture or that of her partner influence her care or that of her child?

8. *Occupational history*
   - Occupation
   - Physical demands (Does she stand all day, or are there opportunities to sit and elevate her legs? Any heavy lifting?)
   - Exposure to chemicals or other harmful substances
   - Opportunity for regular meals and breaks for nutritious snacks
   - Provision for maternity or family leave

9. *Partner's history*
   - Presence of genetic conditions or diseases in him or in his family history
   - Age
   - Significant health problems
   - Previous or present alcohol intake, drug use, or tobacco use
   - Blood type and Rh factor
   - Occupation
   - Educational level; methods by which he learns best
   - Attitude toward the pregnancy

10. *Personal information about the woman (Social history)*
    - Age
    - Educational level; methods by which she learns best

- Race or ethnic group (to identify need for prenatal genetic screening and racially or ethnically related risk factors)
- Housing; stability of living conditions
- Economic level
- Acceptance of pregnancy, whether intended or unintended
- Any history of emotional or physical deprivation or abuse of herself or children or any abuse in her current relationship (Ask specifically whether she has been hit, slapped, kicked, or hurt within the past year or since she has been pregnant. Ask whether she is afraid of her partner or anyone else. If yes, of whom is she afraid? [Note: Ask these questions when the woman is alone.])
- History of emotional problems
- Support systems
- Personal preferences about the birth (expectations of both the woman and her partner, presence of others, and so on) (See Chapter 8 ∞)
- Plans for care of child following birth
- Feeding preference for the baby (breast milk or formula?)

Obtaining Data

A questionnaire is used in many instances to obtain information. The woman should complete the questionnaire in a quiet place with a minimum of distractions. The nurse can obtain further information in an interview, which allows the pregnant woman to clarify her responses to questions and gives the nurse and client the opportunity to begin developing rapport.

The expectant father or partner can be encouraged to attend the prenatal examinations. He or she is often able to contribute to the history and may use the opportunity to ask questions or express concerns that are important to him or her.

Prenatal High-Risk Screening

Risk factors are any findings that suggest the pregnancy may have a negative outcome, for either the woman or her unborn child. Screening for risk factors is an important part of the prenatal assessment. Many risk factors can be identified during the initial assessment; others may be detected during subsequent prenatal visits. It is important to identify high-risk pregnancies early so that appropriate interventions can be started promptly. Not all risk factors threaten a pregnancy equally; thus many agencies use a scoring sheet to determine the degree of risk. Information must be updated throughout pregnancy as necessary. Any pregnancy may begin as low risk and change to high risk because of complications.

Table 10–1 identifies the major risk factors currently recognized. The table also identifies maternal and fetal or newborn implications if the risk is present in the pregnancy.

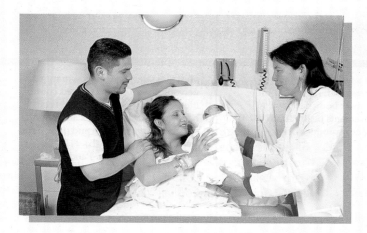

hare

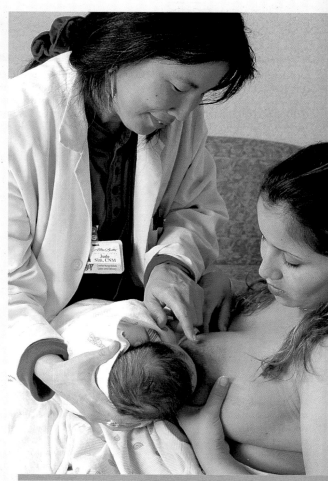

While I'm at the birth center, I check in on Alisa and Richard. Their baby, Lydia Rose, was born 6 hours ago. Alisa has asked for help with breastfeeding. Baby Lydia is a sleepy little one and needs encouragement to latch on and begin feeding.

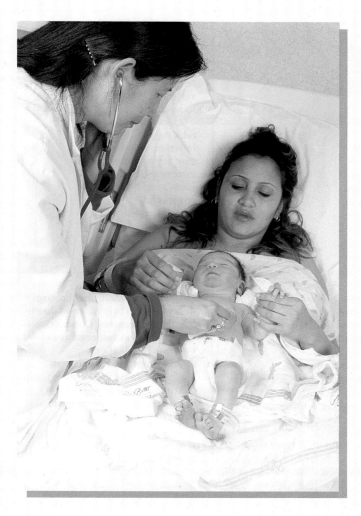

most
r and
l pro-
baby

After baby Lydia has finished nursing, I do a physical assessment. I prefer to do an assessment in the room with the parents. It is such a wonderful opportunity for them to learn about their baby.

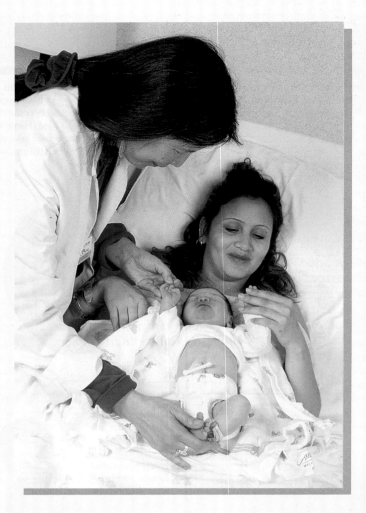

Alisa is fascinated with baby Lydia's tiny fingers and toes. I love being with parents as they explore their baby. Each new baby is such a wonder . . . such a miracle.

Now my attention turns to Alisa. As part of my assessment, I check the position and tone of her fundus. All is well. I head home after a busy, but rewarding, day.

Photographer: Jenny Thomas

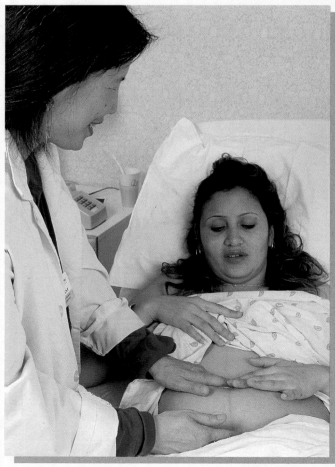

TABLE 10–1	Prenatal High-Risk Factors	
Factor	**Maternal Implications**	**Fetal/Neonatal Implications**
Social–Personal		
Low income level and/or low educational level	Poor antenatal care or late antenatal care Poor nutrition ↑ risk of preeclampsia	Low birth weight Intrauterine growth restriction (IUGR)
Poor diet	Inadequate nutrition/inadequate weight gain ↑ risk anemia ↑ risk preeclampsia	Fetal malnutrition Prematurity Small for gestational age
Living at high altitude	↑ hemoglobin	Prematurity IUGR ↑ hemoglobin (polycythemia)
Multiparity greater than 3	↑ risk antepartum or postpartum hemorrhage	Anemia Fetal death
Weight less than 45.5 kg (100 lb)	Poor nutrition Cephalopelvic disproportion Prolonged labor	IUGR Hypoxia associated with difficult labor and birth
Weight greater than 91 kg (200 lb)	↑ risk hypertension ↑ risk cephalopelvic disproportion ↑ risk diabetes	↓ fetal nutrition ↑ risk macrosomia
Age less than 16	Poor nutrition Poor antenatal care ↑ risk preeclampsia ↑ risk cephalopelvic disproportion	Low birth weight ↑ fetal demise
Age over 35	↑ risk preeclampsia ↑ risk cesarean birth Psychosocial issues	↑ risk congenital anomalies ↑ chromosomal aberrations
Smoking one pack/day or more	↑ risk hypertension ↑ risk cancer	↓ placental perfusion → ↓ O_2 and nutrients available Low birth weight IUGR Preterm birth
Use of addicting drugs	↑ risk poor nutrition ↑ risk of infection with IV drugs ↑ risk HIV, hepatitis C ↑ risk abruptio placentae	↑ risk congenital anomalies ↑ risk low birth weight Neonatal withdrawal Lower serum bilirubin
Excessive alcohol consumption	↑ risk poor nutrition Possible hepatic effects with long-term consumption	↑ risk fetal alcohol syndrome
Preexisting Medical Disorders		
Diabetes mellitus	↑ risk preeclampsia, hypertension Episodes of hypoglycemia and hyperglycemia ↑ risk cesarean birth	Low birth weight Macrosomia Neonatal hypoglycemia ↑ risk congenital anomalies ↑ risk respiratory distress syndrome
Cardiac disease	Cardiac decompensation Further strain on mother's body ↑ maternal death rate	↑ risk fetal demise ↑ perinatal mortality
Anemia: hemoglobin less than 11 g/dL less than 32% hematocrit	Iron deficiency anemia Low energy level Decreased oxygen-carrying capacity	Fetal death Prematurity Low birth weight
Hypertension	↑ vasospasm ↑ risk CNS irritability → convulsions ↑ risk CVA ↑ risk renal damage	↓ placental perfusion → low birth weight Preterm birth
Thyroid disorder Hypothyroidism Hyperthyroidism	↑ infertility ↓ BMR, goiter, myxedema ↑ risk postpartum hemorrhage ↑ risk preeclampsia Danger of thyroid storm	↑ spontaneous abortion ↑ risk congenital goiter Mental retardation → cretinism ↑ incidence congenital anomalies ↑ incidence preterm birth ↑ tendency to thyrotoxicosis
Renal disease (moderate to severe)	↑ risk renal failure	↑ risk IUGR ↑ risk preterm birth

MyNursingKit | Association of Women's Health, Obstetric and Neonatal Nurses

(Continued)

TABLE 10–1 Prenatal High-Risk Factors *(Continued)*

Factor	Maternal Implications	Fetal/Neonatal Implications
DES exposure	↑ infertility, spontaneous abortion ↑ cervical incompetence ↑ risk breech presentation	↑ spontaneous abortion ↑ risk preterm birth
Obstetric Considerations		
Previous pregnancy		
Stillborn	↑ emotional/psychologic distress	↑ risk IUGR ↑ risk preterm birth
Habitual abortion	↑ emotional/psychologic distress ↑ possibility diagnostic workup	↑ risk abortion
Cesarean birth	↑ possibility repeat cesarean birth Risk of uterine rupture	↑ risk preterm birth ↑ risk respiratory distress
Rh or blood group sensitization	↑ financial expenditure for testing	Hydrops fetalis Icterus gravis Neonatal anemia Kernicterus Hypoglycemia
Large baby	↑ risk cesarean birth ↑ risk gestational diabetes ↑ risk instrument-assisted birth	Birth injury Hypoglycemia
Current pregnancy		
Rubella (first trimester)		Congenital heart disease Cataracts Nerve deafness Bone lesions Prolonged virus shedding
Rubella (second trimester)		Hepatitis Thrombocytopenia
Cytomegalovirus		IUGR Encephalopathy
Herpesvirus type 2	Severe discomfort Concern about possibility of cesarean birth, fetal infection	Neonatal herpesvirus type 2 Hepatitis with jaundice Neurologic abnormalities
Syphilis	↑ incidence abortion	↑ fetal demise Congenital syphilis
Urinary tract infection	↑ risk preterm labor Uterine irritability	↑ risk preterm birth
Abruptio placentae and placenta previa	↑ risk hemorrhage Bed rest Extended hospitalization	Fetal/neonatal anemia Intrauterine hemorrhage ↑ fetal demise
Preeclampsia/eclampsia	See hypertension	↓ placental perfusion → low birth weight
Multiple gestation	↑ risk postpartum hemorrhage	↑ risk preterm birth ↑ risk fetal demise
Elevated hematocrit (greater than 41%)	Increased viscosity of blood	Fetal death rate five times normal rate
Spontaneous premature rupture of membranes	↑ uterine infection	↑ risk preterm birth ↑ fetal demise

Initial Prenatal Assessment

The prenatal assessment focuses on the woman holistically by considering physical, cultural, and psychosocial factors that influence her health. At the initial visit the woman may be concerned primarily with the diagnosis of pregnancy. However, during this visit she and her primary support person are also evaluating the health team she has chosen. The establishment of the nurse–client relationship will help the woman evaluate the health team and also provide the nurse with a basis for developing an atmosphere that is conducive to interviewing, support, and education. Because many women are excited and anxious at the first antepartal visit, the initial psychosocial–cultural assessment is general.

As part of the initial psychosocial–cultural assessment, the nurse discusses with the woman any religious or spiritual, cultural, or socioeconomic factors that influence the woman's expectations of the childbearing experience. It is especially helpful if the nurse is familiar with common practices of the members of various religious and cultural groups who reside in the community. Gathering these data in a tactful, caring way can help make the childbearing woman's experience a positive one.

After obtaining the history, the nurse prepares the woman for the physical examination. The physical examination begins with assessment of vital signs; then the woman's body is examined. The pelvic examination is performed last.

Before the examination, the woman should provide a clean urine specimen. When her bladder is empty, the woman is more comfortable during the pelvic examination and the examiner can palpate the pelvic organs more easily. After the woman has emptied her bladder, the nurse asks her to disrobe and gives her a gown and sheet or some other protective covering.

Increasing numbers of nurses, such as CNMs and other nurses in advanced practice, are prepared to perform complete physical examinations. The nurse who has not yet fully developed advanced assessment skills assesses the woman's vital signs, explains the procedures to allay apprehension, positions her for examination, and assists the examiner as necessary. Each nurse is responsible for operating at the expected standard for someone with that individual nurse's skill and knowledge base.

Thoroughness and a systematic procedure are the most important considerations when performing the physical portion of an antepartal examination. To promote completeness, the Assessment Guide: Initial Prenatal Assessment, starting on page 206, is organized in three columns that address the areas to be assessed (and normal findings), the variations or alterations that may be observed, and nursing responses to the data. The nurse should be aware that certain organs and systems are assessed concurrently with others during the physical portion of the examination.

Nursing interventions based on assessment of the normal physical and psychosocial changes of pregnancy, evaluation of the cultural influences associated with pregnancy, and client teaching and counseling needs that have been mutually defined are discussed further in Chapter 11 ∞.

HINTS FOR PRACTICE

In a clinic or office setting, gowns and goggles for the healthcare provider are usually not necessary because splashing of body fluids is unlikely. Gloves are worn for procedures that involve contact with body fluids such as drawing blood for labwork, handling urine specimens, and conducting pelvic examinations. Because of the increasing incidence of latex allergies, it is becoming more common for nonlatex gloves to be used.

CULTURAL PERSPECTIVES

Using Cultural Information Effectively

Although it is important to avoid stereotyping, race and ethnicity may provide valuable starting information about cultural, behavioral, environmental, and medical factors that might affect a pregnant woman's health (American College of Obstetricians and Gynecologists [ACOG], 2005a). With this general knowledge as a framework, it is essential to ask the woman about specific practices to determine their meaning for her.

Determination of Due Date

Childbearing families generally want to know the "due date," or the date around which childbirth will occur. Historically the due date has been called the *estimated date of confinement (EDC)*. The concept of confinement is, however, rather negative, and many caregivers avoid it by referring to the due date as the EDD or estimated date of delivery. Childbirth educators often stress that babies are not "delivered" like a package; they are born. In keeping with a view that emphasizes the normalcy of the process, this text refers to the due date as the **estimated date of birth (EDB)**.

To calculate the EDB it is helpful to know the date of the LMP. However, some women have episodes of irregular bleeding or fail to keep track of menstrual cycles. Thus other techniques also help to determine how far along a woman is in her pregnancy—that is, at how many weeks' gestation she is. Techniques that can be used include evaluating uterine size, determining when quickening occurs, and auscultating fetal heart rate with a Doppler device or ultrasound and later a fetoscope.

Nägele's Rule

The most common method of determining the EDB is **Nägele's rule**. To use this method, one begins with the first day of the last menstrual period, subtracts 3 months, and adds 7 days. For example:

First day of LMP	November 21
Subtract 3 months	−3 months
	August 21
Add 7 days	+7 days
EDB	August 28

It is simpler to change the months to numeric terms:

November 21 becomes	11−21
Subtract 3 months	−3
	8−21
Add 7 days	+7
EDB	August 28

ASSESSMENT GUIDE   INITIAL PRENATAL ASSESSMENT

Physical Assessment/ Normal Findings	Alterations and Possible Causes*	Nursing Responses to Data†
Vital Signs		
Blood Pressure (BP): Less than or equal to 135/85 mm Hg	High BP (essential hypertension; renal disease; pregestational hypertension, apprehension or anxiety associated with pregnancy diagnosis, exam, or other crises; preeclampsia if initial assessment not done until after 20 weeks' gestation)	BP greater than 140/90 requires immediate consideration; establish woman's BP; refer to healthcare provider if necessary. Assess woman's knowledge about high BP; counsel on self-care and medical management
Pulse: 60–90 beats/min; rate may increase 10 beats/min during pregnancy	Increased pulse rate (excitement or anxiety, cardiac disorders)	Count for 1 full minute; note irregularities.
Respirations: 12–22 breaths/min (or pulse rate divided by four); pregnancy may induce a degree of hyperventilation; thoracic breathing predominant	Marked tachypnea or abnormal patterns	Assess for respiratory disease.
Temperature: 36.2°C–37.6°C (97°F–99.6°F)	Elevated temperature (infection)	Assess for infection process of disease state if temperature is elevated; refer to healthcare provider.
Weight		
Depends on body build	Weight less than 45 kg (100 lb) or greater than 91 kg (200 lb); rapid, sudden weight gain (preeclampsia)	Evaluate need for nutritional counselling; obtain information on eating habits, cooking practices, food regularly eaten, income limitations, need for food supplements, pica and other abnormal food habits. Note initial weight to establish baseline for weight gain throughout pregnancy.
Skin		
Color: Consistent with racial background; pink nail beds	Pallor (anemia); bronze, yellow (hepatic disease; other causes of jaundice)	The following tests should be performed: complete blood count (CBC), bilirubin level, urinalysis, and blood urea nitrogen (BUN).
	Bluish, reddish, mottled; dusky appearance or pallor of palms and nail beds in dark-skinned women (anemia)	If abnormal, refer to healthcare provider.
Condition: Absence of edema (slight edema of lower extremities is normal during pregnancy)	Edema (preeclampsia); rashes, dermatitis (allergic response)	Counsel on relief measures for slight edema. Initiate preeclampsia assessment; refer to healthcare provider.
Lesions: Absence of lesions	Ulceration (varicose veins, decreased circulation)	Further assess circulatory status; refer to healthcare provider if lesion is severe.
Spider nevi common in pregnancy	Petechiae, multiple bruises, ecchymosis (hemorrhagic disorders; abuse)	Evaluate for bleeding or clotting disorder. Provide opportunities to discuss abuse if suspected.
	Change in size or color (carcinoma)	Refer to healthcare provider.
Moles		
Pigmentation: Pigmentation changes of pregnancy include linea nigra, striae gravidarum, melasma		Assure woman that these are normal manifestations of pregnancy and explain the physiologic basis for the changes.
Café-au-lait spots	Six or more (Albright syndrome or neurofibromatosis)	Consult with healthcare provider.
Nose		
Character of mucosa: Redder than oral mucosa; in pregnancy nasal mucosa is edematous in response to increased estrogen, resulting in nasal stuffiness (rhinitis of pregnancy) and nosebleeds	Olfactory loss (first cranial nerve deficit)	Counsel woman about possible relief measures for nasal stuffiness and nosebleeds (epistaxis); refer to healthcare provider for olfactory loss.
*Possible causes of alterations are identified in parentheses.		†This column provides guidelines for further assessment and initial intervention.

ASSESSMENT GUIDE   INITIAL PRENATAL ASSESSMENT *(Continued)*

Physical Assessment/ Normal Findings	Alterations and Possible Causes*	Nursing Responses to Data†
Mouth		
May note hypertrophy of gingival tissue because of estrogen	Edema, inflammation (infection); pale in color (anemia)	Assess hematocrit for anemia; counsel regarding dental hygiene habits. Refer to healthcare provider or dentist if necessary. Routine dental care appropriate during pregnancy (no X-ray studies, no nitrous anesthesia).
Neck		
Nodes: Small, mobile, nontender nodes	Tender, hard, fixed, or prominent nodes (infection, carcinoma)	Examine for local infection; refer to healthcare provider.
Thyroid: Small, smooth, lateral lobes palpable on either side of trachea; slight hyperplasia by third month of pregnancy	Enlargement or nodule tenderness (hyperthyroidism)	Listen over thyroid for bruits, which may indicate hyperthyroidism. Question woman about dietary habits (iodine intake). Ascertain history of thyroid problems; refer to healthcare provider.
Chest and Lungs		
Chest: Symmetric, elliptic, smaller anteroposterior (AP) than transverse diameter	Increased AP diameter, funnel chest, pigeon chest (emphysema, asthma, chronic obstructive pulmonary disease [COPD])	Evaluate for emphysema, asthma, pulmonary disease (COPD).
Ribs: Slope downward from nipple line	More horizontal (COPD) angular bumps rachitic rosary (vitamin C deficiency)	Evaluate for COPD. Evaluate for fractures. Consult healthcare provider. Consult nutritionist.
Inspection and palpation: No retraction or bulging of intercostal spaces (ICS) during inspiration or expiration; symmetric expansion.	ICS retractions with inspirations, bulging with expiration; unequal expansion (respiratory disease)	Do thorough initial assessment. Refer to healthcare provider.
Tactile fremitus	Tachypnea, hyperpnea, Cheyne-Stokes respirations (respiratory disease)	Refer to healthcare provider.
Percussion: Bilateral symmetry in tone	Flatness of percussion, which may be affected by chest wall thickness	Evaluate for pleural effusions, consolidations, or tumor.
Low-pitched resonance of moderate intensity	High diaphragm (atelectasis or paralysis), pleural effusion	Refer to healthcare provider.
Auscultation: Upper lobes: bronchovesicular sounds above sternum and scapulas; equal expiratory and inspiratory phases	Abnormal if heard over any other area of chest	Refer to healthcare provider.
Remainder of chest: Vesicular breath sounds heard; inspiratory phase longer (3:1)	Rales, rhonchi, wheezes; pleural friction rub; absence of breath sounds; bronchophony, egophony, whispered pectoriloquy	Refer to healthcare provider.
Breasts		
Supple: Symmetric in size and contour; darker pigmentation of nipple and areola; may have supernumerary nipples, usually 5–6 cm below normal nipple line	"Pigskin" or orange-peel appearance, nipple retractions, swelling, hardness (carcinoma); redness, heat, tenderness, cracked or fissured nipple (infection)	Encourage monthly self-examination; instruct woman how to examine her own breasts.
Axillary nodes unpalpable or pellet sized	Tenderness, enlargement, hard node (carcinoma); may be visible bump (infection)	Refer to healthcare provider if evidence of inflammation.
	*Possible causes of alterations are identified in parentheses.	†This column provides guidelines for further assessment and initial intervention.

(Continued)

ASSESSMENT GUIDE INITIAL PRENATAL ASSESSMENT *(Continued)*

Physical Assessment/ Normal Findings	Alterations and Possible Causes*	Nursing Responses to Data†
Breasts (Continued)		
Pregnancy changes:		Discuss normalcy of changes and their meaning with the woman. Teach and/or institute appropriate relief measures. Encourage use of supportive, well-fitting brassiere.
1. Size increase noted primarily in first 20 weeks.		
2. Become nodular.		
3. Tingling sensation may be felt during first and third trimester; woman may report feeling of heaviness.		
4. Pigmentation of nipples and areolae darkens.		
5. Superficial veins dilate and become more prominent.		
6. Striae seen in multiparas.		
7. Tubercles of Montgomery enlarge.		
8. Colostrum may be present after 12th week.		
9. Secondary areola appears at 20 weeks, characterized by series of washed-out spots surrounding primary areola.		
10. Breasts less firm, old striae may be present in multiparas.		
Heart		
Normal rate, rhythm, and heart sounds	Enlargement, thrills, thrusts, gross irregularity or skipped beats, gallop rhythm or extra sounds (cardiac disease)	Complete an initial assessment. Explain normal pregnancy-induced changes. Refer to healthcare provider if indicated.
Pregnancy changes:		
1. Palpitations may occur due to sympathetic nervous system disturbance.		
2. Short systolic murmurs that increase in held expiration are normal due to increased volume.		
Abdomen		
Normal appearance, skin texture, and hair distribution; liver nonpalpable; abdomen nontender	Muscle guarding (anxiety, acute tenderness); tenderness, mass (ectopic pregnancy, inflammation, carcinoma)	Assure woman of normalcy of diastasis. Provide initial information about appropriate prenatal and postpartum exercises. Evaluate woman's anxiety level. Refer to healthcare provider if indicated.
Pregnancy changes:		
1. Purple striae may be present (or silver striae on a multipara) as well as linea nigra.		
2. Diastasis of the rectus muscles late in pregnancy.		
3. Size: Flat or rotund abdomen; progressive enlargement of uterus due to pregnancy. 10–12 weeks: Fundus slightly above symphysis pubis. 16 weeks: Fundus halfway between symphysis and umbilicus. 20–22 weeks: Fundus at umbilicus. 28 weeks: Fundus three finger breadths above umbilicus. 36 weeks: Fundus just below ensiform cartilage.	Size of uterus inconsistent with length of gestation (intrauterine growth restriction [IUGR], multiple pregnancy, fetal demise, hydatidiform mole)	Reassess menstrual history regarding pregnancy dating. Evaluate increase in size using McDonald's method. Use ultrasound to establish diagnosis.

*Possible causes of alterations are identified in parentheses.

†This column provides guidelines for further assessment and initial intervention.

ASSESSMENT GUIDE INITIAL PRENATAL ASSESSMENT *(Continued)*

Physical Assessment/ Normal Findings	Alterations and Possible Causes*	Nursing Responses to Data†
Abdomen (Continued)		
4. Fetal heart rate: 110–160 beats/min may be heard with Doppler at 10–12 weeks' gestation; may be heard with fetoscope at 17–20 weeks.	Failure to hear fetal heartbeat with Doppler (fetal demise, hydatidiform mole)	Refer to healthcare provider. Administer pregnancy tests. Use ultrasound to establish diagnosis.
5. Fetal movement palpable by a trained examiner after the 18th week.	Failure to feel fetal movements after 20 weeks' gestation (fetal demise, hydatidiform mole)	Refer to healthcare provider for evaluation of fetal status.
6. Ballottement: During fourth to fifth month fetus rises and then rebounds to original position when uterus is tapped sharply.	No ballottement (oligohydramnios)	Refer to healthcare provider for evaluation of fetal status.
Extremities		
Skin warm, pulses palpable, full range of motion; may be some edema of hands and ankles in late pregnancy; varicose veins may become more pronounced; palmar erythema may be present	Unpalpable or diminished pulses (arterial insufficiency); marked edema (preeclampsia)	Evaluate for other symptoms of heart disease; initiate follow-up if woman mentions that her rings feel tight. Discuss prevention and self-treatment measures for varicose veins; refer to healthcare provider if indicated.
Spine		
Normal spinal curves: Concave cervical, convex thoracic, concave lumbar	Abnormal spinal curves; flatness, kyphosis, lordosis	Refer to healthcare provider for assessment of cephalopelvic disproportion (CPD).
In pregnancy, lumbar spinal curve may be accentuated	Backache	May have implications for administration of spinal anesthetics; see Chapter 20 ∞ for relief measures.
Shoulders and iliac crests should be even	Uneven shoulders and iliac crests (scoliosis)	Refer very young women to healthcare provider; discuss back-stretching exercise with older women.
Reflexes		
Normal and symmetric	Hyperactivity, clonus (preeclampsia)	Evaluate for other symptoms of preeclampsia.
Pelvic Area		
External female genitals: Normally formed with female hair distribution; in multiparas, labia majora loose and pigmented; urinary and vaginal orifices visible and appropriately located	Lesions, hematomas, varicosities, inflammation of Bartholin's glands; clitoral hypertrophy (masculinization)	Explain pelvic examination procedure. Encourage woman to minimize her discomfort by relaxing her hips. Provide privacy.
Vagina: Pink or dark pink, vaginal discharge odorless, nonirritating; in multiparas, vaginal folds smooth and flattened; may have episiotomy scar	Abnormal discharge associated with vaginal infections	Obtain vaginal smear. Provide understandable verbal and written instructions about treatment for woman and partner, if indicated.
Cervix: Pink color; os closed except in multiparas, in whom os admits fingertip	Eversion, reddish erosin, nabothian or retention cysts, cervical polyp; granular area that bleeds (carcinoma of cervix); lesions (herpes, human papilloma virus [HPV]); presence of string or plastic tip from cervix (intrauterine device [IUD] in uterus)	Provide woman with a hand mirror and identify genital structures for her; encourage her to view her cervix if she wishes. Refer to healthcare provider if indicated. Advise woman of potential serious risks of leaving an IUD in place during pregnancy; refer to healthcare provider for removal.
Pregnancy changes:		
1–4 weeks' gestation: Enlargement in anteroposterior diameter		

*Possible causes of alterations are identified in parentheses.

†This column provides guidelines for further assessment and initial intervention.

(Continued)

ASSESSMENT GUIDE   INITIAL PRENATAL ASSESSMENT *(Continued)*

Physical Assessment/ Normal Findings	Alterations and Possible Causes*	Nursing Responses to Data†
4–6 weeks' gestation: Softening of cervix (Goodell's sign); softening of isthmus of uterus (Hegar's sign); cervix takes on bluish coloring (Chadwick's sign)	Absence of Goodell's sign (inflammatory conditions, carcinoma)	Refer to healthcare provider.
8–12 weeks' gestation: Vagina and cervix appear bluish violet in color (Chadwick's sign)	Fixed (pelvic inflammatory disease [PID]); nodular surface (fibromas)	Refer to healthcare provider.
Uterus: Pear shaped, mobile; smooth surface		
Ovaries: Small, walnut shaped, nontender (ovaries and Fallopian tubes are located in the adnexal areas)	Pain on movement of cervix (PID); enlarged or nodular ovaries (cyst, tumor, tubal pregnancy, corpus luteum of pregnancy)	Evaluate adnexal areas; refer to healthcare provider.

Pelvic Measurements

Internal measurements:	Measurement below normal	Vaginal birth may not be possible if deviations are present.
1. Diagonal conjugate at least 11.5 cm (Figure 15–7)		
2. Obstetric conjugate estimated by subtracing 1.5–2 cm from diagonal conjugate	Disproportion of pubic arch	
3. Inclination of sacrum	Abnormal curvature of sacrum	
4. Motility of coccyx; external intertuberosity diameter greater than 8 cm	Fixed or malposition of coccyx	

Anus and Rectum

No lumps, rashes, excoriation, tenderness; cervix may be felt through rectal wall	Hemorrhoids, rectal prolapse; nodular lesion (carcinoma)	Counsel about appropriate prevention and relief measures; refer to healthcare provider for further evaluation.

Laboratory Evaluation

Hemoglobin: 12–16 g/dl; women residing in areas of high altitude may have higher levels of hemoglobin	Less than 11 g/dl (anemia)	Note: Wear nonlatex gloves when drawing blood. Hemoglobin less than 12 g/dl requires nutritional counseling; less than 11 g/dl requires iron supplementation.
ABO and Rh typing: Normal distribution of blood types	Rh negative	If Rh negative, check for presence of anti-Rh antibodies. Check partner's blood type; if partner is Rh positive, discuss with woman the need for antibody titers during pregnancy, management during the intrapartal period, and possible need for Rh immune globulin. (See Chapter 16 ∞).

Complete Blood Count (CBC)

Hematocrit: 38%–47% physiologic anemia (pseudoanemia) may occur	Marked anemia or blood dyscrasias	Perform CBC and Schilling differential cell count.
Red blood cells (RBC): 4.2–5.4 million/ microliter		
White blood cells (WBC): 5,000–12,000/microliter	Presence of infection; may be elevated in pregnancy and with labor	Evaluate for other signs of infection.

*Possible causes of alterations are identified in parentheses.

†This column provides guidelines for further assessment and initial intervention.

ASSESSMENT GUIDE INITIAL PRENATAL ASSESSMENT (Continued)

Physical Assessment/ Normal Findings	Alterations and Possible Causes*	Nursing Responses to Data†
Differential Neutrophils: 40%–60% Bands: up to 5% Eosinophils: 1%–3% Basophils: up to 1% Lymphocytes: 20%–40% Monocytes: 4%–8%		
First trimester aneuploidy screening (testing to detect conditions related to abnormal chromosome number); If nuchal translucency (NT) testing is available, offer first-trimester screening for Down syndrome using nuchal translucency and serum markers (PAPP-A and free β-hCG). Normal range. **Integrated screening:** combines first-trimester aneuploidy screening results with second-trimester quad screen to detect aneuploidy and neural tube defects; may be used in areas in which NT testing is not available. (See discussion in Subsequent Prenatal Assessment Guide.)	Increased nuchal translucency, elevated β-hCG, and reduced PAPP-A (Down syndrome, trisomy 18, trisomy 13, Turner syndrome)	If findings are positive, genetic counseling and diagnostic testing using chorionic villus sampling (CVS) or second-trimester amniocentesis is offered (ACOG, 2007).
Syphilis tests: Serologic tests for syphilis (STS), complement fixation test, venereal disease research laboratory (VDRL) test—nonreactive	Positive reaction STS—tests may have 25%–45% incidence of biologic false-positive results; false results may occur in individuals who have acute viral or bacterial infections, hypersensitivity reactions, recent vaccinations, collagen disease, malaria, or tuberculosis	Positive results may be confirmed with the fluorescent treponemal antibody-absorption (FTA-ABS) test; all tests for syphilis give positive results in the secondary stage of the disease; antibiotic tests may cause negative test results.
Gonorrhea culture: Negative	Positive	Refer for treatment.
Urinalysis (u/a): Normal color, specific gravity; pH 4.6–8	Abnormal color (porphyria, hemoglobinuria, bilirubinemia): alkaline urine (metabolic alkalemia, *Proteus* infection, old specimen)	Repeat u/a; refer to healthcare provider.
Negative for protein, red blood cells, white blood cells, casts	Positive findings (contaminated specimen, kidney disease)	Repeat u/a; refer to healthcare provider.
Glucose: Negative (small degree of glycosuria may occur in pregnancy)	Glycosuria (low renal threshold for glucose, diabetes mellitus)	Assess blood glucose level; test urine for ketones.
Rubella titer: Hemagglutination-inhibition (HAI) test–1:10 or above indicates woman is immune	HAI titer less than 1:10	Immunization will be given on postpartum or within 6 weeks after childbirth. Instruct woman whose titers are less than 1:10 to avoid children who have rubella.
Hepatitis B screen for hepatitis B surface antigen (HbsAg): negative	Positive	If negative, consider referral for hepatitis B vaccine. If positive, refer to physician. Infants born to women who test positive are given hepatitis B immune globulin soon after birth followed by first dose of hepatitis B vaccine.
HIV screen: Offered to all women; encouraged for those at risk; negative	Positive	Refer to healthcare provider.
	*Possible causes of alterations are identified in parentheses.	†This column provides guidelines for further assessment and initial intervention.

(Continued)

ASSESSMENT GUIDE INITIAL PRENATAL ASSESSMENT *(Continued)*

Physical Assessment/ Normal Findings	Alterations and Possible Causes*	Nursing Responses to Data†
Illicit drug screen: Offered to all women; negative	Positive	Refer to healthcare provider.
Sickle-cell screen for clients of African descent: Negative	Positive; test results would include a description of cells	Refer to healthcare provider.
Pap smear: Negative	Test results that show atypical cells	Refer to healthcare provider. Discuss with the woman the meaning of the findings and the importance of follow-up.

Cultural Assessment	Variations to Consider*	Nursing Responses to Data†
Determine the woman's fluency in written and oral English.	Woman may be fluent in language other than English.	Work with a knowledgeable translator to provide information and answer questions.
Ask the woman how she prefers to be addressed.	Some women prefer informality; others prefer to use titles.	Address the woman according to her preference. Maintain formality in introducing oneself if that seems preferred.
Determine customs and practices regarding prenatal care:	Practices are influenced by individual preference, cultural expectations, or religious beliefs.	Honor a woman's practices and provide for specific preferences unless they are contraindicated because of safety.
• Ask the woman if there are certain practices she expects to follow when she is pregnant.	Some women believe that they should perform certain acts related to sleep, activity, or clothing.	Have information printed in the language of different cultural groups that live in the area.
• Ask the woman if there are any activities she cannot do while she is pregnant.	Some women have restrictions or taboos they follow related to work, activity, sexual, environmental, or emotional factors.	
• Ask the woman whether there are certain foods she is expected to eat or avoid while she is pregnant. Determine whether she has lactose intolerance.	Foods are an important cultural factor. Some women may have certain foods they must eat or avoid; many women have lactose intolerance and have difficulty consuming sufficient calcium.	Respect the woman's food preferences, help her plan an adequate prenatal diet within the framework of her preferences, and refer to a dietitian if necessary.
• Ask the woman whether the gender of her caregiver is of concern.	Some women are comfortable only with a female caregiver.	Arrange for a female caregiver if it is the woman's preference.
• Ask the woman about the degree of involvement in her pregnancy that she expects or wants from her support person, mother, and other significant people.	A woman may not want her partner involved in the pregnancy. For some the role falls to the woman's mother or a female relative or friend.	Respect the woman's preferences about her partner or husband's involvement; avoid imposing personal values or expectations.
• Ask the woman about her sources of support and counseling during pregnancy.	Some women seek advice from a family member, *curandera*, tribal healer, and so forth.	Respect and honor the woman's sources of support.
Psychologic Status		
Excitement and/or apprehension, ambivalence	Marked anxiety (fear of pregnancy diagnosis, fear of medical facility)	Establish lines of communication. Active listening is useful. Establish trusting relationship. Encourage woman to take active part in her care.
	Apathy; display of anger with pregnancy diagnosis	Establish communication and begin counseling. Use active listening techniques.
Educational Needs		
May have questions about pregnancy or may need time to adjust to reality of pregnancy		Establish educational, supporting environment that can be expanded throughout pregnancy.

*Possible causes of alterations are identified in parentheses.

†This column provides guidelines for further assessment and initial intervention.

ASSESSMENT GUIDE   INITIAL PRENATAL ASSESSMENT *(Continued)*

Cultural Assessment	Variations to Consider*	Nursing Responses to Data†
Support System		
Can identify at least two or three individuals with whom woman is emotionally intimate (partner, parent, sibling, friend)	Isolated (no telephone, unlisted number); cannot name a neighbor or friend whom she can call upon in an emergency; does not perceive parents as part of her support system	Institute support system through community groups. Help woman to develop trusting relationship with healthcare professionals.
Family Functioning		
Emotionally supportive Communications adequate Mutually satisfying Cohesiveness in times of trouble	Long-term problems or specific problems related to this pregnancy, potential stressors within the family, pessimistic attitudes, unilateral decision making, unrealistic expectations of this pregnancy or child	Help identify the problems and stressors, encourage communication, and discuss role changes and adaptations.
Economic Status		
Source of income is stable and sufficient to meet basic needs of daily living and medical needs	Limited prenatal care; poor physical health; limited use of healthcare system; unstable economic status	Discuss available resources for health maintenance and the birth. Institute appropriate referral for meeting expanding family's needs—food stamps and so forth.
Stability of Living Conditions		
Adequate, stable housing for expanding family's needs	Crowded living conditions; questionable supportive environment for newborn	Refer to appropriate community agency. Work with family on self-help ways to improve situation.
	*Possible causes of alterations are identified in parentheses.	†This column provides guidelines for further assessment and initial intervention.

A gestation calculator or wheel permits the caregiver to calculate the EDB even more quickly (Figure 10–2 ■).

If a woman with a history of menses every 28 days remembers her LMP and was not taking oral contraceptives before becoming pregnant, Nägele's rule may be a fairly accurate determiner of the EDB. However, *ovulation usually occurs 14 days before the onset of the next menses, not 14 days after the previous menses.* Consequently, if her cycle is irregular, or more than 28 days long, the time of ovulation may be delayed. If she has been using oral contraceptives, ovulation may be delayed several weeks following her last menses. Then, too, a postpartum woman who is breastfeeding may resume ovulating but be amenorrheic for a time, making calculation impossible. Thus Nägele's rule, although helpful, is not foolproof.

Uterine Assessment

Physical Examination

When a woman is examined in the first 10 to 12 weeks of her pregnancy and her uterine size is compatible with her menstrual history, uterine size may be the single most important clinical method for dating her pregnancy. In many

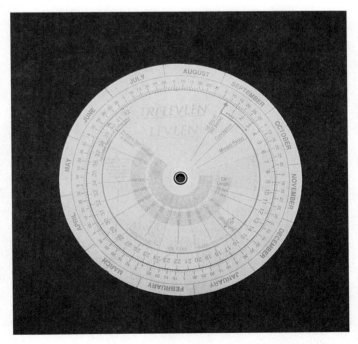

FIGURE 10–2 The EDB wheel can be used to calculate the due date. To use it, place the arrow labeled "1st day of last period" on the date of the woman's LMP. Then read the EDB at the arrow labeled 40. In this case the LMP is September 8th and the EDB is June 17th.

cases, however, women do not seek maternity care until well into their second trimester, when it becomes much more difficult to evaluate specific uterine size. In obese women it is difficult to determine uterine size early in a pregnancy because the uterus is more difficult to palpate.

Fundal Height

Fundal height may be used as an indicator of uterine size, although this method is less accurate late in pregnancy. A centimeter tape measure is used to measure the distance abdominally from the top of the symphysis pubis to the top of the uterine fundus (McDonald's method) (Figure 10–3 ■). Fundal height in centimeters correlates well with weeks of gestation between 22 to 24 weeks and 34 weeks. Thus, at 26 weeks' gestation, fundal height is probably about 26 cm. If the woman is very tall or very short, fundal height will differ. To be most accurate, fundal height should be measured by the same examiner each time. The woman should have voided within 30 minutes of the exam and should lie in the same position each time. In the third trimester, variations in fetal weight decrease the accuracy of fundal height measurements.

A lag in progression of measurements of fundal height from month to month and week to week may signal intrauterine growth restriction (IUGR). A sudden increase in fundal height may indicate twins or hydramnios (excessive amount of amniotic fluid).

Assessment of Fetal Development

Quickening

Fetal movements felt by the mother, called *quickening,* may indicate that the fetus is nearing 20 weeks' gestation. However, quickening may be experienced between 16 and 22 weeks' gestation, so this method is not completely accurate.

Fetal Heartbeat

The ultrasonic Doppler device (Figure 10–4 ■) is the primary tool for assessing fetal heartbeat. It can detect fetal heartbeat, on average, at 8 to 12 weeks' gestation. If an ultrasonic Doppler is not available, a fetoscope may be used, although in current practice it is seldom necessary. The fetal heartbeat can be detected by fetoscope as early as week 16 and almost always by 19 or 20 weeks' gestation.

Ultrasound

In the first trimester, ultrasound scanning can detect a gestational sac as early as 5 to 6 weeks after the LMP, fetal heart activity by 6 to 7 weeks, and fetal breathing movement by 10 to 11 weeks of pregnancy. Crown-to-rump measurements can be made to assess fetal age until the fetal head can be visualized clearly. Biparietal diameter (BPD) can then be used. BPD measurements can be made by approximately 12 to 13 weeks and are most accurate between 20 and 30 weeks, when

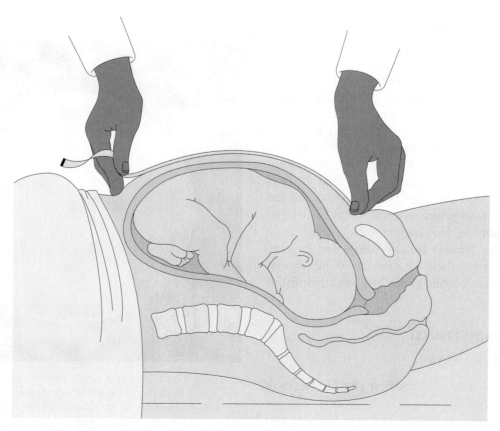

FIGURE 10–3 A cross-sectional view of fetal position when McDonald's method is used to assess the fundal height.

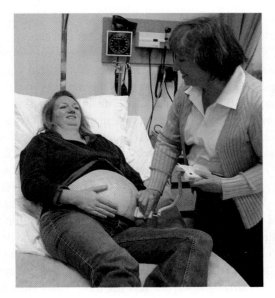

FIGURE 10–4 Listening to the fetal heartbeat with a Doppler device.

rapid growth in the biparietal diameter occurs. (See Chapter 16 ∞ for discussion of fetal ultrasound scanning.)

Assessment of Pelvic Adequacy (Clinical Pelvimetry)

The pelvis can be assessed vaginally to determine whether its size is adequate for a vaginal birth. This procedure, *clinical pelvimetry,* is performed by physicians or by advanced-practice nurses such as certified nurse–midwives or nurse practitioners. Some caregivers assess pelvic adequacy as part of the initial physical examination. Others wait until later in the pregnancy, when hormonal effects are greatest and it is possible to make some determination of fetal size. For a detailed description of clinical pelvimetry, readers are referred to a nurse–midwifery text. This section provides basic information about the assessment of the inlet and outlet (see Figures 10–5 ■ and 10–6 ■), which were described in Chapter 3 ∞.

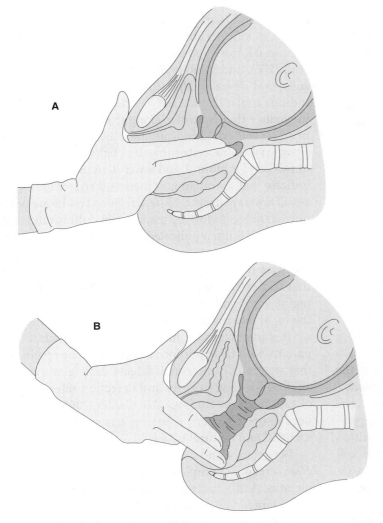

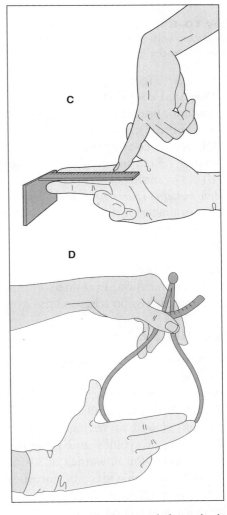

FIGURE 10–5 Manual measurement of inlet and outlet. *A,* Estimation of the diagonal conjugate, which extends from the lower border of the symphysis pubis to the sacral promontory. *B,* Estimation of the anteroposterior diameter of the outlet, which extends from the lower border of the symphysis pubis to the tip of the sacrum. *C* and *D,* Methods that may be used to check the manual estimation of anteroposterior measurements.

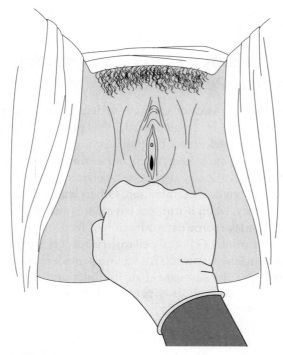

FIGURE 10–6 Use of a closed fist to measure the outlet. Most examiners know the distance between their first and last proximal knuckles. If they don't, they can use a measuring device.

1. *Pelvic inlet (Figure 10–5)*
   - **Diagonal conjugate** (the distance from the lower posterior border of the symphysis pubis to the sacral promontory), at least 11.5 cm
   - **Obstetric conjugate** (a measurement approximately 1.5 cm smaller than the diagonal conjugate), 10 cm or more
2. *Pelvic outlet (Figures 10–5 and 10–6)*
   - Anteroposterior diameter, 9.5 to 11.5 cm
   - Transverse diameter (bi-ischial or intertuberous diameter), 8 to 10 cm

The pelvic cavity (midpelvis) cannot be accurately measured by clinical examination. Examiners estimate its adequacy. However, that discussion is beyond the scope of this text.

Screening Tests

Many screening tests are routinely performed either at the initial prenatal visit or at a specified time during pregnancy. These tests include a Pap smear, a complete blood count, hemoglobin, Rubella titer, ABO and Rh typing, and a hepatitis B screen as well as testing for sexually transmitted infections such as syphilis and gonorrhea. A sickle cell screen is provided for all women of African or Latino descent. Prenatal screening for cystic fibrosis should be offered to all couples regardless of ethnicity or race (ACOG, 2005b).

The urine is screened for abnormal findings initially and at each prenatal visit. In addition, a urine culture at 12 to 16 weeks of pregnancy is recommended for all pregnant women to detect asymptomatic bacteriuria (U.S. Preven-

tive Services Task Force, 2004). Other tests such as HIV screen and a drug screen are offered to all women.

ACOG (2007) recommends that all pregnant women, regardless of age, be offered screening for fetal chromosome anomalies (*aneuploidy*) including Down syndrome, trisomy 18, trisomy 13, and Turner syndrome. First trimester screening is available at many centers using ultrasound assessment of the thickness of the fetal nuchal fold (called *nuchal translucency* [NT]) combined with serum screening for free β-hCG and for pregnancy-associated plasma protein A (PAPP-A). Increased NT, elevated free β-hCG, and reduced PAPP-A suggest aneuploidy. Women with these findings should be offered genetic counseling and chorionic villus sampling or second trimester amniocentesis for diagnosis (ACOG, 2007). If these tests are all negative no further testing is indicated. Instead, during the second trimester, the woman is simply offered a test for maternal serum alpha-fetoprotein to detect the risk of neural tube defects.

The *quadruple screen* (quad screen) is a safe, useful screening test performed on the mother's serum between weeks 15 and 20 of pregnancy. The test is used to detect levels of specific serum markers—alpha-fetoprotein (AFP), human chorionic gonadotropin (hCG), unconjugated estriol (UE), and inhibin-A (a placental hormone). Test results that reveal higher than normal AFP levels might indicate a fetal neural tube defect, a multiple gestation, or a pregnancy that is farther along than believed. Lower than normal AFP could indicate that the woman is at risk for Down syndrome or trisomy 18. Higher than normal levels of hCG and inhibin-A and lower than normal UE may also indicate that a woman is at increased risk of having a baby with Down syndrome. If the screening results are not in the normal range, follow-up testing using ultrasound and amniocentesis is often indicated (Cleveland Clinic, 2006).

NT evaluation requires a skilled ultrasonographer and specialized training. In areas where NT is not available, first trimester free β-hCG screening and PAPP-A screening may be combined with second trimester quad screening in an integrated approach to detection of aneuploidy.

It is important for healthcare professionals to provide parents with factual information about the results of tests that detect chromosomal defects or fetal anomalies including the false-positive and detection rates and the implications of the findings (Nicolaides, 2005). Parents then need to decide on any course of action based on their own spiritual and cultural beliefs.

Between 24 and 28 weeks' gestation a 50 g 1-hour glucose screen is completed to detect gestational diabetes mellitus. Additional testing is indicated if abnormal results are obtained (see Chapter 15 ∞).

Group B streptococcus (GBS) can cause serious problems for a newborn. Consequently rectal and vaginal swabs of the mother are obtained at 35 to 37 weeks' gestation to screen for the infection.

Subsequent Client History

At subsequent prenatal visits the nurse continues to gather data about the course of the pregnancy to date and the woman's responses to it. The nurse also asks about the adjustment of the support person and of other children, if any, in the family. As pregnancy progresses the nurse inquires about the preparations the family has made for the new baby.

The nurse asks specifically whether the woman has experienced any discomfort, especially the kinds of discomfort that are often seen at specific times during a pregnancy. The nurse inquires about physical changes that relate directly to the pregnancy, such as fetal movement. The nurse also asks about the danger signs of pregnancy (see Key Facts to Remember: Danger Signs in Pregnancy). (Note: Many of the danger signs indicate conditions that are potential complications. These conditions are discussed in the at-risk chapters, which are presented later in this text.)

Other pertinent information includes any exposure to contagious illnesses, medical treatment and therapy prescribed for nonpregnancy problems since the last visit, and any prescription or over-the-counter medications or herbal supplements that were not prescribed as part of the woman's prenatal care.

Periodic prenatal examinations offer the nurse an opportunity to assess the childbearing woman's psychologic needs and emotional status. If the woman's partner attends the antepartal visits, the nurse can also identify his needs and concerns. The interchange between the nurse and the woman or her partner will be facilitated if it takes place in a friendly, trusting environment. The woman should have sufficient time to ask questions and air concerns. If the nurse provides the time and demonstrates genuine interest, the woman will be more at ease bringing up questions that she may believe are silly or has been afraid to verbalize. The nurse who has an accurate understanding of all the changes of pregnancy is most able to answer questions and provide information. See the foldout color chart, "Maternal–Fetal Development," in the middle of the book for vivid illustrations of some of this information.

The nurse should also be sensitive to religious or spiritual, cultural, and socioeconomic factors that may influence a family's response to pregnancy, as well as to the woman's expectations of the healthcare system. The nurse can avoid stereotyping clients simply by asking each woman about her expectations for the antepartal period. Although many women's responses may reflect what are thought to be traditional norms, other women will have decidedly different views or expectations that represent a blending of beliefs or cultures.

During the antepartal period, it is essential to begin assessing the readiness of the woman and her partner (if possible) to assume their responsibilities as parents successfully. Table 10–2 identifies areas for assessment of parenting ability.

EVIDENCE IN ACTION

Periodontal disease and urinary tract infections are associated with an increase in the risk of preeclampsia.
(Systematic review and meta-analysis)
(Conde-Agudelo, Villar, & Lindheimer, 2008)

◇ KEY FACTS TO REMEMBER

Danger Signs in Pregnancy

The woman should report the following danger signs in pregnancy immediately.

DANGER SIGN	POSSIBLE CAUSE
Sudden gush of fluid from vagina	Premature rupture of membranes
Vaginal bleeding	Abruptio placentae, placenta previa
	Lesions of cervix or vagina, "bloody show"
Abdominal pain	Premature labor, abruptio placentae
Temperature above 38.3°C (101°F) and chills	Infection
Dizziness, blurring of vision, double vision, spots before eyes	Hypertension, preeclampsia
Persistent vomiting	Hyperemesis gravidarum
Severe headache	Hypertension, preeclampsia
Edema of hands, face, legs, and feet	Preeclampsia
Muscular irritability, convulsions	Preeclampsia, eclampsia
Epigastric pain	Preeclampsia, ischemia in major abdominal vessel
Oliguria	Renal impairment, decreased fluid intake
Dysuria	Urinary tract infection
Absence of fetal movement	Maternal medication, obesity, fetal death

Subsequent Prenatal Assessment

The Assessment Guide: Subsequent Prenatal Assessment, starting on page 220, provides a systematic approach to the regular physical examinations the pregnant woman should undergo for optimal antepartal care and also provides a model for evaluating both the pregnant woman and the expectant father, if he is involved in the pregnancy.

HINTS FOR PRACTICE

When assessing blood pressure, have the pregnant woman sit up with her arm resting on a table so that her arm is at the level of her heart. Expect a decrease in her blood pressure from baseline during the second trimester because of normal physiologic changes. If this decrease does not occur, evaluate further for signs of preeclampsia.

TABLE 10-2	Guide to Prenatal Assessment of Parenting

Areas Assessed	Sample Questions

I. Perception of complexities of mothering

   A. Desires baby for itself
      Positive:
      1. Feels positive about pregnancy
      Negative:
      1. Wants baby to meet own needs such as someone to love her, someone to get her out of unhappy home

   1. Did you plan on getting pregnant?
   2. How do you feel about being pregnant?
   3. Why do you want this baby?

   B. Expresses concern about impact of mothering role on other roles (wife, career, school)
      Positive:
      1. Realistic expectations of how baby will affect job, career, school, and personal goals
      2. Interested in learning about child care
      Negative:
      1. Feels pregnancy and baby will make no emotional, physical, or social demands on self
      2. Has no insight that mothering role will affect other roles or lifestyle

   1. What do you think it will be like to take care of a baby?
   2. How do you think your life will be different after you have your baby?
   3. How do you feel this baby will affect your job, career, school, and personal goals?
   4. How will the baby affect your relationship with your boyfriend or husband?
   5. Have you done any reading, baby-sitting, or made any things for a baby?

   C. Gives up routine habits because "not good for baby" (e.g., quits smoking, adjusts time schedule)
      Positive:
      1. Gives up routines not good for baby (quits smoking, adjusts eating habits)

II. Attachment

   A. Strong feelings regarding sex of baby. Why?
      Positive:
      1. Verbalizes positive thoughts about the baby
      Negative:
      1. Baby will be like negative aspects of self and partner

   1. Why do you prefer a certain sex? (Is reason inappropriate for a baby?)
   2. Note comments client makes about baby not being normal and why client feels this way.

   B. Interested in data regarding fetus (e.g., growth and development, heart tones)
      Positive:
      1. As above
      Negative:
      1. Shows no interest in fetal growth and development, quickening, and fetal heart tones
      2. Expresses negative feelings about fetus by rejecting counseling regarding nutrition, rest, hygiene

   C. Fantasies about baby
      Positive:
      1. Follows cultural norms regarding preparation
      2. Time of attachment behaviors appropriate to her history of pregnancy loss
      Negative:
      1. Bonding conditional depending on sex, age of baby, and/or labor and birth experience
      2. Woman considers only own needs when making plans for baby
      3. Exhibits no attachment behaviors after critical period of previous pregnancy
      4. Failure to follow cultural norms regarding preparation

   1. What did you think or feel when you first felt the baby move?
   2. Have you started preparing for the baby?
   3. What do you think your baby will look like—what age do you see your baby at?
   4. How would you like your new baby to look?

III. Acceptance of child by significant others

   A. Acknowledges acceptance by significant other of the new responsibility inherent in child
      Positive:
      1. Acknowledges unconditional acceptance of pregnancy and baby by significant others
      2. Partner accepts new responsibility inherent with child
      3. Timely sharing of experience of pregnancy with significant others
      Negative:
      1. Significant others not supportively involved with pregnancy
      2. Conditional acceptance of pregnancy depending on sex, race, age of baby
      3. Decision making does not take in needs of fetus (e.g., spends food money on new car)
      4. Takes no/little responsibility for needs of pregnancy, woman/fetus

   1. How does your partner feel about this pregnancy?
   2. How do your parents feel?
   3. What do your friends think?
   4. Does your partner have a preference regarding the baby's sex? Why?
   5. How does your partner feel about being a father?
   6. What do you think he'll be like as a father?
   7. What do you think he'll do to help you with child care?
   8. Have you and your partner talked about how the baby might change your lives?
   9. Who have you told about your pregnancy?

Areas Assessed	Sample Questions

TABLE 10–2 Guide to Prenatal Assessment of Parenting *(Continued)*

B. Concrete demonstration of acceptance of pregnancy/baby by significant others (e.g., baby shower, significant other involved in prenatal education)
Positive:
1. Baby shower
2. Significant other attends prenatal class with client

1. Note if partner attends clinic with client (degree of interest; e.g., listens to heart tones). Significant other plans to be with client during labor and birth.
2. Is your partner contributing financially?

IV. Ensures physical well-being
  A. Concerns about having normal pregnancy, labor and birth, and baby
  1. Preparing for labor and birth, attends prenatal classes, interested in labor and birth
  2. Aware of danger signs of pregnancy
  3. Seeks and uses appropriate health care (e.g., time of initial visit, keeps appointments, follows through on recommendations)
  Negative:
  1. Denies signs and symptoms that might suggest complications of pregnancy
  2. Verbalizes extreme fear of labor and birth—refuses to talk about labor and birth
  3. Misses appointments, fails to follow instructions, refuses to attend prenatal classes
  B. Family/client decisions reflect concern for health of mother and baby (e.g., use of finances, time)
  Positive:
  1. As above

1. What have you heard about labor and birth?
2. Note data about client's reaction to prenatal class.

Note: When "Negative" is not listed in a section, the reader may assume that negative is the absence of positive responses.
Source: Modified and used with permission of the Minneapolis Health Dept, Minneapolis, MN.

The woman's individual needs and the assessment of her risks should determine the frequency of subsequent visits. Generally the recommended frequency of antepartal visits is as follows:

- Every 4 weeks for the first 28 weeks' gestation
- Every 2 weeks until 36 weeks' gestation
- After week 36, every week until childbirth

During the subsequent antepartal assessments, most women demonstrate ongoing psychologic adjustment to pregnancy. However, some women may exhibit signs of possible psychologic problems such as the following:

- Increasing anxiety
- Inability to establish communication
- Inappropriate responses or actions
- Denial of pregnancy
- Inability to cope with stress
- Intense preoccupation with the sex of the baby
- Failure to acknowledge quickening
- Failure to plan and prepare for the baby (e.g., living arrangements, clothing, and feeding methods)
- Indications of substance abuse

If the woman's behavior indicates possible psychologic problems, the nurse can provide ongoing support and counseling and also refer the woman to appropriate professionals.

ASSESSMENT GUIDE SUBSEQUENT PRENATAL ASSESSMENT

Physical Assessment/ Normal Findings	Alterations and Possible Causes*	Nursing Responses to Data†
Vital Signs		
Temperature: 36.2°C–37.6°C (97°F–99.6°F)	Elevated temperature (infection)	Evaluate for signs of infection. Refer to healthcare provider.
Pulse: 60–90/min Rate may increase 10 beats/min during pregnancy	Increased pulse rate (anxiety, cardiac disorders)	Note irregularities. Assess for anxiety and stress.
Respiration: 12–22/min	Marked tachypnea or abnormal patterns (respiratory disease)	Refer to healthcare provider.
Blood pressure: Less than or equal to 135/85 (falls in second trimester)	Greater than 140/90 or increase of 30 mm systolic and 15 mm diastolic (preeclampsia)	Assess for edema, proteinuria, and hyperreflexia. Refer to healthcare provider. Schedule appointments more frequently.
Weight Gain		
First trimester: 1.6–2.3 kg (3.5–5 lb)	Inadequate weight gain (poor nutrition, nausea, IUGR)	Discuss appropriate weight gain.
Second trimester: 5.5–6.8 kg (12–15 lb)	Excessive weight gain (excessive caloric intake, edema, preeclampsia)	Provide nutritional counseling. Assess for presence of edema or anemia.
Third trimester: 5.5–6.8 kg (12–15 lb)		
Edema		
Small amount of dependent edema, especially in last weeks of pregnancy	Edema in hands, face, legs, and feet (preeclampsia)	Identify any correlation between edema and activities, blood pressure, or proteinuria: Refer to healthcare provider if indicated.
Uterine Size		
See "Assessment Guide: Initial Prenatal Assessment" for normal changes during pregnancy	Unusually rapid growth (multiple gestation, hydatidiform mole, hydramnios, miscalculation of EDB)	Evaluate fetal status. Determine height of fundus (page 214). Use diagnostic ultrasound.
Fetal Heartbeat		
120–160/min Funic souffle	Absence of fetal heartbeat after 20 weeks' gestation (maternal obesity, fetal demise)	Evaluate fetal status.
Laboratory Evaluation		
Hemoglobin: 12–16 g/dl Pseudoanemia of pregnancy	Greater than 11 g/dl (anemia)	Provide nutritional counseling. Hemoglobin is repeated at 7 months' gestation. Women of Mediterranean heritage need a close check on hemoglobin because of possibility of thalassemia.
Quad marker screen: Blood test performed at 15–20 weeks' gestation. Evaluates four factors—maternal serum alpha-fetoprotein (MSAFP), unconjugated estriol (UE), hCG, and inhibin-A: normal levels	Elevated MSAFP (neural tube defect, underestimated gestational age, multiple gestation). Lower than normal MSAFP (Down syndrome, trisomy 18). Higher than normal hCG and inhibin-A (Down syndrome). Lower than normal UE (Down syndrome).	Recommended for all pregnant women; especially indicated for women with any of the following risk factors: age 35 and over, family history of birth defects, previous child with a birth defect; insulin-dependent diabetes prior to pregnancy (Cleveland Clinic, 2004). If quad screen abnormal further testing such as ultrasound or amniocentesis may be indicated.

*Possible causes of alterations are identified in parentheses.

†This column provides guidelines for further assessment and initial intervention.

ASSESSMENT GUIDE INITIAL PRENATAL ASSESSMENT *(Continued)*

Physical Assessment/ Normal Findings	Alterations and Possible Causes*	Nursing Responses to Data†
Laboratory Evaluation (Continued)		
Indirect Coombs test done on Rh negative women: Negative (done at 28 weeks' gestation)	Rh antibodies present (maternal sensitization has occurred)	If Rh negative and unsensitized, Rh immune globulin given (see Chapter 20 ∞). If Rh antibodies present, Rh immune globulin not given; fetus monitored closely for isoimmune hemolytic disease. Discuss implications of GDM. Refer for a diagnostic 100 g oral glucose tolerance test.
50-g 1-hour glucose screen (done between 24 and 28 weeks' gestation)	Plasma glucose level greater than 140 mg/dl (gestational diabetes mellitus [GDM]) *Note:* Some facilities use level greater than 130 mg/d, which identifies 90% of women with GDM (American Diabetes Association, 2004)	
Urinalysis: See "Assessment Guide: Initial Prenatal Assessment" for normal findings	See "Assessment Guide: Initial Prenatal Assessment" for deviations	Repeat urinalysis at 7 months' gestation. Repeat dipstick test at each visit.
Protein: Negative	Proteinuria, albuminuria (contamination by vaginal discharge, urinary tract infection, preeclampsia)	Obtain dipstick urine sample. Refer to healthcare provider if deviations are present.
Glucose: Negative *Note:* Glycosuria may be present due to physiologic alterations in glomerular filtration rate and renal threshold	Persistent glycosuria (diabetes mellitus)	Refer to healthcare provider.
Screening for Group B streptococcus (GBS): Rectal and vaginal swabs obtained at 35–37 weeks' gestation for all pregnant women (Centers for Disease Control and Prevention [CDC], 2002).	Positive culture (maternal infection)	Explain maternal and fetal/neonatal risks (see Chapter 20 ∞). Refer to healthcare provider for therapy.

Cultural Assessment	Variations to Consider*	Nursing Responses to Data†
Determine the mother's (and family's) attitudes about the sex of the unborn child.	Some women have no preference about the sex of the child; others do. In many cultures, boys are especially valued as firstborn children.	Provide opportunities to discuss preferences and expectations; avoid a judgmental attitude to the response.
Ask about the woman's expectations of childbirth. Will she want someone with her for the birth? Whom does she choose? What is the role of her partner?	Some women want their partner present for labor and birth; others prefer a female relative or friend. Some women expect to be separated from their partner once cervical dilation has occured.	Provide information on birth options but accept the woman's decision about who will attend.
Ask about preparations for the baby. Determine what is customary for the woman.	Some women may have a fully prepared nursery; others may not have a separate room for the baby.	Explore reasons for not preparing for the baby. Support the mother's preferences and provide information about possible sources of assistance if the decision is related to a lack of resources.
Expectant Mother **Psychologic Status**	Increased stress and anxiety	Encourage woman to take an active part in her care.

*Possible causes of alterations are identified in parentheses.

†This column provides guidelines for further assessment and initial intervention.

(Continued)

ASSESSMENT GUIDE   INITIAL PRENATAL ASSESSMENT (Continued)

Cultural Assessment	Variations to Consider*	Nursing Responses to Data†
Expectant Mother (Continued)		
First trimester: Incorporates idea of pregnancy; may feel ambivalent, especially if she must give up desired role; usually looks for signs of verification of pregnancy, such as increase in abdominal size or fetal movement	Inability to establish communication; inability to accept pregnancy; inappropriate response or actions; denial of pregnancy; inability to cope	Establish lines of communication. Establish a trusting relationship. Counsel as necessary. Refer to appropriate professional as needed.
Second trimester: Baby becomes more real to woman as abdominal size increases and she feels movement; she begins to turn inward, becoming more introspective		
Third trimester: Begins to think of baby as separate being; may feel restless and may feel that time of labor will never come; remains self-centered and concentrates on preparing place for baby		
Educational needs: **Self-care measures and knowledge about the following:**	Inadequate information	Provide information and counseling.
Health promotion		
Breast care		
Hygiene		
Rest		
Exercise		
Nutrition		
Relief measures for common discomforts of pregnancy		
Danger signs in pregnancy (see Table 15–3)		
Sexual activity: Woman knows how pregnancy affects sexual activity	Lack of information about effects of pregnancy and/or alternative positions during sexual intercourse	Provide counseling.
Preparation for parenting: Appropriate preparation	Lack of preparation (denial, failure to adjust to baby, unwanted child)	Counsel. If lack of preparation is due to inadequacy of information, provide information.
Preparation for Childbirth: **Client aware of the following:**		If couple chooses particular technique refer to classes (see page 176 in Chapter 8 ∞ for description of childbirth preparation techniques).
1. Prepared childbirth techniques		
2. Normal processes and changes during childbirth		Encourage prenatal class attendance. Educate woman during visits based on current physical status. Provide reading list for more specific information.
3. Problems that may occur as a result of drug and alcohol use and of smoking	Continued abuse of drugs and alcohol; denial of possible effect on self and baby	Review danger signs that were presented on initial visit.
Woman has met other physician or nurse–midwife who may be attending her birth in the absence of primary caregiver	Introduction of new individual at birth may increase stress and anxiety for woman and partner	Introduce woman to all members of group practice.
Impending Labor: **Client knows signs of impending labor:**	Lack of information	Provide appropriate teaching, stressing importance of seeking appropriate medical assistance.

*Possible causes of alterations are identified in parentheses.

†This column provides guidelines for further assessment and initial intervention.

ASSESSMENT GUIDE — INITIAL PRENATAL ASSESSMENT (Continued)

Cultural Assessment	Variations to Consider*	Nursing Responses to Data†
Expectant Mother (Continued) 1. Uterine contractions that increase in frequency, duration, and intensity 2. Bloody show 3. Expulsion of mucous plug 4. Rupture of membranes		
Expectant Father **Psychologic Status** **First trimester:** May express excitement over confirmation of pregnancy and of his virility; concerns move toward providing for financial needs; energetic, may identify with some discomforts of pregnancy and may even exhibit symptoms	Increasing stress and anxiety; inability to establish communication; inability to accept pregnancy diagnosis; withdrawal of support; abandonment of the mother	Encourage expectant father to come to prenatal visits. Establish line of communication. Establish trusting relationship.
Second trimester: May feel more confident and be less concerned with financial matters; may have concerns about wife's changing size and shape, her increasing introspection		Counsel. Let expectant father know that it is normal for him to experience these feelings.
Third trimester: May have feelings of rivalry with fetus, especially during sexual activity; may make changes in his physical appearance and exhibit more interest in himself; may become more energetic; fantasizes about child but usually imagines older child; fears mutilation and death of woman and child		Include expectant father in pregnancy activities as he desires. Provide education, information, and support. Increasing numbers of expectant fathers are demonstrating desire to be involved in many or all aspects of prenatal care, education, and preparation.
	*Possible causes of alterations are identified in parentheses.	†This column provides guidelines for further assessment and initial intervention.

CHAPTER HIGHLIGHTS

- A complete history forms the basis of prenatal care and is reevaluated and updated as necessary throughout the pregnancy.
- The initial prenatal assessment is a careful and thorough physical examination and cultural and psychosocial assessment designed to identify variations and potential risk factors.
- Laboratory tests completed at the initial visit, such as a complete blood count, ABO and Rh typing, urinalysis, Pap smear, Chlamydia culture, testing for syphilis (Venereal Disease Research Laboratory [VDRL], rapid plasma regain [RPR], or other serology test), gonorrhea culture, rubella titer, various blood screens, and tuberculin test (PPD) for women in high-risk groups with no known history of a positive test provide information about the woman's health during early pregnancy and also help detect potential problems.
- The estimated date of birth (EDB) can be calculated by using Nägele's rule. Using this approach, one begins with the first day of the last menstrual period, subtracts 3 months, and adds 7 days. A gestational calculator or wheel may also be used to calculate the EDB.
- Accuracy of the EDB may be evaluated by physical exam to assess uterine size, measurement of fundal height, and ultrasound. Perception of quickening and auscultation of fetal heartbeat are also helpful in confirming the gestation of a pregnancy.
- The diagonal conjugate is the distance from the lower posterior border of the symphysis pubis to the sacral promontory. The obstetric conjugate is estimated by subtracting 1.5 cm from the length of the diagonal conjugate.
- The nurse begins evaluating the woman psychosocially during the initial prenatal assessment. This assessment continues and is modified throughout the pregnancy.
- Religious, cultural, and ethnic beliefs may strongly influence the woman's attitudes and apparent cooperation with care during pregnancy.

EXPLORE PEARSON **mynursingkit**™

MyNursingKit is your one stop for online chapter review materials and resources. Prepare for success with additional NCLEX®-style practice questions, interactive assignments and activities, web links, animations and videos, and more!

Register your access code from the front of your book at
www.mynursingkit.com

CHAPTER REFERENCES

American College of Obstetricians and Gynecologists. (2005a). *Racial and ethnic disparities in women's health* (ACOG Committee Opinion No. 317). Washington, DC: Author.

American College of Obstetricians and Gynecologists. (2005b). *Update on carrier screening for cystic fibrosis* (ACOG Committee Opinion No. 325). Washington, DC: Author.

American College of Obstetricians and Gynecologists. (2007). *Screening for fetal chromosomal abnormalities* (ACOG Practice Bulletin No. 77). Washington, DC: Author.

Cleveland Clinic. (2006). *Quad marker screen.* Retrieved December 31, 2007, from www.cchs. net/health/health-info/docs/0300/0386.asp? index=4698

Conde-Agudelo, A., Villar, J., & Lindheimer, M. (2008). Maternal infection and risk of preeclampsia: Systematic review and meta-analysis. *American Journal of Obstetrics & Gynecology, January,* 7–22.

Cunningham, F. G., Leveno, K. J., Bloom, S. L., Hauth, J. C., Gilstrap III, L. C., & Wenstrom, K. D. (2005). *Williams obstetrics* (22nd ed.). New York: McGraw-Hill.

Nicolaides, K. H. (2005). First-trimester screening for chromosomal abnormalities. *Seminars in Perinatology, 29,* 190–194.

U.S. Preventive Services Task Force. (2004). Recommendation statement: Screening for asymptomatic bacteriuria. Retrieved December 31, 2007, from http://www.ahrq.gov

Varney, H., Kriebs, J. M., & Gegor, C. L. (2004). *Varney's midwifery* (4th ed.). Sudbury, MA: Jones and Bartlett.

CHAPTER 11

The Expectant Family: Needs and Care

In my role, I have a very special opportunity to help women and their loved ones prepare for their new baby. I give them information about what to expect and answer their questions so that they can make more informed decisions. Sometimes I have to stop and remind myself to be clear about information that is important for any pregnant woman. Otherwise I might make the mistake of trying to impose my values. It is all too easy to view my way as the only way. When I do that, I fail them and I fail myself.

—A Registered Nurse Working in a Prenatal Clinic at an Inner-City Hospital

LEARNING OUTCOMES

11-1. Describe the most appropriate nursing care to help maintain the well-being of the expectant father and siblings during a family's pregnancy.

11-2. Examine the significance of cultural considerations in managing nursing care during pregnancy.

11-3. Explain the causes of the common discomforts of pregnancy in each of the three trimesters.

11-4. Describe appropriate measures and interventions to alleviate the common discomforts of pregnancy.

11-5. Describe self-care measures that a pregnant woman can take to maintain and promote her well-being during pregnancy.

11-6. Examine the concerns that the expectant couple may have about sexual activity.

11-7. Describe the medical risks and special concerns of the older expectant woman and her partner in managing nursing care to this population.

KEY TERMS

Fetal alcohol syndrome **248**
Fetal movement record (FMR) **237**
Kegel exercises **243**
Leukorrhea **233**
Lightening **236**
Pelvic tilt **243**
Ptyalism **233**
Teratogen **247**

From the moment a woman finds out she is pregnant, she faces a future marked by dramatic changes. Her appearance will alter. Her relationships will change. Even her psychologic state will be affected. In coping with these changes she will need to make adjustments in her daily life. So, too, will her family. The roles and responsibilities of family members may be altered as the woman's ability to perform certain activities changes. The family also must adapt psychologically to the expected arrival of a new member.

The expectant woman and her family will probably have many questions about the pregnancy and its impact on all of them, especially if this is a first pregnancy. In addition, the daily activities and healthcare practices of the woman become of concern when she and her family realize that what she does can affect the well-being of the unborn child. Nurses caring for pregnant women need a clear understanding of pregnancy to be effective in implementing the nursing process as they plan and provide care. With this need in mind, Chapter 9 ∞ provided a database for the nurse by presenting material related to the normal physical, social, cultural, and psychologic changes of pregnancy. Chapter 10 ∞ then used that database to begin a discussion of nursing care management by focusing on client assessment. This chapter further addresses nursing care management as it relates to the needs of the expectant woman and her loved ones.

Nursing Care During the Prenatal Period

The nurse may see a pregnant woman only once every 4 to 6 weeks during the first several months of her pregnancy. Therefore a written care plan or clinical pathway that incorporates the database, nursing diagnoses, and client goals is essential to ensure continuity of care.

Nursing Diagnosis

The nurse can anticipate that, for many women with a low-risk pregnancy, certain nursing diagnoses will be made more frequently than others. The diagnoses will, of course, vary from woman to woman and according to the time in the pregnancy. Examples of common nursing diagnoses include the following:

- Constipation related to the physiologic effects of pregnancy
- Ineffective Sexuality Patterns related to discomfort during late pregnancy

After formulating an appropriate diagnosis, the nurse and woman establish related goals to guide the nursing plan and interventions.

Nursing Plan and Implementation

Once nursing diagnoses have been identified, the next step is to establish priorities of nursing care. Sometimes priorities of care are based on the most immediate needs or concerns expressed by the woman. For example, during the first trimester, when she is experiencing nausea or is concerned about sexual intimacy with her partner, the woman is not likely to want to hear about labor and birth. At other times priorities may develop from findings during a prenatal examination. For example, a woman who is showing signs of preeclampsia (a pregnancy complication discussed in Chapter 15 ∞) may feel physically well and find it hard to accept the nurse's emphasis on the need for frequent rest periods. It then becomes the responsibility of medical and nursing professionals to help the woman and her family to understand the significance of a problem and to plan interventions to deal with it.

Community-Based Nursing Care

Prenatal care, especially for women with low-risk pregnancies, is community based, typically in a clinic or a private office. The healthcare community recognizes the value of providing a primary care nurse in these settings to coordinate holistic care for each childbearing family. The nurse in a clinic or health maintenance organization may be the only source of continuity for the woman, who may see a different physician or certified nurse–midwife at each visit. The nurse can be extremely effective in working with the expectant family by answering questions; providing complete information about pregnancy, prenatal healthcare activities, and community resources; and supporting the healthcare activities of the woman and her family.

Communities often have a wealth of services and educational opportunities available for pregnant women and their families, and the knowledgeable nurse can help expectant mothers to assess and access these services. This approach supports the family's assumption of equal responsibility with healthcare providers in working toward their common goal of a positive birth experience. See Key Facts to Remember: Key Antepartal Nursing Interventions.

Throughout the prenatal period, the nurse shares information with the family, both verbally and through written materials. This information is designed to help the family carry out self-care and wellness measures as needed and to report changes that may indicate a health problem. The nurse also provides anticipatory guidance to help the family plan for changes that will occur after childbirth. The expectant couple is encouraged to identify and discuss issues that could be sources of postpartal stress. Issues to be addressed beforehand may include the sharing of infant and household chores, help in the first few days after childbirth, options for baby-sitting to allow the mother (and couple) some free time, the mother's return to work after the baby's birth, and sibling rivalry. Couples resolve these issues in different ways, but postpartal adjustment tends to be easier for couples who agree on the issues beforehand than for couples who do not confront and resolve these issues.

HOME CARE   Home care can be of benefit to any pregnant woman, but it is especially effective in removing barriers for women who have difficulty accessing health care. These barriers may include lack of locally available healthcare facilities, problems with transportation to the facility, or schedule conflicts with available appointment times because of employment hours or family responsibilities.

In-home nursing assessments vary according to the experience and preparation of the nurse and include current history, vital signs, weight, urine screen, physical activity, dietary intake, reflexes, tests of fetal well-being, and cervical examinations, if indicated. Once the assessments are completed, the nurse can determine the level of follow-up home care or telephone contact needed.

A prenatal home care visit or phone contact can also be useful for women who anticipate a short inpatient stay after childbirth. At the prenatal contact, the nurse explains the postpartum program and answers any questions the woman or her family have. See Chapter 31 ∞ for further discussion of home care of the childbearing family.

Currently home care is most often used for women with prenatal complications that can be managed without hospitalization if effective nursing assessment and care are provided in the home (see Chapters 14 and 15 ∞).

Care of the Pregnant Woman's Family

The problems and concerns of the pregnant woman, the relief of her discomforts, and the maintenance of her physical, psychologic, and spiritual health receive much attention. However, her well-being is intertwined with the well-being of those to whom she is closest. Thus the nurse addresses the needs of the woman's family to help maintain the integrity of the family unit.

Care of the Father

Although the father of the baby is present in most cases, his presence cannot be assumed. If he is not part of the family structure, it is important to assess the woman's support system to determine which significant persons in her life will play a major role during this childbearing experience.

Anticipatory guidance of the expectant father, if he is involved in the pregnancy, is a necessary part of any plan of care. He may need information about the anatomic, physiologic, and emotional changes that occur during and after pregnancy, the couple's sexuality and sexual response, and the reactions that he is experiencing. He may wish to express his feelings about breastfeeding versus formula feeding, the sex of the child, his ability to parent, and other topics.

If it is culturally acceptable to the couple and personally acceptable to him, the nurse refers the couple to expectant parents' classes, such as those described in Chapter 8 ∞. These classes provide valuable information about pregnancy and childbirth, using a variety of teaching strategies such as discussion, films, demonstrations with educational models, and written handouts. Some classes even give the father the opportunity to get a "feel" for pregnancy by wearing a pregnancy simulator (Figure 11–1 ■). Such classes also offer the couple an opportunity to gain support from other couples.

The nurse assesses the father's intended degree of participation during labor and birth and his knowledge of what to expect. If the couple prefers that his participation be minimal or restricted, the nurse must support the decision.

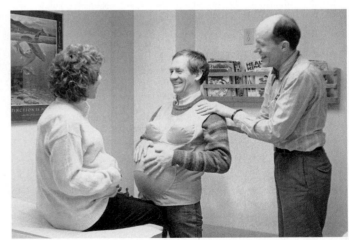

FIGURE 11–1 The Empathy Belly® is a pregnancy simulator that allows males and females to experience 20 of the symptoms of pregnancy. The "belly," which weighs 33 lb, produces symptoms such as shortness of breath, bladder pressure, shift in the center of gravity with resulting waddling gait, increased lordosis and backache, and fatigue. It also can simulate fetal kicking movements.
Source: Photograph courtesy of Birthways, Inc. at empathybelly.org

With this type of consideration and collaboration, the father is less apt to develop feelings of alienation, helplessness, and guilt during the pregnancy. As the couple's relationship is strengthened and the father's self-esteem increases, he is better able to provide physical and emotional support to his partner during labor and birth.

Care of Siblings and Other Family Members

The responses of siblings and other family members to the pregnancy are discussed in Chapter 9 ∞. These responses may include feelings of insecurity and even hostility. Thus, in the plan for prenatal care, the nurse incorporates a discussion about the negative feelings some children develop when anticipating the arrival of a sibling. Parents may be distressed to see an older child regress to "babyish" behavior or become aggressive toward the newborn. Parents who are unprepared for the older child's feelings of insecurity, anger, jealousy, and rejection may respond inappropriately in their confusion and surprise. The nurse emphasizes that open communication between parents and children (or acting out feelings with a doll if the child is too young to verbalize) helps children master their feelings. Children may feel less

---

TABLE 11–1	Cultural Beliefs and Practices During Pregnancy

Here are a few examples of cultural beliefs and practices related to pregnancy. It is important not to make assumptions about a client's beliefs, because cultural norms vary greatly within a culture and from generation to generation. The nurse should observe the client carefully and take the time to ask questions. Clients will benefit greatly from the nurse's increased awareness of their cultural beliefs and practices.

Belief or Practice	Nursing Consideration
Home Remedies Pregnant women of Native American background may use herbal remedies. An example is the dandelion, which contains a milky juice in its stem believed to increase breast milk flow in mothers who choose to breastfeed (Spector, 2004). Clients of Chinese descent may drink ginseng tea for faintness after childbirth or as a sedative when mixed with bamboo leaves. Some people of African heritage may use self-medication for pregnancy discomforts—for example, laxatives to prevent or treat constipation (Spector, 2009).	Find out what medications and home remedies your client is using, and counsel your client regarding overall effects. It is common for individuals to avoid telling healthcare workers about home remedies; the client may feel this will be judged unfavorably. Phrase your questions in a sensitive, accepting way.
Nutrition Some women of Italian background may believe that it is necessary to satisfy desires for certain foods in order to prevent congenital anomalies. Also, they may believe that they must eat food that they smell, or else the fetus will move "inside," which will result in a miscarriage. Pregnant women of African descent may continue the tradition of eating clay, dirt, or starch, which they believe will benefit the mother and fetus (Spector, 2009).	Discuss the client's beliefs and practices in regard to nutrition during pregnancy. Obtain a diet history from the client. Discuss the importance of a well-balanced diet during pregnancy, with consideration of the client's cultural beliefs and practices. In some cases, you might want to suggest remedies that may be more effective—for example, eating high-fiber foods to reduce constipation. If the home remedy is not harmful, there is no reason to ask a client to discontinue this practice.
Alternative Healthcare Providers Pregnant women of Mexican background may choose to seek out the care of a *partera* (midwife) for prenatal and intrapartal care. A partera speaks their language, shares a similar culture, and can care for pregnant women at home or in a birthing center instead of a hospital. Some people in Hispanic-American communities may use the *curandero*, the folk healer. The *curandero* frequently uses herbs, massage, and religious artifacts for treatment (Spector, 2009).	Discuss the variety of choices of healthcare providers available to the pregnant woman. Contrast the benefits and risks of different settings for prenatal care and birth. Provide reassurance that the goal of health care during pregnancy and birth is a healthy outcome for mother and baby, with respect for the specific cultural beliefs and practices of the client.
Exercise Pregnant women of Italian descent may fear changing their body position in certain ways because they believe this may cause the fetus to develop abnormally (Spector, 2009). Some people of European, African, and Mexican descent believe that reaching over the head during pregnancy can harm the baby.	Ask your client whether there are any activities she is afraid to do because of the pregnancy. Assure her that reaching over her head will not harm the baby, and evaluate other activities to their effect on the pregnancy.
Spirituality Navajo Indians are aware of the mind–soul connection and may try to follow certain practices to have a healthy pregnancy and birth. Practices could include focus on peace and positive thoughts as well as certain types of prayers and ceremonies. A traditional healer may assist them (Purnell & Paulanka, 2005). Some people of European background may tend to pay more attention to spirituality in their life to alleviate fears and ensure a safe birth.	Encourage the use of support systems and spiritual aids that provide comfort for the mother.

neglected and more secure if they know that their parents are willing to help with their anger and aggressiveness.

The nurse also addresses the couple's expectations of the grandparents, and encourages the couple to explore ways of dealing with any conflicts that may arise over childrearing approaches. Couples resolve these issues in different ways; however, postpartal adjustment is easier for a couple who acknowledges potential problems and develops a strategy beforehand than for a couple who does not confront and resolve these issues.

Cultural Considerations in Pregnancy

As discussed in Chapter 9 ∞, actions during pregnancy are often determined by cultural beliefs. Table 11–1 presents activities encouraged or forbidden during pregnancy by some specific cultures. The table is not meant to be all-inclusive, nor is it meant to imply that all members of a given culture hold these beliefs. Rather, it offers a few examples of cultural activities that may be important to some clients during the prenatal period.

In working with clients of other cultures, the health professional should be open to and respectful of other beliefs. Culturally competent nurses recognize that each childbearing family, shaped by culture and life experience, has expectations of both its members and the healthcare system during pregnancy and birth.

Language barriers often pose a challenge in providing effective prenatal nursing care. When possible, it is important to have an interpreter—family member, friend, or staff person—present at prenatal visits so the nurse can provide basic information about pregnancy and prenatal care. The nurse should also provide opportunities for the woman to ask questions or express concerns. It is essential to have printed material available in the woman's language. See Nursing Care Plan: Language Barriers at First Prenatal Visit.

CULTURAL PERSPECTIVES

Pregnant Women of African American Heritage

In caring for pregnant women of African American heritage, it is helpful to consider the following general points (Purnell & Paulanka, 2005):

- Pregnant African American women may be guided by their extended family into common practices such as geophagia, the ingestion of dirt or clay, which is believed to reduce mineral deficiencies. This practice has implications for the focus of teaching that a nurse offers.
- Many African American families are matriarchal. Women are respected and heeded in decision making and often stress good behavior and firm parenting with their children, especially to keep them safe in dangerous situations.
- Three-generation extended families are common, and the grandmother is often highly respected for her wisdom. She may play a critical role in the care of the children.
- Certain taboos may exist, such as the belief in the necessity to avoid taking pictures during pregnancy to prevent stillbirths. Some women of African American descent may also believe that the purchase of infant clothing or supplies can result in a stillbirth. Thus they may appear to be unprepared for the arrival of the baby.

Nursing Care Plan Language Barriers at First Prenatal Visit

CLIENT SCENARIO

Martina de Herrara and her husband arrived in the United States from Puerto Rico 6 months ago. This is her first prenatal visit since her pregnancy was confirmed 2 days ago. Martina's first child is 3 years old and was born in Puerto Rico. Their families live in Puerto Rico but Martina's mother has come to visit and help her get settled in their new home. Martina's husband speaks some English but is unable to attend the prenatal visit so she has brought her mother to the prenatal clinic. Spanish is Martina's native language. Both women speak very little English and seem uncomfortable as they wait for the physician. The nurse needs to complete a health history, collect some lab specimens, and get Martina scheduled for her next appointment.

ASSESSMENT

Subjective: Shaking head side to side, no eye contact, anxious

Objective: BP 128/82, pulse 84, respirations 16, height 5'4", weight 140 lb, urine negative for protein and glucose

---

Nursing Diagnosis	Ineffective Health Maintenance related to alteration in verbal and written communication skills*
Client Goal	The client will demonstrate understanding of health information received during prenatal visits.
AEB:	• Uses an interpreter to translate instructions. • Points to pictures and translated phrases on posters. • Uses hand gestures.

(Continued on next page)

Nursing Care Plan **Language Barriers at First Prenatal Visit** (Continued)

NURSING INTERVENTIONS	RATIONALES
1. Refer to posters with pictures to explain routine care and procedures during the prenatal exam.	*Rationale:* Posters help put words into visual images and are helpful in communicating information to the client.
2. Use teaching models to demonstrate procedures.	*Rationale:* Visual aids help to communicate information during the exam. Teaching models may include: plastic pelvis, knitted uterus, fetal model, breast model, birth control devices, ultrasound equipment, amniohook, fetal scalp electrode, and intrauterine pressure catheter.
3. Provide brochures about prenatal care in client's native language.	*Rationale:* Printed material should be available to clients in their native language. This reinforces information that was discussed during the visit and may be used as a reference at home. It also helps the family to understand what the client will experience during the pregnancy and at each visit.
4. Schedule an interpreter during prenatal visits.	*Rationale:* If a family member cannot translate the health information to the client then an independent interpreter should be provided. When an interpreter is used the nurse should be sure that the interpreter is translating the information received from the client and not answering the questions for the client.
5. Refer the client to prenatal classes taught in her native language.	*Rationale:* Prenatal classes taught in the same language as the client allow the client to receive health information that is easily understood, which will provide a better understanding of what to expect during prenatal visits and during labor and childbirth. A tour of the birthing unit may also be helpful. Prenatal classes may also provide a social outlet for clients.
6. Involve other members of the healthcare team to assist with prenatal care.	*Rationale:* Differences between cultures may not only involve verbal communication (language) but may also involve dietary differences as well as nonverbal expressions, usage of time, space (territorial), and silence. Usage of medication and receiving blood and blood products may also be driven by cultural beliefs. Social workers who are familiar with the client's cultural beliefs may help the client adjust to different healthcare practices while providing suggestions to adjust medical care that is more in line with the client's cultural beliefs. Dietitians may help the client plan meals that are more aligned to cultural practices while meeting the nutritional needs of pregnancy.

Evaluation of Client Goals

- Client responds appropriately to the nurse by using an interpreter.
- Client demonstrates understanding by pointing to pictures and phrases on posters.
- Client uses hand gestures to demonstrate understanding.

CRITICAL THINKING QUESTION

1. The nurse has arranged for an interpreter to attend the prenatal visit for a client who speaks Spanish. The woman has brought her mother, who speaks very little English, to the appointment. How can the nurse be assured that the information given is coming from the client?

Answer: The environment should be comfortable and relaxed. Friendly handshakes and smiles may help put the woman at ease. This may encourage a better exchange of information, which in turn assists the nurse in understanding the client's needs during the exam. Before the exam begins and before health information is collected, the nurse should let the interpreter know that the information should come from the woman herself. The interpreter only translates the conversation.

*For your reference, this care plan is an example of how one nursing diagnosis might be addressed.

Relief of the Common Discomforts of Pregnancy

The common discomforts of pregnancy result from physiologic and anatomic changes and are fairly specific to each of the three trimesters. Health professionals often refer to these discomforts as minor, but they are not minor to the pregnant woman. They can make her quite uncomfortable and, if they are unexpected, anxious. Table 11–2 identifies the common discomforts of pregnancy, their possible causes, and the self-care measures that might relieve the discomfort.

HINTS FOR PRACTICE

At each prenatal visit, focus your teaching on changes or possible discomforts the woman might encounter during the coming month and the next trimester. If the pregnancy is progressing normally, spend a few minutes describing her baby at that particular stage of development.

TABLE 11–2	Self-Care Measures for Common Discomforts of Pregnancy	
Discomfort	Influencing Factors	Self-Care Measures
First Trimester		
Nausea and vomiting	Increased levels of human chorionic gonadotropin Changes in carbohydrate metabolism Emotional factors Fatigue	Avoid odors or causative factors. Eat dry crackers or toast before arising in morning. Have small but frequent meals. Avoid greasy or highly seasoned foods. Take dry meals with fluids between meals. Drink carbonated beverages.
Urinary frequency	Pressure of uterus on bladder in both first and third trimesters	Void when urge is felt. Increase fluid intake during the day. Decrease fluid intake *only* in the evening to decrease nocturia.
Fatigue	Specific causative factors unknown May be aggravated by nocturia due to urinary frequency	Plan time for a nap or rest period daily. Go to bed earlier. Seek family support and assistance with responsibilities so that more time is available to rest.
Breast tenderness	Increased levels of estrogen and progesterone	Wear well-fitting, supportive bra.
Increased vaginal discharge	Hyperplasia of vaginal mucosa and increased production of mucus by the endocervical glands due to the increase in estrogen levels	Promote cleanliness by daily bathing. Avoid douching, nylon underpants, and pantyhose; cotton underpants are more absorbent; powder can be used to maintain dryness if not allowed to cake.
Nasal stuffiness and nosebleed (epistaxis)	Elevated estrogen levels	May be unresponsive, but cool-air vaporizer may help; avoid use of nasal sprays and decongestants.
Ptyalism (excessive, often bitter salivation)	Specific causative factors unknown	Use astringent mouthwashes, chew gum, or suck hard candy.
Second and Third Trimesters		
Heartburn (pyrosis)	Increased production of progesterone, decreasing gastrointestinal motility and increasing relaxation of cardiac sphincter, displacement of stomach by enlarging uterus, thus regurgitation of acidic gastric contents into the esophagus	Eat small and more frequent meals. Use low-sodium antacids. Avoid overeating, fatty and fried foods, lying down after eating, and sodium bicarbonate.
Ankle edema	Prolonged standing or sitting Increased levels of sodium due to hormonal influences Circulatory congestion of lower extremities Increased capillary permeability Varicose veins	Practice frequent dorsiflexion of feet when prolonged sitting or standing is necessary. Elevate legs when sitting or resting. Avoid tight garters or restrictive bands around legs.
Varicose veins	Venous congestion in the lower veins that increases with pregnancy Hereditary factors (weakening of walls of veins, faulty valves) Increased age and weight gain	Elevate legs frequently. Wear supportive hose. Avoid crossing legs at the knees, standing for long periods, garters, and hosiery with constrictive bands.

(Continued)

TABLE 11–2	Self-Care Measures for Common Discomforts of Pregnancy *(Continued)*	
Discomfort	Influencing Factors	Self-Care Measures
Second and Third Trimesters		
Hemorrhoids	Constipation (see following discussion) Increased pressure from gravid uterus on hemorrhoidal veins	Avoid constipation. Apply ice packs, topical ointments, anesthetic agents, warm soaks, or sitz baths; gently reinsert into rectum as necessary.
Constipation	Increased levels of progesterone, which cause general bowel sluggishness Pressure of enlarging uterus on intestine Iron supplements Diet, lack of exercise, and decreased fluids	Increase fluid intake, fiber in the diet, and exercise. Develop regular bowel habits. Use stool softeners as recommended by physician.
Backache	Increased curvature of the lumbosacral vertebrae as the uterus enlarges Increased levels of hormones, which cause softening of cartilage in body joints Fatigue Poor body mechanics	Use proper body mechanics. Practice the pelvic-tilt exercise. Avoid uncomfortable working heights, high-heeled shoes, lifting heavy loads, and fatigue.
Leg cramps	Imbalance of calcium/phosphorus ratio Increased pressure of uterus on nerves Fatigue Poor circulation to lower extremities Pointing the toes	Practice dorsiflexion of feet to stretch affected muscle. Evaluate diet. Apply heat to affected muscles. Arise slowly from resting position.
Faintness	Postural hypotension Sudden change of position causing venous pooling in dependent veins Standing for long periods in warm area Anemia	Avoid prolonged standing in warm or stuffy environments. Evaluate hematocrit and hemoglobin.
Dyspnea	Decreased vital capacity from pressure of enlarging uterus on the diaphragm	Use proper posture when sitting and standing. Sleep propped up with pillows for relief if problem occurs at night.
Flatulence	Decreased gastrointestinal motility leading to delayed emptying time Pressure of growing uterus on large intestine Air swallowing	Avoid gas-forming foods. Chew food thoroughly. Get regular daily exercise. Maintain normal bowel habits.
Carpal tunnel syndrome	Compression of median nerve in carpal tunnel of wrist Aggravated by repetitive hand movements	Avoid aggravating hand movements. Use splint as prescribed. Elevate affected arm.

First Trimester

The dramatic hormonal changes of the first trimester account for many of the discomforts experienced in this period. These discomforts tend to abate by the beginning of the fourth month of pregnancy.

Nausea and Vomiting

Nausea and vomiting of pregnancy (NVP) are early, very common symptoms occurring in 70% to 85% of pregnant women (American College of Obstetricians and Gynecologists [ACOG], 2004). These symptoms appear sometime after the first missed menstrual period and usually cease by the fourth missed menstrual period. Some women develop an aversion to specific foods, many experience nausea upon arising in the morning, and others experience nausea throughout the day or in the evening.

The exact cause of NVP is unknown, but it is thought to be multifactorial. An elevated human chorionic gonadotropin (hCG) level is believed to be a major factor, but changes in carbohydrate metabolism, fatigue, and emotional factors may also play a role. Research suggests that pregnant women should start taking a multivitamin before reaching 6 weeks' gestation to reduce the effects of NVP (ACOG, 2004).

In addition to the self-care measures identified in Table 11–2, certain complementary therapies may be useful. For example, many women find that acupressure applied to pressure points in the wrists is helpful (see Figure 11–2 ■). Ginger may also relieve NVP. (See Complementary and Alternative Therapies: Ginger for Morning Sickness.) Pyridoxine (vitamin B_6) or vitamin B_6 plus doxylamine (Unisom), an over-the-counter antihistamine, is considered a first-line treatment. Antihistamine H_1 receptor blockers, benzamines, and phenothiazines are considered safe and effective for treating refractory cases. In severe cases, methylprednisolone, a steroid, may be used, but as a last resort because it poses a potential risk to the fetus (ACOG, 2004).

A woman should be advised to contact her healthcare provider if she vomits more than once a day or shows signs

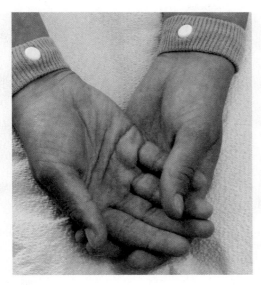

FIGURE 11–2 Acupressure wristbands are sometimes used to help relieve nausea during early pregnancy.

of dehydration such as dry mouth and concentrated urine. In such cases, the physician/certified nurse–midwife might order an antiemetic such as promethazine (Phenergan). However, antiemetics should be avoided if possible during this time because of possible harmful effects on embryonic development.

Urinary Frequency

Urinary frequency, a common discomfort of pregnancy, occurs early in pregnancy and again during the third trimester because of pressure of the enlarging uterus on the bladder. Although frequency is considered normal during the first and third trimesters, the woman is advised to report to her healthcare provider signs of bladder infection such as pain, burning with voiding, or blood in the urine. Fluid intake should never be decreased to prevent frequency. The woman needs to maintain an adequate fluid intake—at least 2,000 ml (eight to ten 8 oz glasses) per day. She should

COMPLEMENTARY AND ALTERNATIVE THERAPIES

Ginger for Morning Sickness

Women who experience nausea and vomiting of pregnancy (NVP) often try alternative approaches to relieve their symptoms because they are reluctant to take medication for fear of harming their fetus. Ginger, long used in traditional Chinese medicine for a variety of maladies ranging from gastrointestinal problems to headaches, is becoming an increasingly popular treatment for NVP and its safety has been demonstrated in clinical trials (White, 2007). Ginger is available in a variety of forms including the fresh root, capsules, tea, candy, cookies, crystals, inhaled powdered ginger, and sugared ginger (Lie, 2004). In the first trimester, the daily dosage should not exceed 2 g of dried ginger or 1 g of ginger syrup (Born & Barron, 2005).

also be encouraged to empty her bladder frequently (about every 2 hours while awake).

Fatigue

Marked fatigue is so common in early pregnancy that it is considered a presumptive sign of pregnancy. It is aggravated if the woman has to arise each night because of urinary frequency. Typically it resolves after the first trimester.

Breast Tenderness

Sensitivity of the breasts occurs early and continues throughout the pregnancy. Increased levels of estrogen and progesterone contribute to soreness and tingling of the breasts and increased sensitivity of the nipples.

Increased Vaginal Discharge

Increased whitish vaginal discharge, called **leukorrhea**, is common in pregnancy. It occurs as a result of hyperplasia of the vaginal mucosa and increased mucus production by the endocervical glands. The increased acidity of the secretions encourages the growth of *Candida albicans*, so the woman is more susceptible to monilial vaginitis.

Nasal Stuffiness and Epistaxis

Once pregnancy is well established, elevated estrogen levels may produce edema of the nasal mucosa, which results in nasal stuffiness, nasal discharge, and obstruction. *Epistaxis* (nosebleeds) may also result. Cool-air vaporizers and normal saline nasal sprays may help, but the problem is often unresponsive to treatment. Women experiencing these problems find it difficult to sleep and may resort to using medicated nasal sprays and decongestants. Such interventions may provide initial relief but can actually increase nasal stuffiness over time. Pregnant women should avoid using any medications, if possible.

Ptyalism

Ptyalism is a rare discomfort of pregnancy in which excessive, often bitter saliva is produced. The cause is unknown, and effective treatments are limited.

Second and Third Trimesters

It is more difficult to classify discomforts as specifically occurring in the second or third trimesters because many problems represent individual variations in women. The discomforts discussed in this section usually do not appear until the third trimester in primigravidas but may occur earlier with each succeeding pregnancy.

Heartburn (Pyrosis)

Heartburn (pyrosis) is the regurgitation of acidic gastric contents into the esophagus. It creates a burning sensation in the esophagus and sometimes leaves a bad taste in the mouth. Heartburn appears to be primarily a result of the displacement of the stomach by the enlarging uterus. The increased production of progesterone in pregnancy, decreases in gastrointestinal motility, and relaxation of the cardiac (gastroesophageal) sphincter also contribute to heartburn.

Liquid forms of low-sodium antacids are often most effective in providing relief. Women should be advised that antacids containing aluminum alone may cause constipation, whereas diarrhea is associated with antacids containing magnesium alone. Thus a combined antacid such as Maalox is often recommended. Sodium bicarbonate (baking soda) and Alka-Seltzer should be avoided because they may lead to electrolyte imbalance.

If maternal heartburn is severe, not relieved by antacids, and accompanied by gastrointestinal reflux, an antisecretory agent (H$_2$ blocker) such as ranitidine (Zantac), cimetidine (Tagamet), or omeprazole (Losec) may be indicated. Research to date has not linked them with an excessive risk of birth defects, preterm birth, or intrauterine growth restriction.

Ankle Edema

Most women experience ankle edema in the last part of pregnancy because of the increasing difficulty of venous return from the lower extremities. Prolonged standing or sitting and warm weather increase the edema. It is also associated with varicose veins. Ankle edema becomes a concern only when accompanied by hypertension or proteinuria or when the edema is not postural in origin.

Varicose Veins

Varicose veins are a result of weakening of the walls of veins or faulty functioning of the valves. Poor circulation in the lower extremities predisposes individuals to varicose veins in the legs and thighs, as does prolonged standing or sitting. Pressure of the gravid uterus on the pelvic veins prevents good venous return and may therefore aggravate existing problems or contribute to obvious changes in the veins of the legs (Figure 11–3 ■).

Treatment of varicose veins by surgery or injection is not generally recommended during pregnancy (Cunningham et al., 2005). The woman can be advised that treatment may be needed after she gives birth because the problem will be aggravated by subsequent pregnancies.

Although they are less common, varicosities in the vulva and perineum may also develop. They produce aching and a sense of heaviness. Wearing one of the foam rubber commercial products that is placed across the perineum and held in place by a sanitary pad type belt can provide support for vulvar varicosities (Cunningham et al., 2005). Elevation of only the legs aggravates vulvar varicosities by creating stasis of blood in the pelvic area. Therefore, it is im-

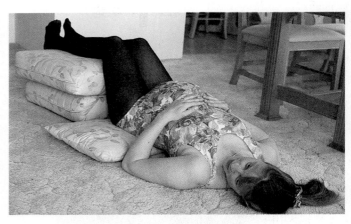

FIGURE 11–3 Swelling and discomfort from varicosities can be decreased by lying down with the legs and one hip elevated (to avoid compression of the vena cava).

portant that the pelvic area also be elevated to promote venous drainage into the trunk of the body. The woman may best relieve uterine pressure on the pelvic veins by resting on her side. Blocks may also be placed under the foot of her bed to elevate it slightly.

Flatulence

Flatulence results from decreased gastrointestinal motility, leading to delayed emptying, and from pressure on the large intestine by the growing uterus. Air swallowing may also contribute to the problem.

Hemorrhoids

Hemorrhoids are varicosities of the veins in the lower rectum and the anus. During pregnancy, the gravid uterus presses on the veins and interferes with venous circulation. In addition, the straining that accompanies constipation is frequently a contributing cause of hemorrhoids.

Some women may not be bothered by hemorrhoids until the postpartum, when pushing during the second stage of labor causes them to appear. These hemorrhoids usually become asymptomatic a few days after childbirth. Symptoms of hemorrhoids include itching, swelling, pain, and bleeding. Women who have had hemorrhoids before pregnancy will probably experience difficulties with them during pregnancy as well.

It is possible to find relief by gently reinserting the hemorrhoid. To do this, the woman lies on her side, places some lubricant on her finger, and presses against the hemorrhoids, pushing them inside. She holds them in place for 1 to 2 minutes and then gently withdraws her finger. The anal sphincter should then hold them inside the rectum. The woman will find it especially helpful if she can maintain a side-lying (Sims') position for a time, so this method is best done before bed or before a daily rest period.

The woman should contact her healthcare provider if the hemorrhoids become hardened and noticeably tender to touch. Rectal bleeding that is more than spotting following defecation should also be reported.

Constipation

Conditions that predispose the pregnant woman to constipation include general bowel sluggishness caused by increased progesterone and steroid metabolism; displacement of the intestines, which increases with the growth of the fetus; and the oral iron supplements most pregnant women need. In severe or preexisting cases of constipation, the woman may need stool softeners, mild laxatives, or suppositories as recommended by her caregiver.

Backache

Over 50% of women experience backache during pregnancy (Johnson, Gregory, & Niebyl, 2007). Backache is due primarily to exaggeration of the lumbosacral curve that occurs as the uterus enlarges and becomes heavier. Maintaining good posture and using proper body mechanics throughout pregnancy can help prevent backache. The pregnant woman is advised to avoid bending over at the waist to pick up objects and should bend from the knees instead (Figure 11–4 ■). She should place her feet 12 to 18 inches apart to maintain body balance. If the woman uses work surfaces that require her to bend, the nurse can advise the woman to adjust the height of the surfaces.

Leg Cramps

Leg cramps are painful muscle spasms in the gastrocnemius muscles. They occur most frequently after the woman has gone to bed at night but may occur at other times. Extension of the foot can often cause leg cramps. The nurse should warn the pregnant woman not to extend the foot during childbirth preparation exercises or during rest periods. The exact cause of leg cramps is not known, but pressure of the enlarged uterus on pelvic nerves or blood vessels leading to the legs may be a contributing factor (Varney et al., 2004), especially during the third trimester.

The woman can achieve immediate relief of the muscle spasm by stretching the muscle. With the woman lying on her back, another person presses the woman's knee down to straighten her leg while pushing her foot toward her leg. The woman may also stand and put her foot flat on the floor. Massage and warm packs can alleviate the discomfort

---

EVIDENCE-BASED PRACTICE

Preventing and Treating Back Pain in Pregnancy

Clinical Question

What are interventions that can prevent back pain in pregnancy? How can back pain be safely treated during the prenatal period?

The Evidence

A descriptive study of the prevalence of prenatal back pain revealed that more than two-thirds of pregnant women report back pain during pregnancy. Of these, 21% described the pain as "severe," 80% reported it interfered with sleep, and 75% took pain medication for relief. Unfortunately, 85% of these women reported they had not been offered any treatment for their pain. A systematic review of randomized trials revealed very little research dealing specifically with prevention of back pain. Eight studies examined the effects of exercise, physical therapy, acupuncture, and the use of sleep pillows to treat the pain. This aggregation of randomized trials comparing pain interventions to standard prenatal care represents the strongest level of evidence for practice.

What Is Effective?

Exercises to strengthen the lower back, including pelvic tilt exercises, reduced pain intensity. Water aerobics reduced pain severity and also decreased the number of missed work days because of pain. Acupuncture reduced pain intensity and provided relief from evening pain, and so helped with sleep. Supporting the back with standard bed pillows did not demonstrate any therapeutic effect. Mothers who received standard prenatal care with no back pain interventions reported more use of analgesics than mothers who used these treatments.

What Is Inconclusive?

How much pain relief is achieved by these methods, and how long the pain relief is sustained, is unclear. Aside from learning strengthening exercises, the benefits of physical therapy for back pain in pregnancy were inconclusive. It is not known if any of these interventions can prevent back pain from starting in the first place.

Best Practice

You should ask your clients if they are experiencing back pain during pregnancy, as most women do. Offer treatments that have been shown to be effective, such as strengthening exercises and water aerobics. The latter may help women miss less work and enable them to continue normal daily activities. Women who are considering acupuncture can be encouraged to pursue this option, as it has been shown to provide relief from pain, particularly in the evening. Helping mothers use these interventions may reduce their reliance on pharmacologic pain relievers.

References

Granath, A., Hellgren, M., & Gunnarsson, R. (2006). Water aerobics reduces sick leave due to low back pain during pregnancy. *JOGNN: Journal of Obstetric, Gynecologic, & Neonatal Nursing, 35*(4), 465–471.

Pennick, R., & Young, G. (2007). Interventions for preventing and treating pelvic and back pain in pregnancy. *Cochrane Database of Systematic Reviews,* 4.

Skaggs, C., Prather, H., Gross, G., George, J., Thompson, P., & Nelson, D. (2007). Back and pelvic pain in an underserved United States pregnant population: A preliminary descriptive survey. *Journal of Manipulative & Physiological Therapeutics, 30*(2), 130–134.

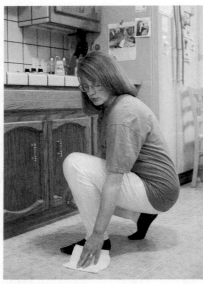

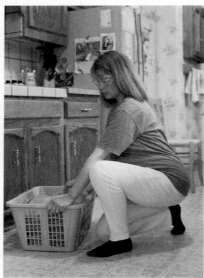

FIGURE 11–4 When picking up objects from floor level or lifting objects, the pregnant woman needs to use proper body mechanics.

of leg cramps (Figure 11–5 ■). In addition, to help prevent leg cramps, the caregiver may recommend a diet that includes daily portions of both calcium and phosphorus.

Faintness

Many pregnant women occasionally feel faint, especially in warm, crowded areas. Faintness is caused by a combination of changes in blood volume, and postural hypotension caused by pooling of blood in the dependent veins. Sudden change of position or standing for prolonged periods can also cause this sensation, and fainting can occur.

If a woman begins to feel faint from prolonged standing or from being in a stuffy room, she should sit down and lower her head between her knees. If this procedure does not help, the woman can be assisted to an area where she can lie down and get fresh air. When arising from a resting position, it is important that she move slowly. Women whose jobs re-

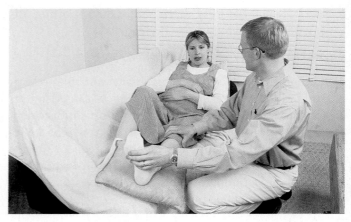

FIGURE 11–5 The expectant father can help relieve the woman's leg cramps by flexing her foot and straightening her leg.

quire standing in one place for long periods should march in place regularly to increase venous return from the legs.

Shortness of Breath (Dyspnea)

Shortness of breath occurs as the uterus rises into the abdomen and causes pressure on the diaphragm. This problem worsens in the last trimester because the enlarged uterus presses directly on the diaphragm, decreasing vital capacity. The primigravida experiences considerable relief from shortness of breath in the last few weeks of pregnancy, when **lightening** occurs, and the fetus and uterus move down in the pelvis. Because the multigravida does not usually experience lightening until labor, she tends to feel short of breath throughout the latter part of her pregnancy.

Difficulty Sleeping

Many physical factors in late pregnancy may make sleeping difficult. The enlarged uterus may make it difficult to find a comfortable position for sleep, and an active fetus may aggravate the problem. Other discomforts of pregnancy such as urinary frequency, shortness of breath, and leg cramps may also be contributing factors.

Round Ligament Pain

As the uterus enlarges during pregnancy, the round ligaments stretch and hypertrophy as the uterus rises up in the abdomen. Round ligament pain is attributed to this stretching. The woman may feel concern when she first experiences round ligament pain, because it is often intense and causes a "grabbing" sensation in the lower abdomen and inguinal area. The nurse should warn the pregnant woman of this possible discomfort. Once the caregiver has determined that the cause of the pain is not a medical complication such as appendicitis, the woman may find that applying a heating pad to the abdomen brings relief. Figure 3–6 shows the location of the round ligaments.

Carpal Tunnel Syndrome

Carpal tunnel syndrome, characterized by numbness and tingling of the hand near the thumb, occurs in about 25% to 50% of pregnant women (Johnson et al., 2007). It is caused by compression of the median nerve in the carpal tunnel of the wrist. The syndrome is aggravated by repetitive hand movements such as typing and may disappear following childbirth. Treatment usually involves splinting and avoiding aggravating movements. Surgery is indicated in severe cases if more conservative approaches are not effective.

Promotion of Self-Care During Pregnancy

Nurses can help promote maternal and fetal well-being by providing expectant couples with accurate, complete information about health behaviors and issues that can affect pregnancy and childbirth.

Fetal Activity Monitoring

Many caregivers encourage pregnant women to monitor their unborn child's well-being by regularly assessing fetal activity beginning at 28 weeks' gestation. Vigorous fetal activity generally provides reassurance of fetal well-being, whereas a marked decrease in activity or cessation of movement may indicate possible fetal compromise that requires immediate evaluation. Fetal activity is affected by fetal sleep, sound, time of day, blood glucose levels, cigarette smoking, and some illicit drugs such as crack and cocaine. At times a healthy fetus may be minimally active or inactive.

A variety of methods for tracking fetal activity have been developed. They focus on having the woman keep a **fetal movement record (FMR)** such as the Cardiff Count-to-Ten method (Figure 11–6 ■). An FMR is a noninvasive technique that enables the pregnant woman to monitor and record movements easily and without expense. See Client Teaching: What to Tell the Pregnant Woman About Assessing Fetal Activity.

Client Teaching WHAT TO TELL THE PREGNANT WOMAN ABOUT ASSESSING FETAL ACTIVITY

Content

Explain that fetal movements are first felt around 18 weeks' gestation. From that time the fetal movements get stronger and easier to detect. A slowing or stopping of fetal movement may be an indication that the fetus needs some attention and evaluation.

Explain the procedure for the Cardiff Count-to-Ten method or for the Daily Fetal Movement Record (DFMR). For both methods, advise the woman to

- Beginning at about 28 weeks' gestation, keep a daily record of fetal movement.
- Try to begin counting at about the same time each day, about 1 hour after a meal if possible.
- Lie quietly in a side-lying position.

Using the Cardiff card, have the woman place an X for each fetal movement until she has recorded 10. Movement varies considerably, but most women feel fetal movement at least 10 times in 3 hours (see Figure 11–6).

Using the DFMR, have the woman count three times a day for 20 to 30 minutes each session. If there are fewer than three movements in a session, have the woman count for 1 hour or more.

Explain when to contact the care provider:

- If there are fewer than 10 movements in 3 hours
- If overall the fetus's movements are slowing, and it takes much longer each day to note 10 movements
- If there are no movements in the morning
- If there are fewer than 3 movements in 8 hours

Teaching Method

Describe procedures and demonstrate how to assess fetal movement. Sit beside the woman and show her how to place her hand on the fundus to feel fetal movement.

Provide a written teaching sheet for the woman's use at home.

Demonstrate how to record fetal movements on a Cardiff Count-to-Ten scoring card or on a DFMR.
Watch the woman fill out the record as examples are provided. Encourage her to complete the record each day and bring it with her to each prenatal visit. Assure her that the record will be discussed at each prenatal visit, and questions may be addressed at that time if desired.

Provide the woman with a name and phone number in case she has further questions.

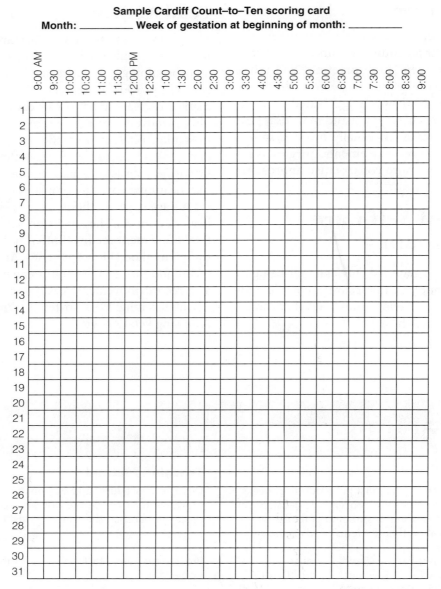

FIGURE 11—6 An adaptation of the Cardiff Count-to-Ten scoring card for fetal movement assessment.

Breast Care

Whether the pregnant woman plans to formula-feed or breastfeed her infant, support of the breasts is important to promote comfort, retain breast shape, and prevent back strain, particularly if the breasts become large and pendulous. The sensitivity of the breasts in pregnancy is frequently relieved by good support.

A well-fitting, supportive brassiere has the following qualities:

- The straps are wide and do not stretch (elastic straps soon lose their tautness with the weight of the breasts and frequent washing).
- The cup holds all breast tissue comfortably.

- The brassiere has tucks or other devices that allow it to expand, thus accommodating the enlarging chest circumference.
- The brassiere supports the nipple line approximately midway between the elbow and shoulder but is not pulled up in the back by the weight of the breasts.

Cleanliness of the breasts is important, especially as they begin producing colostrum. If colostrum crusts on the nipples, it can be removed with warm water. The woman planning to breastfeed is advised not to use soap on her nipples because of its drying effect.

Some women have flat or inverted nipples. True nipple inversion, which is rare, is usually diagnosed during the initial prenatal assessment. Breast shields designed to correct

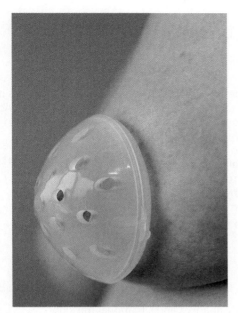

FIGURE 11–7 This breast shield is designed to increase the protractility of inverted nipples. Worn the last 3 to 4 months of pregnancy, it exerts gentle pulling pressure at the edge of the areola, gradually forcing the nipple through the center of the shield. It may be used after birth if necessary.

inverted nipples are effective for some women but others gain no benefit from them (Figure 11–7 ■). For further discussion of inverted nipples, see Chapter 27 ∞.

Clothing

Traditionally maternity clothes have been constructed with fuller lines to allow for the increase in abdominal size during pregnancy. However, maternity wear has changed in recent years and now also includes clothes that are more fitted, with little attempt to hide the pregnant abdomen. Maternity clothing can be expensive, however, and is worn for a relatively short time. Women can economize by sharing clothes with friends, sewing their own garments, or buying used maternity clothes.

High-heeled shoes tend to aggravate back discomfort by increasing the curvature of the lower back. They are best avoided if the woman experiences backache or has problems with balance. Shoes should fit properly and feel comfortable.

Bathing

Because perspiration and mucoid vaginal discharge increase during pregnancy, hygiene is important. Practices related to cleansing the body are often influenced by cultural norms; thus a pregnant woman may choose to cleanse only some portions of her body daily or may elect to take daily showers or tub baths. Caution is needed during tub baths because balance becomes a problem in late pregnancy. Rub-

ber mats and hand grips are important safety devices. Moreover, vasodilation caused by warm water may make the woman feel faint when she attempts to get out of the tub. Thus she may require assistance, especially during the last trimester. During the first trimester, pregnant women should avoid hyperthermia associated with the use of a hot tub or Jacuzzi, as it may increase risk for miscarriage or neural tube defects (Cunningham et al., 2005).

Employment

Pregnant women who have no complications can usually continue to work until they go into labor (American Academy of Pediatrics & ACOG, 2008). Although pregnant women who are employed in jobs that require prolonged standing (more than 5 hours) do have a higher incidence of preterm birth, this has no effect on fetal growth (Saade, 2007).

Overfatigue, excessive physical strain, fetotoxic hazards in the environment, and medical or obstetric complications are the major deterrents to employment during pregnancy. In the last half of pregnancy, occupations involving balance should be adjusted to protect the mother.

Fetotoxic hazards are always a concern to the expectant couple. The pregnant woman (or the woman contemplating pregnancy) who works in industry should contact her company physician or nurse about possible hazards in her work environment and should do her own reading and research on environmental hazards as well. Similarly, her partner can seek information about hazards in his workplace that might affect his sperm. See Nursing Care Plan: The Economically Disadvantaged Woman.

Travel

If medical or pregnancy complications are not present, there are no restrictions on travel. Pregnant women are advised to avoid travel if there is a history of bleeding or preeclampsia or if multiple births are anticipated.

Travel by automobile can be especially fatiguing, aggravating many of the discomforts of pregnancy. The pregnant woman needs frequent opportunities to get out of the car and walk. (A good pattern is to stop every 2 hours and walk around for approximately 10 minutes.) She should wear both lap and shoulder belts; the lap belt should fit snugly and be positioned under the abdomen and across the upper thighs. The shoulder strap should rest comfortably between the woman's breasts. Seat belts play an important role in preventing fetal and maternal morbidity and mortality with subsequent fetal death (Cesario, 2007). Fetal death in car accidents is also caused by placental separation (abruptio placenta) as a result of uterine distortion. Use of the shoulder belt decreases the risk of traumatic flexion of the woman's body, thereby decreasing the risk of placental separation.

Nursing Care Plan The Economically Disadvantaged Woman

CLIENT SCENARIO

Carol is 5 months pregnant when she visits the employee health nurse at the company where she works. Although she previously stayed at home caring for her 4-year-old son, Carol was recently divorced and is now working part time to handle the expenses she faces as a single parent. A close friend cares for her son while she works. Because her employer does not provide health insurance to part-time employees, Carol is looking for a full-time position that will include health insurance; however, with a limited employment history it is difficult for her to meet the hiring requirements for most jobs. Because she has not received any child support since the divorce, she is now behind on her mortgage and car payments. Being a divorced single parent and adjusting to the burden of a part-time job has placed stress on Carol and her pregnancy. During her first pregnancy, she had one hospital admission because of preterm labor. Carol is determined to pursue full-time employment and gain access to healthcare benefits so that she can begin prenatal care as soon as possible.

ASSESSMENT

Subjective: States that she has not received child support and describes outstanding debts

Objective: Part-time employment with no benefits and no prenatal care

Nursing Diagnosis	Altered Family Process related to insufficient family finances and situational transition*
Client Goal	The client will identify and use government and community resources to assist with financial support to maintain health and well-being.
AEB:	• Acquires health insurance. • Receives prenatal care. • Accesses community agencies for assistance. • Acquires and maintains full-time employment.

NURSING INTERVENTIONS

1. Assess financial resources.

2. Refer client to a financial counselor who provides services to women at no charge or on a sliding scale basis.

3. Provide a listing of agencies that offer information about housing assistance, access to food pantries, clothing distribution centers, and free health clinics within the community.

4. Assist the client with the Medicaid application process.

5. Refer the client to the Women, Infants, and Children (WIC) program.

RATIONALES

Rationale: Identifies clients who have limited resources to provide for adequate housing, medical care, and/or child care. Pregnant women who are economically disadvantaged may also suffer physical and psychologic problems.

Rationale: A financial counselor who is knowledgeable about financial support services in the community will be able to direct the client to appropriate agencies that assist in meeting the needs of economically disadvantaged women.

Rationale: Educating the woman about community resources enables her to access care that best meets her needs to promote health and well-being for herself and her family.

Rationale: Medicaid provides health care to low-income people and also finances maternity care. Women who receive adequate prenatal care have a greater chance for a positive birth outcome. Inadequate prenatal care or lack of care places the client at risk for having a low-birth-weight newborn and is also a risk factor for infant morbidity and mortality. The application process can be lengthy and frustrating; therefore assistance and support are needed.

Rationale: WIC is a health and nutrition program that is available to pregnant women, to mothers who are breastfeeding, and to children until the age of 5. Supplemental food is provided to participants; formula also is provided to women who are not breastfeeding. The WIC program also provides access to healthcare services. Women with household incomes that are less than the poverty level can qualify for WIC benefits.

(Continued on next page)

Nursing Care Plan The Economically Disadvantaged Woman (Continued)

6. Encourage the client to investigate job-training programs within local businesses.

Rationale: Job training may lead to a permanent full-time position with long-term employment possibilities. Full benefits, including health insurance, are usually provided to full-time employees. Another benefit may include a tuition reimbursement program for employees who want to return to school to obtain a college degree. Some employers offer support for childcare needs through referral programs or offer financial assistance.

7. Encourage the client to report lack of child support payments to the Department of Health and Human Services.

Rationale: A woman's standard of living is often decreased after divorce. This makes it especially hard when the woman has sole custody of the children and child support payments are not received. The United States Department of Justice actively investigates and prosecutes individuals who cross state lines to avoid paying child support.

Evaluation of Client Goals

• Client is enrolled in Medicaid and attends monthly prenatal appointments.
• Client is enrolled in a job-training program and will begin full-time employment at the end of training.

CRITICAL THINKING QUESTIONS

1. Describe ways a nurse can become involved in the community that would have a positive impact on economically disadvantaged women.

Answer: Nurses who are involved in community services and aware of the resources that these services provide can be a great asset to low-income families and impoverished women. Another way the nurse can make a difference in the lives of economically disadvantaged women is by supporting and voting for community leaders who support and lobby for increases in funding of various programs. Nurses can also use examples from client situations as part of a rationale that would support an increased need for funding various programs to benefit women and children.

2. A community health nurse is counseling a homeless pregnant woman in a free clinic. What are some of the challenges that healthcare providers might face as they care for this population of women?

Answer: Healthcare providers face many challenges as they support and assist homeless women. Because of limited resources and a lack of adequate funding for programs, homeless women are more likely to have inadequate prenatal care, limited access to health care in general, poor nutrition, and temporary or unsuitable living conditions. They are also at risk for illnesses and diseases that might jeopardize the health of the woman and her fetus during pregnancy, which may eventually lead to poor birth outcomes.

*For your reference, this care plan is an example of how one nursing diagnosis might be addressed.

As pregnancy progresses, long-distance trips are best taken by plane or train. Before flying the woman should check with her airline to see if they have any travel restrictions. To avoid the development of phlebitis or blood clots, pregnant women should drink plenty of fluid to avoid dehydration and hemoconcentration. They should also walk about the plane at regular intervals and change position frequently (Saade, 2007). Support stockings are also recommended (Johnson et al., 2007). Currently flying is considered safe up to 36 weeks' gestation in the absence of any complications. However, those women who have medical or obstetric complications such as poorly controlled diabetes, sickle cell disease, or preeclampsia, and those women with placental abnormalities or who are at risk for preterm birth are advised to avoid flying during pregnancy (ACOG, 2004). Availability of medical care at the destination is an important factor for the near-term woman who travels.

Activity and Rest

Exercise during pregnancy helps maintain maternal fitness and muscle tone, leads to improved self-image, promotes regular bowel function, increases energy, improves sleep, relieves tension, helps control weight gain, and is associated with improved postpartum recovery. Regular aerobic exercise maintains or improves a pregnant woman's general fitness and body image (Kramer, 2006). Normal participation in exercise can continue throughout an uncomplicated pregnancy and, in fact, is encouraged.

The woman can check with her certified nurse–midwife or physician about taking part in strenuous sports, such as skiing and horseback riding. In general, however, the skilled sportswoman is no longer discouraged from participating in these activities if her pregnancy is uncomplicated. However, pregnancy is not the appropriate time to learn a new sport.

Certain conditions contraindicate exercise. These conditions include rupture of the membranes, preeclampsia–eclampsia, incompetent cervix or cerclage placement, persistent vaginal bleeding in the second and third trimesters, risk factors for preterm labor or a history of preterm labor in the prior or current pregnancy, placenta previa after 26 weeks' gestation, and chronic medical conditions that might be negatively impacted by vigorous exercise such as significant heart disease (ACOG, 2002).

The following guidelines are helpful in counseling pregnant women about exercise:

- Even mild to moderate exercise is beneficial during pregnancy. Regular exercise—at least 30 minutes of moderate exercise daily or at least most days—is preferred (Penney, 2008).
- After the first trimester women should avoid exercising in the supine position. In most pregnant women, the supine position is associated with decreased cardiac output. Because uterine blood flow is reduced during exercise as blood is shunted from the visceral organs to the muscles, the remaining cardiac output is further decreased. Similarly, women should also avoid standing motionless for prolonged periods (ACOG, 2002; Penney, 2008).
- Because decreased oxygen is available for aerobic exercise during pregnancy, women should modify the intensity of their exercise based on their symptoms, should stop when they become fatigued, and should avoid exercising to the point of exhaustion. Non-weight-bearing exercises such as swimming and cycling are recommended because they decrease the risk of injury and provide fitness with comfort.
- As pregnancy progresses and the center of gravity changes, especially in the third trimester, women should avoid exercises in which the loss of balance could pose a risk to mother or fetus. Similarly, women should avoid any type of exercise that might result in even mild abdominal trauma.
- A normal pregnancy requires an additional 300 kcal per day. Women who exercise regularly during pregnancy should be careful to ensure that they consume an adequate diet.
- To augment heat dissipation, especially during the first trimester, pregnant women who exercise should wear clothing that is comfortable and loose, ensure adequate hydration, and avoid the prolonged overheating associated with vigorous exercise in hot, humid weather be-

cause of the possible teratogenic effects of hyperthermia on the fetus (Berk, 2004). For the same reason, pregnant women are advised to avoid hot tubs and saunas.

- As a result of the cardiovascular changes of pregnancy, heart rate is not an accurate indicator of the intensity of exercise for pregnant women (Wolfe & Weissgerber, 2003). If a pregnant, exercising woman is unable to maintain a conversation, then the exercise effort is too high (Saade, 2007).

The nurse may also suggest that the woman wear a supportive bra and appropriate shoes when exercising. She should be advised to warm up and stretch to help prepare the joints for activity and cool down with a period of mild activity to help restore circulation and avoid pooling of blood. A moderate, rhythmic exercise routine involving large muscle groups such as swimming, cycling, or brisk walking is best. Jogging or running is acceptable for women already conditioned to these activities as long as they avoid exercising at maximum effort and overheating.

During exercise, warning signs include pain of any kind, decreased or absent fetal movement, difficulty walking, dizziness, headache, muscle weakness, dyspnea before exertion, uterine contractions, vaginal bleeding, or fluid loss from the vagina (ACOG, 2002). The woman should stop exercising if these symptoms occur and modify her exercise program. If the symptoms persist, the woman should contact her caregiver.

Adequate rest in pregnancy is important for both physical and emotional health. Women need more sleep throughout pregnancy, particularly in the first and last trimesters, when they tire easily. Without adequate rest, pregnant

COMPLEMENTARY AND ALTERNATIVE THERAPIES

Yoga During Pregnancy

The following advice is important for women who practice yoga during pregnancy (Fontaine, 2005):

- During pregnancy, some yoga poses or positions are contraindicated. In particular pregnant women should avoid those poses that put pressure on the uterus as well as any extreme stretching positions.
- Because of the changed center of gravity that occurs as pregnancy progresses, women need to be especially careful to maintain balance when doing stretching.
- Pregnant women should avoid stomach-lying for any poses. After 20 weeks' gestation, women should lie on their left side rather than their back for floor positions.
- Pregnant women should immediately stop any pose that is uncomfortable.
- Warning signs that indicate the need to contact the physician or certified nurse–midwife immediately include the following: dizziness, extreme shortness of breath, sudden swelling, vaginal bleeding.

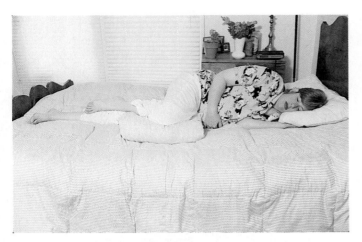

FIGURE 11–8 Position for relaxation and rest as pregnancy progresses.

women have less resilience. Finding time to rest during the day may be difficult for women who work outside the home or who have small children. The nurse can help the expectant mother examine her daily schedule to develop a realistic plan for short periods of rest and relaxation.

Sleeping becomes more difficult during the last trimester because of the enlarged abdomen, increased frequency of urination, and greater activity of the fetus. Finding a comfortable position becomes difficult for the pregnant woman. Figure 11–8 ■ shows a position most pregnant women find comfortable. Progressive relaxation techniques similar to those taught in prepared childbirth classes can help prepare the woman for sleep.

Exercises to Prepare for Childbirth

Certain exercises help strengthen muscle tone in preparation for birth and promote more rapid restoration of muscle tone after birth. Some physical changes of pregnancy can be minimized by faithfully practicing prescribed body-conditioning exercises. Many body-conditioning exercises for pregnancy are taught; a few of the more common ones are discussed here.

TEACHING TIP

Handouts are a valuable tool for providing information, as are pictures. When combined, they are especially useful. Develop a handout that describes the correct way to perform prenatal exercises and include drawings or photos. For exercises that may be new to a woman, such as the pelvic tilt, provide a handout for later reference, but also demonstrate it and have the woman do a return demonstration.

The **pelvic tilt**, or pelvic rocking, is an exercise that helps prevent or reduce back strain as it strengthens abdominal muscles. To do the pelvic tilt in early pregnancy, the woman lies on her back and puts her feet flat on the floor. This flexes

the knees and helps prevent strain or discomfort. She decreases the curvature in her back by pressing her spine toward the floor. With her back pressed to the floor, the woman tightens her abdominal muscles as she tightens and tucks in her buttocks. In the second and third trimesters of pregnancy, the woman can also perform the pelvic tilt on her hands and knees (Figure 11–9 ■), while sitting in a chair, or while standing with her back against a wall. The body alignment that results when the pelvic tilt is done correctly should be maintained as much as possible throughout the day.

HINTS FOR PRACTICE

Doing the pelvic rock on hands and knees may aggravate back strain. Teach women with a history of minor back problems to do the pelvic rock only in the standing position.

Abdominal Exercises

A basic exercise to increase abdominal muscle tone is tightening abdominal muscles with each breath. It can be done in any position, but it is best learned in early pregnancy. The woman lies supine with knees flexed and feet flat on the floor. The woman expands her abdomen and slowly takes a deep breath. Exhaling slowly, she gradually pulls in her abdominal muscles until they are fully contracted. She relaxes for a few seconds and then repeats the exercise. The pregnant woman should avoid the supine position after the first trimester.

Partial sit-ups strengthen abdominal muscle tone and are best done according to individual comfort levels. In early pregnancy partial sit-ups must be done with the knees flexed and the feet flat on the floor to avoid strain on the lower back. The woman stretches her arms toward her knees as she slowly pulls her head and shoulders off the floor to a comfortable level (if she has poor abdominal muscle tone, she may not be able to pull up very far). She then slowly returns to the starting position, takes a deep breath, and repeats the exercise while exhaling. To strengthen the oblique abdominal muscles, she repeats the process but stretches the left arm to the side of her right knee, returns to the floor, takes a deep breath, and then while exhaling reaches with the right arm to the left knee. During the second and third trimesters these exercises can be done on a large exercise ball. They can be done approximately five times in a sequence, and the sequence can be repeated at other times during the day as desired. It is important to do the exercises slowly to prevent muscle strain and overtiring.

Perineal Exercises

Perineal muscle tightening, also called **Kegel exercises**, strengthens the pubococcygeus muscle and increases its

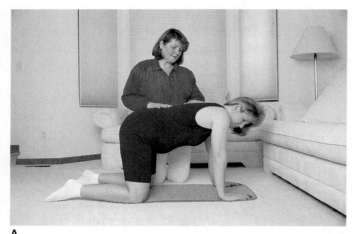

A

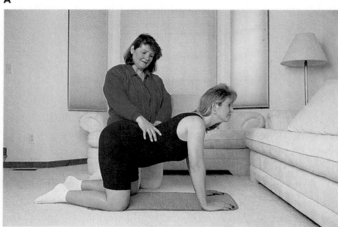

B

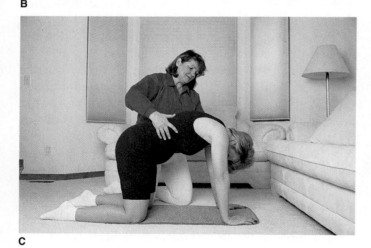

C

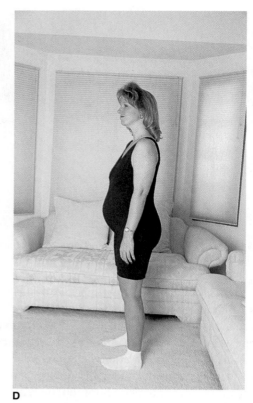

D

FIGURE 11–9 *A,* Starting position when the pelvic tilt is done on hands and knees. The back is flat and parallel to the floor, the hands are below the head, and the knees are directly below the buttocks. *B,* A prenatal yoga instructor offers pointers for proper positioning for the first part of the tilt: head up, neck long and separated from the shoulders, buttocks up, and pelvis thrust back, allowing the back to drop and release on an inhaled breath. *C,* The instructor helps the woman assume the correct position for the next part of the tilt. It is done on a long exhalation, allowing the pregnant woman to arch her back, drop her head loosely, push away from her hands, and draw in the muscles of her abdomen to strengthen them. Note that in this position the pelvis and buttocks are tucked under, and the buttock muscles are tightened. *D,* Proper posture. The knees are slightly bent but not locked, the pelvis and buttocks are tucked under, thereby lengthening the spine and helping support the weighty abdomen. With her chin tucked in, this woman's neck, shoulders, hips, knees, and feet are all in a straight line perpendicular to the floor. Her feet are parallel. This is also the starting position for doing the pelvic tilt while standing.

elasticity (Figure 11–10 ■). The woman can feel the specific muscle group to be exercised by stopping urination midstream. Doing Kegel exercises while urinating is discouraged, however, because this practice has been associated with urinary stasis and urinary tract infection.

Childbirth educators sometimes use the following technique to teach Kegel exercises. They tell the woman to think of her perineal muscles as an elevator. When she relaxes, the elevator is on the first floor. To do the exercises, she contracts, bringing the elevator to the second,

third, and fourth floors. She keeps the elevator on the fourth floor for a few seconds, and then gradually relaxes the area. If the exercise is properly done, the woman does not contract the muscles of the buttocks and thighs.

Kegel exercises can be done at almost any time. Some women use ordinary events—for instance, stopping at a red light—as a cue to remember to do the exercise. Others do Kegel exercises while waiting in a checkout line, talking on the telephone, or watching television.

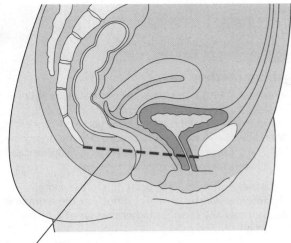

Pubococcygeus muscle with good tone

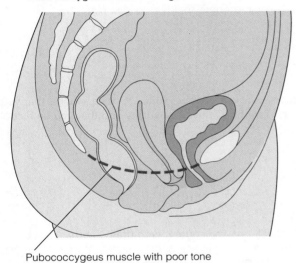

Pubococcygeus muscle with poor tone

FIGURE 11–10 Kegel exercises. The woman tightens the pubococcygeus muscle to improve support to the pelvic organs.

Inner Thigh Exercises

The nurse can advise the pregnant woman to assume a cross-legged sitting position when possible. This "tailor sit" stretches the muscles of the inner thighs in preparation for labor and birth.

Sexual Activity

As a result of the physiologic, anatomic, and emotional changes of pregnancy, couples usually have many questions and concerns about sexual activity during pregnancy. Often these questions are about possible injury to the baby or the woman during intercourse and about changes in the desire each partner feels.

In the past, couples were often warned to avoid sexual intercourse during the last 6 to 8 weeks of pregnancy to prevent complications such as infection or premature rupture of the membranes. However, these fears seem to be un-

founded. In a healthy pregnancy, there is no medical reason to limit sexual activity. Intercourse is contraindicated for medical reasons such as threatened spontaneous abortion or risk of preterm labor (Cunningham et al., 2005).

The expectant mother may experience changes in sexual desire and response. Often these changes are related to the various discomforts that occur throughout pregnancy. For instance, during the first trimester fatigue or nausea and vomiting may decrease desire, and breast tenderness may make the woman less responsive to fondling of her breasts. During the second trimester, many of the discomforts have lessened, and, with the vascular congestion of the pelvis, the woman may experience greater sexual satisfaction than she experienced before pregnancy.

During the third trimester, interest in coitus may again decrease as the woman becomes more uncomfortable and fatigued. In addition, shortness of breath, painful pelvic ligaments, urinary frequency, leg cramps, and decreased mobility may lessen sexual desire and activity. If they are not already doing so, the couple should consider coital positions other than male superior, such as side-by-side, female superior, and vaginal rear entry.

Sexual activity does not have to include intercourse. Many of the nurturing and sexual needs of the pregnant woman can be satisfied by cuddling, kissing, and being held. The warm, sensual feelings that accompany these activities can be an end in themselves. Her partner, however, may choose to masturbate more frequently than before.

The sexual desires of men are also affected by many factors in pregnancy. These factors include the previous relationship with the partner, acceptance of the pregnancy, attitudes toward the partner's change of appearance, and concern about hurting the expectant mother or baby. Some men find it difficult to view their partners as sexually appealing while they are adjusting to the concept of them as mothers. Other men find their partners' pregnancies arousing and experience feelings of increased happiness, intimacy, and closeness.

The expectant couple should be aware of their changing sexual desires, the normality of these changes, and the importance of communicating these changes to each other so that they can make nurturing adaptations. The nurse has an important role in helping the expectant couple adapt. It is important that the couple feel free to express concerns about sexual activity and that the nurse be able to respond and give anticipatory guidance in a comfortable manner. See Client Teaching: Sexual Activity During Pregnancy.

Dental Care

Proper dental hygiene is important in pregnancy because ensuring a healthy oral environment is essential to overall health. In spite of such discomforts as nausea and vomiting,

Client Teaching SEXUAL ACTIVITY DURING PREGNANCY

Content

Begin by explaining that the pregnant woman may experience changes in desire during the course of pregnancy. During the first trimester, discomforts such as nausea, fatigue, and breast tenderness may make intercourse less desirable for many women.

In the second trimester, as symptoms decrease, desire may increase. In the third trimester, discomfort and fatigue may lead to decreased desire in the woman.

Explain that men may notice changes in their level of desire, too. Among other things, this change may be related to feelings about their partner's changing appearance, their belief about the acceptability of sexual activity with a pregnant woman, or concern about hurting the woman or fetus. Some men find the changes of pregnancy erotic; others must adjust to the notion of their partners as mothers.

Explain that the woman may notice that orgasms are much more intense during the last weeks of pregnancy and may be followed by cramping. Because of the pressure of the enlarging uterus on the vena cava, the woman should not lie flat on her back for intercourse after about the fourth month. If the couple prefers that position, a pillow should be placed under her right hip to displace the uterus. Alternate positions such as side-by-side, female superior, or vaginal rear entry may become necessary as her uterus enlarges.

Stress that sexual activities that both partners enjoy are generally acceptable. It is not advisable for couples who favor anal sex to go from anal penetration to vaginal penetration because of the risk of introducing *Escherichia coli* into the vagina.

Suggest that alternative methods of expressing intimacy and affection such as cuddling, holding and stroking each other, and kissing may help maintain the couple's feelings of warmth and closeness. If the man feels desire for further sexual release, his partner may help him masturbate to ejaculation, or he may prefer to masturbate in private.

Advise the woman who is interested in masturbation as a form of gratification that the orgasmic contractions may be especially intense in later pregnancy.

Stress that sexual intercourse is contraindicated once the membranes are ruptured or if bleeding is present. Women with a history of preterm labor may be advised to avoid intercourse because the oxytocin that is released with orgasm stimulates uterine contractions and may trigger preterm labor. Because oxytocin is also released with nipple stimulation, fondling the breasts may also be contraindicated in those cases.

A discussion of sexuality and sexual activity should stress the importance of open communication so that the couple feels comfortable expressing feelings, preferences, and concerns.

Teaching Method

Universal statements that give permission, such as "Many couples experience changes in sexual desire during pregnancy. What kind of changes have you experienced?" are often effective in starting discussion. Depending on the woman's (or couple's) level of knowledge and sophistication, part or all of this discussion may be necessary.

If the partner is present, approach him in the same nonjudgmental way used above. If not, ask the woman if she has noticed any changes in her partner or if he has expressed any concerns.

Deal with any specific questions about the physical and psychologic changes that the couple may have.

Discussion about various sexual activities requires that you be comfortable with your sexuality and that you be tactful.

The couple may be content with these approaches to meeting their sexual needs, or they may require assurance that such approaches are indeed "normal."

An explanation of the contraindications accompanied by their rationale provides specific guidelines that most couples find helpful.

Some couples are skilled at expressing their feelings about sexual activity. Others find it difficult and can benefit from specific suggestions. The nurse should provide opportunities for discussion throughout the talk.

Specific handouts on sexual activity are also helpful for couples and may address topics that were not discussed.

gum hypertrophy and tenderness, possible ptyalism, and heartburn, it is important for pregnant women to maintain regular oral hygiene by brushing at least twice a day and flossing daily.

The nurse can encourage the pregnant woman to have a dental checkup early in her pregnancy. General dental repair and extractions can be done during pregnancy, preferably under local anesthetic. Dental treatment is safe throughout pregnancy; however, the second trimester is considered the most appropriate time for dental treatment because the risk of pregnancy loss tends to be lower and the woman tends to be more comfortable (Russell & Mayberry, 2008). The woman should inform her dentist of her pregnancy so that she is not exposed to teratogenic substances. Dental x-ray examinations and extensive dental work need to be delayed until after the birth when possible.

Immunizations

All women of childbearing age need to be aware of the risks of receiving certain immunizations if pregnancy is possible. Immunizations with attenuated live viruses, such as rubella vaccine, should not be given in pregnancy because of the teratogenic effect of the live viruses on the developing embryo. The most current recommendations on vaccines related to pregnancy should be obtained from the Centers for Disease Control and Prevention website.

Complementary and Alternative Therapy

As discussed in Chapter 2 ∞, many women are electing to use complementary and alternative medicine (CAM) such as homeopathy, herbal medicine, acupressure and acupuncture, biofeedback, therapeutic touch, massage, and chiropractic as part of a holistic approach to their healthcare regimens. The nurse should inquire about the use of CAM as part of a routine antepartal assessment. Nurses working with pregnant women and childbearing families need to develop a general understanding of the more commonly used therapies to be able to answer basic questions and to provide resources as needed.

It is important for the pregnant woman to understand that herbs are considered dietary supplements and are not regulated as prescription or over-the-counter drugs are through the FDA. Herbal products have not been studied for potential harmful effects on the fetus during pregnancy and therefore should be avoided, particularly in the first trimester (Born & Barron, 2005). The website of the National Center for Complementary and Alternative Medicine is a reliable source of information about herbs, homeopathic remedies, and other alternative options.

Teratogenic Substances

Substances that adversely affect the normal growth and development of the fetus are called **teratogens** (see Chapter 4 ∞). Many substances are known or suspected teratogens, including, for example, certain medications, psychotropic drugs, and alcohol. The harmful effects of others, such as some pesticides or exposure to x-rays in the first trimester of pregnancy, have also been documented. It is essential to provide pregnant women with information about recognized teratogens and environmental risks.

Medications

The use of medications during pregnancy, including prescriptions, over-the-counter drugs, and herbal remedies, is of great concern because maternal drug exposure is thought to account for at least 10% of birth defects (Black & Hill, 2003). Many pregnant women need medication for therapeutic purposes, such as the treatment of infections, allergies, or other pathologic processes. In these situations, the problem can be complex. Known teratogenic agents are not prescribed and usually can be replaced by medications considered safe. Even when a woman is highly motivated to avoid taking any medications, she may have taken potentially teratogenic medications before her pregnancy was confirmed, especially if she has an irregular menstrual cycle.

The greatest potential for gross abnormalities in the fetus occurs during the first trimester of pregnancy, when fetal organs are first developing. The classic period of teratogenesis in a woman with a 28-day cycle extends from day 31 after the LMP (17 days after fertilization) to day 71 (54 days after fertilization) (Niebyl & Simpson, 2007). Many factors influence teratogenic effects, including the specific type of teratogen and the dose, the stage of embryonic development, and the genetic sensitivity of the mother and fetus. For example, the commonly prescribed acne medication isotretinoin (Accutane) is associated with a high incidence of spontaneous abortion and congenital malformations if taken early in pregnancy.

To provide information for caregivers and clients, the U.S. Food and Drug Administration (FDA) has developed the following classification system for medications administered during pregnancy:

Category A: Controlled studies in women have demonstrated no associated fetal risk. Few drugs fall into this category.
Category B: Animal studies show no risk, but there are no controlled studies in women, or animal studies indicate a risk, but controlled human studies fail to demonstrate a risk. The penicillins fall into this category.
Category C: Either (1) no adequate animal or human studies are available or (2) animal studies show teratogenic effects, but no controlled studies in women are available.

Many drugs fall into this category, which, because of the lack of information, is a problematic one for caregivers. Epinephrine, beta-blockers, and zidovudine (a drug used to decrease perinatal transmission of human immunodeficiency virus) fall into this category.

Category D: Evidence of human fetal risk exists, but the benefits of the drug in certain situations are thought to outweigh the risks. Examples of drugs in this category include tetracycline, vincristine, lithium, and hydrochlorothiazide.

Category X: The demonstrated fetal risks clearly outweigh any possible benefit. Examples of drugs in this category include isotretinoin (Accutane), the acne medication, which can cause multiple central nervous system (CNS), facial, and cardiovascular anomalies.

If a woman has taken a drug in category D or X, she should be informed of the risks associated with that drug and of her alternatives. Similarly, a woman who has taken a drug in the safer categories can be reassured (Cunningham et al., 2005).

This system, although useful, has been criticized because the use of letters suggests a risk grading that is not necessarily accurate. More importantly, not all drugs in a category have the same risk level. Currently the FDA is working to develop a new labeling system (Cunningham et al., 2005).

Although the first trimester is the critical period for teratogenesis, some medications are known to have a teratogenic effect when taken in the second and third trimesters. For example, tetracycline taken in late pregnancy is commonly associated with staining of teeth in children and has been shown to depress skeletal growth, especially in premature infants. Sulfonamides taken in the last few weeks of pregnancy are known to compete with bilirubin attachment of protein-binding sites, increasing the risk of jaundice in the newborn (Niebyl & Simpson, 2007).

Pregnant women need to avoid all medication—prescribed, homeopathic, or over-the-counter—if possible. If no alternative exists, it is wisest to select a well-known medication rather than a newer drug whose potential teratogenic effects may not be known. When possible, the oral form of a drug should be used, and it should be prescribed in the lowest possible therapeutic dose for the shortest time possible. Finally, the caregiver needs to consider the multiple components of the medication. Caution is the watchword for nurses caring for pregnant women who have been taking medications. It is essential that pregnant women check with their certified nurse–midwives or physicians about any herbs or medications they were taking when pregnancy occurred and about any nonprescription drugs they are thinking of using. The advantage of using a particular medication must outweigh the risks. Any medication with possible teratogenic effects is best avoided.

Tobacco

In the United States, smoking during pregnancy is one of the most significant, modifiable causes of poor pregnancy outcomes. Smoking during pregnancy has a strong association with low-birth-weight infants. In addition, mothers who smoke have an increased risk of preterm birth, premature rupture of the membranes, fetal demise, placentae previa, abruptio placentae, premature rupture of membranes, and preterm birth (Hartmann, Wechter, Payne et al., 2007). Pregnant women who smoke as well as participate in other unhealthy behaviors, such as alcohol use, further increase their risk for low-birth-weight infants (Okah, Cai, & Hoff, 2005). Research also links maternal smoking, both during pregnancy and afterward, with an increased risk of sudden infant death syndrome (SIDS). Maternal smoking exposes young children to other risks of secondhand smoke including middle ear infections, acute and chronic respiratory tract illnesses, and behavioral and learning disabilities (Albrecht et al., 2004).

The specific mechanism of smoking's effect on the fetus is not known. However, the ingredients in cigarette smoke, such as carbon monoxide, nicotine, lead, and cotinine, are toxic to the fetus and decrease the availability of oxygen to maternal and fetal tissues (Cunningham et al., 2005).

In response to public health education campaigns in the United States, smoking during pregnancy has decreased significantly. In fact, approximately 46% of women who smoke quit during pregnancy. Unfortunately, 60% to 80% of women who quit smoking during their pregnancy resume smoking within a year after childbirth (ACOG, 2005). This finding suggests that although women are aware of the potential impact of smoking on the fetus, they may be less knowledgeable about the effects of passive smoke on the baby.

Any decrease in smoking during pregnancy most likely improves fetal outcome, and researchers continue to explore approaches designed to help women quit smoking. Pregnancy may be a difficult time for a woman to stop smoking, but the nurse should encourage her to reduce the number of cigarettes she smokes daily. The perceived need to protect her unborn child may increase her motivation.

Alcohol

Fetuses of women who drink heavily are at increased risk of developing **fetal alcohol syndrome** (Chapter 28 ∞). In fact, currently fetal alcohol syndrome, which is characterized by growth retardation, facial anomalies, and central nervous system dysfunction of varying severity, is the most common preventable cause of mental retardation in the United States. Moreover, women who have more than three drinks per week have an increased risk for miscarriage while those who have five or more drinks per week increase their risk for intrauterine death by two to three times that of women who are nondrinkers (Wisner, Sit, Reynolds, et al., 2007).

The effects of moderate intake of alcohol during pregnancy are unclear. Research indicates an increased incidence of lowered birth weight and some neurologic effects, such as attention deficit disorder. Evidence suggests that the risk of teratogenic effects increases proportionately with increased average daily intake of alcohol. Recent research also indicates that young adults who had heavy exposure to alcohol in utero are more likely to be problem drinkers than those who were not heavily exposed (Baer, Sampson, Barr et al., 2003).

Although an occasional drink during pregnancy does not carry any known risk, no safe level of drinking during pregnancy has been identified; thus caregivers recommend that pregnant women abstain from all alcohol during pregnancy. In most cases, once a woman becomes aware of her pregnancy, she decreases her consumption of alcohol. However, the alcohol consumed after conception and before pregnancy is diagnosed remains a cause for concern.

Assessment of alcohol intake is a major part of every woman's medical history, with questions asked in a direct, nonjudgmental manner. All women need to be counseled about the role of alcohol in pregnancy. If heavy consumption is involved, the nurse can refer the pregnant woman immediately to an alcoholic treatment program. Counselors in these programs need to be made aware of a woman's pregnancy before drug therapy is suggested, because certain drugs may be harmful to the developing fetus. For example, the drug disulfiram (Antabuse), often used in conjunction with alcohol treatment, is suspected to be a teratogenic agent.

Caffeine

Current research reveals no evidence that moderate caffeine intake has teratogenic effects in humans nor is it linked to IUGR, low birth weight, or preterm birth. However, high caffeine intake may be linked to an increased risk of miscarriage (Weng, Odouli, & Li, 2008). In addition, an increased risk of decreased birth weight has been found in infants of mothers who consume at least 600 mg of caffeine daily (Bracken, Triche, Belanger et al., 2003). (The average cup of brewed coffee has 100 mg, a 12-oz can of cola has about 50 mg, and a cup of tea has about 50 mg.) Until more definitive data are available, nurses can advise women about common sources of caffeine, including coffee, tea, colas, and chocolate, and suggest that they limit their caffeine intake to about 300 mg/day (Niebyl & Simpson, 2007).

> **EVIDENCE IN ACTION**
>
> *Any amount of alcohol consumption during pregnancy increases the risk for fetal central nervous system dysfunction.*
> (Advisory, evidence and recommendation) (U.S. Surgeon General's Advisory, 2005; Bailey & Sokol, 2008).

Marijuana

The prevalence of marijuana use in our society raises many concerns about its effect on the fetus, but, to date, no teratogenic effects of marijuana use during pregnancy have been documented (Schempf, 2007). Research on marijuana use in pregnancy is difficult, however, because it is an illegal drug. Unreliability of reporting, lack of a representative population, inability to determine strength or composition of the marijuana used (including the presence of herbicides), and use of other drugs at the same time are major factors complicating the research being done.

Cocaine

A woman who uses cocaine during pregnancy is at increased risk for acute myocardial infarction, cardiac arrhythmias, ruptured ascending aorta, seizures, cerebrovascular accidents, hyperthermia, bowel ischemia, and sudden death (Cunningham et al., 2005). Cocaine use during pregnancy has been related to abruptio placentae, premature rupture of the membranes, preterm birth, low birth weight, neonatal irritability, and neonatal depression (Schempf, 2007) as well as SIDS and developmental delays as a toddler (King, 2003). Several congenital anomalies in the newborn have also been linked to maternal cocaine use, including, for example, genitourinary anomalies, congenital heart defects, limb reduction defects, and CNS anomalies (Cunningham et al., 2005).

As the number of women of childbearing age using cocaine increases, healthcare providers must be alert to early signs of cocaine use. It is often difficult for a nurse or physician to face the fact that a client is using cocaine, but ongoing alertness and an open, nonjudgmental approach are important in early detection. Urine screening for cocaine is valuable, but because cocaine is metabolized rapidly, the drug screen is negative within 24 to 48 hours after cocaine use. Thus it is probable that many expectant mothers who use cocaine are not identified.

Evaluation

Throughout the antepartal period, evaluation is an ongoing and essential part of effective nursing care. As nurses ask questions of the pregnant woman and her family or make observations of physical changes, they are evaluating the results of previous interventions. In evaluating the effectiveness of the interactions, nurses can try creative solutions if they are logical and carefully thought out. Creative solutions are especially important in dealing with families from other cultures. If a practice is important to a woman and not harmful, the culturally competent nurse will not discourage it.

MyNursingKit | Abstracts of the Cochrane Review

In completing an evaluation, the nurse also recognizes situations that require referral for further evaluation. For example, a woman who has gained 4 lb in a single week does not require counseling about nutrition; she needs further assessment for preeclampsia. The nurse who has a sound knowledge of theory will recognize this need and act immediately. The ongoing and cyclic nature of the nursing process is especially evident in the prenatal setting. Throughout the course of pregnancy, however, certain criteria can be used to determine the quality of care provided. In essence, nursing care has been effective if the following occur:

- The common discomforts of pregnancy are quickly identified and are relieved or lessened effectively.
- The woman is able to discuss the physiologic and psychologic changes of pregnancy.
- The woman implements self-care measures, if they are indicated, during pregnancy.
- The woman avoids substances and situations that pose a risk to her well-being or that of her child.
- The woman seeks regular prenatal care.

Care of the Expectant Couple over Age 35

Today an increasing number of women are choosing to have their first baby after age 35. In fact, in the United States in 2005, 14.4% of all live births occurred to women age 35 or older. Moreover, the birth rates for women between the ages of 35 and 39 (46.3 births per 1,000 women) and between 40 and 44 (9.1 per 1,000) are the highest in more than three decades (Martin, Hamilton, Sutton et al., 2007). Many factors have contributed to this trend, including the following:

- Availability of effective birth control methods
- Availability of expanded roles and career options for women
- Increased number of women obtaining advanced education, pursuing careers, and delaying parenthood until they are established professionally
- Increased incidence of later marriage and second marriage
- High cost of living, which causes some young couples to delay childbearing until they are more secure financially
- Increased number of women in this older reproductive age group because of the baby boom between 1946 and 1964
- Increased availability of specialized fertilization procedures, which offer opportunities for women who had previously been considered infertile

There are advantages to having a first baby after age 35. Single women or couples who delay childbearing until they are older tend to be well educated and financially se-

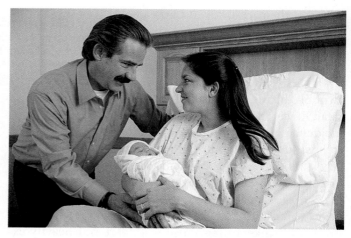

FIGURE 11–11 For many older couples, the decision to have a child may be very rewarding.

cure. In fact, over 40% of women age 30 or older who gave birth in 2005 had a bachelor's degree or higher (Martin et al., 2007). Moreover, their decision to have a baby is usually deliberately and thoughtfully made (Figure 11–11 ■). Because of their greater life experiences, they also tend to be more aware of the realities of having a child and what it means to have a baby at their age. Many of the women have experienced fulfillment in their careers and feel secure enough to take on the added responsibility of a child. Some women are ready to make a change in their lives, desiring to stay home with a new baby. Those who plan to continue working typically are able to afford good child care. See Key Facts to Remember: Pregnancy in Women over Age 35.

Medical Risks

In the United States and Canada over the past 30 years, the risk of death has declined dramatically for women of all ages because of advances in maternal health and obstetrical practice. However, the risk of maternal death is significantly higher for women over age 35, and even higher for

---

◆

KEY FACTS TO REMEMBER

Pregnancy in Women over Age 35

- Couples who choose pregnancy at a later age are usually financially secure and have made a thoughtful planned choice.
- The decreased fertility of women over age 35 may make conception more difficult.
- The incidence of Down syndrome increases somewhat in women over age 35 and significantly in those over age 40.
- The couple may choose to have amniocentesis or chorionic villus sampling to gain information about the health of their fetus.

women age 40 and older. This is true regardless of a woman's parity, the time at which she begins prenatal care, and her level of education (Callaghan & Berg, 2003).

Women over age 35 and, even more, women over age 40 are more likely to have chronic medical conditions that can complicate a pregnancy. Preexisting medical conditions such as hypertension or diabetes probably play a more significant role than age in maternal well-being and the outcome of pregnancy. The incidence of low-birth-weight infants, very preterm births, and perinatal death is higher among women age 35 or older (Delbaere, Verstralen, Goetgeluk et al., 2007). In addition, the rate of miscarriage is significantly higher in older women. Women over age 35 who become pregnant also have an increased risk for gestational diabetes mellitus, hypertension, placenta previa, difficult labor, and newborn complications (March of Dimes [MOD], 2006).

The cesarean birth rate is also increased in pregnant women over age 35. This practice may be related to pregnancy complications as well as to increased concern by the woman and physician about the pregnancy outcome (MOD, 2006).

The risk of conceiving a child with Down syndrome increases with age, especially over age 35. ACOG (2007) recommends that all pregnant women, regardless of age, be offered screening for Down syndrome. More and more facilities are now able to do first trimester ultrasound assessment of the thickness of the fetal nuchal fold (called *nuchal translucency* [NT]) combined with serum screens of free ß-hCG and pregnancy-associated plasma protein A (PAPP-A). This combination is useful in detecting Down syndrome, trisomy 18, and trisomy 13. If the screening results are not in the normal range, follow-up testing using ultrasound and amniocentesis are offered to the family (Cleveland Clinic, 2006). These tests are often combined with a *quad screen*, which is performed between 15 and 20 weeks' gestation. See Chapter 10 ∞.

Amniocentesis is routinely offered to all women over age 35 to permit the early detection of several chromosomal abnormalities, including Down syndrome. Routine genetic testing has not been offered to couples in whom there is only advanced paternal age because there is not sufficient evidence to determine a specific paternal age at which to start genetic testing. However, advanced paternal age affects autosomal dominant inherited diseases, such as neurofibromatosis, achondroplasia, and Marfan syndrome. Early pregnancy loss can be increased as a result of these mutations (Cunningham et al., 2005). Additionally, advanced paternal age increases the risk for late fetal death, especially if the father is 50 or older at the time of conception (Andersen, Hansen, Andersen, & Smith, 2004).

Special Concerns of the Expectant Couple over Age 35

No matter what their age, most expectant couples have concerns regarding the well-being of the fetus and their ability to parent. Expectant parents over age 35 often have additional concerns related to their age, especially the closer they are to age 40. Some couples are concerned about whether they will have enough energy to care for a new baby. Of greater concern is their ability to deal with the needs of the child as they age.

The financial concerns of the older couple are usually different from those of the younger couple. The older couple is generally more financially secure than the younger couple. However, when their "baby" is ready for college, the older couple may be close to retirement and might not have the means to provide for their child.

While considering their financial future and future retirement, the older couple may be forced to face their own mortality. Certainly the realization of one's mortality is not uncommon in midlife, but instead of confronting this issue at 40 to 45 years of age or later, the older expectant couple may confront the issue earlier as they consider what will happen as their child grows.

Older couples facing pregnancy following a late or second marriage or after therapy for infertility may find themselves somewhat isolated socially. They may feel different because they are often the only couple in their peer group expecting their first baby. In fact, many of their peers are likely to be parents of adolescents or young adults and may be grandparents as well.

The response of older couples who already have children to learning that the woman is pregnant may vary greatly depending on whether the pregnancy was planned or unexpected. Other factors influencing their response include their children's, family's, and friends' attitudes toward the pregnancy; the impact on their lifestyle; and the financial implications of having another child. Sometimes couples who had previously been married to other mates will choose to have a child together. The concept of blended family applies to situations in which "her" children, "his" children, and "their" children come together as a new family group.

Healthcare professionals may treat the older expectant couple differently than they would a younger couple. Older women may be offered more medical procedures, such as amniocentesis and ultrasound, than younger women. An older woman may be discouraged from using a birthing room or birthing center even if she is healthy because her age is considered to put her at risk.

The woman who has delayed pregnancy may be concerned about the limited amount of time that she has to bear children. When pregnancy does not occur as quickly as she had hoped, the older woman may become increasingly anxious as time ticks away on her "biological clock." When an older woman becomes pregnant but experiences a spontaneous abortion, her grief for the loss of her unborn child is exacerbated by her anxiety about her ability to conceive again in the time remaining to her.

Nursing Care Management

Nursing Assessment and Diagnosis

In working with a woman in her late 30s or 40s who is pregnant, the nurse makes the same assessments as are indicated in caring for any woman who is pregnant. The nurse assesses physical status, the woman's understanding of pregnancy and the changes that accompany it, the couple's attitudes about the pregnancy and their expectations of the impact a baby will have on their lives, any health teaching needs, the degree of support the woman has available to her, and the woman's knowledge of infant care.

The nursing diagnoses applicable to pregnant women in general apply to pregnant women over age 35. Examples of other nursing diagnoses that may apply include the following:

- *Decisional Conflict* related to unexpected pregnancy
- *Moderate Anxiety* related to uncertainty about fetal well-being

Nursing Plan and Implementation

Once an older couple has made the decision to have a child, it is the nurse's responsibility to respect and support the couple in this decision. As with any client, the nurse needs to discuss risks, identify concerns, and promote strengths. The woman's age should not be made an issue. It is helpful in promoting a sense of well-being for the nurse to treat the pregnancy as normal unless specific health risks are identified.

As the pregnancy continues, the nurse identifies and discusses concerns the woman may have related to her age or to specific health problems. The older woman who has made a conscious decision to become pregnant often has carefully thought through potential problems and may actually have fewer concerns than a younger woman or one with an unplanned pregnancy.

Childbirth education classes are important in promoting adaptation to the event of childbirth for expectant couples of any age. However, older expectant couples, who are still in the minority, often feel uncomfortable in classes in which most of the participants are much younger. Consequently, classes for expectant parents over age 35 are now available in many communities.

Women who are over age 35 and having their first baby tend to be better educated than other healthcare consumers. These clients frequently know the kind of care and services they want and may be assertive in their interactions with the healthcare system. The nurse should neither be intimidated by these individuals nor assume that anticipatory guidance and support are not needed. Instead, the nurse should support the couple's strengths and be sensitive to their needs.

For couples who decide to have amniocentesis, the first few months of pregnancy are a difficult time. Amniocentesis cannot be done until week 14 of pregnancy, and the chromosomal studies take roughly 2 weeks to complete. Their fear that the fetus is at risk may delay the successful completion of the psychologic tasks of early pregnancy.

The nurse can support couples who decide to have amniocentesis by providing information and answering questions about the procedure and by providing comfort and emotional support during the amniocentesis. If the results indicate that the fetus has Down syndrome or another genetic abnormality, the nurse can ensure that the couple has complete information about the condition, its range of possible manifestations, and its developmental implications.

Evaluation

Anticipated outcomes of nursing care include the following:

- The woman and her partner are knowledgeable about the pregnancy and express confidence in their ability to make appropriate healthcare choices.
- The expectant couple (and their children) are able to cope with the pregnancy and its implications for the future.
- The woman receives effective health care throughout her pregnancy and during birth and the postpartum period.
- The woman and her partner develop skills in child care and parenting.

CHAPTER HIGHLIGHTS

- Provision of anticipatory guidance about childbirth, the postpartum period, and childrearing is a primary responsibility of the nurse caring for women in an antepartal setting.

- The nurse assesses the expectant father's knowledge level and intended degree of participation and then works with the couple to help ensure a satisfying experience.
- Culturally based practices and proscribed activities may have an impact on the childbearing family.

- The common discomforts of pregnancy occur as a result of physiologic and anatomic changes. The nurse provides the woman with information about self-care activities aimed at reducing or relieving discomfort.
- To make self-care choices and acquire desired healthful habits, a pregnant woman requires accurate information about a range of subjects, from exercise to sexual activity and from bathing to immunization.
- Teratogenic substances are those that adversely affect the normal growth and development of the fetus.
- A pregnant woman should avoid taking prescribed medications or using over-the-counter preparations during pregnancy.
- Evidence exists that smoking, consuming alcohol, or using "social" drugs such as marijuana or cocaine during pregnancy may be harmful to the fetus.

- Maternal assessment of fetal activity keeps the woman "in touch" with her fetus and provides ongoing assessment of fetal status.
- Childbirth among women over age 35 is becoming increasingly common. It poses fewer health risks than previously believed and seems to offer advantages for the woman or couple who make the choice.
- A major risk for the older expectant couple relates to the increased incidence of Down syndrome in children born to women over age 35. Amniocentesis can provide information as to whether the fetus has Down syndrome. The couple can then decide whether they wish to continue the pregnancy.

EXPLORE mynursingkit

MyNursingKit is your one stop for online chapter review materials and resources. Prepare for success with additional NCLEX®-style practice questions, interactive assignments and activities, web links, animations and videos, and more!

Register your access code from the front of your book at
www.mynursingkit.com

CHAPTER REFERENCES

Albrecht, S. A., Maloni, J. A., Thomas, K. K., Jones, R., Halleran, J., & Osborne, J. (2004). Smoking cessation for pregnant women who smoke: Scientific basis for practice: AWHONN's SUCCESS Project. *Journal of Obstetric, Gynecologic, and Neonatal Nursing, 33*(3), 298–305.

American Academy of Pediatrics and the American College of Obstetricians and Gynecologists. (2008). *Guidelines for perinatal care* (6th ed.). Elk Grove Village, IL: Author.

American College of Obstetricians and Gynecologists (ACOG). (2002). *Exercise during pregnancy and the postpartum period* (ACOG Technical Bulletin No. 267). Washington, DC: Author.

American College of Obstetricians and Gynecologists (ACOG). (2004). *Diagnosis and treatment of nausea and vomiting in pregnancy* (ACOG Practice Bulletin No. 52). Washington, DC: Author.

American College of Obstetricians and Gynecologists (ACOG). (2005). *Smoking cessation during pregnancy* (Committee Opinion No. 316). Washington, DC: Author.

American College of Obstetricians and Gynecologists (ACOG). (2007). *Screening for fetal chromosomal abnormalities.* (ACOG Practice Bulletin No. 77). Washington, DC: Author.

Andersen, A. N., Hansen, K. D., Andersen, P. K., & Smith, G. D. (2004). Advanced paternal age and risk of fetal death: A cohort study.

American Journal of Epidemiology, 160(12), 1214–1222.

Baer, J. S., Sampson, P. D., Barr, H. M., et al. (2003). A 21-year longitudinal analysis of the effects of prenatal alcohol exposure on young adult drinking. *Archives of General Psychiatry, 60*(4), 377–385.

Bailey, B. A., & Sokol, R. J. (2008). Pregnancy and alcohol use: Evidence and recommendations for prenatal care. *Clinical Obstetrics and Gynecology, 51*(2), 436–444.

Berk, B. (2004). Recommended exercise during and after pregnancy: What the evidence says. *The International Journal of Childbirth Education, 19*(2), 18–22.

Black, R. A., & Hill, D. A. (2003). Over-the-counter medications in pregnancy. *American Family Physician, 67*(12), 2517–2524.

Born, D., & Barron, M. L. (2005). Herb use in pregnancy. *American Journal of Maternal Child Nursing, 30*(3), 201–206.

Bracken, M. B., Triche, E. W., & Belanger, K., et al. (2003). Association of maternal caffeine consumption with decrements in fetal growth. *American Journal of Epidemiology, 157*(5), 456–466.

Callaghan, W. M., & Berg, C. J. (2003). Pregnancy-related mortality among women aged 35 years and older, United States, 1991–1997. *Obstetrics and Gynecology, 102*(5, Pt 1), 1015–1021.

Cesario, S. K. (2007). Seat belt use in pregnancy. *Nursing for Women's Health, 11*(5), 474–481.

Cleveland Clinic. (2006). Quad marker screen. Retrieved May 27, 2008 from http://my. clevelandclinic.org/services/quad_marker_ screen/hic_quad_marker_screen.aspx

Cunningham, F. G., Leveno, K. J., Bloom, S. L., Hauth, J. C., Gilstrap III, L. C., & Wenstrom. K. D. (2005). *Williams obstetrics* (22nd ed.). New York: McGraw-Hill.

Delbaere, I., Verstraelen, H., Goetgeluk, S., Martens, G., DeBacker, G., & Temmerman, M. (2007). Pregnancy outcome in primiparae of advanced maternal age. *European Journal of Obstetrics, Gynecology, and Reproductive Biology, 135*(1), 41–46.

Fontaine, K. L. (2005). *Healing practices: Alternative therapies for nursing* (2nd ed.). Upper Saddle River, NJ: Prentice Hall.

Hartmann, K. E., Wechter, M. E., Payne, P., Salisbury, K., Jackson, R. D., & Melvin, C. L. (2007). Best practice smoking cessation and resource needs of prenatal care providers. *Obstetrics & Gynecology, 110*(4), 765–770.

Johnson, T. R. B., Gregory, K. D., & Niebyl, J. R. (2007). Preconception and prenatal care: Part of the continuum. In S. G. Gabbe, J. R. Niebyl, & J. L. Simpson (Eds.), *Obstetrics: Normal and problem pregnancies* (5th ed.). New York: Churchill-Livingstone.

King, D. E. (2003). Statistics: Cocaine use and infant development. *The International Journal of Childbirth Education, 18*(2), 15.

Kramer, M. S. (2006). Aerobic exercise for women during pregnancy. *Cochrane Library* (1), (Article 2006 No.CD000180).

Lie, D. (2004). Ginger helpful for nausea and vomiting of pregnancy. Medscape CME offering. Retrieved January 13, 2004, from www. medscape.com/viewarticle/466746_print

March of Dimes. (2006). Pregnancy after 35. Retrieved January 16, 2006, from www. marchofdimes.com/printableArticles/ 14332_1155.asp

Martin, J. A., Hamilton, B. E., Sutton, P. D., Ventura, S. J., Menacker, F., Kirmeyer, S., & Munson, M. L. (2007). Births: Final data for 2005. *National Vital Statistics Reports, 56*(6), 1–108.

Niebyl, J. R., & Simpson, J. L. (2007). Drugs and environmental agents in pregnancy and lactation: Embryology, teratology, epidemiology. In S. G. Gabbe, J. R. Niebyl, & J. L. Simpson (Eds.), *Obstetrics: Normal and problem pregnancies* (5th ed.). New York: Churchill-Livingstone.

Okah, F. A., Cai, J., & Hoff, G. L. (2005). Term gestation low birth weight and health

compromising behaviors during pregnancy. *Obstetrics and Gynecology, 105*(3), 543–550.

Penney, D. S. (2008). The effects of vigorous exercise during pregnancy. (2008). *Journal of Midwifery and Women's Health, 53*(2), 155–159.

Purnell, L. D., & Paulanka, B. J. (2005). *Guide to culturally competent health care.* Philadelphia: F. A. Davis.

Russell, S. L., & Mayberry, L. J. (2008). Pregnancy and oral health. *MCN: The American Journal of Maternal/Child Nursing, 33*(1), 32–37.

Saade, G. R. (2007). Occupational hazards. *Contemporary OB/Gyn, 52*(3), 59–68.

Schempf, A. H. (2007). Illicit drug use and neonatal outcomes: A critical review. *Obstetrical & Gynecological Survey, 62*(11), 749–757.

U. S. Surgeon General. (21). *U.S. Surgeon General Releases Advisory on Alcohol Use in Pregnancy.* Retrieved March 20, 2008, from http://www.hhs.gov/surgeongeneral/ pressreleases/sg02222005.html

Spector, R. E. (2009). *Cultural diversity in health and illness* (7th ed.). Upper Saddle River, NJ: Pearson/Prentice Hall.

Varney, H., Kriebs, J. M., & Gegor, C. L. (2004). *Varney's midwifery* (4th ed.). Sudbury, MA: Jones and Bartlett.

Weng, X., Odouli, R., & Li, D-K. (2008). Maternal caffeine consumption during pregnancy and the risk of miscarriage: A prospective cohort study. *American Journal of Obstetrics & Gynecology, 198*, 279.e1–279.e8.

White, B. (2007). Ginger: An overview. *American Family Physician, 75*, 1689–1691.

Wisner, K. L., Sit, D. K. Y., Reynolds, S. K., Altemus, M., Bogen, D. L., Sunder, K. R., et al. (2007). Psychiatric disorders. In S. G. Gabbe, J. R. Niebyl, & J. L. Simpson (Eds.), *Obstetrics: Normal and problem pregnancies* (5th ed.). Philadelphia: Churchill Livingstone.

Wolfe, L. A., & Weissgerber, T. L. (2003). Clinical physiology of exercise in pregnancy: A literature review. *Journal of Obstetrics and Gynaecology Canada, 25*(6), 473–483.

CHAPTER 12

Maternal Nutrition

When I was a nursing student I thought nutrition was boring—was I wrong! Now I know how important good nutrition is to every aspect of life, but especially to pregnancy, and I find it endlessly fascinating. When my enthusiasm sparks a response in a pregnant woman I am meeting with, I feel that I am having a long-term impact on the woman's life and hopefully on her family, too.

—A Nurse Working as a Patient Educator

LEARNING OUTCOMES

12-1. Describe the recommended levels of weight gain during pregnancy when providing nursing care for pregnant women.

12-2. Explain the significance of specific nutrients in the diet of the pregnant woman.

12-3. Compare nutritional needs during pregnancy, the postpartum period, and lactation with nonpregnant requirements.

12-4. Plan adequate prenatal vegetarian diets based on the nutritional requirements of pregnancy.

12-5. Explain the ways in which various physical, psychosocial, and cultural factors can affect nutritional intake and status in the nursing care management of pregnant women.

12-6. Compare recommendations for weight gain and nutrient intakes in the pregnant adolescent with those for the mature pregnant adult.

12-7. Examine the basic factors a nurse should consider when offering nutritional counseling to a pregnant adolescent.

12-8. Compare nutritional counseling issues for breastfeeding and formula-feeding mothers.

12-9. Apply the nursing process to support an optimal diet for the pregnant or postpartal woman.

KEY TERMS

Adequate intake (AI) 256
Calorie (cal) 260
Dietary reference intakes (DRIs) 256
Folic acid 264
Kilocalorie (kcal) 260

A woman's nutritional status before and during pregnancy can significantly influence her health and that of her fetus. In most prenatal clinics and offices, nurses offer nutritional counseling directly or work closely with the nutritionist in providing nutritional assessment and teaching.

This chapter focuses on the nutritional needs of a pregnant woman. Special sections consider the nutritional needs of the pregnant adolescent and the woman after giving birth.

The following factors influence a woman's ability to achieve good prenatal nutrition:

- *General nutritional status before pregnancy.* Nutritional deficits such as folic acid deficiency present at the time of conception and during the early prenatal period may influence the outcome of the pregnancy.
- *Maternal age.* An expectant adolescent must meet her own growth needs in addition to the nutritional needs of pregnancy.
- *Maternal parity.* The mother's nutritional needs and the outcome of the pregnancy are influenced by the number of pregnancies she has had and the interval between them.

Fetal growth occurs in three overlapping stages: (1) growth by increase in cell number, (2) growth by increases in cell number and cell size, and (3) growth by increase in cell size alone. Nutritional problems that interfere with cell division may have permanent consequences. If the nutritional insult occurs when cells are mainly enlarging, the changes are usually reversible when normal nutrition resumes.

Growth of fetal and maternal tissues requires increased quantities of essential dietary components. These are listed in the **dietary reference intakes (DRIs)** as specific allowances for pregnant and lactating women (Table 12–1). The DRIs are subdivided into the **recommended dietary allowance (RDA)** and **adequate intake (AI)**. An RDA is the daily dietary intake that is considered sufficient to meet the nutritional requirements of nearly all individuals in a specific life stage and gender group. An AI is a value cited for a nutrient when there is not sufficient data to calculate an estimated average requirement. Most of the recommended nutrients can be obtained by eating a well-balanced diet each day. The basic food groups, nutrients provided, and recommended amounts during pregnancy and lactation are presented in Table 12–2.

TABLE 12–1 Dietary Reference Intakes (DRIs) for Nonpregnant Females and for Pregnant and Lactating Females

	>Age	Vitamin A (mcg/d)	Vitamin D (mcg/d)	Vitamin E (mg/d α-tocopherol)	Vitamin K (mcg/d)	Vitamin C (mg/d)	Thiamine (mg/d)	Riboflavin (mg/d)	Niacin (mg/d)
Females	9–13 y	600	5*	11	60*	45	0.9	0.9	12
	14–18 y	700	5*	15	75*	65	1.0	1.0	14
	19–30 y	700	5*	15	90*	75	1.1	1.1	14
	31–50 y	700	5*	15	90*	75	1.1	1.1	14
	51–70 y	700	10*	15	90*	75	1.1	1.1	14
	>70 y	700	15*	15	90*	75	1.1	1.1	14
Pregnancy	≤18 y	750	5*	15	75*	80	1.4	1.4	18
	19–30 y	770	5*	15	90*	85	1.4	1.4	18
	31–50 y	770	5*	15	90*	85	1.4	1.4	18
Lactation	≤18 y	1200	5*	19	75*	115	1.4	1.6	17
	19–30 y	1300	5*	19	90*	120	1.4	1.6	17
	31–50 y	>1300	5*	19	90*	120	1.4	1.6	17

*Values are adequate intakes (AIs) rather than recommended dietary allowances (RDAs). All other values on the chart are RDAs.

Source: All data from the Institute of Medicine (1997–2001). Dietary reference intakes, Washington, DC: National Academy Press. Also available at www.nap.edu.

Maternal Weight Gain

Maternal weight gain is an important factor in fetal growth and infant birth weight. The optimal weight gain depends on the woman's weight for height (body mass index [BMI]) and her prepregnant nutritional state. An adequate weight gain indicates an adequate caloric intake. It does not, however, ensure that the woman has a sufficient nutrient intake. The pregnant woman must maintain the nutritional quality of her diet as her weight gain progresses.

The Institute of Medicine (IOM) (1992) recommends weight gains in terms of optimum ranges. Its recommendations are as follows:

- Underweight woman: 12.5–18 kg (28–40 lb)
- Normal-weight woman: 11.5–16 kg (25–35 lb)
- Overweight woman: 7–11.5 kg (15–25 lb)
- Obese woman: more than or equal to 7.0 kg (15 lb)

The average maternal weight gain is distributed as follows:

5.0 kg (11 lb)	Fetus, placenta, amniotic fluid
0.9 kg (2 lb)	Uterus
1.8 kg (4 lb)	Increased blood volume
1.4 kg (3 lb)	Breast tissue
2.3–4.5 kg (5–10 lb)	Maternal stores

The pattern of weight gain is important. The ideal pattern for a normal-weight woman consists of a gain of 1.6 to 2.3 kg (3.5 to 5 lb) during the first trimester, followed by a gain of about 0.5 kg (1 lb) per week during the second and third trimesters. The rate of weight gain in the second and third trimesters needs to be slightly higher for underweight women and slightly lower (0.7 lb per week [.3 kg]) for overweight women (IOM, 1990). A normal-weight woman who is expecting twins is advised to gain about 1.5 lb (.7 kg) per week during the second and third trimesters of her pregnancy. Inadequate maternal weight gain has been associated with preterm birth and its associated problems for the newborn (Salzberg, 2002).

Obesity is becoming a major health problem in many developed countries, and more and more women are entering pregnancy already overweight or obese. Obese pregnant women are at an increased risk for medical and pregnancy-related complications such as spontaneous abortion, gestational diabetes, preeclampsia, labor induction, and cesarean birth. They also have a higher incidence of fetal anomalies. They should be considered high risk and counseled accordingly (Morin & Reilly, 2007).

Maternal obesity also has implications for children. The children of overweight and obese mothers are predisposed to developing obesity and its related health concerns. In fact, the child of an overweight mother is three times more likely to be overweight by the age of 7 than a child of a normal-weight mother (Reece, 2008).

Because of the association between maternal weight gain and pregnancy outcome, most caregivers pay close attention to weight gain during pregnancy (Figure 12–1 ■). Weight gain charts can be useful in monitoring the rate and pattern of weight gain over time.

EVIDENCE IN ACTION

Maternal obesity and high body mass increases the risk for a cesarean birth. (Meta-analysis) (Chu, Kim, Schmid, Dietz, Callaghan, Lau, & Curtis, 2007)

Vitamin B$_6$ (mg/d)	Folate (mcg/d)	Vitamin B$_{12}$ (mcg/d)	Calcium (mg/d)	Phosphorus (mg/d)	Magnesium (mg/d)	Iron (mg/d)	Zinc (mg/d)	Iodine (mcg/d)	Selenium (mcg/d)
1.0	300	1.8	1300*	1250	240	8	8	120	40
1.2	400	2.4	1300*	1250	360	15	9	150	55
1.3	400	2.4	1000*	700	310	18	8	150	55
1.3	400	2.4	1000*	700	320	18	8	150	55
1.5	400	2.4	1200*	700	320	8	8	150	55
1.5	400	2.4	1200*	700	320	8	8	150	55
1.9	600	2.6	1300*	1250	400	27	12	220	60
1.9	600	2.6	1000*	700	350	27	11	220	60
1.9	600	2.6	1000*	700	360	27	11	220	60
2.0	500	2.8	1300*	1250	360	10	13	290	70
2.0	500	2.8	1000*	700	310	9	12	290	70
2.0	500	2.8	1000*	700	320	9	12	290	70

TABLE 12–2 Daily Food Plan for Pregnancy and Lactation

Food Group	Nutrients Provided	Food Source	Recommended Daily Amount During Pregnancy	Recommended Daily Amount During Lactation
Dairy products	Protein; riboflavin; vitamins A, D, and others; calcium; phosphorus; zinc; magnesium	Milk—whole, 2%, skim, dry, buttermilk	Four (8 oz) cups (five for teenagers) used plain or with flavoring, in shakes, soups, puddings, custards, cocoa	Four (8 oz) cups (five for teenagers); equivalent amount of cheese, yogurt, and so forth
		Cheeses—hard, semisoft, cottage	Calcium in 1 cup milk equivalent to 1½ cups cottage cheese, 1½ oz hard or semisoft cheese, 1 cup yogurt, 1½ cups ice cream (high in fat and sugar)	
		Yogurt—plain, low-fat		
		Soybean milk—canned, dry		
Meat and meat alternatives	Protein; iron; thiamine, niacin, and other vitamins; minerals	Beef, pork, veal, lamb, poultry, animal organ meats, fish, eggs; legumes; nuts, seeds, peanut butter, grains in proper vegetarian combination (vitamin B$_{12}$ supplement needed)	Three servings (one serving = 2 oz), combination in amounts necessary for same nutrient equivalent (varies greatly)	Two servings
Grain products, whole grain or enriched	B vitamins; iron; whole grain also has zinc, magnesium, and other trace elements; provides fiber	Breads and bread products such as cornbread, muffins, waffles, hotcakes, biscuits, dumplings, cereals, pastas, rice	Six to 11 servings daily: one serving = one slice bread, ¾ cup or 1 oz dry cereal, ½ cup rice or pasta	Same as for pregnancy
Fruits and fruit juices	Vitamins A and C; minerals; raw fruits for roughage	Citrus fruits and juices, melons, berries, all other fruits and juices	Two to four servings (one serving for vitamin C): one serving = one medium fruit, ½–1 cup fruit, 4 oz orange or grapefruit juice	Same as for pregnancy
Vegetables and vegetable juices	Vitamins A and C; minerals; provides roughage	Leafy green vegetables; deep yellow or orange vegetables such as carrots, sweet potatoes, squash, tomatoes; green vegetables such as peas, green beans, broccoli; other vegetables such as beets, cabbage, potatoes, corn, lima beans	Three to five servings (one serving of dark green or deep yellow vegetable for vitamin A): one serving = ½–1 cup vegetable, two tomatoes, one medium potato	Same as for pregnancy
Fats	Vitamins A and D; linoleic acid	Butter, cream cheese, fortified table spreads; cream, whipped cream, whipped toppings; avocado, mayonnaise, oil, nuts	As desired in moderation (high in calories): one serving = 1 tbsp butter or enriched margarine	Same as for pregnancy
Sugar and sweets		Sugar, brown sugar, honey, molasses	Occasionally, if desired	Same as for pregnancy
Desserts		Nutritious desserts such as puddings, custards, fruit whips, and crisps; other rich, sweet desserts and pastries	Occasionally, if desired	Same as for pregnancy
Beverages	Fluid	Coffee, decaffeinated beverages, tea, bouillon, carbonated drinks	As desired, in moderation	Same as for pregnancy
Miscellaneous		Iodized salt, herbs, spices, condiments	As desired	Same as for pregnancy

Note: The pregnant woman should eat regularly, three meals a day, with nutritious snacks of fruit, cheese, milk, or other foods between meals if desired. (More frequent but smaller meals are also recommended.) Between 4 to 6 (8 oz) glasses of water and a total of 8 to 10 (8 oz) cups total fluid intake should be consumed daily. Water is an essential nutrient.

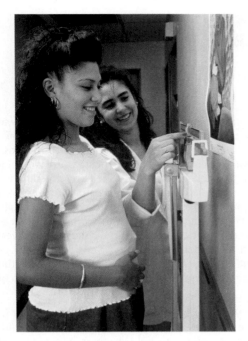

FIGURE 12–1 It is important to monitor a pregnant woman's weight over time.
Source: Michael Newman/Photo Edit

Excessive weight gain during pregnancy also has long-term implications because weight gain during pregnancy is by far the most important predictor of the amount of weight that a woman will retain following childbirth (Walker, 2007). Counseling the pregnant woman to eat a variety of nutrients from each of the food groups places less emphasis on the amount of her weight gain and more on the quality of her intake. It may also be helpful to encourage her to begin a simple exercise program such as walking. The newly designed food group pyramid, renamed MyPyramid in 2005, offers users a colorful plan that emphasizes variety, proportionality, moderation, and physical activity. It is also designed to help guide individuals to make healthier choices (Figure 12–2 ■).

HINTS FOR PRACTICE

Weight varies with time of day, amount of clothing, inaccurate scale adjustment, or weighing error. Do not overemphasize a single weight but pay attention to the overall pattern of weight gain.

Nutritional Requirements

The RDA for almost all nutrients increases during pregnancy, although the amount of increase varies with each nutrient. These increases reflect the additional requirements of both the mother and the developing fetus (see Table 12–1). Folic acid and iron are the only nutritional supplements generally recommended during pregnancy. The increased need for other vitamins and minerals can usually be met with an adequate diet. To avoid possible deficiencies, however, most healthcare professionals recommend a daily vitamin supplement.

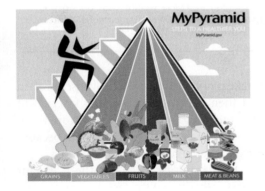

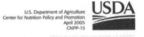

FIGURE 12–2 MyPyramid: Steps to a Healthier You identifies the basic food groups and provides guidance about healthful eating. Grains, vegetables, fruits, and dairy products are emphasized with slightly less emphasis on protein. The narrow yellow bar is designated for fats, sugar, and salt. People are encouraged to have most of their fat intake come from fish, nuts, and vegetable oils while limiting solid fats like butter, margarine, shortening, and lard. The emphasis is also placed on limiting added sugars, which contribute calories but few, if any, nutrients.
Source: U.S. Department of Agriculture; U.S. Department of Health and Human Services.

EVIDENCE-BASED PRACTICE

Managing Excessive Weight Gain of Pregnancy

Clinical Question

How can excessive weight gain in pregnancy be prevented? How can it be managed if it occurs?

The Evidence

Excessive prenatal weight gain is a serious condition that impacts not only a mother's physical and mental health but also the future health of her babies. Up to 20% of women may retain excessive weight after pregnancy, increasing their vulnerability to a host of lifelong health problems. The Association of Women's Health, Obstetric, and Neonatal Nurses published an integrative review of research related to preventing and treating excessive weight gain in pregnancy. Seven studies were evaluated in an integrative review that focused on either prenatal prevention or postnatal interventions aimed at reducing long-term weight gain. Integrative reviews combine multiple research designs and represent the strongest level of evidence for holistic professions such as nursing.

What Is Effective?

Women who are overweight before pregnancy, African-American women, and women who have been treated for infertility are the most vulnerable to excessive gestational weight gain. Prenatal prevention activities are not as successful as postnatal interventions in managing long-term weight change. Interventions that began immediately after birth and lasted at least 10 weeks have the greatest success. Weight losses for women ranged from 4.8 to 7.8 kg, with larger losses associated with longer interventions. Each successful program included the use of reduced-calorie diets, exercise, behavioral coaching, and motivational content.

What Is Inconclusive?

Contrary to commonly held belief, breastfeeding was not shown to be protective against weight retention after pregnancy. Although exclusive breastfeeding for 6 months postpartum was associated with a small postpartum weight loss in one study, these effects were not seen if breastfeeding was not exclusive or was discontinued early. Postpartum interventions, although found efficacious, were tested almost exclusively with White women, so success with women of other ethnic backgrounds is not assured. Culturally sensitive interventions may need to be developed for women from specific ethnic communities. None of the studies mentioned postpartum depression and any impact it might have on weight outcomes.

Best Practice

Although you may be able to identify women at risk for excessive prenatal weight gain, it may be a difficult condition to prevent. Interventions to help mothers lose excess weight should begin immediately after birth and should include low-calorie diets of 1500 calories per day and an exercise component equal to walking 2 miles five times a week. Behavioral content delivered through group meetings and motivational content via telephone contact supplement the mother's physical efforts. Longer programs, lasting at least 10 weeks, are the most successful.

References

Smith, S., Hulsey, T., & Goodnight, W. (2008). Effects of obesity on pregnancy. *JOGNN: The Journal of Obstetric, Gynecologic, and Neonatal Nursing, 37*(2),176–184.

Walker, L. (2007). Managing excessive weight gain during pregnancy and the postpartum period. *JOGNN: The Journal of Obstetric, Gynecologic, and Neonatal Nursing, 36*(5), 490–500.

Calories

The term **calorie (cal)** designates the amount of heat required to raise the temperature of 1 g of water 1°C. The **kilocalorie (kcal)** is equivalent to 1000 cal and is the unit used to express the energy value of food.

The RDA for energy requirements during pregnancy recommends no increase during the first trimester but an increase of 300 kcal/day during the second and third trimesters. Prepregnant weight, height, maternal age, health status, and activity level all influence caloric needs, and weight should be monitored regularly during the pregnancy. Client Teaching: Helping the Pregnant Woman Add 300 Kcal to Her Diet (page 261) offers suggestions for providing basic nutritional information to pregnant women.

Carbohydrates

Carbohydrates provide the body's primary source of energy as well as the fiber necessary for proper bowel functioning. If the total caloric intake is not adequate, the body uses protein for energy. Protein then becomes unavailable for growth needs. In addition, protein breakdown leads to ketosis. Ketosis can be a problem, especially in diabetic women, because of glycosuria, reduced alkaline reserves, and lipidemia.

The carbohydrate and caloric needs of the pregnant woman increase, especially during the last two trimesters. Carbohydrate intake promotes weight gain and growth of the fetus, placenta, and other maternal tissues. Dairy products, fruits, vegetables, and whole-grain cereals and breads all contain carbohydrates and other important nutrients.

Protein

Protein supplies the amino acids (nitrogen) required for hyperplasia and hypertrophy of maternal tissues, such as the uterus and breasts, and to meet fetal needs. The fetus makes its greatest demands during the last half of pregnancy, when fetal growth is greatest. Protein also contributes to the body's overall energy metabolism.

Client Teaching HELPING THE PREGNANT WOMAN ADD 300 KCAL TO HER DIET

Content

Describe the basic food groups, which include the following:

Grains: 6 to 11 servings (one serving = 1 slice bread, ½ hamburger roll, 1 oz dry cereal, 1 tortilla, ½ cup pasta, rice, grits)

Fruits: Two to four servings; one should be a good source of vitamin C (one serving = 1 medium-sized piece of fruit, ½ cup juice)

Vegetables: Three to five servings (one serving = 1 cup raw vegetable, 1 cup green leafy vegetable, ½ cup cooked vegetable)

Dairy: Two to three servings (one serving = 1 cup milk or yogurt, 1.5 oz hard cheese, 2 cups cottage cheese, 1 cup pudding made with milk)

Meats and alternatives: Two to three servings (one serving = 2 oz cooked lean meat, poultry, or fish; 2 eggs; ½ cup cottage cheese; 1 cup cooked legumes [kidney, lima, garbanzo, or soybeans, split peas]; 6 oz tofu; 2 oz nuts or seeds; 4 tbsp peanut butter)

Point out that not all foods that are nutritionally equivalent have the same number of calories; it is important to consider that when making food choices.

Explain the Food Guide Pyramid

The Food Guide Pyramid is designed to represent the food groups needed to make a balanced diet. The grain, fruit, and vegetable groups are at the base of the pyramid and should account for the majority of the food selections. Fewer servings of dairy and meat or meat alternative are required in the diet, and these groups fall in the middle portion of the pyramid. The very top of the pyramid represents fats, oils, and sweets. These items do not have a high nutritional value and should be used sparingly.

Emphasize that a woman only has to add 300 kcal/day during pregnancy. This can be achieved by adding two milk servings and one serving of meat or alternative. Because of the varying caloric value, a woman needs to consider the advisability of using low-fat milk, lean cuts of meat, or fish broiled or baked instead of fried.

Foods can be combined. For example, 1 cup spaghetti with a 2 oz meatball would count as 1 serving meat, ¾ cup spaghetti = 1 grain, and ¼ cup tomato sauce = ½ serving vegetable.

Teaching Method

Ask woman if she has received nutritional information using this approach before. Discuss her understanding of it. Use that information to plan the amount of detail you will use.

Use a chart or colorful handout to explain the basic food groups and to give examples of equivalent foods.

Use a calorie-counting guide to compare the calories in a variety of foods that are equivalent, such as 2 oz beef and 2 oz fish or 1 cup low-fat milk and 1 cup whole milk.

Use a similar approach to evaluate the calories in fats, oils, and sweets, but also evaluate their nutrient content, especially levels of nutrients such as vitamin C, iron, and calcium.

In planning the woman's diet to get optimum nutrition without too many additional calories, it is often helpful to ask her to plan and evaluate a sample menu.

Provide handouts on which the woman can list the foods she has eaten and check off the corresponding nutrient categories. Have her bring her completed handouts to a subsequent visit.

The protein requirement for the pregnant woman is 60 g/day, an increase of 14 g over nonpregnant levels. Animal products such as meat, fish, poultry, and eggs are sources of high-quality protein. Dairy products are also important protein sources. A quart of milk supplies 32 g of protein, more than half the average daily protein requirement. Milk can be incorporated into the diet in a variety of dishes, including soups, puddings, custards, sauces, and yogurt. Beverages such as hot chocolate and milk-and-fruit drinks can also be included, but they are high in calories. Various kinds of hard and soft cheeses and cottage cheese are excellent protein sources, although cream cheese is categorized as a fat source only.

Women who have allergies to milk, are lactose intolerant, or practice vegetarianism may find soy milk acceptable. Soy milk can be used in cooked dishes or as a beverage. Tofu, or soybean curd, can replace cottage cheese.

Fat

Fats are valuable sources of energy for the body. Fats are more completely absorbed during pregnancy, resulting in a marked increase in serum lipids, lipoproteins, and cholesterol and decreased elimination of fat through the bowel. Fat deposits in the fetus increase from about 2% at midpregnancy to almost 12% at term. However, fat requirements are unchanged during pregnancy and should account for about 30% of daily caloric intake, of which less than 10% should be saturated fat.

Minerals

Increased minerals needed for the growth of new tissue during pregnancy are obtained by improved mineral absorption and an increase in mineral allowances.

Calcium and Phosphorus

Calcium and phosphorus are involved in the mineralization of fetal bones and teeth as well as acid–base buffering. Calcium is absorbed and used more efficiently during pregnancy. Some calcium and phosphorus are required early in pregnancy, but most fetal bone calcification occurs during the last 2 to 3 months. Teeth begin to form at about 8 weeks' gestation and are formed by birth. The 6-year molars begin to calcify just before birth.

The identified adequate intake for calcium for the pregnant or lactating woman 19 years of age or older is 1000 mg per day. It is 1300 mg/day for pregnant women under age 19. If calcium intake is low, fetal needs will be met at the mother's expense by demineralization of maternal bone.

A diet that includes 4 cups of milk or an equivalent alternative (such as calcium-fortified soy milk or orange juice) and a variety of other foods will provide sufficient calcium. Smaller amounts of calcium are supplied by legumes, nuts, dried fruits, and dark green leafy vegetables (such as kale, cabbage, collards, and turnip greens); however, the calcium in these foods is absorbed more efficiently than the calcium in dairy foods. Note that some of the calcium in beet greens, spinach, and chard is bound with oxalic acid, which makes it less available to the body.

The RDA for phosphorus does not change from that of the nonpregnant woman age 19 or older: 700 mg per day. Similarly for females age 18 and younger it remains stable at 1250 mg per day. Phosphorus is readily supplied through calcium- and protein-rich foods.

Iodine

Iodine is an essential part of the thyroid hormone thyroxine. Inorganic iodine is excreted in the urine during pregnancy. Enlargement of the thyroid gland may occur if iodine is not replaced by adequate dietary intake or an additional supplement. Moreover, cretinism may occur in the infant if the mother has a severe iodine deficiency. The iodine requirement of 220 mcg per day can be met by using iodized salt. When sodium is restricted, the physician may prescribe an iodine supplement.

Sodium

The sodium ion is essential for proper metabolism and the regulation of fluid balance. Sodium intake in the form of salt is never entirely curtailed during pregnancy, even when hypertension or preeclampsia is present. The pregnant woman may season food to taste during cooking but should avoid using extra salt at the table. She can avoid excessive intake by eliminating salty foods such as potato chips, ham, sausages, and sodium-based seasonings.

Zinc

Zinc is involved in protein metabolism and the synthesis of DNA and RNA. It is essential for normal fetal growth and development as well as milk production during lactation. The RDA during pregnancy for women age 19 and older is 11 mg per day. This increases to 12 mg during lactation. Sources include meats, shellfish, poultry, whole grains, and legumes.

Magnesium

Magnesium is essential for cellular metabolism and bone mineralization. The RDA for pregnancy is 320 mg/day. Good sources include milk, whole grains, dark green vegetables, nuts, and legumes.

Iron

Iron requirements increase during pregnancy because of the growth of the fetus and placenta and the expansion of maternal blood volume. Anemia in pregnancy is mainly caused by low iron stores, although it may also be caused by inadequate intake of other nutrients such as vitamins B_6 and B_{12}, folic acid, ascorbic acid, copper, and zinc. Iron deficiency anemia is defined as a decrease in the oxygen-carrying capacity of the blood. Anemia leads to a significant reduction in hemoglobin in the volume of packed red cells per deciliter of blood (hematocrit) or in the number of erythrocytes. Iron deficiency anemia in pregnancy is associated with an increased incidence of low-birth-weight infants and preterm birth (National Institutes of Health [NIH], 2007a).

Fetal demands for iron further contribute to symptoms of anemia in the pregnant woman. The fetal liver stores iron, especially during the third trimester. The infant needs this stored iron during the first 4 months of life to compensate for the normally inadequate levels of iron in breast milk and non-iron-fortified formulas.

To prevent anemia, the woman must balance iron requirements and intake. Adequate iron intake is a problem for nonpregnant women and a greater one for pregnant women. By carefully selecting foods high in iron, the woman can increase her daily iron intake considerably. Lean meats, dark green leafy vegetables, eggs, and whole-grain and enriched breads and cereals are the usual food sources of iron. Other iron sources include dried fruits, legumes, shellfish, and molasses.

Iron absorption is generally higher for animal products than for vegetable products. However, the woman can enhance absorption of iron from nonmeat sources by combining them with meat or a food rich in vitamin C. The RDA for iron during pregnancy is 27 mg/day, but the most iron that can be reasonably obtained through diet is about 15 to 18 mg/day. Thus the pregnant woman needs a supplement of simple iron salt, such as ferrous gluconate, ferrous fumarate, or ferrous sulfate. The amount necessary is provided by most prenatal vitamins. Unfortunately iron supplements often cause gastrointestinal discomfort, especially if taken on an empty stomach. Consequently, caregivers often begin iron supplements in the second trimester after the incidence of nausea and vomiting subsides. Iron supplements may also cause constipation, so an adequate intake of fluid and fiber is especially important in pregnancy.

Vitamins

Vitamins are organic substances necessary for life and growth. They are found in small amounts in specific foods and generally cannot be synthesized by the body in adequate amounts.

Vitamins are grouped according to solubility. Vitamins that dissolve in fat are A, D, E, and K; those soluble in water include vitamin C and the B complex. An adequate intake of all vitamins is essential during pregnancy; however, several are required in larger amounts to fulfill specific needs.

Fat-Soluble Vitamins

Fat-soluble vitamins A, D, E, and K are stored in the liver and thus are available if the dietary intake becomes inadequate. The major complication related to these vitamins is not deficiency but toxicity caused by overdose. Unlike water-soluble vitamins, excess amounts of vitamins A, D, E, and K are not excreted in the urine. Symptoms of vitamin toxicity include nausea, gastrointestinal upset, dryness and cracking of the skin, and loss of hair.

VITAMIN A   Vitamin A is involved in the growth of epithelial cells, which line the entire gastrointestinal tract and compose the skin. Vitamin A plays a role in the metabolism of carbohydrates and fats. In the absence of vitamin A, the body cannot synthesize glycogen, and the body's ability to handle cholesterol is also affected. The protective layer of tissue surrounding nerve fibers does not form properly if vitamin A is lacking.

Probably the best known function of vitamin A is its effect on vision in dim light. A person's ability to see in the dark depends on the eye's supply of retinol, a form of vitamin A. In this manner, vitamin A prevents night blindness. Vitamin A is associated with the formation and development of healthy eyes in the fetus.

If maternal stores of vitamin A are adequate, the overall effects of pregnancy on the woman's vitamin A requirements are not remarkable. The blood serum level of vitamin A decreases slightly in early pregnancy, rises in late pregnancy, and falls before the onset of labor. The RDA for vitamin A is 770 mcg per day for pregnant women age 19 and older.

Although routine supplementation with vitamin A is not recommended, supplementation with 5000 international units is indicated for women whose dietary intake may be inadequate, specifically strict vegetarians and recent emigrants from countries where deficiency of vitamin A is endemic.

Rich plant sources of vitamin A include deep green, deep orange, and yellow vegetables. Animal sources include egg yolk, cream, butter, and fortified margarine and milk.

VITAMIN D   Vitamin D is critical for the absorption and use of calcium and phosphorus in skeletal development. Vitamin D prevents osteomalacia in adults and rickets in children. To supply the needs of the developing fetus, the pregnant woman should have a vitamin D intake of 5 mcg/day. Main food sources of vitamin D include fortified milk, margarine, butter, liver, and egg yolks. Drinking a quart of milk daily provides the vitamin D needed during pregnancy. Exposure to the ultraviolet rays of sunlight is also an important source of vitamin D. However, season, time of day, latitude, smog, cloud cover, and sun screens affect UV ray exposure. (Note: It is still important to use sunscreens routinely.) For example, the average amount of sunlight in Boston and in points further north is insufficient to produce significant synthesis of vitamin D from November through February. Thus it is vital for people with limited sun exposure to consume a diet that contains good sources of vitamin D (NIH, 2007b).

Excessive intake of vitamin D is not usually a result of eating but of taking high-potency vitamin preparations. Overdoses during pregnancy can cause hypercalcemia, or high blood calcium levels, because of withdrawal of calcium from the skeletal tissue. Symptoms of toxicity are excessive thirst, loss of appetite, vomiting, weight loss, irritability, and high blood calcium levels.

VITAMIN E   The major function of vitamin E, or tocopherol, is antioxidation. Vitamin E takes on oxygen, thus preventing another substance from undergoing chemical change. For example, vitamin E helps spare vitamin A by preventing its oxidation in the intestinal tract and in the tissues. It decreases the oxidation of polyunsaturated fats, thus helping to retain the flexibility and health of the cell membrane. In protecting the cell membrane, vitamin E affects the health of all cells in the body.

Vitamin E is also involved in certain enzymatic and metabolic reactions. It is an essential nutrient for the synthesis of nucleic acids required in the formation of red blood cells in the bone marrow. Vitamin E is beneficial in treating certain types of muscular pain and intermittent claudication, in surface healing of wounds and burns, and in protecting lung tissue from the damaging effects of smog. These functions may help explain the abundant claims and cures attributed to vitamin E, many of which have not been scientifically proved.

The recommended intake of vitamin E is unchanged at 15 mg/day. Vitamin E is widely distributed in foodstuffs, especially vegetable fats and oils, whole grains, greens, and eggs.

Some pregnant women use vitamin E oil on the abdominal skin to make it supple and possibly prevent permanent stretch marks. It is questionable whether taking high doses internally will accomplish this goal or satisfy any other claims related to vitamin E's role in reproduction or virility. Excessive intake of vitamin E has been associated with abnormal coagulation in the newborn.

VITAMIN K Vitamin K, or menadione (as used synthetically in medicine), is an essential factor for the synthesis of prothrombin; its function is thus related to normal blood clotting. Synthesis occurs in the intestinal tract by the *Escherichia coli* bacteria normally inhabiting the large intestine. However, the body's need for vitamin K is not totally met by synthesis. Green leafy vegetables and liver are excellent sources. The RDA for vitamin K does not increase during pregnancy.

Intake of vitamin K is usually adequate in a well-balanced prenatal diet. Secondary problems may arise if an illness is present that results in malabsorption of fats or if antibiotics are used for an extended period, which would inhibit vitamin K synthesis by destroying intestinal *E. coli*.

Water-Soluble Vitamins

Water-soluble vitamins are excreted in the urine. Because only small amounts are stored, there is little protection from dietary inadequacies. Thus adequate amounts must be ingested daily. During pregnancy, the concentration of water-soluble vitamins in the maternal serum falls, whereas high concentrations are found in the fetus.

VITAMIN C The RDA for vitamin C (ascorbic acid) increases in pregnancy from 75 to 85 mg per day. The major function of vitamin C is to aid in the formation and devel-

opment of connective tissue and the vascular system. Ascorbic acid is essential to the formation of collagen, which binds cells together. If the collagen begins to disintegrate because of a lack of ascorbic acid, cell functioning is disturbed and cell structure breaks down, resulting in muscular weakness, capillary hemorrhage, and eventual death. These are symptoms of scurvy, the disease caused by vitamin C deficiency. Infants fed mainly cow's milk become deficient in vitamin C, and they are the main population that develops these symptoms. Surprisingly, newborns of women who have taken megadoses of vitamin C may experience a rebound form of scurvy.

Maternal plasma levels of vitamin C progressively decline during pregnancy, with values at term being about half those at midpregnancy. It appears that ascorbic acid concentrates in the placenta; levels in the fetus are 50% or more above maternal levels.

A nutritious diet should meet the pregnant woman's needs for vitamin C without additional supplementation. Common food sources of vitamin C include citrus fruit, tomatoes, cantaloupe, strawberries, potatoes, broccoli, and other leafy greens. Ascorbic acid is readily destroyed by water and oxidation. Therefore, foods containing vitamin C must be stored and cooked properly.

THE B VITAMINS The B vitamins include thiamine (B_1), riboflavin (B_2), niacin, folic acid, pantothenic acid, vitamin B_6, and vitamin B_{12}. These vitamins serve as vital coenzyme factors in many reactions such as cell respiration, glucose oxidation, and energy metabolism. The quantities needed, therefore, invariably increase as caloric intake increases to meet the metabolic and growth needs of the pregnant woman.

The thiamine requirement increases from the prepregnant level of 1.1 mg/day to 1.4 mg/day. Sources of thiamine include pork, liver, milk, potatoes, and enriched breads and cereals.

Riboflavin deficiency is manifested by cheilosis (fissures and cracks of the lips and corners of the mouth) and other skin lesions. During pregnancy women may excrete less riboflavin and still require more because of increased energy and protein needs. An additional 0.3 mg/day, to 1.4 mg/day is recommended for pregnant women age 19 and older. Sources of riboflavin include milk, liver, eggs, enriched breads, and cereals.

Niacin intake should increase 4 mg/day during pregnancy to 18 mg. Sources of niacin include meat, fish, poultry, liver, whole grains, enriched breads, cereals, and peanuts.

Folic acid, or folate, is required for normal growth, reproduction, and lactation and prevents the macrocytic, megaloblastic anemia of pregnancy. Megaloblastic anemia caused by folate deficiency is rarely found in the United States, but it does occur.

Even more significantly, an inadequate intake of folic acid has been associated with neural tube defects (NTDs) (spina bifida, meningomyelocele) in the fetus or newborn. Although these defects are considered multifactorial (see Chapter 7 ∞), research indicates that 50% to 70% of spina bifida and anencephaly could be prevented by adequate intake of folic acid (CDC & Pan American Health Organization, 2003). Consequently experts recommend that all women of childbearing age (15 to 45 years) consume 400 mcg of folic acid daily because half of all U.S. pregnancies are unplanned and NTDs occur very early in pregnancy (3 to 4 weeks after conception), before most women realize they are pregnant (National Center on Birth Defects and Developmental Disabilities, 2005). The best food sources of folates are fresh green leafy vegetables, liver, peanuts, and whole-grain breads and cereals. Folic acid can be made inactive by oxidation, ultraviolet light, and heating. It can easily be lost during improper storage and cooking. To prevent unnecessary loss, foods should be stored covered to protect them from light, cooked with only a small amount of water, and not overcooked.

No allowance has been set for pantothenic acid in pregnancy, but 5 mg/day is considered a safe, adequate intake. Sources include meats, egg yolk, legumes, and whole-grain cereals and breads.

Vitamin B_6 (pyridoxine) is associated with amino acid metabolism; thus a higher-than-average protein intake requires increased pyridoxine intake. The RDA for vitamin B_6 during pregnancy is 1.9 mg/day, an increase of 0.6 mg over the allowance for nonpregnant women. Generally, the slightly increased need can be supplied by dietary sources, which include wheat germ, yeast, fish, liver, pork, potatoes, and lentils.

Vitamin B_{12}, or cobalamin, plays a role in the synthesis of DNA and red blood cells. It also is important in maintaining the myelin sheath of nerve cells. B_{12} is the cobalt-containing vitamin found only in animal sources. Women of reproductive age rarely have a B_{12} deficiency. Vegetarians (see later discussion on vegetarian diets) can develop a deficiency, however, so it is essential that their dietary intake be supplemented with this vitamin. Occasionally vitamin B_{12} levels decrease during pregnancy but increase again after childbirth. The RDA during pregnancy is 2.6 mcg/day, an increase of 0.2 mcg. A deficiency may be because of a congenital inability to absorb vitamin B_{12}, resulting in pernicious anemia. Infertility is a complication of this type of anemia.

HINTS FOR PRACTICE

More women are consuming over-the-counter (OTC) vitamin, mineral, and food supplements today than in the past. Ask about the use of any over-the-counter supplements to help avoid potentially harmful excess intakes.

Fluid

Water is essential for life, and it is found in all body tissues. Water is necessary for many biochemical reactions. It also serves as a lubricant, as a medium of transport for carrying substances in and out of the body, and as an aid in temperature control. A pregnant woman should consume at least 8 to 10 (8 oz) glasses of fluid each day, of which 4 to 6 glasses should be water.

Because of their sodium content, diet sodas should be consumed in moderation. Caffeinated beverages have a diuretic effect, which is counterproductive to increasing fluid intake.

Vegetarianism

Vegetarianism is the dietary choice of many people for religious, health, or ethical reasons. There are several types of vegetarians. **Lacto-ovovegetarians** include milk, dairy products, and eggs in their diets. **Lactovegetarians** include dairy products but no eggs in their diets. **Vegans** are "pure" vegetarians who will not eat any food from animal sources.

The expectant woman who is vegetarian must eat the proper combination of foods to obtain adequate nutrients. If her diet allows, a woman can obtain ample and complete proteins from dairy products and eggs. Plant protein quality can be improved if it is consumed with these animal proteins.

If the woman follows a vegan diet, careful planning is necessary to obtain complete proteins and sufficient calories. An adequate, pure vegan diet contains protein from unrefined grains (brown rice, whole wheat), legumes (beans, split peas, lentils), nuts in large quantities, and a variety of cooked and fresh vegetables and fruits. Adequate dietary protein can be obtained by consuming a varied diet with complementary amino acids, which together provide complete proteins. Complete proteins can be obtained by eating different types of plant-based proteins such as beans and rice, peanut butter on whole-grain bread, and whole-grain cereal with soy milk, either in the same meal or over a day. Seeds may provide adequate protein in the vegetarian diet if the quantity is large enough. Obtaining sufficient calories to ensure adequate weight gain can be difficult because vegan diets tend to be high in fiber and therefore filling. Figure 12–3 ■ depicts the vegetarian food pyramid.

Both lacto-ovovegetarians and vegans should eat four servings of vitamin B_{12}-fortified foods (meat substitutes, tofu, cereals, soy milk, and nutritional yeast) daily. A daily supplement of vitamin B_{12} is also recommended during pregnancy and while breastfeeding (Penney & Miller, 2008).

The best sources of iron and zinc are animal products; consequently vegan diets may also be low in these minerals. In addition, a high fiber intake may reduce mineral (calcium, iron, and zinc) bioavailability. Thus pregnant

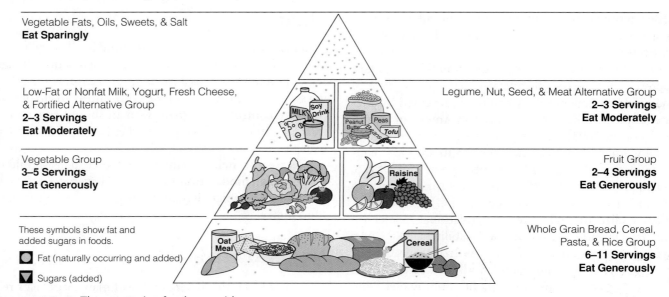

FIGURE 12–3 The vegetarian food pyramid.
Source: Adapted from The Health Connection, 55 West Oak Ridge Drive, Hagerstown, MD 21740-7390.

vegetarians are advised to have about 1200 to 1500 mg/day of calcium, which is higher than recommended levels for women who are omnivores. Vitamin D supplements may be indicated for women who do not have adequate exposure to sunlight (Penney & Miller, 2008).

To achieve optimum nutrition, the nurse should emphasize the use of foods that are nutrient-dense and that provide a balanced diet. A vegetarian food group guide appears in Table 12–3.

Factors Influencing Nutrition

It is important to consider the many factors that affect a client's nutrition. What environmental risks should the woman consider? What are the age, lifestyle, and culture of the pregnant woman? What food beliefs and habits does she have? What a person eats is determined by availability, economics, and symbolism. These factors and others influence the expectant mother's acceptance of the nurse's intervention.

Common Discomforts of Pregnancy

Gastrointestinal functioning can be altered at various times throughout pregnancy, resulting in discomforts such as nausea, vomiting, heartburn, and constipation. Although these changes can be uncomfortable for the woman, they are seldom a major problem. These discomforts, as well as dietary modifications that may provide relief, are discussed in Chapter 11 ∞.

Use of Artificial Sweeteners

Foods and beverages that contain artificial sweeteners are increasingly available. Sweeteners classified as Generally Recognized as Safe (GRAS) by the Food and Drug Administration are acceptable for use during pregnancy. As with other foods, moderation should be exercised when using artificial sweeteners, such as saccharin, which can cross the placenta and may remain in fetal tissues. Aspartame also appears to be safe if taken within FDA guidelines. Women affected by

TABLE 12–3	Vegetarian Food Groups			
Food Group	Mixed Diet	Lacto-ovovegetarian	Lactovegetarian	Vegan
Grain	Bread, cereal, rice, pasta	Bread, cereal, rice, pasta	Bread, cereal, rice, pasta	Bread, cereal, rice, pasta
Fruit	Fruit, fruit juices	Fruit, fruit juices	Fruit, fruit juices	Fruit, fruit juices
Vegetable	Vegetables, vegetable juices	Vegetables, vegetable juices	Vegetables, vegetable juices	Vegetables, vegetable juices
Dairy and dairy alternatives	Milk, yogurt, cheese	Milk, yogurt, cheese	Milk, yogurt, cheese	Fortified soy milk, rice milk
Meat and meat alternatives	Meat, fish, poultry, eggs, legumes, tofu, nuts, nut butters	Eggs, legumes, tofu, nuts, nut butters	Legumes, tofu, nuts, nut butters	Legumes, tofu, nuts, nut butters

COMPLEMENTARY AND ALTERNATIVE THERAPIES

Nutritional Content of Herbs

Several herbs are good sources of various vitamins and minerals. Like other "whole" foods, herbs contain all the necessary nutrients and enzymes to increase bioavailability versus isolated substances (such as in vitamin and mineral supplements):

Dandelion root and herb: Contains high concentrations of vitamins A and C, beta carotene, and potassium (Blumenthal, 2000).

Oat straw: Rich in calcium and magnesium, plus iron, manganese, and zinc (Blumenthal, 2000; Skidmore-Roth, 2004). Note that this is the same plant from which we derive oatmeal.

Raspberry leaf: Contains vitamin C and naturally chelated iron (Skidmore-Roth, 2004).

phenylketonuria (PKU) should avoid aspartame, as phenylalanine intake needs to be monitored. Splenda, or sucralose, is the newest artificial sweetener to become available to the public. Tests have shown Splenda to have no effects on fetal or neonatal development, and support the safety of sucralose for use in pregnant or lactating women.

Mercury in Fish

Fish and shellfish are important parts of a healthy diet, but nearly all contain traces of mercury. Although this is not a concern for most people, some fish and shellfish contain higher levels of mercury than others, and mercury can pose a threat to the developing nervous system of a fetus or young child. Mercury exposure can have a negative effect on cognitive functioning resulting in deficiencies in language, attention, motor function, memory, and visual–spatial abilities (Huffling, 2006). Because of this, the U.S. government has issued the following guidelines for women who are pregnant or who may become pregnant, breastfeeding mothers, and young children (U.S. Department of Health and Human Services & U.S. Environmental Protection Agency, 2004).

- Do not eat swordfish, shark, tilefish, or king mackerel because these fish contain high levels of mercury.
- Eat up to 12 oz/week (two average meals) of a variety of shellfish and fish that are lower in mercury. (Commonly eaten fish that are lower in mercury include canned light tuna, shrimp, salmon, catfish, and pollack. Albacore [white] tuna has more mercury than canned light tuna; therefore only 6 oz/week of albacore tuna is recommended.)
- Check local advisories about the mercury content of fish caught locally by family and friends. If no information is available, limit fish caught in local areas to 6 oz/week and avoid consuming additional fish that week.

Seafood is an important source of omega-3 fatty acids, which are essential for neural development in the fetus. Research suggests that low maternal seafood consumption is linked to suboptimum outcomes for verbal IQ, fine motor skills, communication, and social development in the child (Hibbeln, 2007). Consequently women need information about the importance of seafood in their diet and the need to consume seafood that is low in mercury.

Foodborne Illnesses

Salmonella

Because of the risk of *Salmonella* contamination in raw eggs, pregnant women are advised to avoid eating or tasting foods that may contain raw or lightly cooked eggs. These foods include, for example, cake batter, homemade eggnog, sauces made with raw eggs such as Caesar salad dressing, and homemade ice cream (Food and Drug Administration [FDA], 2005).

Listeriosis

Listeria monocytogenes is another bacterium that poses a threat to an expectant mother and her fetus. Listeria is especially challenging because the organism can be found in refrigerated, ready-to-eat foods such as unpasteurized milk and dairy products, meat, poultry, and seafood. To prevent listeriosis, pregnant women should be advised to do the following (Food and Drug Administration, 2005):

- Maintain refrigerator temperature at 40°F (4°C) or below and the freezer at 0°F (−18°C).
- Refrigerate or freeze prepared foods, leftovers, and perishables within 2 hours after eating or preparation.
- Do not eat hot dogs, deli meats, or luncheon meats unless they are reheated until they are steaming hot.
- Avoid soft cheeses such as feta, brie, Camembert, blue veined cheeses, queso fresco, or queso blanco (a soft cheese often used by Hispanic women in their cooking) unless the label clearly states that they are made with pasteurized milk.
- Do not eat refrigerated pates or meat spreads or foods that contain raw (unpasteurized) milk or drink unpasteurized milk.
- Avoid eating refrigerated smoked seafood such as salmon, trout, cod, tuna, or mackerel unless it is in a cooked dish such as a casserole. Canned or shelf-stable pates, meat spreads, and smoked seafood are considered safe to eat.

Hepatitis E

Hepatitis E is a viral infection found most often in developing countries. This disease is spread through the feces of infected people or animals. It is transmitted most often through unclean drinking water but it can also be contracted by eating contaminated food. Hepatitis E is often more severe in pregnant women, especially during the third trimester, and may lead to maternal death (Bazaco, Albrecht, & Malek, 2008).

To prevent hepatitis E, pregnant women should wash their hands thoroughly after using the bathroom, changing diapers, or handling raw foods. When traveling to areas where the quality of the water is uncertain, they should avoid eating raw foods, unpeeled fruit, and uncooked fish. They should also avoid drinking tap water or using ice made with tap water. Rather, they should use bottled or boiled water for drinking, tooth brushing, and formula preparation (Bazaco et al., 2008).

Lactase Deficiency (Lactose Intolerance)

Some individuals have difficulty digesting milk and milk products. This condition, known as **lactase deficiency** or **lactose intolerance**, results from an inadequate amount of the enzyme lactase, which breaks down the milk sugar lactose into smaller digestible substances.

Lactase deficiency is found in most adults of African, Mexican, Native American, Ashkenazic Jewish, and Asian descent and, indeed, in many other adults worldwide. People who are not affected are mainly of northern European heritage. Symptoms include abdominal distention, discomfort, nausea, vomiting, loose stools, and cramps.

In counseling pregnant women who might be intolerant of milk and milk products, the nurse should be aware that even one glass of milk can produce symptoms. Milk in cooked form, such as custards, is sometimes tolerated, as are cultured or fermented dairy products such as buttermilk, some cheeses, and yogurt. Lactase deficiency need not be a problem for pregnant women because the enzyme is available over the counter in tablets or drops. Lactase-treated milk is also available commercially in most large grocery stores.

Cultural, Ethnic, and Religious Influences

Cultural, ethnic, and occasionally religious backgrounds determine one's experiences with food and influence food preferences and habits (Figure 12–4 ■). People of different nationalities are accustomed to eating different foods because of the kinds of foodstuffs available in their countries of origin. The way food is prepared varies, depending on the customs and traditions of the ethnic and cultural group. In addition, the laws of certain religions sanction particular foods, prohibit others, and direct the preparation and serving of meals (see Cultural Perspectives: The Kosher Diet as an example).

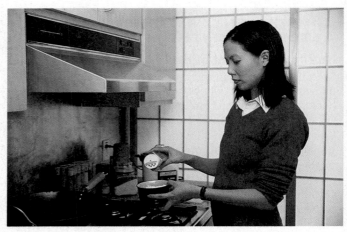

FIGURE 12–4 Cultural factors affect food preferences and habits.

CULTURAL PERSPECTIVES

The Kosher Diet

The kosher diet followed by many Jewish people forbids the eating of pig products and shellfish. Certain cuts of meat from sheep and cattle are allowed as are fish with fins and scales. In addition, many Jews believe that meat and milk should not be mixed and eaten at the same meal.

In each culture, certain foods have symbolic significance. Generally these symbolic foods are related to major life experiences such as birth, death, or developmental milestones. Although generalizations have been made about the food practices of ethnic and religious groups, there are many variations. The extent to which individuals continue to consume traditional ethnic foods and follow food-related ethnic customs is affected by the extent of exposure to other cultures; the availability, quality, and cost of traditional foods; and the recency of immigration.

When working with pregnant women from any ethnic background, it is important for the nurse to understand the impact of the woman's cultural and spiritual beliefs on her eating habits and to identify any beliefs she may have about food and pregnancy. Talking with the client can help the nurse determine the level of influence that traditional food customs exert. The nurse can then provide dietary advice that is meaningful to the woman and her family.

Psychosocial Factors

The nurse should be aware of the various psychosocial factors that influence a woman's food choices. The sharing of food has long been a symbol of friendliness, warmth, and social acceptance in many cultures. Some foods and food practices are associated with status. Some foods are prepared "just for company"; others are served only on special occasions or holidays.

Socioeconomic level may be a determinant of nutritional status. Poverty-level families cannot afford the same foods that higher-income families can. Thus pregnant women with low incomes are frequently at risk for poor nutrition.

Knowledge about the basic components of a balanced diet is essential. Often educational level is related to economic status, but even people on very limited incomes can prepare well-balanced meals if their knowledge of nutrition is adequate.

The expectant woman's attitudes and feelings about her pregnancy influence her nutritional status. For example, foods may be used as a substitute for the expression of emotions, such as anger or frustration, or as a way of expressing feelings of joy. The woman who is depressed or does not wish to be pregnant may manifest these feelings in loss of appetite or overindulgence in certain foods.

Eating Disorders

Two serious eating disorders, *anorexia nervosa* and *bulimia nervosa*, develop most commonly in adolescent girls and young women. Both conditions are psychiatric disorders that can have a major impact on physiologic well-being.

Anorexia nervosa is an eating disorder characterized by an extreme fear of weight gain and fat. People with this problem have distorted body images and perceive themselves as fat even when they are extremely underweight. Their dietary intake is very restrictive in both variety and quantity. They may also engage in excessive exercise to prevent weight gain. Individuals with anorexia nervosa are often amenorrheic because they have too little body fat to sustain the levels of estrogen needed to maintain the female reproductive cycle.

Bulimia is characterized by bingeing (secretly consuming large amounts of food in a short time) and purging. Self-induced vomiting is the most common method of purging; laxatives and/or diuretics may also be used. Individuals with bulimia nervosa often maintain normal or near-normal weight for their height, so it is difficult to know whether bingeing and purging occur.

Women with eating disorders who become pregnant are at risk for a variety of complications. The consequences of the restricting, bingeing, and purging behaviors characteristic of eating disorders can result in a lack of nutrients available for the fetus. They are at increased risk for miscarriage, hyperemesis gravidarum, preeclampsia, and birth complications, whereas their infants have an increased incidence of preterm birth, low birth weight, low Apgar scores, and intrauterine death (Martos-Ordonez, 2005). Women with eating disorders also are at higher risk for cesarean birth and postpartum depression (Zerbe, 2007).

Pregnancy can be an especially difficult time for the woman with an eating disorder, even if she has long desired a child. The consumption of additional food and the expectations that she will gain additional weight can result in feelings of fear, anxiety, depression, and guilt. Women with eating disorders also have high rates of depression postpartally (Martos-Ordonez, 2005).

When working with a pregnant woman with an eating disorder, education and individualized meal plans can help the woman increase her dietary intake while maintaining a sense of control. A multidisciplinary approach to treatment, involving medical, nursing, psychiatric, and dietetic practitioners, is indicated. Pregnant women with eating disorders need to be closely monitored and supported throughout their pregnancies.

Pica

Pica is the craving for and persistent eating of nonnutritive substances such as soil or clay (geophagia), powdered laundry starch or corn starch (amylophagia), soap, baking powder, freezer frost, ice (pagophagia), charcoal, burnt matches, or ashes that are not ordinarily considered edible or nutritionally valuable. Pica appears to occur worldwide but it is underreported because women are often embarrassed to discuss it. In the United States, pica is more common among economically disadvantaged women, women of African American descent, women who live in rural areas, women who practiced pica before pregnancy, women whose culture encourages pica as important for fertility, and women who have family members who also practice pica (Corbett, Ryan, & Weinrich, 2003).

Iron deficiency anemia is the most common concern in pica. The ingestion of laundry starch or certain types of clay may contribute to iron deficiency because they interfere with iron absorption. The ingestion of large quantities of clay could fill the intestine and cause fecal impaction, and the ingestion of starch may be associated with excessive weight gain. Lead poisoning, one of the most serious complications that can result from geophagia, may affect both the mother and her fetus. It can result in impaired cognitive functioning, kidney damage, and encephalopathy. Consequently blood lead levels should be determined in cases of diagnosed or suspected geophagia (Mills, 2007).

Nurses should be aware of pica and its implications for the woman and fetus. Assessment for pica is an important part of a nutritional history. However, a woman may be embarrassed about her cravings or reluctant to discuss them for fear of criticism. Using a nonjudgmental approach, the nurse can provide the woman with information that is useful in helping her to decrease or eliminate this practice. Some women are able to switch to eating nonfat powdered milk instead of powdered laundry starch and frozen fruit juice instead of ice. Others find that sucking on hard lemon or mint candies helps decrease the craving (Salzberg, 2002).

Nutritional Care of the Pregnant Adolescent

Nutritional care of the pregnant adolescent is of particular concern to healthcare professionals. Many adolescents are nutritionally at risk because of a variety of complex and interrelated emotional, social, and economic factors. Important nutrition-related factors to assess in pregnant adolescents include low prepregnant weight, low weight gain during pregnancy, young age at menarche, smoking, excessive prepregnant weight, anemia, unhealthy lifestyle (drugs or alcohol use), chronic disease, and history of an eating disorder.

Estimates of the nutritional needs of adolescents are generally determined by using the DRI for nonpregnant teenagers (ages 11 to 14 or 15 to 18) and adding nutrient amounts recommended for all pregnant women (see Table 12–1). If mature (more than 4 years since menarche), the pregnant adolescent's nutritional needs approach those reported for pregnant adults. However, adolescents who become pregnant less than 4 years after menarche are at high biologic risk because of their physiologic and anatomic immaturity. They are more likely than older adolescents to still be growing, which can impact the fetus's development. Thus young adolescents (age 14 and under) need to gain more weight than older adolescents (18 years and older) to produce babies of equal size.

In determining the optimal weight gain for the pregnant adolescent, the nurse adds the recommended weight gain for an adult pregnancy to that expected during the postmenarcheal year in which the pregnancy occurs. If the teenager is underweight, additional weight gain is recommended to bring her to a normal weight for her height.

Specific Nutrient Concerns

Caloric needs of pregnant adolescents vary widely. Major factors in determining caloric needs include whether growth has been completed and the physical activity level of the individual. Figures as high as 50 kcal/kg have been suggested for young, pregnant adolescents who are very active physically. A satisfactory weight gain usually confirms an adequate caloric intake.

An inadequate iron intake is a major concern with the adolescent diet. Iron needs are high for the pregnant teen because of the requirement for iron by the enlarging maternal muscle mass and blood volume. Iron supplements—providing between 30 and 60 mg of elemental iron—are definitely indicated.

Calcium is another nutrient that demands special attention from pregnant adolescents. Inadequate intake of calcium is frequently a problem in this age group. Adequate calcium intake is necessary to support normal growth and development of the fetus as well as growth and maintenance of calcium stores in the adolescent. An extra serving of dairy products is usually suggested for teenagers. Calcium supplementation is indicated for teens with an aversion to milk, unless other dairy products or significant calcium sources are consumed in sufficient quantities.

Because folic acid plays a role in cell reproduction, it is also an important nutrient for pregnant teens. As previously indicated, a supplement is usually recommended for all pregnant females, whether adult or teenager.

Other nutrients and vitamins must be considered when evaluating the overall nutritional quality of the teenager's diet. Nutrients that have frequently been found to be deficient in this age group include zinc and vitamins A, D, and B_6. Inclusion of a wide variety of foods—especially fresh and lightly processed foods—is helpful in obtaining adequate amounts of trace minerals, fiber, and other vitamins.

Dietary Patterns

Healthy adolescents often have irregular eating patterns. Many skip breakfast, and most tend to be frequent snackers. Teens rarely follow the traditional three-meals-a-day pattern. Their day-to-day intake often varies drastically, and they eat food combinations that may seem bizarre to adults. Despite these practices, adolescents usually achieve a better nutritional balance than most adults would expect.

In assessing the diet of the pregnant adolescent, the nurse should consider the eating pattern over time, not simply a single day's intake. Once the pattern is identified, counseling can be directed toward correcting deficiencies.

Counseling Issues

Counseling about nutrition and healthy eating practices is an important element of care for pregnant teenagers that nurses can effectively provide in a community setting. This counseling may be individualized, involve other teens, or provide a combination of both approaches. If an adolescent's family member does most of the meal preparation, it may be useful to include that person in the discussion if the adolescent agrees. Involving the expectant father in counseling may also be beneficial. Clinics and schools often offer classes and focused activities designed to address this topic.

The pregnant teenager will soon become a parent, and her understanding of nutrition will influence not only her well-being but also that of her child. However, teens tend to live in the present, and counseling that stresses long-term changes may be less effective than more concrete approaches. In many cases group classes are effective, especially those with other teens. In a group atmosphere, adolescents often work together to plan adequate meals including foods that are special favorites.

Postpartum Nutrition

Nutritional needs change following childbirth. Nutrient requirements vary depending on whether the mother decides to breastfeed. An assessment of postpartal nutritional status is necessary before nutritional guidance is given.

Postpartum Nutritional Status

Postpartal nutritional status is determined primarily by assessing the new mother's weight, hemoglobin and hematocrit levels, clinical signs, and dietary history. After birth there is a weight loss of approximately 10 to 12 lb (4.5 kg to 5.4 kg). Additional weight loss is most rapid during the next few weeks as the body adjusts to the completion of pregnancy. Weight stabilization may take 6 months or longer.

The amount of weight gained during pregnancy is a major determinant of weight loss after childbirth. Generally, women who gain excessive weight during pregnancy are more likely to sustain a weight gain 1 year following childbirth, putting them at increased risk of long-term overweight or obesity (Johnson, Gerstein, Evans, & Woodward-Lopez, 2006).

The mother's weight should be considered in terms of ideal weight, prepregnancy weight, and weight gain during pregnancy. Women who desire information about weight reduction can be referred to a dietitian for individual counseling or to community-based educational programs. Educational programs need to address a variety of issues such as the significance of the quality of food eaten rather than the quantity; the importance of regular physical activity in improving health, building lean muscle mass, and increasing metabolism; and the value of meal planning to ensure that healthy foods are readily available and to avoid pitfalls such as opting for fast foods, which are often high in fat (Smith, Hulsey, & Goodnight, 2008).

Hemoglobin and erythrocyte levels should return to normal within 2 to 6 weeks after childbirth. Hematocrit levels gradually rise because of hemoconcentration as extracellular fluid is excreted. Iron supplements are generally continued for 2 to 3 months following childbirth to replenish stores depleted by pregnancy.

The nurse assesses clinical symptoms the new mother may be experiencing. Constipation, in particular, is a common problem following birth. The nurse can encourage the woman to maintain a high fluid intake to keep the stool soft. Dietary sources of fiber, such as whole grains, fruits, and vegetables, are also helpful in preventing constipation.

The nurse obtains specific information on dietary intake and eating habits directly from the woman. Visiting the mother during mealtimes provides an opportunity for unobtrusive nutritional assessment. Which foods has the woman selected? Is her diet nutritionally sound? A comment focusing on a positive aspect of her meal selection may initiate a discussion of nutrition.

The nurse needs to inform the dietitian of any woman whose cultural or religious beliefs require specific foods so appropriate meals can be prepared for her. The nurse may also refer women with unusual eating habits or numerous questions about good nutrition to the dietitian. In addition, the nurse provides literature on nutrition so that the woman will have a source of appropriate information at home.

During the childbearing years the risk for obesity becomes especially problematic for women. Consequently it is critical to use the postpartum period to change behaviors and help promote effective weight management in women (Krummel, 2007).

Nutritional Care of Formula-Feeding Mothers

After birth, the formula-feeding mother's dietary requirements return to prepregnancy levels (see Table 12–1). If the mother has a good understanding of nutritional principles, it is sufficient to advise her to reduce her daily caloric intake by about 300 kcal and to return to prepregnancy levels for other nutrients.

If the mother has a limited understanding of nutrition, now is the time to teach her the basic principles and the importance of a well-balanced diet. Her eating habits and dietary practices will eventually be reflected in the diet of her child.

If the mother has gained excessive weight during pregnancy (or perhaps was overweight before pregnancy) and wishes to lose weight, a referral to the dietitian is appropriate. The dietitian can design weight-reduction diets to meet nutritional needs and food preferences. Weight loss goals of 1 to 2 lb (.45 kg to .9 kg)/week are usually suggested.

In addition to meeting her own nutritional needs, the new mother is usually interested in learning how to provide for her infant's nutritional needs. A discussion of infant feeding that includes topics such as selecting infant formulas, formula preparation, and vitamin and mineral supplementation is appropriate and generally well received.

Nutritional Care of Breastfeeding Mothers

Nutrient needs are increased during breastfeeding. Table 12–1 lists the RDA during breastfeeding for specific nutrients. Table 12–2 provides a sample daily food guide for lactating women. It is especially important for the breastfeeding mother to consume sufficient calories, because inadequate caloric intake can reduce milk volume. However, milk quality generally remains unaffected. The breastfeeding mother should increase her calories by about 200 kcal over her pregnancy requirement, or 500 kcal over her prepregnancy requirement. This results in a total of about 2500 to 2700 kcal per day for most women.

Because protein is an important ingredient in breast milk, an adequate intake while breastfeeding is essential. An intake of 65 g/day during the first 6 months of breastfeeding and 62 g/day during the second 6 months is recommended. As in pregnancy, it is important to consume adequate nonprotein calories to prevent the use of protein as an energy source.

Calcium is an important ingredient in milk production, and requirements during lactation remain the same as during pregnancy—an increase of 1000 mg/day. If the intake of calcium from food sources is not adequate, calcium supplements are recommended.

Because iron is not a principal mineral component of milk, the needs of lactating women are not substantially different from those of nonpregnant women. As previously mentioned, however, supplementation for 2 to 3 months after childbirth is advisable to replenish maternal stores depleted by pregnancy.

Liquids are especially important during lactation, because inadequate fluid intake may decrease milk volume. Fluid recommendations while breastfeeding are 8 to 10 (8 oz) glasses daily, including water, juice, milk, and soups.

In addition to counseling nursing mothers on how to meet their increased nutrient needs during breastfeeding, it is important to discuss a few issues related to infant feeding. For example, many mothers are concerned about how specific foods they eat will affect their babies during breastfeeding. Generally the nursing mother need not avoid any foods except those to which she might be allergic. Occasionally, however, some nursing mothers find that their babies are affected by certain foods; that is, they may cause the infant to be colicky after nursing, or to develop a skin rash. Onions, turnips, cabbage, chocolate, spices, and seasonings are common offenders. The best advice to give the nursing mother is to avoid those foods she suspects cause distress in her infant. For the most part, however, she should be able to eat any nourishing food she wants without fear that her baby will be affected. For further discussion of successful infant feeding, see Chapter 27 ∞.

Nursing Care Management

Nursing Assessment and Diagnosis

The nurse needs to assess nutritional status in order to plan an optimal diet with each woman. From the woman's chart and by interviewing her, the nurse gathers information about the following:

- Woman's height and weight, as well as her weight gain during pregnancy
- Pertinent laboratory values, especially hemoglobin and hematocrit
- Clinical signs that have possible nutritional implications, such as constipation, anorexia, or heartburn
- Dietary history to evaluate the woman's views on nutrition as well as her specific nutrient intake

The nurse can obtain a dietary history by asking the woman to complete a 24-hour diet recall, in which she lists everything she has eaten in the last 24 hours, including foods, fluids, and any supplements. At least 3 days of recall should be done to compensate for daily variations. Diet may also be evaluated using a food frequency questionnaire. The questionnaire lists common categories of foods and asks the woman how frequently in a day (or a week) she consumes food from the list. Common categories include vegetables, fruits, milk or cheese, meat or poultry, fish, desserts or sweets, coffee or tea, and alcohol. This method may be less reliable because it requires a person to be accurate about intake.

While gathering data, the nurse has an opportunity to discuss important aspects of nutrition within the context of the family's needs and lifestyle. The nurse also seeks information about psychologic, cultural, and socioeconomic factors that may influence food intake.

The nurse can use a nutritional questionnaire to gather and record important facts. This information provides a database the nurse can use to develop an intervention plan to fit the woman's individual needs.

Once the nurse obtains the data, he or she begins to analyze the information, formulate appropriate nursing diagnoses, and, with the woman, develop goals and desired outcomes. For a woman during the first trimester, for example, the diagnosis may be *Imbalanced Nutrition: Less than Body Requirements related to nausea and vomiting*. In other cases, the diagnosis may be related to excessive weight gain. In such situations the diagnosis might be *Imbalanced Nutrition: More than Body Requirements related to excessive caloric intake*. Although these diagnoses are broad, the nurse needs to be specific in addressing issues such as inadequate intake of nutrients including iron, calcium, or folic acid; problems with nutrition because of a limited food budget; problems related to physiologic alterations including anorexia, heartburn, or nausea; and behavioral problems related to excessive dieting, binge eating, and so on. At other times the diagnosis *Health-Seeking Behaviors* may seem most appropriate, especially if the woman asks for information about nutrition.

Nursing Plan and Implementation

After determining the nursing diagnosis, the nurse can plan an approach to address any nutritional deficiencies or improve the overall quality of the diet. To be truly effective, this plan must be made in cooperation with the woman. The following example demonstrates ways in which the nurse can plan with the woman based on the nursing diagnosis.

Diagnosis: Imbalanced Nutrition: Less than Body Requirements related to low intake of calcium

Client goal: The woman will increase her daily intake of calcium to the DRI level.

Implementation:

1. Plan with the woman how to add more milk or dairy products to the diet (specify amounts).
2. Encourage the use of other calcium sources such as leafy greens and legumes.
3. Plan for the addition of powdered milk in cooking and baking.
4. If none of the preceding options are realistic or acceptable, consider the use of calcium supplements.

Most families can benefit from guidance about food purchasing and preparation. Women should be advised to plan food purchases thoughtfully by preparing general menus and a list before shopping. It is also helpful to advise clients to monitor sales, compare brands, and be cautious when purchasing "convenience" foods, which tend to be expensive. Other techniques for keeping food costs down without jeopardizing quality include buying food in season, using bulk foods when appropriate, using whole-grain or enriched products, buying lower-grade eggs (grading has no relation to the egg's nutritional value but indicates color of the shell, delicacy of flavor, and so forth), and avoiding foods from specialty shops and foods in elaborate packaging.

Community-Based Nursing Care

Good nutrition during pregnancy begins with good nutrition before conception. Nurses can help women planning a pregnancy to evaluate their nutritional status and make improvements if necessary.

The American Dietetic Association (2008) has issued a position statement addressing nutrition and lifestyle during pregnancy. During pregnancy, to optimize maternal health and reduce the risk of birth defects, the following activities are important:

- Achieve appropriate weight gain
- Participate in regular physical activity (at least 30 minutes of moderate, safe activity on most, if not all, days)
- Consume a variety of healthy foods using MyPyramid as a guideline
- Take appropriate vitamin and mineral supplements
- Avoid alcohol, tobacco, and other harmful substances
- Follow safe food handling practices

Food is a significant portion of a family's budget, and meeting nutritional needs may be a challenge for families on limited incomes. Community-based services offered through clinics, local agencies, schools, and volunteer organizations are effective in addressing these needs. Increasingly nurses play an important role in managing such community-based services, especially those focusing on client education. In addition, most communities offer special assistance to qualifying families to meet their nutritional needs. The Food Stamp Program provides stamps or coupons for participating households whose net monthly income is below a specified level. These stamps can be used to purchase food for the household each month.

The Special Supplemental Food Program for Women, Infants, and Children (WIC) is designed to assist pregnant or breastfeeding women with low incomes and their children under 5 years of age. The program provides food assistance, nutrition education, and referrals to healthcare providers. The food distributed, including dried beans and peas, peanut butter, eggs, cheese, milk, fortified adult and infant cereals, juice, and iron-fortified formula, is designed to provide good sources of iron, protein, and certain vitamins and minerals for individuals with an inadequate diet. Participation in the WIC program during pregnancy and infancy is associated with a reduced risk of infant death.

Evaluation

Once a plan has been developed and implemented, the nurse and client may wish to identify ways of evaluating its effectiveness. Evaluation may involve keeping a food journal, writing out weekly menus, returning for weekly weigh-ins, and the like. If anemia is a special problem, periodic hematocrit assessments are also indicated. Key Facts to Remember: Prenatal Nutrition summarizes key points that the pregnant woman should thoroughly understand.

Women with serious nutritional deficiencies are referred to a dietitian. The nurse can then work closely with the dietitian and the client to improve the pregnant woman's health by modification of her diet.

KEY FACTS TO REMEMBER

Prenatal Nutrition

- The pregnant woman should eat regularly, three meals a day, and snack on fruits, cheese, milk, or other nutritious foods between meals if desired.
- More frequent but smaller meals are recommended.
- The woman should diet *only* under the guidance of her primary healthcare provider.
- Water is an essential nutrient. The woman should drink 4 to 6 (8 oz) glasses of water and a total of 8 to 10 glasses of fluid daily.
- If the diet is adequate, iron is the only supplement necessary during pregnancy.
- A multivitamin supplement is indicated for women with a poor diet and for those at high nutritional risk.
- To avoid possible deficiencies, many caregivers also recommend a daily vitamin supplement.
- Taking megadoses of vitamins during pregnancy is unnecessary and potentially dangerous.

- Maternal weight gains averaging 11.5 to 16 kg (25 to 35 lb) for a normal-weight woman are associated with the best reproductive outcomes.
- If the diet is adequate, folic acid and iron are the only supplements generally recommended during pregnancy.
- Because of the risk of neural tube defects, a national campaign is underway to encourage all women of childbearing age to take a 0.4 mg supplement of folic acid daily.
- Women should not undertake caloric restriction to reduce weight during pregnancy.
- It is most healthful for pregnant women to eat regularly and choose a wide variety of foods, especially fresh and lightly processed foods.
- Taking megadoses of vitamins during pregnancy is unnecessary and potentially dangerous.
- In vegetarian diets, special emphasis is placed on obtaining ample protein, calories, calcium, iron, vitamin D, vitamin B_{12}, and zinc through food sources or supplementation if necessary.
- Pregnant women should avoid eating fish which contain high levels of mercury such as swordfish, shark, tilefish, or king mackerel and limit their intake of fish that are lower in mercury.
- Food safety and sanitation should be a priority when preparing and storing food; foods that are known to cause foodborne illness should be avoided during pregnancy.

- Evaluation of physical, psychosocial, and cultural factors that affect food intake is essential before the nurse can determine nutritional status and plan nutritional counseling.
- The EPA and the FDA have issued a joint recommendation about the consumption of fish and shellfish by women who are pregnant, may become pregnant, or are breastfeeding, and by young children. This recommendation focuses on mercury in fish and shellfish because of the negative effects of mercury on the developing nervous system of a fetus or young child.
- Adolescents who become pregnant less than 4 years after menarche have higher nutritional needs than older pregnant adolescents and are considered to be at high biologic risk.
- Weight gains during adolescent pregnancy need to accommodate recommended gains for a normal pregnancy plus necessary gains because of maternal growth.
- After giving birth, the formula-feeding mother's dietary requirements return to prepregnancy levels.
- Breastfeeding mothers need an adequate calorie and fluid intake to maintain ample milk volume.

CHAPTER REFERENCES

American Dietetic Association. (2008). Position of the American Dietetic Association: Nutrition and lifestyle for a healthy pregnancy outcome. *Journal of the American Dietetic Association, 108*(3), 553–561.

Bazaco, M. C., Albrecht, S. A., & Malek, A. M. (2008). Preventing foodborne infection in pregnant women and infants. *Nursing for Women's Health, 12*(1), 46–54.

Blumenthal, M. (2000). *Herbal medicine: Expanded commission E monographs.* Austin, TX: American Botanical Council.

Centers for Disease Control and Prevention & the Pan American Health Organization. (2003). The prevention of neural tube defects with folic acid. Retrieved April 26, 2004, from www.cdc.

gov/Images_Video_and_Audio/Images/ Birth_Defects/Folic_Acid/ntd_dave.pdf

Chu, S. Y., Kim, S. Y., Schmid, C. H., Dietz, P. M., Callaghan, W. M., Lau, J., et al. (2007). Maternal obesity and risk of cesarean delivery: A meta-analysis. *Obesity Reviews, 8*(5), 385–394.

Corbett, R. W., Ryan, C., & Weinrich, S. P. (2003). Pica in pregnancy. *American Journal of Maternal-Child Nursing, 28*(3), 183–189.

Food and Drug Administration (FDA). (2005). *Food safety for mothers-to-be: Educator's resources guide.* College Park, MD: Center for Food Safety and Applied Nutrition.

Hibbeln, J. R. (2007). Maternal seafood consumption in pregnancy and neurodevelopment outcomes in childhood

(ALSPAC Study): An observational cohort study. *Lancet, 369*(9561), 578–585.

Huffling, K. (2006). The effects of environmental contaminants in food on women's health. *Journal of Midwifery and Women's Health, 51*(1), 19–25.

Institute of Medicine, Subcommittee for a Clinical Application Guide. (1992). *Nutrition during pregnancy and lactation: An implementation guide.* Washington, DC: National Academy Press.

Institute of Medicine, Subcommittee on Dietary Intake and Nutrient Supplements During Pregnancy, Committee on Nutrition Status During Pregnancy and Lactation, Food and Nutrition Board. (1990). *Nutrition during* pregnancy: Weight gain and nutrient supplements. Washington, DC: National Academy Press.

Johnson, D. B., Gerstein, D. E., Evans, A. E., & Woodward-Lopez, G. (2006). Preventing obesity: A life cycle perspective. *Journal of the American Dietetic Association, 106*(1), 97–102.

Krummel, D. A. (2007). Postpartum weight control: A vicious cycle. *Journal of the American Dietetic Association, 107*(1), 37–41.

Martos-Ordonez, C. (2005). Pregnancy in women with eating disorders: A review. *British Journal of Midwifery, 13*(7), 446–448.

Mills, M. E. (2007). Craving more than food: The implications of pica in pregnancy. *Nursing for Women's Health, 11*(3), 266–273.

Morin, K. H., & Reilly, L. (2007). Caring for obese pregnant women. *Journal of Obstetric, Gynecologic & Neonatal Nursing, 36*(5), 480–489.

National Center on Birth Defects and Developmental Disabilities. (2005). *Folic acid: Frequently asked questions (FAQs).* Retrieved January 3, 2008, from www.cdc.gov/ncbddd/folicacid/faqs.htm

National Institutes of Health. (2007a). *Dietary supplement fact sheet: Iron.* Retrieved January 3, 2008, from www.ods.od.nih.gov/factsheets/iron.asp

National Institutes of Health. (2007b). *Dietary supplement fact sheet: Vitamin D.* Retrieved January 3, 2008, from www.ods.od.nih.gov/factsheets/vitamind.asp

Penney, D. S., & Miller, K. G. (2008). Nutritional counseling for vegetarians during pregnancy. *Journal of Midwifery & Women's Health, 53,* 37–44.

Reece, E. A. (2008). Perspectives on obesity, pregnancy and birth outcomes in the United States: The scope of the problem. *American Journal of Obstetrics and Gynecology, 198*(1), 23–27.

Salzberg, H. S. (2002). Nutrition in pregnancy. In J. J. Sciarra (Ed.), *Gynecology and obstetrics: Vol. 2* (chap 7). Philadelphia: Lippincott Williams & Wilkins.

Skidmore-Roth, L. (2004). *Mosby's handbook of herbs and natural supplements* (2nd ed.). St. Louis, MO: Mosby.

Smith, S. A., Hulsey, T., & Goodnight, W. (2008). Effects of obesity on pregnancy. *JOGNN: Journal of Obstetric, Gynecologic, and Neonatal Nursing, 37*(2), 176–184.

U.S. Department of Health and Human Services & U.S. Environmental Protection Agency. (2004). *What you need to know about mercury in fish and shellfish.* Retrieved April 24, 2004, from www.cfsan.fda.gov/~dms/admehg3.html

Walker, L. O. (2007). Managing excessive weight gain during pregnancy and the postpartum period. *Journal of Obstetric, Gynecologic & Neonatal Nursing, 36*(5), 490–500.

Zerbe, K. J. (2007). Eating disorders in the 21st century: Identification, management, and prevention in obstetrics and gynecology. *Best Practice & Research in Clinical Obstetrics and Gynaecology, 21*(2), 331–343.

CHAPTER 13

Adolescent Pregnancy

Sometimes I get discouraged by the terrible reality of children having children. On days when that feeling hits I have to give myself a mental shake and get back into the thick of things. Clinics like ours do make a difference for pregnant teens—we listen, we teach, we care, we accept people where they are, and we never lose sight of the importance of helping the young women who turn to us succeed.

—A Registered Nurse Working in an Adolescent Pregnancy Clinic

LEARNING OUTCOMES

13-1. Describe the scope of the problem and impact of adolescent pregnancy.

13-2. Examine factors contributing to adolescent pregnancy in the nursing care management of this population.

13-3. Assess the physical, psychologic, and sociologic risks faced by a pregnant adolescent.

13-4. Analyze the characteristics of the fathers of children born to adolescent mothers.

13-5. Explain the range of reactions to the adolescent's pregnancy from the adolescent's family and social network.

13-6. Formulate a plan of care to meet the needs of a pregnant adolescent.

13-7. Examine successful community approaches to prevention of adolescent pregnancy.

KEY TERMS

Early adolescence **277**
Emancipated minors **283**
Late adolescence **277**
Middle adolescence **277**

Pregnancy is a challenging time for a woman as she adjusts to the physical and psychologic changes she experiences and prepares to assume a new role. Typically this challenge is even greater if the expectant mother is an adolescent, in part because her physical development and the developmental tasks of adolescence are incomplete. She is not prepared physically, psychologically, or economically for parenthood. Thus both she and her child are at high risk.

In the United States each year about 750,000 teenage girls (ages 15 to 19) become pregnant, and 8 out of 10 of these pregnancies are unplanned (National Campaign to Prevent Teen and Unplanned Pregnancy [NCPTUP], 2006). Of these pregnancies, about one-third (34%) are terminated by therapeutic abortion (Alan Guttmacher Institute [AGI], 2006b). Thus more than half the teens who become pregnant give birth and keep their babies.

The U.S. birth rate (number of births per 1000 women) for adolescents ages 15 to 19 dropped steadily from 1991 to 2005, which was an encouraging trend. In 2006, however, the overall birth rate for teens ages 15 to 19 rose 3% to 41.9 per 1000 women, which was still significantly lower than the 1991 rate of 61.8 per 1000 women (Hamilton, Martin, & Ventura, 2007). The United States continues to have the highest adolescent birth rates among industrialized nations (NCPTUP, 2006). The incidence of sexual activity among teens in many other countries is as high as it is in the United States. However, these countries may have lower adolescent pregnancy rates because of family influences, a greater openness about sexuality, better access to contraceptives, and a more comprehensive approach to sex education.

This chapter explores the issue of adolescent pregnancy and the role of the nurse in meeting the special needs and concerns of pregnant adolescents and their families. It concludes with a discussion of efforts to prevent adolescent pregnancy.

Overview of Adolescence

Physical Changes

Puberty—that period during which an individual becomes capable of reproduction—is a maturational process that can last from 1.5 to 6 years. The major physical changes of puberty include a growth spurt, weight change, and the appearance of secondary sexual characteristics. *Menarche,* or the time of the first menstrual period, usually occurs in the last half of this maturational process, with the average age between 12 and 13.

The initial menstrual cycles are usually irregular and often anovulatory, although they are not always so. Thus

contraception is important during this time for all adolescents who are sexually active.

Psychosocial Development

Many writers have described the developmental tasks of adolescence, based on a variety of classic theories. The following are major developmental tasks of this period (Steinberg, 2005).

- Developing a sense of identity
- Gaining autonomy and independence
- Developing intimacy in a relationship
- Developing comfort with one's own sexuality
- Developing a sense of achievement

Resolution of these tasks occurs over time in a developmental process reflected in the behaviors of youths during early, middle, and late adolescence. Although average ages for the completion of tasks have been identified, these ages are somewhat arbitrary and are affected by many factors, including culture, religion, and socioeconomic status.

In **early adolescence** (age 14 and under) teens still see their parents as authority figures. However, they begin the process of gaining independence from the family by spending more time with friends. Conformity to peer group standards is important to teens. Adolescents in this phase are very egocentric and are concrete thinkers, with only minimal ability to see themselves in the future or foresee the consequences of their behavior. Teens perceive their locus of control as external; that is, their destiny is controlled by others such as parents and school authorities.

Middle adolescence (ages 15 to 17 years) is the time for challenges. Experimentation with drugs, alcohol, and sex is a common avenue for rebellion. Middle adolescents seek independence and turn increasingly to a peer group. They are beginning to move from concrete thinking to formal operational thought but are not yet able to anticipate the long-term implications of all their actions. These years are often a time of great turmoil for families as adolescents struggle for independence and challenge family values and expectations.

In **late adolescence** (ages 18 to 19 years) teens are more at ease with their individuality and decision-making abilities. They can think abstractly and anticipate consequences. Late adolescents are capable of formal operational thought. They are learning to solve problems, to conceptualize, and to make decisions. Such abilities help these teens to see themselves as having control, which leads to the ability to understand and accept the consequences of their behavior.

MyNursingKit | March of Dimes

Factors Contributing to Adolescent Pregnancy

Socioeconomic and Cultural Factors

Poverty is a major risk factor for adolescent pregnancy. Adolescents who do not have access to middle-class opportunities tend to maintain their pregnancies, because they see pregnancy as their only option for adult status; 85% of births to unmarried teens occur among those adolescents from poor or low-income families (Alan Guttmacher Institute, 2006a). Not surprisingly, research indicates that the more time high-school students spend without adult supervision, the greater their level of sexual activity.

In the United States, the adolescent birth rate is higher among African American teens (63.7 per 1000) and Hispanic teens (83 births per 1000) than among white teens (26.6 per 1000). However, until 2006 these pregnancy rates had been declining (Hamilton et al., 2007). To some degree, the higher teenage pregnancy rate in these groups reflects the impact of poverty, as a disproportionately higher number of African American and Hispanic youths live in poverty.

Low educational achievement is another major risk factor for adolescent pregnancy. Teenage girls who participate in after-school activities are less likely to be sexually experienced than girls who do not participate (Cohen et al., 2002). Similarly, compared with other teens, teens with future goals (i.e., college or job) tend to use birth control more consistently; if they become pregnant, they are also more likely to have abortions.

The younger the teen when she first gets pregnant, the more likely she is to have another pregnancy in her teens. Moreover, the likelihood of repeat pregnancies increases when the teen is living with a sexual partner and has dropped out of school. Daughters and sisters of women who had a baby in their early teens tend to have intercourse earlier and are at higher risk for teen pregnancy themselves (Short & Rosenthal, 2003).

Internationally, adolescent women are more likely to welcome a pregnancy in a country (1) in which Islam is the predominant religion, (2) where large families are desired, (3) where social change is slow in coming, and (4) where most childbearing occurs within marriage. Early pregnancy is less desired in countries in which the reverse is true.

High-Risk Behaviors

Developmentally, adolescents, especially younger ones, are not yet able to foresee the consequences of their actions. As a result, they may have a sense of invulnerability that leads to the mistaken idea that harm will not befall them. This sense of invulnerability may also result in an overly optimistic view of the risks associated with their actions (King-Jones, 2008).

Among American adolescents there is tremendous peer pressure to become sexually active during the teen years. Premarital sexual activity is commonplace, and teenage pregnancy is more socially acceptable today than it was in the past. In fact, nearly half (46%) of all teens, ages 15 to 19, have had sex at least once (AGI, 2006a). Sexual innuendo permeates every aspect of the popular media, including music, music videos, television, and movies, but issues of sexual responsibility are commonly ignored.

High-risk sexual behaviors, including for example multiple partners and lack of contraceptive use, are of concern. Research indicates that young people ages 15 to 24 comprise 25% of the sexually experienced population in the United States; however, they account for 48% of the new cases of sexually transmitted infections (STIs). This is particularly worrisome because many STIs, including HIV, are asymptomatic. Thus apparently healthy young people who are infected may not have a reason to seek health care (Weinstock, Berman, & Cates, 2004).

Worldwide, people younger than 25 years of age account for the greatest proportion of STIs. Moreover, estimates suggest that 6000 young people are infected with HIV *daily* (Bearinger, Sieving, Ferguson, & Sharma, 2007).

Statistics have demonstrated an increased use of condoms among the adolescent population, probably because of the tremendous educational efforts related to the human immunodeficiency virus. Among currently sexually active students, 62.8% report using a condom during their last sexual intercourse (Eaton, Kann, Kinchen et al., 2006). Nevertheless, adolescents remain inconsistent contraceptive users. Contraceptive use is more consistent in situations in which teens discuss contraception before having sex, when they have waited a longer time after starting a relationship to have sex with that person, and when they use dual methods of contraception (Manlove, Ryan, & Franzetta, 2003).

Many teens lack accurate and adequate knowledge about contraceptive options. This is a common topic of sex-education programs; however, debate continues about the appropriateness of such programs in schools. Proponents advocate early sex education to provide teens with the knowledge they need to avoid unwanted pregnancy and the risk of sexually transmitted infection. Opponents

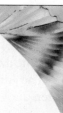

CULTURAL PERSPECTIVES

Throughout the world, the higher a woman's educational level, the more likely she is to delay marriage and childbirth.

believe that sex education is the responsibility of parents and worry that sex education in the schools will promote sexual activity. However, a review of research on sex education reveals that it does not increase initiation of sexual activity at an earlier age (Doniger, Adams, Utter et al., 2001). Other factors affecting the use of contraception include access or availability, cost of supplies, and concern about confidentiality.

Psychosocial Factors

Family dysfunction and poor self-esteem are also major risk factors for adolescent pregnancy. Some young teenagers deliberately plan to get pregnant. The adolescent girl may use pregnancy for various subconscious or conscious reasons: to punish her father and/or mother, to escape from an undesirable home situation, to gain attention, or to feel that she has someone to love and to love her. Pregnancy may also be a young woman's form of acting out. In some circumstances, pregnancy could represent an important milestone that leads to positive lifestyle changes and healthier behaviors (Klima, 2003).

Teenage pregnancy can result from an incestuous relationship. In the very young adolescent, incest or sexual abuse should be suspected as a possible cause of pregnancy. More teens who become pregnant, compared with teens who have not been pregnant, have been physically, emotionally, or sexually abused. In fact, maltreatment of any kind is a high-risk contributor to early teen pregnancy (Montgomery, 2003). Teenage pregnancy could also be caused by other nonvoluntary sexual experiences such as acquaintance rape.

Risks to the Adolescent Mother

Physiologic Risks

Adolescents over age 15 who receive early, thorough prenatal care are at no greater risk during pregnancy than women over age 20. Unfortunately adolescents typically begin prenatal care later in pregnancy than any other age group. Thus risks for pregnant adolescents include preterm births, low-birth-weight infants, cephalopelvic disproportion, iron deficiency anemia, and preeclampsia–eclampsia and its sequelae. In the adolescent age group, prenatal care is the critical factor that most influences pregnancy outcome.

Teenagers ages 15 to 19 have a high incidence of sexually transmitted infections, including genital herpes, syphilis, and gonorrhea. The incidence of chlamydial infection is also increased in this age group. The presence of such infections during a pregnancy greatly increases the risk to the fetus (refer to Chapter 15 ∞). Other problems seen in adolescents are cigarette smoking and drug use. By the time pregnancy is confirmed in young women, the fetus may already have been harmed by these substances.

Psychologic Risks

The major psychologic risk to the pregnant adolescent is the interruption of her developmental tasks. Adding the tasks of pregnancy to her other developmental tasks creates an overwhelming amount of psychologic work, the completion of which will affect the adolescent's and her newborn's futures. Table 13–1 suggests typical behaviors of the early, middle, and late adolescent when she becomes aware of her pregnancy. In reviewing these behaviors, the nurse should realize that other factors may influence individual response.

Sociologic Risks

Being forced into adult roles before completing adolescent developmental tasks causes a series of events that affects the adolescent's entire life. These events may result in a prolonged dependence on parents, lack of stable relationships with the opposite sex, and lack of economic and social stability.

Many teenage mothers drop out of school during their pregnancy and then are less likely to complete their schooling. Similarly they are less likely to go to college, more likely to have big families, and more likely to be single. Lack of education in turn reduces the quality of jobs available. Childbearing at an early age is a strong predictor that the adolescent mother's children will live in poverty (Kirby, 2007).

Adolescent mothers frequently fail to establish a stable family, especially if they have a second child while still in their teens. Their family structure tends to be a single-parent, matriarchal structure, often the same type in which the adolescents themselves were raised.

Some pregnant adolescents choose to marry the father of the baby, who may also be a teenager. Unfortunately, the majority of adolescent marriages end in divorce. This fact should not be surprising because pregnancy and marriage interrupt the adolescents' childhood and basic education. Lack of maturity in dealing with an intimate relationship also contributes to marital breakdown in this age group.

Studies suggest that 16% to 37% of pregnant teens experience domestic violence. This rate is higher than that estimated for pregnant adults and suggests that teens are more susceptible to such victimization than pregnant adults (Scheiman & Zeoli, 2003). Dating violence is often an issue for teens, especially for younger girls dating older boys. These younger teens may interpret such actions as hitting, pushing, and making verbal threats as signs of love and caring, and a deep commitment to the relationship

TABLE 13–1	Initial Reaction to Awareness of Pregnancy	
Age	Adolescent Behavior	Nursing Implications
Early adolescent (14 and under)	Fears rejection by family and peers. Enters healthcare system with an adult, most likely mother (parents still seen as locus of control). Value system still closely reflects that of parents, so still turns to parents for decision or approval of decision. Pregnancy probably is not the result of intimate relationship. Is self-conscious about normal adolescent changes in body. Self-consciousness and low self-esteem likely to increase with rapid breast enlargement and abdominal enlargement of pregnancy.	Be nonjudgmental in approach to care. Focus on needs and concerns of adolescent, but if parent accompanies daughter, include parent in plan of care. Encourage both to express concerns and feelings regarding pregnancy and options: abortion, maintaining pregnancy, adoption. Be realistic and concrete in discussing implications of each option. During physical exam of adolescent, respect increased sense of modesty. Explain in simple and concrete terms physical changes that are produced by pregnancy versus puberty. Explain each step of physical exam in simple and concrete terms.
Middle adolescent (15–17 years)	Fears rejection by peers and parents. Unsure in whom to confide. May seek confirmation of pregnancy on own with increased awareness of options and services, such as over-the-counter pregnancy kits, Planned Parenthood, and Birthright. If in an ongoing, caring relationship with partner (peer), adolescent may choose him as confidant. Economic dependence on parents may determine if and when parents are told. Future educational plans and perception of parental support or lack of support are significant factors in decision regarding termination or maintenance of the pregnancy. Possible conflict in parental and own developing value system.	Be nonjudgmental in approach to care. Reassure the adolescent that confidentiality will be maintained. Help adolescent identify significant individuals in whom she can confide to help make a decision about the pregnancy. Be aware of state laws regarding requirement of parental notification if abortion is intended. Also be aware of state laws regarding requirements for marriage: usually, minimum age for both parties is 18; 16- and 17-year-olds are, in most states, allowed to marry only with consent of parents. Encourage adolescent to be realistic about parental response to pregnancy.
Late adolescent (18–19 years)	Most likely to confirm pregnancy on own and at an earlier date because of increased acceptance and awareness of consequences of behavior. Likely to use pregnancy kit for confirmation. Relationship with father of baby, future educational plans, and own value system are among significant determinants of decision about pregnancy.	Be nonjudgmental in approach to care. Reassure the adolescent that confidentiality will be maintained. Encourage adolescent to identify significant individuals in whom she can confide. Refer to counseling as appropriate. Encourage adolescent to be realistic about parental response to pregnancy.

that will ultimately produce long-term positive results (Glass, Fredland, Campbell et al., 2003).

The increased incidence of maternal complications, premature birth, and low-birth-weight babies among adolescent mothers also has an impact on society because many of these mothers are on welfare. The need for increased financial support for good prenatal care and nutritional programs remains critical.

Table 13–2 identifies the early adolescent's response to the developmental tasks of pregnancy. Middle and older adolescents respond differently, reflecting their progression through the developmental tasks. In addition to her maturational level, the amount of nurturing the pregnant adolescent receives is a critical factor in the way she handles pregnancy and motherhood.

Risks for Her Child

Children of adolescent parents are at a disadvantage in many ways because teens are not developmentally or economically prepared to be parents. In general, children of teenage mothers are found to be at a developmental disadvantage compared with children whose mothers were older at the time of their birth. Many factors contribute to these differences, especially the adverse social and economic conditions many teenage mothers face. These factors result in high rates of family instability, disadvantaged neighbor-

hoods, and high rates of behavior problems. In addition, these children do not do as well in school and are less likely to complete high school. Children born to adolescent mothers also have higher rates of abuse and neglect (National Campaign to Prevent Teen Pregnancy [NCPTP], 2004).

Partners of Adolescent Mothers

Approximately two-thirds of the fathers of infants born to adolescent mothers are not teens but rather are 20 years of age or older. In particular, teens in poorer, recently immigrated populations have considerably older partners (Males, 2004).

Adolescent males tend to become sexually active at an earlier age than females, and they have more sexual partners in their teenage years (Marcell, Raine, & Eyre, 2003). When the father is an adolescent, he, too, has uncompleted developmental tasks for his age group and is no better prepared psychologically than his female counterpart to deal with the consequences of pregnancy. Consequently, the adolescent who attempts to assume his responsibility as a father faces many of the same psychologic and sociologic risks as the adolescent mother. The mother and father are generally from similar socioeconomic backgrounds and have similar educational levels.

TABLE 13–2	**The Early Adolescent's Response to the Developmental Tasks of Pregnancy**		
Stage	**Developmental Tasks of Pregnancy**	**Early Adolescent's Response to Pregnancy**	**Nursing Implications**
First trimester	Pregnancy confirmation. Seeking early prenatal care as a confirmation tool. Begins to evaluate her diet and general health habits. Initial ambivalence common. Usually supportive partner.	May delay confirmation of pregnancy until late part of first trimester or later. Reasons for delay may include lack of awareness that she is pregnant, fear of confiding in anyone, or denial. Rapid enlargement and sensitivity of breasts are embarrassing and frightening to early adolescent—may be perceived as changes of puberty. If confiding in mother, may be experiencing family turmoil in response to pregnancy.	Emphasize need for good nutrition as important for her well-being as much as infant's (prevention of preeclampsia and anemia). Use simple explanations and lots of audiovisuals. Have adolescent listen to fetal heart rate (FHR) with Doppler.
Second trimester	Changes in physical appearance begin, and fetal movement is experienced, causing pregnancy to be experienced as a reality. Begins wearing maternity clothes to accommodate the physical changes. As a result of quickening she perceives her fetus as a real baby and begins preparing for the maternal role and new relationships with her partner and members of her family.	Some teenagers may delay validation of pregnancy until now, with family turmoil occurring at this time. Abdominal enlargement and quickening may be perceived as loss of control over body image. May try to maintain prepregnant weight and wear restrictive clothing to control and conceal changing body. Becomes dependent on her own mother for support. Egocentric; unable to develop a maternal role at this time.	Continue to discuss importance of good nutrition and adequate weight gain as previously noted. Discuss ways of utilizing common teenage clothing (large sweatshirts, blouses) to promote comfort but preserve adolescent image to some degree. Discuss plans being made for baby, continued educational plans, and role of teen's parents.
Third trimester	At end of second trimester begins to view fetus as separate from self. Buys baby clothes and supplies. Prepares a place for the baby. Realistic about what baby is like. Prepares to give birth to infant. Anxiety increases as labor and birth approach; adolescent has concerns about well-being of fetus.	May focus on "wanting it to be over." May have trouble individuating fetus. May have fantasies, dreams, or nightmares about childbirth. Natural fears of labor and birth greater than with older primigravida. Probably has not been in a hospital, and may associate this with negative experiences. Explain physiologic changes of pregnancy versus those associated with puberty. Explain that ambivalence is normal with any pregnancy, but recognize it as a much greater concern with adolescent pregnancy.	Assess whether adolescent is preparing for baby by buying supplies and preparing a place in the home. Childbirth education important. Provide hospital tour. Assess for discomforts of pregnancy, such as heartburn and constipation. Adolescent may be uncomfortable mentioning these and other problems.

Although not married, many adolescent couples are involved in meaningful relationships. Adolescent fathers may be involved in the pregnancy and be present for the birth. In situations in which the adolescent father wants to assume some responsibility, healthcare providers should support him in his decision. It is important, however, that the pregnant adolescent have the opportunity to decide whether she wants the father to participate in her health care.

The lack of responsibility shown by some unwed fathers has caused a shift in cultural and community attitudes. Fathers are being included on birth certificates far more frequently today than in the past. This inclusion helps ensure the fathers' rights and encourages them to meet their responsibilities to their children. In addition, legal paternity gives children access to military and social security benefits and to medical information about their fathers.

In some situations, the pregnant adolescent female may not want to identify or contact the baby's father, and the male may not readily acknowledge paternity. Those situations include rape, exploitative sexual relations, incest, and casual sexual relations. If healthcare providers suspect any of the first three causes, further investigation into the situation is important for the well-being of the pregnant adolescent, and referral to other resources should be made

as appropriate. If the adolescents perceive that they have a caring relationship, the adolescent father may want to be supportive and protective but may not understand the physical and psychologic changes that his partner is experiencing. The young man will need education about pregnancy, childbirth, child care, and parenting.

Even if the adolescent father has been included in the health care of the young woman throughout the pregnancy, it is not unusual for her to want her mother as her primary support person during labor and birth. Younger adolescents are especially likely to choose their mothers for this role. It is important both to support the pregnant adolescent's wishes and to acknowledge and support the adolescent father's wishes as appropriate.

As a part of counseling, the nurse should assess the young man's stressors, his support systems, his plans for involvement in the pregnancy and childbearing, and his future plans. He should be referred to social services for an opportunity for counseling regarding his educational and vocational future. When the father is involved in the pregnancy, the young mother feels less deserted, more confident in her decision making, and better able to discuss her future. Relationships between fathers, teenage mothers, and their infants appear prone to deterioration over time.

Research suggests, however, that many young fathers genuinely want to be involved with their children and would have more contact and input if they could. Issues such as conflicts with the teen mother or maternal grandparents and a lack of financial resources may act as barriers for the young father (Bunting & McAuley, 2004).

Reactions of Family and Social Network to Adolescent Pregnancy

The reactions of family members and support groups to adolescent pregnancy are as varied as the motivation and cause of the pregnancy. In families that foster their children's educational and career goals, adolescent pregnancy is often a shock. Anger, shame, and sorrow are common reactions. The majority of pregnant adolescents from these families are likely to use contraception or choose abortion, with the exception of teens whose cultural and religious beliefs prevent them from seeking abortions.

Some adolescent fathers also face negative reactions from people, including their own families and the families of their young partners. They may experience others' anger, shame, and disappointment. Their relationships with their peers may be altered as well.

In populations in which adolescent pregnancy is more prevalent and more socially acceptable, family and friends may be more supportive of the adolescent parents. In many cases, the teen's friends and mother are present at the birth. The expectant couple may also have friends who are already teen parents. Some male partners of these adolescent mothers see pregnancy and the birth of a baby as signs of adult status and increased sexual prowess—a source of pride.

The mother of the pregnant adolescent is usually among the first to be told about the pregnancy. She typically becomes involved with decision making, especially with the young adolescent, about issues such as maintaining the pregnancy, abortion, and dealing with the father-to-be and his family.

Once the pregnant adolescent decides how to proceed, it is often the mother who helps the teen access health care and accompanies her to her first prenatal visit. If the pregnancy is maintained, the mother may participate in prenatal care and classes and can be an excellent source of support for her daughter. She should be encouraged to participate if the mother–daughter relationship is positive. If the baby's father is involved in the pregnancy, he and the pregnant adolescent's mother may be able to work together to support the teenage mother. The nurse can update the pregnant adolescent's mother on childbearing practices to clarify any misconceptions she might have. During labor and birth, the mother may be a key figure for her daughter, offering her reassurance and instilling confidence. The

younger the adolescent when she gives birth, the more she needs her mother's support. Children of adolescent parents experience more negative outcomes, including more aggressive behavior at a younger age, when the adolescent is in constant conflict with her mother and becomes less involved in parenting.

Nursing Care Management

Nursing Assessment and Diagnosis

The nurse begins her care of the pregnant adolescent by establishing a database to plan interventions for the adolescent mother-to-be and family. Areas of assessment include a history of family and personal physical health, developmental level and impact of pregnancy, and emotional and financial support. The nurse also assesses the family and social support network and the father's degree of involvement in the pregnancy.

As with all pregnant women, it is important to have information on the teen's general physical health. This may be the first time the adolescent has ever provided a health history. Consequently, the nurse may find it helpful to ask specific questions and give examples if the young woman appears confused about a question. The nurse may find that the teen's mother is best able to answer questions about family history because the adolescent is often unaware of this information.

The following areas should be assessed:

- Family and personal health history
- Medical history
- Menstrual history
- Obstetric and gynecologic history
- Substance abuse history

It is important to assess the maturational level of the pregnant teen and her partner if he is involved. The adolescent's development level and the impact of pregnancy are reflected in the degree of recognition she displays of the realities and responsibilities involved in teenage pregnancy and parenting. The mother's self-concept (including body image), her relationship with the significant adults in her life, her attitude toward her pregnancy, and her coping methods in the situation are just a few of the significant factors that need to be assessed. The nurse assesses the adolescent's knowledge of, attitude toward, and anticipated ability to care for the coming baby.

The socioeconomic status of the pregnant adolescent often places the baby at risk throughout life, beginning with conception. Thus it is essential to assess family and social support systems, as well as the extent of financial support available.

The nursing diagnoses applicable to pregnant women in general also apply to pregnant adolescents. Other nursing diagnoses are influenced by the adolescent's age, support systems, socioeconomic situation, health, and maturity. Examples of nursing diagnoses specific to the pregnant adolescent include the following:

- *Imbalanced Nutrition: Less than Body Requirements* related to poor eating habits
- *Risk for Situational Low Self-Esteem* related to unanticipated pregnancy

Nursing Plan and Implementation

Early, thorough prenatal care is the strongest and most critical determinant for reducing risk for the adolescent mother and her newborn. When an adolescent presents for health care, her needs must be met and she must be treated as an individual who can make decisions about her own health care.

Community-Based Nursing Care

Nurses who work with adolescent girls can help them by providing information and guidance that enables each teen to make choices that are based on and lead to the attainment of four goals (Short & Rosenthal, 2003):

- Developing a positive attitude about her body and its physical changes
- Accepting and feeling comfortable about desire, arousal, and sexual feelings
- Feeling comfortable about sexual behavior
- Practicing safer-sex behaviors (for sexually experienced adolescents)

If pregnancy occurs, early, thorough prenatal care is the strongest and most critical determinant for reducing risk for the adolescent mother and her newborn. The nurse needs to understand the special needs of the adolescent mother to meet this challenge successfully. See Key Facts to Remember: The Pregnant Adolescent.

Many new and innovative community-based programs have evolved to provide care for high-risk clients and their partners throughout the childbearing experience and beyond. Nurses in community-based agencies can help adolescents access the healthcare system as well as social services and other support services (e.g., food banks and the Women, Infants, and Children [WIC] program). These nurses are also involved extensively in counseling and client teaching.

Community programs providing educational materials and group classes can be an important adjunct to routine prenatal care. Helping pregnant adolescents understand the importance of finding a healthcare provider they are comfortable with, maintaining scheduled appointments, childbirth and labor preparation, and other health-promoting content may be included. Many adolescents prefer group activities; these may be helpful forums to exchange ideas and

---

◆ KEY FACTS TO REMEMBER
The Pregnant Adolescent

- The rate of adolescent pregnancy in the United States is among the highest of all the world's developed countries.
- Early, regular, and excellent prenatal care can prevent many of the risks associated with adolescent pregnancy, especially for the young adolescent.
- Prenatal education especially designed for adolescents also plays a significant role in increasing an adolescent's knowledge and in decreasing maternal and perinatal complications.

---

help them cope with the demands of pregnancy and adolescence (Montgomery, 2003).

Issues of Confidentiality and Consent to Care

Most states in the United States have passed legislation that confirms the right of some minors to assume the rights of adults. These adolescents are referred to as **emancipated minors**. An adolescent may be considered emancipated if he or she is self-supporting and living away from home, married, pregnant, a parent, or in the military service. Even if a minor has not become formally "emancipated," all 50 states permit confidential testing and treatment for STIs but only half (25 states) explicitly permit minors (12 and older) to consent to contraception without a parent's knowledge or consent. Currently 32 states explicitly allow minors to consent to prenatal care; three states specify that "mature" minors can consent, whereas the remaining 15 states have no relevant law or policy (AGI, 2008a). All states either explicitly allow minors to give consent for their children's medical care or have no explicit policy about it (AGI, 2008b). If a pregnant minor is considered emancipated, she is entitled to confidentiality in her dealings with healthcare providers. Only with her agreement can other adults, including her parents, be included in communication.

Development of a Trusting Relationship with the Pregnant Adolescent

The first visit to the clinic or caregiver's office may make the young woman feel anxious and vulnerable. Making this first experience as positive as possible for the young woman will encourage her to return for follow-up care and to cooperate with her caregivers and will help her recognize how important health care is for her and her baby.

Depending on the adolescent's age, this may be her first pelvic examination, which is an anxiety-provoking experience for any woman. The nurse can provide explanations during the procedure. A gentle and thoughtful examination technique will help the young woman to relax.

Developing a trusting relationship with the pregnant adolescent is essential. Honesty and respect for the individual and a caring attitude promote self-esteem. In developing a trusting relationship with the young woman, the nurse's attitudes about self-care and responsibility affect the adolescent's maturation process.

Promotion of Self-Esteem and Problem-Solving Skills

The nurse assists the adolescent in her decision-making and problem-solving skills so that she can proceed with her developmental tasks and begin to assume responsibility for her life and that of her newborn. Many adolescents are not aware of all the legally available options to deal with an unplanned pregnancy. In an open, nonjudgmental way, without imposing personal values, the nurse can educate the teen about her alternatives: maintaining or terminating the pregnancy and parenting the infant or relinquishing the infant for adoption. The nurse can encourage the young woman to share her feelings about each alternative and the projected consequences as they relate to her situation in life. The nurse can also provide information about community resources available to help with each alternative. Once the adolescent has decided on a course of action, healthcare providers should respect her decision and support her efforts to achieve her goals.

If the adolescent chooses to continue her pregnancy, the nurse summarizes what she can expect over the prenatal period and provides a thorough explanation and rationale for each procedure as it occurs. This overview fosters the adolescent's understanding and gives her some measure of control (Figure 13–1 ■).

Early adolescents tend to be egocentric and oriented to the present. They may not regard as important the fact that their health and habits affect the fetus. Thus it is often helpful to emphasize the effects of these practices on the clients themselves. Early adolescents also need help in problem solving and in visualizing the future so they can plan effectively.

Middle adolescents are developing the ability to think abstractly and can recognize that actions may have long-term consequences. They may not yet have acquired assertive communication skills, however, and may be reluctant to ask questions. Thus the nurse should ask teens

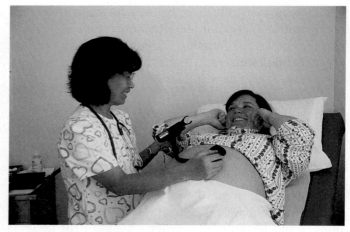

FIGURE 13–1 The nurse gives a young mother an opportunity to listen to her baby's heartbeat.

directly if they have questions. Middle adolescents can absorb more detailed health teaching and apply it.

Late adolescents can usually think abstractly, plan for the future, and function in a manner comparable to older pregnant women. They can also handle complex information and apply it.

Promotion of Physical Well-Being

Baseline weight and blood pressure measurements are valuable in assessing weight gain and predisposition to pregnancy-induced hypertension. The nurse can encourage the adolescent to take part in her care by measuring and recording her own weight. The nurse may use this time as an opportunity for assisting the young woman in problem solving and encourage her to ask herself the following questions: "Have I gained too much or too little weight?" "What influence does my diet have on my weight?" "How can I change my eating habits?"

Another way to introduce the subject of nutrition is during measurement of baseline and subsequent hemoglobin and hematocrit values. Because the adolescent is at risk for anemia, she will need education regarding the importance of iron in her diet. Indeed, basic education about nutrition is a critical component of care for pregnant teens.

Preeclampsia–eclampsia is the most prevalent medical complication of pregnant adolescents. Blood pressure readings of 140/90 mm Hg are not acceptable as the determinant of preeclampsia in adolescents. Women ages 14 to 20 years without evidence of high blood pressure usually have diastolic readings between 50 and 66 mm Hg. Gradual increases from the prepregnant diastolic readings, along with excessive weight gain, must be evaluated as precursors to preeclampsia. Establishment of baseline readings is one reason why early prenatal care is vital to the management of the pregnant adolescent.

Adolescents have an increased incidence of sexually transmitted infections (STIs). The initial prenatal examination should include gonococcal and chlamydial cultures; wet-mount prep for *Candida, Trichomonas,* and *Gardnerella;* and tests for syphilis. Education about STIs is important, as is careful observation of herpetic lesions or other symptoms throughout a young woman's pregnancy. Although today's teens are knowledgeable about HIV/AIDS, they know much less about other STIs, especially with regard to symptoms and risk reduction. If the adolescent's history indicates that she is at increased risk for HIV, she should be given information about it and offered HIV screening.

The nurse should discuss substance abuse with the adolescent. It is important to review the risks associated with the use of tobacco, caffeine, drugs, and alcohol. The young woman should be aware of the ways that these substances affect both her development and that of her fetus.

Ongoing care should include the same assessments that an older pregnant woman receives. The nurse should pay special attention to evaluating fetal growth by determining when quickening occurs and by measuring fundal height, fetal heart rate, and fetal movement. The corresponding dates of auscultating fetal heart tones with the date of last menstrual period and quickening can be helpful in determining correct estimates of time of birth. If there is a question of size–date discrepancy by 2 cm either way when assessing fundal height, an ultrasound is warranted to establish fetal age so that instances of intrauterine growth restriction can be diagnosed and treated early.

Promotion of Family Adaptation

The nurse assesses the family situation during the first prenatal visit and discovers the level of involvement the adolescent desires from each of her family members and the father of the child, as well as her perception of their present support. A sensitive approach to the daughter–mother relationship helps motivate their communication. If the mother and daughter agree, the mother should be included in the client's care. Pregnancy may change a teen's relationship with her mother from one of antagonism to one of understanding and empathy. The opportunity to renew or establish a positive relationship with their mothers is welcomed by most teens. It symbolizes approval, acceptance, and support from the individual who would serve as her role model for mothering.

The nurse should also help the mother assess and meet her daughter's needs. Some adolescents become more dependent during pregnancy, and some become more independent. The mother can ease and encourage her daughter's self-growth by understanding how best to respond to and support the adolescent.

The adolescent's relationship with her father is also affected by her pregnancy. The nurse can provide information to the father and encourage his involvement to whatever degree is acceptable to both daughter and father.

Finally, the father of the adolescent's infant should not be forgotten in promoting the family's adaptation to the pregnancy. He should be included in prenatal visits, classes, health teaching, and in the birth itself to the extent that he wishes and that is acceptable to the teenage mother. He should also have the opportunity to express his feelings and concerns and to have his questions answered.

Facilitation of Prenatal Education

Some school systems are currently attempting to meet prenatal education needs in a variety of ways. The most effective method appears to be mainstreaming the pregnant adolescent in academic classes with her peers and adding classes appropriate to her needs during pregnancy and initial parenting experiences. Classes about growth and development beginning with the newborn and early infancy periods can help teenage parents to develop realistic expectations of their infants and may help decrease child abuse. Mainstreaming pregnant adolescents in school is also an ideal way to help them complete their education while learning the skills they need to cope with childbearing and parenting. Vocational guidance in this setting is also beneficial as they plan for their futures.

Most childbirth educators believe that prenatal classes with other teens are preferable, even though these classes can be challenging to teach (Figure 13–2 ■). Attendance may be sporadic. The pregnant teen may be accompanied by her mother, her boyfriend, or a girlfriend. Those who bring girlfriends may bring a different one each time, and giggling and side conversations may occur. Such activity reflects the teen's short attention span and is fairly typical. Thus to keep the attention of the participants, it is important to use a variety of teaching strategies including age-appropriate audiovisual aids, demonstrations, and games.

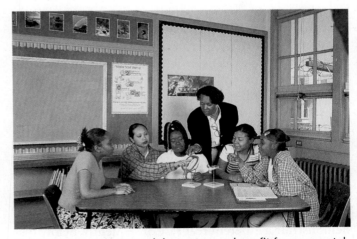

Figure 13–2 Young adolescents may benefit from prenatal classes designed specifically for them.

Goals for prenatal classes may include some or all of the following:

- Providing anticipatory guidance about pregnancy
- Preparing participants for labor and birth
- Helping participants identify the problems and conflicts of teenage pregnancy and parenting
- Promoting increased self-esteem
- Providing information about available community resources
- Helping participants develop adaptive coping skills

Although parenting topics are sometimes included in prenatal classes for adolescents, teens may not retain the information because they tend to be present oriented. Parenting skills are crucial, but adolescents generally are not ready to learn about these skills until birth makes the newborn—and thus parenting—a reality.

Hospital-Based Nursing Care

The adolescent's mother is often present during the teen's labor and birth. The baby's father may also be involved. Close girlfriends may arrive soon after the teen is admitted. It is important on admission for the nurse to ask the pregnant adolescent who will be her primary support person in labor and who she wants involved in the labor and birth. This information may also be included on her prenatal record.

The adolescent in labor has the same care needs as any pregnant woman. However, she may require more sustained care. Adolescents need their caregiver to provide education to guide their choices. The nurse must be readily available and should answer questions simply and honestly, using lay terminology. The nurse can also help the adolescent's support people understand their roles in assisting the teen. If the baby's father is involved, the nurse can encourage him to work within his own level of comfort to play an active role in all phases of the birth process, perhaps by supporting the teen's relaxation techniques, feeding her ice chips, timing her contractions, and coaching her with her breathing. The nurse can also recommend handholding, back rubs, and supportive touching.

During the postpartum period, most teens do not foresee that they will become sexually active in the near future and are often adamant that they will not become pregnant again for a long time. However, the statistics demonstrate a different reality. Consequently, before discharge, the nurse's teaching should include information

---

EVIDENCE IN ACTION

To encourage breastfeeding in adolescent mothers, it is suggested that health care providers provide positive interpersonal relationships and in-person experiences.
(Systematic review) (Hall Moran, Edwards, Dykes, & Downe, 2007)

EVIDENCE IN ACTION

The opinion of the American College of Obstetricians and Gynecologists (ACOG) is that the benefits and convenience of long-acting contraceptives make them an appropriate choice for sexually active adolescents.
(Opinion for practice) (Tolaymat & Kaunitz, 2007).

---

about the resumption of ovulation and the importance of contraception. It is especially helpful to provide this information to both the adolescent mother and her sexual partner.

Several safe and effective contraceptive options are available for adolescents. Condoms are by far the most common method of contraception among teens and, when used consistently and correctly, they offer the added advantage of protection against STIs. Increasingly, experts are recommending a dual approach to prevent pregnancy and STIs—a condom combined with a second method of contraception, typically a hormonal method such as a combined oral contraceptive (Hillard, 2005; WHO, 2004). The American College of Obstetricians and Gynecologists (ACOG) (2007) has issued a committee opinion supporting the use of intrauterine devices (IUDs) as a safe, first-line contraceptive choice for adolescents. ACOG (2007) reports that the IUD does not increase the adolescent's risk of PID or affect her fertility.

As part of discharge planning, the nurse should ensure that the teen is aware of community resources available to assist her and her family. Postpartum classes, especially with peers, can be particularly beneficial. Such classes address a variety of topics including postpartum adaptation, infant and child development, and parenting skills.

Evaluation

Expected outcomes of nursing care include the following:

- A trusting relationship is established with the pregnant adolescent.
- The adolescent is able to use her problem-solving abilities to make appropriate choices.
- The adolescent follows the recommendations of the healthcare team and receives effective health care throughout her pregnancy, the birth, and the postpartum period.
- The adolescent, her partner (if he is involved), and their families are able to cope successfully with the effects of the pregnancy.
- The adolescent is able to discuss pregnancy, prenatal care, and childbirth.
- The adolescent demonstrates developmental and pregnancy progression within established normal parameters.
- The adolescent develops skill in child care and parenting.

Prevention of Adolescent Pregnancy

At the individual level, balanced, realistic sexuality education, which includes information on both abstinence and contraception, can delay teens' onset of sexual activity, increase the use of contraception by sexually active teens, and reduce the number of their sexual partners. The American Academy of Pediatrics (2007) has issued a policy statement on contraception and adolescents that addresses the role of healthcare providers in working with adolescents. The statement stresses the importance of encouraging abstinence, although it also provides counseling on risk-reduction approaches including the use of latex condoms for every act of sexual intercourse. It also emphasizes the need to ensure ready access to contraceptive services and appropriate follow-up.

At the national level, a major effort to prevent teen pregnancy was initiated in 1996 with the organization of the National Campaign to Prevent Teen Pregnancy (NCPTP) (now the National Campaign to Prevent Teen and Unplanned Pregnancy [NCPTUP]). Its purpose is to reduce teenage pregnancy by one-third between 2006 and 2015 (NCPTUP, 2006). The National Campaign is a private, nonprofit organization made up of a broad spectrum of religious, political, social, human services, health, and academic organizations. The Association of Women's Health, Obstetric, and Neonatal Nurses (AWHONN) is one of the many professional organizations that joined this group and made a commitment to focus on adolescent pregnancy prevention.

One of the first actions of the National Campaign was to commission a task force to do a comprehensive review of the incidence of adolescent pregnancy and its impact in the United States. At the same time, another task force was commissioned to review the research on the effectiveness of pregnancy prevention programs. The purpose of these task forces was to provide accurate information based on fact and research. Not surprisingly, the task forces have found that adolescent pregnancy is a multifaceted problem with no easy answers. The best approach is local and is based on strong, community-wide involvement with a variety of programs directed at the multiple causes of the problem. Three interventions that have shown promising results are accurate, balanced, and realistic sexuality education; youth development programs that build on the assets and strengths of young people; and confidential and low-cost access to contraceptive services (Advocates for Youth, 2005).

A problem in local communities continues to be conflict among different groups about how to approach adolescent pregnancy prevention. Many parents advocate an "abstinence-plus" approach that stresses abstinence as the best approach but includes information on condoms and contraception for those teens who do not abstain.

Interestingly, recent research suggests that only 7% of people in the United States believe that sex education should not be provided in schools. Moreover, controversy about the type of sex education offered in schools seems to have decreased. Nearly three-fourths (74%) of principals surveyed state that they have not had any recent discussions or debate (in school board, PTA, or other public meetings) about what should be taught (National Public Radio [NPR], Kaiser Family Foundation, & John F. Kennedy School of Government, 2004).

Most Americans support providing education in junior and senior high schools with information about protection against unplanned pregnancy and STIs. Youth development programs that focus on meeting needs of adolescents by building on young people's capacities, assisting them to cultivate their own talent and to increase their feelings of self-worth, ease their transition into adulthood and can reduce sexual risk behaviors and unintended teen pregnancy (Advocates for Youth, 2005).

The National Campaign's task forces have also identified characteristics shared by all successful programs, regardless of the type of offering or community. Effective adolescent pregnancy prevention programs are long term and intensive. They also involve adolescents in program planning, include good role models from the same cultural and racial backgrounds, and focus on the adolescent male. Survey data from a representative sample of teens and adults provides some additional interesting insights (NCPTUP, 2004).

- Parents tend to underestimate their influence on their adolescents. Teens report that their parents, and not their friends, have the most influence on the teens' decisions about sex. However, a preponderance of teens also report that it would be easier to deal with issues related to sexuality and teen pregnancy if they could have more honest, open conversations with their parents.
- Teens' expressed attitudes about sexual activity reflect more cautious values and attitudes than generally believed. Teens report that their values, morals, religious beliefs, and concern for their future influence their decisions about sex more than concerns about becoming pregnant or developing a sexually transmitted infection.
- Almost all the adults and teens surveyed said that society should give teens a strong message that they should not have sex until they are at least out of high school.
- The majority of both groups advocate a message stressing abstinence while also providing information about contraception. They rejected the notion that such an approach sends a "mixed message."
- Teens want more information about sexuality, abstinence, and contraception.
- Teens tend to overestimate the percentage of their classmates and peers who have had sex.

In summary, although it is sometimes difficult for adults, it is important to address topics related to healthy relationships, abstinence, birth control, responsible sexual behavior, and the possible consequences of unsafe practices honestly and in a way that reflects adolescents' knowledge level, perspectives, and personal experience.

Discussion about teenage pregnancy needs to reflect an awareness of teens' priorities related to the costs and rewards of having a baby. All such discussions need to be honest, frank, and open and based on a recognition of the teen's developmental level (Herman, 2008).

CHAPTER HIGHLIGHTS

- Although the U.S. birth rate (number of births per 1000 women) for adolescents ages 15 to 19 dropped steadily from 1991 to 2005, it rose 3% in 2006 to 41.9 per 1000 females. Although this rate is significantly lower than the 1991 rate of 61.8, the United States continues to have the highest adolescent birth rates among industrialized nations.
- Many factors contribute to the high teenage pregnancy rate, including earlier age at first experience with sexual intercourse, lack of knowledge about conception, lack of easy access to contraception, lessened stigma associated with adolescent pregnancy in some populations, poverty, early school failure, and early childhood sexual abuse.
- Physical risks of adolescent pregnancy include preterm births, low-birth-weight infants, cephalopelvic disproportion, iron deficiency anemia, and preeclampsia–eclampsia and its sequelae.
- In the adolescent age group, prenatal care is the critical factor that most influences pregnancy outcome.

- The major psychologic risk the pregnant adolescent faces is the interruption of her own developmental tasks.
- In general, the children of teenage mothers are found to be at a developmental disadvantage compared with children whose mothers were older at the time of their birth.
- Almost half of the fathers of infants of adolescent mothers are age 20 or older but are often similar to adolescent fathers psychosocially and no more likely to be able to support the mother.
- Factors affecting an adolescent's response to pregnancy include her degree of achievement of the developmental tasks of adolescence (which can be closely associated with age), as well as cultural, religious, and socioeconomic factors.
- Often the adolescent has little understanding of pregnancy, childbirth, or parenting. Consequently, education is a primary responsibility of the nurse.
- Adolescent pregnancy prevention programs should be multifaceted, target males as well as females, and involve community-wide approaches.

CHAPTER REFERENCES

Advocates for Youth. (2005). *Teenage pregnancy, the case for prevention: An updated analysis of recent trends and federal expenditures associated with teenage pregnancy.* Retrieved October 7, 2005, from www.advocates for youth.org/publications/coststudy/

Alan Guttmacher Institute. (2006a). *Facts on American teens' sexual and reproductive health.* Retrieved January 11, 2008, from www. guttmacher.org

Alan Guttmacher Institute. (2006b). *U.S. teenage pregnancy statistics: National and state trends and trends by race and ethnicity.* Retrieved January 11, 2008, from www.guttmacher.org

Alan Guttmacher Institute. (2008a). State policies in brief: An overview of minors' consent law. Retrieved January 18, 2008, from www. guttmacher.org

Alan Guttmacher Institute. (2008b). State policies in brief: Minors' rights as parents. Retrieved January 18, 2008, from www.guttmacher.org

American Academy of Pediatrics. (2007). Policy statement: Contraception and adolescents. *Pediatrics, 120*(5), 1135–1148.

American College of Obstetricians and Gynecologists (ACOG). (2007). Intrauterine device and adolescents (Committee Opinion No. 392). Washington, DC: Author.

Bearinger, L. H., Sieving, R. E., Ferguson, J., & Sharma, V. (2007). Global perspectives on the sexual and reproductive health of adolescents: Patterns, prevention, and potential. *The Lancet, 369*, 1220–1229.

Bunting, L., & McAuley, C. (2004). Research review: Teenage pregnancy and parenthood: The role of fathers. *Child and Family Social Work, (9)*, 295–303.

Cohen, D. A., et al. (2002). When and where do youths have sex? The potential role of adult supervision. *Pediatrics, 110*(6), 66–69.

Doniger, A., Adams, E., Utter, C., & Riley, J. (2001). Impact evaluation of the "not me, not now" abstinence-oriented adolescent pregnancy prevention communication program, Monroe County, New York. *Journal of Health Communication, 6*(1), 45–60.

Eaton, D. K., Kann, L., Kinchen, S., Ross, L., Hawkins, J., et al. (2006, June 9). Youth risk behavior surveillance—United States, 2005. *Morbidity and Mortality Weekly Reports, 55*(SS05), 1–108.

Glass, N., Fredland, N., Campbell, J., Yonas, M., Sharps, P., & Kub, J. (2003). Adolescent dating violence: Prevalence, risk factors, health outcomes, and implications for clinical practice. *Journal of Obstetric, Gynecologic, and Neonatal Nursing, 32*(2), 227–238.

Hall Moran, V., Edwards, J., Dykes, F., & Downe, S. (2007). A systematic review of the nature of support for breast-feeding adolescent mothers. *Midwifery, 23,* 157–171.

Hamilton, B. E., Martin, J., & Ventura, S. J. (2007). Births: Preliminary data for 2006. *National Vital Statistics Reports, 56*(7), 1–18.

Herman, J. W. (2008). Adolescent perceptions of teen births. *JOGNN: Journal of Obstetric, Gynecologic, and Neonatal Nursing, 37*(1), 42–50.

Hillard, P. J. A. (2005). Contraceptive behaviors in adolescents. *Pediatric Annals, 34*(10), 794–802.

Key, J. D., Barbosa, G. A., & Owens, V. J. (2001). The second chance club: Repeat adolescent pregnancy prevention with a school-based intervention. *Journal of Adolescent Health, 28*(3), 167–169.

King-Jones, T. C. (2008). Pregnant adolescents: Perils and pearls of communication. *Nursing for Women's Health, 12*(2), 114–119.

Kirby, D. (2007). Emerging answers: Research findings on programs to reduce teen pregnancy and sexually transmitted diseases. The National Campaign to Prevent Teen and Unplanned Pregnancy. Retrieved April 17, 2008 from http://www.thenationalcampaign.org/EA2007/EA2007_sum.pdf

Klima, C. S. (2003). Centering pregnancy: A model for pregnant adolescents. *Journal of Midwifery & Women's Health, 48*(3), 220–225.

Males, M. (2004). Teens and older partners. *Resource Center for Adolescent Pregnancy Prevention (ReCAPP)* Retrieved January 15, 2008, from www.etr.org/recap/research/AuthoredPapOlderPrtnrs0504.htm

Manlove, J., Ryan, S., & Franzetta, K. (2003). Patterns of contraceptive use within teenagers' first sexual relationships. *Perspectives on Sexual and Reproductive Health, 35*(6), 246–255.

Marcell, A. V., Raine, T., & Eyre, S. L. (2003). Where does reproductive health fit into the lives of adolescent males? *Perspectives on Sexual and Reproductive Health, 35*(4), 180–186.

Montgomery, K. S. (2003). Nursing care for pregnant adolescents. *Journal of Obstetric, Gynecologic, and Neonatal Nursing, 32*(2), 249–257.

National Campaign to Prevent Teen Pregnancy. (2004). Survey slices: Highlights from the National Campaign's 2003 Annual Survey.

Retrieved January 22, 2004, from www.teenpregnancy.org

National Campaign to Prevent Teen and Unplanned Pregnancy. (2006). *Teen sexual activity, contraceptive use, pregnancy, and childbearing: General facts and stats.* Retrieved January 11, 2008, from www.teenpregnancy.org

National Public Radio [NPR], Kaiser Family Foundation, & John F. Kennedy School of Government. (2004). NPR/Kaiser/Kennedy School Poll: Sex Education in America. Retrieved April 18, 2004, from www.kff.org

Scheiman, L., & Zeoli, A. M. (2003). Adolescents' experiences of dating and intimate partner violence: "Once is not enough." *Journal of Midwifery and Women's Health, 48*(3), 226–228.

Short, M. B., & Rosenthal, S. L. (2003). Helping teenaged girls make wise sexual decisions. *Contemporary OB/GYN, 48*(5), 84–95.

Steinberg, L. (2005). *Adolescence* (7th ed.). New York: McGraw-Hill.

Tolaymat, L. L., & Kaunitz, A. M. (2007). Long-acting contraceptives in adolescents. *Current Opinion in Obstetrics and Gynecology, 19,* 453–460.

Weinstock, H., Berman, S., & Cates, W. (2004). Sexually transmitted diseases among American youth: Incidence and prevalence estimates, 2000. *Perspectives on Sexual and Reproductive Health, 36*(1), 6–10.

World Health Organization (WHO). (2004). *Adolescent pregnancy: Issues in adolescent health and development.* Geneva, Switzerland: Author.

CHAPTER 14

Assessment of Fetal Well-Being

What makes my job special is the relationships I develop with my patients. Many of the expectant mothers I work with begin coming to our office in early pregnancy and continue on a regular basis until they give birth. I know that some of the diagnostic tests we do can be intimidating, and it's my responsibility to help make those tests understandable. I love connecting with my patients, building a personal relationship with them, and explaining things to them when they have questions or fears. I feel a sense of accomplishment and pride when they feel comfortable enough to express those concerns with me.

—A Perinatal and Genetics Office Nurse

LEARNING OUTCOMES

14-1. Identify pertinent information to be discussed with the woman regarding her own assessment of fetal activity and methods of recording fetal activity.

14-2. Describe the methods, clinical applications, and results of ultrasound in the nursing care management of the pregnant woman.

14-3. Describe the use, procedure, information obtained, and nursing considerations for Doppler velocimetry, nonstress test, contraction stress test, and biophysical profile test.

14-4. Explain the use of amniocentesis as a diagnostic tool.

14-5. Describe the nurse's role and responsibilities in assisting during amniocentesis.

14-6. Compare the advantages and disadvantages of chorionic villus sampling (CVS) to amniocentesis.

KEY TERMS

Amniocentesis **302**
Biophysical profile (BPP) **299**
Chorionic villus sampling (CVS) **305**
Contraction stress test (CST) **300**
First-trimester combined screening **294**
Lecithin/sphingomyelin (L/S) ratio **304**
Nonstress test (NST) **296**
Nuchal translucency testing (NTT) **293**
Phosphatidylglycerol (PG) **304**
Quadruple screen **304**
Surfactant **304**
Ultrasound **292**
Umbilical velocimetry **296**

The past few decades have produced a notable increase in the number of techniques used to assess fetal well-being. From the relatively simple maternal assessment of fetal movement to more complex diagnostic tests guided by ultrasound, each technique is used to obtain accurate and helpful data about the developing fetus. For example, specialized diagnostic tests can provide information about the normal growth of the fetus, the presence of congenital anomalies, the location of the placenta, and fetal lung maturity (Table 14–1). At times just one test is done, and in other circumstances a combination of testing is needed.

Some of these assessment techniques pose risks to the fetus and possibly to the pregnant woman; the risk to both should be considered before deciding to perform the test. The healthcare provider must be certain that the advantages outweigh the potential risks and added expense. In addition, the diagnostic accuracy and applicability of these tests may vary. Although some tests are for screening purposes, meaning that they indicate the fetus *may* be at risk for a certain disorder or abnormality, others are diagnostic, meaning that they can diagnose the abnormality.

Certainly not all high-risk pregnancies require the same tests. Conditions that indicate a pregnancy at risk include the following:

- Maternal age less than 16 or more than 35 years
- Chronic maternal hypertension, preeclampsia, diabetes mellitus, or heart disease
- Presence of Rh alloimmunization
- A maternal history of unexplained stillbirth
- Suspected intrauterine growth restriction (IUGR)
- Pregnancy prolonged past 42 weeks' gestation
- Multiple gestation
- Maternal history of preterm labor
- Previous cervical incompetence

See Chapter 9 ∞ for further discussion of prenatal at-risk factors and Chapters 15 and 16 ∞ for descriptions of various conditions that may threaten the successful completion of pregnancy.

Nursing care for the woman who is undergoing diagnostic testing focuses on outcomes to ensure that she understands the reasons for the test, understands the test

---

TABLE 14–1   Summary of Screening and Diagnostic Tests

Goal	Test	Timing
To validate the pregnancy	Ultrasound: gestational sac volume	5 and 6 weeks after last menstrual period (LMP) by transvaginal ultrasound
To determine how advanced the pregnancy is	Ultrasound: crown–rump length	6 to 10 weeks' gestation
	Ultrasound: biparietal diameter, femur length, abdomen circumference	13 to 40 weeks' gestation
To identify normal growth of the fetus	Ultrasound: biparietal diameter	Most useful from 20 to 30 weeks' gestation
	Ultrasound: head/abdomen ratio	13 to 40 weeks' gestation
	Ultrasound: estimated fetal weight	About 24 to 40 weeks' gestation
To detect congenital anomalies and problems	Nuchal translucency testing	9 to 13 weeks' gestation
	Ultrasound	18 to 40 weeks' gestation
	Chorionic villus sampling	10 to 12 weeks' gestation
	Amniocentesis	15 to 20 weeks' gestation
	Fetoscopy	18 weeks' gestation
	First trimester combination screening test or quadruple test	Generally 15 to 20 weeks' gestation
To localize the placenta	Ultrasound	Usually in third trimester or before amniocentesis
To assess fetal status	Biophysical profile	Approximately 28 weeks to birth
	Maternal assessment of fetal activity	Approximately 28 weeks to birth
	Nonstress test	Approximately 28 weeks to birth
	Contraction stress test	After 28 weeks
To diagnose cardiac problems	Fetal echocardiography	Second and third trimesters
To assess fetal lung maturity	Amniocentesis	33 to 40 weeks
	L/S ratio	33 weeks to birth
	Phosphatidylglycerol	33 weeks to birth
	Phosphatidylcholine	33 weeks to birth
	Lamellar body counts	33 weeks to birth
To obtain more information about breech presentation	Ultrasound	Just before labor is anticipated or during labor

results, and has had support during the test (see Table 14–2). In addition, other objectives include completing the tests without complication and ensuring that the safety of the mother and her unborn child has been maintained.

HINTS FOR PRACTICE

Families undergoing fetal testing experience a wide range of emotions based on personal expectations, past experiences, fears, and cultural norms. Encouraging the family to verbalize concerns, ask questions, and express any apprehensions or fears can help put the family at ease.

Maternal Assessment of Fetal Activity

Clinicians now generally agree that vigorous fetal activity provides reassurance of fetal well-being and that marked decrease in activity or cessation of movement may indicate possible fetal compromise (or even death) requiring immediate follow-up (Gabbe, Niebyl, & Simpson, 2007). The technique is typically used to monitor fetal well-being beginning at approximately 28 gestational weeks. Fetal activity monitoring has been used for some time as a low technology, inexpensive means to evaluate fetal well-being. One study identified 19% of fetuses with intrauter-

ine growth restriction on the basis of an initial report by the mother of decreased fetal movement (Sinha, Sharma, Nallaswamy et al., 2007). A reduction of fetal movement has been associated with fetal hypoxia, fetal growth restriction, and fetal death (Heazell & Frøen, 2008). Another study showed that 5% to 15% of women report decreased fetal movement during their pregnancies (Heazell, Green, Wright, Flenady et al., 2008). Although more research is needed to determine if fetal activity assessment improves neonatal outcomes, the literature does suggest that maternal monitoring does result in a decrease in perinatal mortaility (Frøen, 2004; Heazell & Frøen, 2008; Mangesi & Hofmeyr, 2007). There is no definitive definition of how many movements should occur within a specified time period. The mother is instructed to count fetal movments at the same time each day. If there are less than 10 movements in a 3-hour period or if the amount of movement is significantly less than normal, the woman should immediately notify her healthcare provider. The newest literature suggests that a maternal perception of decreased movement occurring during a 24-hour period should cause concern and warrant antepartum fetal testing (Frøen, 2004; Heazell et al., 2008).

Fetuses spend approximately 10% of their time making gross body movements. Fetal movements are directly related to the infant's sleep–wake cycles and vary from the maternal sleep–wake cycle (Blackburn, 2007). Fetuses may react to maternal hypoglycemia by decreasing their activity level (Mirghani, Weerasinghe, Al-Awar et al., 2005). In women with a multiple gestation, daily fetal movements are significantly higher. After 38 weeks, the fetus spends 75% of its time in a quiet sleep or active sleep state. Other factors affecting fetal movement include sound, cigarette smoking, and drugs.

The expectant mother's perception of fetal movements and her commitment to completing a fetal movement record may vary. When a woman understands the purpose of the assessment, how to complete the form, whom to call with questions, and what to report—and has the opportunity for follow-up during each visit—she generally views completing the fetal movement record as an important activity. The nurse is available to answer questions and clarify areas of concern. (See further discussion and Client Teaching: What to Tell the Pregnant Woman About Assessing Fetal Activity, in Chapter 11 ∞.)

TABLE 14–2	Sample Nursing Approaches to Pretest Teaching

Assess whether the woman knows the reason the screening or diagnostic test is being recommended.

Examples:

"Has your doctor or nurse–midwife told you why this test is necessary?"

"Sometimes tests are done for many different reasons. Can you tell me why you are having this test?"

"What is your understanding about what the test will show?"

Provide an opportunity for questions.

Examples:

"Do you have any questions about the test?"

"Is there anything that is not clear to you?"

Explain the test procedure, paying particular attention to any preparation the woman needs before the test.

Example:

"The test that has been ordered for you is designed to _____." (Add specific information about the particular test. Give the explanation in simple language.)

Validate the woman's understanding of the preparation.

Example:

"Tell me what you will have to do to get ready for this test."

Give permission for the woman to continue to ask questions if needed.

Example:

"I'll be with you during the test. If you have any questions at any time, please don't hesitate to ask."

Ultrasound

Valuable information about the fetus may be obtained from **ultrasound** testing. Intermittent ultrasonic waves (high-frequency sound waves) are transmitted by an alternating current to a transducer, which is applied to the woman's abdomen. The ultrasonic waves deflect off tissues

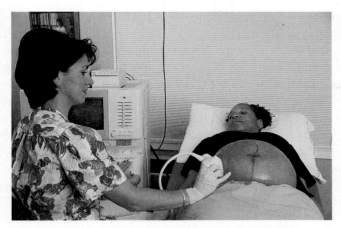

Figure 14–1 Ultrasound scanning permits visualization of the fetus in utero.

within the woman's abdomen, showing structures of varying densities (Figures 14–1 ■ and 14–2 ■).

Diagnostic ultrasound has several advantages. It is noninvasive, painless, and nonradiating to both the woman and the fetus, and it has no known harmful effects to either. Serial studies (several ultrasound tests done over a span of time) may be done for assessment and comparison. Soft-tissue masses (such as tumors) can be differentiated, the fetus can be visualized, fetal growth can be followed (especially in the presence of multiple gestation), cervical length and impending cervical incompetence can be detected, and a number of other potential problems can be averted (Smith, Celik, To et al., 2008; Verburg, Steegers, De Ridder et al., 2008). In addition, the ultrasonographer or physician immediately obtains results.

Future research in fetal well-being will be generated and enhanced by the use of the *four-dimensional ultrasound.* Four-dimensional ultrasound combines the components of three-dimensional ultrasound with a fourth dimension, time, because it monitors live action. The technology produces images of photolike quality, allowing healthcare providers to better visualize fetal structures, and

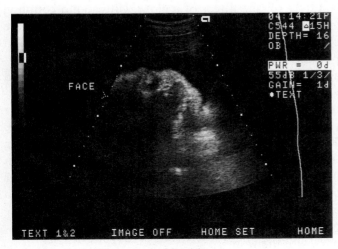

Figure 14–2 Ultrasound of fetal face.

providing better guidance during invasive intrauterine procedures such as amniocentesis and chorionic villus sampling (CVS) (discussed later in this chapter). The use of three- and four-dimensional ultrasound has been helpful in identifying facial anomalies, neural tube defects, and skeletal malformations (Kurjak, Miskovic, Andonotopo et al., 2007). Although ultrasound serves as a useful tool in monitoring the fetus throughout pregnancy, ultrasound has limitations and it cannot guarantee that a fetus does not have certain disorders or defects. Ultrasound is limited by maternal body habits, fetal positioning, and technician or physician skill. Even though fetal problems can be diagnosed via the technology, there are times that abnormalities go unrecognized. A "normal" ultrasound is reassuring for the parents and healthcare team, but it is important that parents realize a normal sonogram is not 100% reliable.

Nuchal Translucency Testing

Nuchal translucency testing (NTT), also known as nuchal testing (NT) or nuchal fold test, is performed at 11 1/7 to 13 6/7 gestational weeks to screen for trisomies 13, 18, and 21 (Wright, Kagan, Molina et al., 2008). Although women over the age of 35 have a higher risk of chromosomal disorders, ACOG (2004) recommends that all women be offered first- and second-trimester screening. The test uses ultrasound to scan the translucent or clear area on the back of the fetal neck, measuring the diameter of the area. Fetuses with certain genetic disorders often have an excess accumulation of fluid that can be seen at the end of the first trimester. The results are computed using the nuchal measurement, exact gestational age, and maternal age. Fetuses that have a nuchal translucency measurement of greater than 3 mm are at risk for trisomies 13, 18, and 21 and should be offered an amniocentesis (to be discussed later). The NTT is a *screening test,* meaning it indicates that a fetus is at risk. Diagnostic testing, such as an amniocentesis, is a *diagnostic test,* which indicates that the fetus has the specific diagnosis.

The NTT test has several advantages over other testing options. It can be performed in the first trimester, early in a pregnancy, to determine if a fetus is *at risk* for chromosomal disorders. Unlike the chorionic villus sampling (CVS) or amniocentesis, it has no risk of spontaneous abortion because it is a noninvasive test. The NTT accurately detects 70% to 80% of fetuses with Down Syndrome (DS) (Scott, 2007). When combined with serum testing, the accuracy level increases. Many women feel anxious during pregnancy. A normal result can provide reassurance to the woman that her baby is most likely without a chromosome disorder.

The disadvantage is that it can provide false positives and is not diagnostic. The combined test has a 5% false positive rate, meaning the test will indicate that the fetus is at risk for Down syndrome when in fact the fetus has normal chromosomes. Women who receive an abnormal test are then counseled to determine if they would like to have an amniocentesis for diagnostic purposes. The choice to proceed with testing is a very personal one. Some women will wish to obtain the test so they will be more prepared for the diagnosis; other women will want to discontinue the pregnancy. Some women may decide not to have additional testing.

Fetuses that have a nuchal translucency measurement above the 99th percentile are also at risk for congenital heart disease (Clur, Mathijssen, Pajkrt et al., 2008). A fetal echocardiogram is ordered in these cases to determine if a cardiac anomaly is also present. Fetuses with a nuchal fold measurement equal to or greater than 6.5 mm had a 27.7% risk of having a congenital heart defect (Clur et al., 2008).

First-trimester combined screening is comprehensive screening testing that includes the NTT and serum screening for pregnancy-associated plasma protein-A (PAPP-A) and free beta human chorionic gonadotropin (BHCG) to determine if a fetus is at risk for trisomies 13, 18, and 21. The combined test is more accurate than a NTT alone because it provides additional data. Using both the NTT and the serum testing, the accuracy rates for diagnosis improves to 91% for accurately assessing the risk of Down Syndrome and 98% for assessing trisomy 18 (Clur et al., 2008).

HINTS FOR PRACTICE

When advising clients that a screening test, such as the NTT, is abnormal, make sure to explain that this does *not* mean their baby definitely has the disorder, but rather indicates that the baby *may* be at risk. It is imperative that parents understand an abnormal NTT, or any type of screening test, is only an indication that more testing is needed to make the actual diagnosis. Advise parents that some women with abnormal test results have normal fetuses and that because the test only screens and does not actually diagnosis the fetus, a fetus that screens within the normal criteria could have an unrecognized anomaly.

Procedures

The two most common methods of ultrasound scanning are transabdominal and transvaginal.

Transabdominal Ultrasound

In the transabdominal approach, a transducer is moved across the woman's abdomen. The woman is often scanned with a full bladder; when the bladder is full, the examiner can assess other structures, especially the vagina and cervix, in relation to the bladder. The ability to see the lower portion of the uterus and cervix is particularly im-

portant when vaginal bleeding is noted and placenta previa is the suspected cause. The woman is advised to drink 1 to 1.5 quarts of water approximately 2 hours before the examination, and she is asked to refrain from emptying her bladder. If the bladder is not sufficiently filled, she is asked to drink three to four (8 oz) glasses of water and is rescanned 30 to 45 minutes later.

Mineral oil or a transmission gel is generously spread over the woman's abdomen, and the sonographer slowly moves a transducer over the abdomen to obtain a picture of the uterus contents. Ultrasound testing takes 20 to 30 minutes. The woman may feel discomfort caused by pressure applied over a full bladder. In addition, if the woman lies on her back during the test, shortness of breath can develop. This may be relieved by elevating her upper body during the test.

Transvaginal Ultrasound

The transvaginal approach uses a probe inserted into the vagina. Once inserted, the transvaginal probe is close to the structures being imaged and so produces a clearer, more defined image. The improved images obtained by transvaginal ultrasound have enabled sonographers to identify structures and fetal characteristics earlier in pregnancy (McAuliffe, Fong, Toi et al., 2005). Internal visualization can also be used as a predictor for preterm birth in high-risk cases (Grimes-Dennis, 2007). Use of the ultrasound to detect shortened cervical length or funneling (a cone-shaped indentation in the cervical os) is helpful in predicting preterm labor, especially in women who have a history of preterm birth (Borrell, 2007).

After the procedure is fully explained to the woman, she is prepared in the same manner as for a pelvic examination: in the lithotomy position, with appropriate drapes to provide privacy and a female attendant in the room. It is important that her buttocks are at the end of the table so that, once inserted, the probe can be moved in various directions. A small, lightweight vaginal transducer is covered with a specially fitted sterile sheath, a condom, or one finger of a glove. Ultrasound coupling gel is then applied to both the inside and outside of the covering, making insertion into the vagina easier and providing a medium for enhancing the ultrasound image. The transvaginal procedure can be accomplished with an empty bladder, and most women do not feel discomfort during the exam. The probe is smaller than a speculum, so insertion is usually completed with ease. The woman may feel the movement of the probe during the exam as various structures are imaged. Some women may want to insert the probe themselves to enhance their comfort, whereas others would feel embarrassed even to be asked. The certified nurse–midwife, physician, or ultrasonographer offers the choice based on personal rapport with the woman.

Clinical Applications

Ultrasound testing can be of benefit in the following ways:

- *Early identification of pregnancy.* Pregnancy may be detected as early as the fifth or sixth week after the last menstrual period (LMP) by assessing the gestational sac and the presence of a fetal heart rate after 6 gestational weeks.
- *Observation of fetal heartbeat and fetal breathing movements (FBMs).* FBMs have been observed as early as week 11 of gestation.
- *Identification of more than one embryo or fetus.*
- *Measurement of the biparietal diameter of the fetal head or the fetal femur length to assess growth patterns.* These measurements help determine the gestational age of the fetus and identify IUGR.
- *Clinical estimations of birth weight.* This assessment helps to identify macrosomia (infants greater than 4000 g at birth) and low-birth-weight infants (infants less than 2500 g at birth). Macrosomia has been identified as a predictor of birth-related trauma and is a risk factor for both maternal and fetal morbidity (Sritippayawan, 2007).
- *Detection of fetal anomalies such as anencephaly and hydrocephalus.*
- *Examination of nuchal translucency in the first trimester to assess for Down syndrome and other fetal structural anomalies* (Piazze, 2007). Nuchal translucency describes an area in the back of the fetal neck that is measured via ultrasound during the first trimester of pregnancy. Fetuses with a nuchal translucency measurement of greater than 3 mm are at risk for certain birth defects, including trisomies 13, 18, and 21.
- *Examination of fetal cardiac structures (echocardiography).*
- *Length of fetal nasal bone.* The length of the fetal nasal bone during the nuchal translucency test is used to indicate a risk factor for Down syndrome. Fetuses with a nonvisualized or shortened nasal bone are more likely to have trisomy 21 than those with a normal length nasal bone (Cusick, Shevell, Duchan et al., 2008).
- *Identification of amniotic fluid index (AFI).* The maternal abdomen is divided into quadrants. The umbilicus is used to divide the upper and lower sections, and the linea nigra divides the right and left sections. The vertical diameter of the largest amniotic fluid pocket in each quadrant is measured. All measurements are totaled to obtain the AFI in centimeters. Women with an AFI of more than 20 cm are considered to have hydramnios, and women with less than 5 cm at term are considered to have oligohydramnios. An AFI between 5 and 20 cm is considered normal. After 39 weeks, the amniotic fluid volume begins to decline (Gabbe et al., 2007). Both hydramnios and oligohydramnios are associated with increased risk to the fetus, including nonreassuring fetal status, intrauterine growth restriction, meconium-stained amniotic fluid, and an increase in admissions to the neonatal intensive care unit (Gumus, 2007).
- *Location of the placenta.* The placenta is located before amniocentesis to avoid puncturing the placenta. Ultrasound is valuable in identifying and evaluating placenta previa (Abramowicz, 2007).
- *Placental grading.* As the fetus matures, the placenta calcifies. These changes can be detected by ultrasound and graded according to the degree of calcification. Placenta grading can be used to identify internal placenta vasculature which can be associated with preeclampsia and chronic hypertension. It can also identify disorders such as fetal growth abnormalities, triploidy, non-immune hydrops, and infections (Abramowicz, 2007).
- *Detection of fetal death.* Inability to visualize the fetal heart beating and the separation of the bones in the fetal head are signs of fetal death.
- *Determination of fetal position and presentation.*
- *Accompanying procedures.* Amniocentesis, chorionic villus sampling, intrauterine procedures, and other procedures will be discussed shortly.

Risks of Ultrasound

Ultrasound has been used clinically for over 40 years; to date no clinical studies verify harmful effects to the mother, the fetus, or the newborn. The use of ultrasound in pregnancy has spanned nearly three generations. Many pregnant clients themselves received diagnostic ultrasound in utero with no adverse effects (Cunningham et al., 2005).

Nursing Care Management

It is important for the nurse to ascertain whether the woman understands why the ultrasound is being suggested and that the ultrasound is an extremely valuable tool although it is not 100% reliable. The nurse provides an opportunity for the woman to ask questions and acts as an advocate if there are questions or concerns that need to be addressed before the ultrasound examination. The nurse discusses the options available to the woman and her partner for fetal evaluation. According to ACOG (2007), the option of fetal evaluation should be offered to all women, regardless of age. This includes both invasive testing, such as amniocentesis and chorionic villus sampling (CVS), and ultrasound screening. The nurse explains the preparation needed and ensures that adequate preparation is done. After the test is completed, the nurse can assist with clarifying or interpreting test results for the woman and her partner.

Doppler Blood Flow Studies (Umbilical Velocimetry)

Umbilical velocimetry, a noninvasive ultrasound test, measures blood flow changes that occur in maternal and fetal circulation in order to assess placental function. An ultrasound beam, like that provided by the pocket Doppler (a handheld ultrasound device), is directed at the umbilical artery (in some cases a maternal vessel such as the arcuate can also be used). The signal is reflected off the red blood cells moving within the vessels and creates a "picture" (waveform) that looks like a series of waves (Figures 14–3 ■ and 14–4 ■). The highest-velocity peak of the waves is the systolic measurement, and the lowest point is the diastolic velocity. To interpret the waveforms, the systolic (S) peak is divided by the end-diastolic (D) component. This calculation is called the S/D ratio. The normal S/D ratio is below 2.6 by 26 weeks' gestation and below 3 at term. A decrease in uteroplacental perfusion (because of narrowing of the vessels) causes an increase in placental bed resistance and a decrease in diastolic flow, resulting in an elevated S/D ratio (Kwon, 2006). Elevations of 3 and above are considered abnormal. Doppler blood flow studies are helpful in assessing and managing pregnancies with suspected uteroplacental insufficiency before asphyxia occurs (Kwon, 2006). Abnormal Doppler flow studies accompanied by a decrease in amniotic fluid have been associated with small for gestational age fetuses, cesarean section for nonreassuring fetal status, 5 min Apgar score of less than 7 (7 to 10 is the normal range), respiratory distress syndrome, NICU admission, and perinatal death (Kwon, 2006).

Doppler blood flow studies are relatively easy to obtain. The woman lies supine with a wedge under the right hip (to promote uteroplacental perfusion). Warmed transducer gel is applied to the abdomen, and a pulsed-wave Doppler device is used to ascertain the blood flow. The Doppler flow study takes about 15 to 20 minutes. Doppler flow studies can be initiated at 16 to 18 weeks' gestation and are then scheduled at regular intervals for women at risk.

Nonstress Test

The **nonstress test (NST)**, a widely used method of evaluating fetal status, may be used alone or as part of a more comprehensive diagnostic assessment called a *biophysical profile (BPP)*. The nonstress test is based on the knowledge that when the fetus has adequate oxygenation and an intact central nervous system, there are accelerations of the fetal heart rate (FHR) with fetal movement. An NST requires an electronic fetal monitor to observe and record these fetal heart rate accelerations (see discussion of accel-

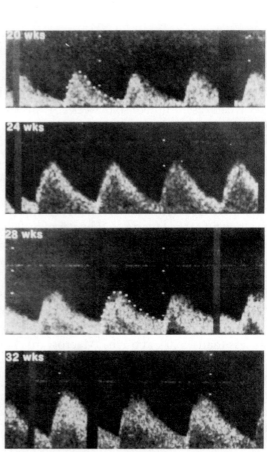

FIGURE 14–3 Serial studies of the umbilical artery velocity waveforms in a normal pregnancy from one client.
Source: AWHONN. (1990). Cundiff, J. L., Haybrich, K. L., & Hinzman, N. G. Umbilical artery Doppler flow studies during pregnancy. *Journal of Obstetric, Gynecologic, and Neonatal Nursing, 19*(6), 475–481 (Figure 3, p. 478). Washington, DC: Author. © 1990 by the Association of Women's Health, Obstetric, and Neonatal Nurses. All rights reserved.

eration in Chapter 18 ∞). A nonreactive NST is fairly consistent in identifying at-risk fetuses (Gabbe et al., 2007). The advantages of the NST are as follows:

- It is quick to perform, permits easy interpretation, and is inexpensive.
- It can be done in an office or clinic setting.
- There are no known side effects.

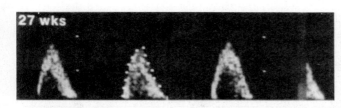

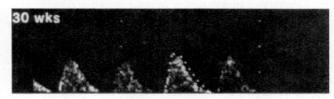

FIGURE 14–4 Two examples of abnormal umbilical artery velocity waveforms taken from a client with intrauterine growth restriction.
Source: AWHONN. (1990). Cundiff, J. L., Haybrich, K. L., & Hinzman, H. G. Umbilical artery Doppler flow studies during pregnancy. *Journal of Obstetric, Gynecologic, and Neonatal Nursing, 19*(6), 475–481 (Figure 4, p. 478). Washington, DC: Author. © 1990 by the Association of Women's Health, Obstetric, and Neonatal Nurses. All rights reserved.

The disadvantages of the NST include the following:

* It is sometimes difficult to obtain a suitable tracing.
* The woman has to remain relatively still for at least 20 minutes.

Procedure for NST

The test can be done with the woman in a reclining chair or in bed in a left-tilted semi-Fowler's or side-lying position. Research has shown that certain maternal positions can help produce more favorable results. Women in left-tilted semi-Fowler's, sitting positions, and left lateral positions have more fetal movement and are more likely to have a reactive tracing. Women should not be placed in a supine position because it is associated with less fetal movement, maternal back pain, and maternal shortness of breath (Alus, Okumus, Mete et al., 2007). An electronic fetal monitor is used to obtain a tracing of the fetal heart rate (FHR) and fetal movement (FM). The nurse places the monitor under the woman's clothing. Privacy should be provided. The examiner puts two elastic belts on the woman's abdomen. One belt holds a device that detects uterine or fetal movement; the other belt holds a device that detects the FHR. As the NST is done, each fetal movement is documented, so that associated or simultaneous FHR changes can be evaluated.

Interpretation of NST Results

Women with a high-risk factor will probably begin having NSTs at 30 to 32 weeks' gestation and at frequent intervals for the remainder of the pregnancy. The results of the NST are interpreted as follows:

* *Reactive test.* A reactive NST shows at least two accelerations of FHR with fetal movements of 15 beats per minute, lasting 15 seconds or more, over 20 minutes (Figure 14–5 ■). This is the desired result. (See Key Facts to Remember: Nonstress Test.)
* *Nonreactive test.* In a nonreactive test, the reactive criteria are not met. For example, the accelerations do not meet the requirements of 15 beats per minute or do not last 15 seconds (Figure 14–6 ■).
* *Unsatisfactory test.* An NST is unsatisfactory if the data cannot be interpreted or there was inadequate fetal activity.

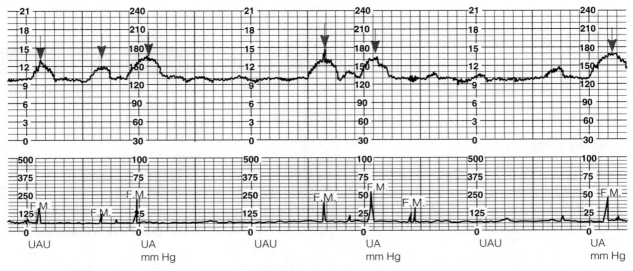

FIGURE 14–5 Example of a reactive nonstress test (NST). Accelerations of 15 bpm lasting 15 seconds with each fetal movement (FM). Top of strip shows FHR; bottom of strip shows uterine activity tracing. Note that FHR increases (above the baseline) at least 15 beats and remains at that rate for at least 15 seconds before returning to the former baseline.

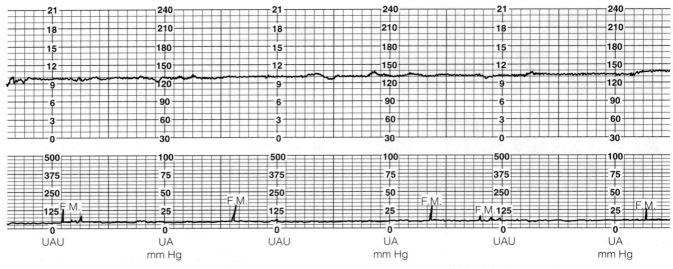

FIGURE 14–6 Example of a nonreactive NST. There are no accelerations of FHR with FM. Baseline FHR is 130 bpm. The tracing of uterine activity is on the bottom of the strip.

KEY FACTS TO REMEMBER

Nonstress Test

Diagnostic value: Demonstrates fetus's ability to respond to its environment by acceleration of FHR with movement.

RESULTS

- *Reactive test:* Accelerations (at least 2) of 15 bpm above the baseline, lasting 15 sec or more in a 20-min window, are present, indicating fetal well-being.
- *Nonreactive test:* Accelerations are not present or do not meet the above criteria indicating that the fetus is at risk or asleep.
- *Unsatisfactory test:* Data cannot be interpreted or there was inadequate fetal activity.

It is important that anyone who performs the NST understand the significance of any decelerations of the FHR during testing. If decelerations are noted, the certified nurse–midwife or physician should be notified for further evaluation of fetal status. (See Chapter 18 ∞ for further discussion of FHR decelerations.)

Clinical Management

The clinical management of potential nonreassuring fetal status may vary somewhat among clinicians depending on the clinical judgment of the care provider. One commonly used protocol is as follows: If the NST is reactive in less than 30 minutes, the test is concluded and rescheduled as indicated by the high-risk condition that is present; if it is nonreactive, the test time is extended for 30 minutes until the results are reactive, and then the test is rescheduled as indicated. It is estimated that 80% to

90% of nonreactive NSTs happen because of fetal sleep states (Gabbe et al., 2007). If the FHR remains nonreactive for longer than 30 minutes, the test is typically repeated after the woman eats or the fetus is stimulated via vibroacoustic stimulation, a foot massage, or palpation. Such measures often wake a fetus so a reactive NST can be obtained. If a reactive test is not obtained within 30 minutes, additional testing (such as diagnostic ultrasound and BPP) or immediate birth is considered; if the NST is nonreactive and spontaneous decelerations of the FHR are present, diagnostic ultrasound and BPP are performed and birth is recommended (Figure 14–7 ■). Many testing guidelines vary in frequency, recommending a retest either once or twice a week, depending upon the at-risk condition that exists. In some situations, such as preterm premature rupture of membranes, testing may be done daily (Cunningham et al., 2005).

Nursing Care Management

The nurse evaluates the woman's understanding of the NST and the possible results. The reasons for the NST and the procedure are reviewed before beginning the test. The nurse administers the NST, interprets the results, and reports the findings to the certified nurse–midwife or physician and the expectant woman.

HINTS FOR PRACTICE

If a nonstress test fails to become reactive, a 3-minute foot massage has been shown to stimulate the fetus and increase fetal activity. It also helps the woman to relax during the test.

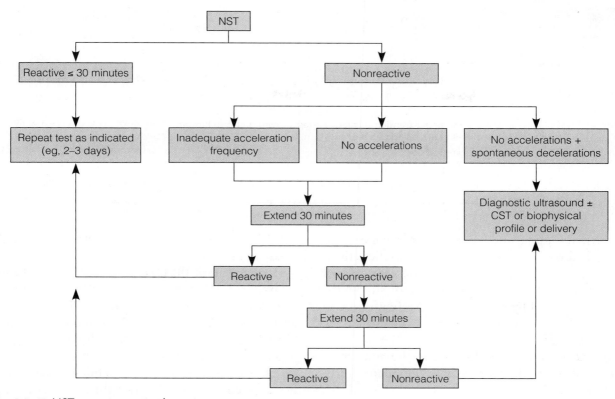

FIGURE 14–7 NST management scheme.
Source: Devoe, L. D. (1989). Nonstress and contraction stress testing. In R. Depp, D. A. Eschenbach, & J. J. Sciarri (Eds.), *Gynecology and obstetrics* (Vol. 3, p. 9, Figure 14–5). Philadelphia: Lippincott.

Fetal Acoustic Stimulation Test and Vibroacoustic Stimulation Test

Acoustic (sound) and vibroacoustic (vibration and sound) stimulation of the fetus can be used as an adjunct to the NST. A handheld, battery-operated device is applied to the woman's abdomen over the area of the fetal head. This device generates a low-frequency vibration and a buzzing sound. These are intended to induce movement and associated accelerations of FHR in fetuses with a nonreactive NST and in fetuses with decreased variability of FHR during labor. (See discussion of variability in Chapter 18 ∞.) The sound stimulus persists for 2 to 5 seconds; if no accelerations occur, it is then repeated at 1-minute intervals up to three times. Whether the fetus responds more to the vibration or to the sound is not known. Two FHR accelerations of 15 beats per minute, lasting 15 seconds, in a 20-minute period indicate a reactive test (Gabbe et al., 2007). In one study, 82% of women perceived fetal movement after acoustic stimulation was performed. In the same study, 67% of women who had reported absent or decreased fetal movement felt movement and 91% had a reactive nonstress test. The test had a better predictive value of identifying fetuses with asphyxia than fetuses who underwent NST alone (Batcha, 2005). Advantages of the fetal acoustic stimulation test (FAST) and the vibroacoustic stimulation test (VST) are as follows:

- Both are noninvasive techniques and are easy to perform.
- Results are rapidly available.
- Time for the NST is shortened.

Biophysical Profile

The **biophysical profile (BPP)** is a comprehensive assessment of five biophysical variables:

1. Fetal breathing movement
2. Fetal movements of body or limbs
3. Fetal tone (extension and flexion of extremities)
4. Amniotic fluid volume (visualized as pockets of fluid around the fetus)
5. Reactive FHR with activity (reactive NST)

The first four variables are assessed by ultrasound scanning; FHR reactivity is assessed with the NST. By combining these five assessments, the BPP helps to either identify the compromised fetus or confirm the healthy fetus and provides an assessment of placental functioning. Specific criteria for normal and abnormal assessments are presented in Table 14–3. A score of 2 is assigned

TABLE 14–3	Criteria for Biophysical Profile Scoring	
Component	Normal (score = 2)	Abnormal (score = 0)
Fetal breathing movements	≥ 1 episode of rhythmic breathing lasting ≥ 30 sec within 30 min	≤ 30 sec of breathing in 30 min
Gross body movements	≥ 3 discrete body or limb movements in 30 min (episodes of active continuous movement considered as single movement)	≤ 2 movements in 30 min
Fetal tone	≥ 1 episode of extension of a fetal extremity with return to flexion, or opening or closing of hand	No movements or extension/flexion
Amniotic fluid volume	Single vertical pocket > 2 cm	Largest single vertical pocket ≤ 2 cm
	AFI > 5 cm	AFI < 5 cm
Nonstress test	≥ 2 accelerations of ≥ 15 beats/min for ≥ 15 sec in 20–40 min	0 or 1 acceleration in 20–40 min

to each normal finding, and 0 to each abnormal one, for a maximum score of 10. The absence of a specific activity is difficult to interpret, because it may be indicative of central nervous system (CNS) depression or simply the resting state of a healthy fetus. Scores of 8 (with normal amniotic fluid) and 10 are considered normal. Such scores have the least chance of being associated with a compromised fetus unless a decrease in the amount of amniotic fluid is noted, in which case the infant's birth may be indicated (Kwon, 2006).

The BPP is indicated when there is risk of placental insufficiency or fetal compromise because of the following:

- Intrauterine growth restriction (IUGR)
- Maternal diabetes mellitus
- Maternal heart disease
- Maternal chronic hypertension
- Maternal preeclampsia or eclampsia
- Maternal sickle cell anemia
- Suspected fetal postmaturity (more than 42 weeks' gestation)
- History of previous stillbirths
- Rh sensitization
- Abnormal estriol excretion
- Hyperthyroidism
- Renal disease
- Nonreactive NST

Contraction Stress Test

The **contraction stress test (CST)** is a means of evaluating the respiratory function (oxygen and carbon dioxide exchange) of the placenta. It enables the healthcare team to identify the fetus at risk for intrauterine asphyxia by observing the response of the FHR to the stress of uterine contractions (spontaneous or induced). During contractions, intrauterine pressure increases. Blood flow to the intervillous space of the placenta is reduced momentarily, thereby decreasing oxygen transport to the fetus. A healthy fetus usually tolerates this reduction well and maintains a steady heart rate. If the placental reserve is insufficient,

fetal hypoxia, depression of the myocardium, and a decrease in FHR occur.

In many areas, the CST has given way to the biophysical profile. It is still used in areas where the availability of other technology is reduced (such as during night shifts) or limited (such as at small community hospitals or birthing centers). It may also be used as an adjunct to other forms of fetal assessment.

The CST is contraindicated in third-trimester bleeding from placenta previa, marginal abruptio placentae or unexplained vaginal bleeding, previous cesarean with classical incision (vertical incision in the fundus of the uterus), premature rupture of the membranes, incompetent cervix, cerclage in place, anomalies of the maternal reproductive organs, history of preterm labor (if being done before term), or multiple gestation.

Procedure

The critical component of the CST is the presence of uterine contractions. They may occur spontaneously (which is unusual before the onset of labor), or they may be induced (stimulated) with oxytocin (Pitocin) administered intravenously (also known as an oxytocin challenge test [OCT]). A natural method of obtaining oxytocin is through the use of breast stimulation (either via nipple self-stimulation or application of an electric breast pump); the posterior pituitary produces oxytocin in response to stimulation of the breasts or nipples.

An electronic fetal monitor is used to provide continuous data about the fetal heart rate and uterine contractions. After a 15-minute baseline recording of uterine activity and FHR, the tracing is evaluated for evidence of spontaneous contractions. If three spontaneous contractions of good quality and lasting 40 to 60 seconds occur in a 10-minute window, the results are evaluated, and the test is concluded. If no contractions occur or they are insufficient for interpretation, oxytocin is administered intravenously or breast self-stimulation or application of an electric breast pump is done to produce contractions of good quality. (See Chapter 23 ∞ for more information on nursing care management of oxytocin induction.) The CST should only be conducted in a setting where tocolytic medications are available if a hyperstimulation pattern occurs or if labor is stimulated from the test.

Interpretation of CST Results

The CST is classified as follows:

- *Negative.* A negative CST shows three contractions of good quality lasting 40 or more seconds in 10 minutes without evidence of late decelerations. This is the desired result. It implies that the fetus can handle the hypoxic stress of uterine contractions.
- *Positive.* A positive CST shows repetitive persistent late decelerations with more than 50% of the contractions (Figure 14–8 ■). This is not a desired result. The hypoxic stress of the uterine contraction causes a slowing of the FHR. The pattern will not improve and will most likely get worse with additional contractions.
- *Equivocal.*
  - An equivocal-suspicious test is where less than 50% of the contractions on strip are late decelerations. Variability is usually good (Gilbert, 2007).
  - An equivocal-hyperstimulation test. Uterine contraction frequency of every 2 minutes or contraction lasting greater than 90 seconds with a late deceleration occurring). When this test result occurs, more information is needed.
- *Unsatisfactory.* The quality of tracing is too poor to accurately interpret FHR with contractions or the frequency of three contractions lasting 40 to 60 seconds occurring in a 10-minute window of time cannot be obtained for endpoint of the test.

Clinical Application

A negative CST implies that the placenta is functioning normally, fetal oxygenation is adequate, and the fetus will probably be able to withstand the stress of labor. If labor does not occur in the ensuing week, further testing is done.

A positive CST with a nonreactive NST presents evidence that the fetus will not likely withstand the stress of labor. A positive CST may be able to identify compromised fetuses earlier than a nonreactive NST because of the stimulated interruption of intervillous blood flow (Gabbe et al., 2007). Although a negative CST is reliable in predicting fetal status, a positive result needs to be verified, such as a biophysical profile. (See Key Facts to Remember: Contraction Stress Test.)

◆

KEY FACTS TO REMEMBER
Contraction Stress Test

Diagnostic value: Demonstrates reaction of FHR to stress of uterine contraction.

RESULTS

- *Negative test:* Stress of uterine contraction shows three contractions of good quality lasting 40 or more seconds in 10 minutes without evidence of late decelerations.
- *Positive test:* Stress of uterine contraction shows repetitive persistent late deceleration with more than 50% of the uterine contractions.
- *Equivocal:* Suspicious test shows inconsistent late decelerations. Hyperstimulation test shows uterine contraction frequency of every 2 minutes or contractions lasting greater than 90 seconds with a late deceleration occurring.

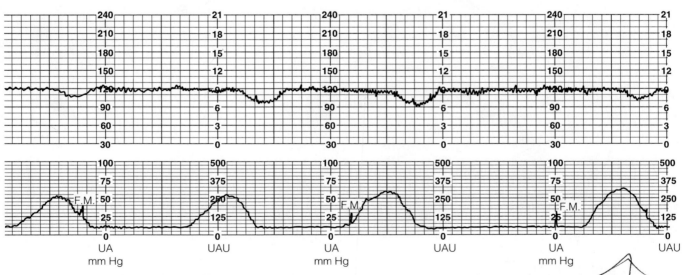

FIGURE 14–8 Example of a positive contraction stress test (CST). Repetitive late decelerations occur with each contraction. Note that there are no accelerations of FHR with three fetal movements (FM). The baseline FHR is 120 bpm. Uterine contractions (bottom half of strip) occurred four times in 12 minutes.

Nursing Care Management

The nurse ascertains the woman's understanding of the CST, the reasons for the test, and the possible results before the test begins. Written consent is required in some settings. In this case, the certified nurse–midwife or physician is responsible for fully informing the woman about the test. The nurse administers the CST, interprets the results, and reports the findings to the certified nurse–midwife or physician and the expectant woman. In some settings, the presence of the CNM or physician is required because there is a risk of initiating labor or hypertonic uterine contractions. Throughout the procedure, the nurse performs critical assessments and provides continual reassurance to the woman and her support person.

HINTS FOR PRACTICE

When offering expectant parents options for fetal evaluation, make sure that the parents understand the differences between *screening* tests, such as the nuchal translucency testing (NTT) and quadruple screen, and *diagnostic* testing, such as the chorionic villus sampling and amniocentesis. Screening tests can be valuable tools to determine if a fetus is at risk; however, a diagnostic test indicates whether or not the fetus actually has the disorder.

Amniotic Fluid Analysis

Amniocentesis is a procedure used to obtain amniotic fluid for genetic testing for fetal abnormalities or to determine fetal lung maturity in the third trimester of pregnancy. During an amniocentesis, the physician scans the uterus using ultrasound to identify the fetal and placental positions and to identify adequate pockets of amniotic fluid. The skin is then cleaned with a betadine solution. The use of a local anesthesia at the needle insertion site is optional. A 22-gauge needle is then inserted into the uterine cavity to withdraw amniotic fluid (Figure 14–9 ■). After 15 to 20 mL of fluid has been removed, the needle is withdrawn and the site is assessed for streaming (movement of fluid), which is an indication of bleeding. The fetal heart rate and maternal vital signs are then assessed. Rh immune globulin is given to all Rh-negative women. The analysis of amniotic fluid provides valuable information about fetal status. Amniocentesis is a fairly simple procedure, although complications do occur on rare occasions (less than 1% of cases). See Clinical Skill: Assisting During Amniocentesis for nursing interventions during amniocentesis.

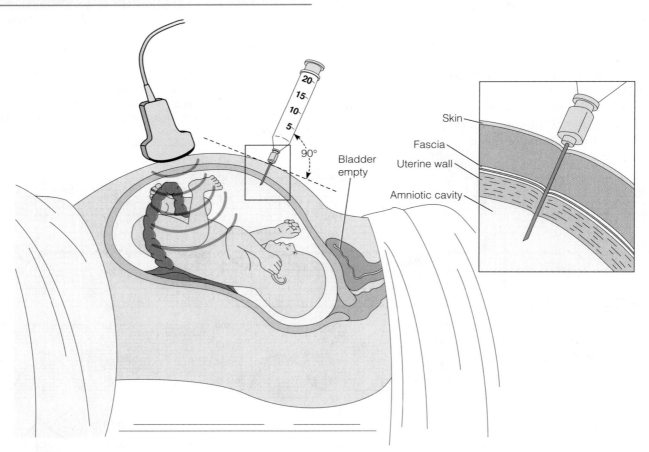

FIGURE 14–9 Amniocentesis. The woman is scanned by ultrasound to determine the placenta site and to locate a pocket of amniotic fluid. The needle is then inserted into the uterine cavity to withdraw amniotic fluid.

Clinical Skill Assisting During Amniocentesis

NURSING ACTION	RATIONALE
Preparation	
• Explain the procedure, the indications for it and reassure the woman.	*Explanation of the procedure decreases anxiety.*
• Determine whether an informed consent has been signed. If not, verify that the woman's doctor has explained the procedure and ask her to sign a consent form.	*It is the physician's responsibility to obtain informed consent. The woman's signature indicates her awareness of risks and gives her consent to the procedure.*
Equipment and Supplies	
Prepare and arrange the following items so they are easily accessible:	*Amniotic fluid must be shielded from light to prevent breakdown of bilirubin.*
• 22-gauge spinal needle with stylet	
• 10 and 20 mL syringes	
• 1% xylocaine	
• Povidone–iodine (Betadine)	
• Three 10-mL test tubes with tops (amber colored or covered with tape)	
Procedure: Sterile Gloves	
1. Obtain baseline vital signs data on maternal BP, temperature, pulse, respirations, and FHR before procedure begins; then monitor BP, pulse, respirations, and FHR every 15 minutes during procedure.	Baseline information is essential to detect any changes in maternal or fetal status that might be related to the procedure.
2. Provide gel for the ultrasound and assist with the real-time ultrasound to assess needle insertion during the procedure as needed.	*Amniocentesis is usually performed laterally in the area of fetal small parts, where pockets of amniotic fluid are often seen. Real-time ultrasound will identify fetal parts and locate pockets of amniotic fluid.*
3. Cleanse the woman's abdomen.	*Cleansing the woman's abdomen before needle insertion helps decrease the risk of infection.*
4. The physician dons gloves, inserts the needle into the identified pocket of fluid, and withdraws a sample.	
5. Obtain the test tubes from the physician.	
6. Label the tubes with the women's correct identification and send to the lab with the appropriate lab slips.	
7. Monitor the woman and reassess her vital signs.	*Monitoring maternal and fetal status postprocedure provides information about response to the procedure and helps detect any complications such as inadvertent fetal puncture.*
• Determine the woman's BP, pulse, respirations, and FHR.	
• Palpate the woman's fundus to assess for uterine contractions.	
• Monitor the woman with an external fetal monitor for 20 to 30 minutes after the amniocentesis.	
• Determine a treatment course to counteract any supine hypotension and to increase venous return and cardiac output.	
8. Assess the woman's blood type and determine any need for Rh immune globulin.	
9. Administer Rh immune globulin if indicated.	*Rh immune globulin is administered prophylactically following an amniocentesis to prevent Rh sensitization in an Rh-negative woman.*
10. Reassure the woman and provide self-care education.	*The woman will know how to recognize changes or symptoms that warrant further evaluation.*
• Instruct the woman to report any of the following changes or symptoms to her primary caregiver:	
a. Unusual fetal hyperactivity or, conversely, any lack of movement	
b. Vaginal discharge—clear drainage or bleeding	
c. Uterine contractions or abdominal pain	
d. Fever or chills	

(Continued on next page)

Clinical Skill Assisting During Amniocentesis (*Continued*)

NURSING ACTION	RATIONALE
11. Encourage the woman to engage in only light activity for 24 hours and to increase her fluid intake.	*A decrease in maternal activity will decrease uterine irritability and increase uteroplacental circulation.*
	Increased hydration will replace the amniotic fluid through the uteroplacental circulation.
12. Complete the client record.	*Provides a permanent record.*
• Record the type of procedure, the date and time, name of the physician who performed the procedure and the disposition of the specimen.	
• Record the maternal–fetal response such as maternal vital signs, level of discomfort, FHR, and presence of contractions, bleeding and fluid leakage, if occurred. Discharge instructions given should be documented.	

Diagnostic Uses of Amniocentesis

A number of studies can be performed on amniotic fluid. These tests can provide information about genetic disorders (see Chapter 7 ∞), fetal health, and fetal lung maturity.

Evaluation of Fetal Health

Concentrations of certain substances in amniotic fluid provide information about the health status of the fetus. The **quadruple screen** is the most widely used test to screen for Down syndrome (trisomy 21), trisomy 18, and neural tube defects (NTDs). The serum test assesses for appropriate levels of alpha-fetoprotein (AFP), human chorionic gonadotropin (hCG), and unconjugated estriol (UE3) and Diameric Inhibin-A. The quadruple screen offers the advantage of being noninvasive but is only a screening test and does not actually diagnose genetic abnormalities (see Chapter 7 ∞). An amniocentesis is 99% accurate in diagnosing genetic abnormalities.

Evaluation of Fetal Maturity

Because gestational age, birth weight, and the rate of development of organ systems do not necessarily correspond, amniotic fluid may also be analyzed to determine the maturity of the fetal lungs. Fetal lung maturity determination is important when making clinical decisions regarding the timing of birth for women who may have complications, such as preeclampsia or diabetes.

LECITHIN/SPHINGOMYELIN (L/S) RATIO The alveoli of the lungs are lined with a substance called **surfactant**, which is composed of phospholipids. Surfactant lowers the surface tension of the alveoli when the newborn exhales. When a newborn with mature pulmonary function takes its first breath, a tremendously high pressure is needed to open the lungs. By lowering the alveolar surface tension, surfactant stabilizes the alveoli, and a certain amount of air always remains in the alveoli during expiration. Thus when the infant exhales, the lungs do not collapse. An infant born before synthesis of surfactant is complete is unable to maintain lung stability. Each breath requires the same effort as the first. This results in underinflation of the lungs and the development of respiratory distress syndrome (RDS).

Fetal lung maturity can be ascertained by determining the **lecithin/sphingomyelin (L/S) ratio**; lecithin and sphingomyelin are two components of surfactant. Early in pregnancy, the sphingomyelin concentration in amniotic fluid is greater than the concentration of lecithin, and so the L/S ratio is low (lecithin levels are low and sphingomyelin levels are high). At about 32 weeks' gestation, sphingomyelin levels begin to fall and the amount of lecithin begins to increase. By 35 weeks' gestation, an L/S ratio of 2:1 (also reported as 2.0) is usually achieved in the normal fetus. A 2:1 L/S ratio indicates that the risk of RDS is very low. Under certain conditions of stress (a physiologic problem in the mother, placenta, and/or fetus, such as hypertension or placental insufficiency), the fetal lungs mature more rapidly (Torrance, Voorbij, Wijnberger et al., 2008).

PHOSPHATIDYLGLYCEROL Phosphatidylglycerol (**PG**) is another phospholipid in surfactant. Phosphatidylglycerol is not present in the fetal lung fluid early in gestation. It appears when fetal lung maturity has been attained, at about 35 weeks' gestation. Because the presence of PG is associated with fetal lung maturity, when it is present the risk of RDS is low. Phosphatidylglycerol determination is also useful in

KEY FACTS TO REMEMBER
Fetal Lung Maturity Values

Diagnostic value: Provides information to help determine fetal lung maturity.

RESULTS
- L/S ratio of 2:1 and presence of PG correlate with 35 weeks' gestation.
- An L/S ratio lower than 2:1 and/or an absence of PG may indicate underinflation of lungs and an increased risk for development of respiratory distress syndrome.
- An LBC over 32,000 counts/uL is predictive of fetal lung maturity.

blood-contaminated specimens. Because PG is not present in blood or vaginal fluids, its presence is reliable in predicting fetal lung maturity. (See Key Facts to Remember: Fetal Lung Maturity Values.)

LAMELLAR BODY COUNT *Lamellar body counts (LBC)* are present in amniotic fluid when phosphatidylglycerol (PG) is present (Karcher, Sykes, Batton et al., 2005). When the LBC is over 32,000 counts/uL, probable lung maturity is assumed. The laboratory analysis for LBC is considerably less costly than the previously discussed tests and can usually be performed at the acute care facility rather than a reference laboratory (Druzin, Smith, Gabbe & Reed, 2007; Karcher et al., 2005).

Chorionic Villus Sampling

Chorionic villus sampling (CVS) involves obtaining a small sample of chorionic villi from the developing placenta. Chorionic villus sampling is performed in some medical centers for first-trimester diagnosis of genetic, metabolic, and deoxyribonucleic acid (DNA) studies. Chorionic villus sampling can be performed either transabdominally or transcervically. The fetal loss rate is the same regardless of the approach used although vaginal spotting is more common with the transcervical approach (ACOG, 2007).

The advantages of this procedure are early diagnosis and short waiting time for results. Whereas amniocentesis is not done until at least 16 weeks' gestation, CVS is typically performed between 10 and 12 weeks. Previous studies that evaluated the use of CVS at 9 weeks found a possible association between limb reduction birth defects and early CVS. Based on these findings, most practitioners do not recommend early CVS before 10 gestational weeks (ACOG, 2007). Risks of CVS include failure to obtain tissue, rupture of membranes, leakage of amniotic fluid, bleeding, intrauterine infec-

tion, maternal tissue contamination of the specimen, and Rh alloimmunization.

Because CVS testing is performed so early in the pregnancy, it cannot detect neural tube defects. Women who desire testing for neural tube defects would need a quadruple screening at 15 to 20 weeks' gestation.

TEACHING TIP

When explaining genetic testing options to expectant parents, inform the mother that even if a CVS shows no chromosomal abnormality, it cannot screen for neural tube defects. Women who have a normal CVS and an abnormal quadruple screen test would be offered amniocentesis. Women with risk factors for neural tube defects may want to consider amniocentesis instead of CVS because it screens for both types of disorders.

Nursing Care Management

The nurse assists the physician during the amniocentesis or CVS and supports the woman undergoing the procedure. Although the physician has explained the procedure in advance so that the woman can give informed consent, the woman is likely to be apprehensive both about the procedure itself and about the information it may reveal. She may become anxious during the procedure and need additional emotional support. The nurse can provide support by further clarifying the physician's instructions or explanations, by relieving the woman's physical discomfort when possible, and by responding verbally and physically to the woman's need for reassurance.

Following the procedure, the nurse reiterates explanations given by the physician and provides opportunities for questions. The nurse reviews the experience with the woman and presents self-care measures. Typically, the woman is monitored for a short time following the procedure. The nurse observes for contraction or uterine activity, amniotic fluid leakage, bleeding, or pain. The woman is advised of the warning signs of complications following the procedure.

Following an amniocentesis, approximately 1% to 2% of women develop complications such as amniotic fluid leakage from the puncture site or vaginal spotting. Approximately 1 in 1000 women develop infection. Needle puncture of the fetus rarely occurs during amniocentesis because of the use of ultrasound technology that allows for continuous visualization of the fetus (ACOG, 2007). Women should be reassured that although the complication rates are low, notification of her healthcare provider is necessary if any of these symptoms develop.

Because fetal loss occurs more commonly before 15 weeks, many practitioners theorize that the loss rates associated with CVS are higher than those associated with amniocentesis. Early amniocentesis before

15 weeks is associated with an increased risk of fetal loss when compared with performing the procedure after 15 weeks. Approximately 1 in 200 fetal losses occur with CVS. When an amniocentesis is performed between 15 to 20 weeks, the risk of fetal loss is 1 in 300 to 1 in 500 (ACOG, 2007).

When an invasive procedure, such as an amniocentesis or a CVS, is performed, the nurse administers RhoGAM to the woman if she is Rh negative to prevent alloimmunization. Documentation should be charted and provided to the woman for future reference.

CHAPTER HIGHLIGHTS

- Maternal assessment of fetal activity can be used as a screening tool to provide information about fetal well-being.
- Ultrasound offers a valuable means of assessing intrauterine fetal growth because the growth can be followed over a period of time. It is noninvasive and painless, allows the certified nurse–midwife or physician to study the gestation serially, is nonradiating to both the woman and her fetus, and has no known harmful effects.
- Nuchal translucency testing is used as a tool to screen for trisomies 13, 18, and 21. It is noninvasive and painless, but is not diagnostic in determining if a fetus has an abnormality.
- First trimester combined screening includes nuchal translucency testing (NTT) and serum tests, which is more accurate than using only the ultrasound screening.
- Doppler blood flow studies are used to assess placental function and sufficiency.
- A nonstress test (NST) is based on the knowledge that the FHR normally increases in response to fetal activity and to sound stimulation. The desired result is a reactive test.
- A fetal biophysical profile (BPP) includes five variables (fetal breathing movement, fetal body movement, fetal tone, amniotic fluid volume, and FHR reactivity) to assess the fetus at risk for intrauterine compromise.
- A contraction stress test (CST) provides a method for observing the response of the FHR to the stress of uterine contractions. The desired result is a negative test.
- Amniocentesis can be used to obtain amniotic fluid for genetic testing or for evaluating fetal lung maturity.
- The quadruple screen measures substances contained in the amniotic fluid that provide information regarding the presence of fetal anomalies, such as neural tube defects and Down syndrome.
- The lecithin/sphingomyelin ratio, presence of phosphatidylglycerol, and level of lamellar body counts can be assessed to determine fetal lung maturity.
- Advantages of CVS include early detection of certain fetal disorders with a decreased waiting time for results. Disadvantages include an increased risk to the fetus, inability to detect neural tube defects, and the potential for repeated invasive procedures.

EXPLORE **PEARSON mynursingkit™**

MyNursingKit is your one stop for online chapter review materials and resources. Prepare for success with additional NCLEX®-style practice questions, interactive assignments and activities, web links, animations and videos, and more!

Register your access code from the front of your book at
www.mynursingkit.com

CHAPTER REFERENCES

Abramowicz, J. S. (2007). In utero imaging of the placenta: Importance for diseases of pregnancy (eng; includes abstract). *Placenta, 28*(Suppl A), S14–22.

Alus, M., Okumus, H., Mete, S., & Guclu, S. (2007, March). The effects of different maternal positions on non-stress test: An experimental study. *Journal Clinical Nursing. 2007, 16*(3), 562–568.

American College of Obstetricians & Gynecologists [ACOG]. (2004). First-trimester screening for fetal aneuploidy (ACOG Committee Opinion No. 296). Washington, DC: Author.

American College of Obstetricians & Gynecologists [ACOG]. (2007). First-trimester screening for fetal aneuploidy (ACOG Practice Bulletin No. 88). Washington, DC: Author.

Batcha, T. M. (2005). The fetal acoustic stimulation test: A reliable and cost effective method of antepartum fetal monitoring. *Ceylon Medical Journal, 50*(4),156–159.

Blackburn, S. T. (2007). *Maternal, fetal, & neonatal physiology: A clinical perspective* (2nd ed.). St. Louis, MO: Saunders.

Borrell, A. (2007). Reliability analysis on ductus venosus assessment at 11–14 weeks' gestation in a high-risk population. *Prenatal Diagnosis, 27*(5), 442–446.

Clur, S. A, Mathijssen, I. B., Pajkrt, E., Cook, A. L., Ottenkamp, J., & Bilardo, C. M. (2008). Structural heart defects associated with an increased nuchal translucency: 9 years experience in a referral centre. *Prenatal Diagnosis, 28*(4), 347–354.

Cunningham, F. G., Leveno, K. J., Bloom, S. L., Hauth, J. C., & Wenstrom, K. D. (2005). *William's obstetrics* (22nd ed.). New York: McGraw Hill.

Cusick, W., Shevell, T., Duchan, L. S., Lupinacci, C. A., Terranova, J., & Crombleholme, W. R.

(2008). Likelihood ratios for fetal trisomy 21 based on nasal bone length in the second trimester: How best to define hypoplasia? *Ultrasound in Obstetrics & Gynecology, 30*(3), 271–274.

Druzin, M. L., Smith, J. F., Gabbe, S. G., & Reed, K. L. (2007). Antepartum fetal evaluation. In S. G. Gabbe, J. R. Niebyl & J. L. Simpson (Eds.). *Obstetrics: Normal and problem pregnancies.* (5th ed. pp. 267–300). Philadelphia, PA: Churchill Livingston/Elsevier.

Frøen, J. F. (2004). A kick from within: Fetal movement counting and the cancelled process in prenatal care. *Journal of Perinatal Medicine, 32*(1), 13–24.

Gabbe, S. G., Niebyl, J. R., & Simpson, J. L. (2007). *Obstetrics: Normal and problem pregnancies pocket companion.* New York: Churchill Livingstone.

Gilbert, E. S. (2007). *Manual of high risk pregnancy & delivery.* (4th ed.). St. Louis: Mosby.

Grimes-Dennis J. (2007). Cervical length and prediction of preterm delivery. *Current Opinion in Obstetrics & Gynecology, 19*(2), 34–46.

Gumus, I. I. (2007). Perinatal outcomes of pregnancies with borderline amniotic fluid index. *Archives of Gynecology and Obstetrics, 276*(1), 17–19.

Heazell, A. E., & Frøen, J. F. (2008). Methods of fetal movement counting and the detection of fetal compromise. *Journal of Obstetrics & Gynaecology, 28*(2), 147–154.

Heazell, A. E., Green, M., Wright, C., Flenady, V., & Frøen, J. F. (2008). Midwives' and obstetricians' knowledge and management of women presenting with decreased fetal movements. *Acta Obstetrics & Gynecology Scandavia, 87*(3), 331–339.

Karcher, R., Sykes, E., Batton, D., Uddin, Z., Ross, G., Hockman, E., & Shade, G. H. Jr. (2005). Gestational age-specific predicted risk of neonatal respiratory distress syndrome using lamellar body count and surfactant-to-albumin ratio in amniotic fluid. *American Journal Obstetrics and Gynecology, 193*(5), 1680–1684.

Kurjak, A., Miskovic, B., Andonotopo, W., Stanojevic, M., Azumendi, G., et al. (2007). How useful is 3D and 4D ultrasound in perinatal medicine? *Journal of Perinatal Medicine, 35*(1), 10–27.

Kwon, J. Y. (2006). Abnormal Doppler velocimetry is related to adverse perinatal outcome for borderline amniotic fluid index during third trimester. *The Journal of Obstetrics and Gynaecology Research, 32*(6), 545–549.

Mangesi, L., & Hofmeyr, G. J. (2007). Fetal movement counting for assessment of fetal wellbeing. *Cochrane Database of Systematic Reviews* 2007, Issue 1. Art. No.: CD004909. DOI: 10.1002/14651858.CD004909.pub2.

McAuliffe, F. M., Fong, K. W., Toi, A., Chitayat, D., Keating, S., & Johnson, J. (2005). Ultrasound detection of fetal anomalies in conjunction with first-trimester nuchal translucency screening: A feasibility study. *American Journal of Obstetrics & Gynecology, 19*(3), Pt. 2, 1260–1265.

Mirghani, H. M., Weerasinghe, S., Al-Awar, S., Abdulla, L., & Ezimokhai, M. (2005). The effect of intermittent maternal fasting on computerized fetal heart tracing. *Journal of Perinatology, 25*(2), 90–92.

Piazze, J. J. (2007). Nuchal translucency as a predictor of adverse pregnancy outcome (eng; includes abstract). *International Journal of Gynaecology and Obstetrics, 98*(1), 5–9.

Scott, A. (2007, June). Nuchal translucency in first trimester Down syndrome screening. *Issues in Emerging Health Technology, 100,* 1–6.

Sinha, D., Sharma, A., Nallaswamy, V., Jayagopal, N., & Bhatti, N. (2007). Obstetric outcome in women complaining of reduced fetal movements. *Journal of Obstetrics & Gynaecology, 27*(1), 41–43.

Smith, G. C., Celik, E., To, M., Khouri, O., & Nicolaides, K. H. (2008). Cervical length at mid-pregnancy and the risk for primary cesarean delivery. *New England Journal of Medicine, 358*(13), 1346–1353.

Sritippayawan, S. (2007). The accuracy of gestation-adjusted projection method in estimating birth weight by sonographic fetal measurements in the third trimester. *Journal of the Medical Association of Thailand, 90*(6), 1058–1067.

Torrance, H. L., Voorbij, H. A., Wijnberger, L. D., van Bel, F., & Visser, G. H. (2008). Lung maturation in small for gestational age fetuses from pregnancies complicated by placental insufficiency or maternal hypertension. *Early Human Development, 84*(7), 465–469.

Verburg, B. O., Steegers, E. A., De Ridder, M., Snijders, R. J., Smith, E., Hofman, A., et al. (2008). New charts for ultrasound dating of pregnancy and assessment of fetal growth: Longitudinal data from a population-based cohort study. *Ultrasound in Obstetrics & Gynecology, 31*(4), 388–396.

Wright, D., Kagan, K. O., Molina, F. S., Gazzoni, A., & Nicolaides, K. H. (2008). A mixture model of nuchal translucency thickness in screening for chromosomal defects. *Ultrasound in Obstetrics & Gynecology, 31*(4), 376–383.

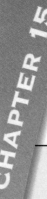

CHAPTER 15

Pregnancy at Risk: Pregestational Problems

When you work on a high-risk maternity unit, it is sometimes easy to get caught up in technology and procedures, but this area is about families—their fears, their pain, their health, their future. We can never lose sight of that reality and remain effective nurses. Never.

—A Maternity Nurse Working with High-Risk Pregnant Women

LEARNING OUTCOMES

15-1. Describe the effects of alcohol and illicit drugs in the nursing care management of the childbearing woman and her fetus/newborn.

15-2. Relate the pathology and clinical treatment of diabetes mellitus in pregnancy to the implications for nursing care.

15-3. Distinguish among the types of anemia associated with pregnancy regarding signs, treatment, and implications for pregnancy.

15-4. Describe acquired immunodeficiency syndrome (AIDS), including care of the pregnant woman who has tested positive for the human immunodeficiency virus (HIV), fetal/neonatal implications, and ramifications for the childbearing family.

15-5. Explain the effects of various heart disorders on pregnancy, including implications for nursing care management in the antepartum, intrapartum, and postpartum periods.

15-6. Delineate the effects of selected pregestational medical conditions on pregnancy.

KEY TERMS

Acquired immunodeficiency syndrome (AIDS)   **324**
Crack   **310**
Gestational diabetes mellitus (GDM)   **314**
Human immunodeficiency virus type 1 (HIV-1)   **323**
Macrosomia   **316**

Even though it is a normal process, for some women pregnancy may become a life-threatening event because of potential or existing complications. These complications can be the result of factors such as age, parity, blood type, socioeconomic status, psychologic health, or preexisting chronic illnesses. Effective prenatal care is directed toward identifying factors that increase a pregnant woman's risk and developing supportive therapies that will promote optimal health for the mother and her fetus.

This chapter focuses on women with pregestational medical disorders and the possible effects of these disorders on the pregnancy.

Care of the Woman with Substance Abuse Problems

Substance abuse occurs when an individual experiences difficulties with work, family, social relations, and health as a result of alcohol or drug use. In general, the rate of illicit drug use among pregnant women is significantly less than the rate among nonpregnant women. Specifically, approximately 4% of pregnant women ages 15 to 44 report having used an illicit drug in the past month as compared with 10% of nonpregnant women (Substance Abuse and Mental Health Services Administration [SAMHSA], 2007). However, illicit drug usage varies significantly by race and by age with higher rates among women ages 18 to 25 than among women ages 26 to 44. Rates are highest among American Indians and Alaskan Natives (13.7%) and lowest among Asians (3.6%). Rates are 9.8% among blacks, 8.5% among whites, and 6.9% among Hispanics (SAMHSA, 2007).

Drugs that are commonly misused include tobacco, alcohol, cocaine, marijuana, amphetamines, barbiturates, hallucinogens, club drugs, heroin, and other narcotics. (Tobacco is discussed in Chapter 11 ∞ as a teratogenic substance.) *Polydrug use* involving multiple substances such as alcohol, tobacco, and illicit drugs is fairly common and contributes to the risks a pregnant woman faces. Table 15–1 identifies common addictive drugs and their effects on the fetus or newborn.

Drug use during pregnancy, particularly in the first trimester, may adversely affect the health of the woman and the growth and development of the fetus. Unfortunately, prenatal drug use may be the most frequently missed diagnosis in all of maternity care. Physicians and nurses may fail to ask women about drug and alcohol use because of their own lack of knowledge, discomfort, or biases. Often substance-abusing women wait until late in pregnancy to seek health care. Moreover, the substance-abusing woman who seeks early prenatal care may not voluntarily reveal her addiction, so caregivers should ask direct, nonjudgmental questions (Chapter 10 ∞) and be alert for a history or physical signs that suggest substance abuse.

Providing effective prenatal care to chemically dependent women presents many challenges for clinicians. However, pregnancy represents a period in most women's lives when they recognize the need for and are receptive to caring interventions.

HINTS FOR PRACTICE

Keep in mind that almost 1 out of 10 women in the United States, regardless of socioeconomic status or ethnic background, is currently abusing a substance. If you consider that possibility with every woman, you will ask the important questions about drug use and be alert for signs of substance abuse.

Substances Commonly Abused During Pregnancy

Alcohol

Alcohol is a central nervous system (CNS) depressant and a potent teratogen. The incidence of alcohol abuse is highest among women ages 20 to 40 years; alcoholism is also seen in teenagers. Among pregnant women ages 15 to 44, 11.8% used alcohol in a given month. This rate is significantly lower than the rate for nonpregnant women of that age (53%) (SAMHSA, 2007). This figure is of concern, however, because birth defects that are related to fetal alcohol exposure can occur in the first 3 to 8 weeks' gestation, often before the woman even knows she is pregnant. Alcohol use among pregnant women tends to decrease by trimester.

The effects of alcohol on the fetus may result in a group of signs known as fetal alcohol spectrum disorders (FASD). The syndrome has characteristic physical and mental abnormalities that vary in severity and combination. (See discussion in Chapter 27 ∞.) There is no definitive answer to how much alcohol a woman can safely consume during pregnancy. Consequently, the expectant woman should avoid alcohol completely. Even low levels of alcohol cannot be recommended (Food and Drug Administration [FDA], 2005).

Chronic abuse of alcohol can undermine maternal health by causing malnutrition (especially folic acid and thiamine deficiencies), bone marrow suppression, increased incidence of infections, and liver disease. As a result of alcohol dependence, a woman may have withdrawal seizures in the intrapartal period as early as 12 to 48 hours after she stops drinking. Delirium tremens (DTs) may occur in the postpartal period, and the newborn may suffer a withdrawal syndrome. The nursing staff in the maternal-newborn unit must be aware of the manifestations of alcohol abuse so they can prepare for the client's special needs. The care regimen includes sedation to decrease irritability and tremors, seizure precautions, intravenous fluid therapy for hydration, and preparation for an addicted newborn. Although high doses

TABLE 15–1 Possible Effects of Selected Drugs of Abuse/Addiction on Fetus and Newborn

Maternal Drug	Effect on Fetus/Newborn
Depressants	
Alcohol	Mental retardation, microcephaly, midfacial hypoplasia, cardiac anomalies, intrauterine growth restriction (IUGR), potential teratogenic effects, fetal alcohol syndrome (FAS), fetal alcohol effects (FAE)
Narcotics	
Heroin	Withdrawal symptoms, convulsions, IUGR, tremors, irritability, sneezing, vomiting, fever, diarrhea, and abnormal respiratory function
Methadone	Fetal distress, meconium aspiration; with abrupt termination of the drug, severe withdrawal symptoms, preterm labor, rapid labor, abruption Withdrawal symptoms
Barbiturates	
Phenobarbital	Withdrawal symptoms Fetal growth restriction
"T's and Blues" (combination of the following)	
Talwin (narcotic)	Safe for use in pregnancy; depresses respiration if taken close to time of birth
Amytal (barbiturate)	See barbiturates
Tranquilizers	
Phenothiazine derivatives	Withdrawal, extrapyramidal dysfunction, delayed respiratory onset, hyperbilirubinemia, hypotonia or hyperactivity, decreased platelet count
Diazepam (Valium)	Hypotonia, hypothermia, low Apgar score, respiratory depression, poor sucking reflex, possible cleft lip
Antianxiety Drugs	
Lithium	Congenital anomalies
Stimulants	
Amphetamines	
Amphetamine sulfate (Benzedrine)	Generalized arthritis, learning disabilities, poor motor coordination, transposition of the great vessels, cleft palate
Dextroamphetamine sulfate (Dexedrine)	Congenital heart defects, biliary atresia, limb reduction defects
Cocaine	Cerebral infarctions, microcephaly, learning disabilities, poor state organization, decreased interactive behavior, CNS anomalies, cardiac anomalies, genitourinary anomalies, sudden infant death syndrome (SIDS)
Nicotine (half to one pack cigarettes/day)	Increased rate of spontaneous abortion, increased incidence of placental abruption, SGA, small head circumference, decreased length, SIDS, attention-deficit/hyperactivity disorder (ADHD) in school-age children
Psychotropics	
PCP ("angel dust")	Withdrawal symptoms Newborn behavioral and developmental abnormalities
LSD	Chromosomal breakage?
Marijuana	IUGR?

of sedatives and analgesics may be necessary for the woman, caution is advised because these medications can cause fetal depression.

Breastfeeding generally is not contraindicated, although alcohol is excreted in breast milk. Excessive alcohol consumption may intoxicate the infant and inhibit the maternal letdown reflex. Discharge planning for the alcohol-addicted mother and newborn needs to be coordinated with the social service department of the hospital.

Cocaine and Crack

Cocaine acts at the nerve terminals to prevent the reuptake of dopamine and norepinephrine, which in turn results in vasoconstriction, tachycardia, and hypertension. Placental vasoconstriction decreases blood flow to the fetus. The onset of cocaine effects occurs rapidly, but the euphoria lasts only about 30 minutes. Euphoria and excitement are usually followed by irritability, depression, pessimism, fatigue, and a strong desire for more cocaine. This pattern often leads the user to take repeated doses to sustain the effect. Cocaine metabolites may be present in the urine of a pregnant woman for as long as 4 to 7 days after use.

Cocaine can be taken by intravenous injection or by snorting the powdered form. **Crack**, a form of freebase cocaine that is made up of baking soda, water, and cocaine mixed into a paste and microwaved to form a rock, can be smoked. Smoking crack leads to a quicker, more intense high because the drug is absorbed through the large surface area of the lungs.

The cocaine user is difficult to identify prenatally. Because cocaine is an illegal substance, many women are reluctant to volunteer information about their drug use. The nurse who is familiar with the woman may recognize subtle signs of cocaine use, including mood swings and appetite changes, and withdrawal symptoms such as depression, irritability, nausea, lack of motivation, and psychomotor changes.

Major adverse maternal effects of cocaine use include seizures and hallucinations, pulmonary edema, cerebral hemorrhage, respiratory failure, and heart problems. Women who use cocaine have an increased incidence of spontaneous abortion, abruptio placentae, preterm birth, and stillbirth (March of Dimes [MOD], 2007).

Exposure of the fetus to cocaine in utero increases the risk of intrauterine growth restriction (IUGR), small head circumference, cerebral infarctions, shorter body length, altered brain development, malformations of the genitourinary tract, and lower Apgar scores. Newborns exposed to cocaine in utero may have neurobehavioral disturbances, marked irritability, an exaggerated startle reflex, labile emotions, and an increased risk of sudden infant death syndrome (SIDS). (See Chapter 25 ∞ for further discussion.) Most children who were exposed to cocaine in utero have normal intelligence. In some cases, cocaine-exposed children have subtle behavioral and learning problems; however, a good home environment seems to help reduce these effects (MOD, 2007).

Cocaine crosses into breast milk and may cause symptoms in the breastfeeding infant, including extreme irritability, vomiting, diarrhea, dilated pupils, and apnea. Thus women who continue to use cocaine after childbirth should avoid nursing.

Marijuana

Perhaps not surprisingly, marijuana is the most widely used illicit drug among women, both pregnant and nonpregnant (SAMHSA, 2007). To date, there is no strong evidence that marijuana has teratogenic effects on the fetus although, following birth, some infants who were regularly exposed to marijuana in utero appear to have withdrawal symptoms including trembling and excessive crying (MOD, 2007). In reality, the impact of heavy marijuana use on pregnancy is difficult to evaluate because of the variety of social factors including, for example, polydrug use that may influence the direct results of marijuana itself.

Phencyclidine (PCP)

Phencyclidine (PCP) is a popular hallucinogen that can be smoked, taken orally, or injected intravenously. The drug causes confusion, delirium, and hallucinations and may produce feelings of euphoria. The greatest risk for the pregnant woman is overdose or psychotic response. Signs of overdose include hypertension, hyperthermia, diaphoresis, and possible coma, which may jeopardize fetal well-being.

MDMA (Ecstasy)

MDMA (methylenedioxymethamphetamine), better known as Ecstasy, is the most commonly used of a group of drugs referred to as *club drugs*, so called because they have become popular among adolescents and young adults who frequent dance clubs and "raves." Other club drugs include flunitrazepam (Rohypnol), gamma hydroxybutyrate (GHB), and ketamine hydrochloride. PCP and LSD are sometimes classified as club drugs as well.

MDMA is the third most widely used illicit drug in the United States after marijuana and amphetamines. MDMA is taken by mouth, usually as a tablet. It produces euphoria and feelings of empathy for others. It has been widely perceived as a "safe" drug because of a relatively low incidence of adverse reactions. However, adverse responses are very unpredictable and their incidence is growing as MDMA use becomes more commonplace (Gamma, Jerome, Liechti et al., 2005). Deaths have occurred among users.

Little is yet known about the effects of MDMA on pregnancy. Preliminary research using rats suggests that prenatal use of MDMA may be associated with long-term impaired memory and learning in the child. However, the impact of the timing of Ecstasy use by the pregnant woman during fetal brain development may be a critical issue (Koprich, Chen, Kanaan et al., 2003).

Heroin

Heroin is an illicit CNS depressant narcotic that alters perception and produces euphoria. It is an addictive drug that is generally administered intravenously. Pregnancy in women who use heroin is considered high risk because of the increased incidence in these women of poor nutrition, iron deficiency anemia, and preeclampsia. Women addicted to heroin also have a higher incidence of sexually transmitted infections because many rely on prostitution to support their drug habit.

The fetus of a heroin-addicted woman is at increased risk for IUGR, meconium aspiration, and hypoxia. The newborn frequently shows signs of heroin addiction such as restlessness; shrill, high-pitched cry; irritability; fist sucking; vomiting; and seizures. Signs of withdrawal usually appear within 72 hours and may last for several days. The newborn may exhibit poor consolability for 3 months or more. These behaviors may interfere with successful maternal attachment and increase the risk for parenting problems or abuse in an already high-risk mother. (See discussion in Chapter 27 ∞.)

Methadone

Methadone is the most commonly used therapy for women who are dependent on opioids such as heroin. Methadone blocks withdrawal symptoms and reduces or eliminates the craving for narcotics. Dosage should be individualized at the lowest possible therapeutic level. Methadone crosses the placenta, but the effects on the newborn are inconsistent and do not seem to indicate as much of a dose-related effect on the newborn as previously believed (Jansson, DiPietro, & Elko, 2005). The therapeutic goal is to use methadone to help the mother recover from illicit drug abuse to optimize her health and that of her baby.

Clinical Therapy

Antepartal care of the pregnant woman with substance abuse problems involves medical, socioeconomic, and legal considerations. A team approach allows for the comprehensive management necessary to provide safe labor and childbirth for the woman and her child.

The management of drug addiction may include hospitalization as necessary to initiate detoxification. "Cold turkey" withdrawal is not advisable during pregnancy because of potential risk to the fetus. Maintenance and support therapy are best individualized to the woman's history and condition. Urine screening is also done regularly throughout pregnancy if the woman has a known or suspected substance abuse problem and should include maternal informed consent. This testing helps to identify the type and amount of drug being abused.

Nursing Care Management

Nursing Assessment and Diagnosis

Because of the prevalence of substance abuse in society today, nurses and other care providers should screen all pregnant women for substance abuse during the health

---

EVIDENCE-BASED PRACTICE

Psychosocial Interventions to Reduce Prenatal Illicit Drug Use

Clinical Question

What non-pharmacological interventions are effective in reducing illicit drug use during the prenatal period?

The Evidence

The use of illicit drugs during pregnancy has potentially serious consequences for the mother and her baby. Women who use drugs during the prenatal period are more likely to have low birth weight and preterm babies. The effect of non-pharmacologic interventions on outcomes was evaluated through a systematic review conducted by the Cochrane group. Outcomes of interest were attendance and retention in drug treatment, drug abstinence, and neonatal condition. Evidence was gathered from the Cochrane Drug and Alcohol Group register, the Cochrane Central Register of Trials, and three nursing/medical databases. Nine trials involving 546 women were included in this review. Two types of treatments were evaluated—contingency management and motivational interviewing. Conclusions drawn from multiple trials and held to the rigorous standards of the Cochrane Review represent the strongest evidence for practice.

What Is Effective?

The most motivating element was the mother's concern for her baby. Informing the mother about possible fetal and neonatal effects and encouraging entrance into drug treatment were most effective. Contingency management was also effective in retaining mothers in treatment programs and supporting abstinence. Contingency management uses positive, supportive reinforcement for continuation of desired behaviors. These reinforcements are generally concrete and have monetary value. Examples of reinforcements were monetary vouchers, gift cards, or giving work and a salary only when abstaining from drug use. Motivational interviewing was not found to be effective. Motivational interviewing is the use of a directive, counseling style aimed at changing behavior. These studies found that motivational interviewing over three to six sessions may actually lead to poorer retention in treatment.

What Is Inconclusive?

The majority of subjects were African American, single, never married, and unemployed. It is unclear whether these findings can be generalized to other population groups. Only two of the studies included nicotine as a targeted drug, and so it is unclear whether these strategies will work for smoking cessation as well. Even when mothers remained abstinent and in treatment, no effect on neonatal outcomes was discovered. More study is needed to determine the specific effects of maternal drug treatment on newborns.

Best Practice

Inform mothers about the effects of their illicit drug use on fetal development and neonatal health. Emphasize to mothers that drug treatment during pregnancy can help them avoid these consequences. You can feel confident using concrete reinforcement to help the mother remain in treatment and abstain from illicit drug use. Directive counseling, on the other hand, is ineffective and may actually decrease the mother's motivation to stay in treatment.

References

Terplan, M., & Lui, S. (2008). Psychosocial interventions for pregnant women in outpatient illicit drug treatment programs compared to other interventions. *Cochrane Database of Systematic Reviews*, Issue 2.

TABLE 15–2 Possible Signs of Substance Abuse

History
- History of vague or unusual medical complaints
- Family history of alcoholism or other addiction
- History of childhood physical, sexual, or emotional abuse
- History of cirrhosis, pancreatitis, hepatitis, gastritis, sexually transmitted infections, or unusual infections such as cellulitis or endocarditis
- History of high-risk sexual behavior
- Psychiatric history of treatment and/or hospitalization

Physical Signs
- Dilated or constricted pupils
- Inflamed nasal mucosa
- Evidence of needle "track marks" or abscesses
- Poor nutritional status
- Slurred speech or staggering gait
- Odor of alcohol on breath

Behavioral Signs
- Memory lapses, mood swings, hallucinations
- Pattern of frequently missed appointments
- Frequent accidents, falls
- Signs of depression, agitation, euphoria
- Suicidal gestures

---

history. Several simple screening tools are available. In addition, the nurse needs to be alert for clues in the history or appearance of the woman that suggest substance abuse (Table 15–2). If abuse is suspected, the nurse needs to ask direct questions, beginning with less threatening questions about use of tobacco, caffeine, and over-the-counter medications. The nurse can then progress to questions about alcohol consumption and finally to questions focusing on past and current use of illicit drugs. The nurse who is matter-of-fact and nonjudgmental in her or his approach is more likely to elicit honest responses.

Nursing assessment of the woman with a known substance abuse problem focuses on the woman's general health status, with specific attention paid to nutritional status, susceptibility to infections, and evaluation of all body systems. The nurse also assesses the woman's understanding of the impact of substance abuse on herself and on her pregnancy.

Nursing diagnoses that may apply to a woman at risk because of substance abuse include the following:

- *Imbalanced Nutrition: Less than Body Requirements* related to inadequate food intake secondary to substance abuse
- *Risk for Infection* related to use of inadequately cleaned syringes and needles secondary to intravenous (IV) drug use
- *Risk for Ineffective Health Maintenance* related to a lack of information about the impact of substance abuse on the fetus

Nursing Plan and Implementation

Prevention of substance abuse during pregnancy is the ideal nursing goal and is best accomplished through education. Unfortunately, many women who abuse substances do not receive regular health care and may not seek care until they are far along in pregnancy.

The nurse's role in providing prenatal care for the woman who abuses substances focuses on ongoing assessment and client teaching. The nurse can provide information about the relationship between substance abuse and existing health problems and the implications for the woman's unborn child. By establishing a relationship of trust and support, the nurse may gain the woman's cooperation. The knowledgeable nurse can discuss possible strategies to help the woman quit (addiction treatment programs, 12-step programs, individual counseling) and suggest a referral for more in-depth assessment by a specialist. Relapse rates are high, even for motivated women, but the nurse's continued support and encouragement are important factors in helping women stop using substances.

Preparation for labor and birth should be part of prenatal planning. Fear, tension, or discomfort may be relieved through nonnarcotic psychologic support and careful explanation of the labor process. If pain medication is necessary, it should not be withheld; the notion that it will contribute to further addiction is mistaken. Preferred methods of pain relief include the use of psychoprophylaxis and regional blocks such as epidurals or local anesthetics such as pudendal block and local infiltration. Immediate intensive care should be available for the newborn, who is often depressed, small for gestational age (SGA), and premature. (For care of the addicted newborn, see Chapter 27 ∞.)

Evaluation

Expected outcomes of nursing care include the following:

- The woman is able to describe the impact of her substance abuse on herself and her unborn child.
- The woman gives birth to a healthy infant.
- The woman agrees to accept a referral to social services (or another appropriate community agency) for follow-up care after discharge.

Care of the Woman with Diabetes Mellitus

Diabetes mellitus (DM), an endocrine disorder of carbohydrate metabolism, results from inadequate production or use of insulin. Insulin, produced by the β-cells of the islets of Langerhans in the pancreas, lowers blood glucose levels by enabling glucose to move from the blood into muscle and adipose tissue cells.

Carbohydrate Metabolism in Normal Pregnancy

In early pregnancy the rise in serum levels of estrogen, progesterone, and other hormones stimulates increased insulin production by the maternal pancreas and increased tissue response to insulin. Thus an anabolic (building up) state exists during the first half of pregnancy, with storage of glycogen in the liver and other tissues.

In the second half of pregnancy, placental secretion of human placental lactogen (hPL) and prolactin (from the decidua), as well as elevated cortisol and glycogen levels, cause increased resistance to insulin and decreased glucose tolerance. This decreased effectiveness of insulin results in a catabolic (destructive) state during fasting periods, such as during the night or after meal absorption. Because increasing amounts of circulating maternal glucose and amino acids are diverted to the fetus, maternal fat is metabolized much more readily during fasting periods than in a nonpregnant woman. As a result of this lipolysis (maternal metabolism of fat), ketones may be present in the urine.

The delicate system of checks and balances that exists between glucose production and glucose use is stressed by the growing fetus, who derives energy from glucose taken solely from maternal stores. This stress is known as the diabetogenic effect of pregnancy. Thus any preexisting disruption in carbohydrate metabolism is augmented by pregnancy, and any diabetic potential may precipitate gestational diabetes mellitus.

Pathophysiology of Diabetes Mellitus

In diabetes mellitus, the pancreas does not produce enough insulin to allow necessary carbohydrate metabolism. Without adequate insulin, glucose does not enter the cells and they become energy depleted. Blood glucose levels remain high (hyperglycemia), and the cells break down their stores of fats and protein for energy. Protein breakdown results in a negative nitrogen balance; fat metabolism causes ketosis.

These pathologic developments cause the four cardinal signs and symptoms of diabetes mellitus: polyuria, polydipsia, polyphagia, and weight loss. *Polyuria* (frequent urination) results because water is not reabsorbed by the renal tubules because of the osmotic activity of glucose. *Polydipsia* (excessive thirst) is caused by dehydration from polyuria. *Polyphagia* (excessive hunger) is caused by tissue loss and a state of starvation, which results from the inability of the cells to use the blood glucose. *Weight loss* (seen with marked hyperglycemia) is because of the use of fat and muscle tissue for energy.

TABLE 15–3 Etiologic Classification of Diabetes Mellitus

I. Type 1 diabetes* (β-cell destruction, usually leading to absolute insulin deficiency)
  A. Immune mediated
  B. Idiopathic
II. Type 2 diabetes* (may range from predominantly insulin resistance with relative insulin deficiency to a predominantly secretory defect with insulin resistance)
III. Other specific types†
IV. Gestational diabetes mellitus

*Clients with any form of diabetes may require insulin treatment at some stage of their disease. Such use of insulin does not classify the client.
†The more detailed classification, which can be found in medical-surgical texts and the original source, provides eight subcategories of type.

Source: Adapted from the 1999 Report of the Expert Committee on the Diagnosis and Classification of Diabetes Mellitus, *Diabetes Care,* Suppl. 5.

Classification

States of altered carbohydrate metabolism have been classified in several ways. Table 15–3 shows the classification of diabetes mellitus based on its cause. This classification contains four main categories: type 1 diabetes, type 2 diabetes, other specific types, and gestational diabetes mellitus (GDM). Type 1 diabetes develops because of β-cell destruction and generally results in an absolute insulin deficiency. Type 2 diabetes, which is the most common form, "may range from predominantly insulin resistance with relative insulin deficiency to a predominantly secretory defect with insulin resistance" (American Diabetes Association [ADA], 2007, p. S43).

Table 15–4 shows White's classification of diabetes in pregnancy. This classification is useful for describing the extent of the disease.

Gestational diabetes mellitus (GDM) is defined as any degree of glucose intolerance that has its onset or is first diagnosed during pregnancy. It complicates about 4% of all pregnancies. Women who are markedly obese, have a prior history of GDM, have glycosuria, or have a strong family history of diabetes are at high risk (ADA, 2007). Diagnosis of GDM is important because even mild diabetes causes increased risk for perinatal morbidity and mortality. Furthermore, with time, many women with GDM progress to overt type 2 diabetes mellitus.

Influence of Pregnancy on Diabetes

Pregnancy can affect diabetes significantly because the physiologic changes of pregnancy can drastically alter insulin requirements. Pregnancy may also alter the progress of vascular disease secondary to DM. Pregnancy can affect diabetes in the following ways.

TABLE 15–4	White's Classification of Diabetes in Pregnancy
Class	**Criterion**
A	Chemical diabetes
B	Maturity onset (age over 20 years), duration under 10 years, no vascular lesions
C_1	Age 10 to 19 years at onset
C_2	10 to 19 years' duration
D_1	Under 10 years at onset
D_2	Over 20 years' duration
D_3	Benign retinopathy
D_4	Calcified vessels of legs
D_5	Hypertension
E	No longer sought
F	Nephropathy
G	Many failures
H	Cardiopathy
R	Proliferating retinopathy
T	Renal transplant (added by Tagatz and colleagues of the University of Minnesota)

Source: White, P. (1978). Classification of obstetric diabetes. *American Journal of Obstetrics and Gynecology, 130,* 228. Used with permission.

[handwritten notes: hPL only present during pregnancy, changes mothers metabolic system, puts a brake on insulin so glucose can go to baby ↑ hypoglycemia → hPL rises insulin available]

- DM may be difficult to control because insulin requirements are changeable.
  1. During the first trimester, the need for insulin frequently decreases. Levels of hPL, an insulin antagonist, are low, fetal needs are minimal, and the woman may consume less food because of nausea and vomiting.
  2. Nausea and vomiting may cause dietary fluctuations and increase the risk of hypoglycemia, formerly called insulin shock.
  3. Insulin requirements begin to rise in the second trimester as glucose use and glucose storage by the woman and fetus increase. Insulin requirements may double or quadruple by the end of pregnancy as a result of placental maturation and hPL production.
  4. Increased energy needs during labor may require increased insulin to balance intravenous glucose.
  5. Usually an abrupt decrease in insulin requirement occurs after the passage of the placenta and the resulting loss of hPL in maternal circulation.
- A decreased renal threshold for glucose leads to a higher incidence of glycosuria.
- The risk of ketoacidosis, which may occur at lower serum glucose levels in the pregnant woman with DM than in the nonpregnant diabetic, increases.
- The vascular disease that accompanies DM may progress during pregnancy.
  1. Hypertension may occur, contributing to vascular changes.
  2. Nephropathy may result from renal impairment, and retinopathy may develop.

Influence of Diabetes on Pregnancy Outcome

The pregnancy of a woman who has diabetes carries a higher risk of complications, especially perinatal mortality and congenital anomalies. This risk has been reduced by the recognition of the importance of tight metabolic control (fasting blood glucose less than 95 mg/dL and 2-hour postprandial glucose less than 120 mg/dL) (ACOG, 2005). New techniques for monitoring blood glucose level, delivering insulin, and monitoring the fetus have also reduced perinatal mortality.

Maternal Risks

The prognosis for the pregnant woman with gestational, type 1, or type 2 diabetes without significant vascular damage is positive. However, diabetic pregnancy still carries a higher risk of complications than normal pregnancy.

Hydramnios, or an increase in the volume of amniotic fluid, occurs in 10% to 20% of pregnant diabetic women. It is thought to be a result of excessive fetal urination because of fetal hyperglycemia (Forsbach-Sanchez et al., 2005). Premature rupture of membranes and onset of labor may occasionally be a problem with hydramnios.

Preeclampsia-eclampsia occurs more often in diabetic pregnancies than in normal pregnancies, especially when vascular changes already exist.

Hyperglycemia can lead to *ketoacidosis* as a result of the increase in ketone bodies (which are acidic) released in the blood from the metabolism of fatty acids. Decreased gastric motility and the contrainsulin effects of hPL also predispose the woman to ketoacidosis. Ketoacidosis usually develops slowly but, if untreated, can lead to coma and death for mother and fetus.

Pregnancy can also worsen retinopathy in women with diabetes. However good control of blood glucose levels lessens the impact and a laser treatment exists that can prevent retinal hemorrhage when indicated. Hence women with preexisting diabetes should be referred to an ophthalmologist for evaluation during pregnancy (ACOG, 2005). The pregnant woman with diabetes is also at increased risk for monilial vaginitis and urinary tract infections because of increased glycosuria, which contributes to a favorable environment for bacterial growth.

Fetal-Neonatal Risks *[handwritten: ↑ fetal urination]*

Many of the problems of the newborn result directly from high maternal plasma glucose levels. In the presence of untreated maternal ketoacidosis, the risk of fetal death increases dramatically.

The incidence of *congenital anomalies* in diabetic pregnancies is 5% to 10% and is the major cause of death among infants of diabetic mothers. Research suggests that this increased incidence is related to multiple factors including high glucose levels in early pregnancy (Wyatt, Frias, Hoyme et al., 2005). Most anomalies involve the heart, central nervous system, and skeletal system. One anomaly, *sacral agenesis,* appears almost exclusively in infants of diabetic mothers. In sacral agenesis, the sacrum and lumbar spine fail to develop and the lower extremities develop incompletely. To reduce the incidence of congenital anomalies, preconception counseling and strict diabetes control before conception are indicated.

Characteristically, infants of diabetic mothers on insulin therapy (or White's classes A, B, and C; see Table 15–3) are large for gestational age (LGA) as a result of the high maternal levels of blood glucose, from which the fetus derives its glucose. These elevated levels continually stimulate the fetal islets of Langerhans to produce insulin. This hyperinsulin state causes the fetus to use the available glucose, which leads to excessive growth (known as **macrosomia**) and fat deposits. If born vaginally, the macrosomic infant is at increased risk for shoulder dystocia and traumatic birth injuries; thus cesarean birth may be indicated if birth weight is expected to exceed 4500 g (ACOG, 2005).

After birth the umbilical cord is severed and the generous maternal blood glucose supply eliminated. However, continued islet cell hyperactivity leads to excessive insulin levels and depleted blood glucose (hypoglycemia) in 2 to 4 hours. Macrosomia can be significantly reduced by strict maternal blood glucose control.

Infants of mothers with advanced diabetes (vascular involvement) may demonstrate *intrauterine growth restriction.* IUGR occurs because vascular changes in the diabetic woman decrease the efficiency of placental perfusion and the fetus is not as well sustained in utero.

Respiratory distress syndrome appears to result from inhibition, by high levels of fetal insulin, of some fetal enzymes necessary for surfactant production. *Polycythemia* (excessive number of red blood cells) in the newborn is due primarily to the diminished ability of glycosylated hemoglobin in the mother's blood to release oxygen. *Hyperbilirubinemia* is a direct result of the inability of immature liver enzymes to metabolize the increased bilirubin resulting from the polycythemia.

Clinical Therapy

All pregnant women, regardless of risk factors, should have their risk for GDM assessed at the first prenatal visit. Women at low or normal risk should be screened for gestational diabetes at 24 to 28 weeks' gestation using a non-fasting 1-hour, 50 g oral glucose tolerance test (OGTT). Women with risk factors such as marked obesity, history of diabetes in a first-degree relative; a prior macrosomic, malformed, or stillborn infant; hypertension; or glucosuria should be screened earlier in pregnancy (Perkins, Dunn, & Jagasia, 2007).

To do the 1-hour OGTT, the woman ingests a 50 g oral glucose solution at any time during the day. One hour later a blood sample is obtained. If the level exceeds 130 to 140 mg/dL (depending on the lab used), a 3-hour oral glucose tolerance test (OGTT) is necessary (ADA, 2007). To do this test, the woman eats a high-carbohydrate (at least 150 g of carbohydrates daily) diet for 3 days before her scheduled test. She then ingests a 100 g oral glucose solution in the morning after an overnight fast. Plasma glucose levels are determined fasting and at 1, 2, and 3 hours. Gestational diabetes is diagnosed if two or more of the following values are equaled or exceeded.

Fasting	95 mg/dL
1 hour	180 mg/dL
2 hour	155 mg/dL
3 hour	140 mg/dL

Laboratory Assessment of Long-Term Glucose Control

Measurement of glycosylated hemoglobin levels provides information about the long-term (previous 4 to 8 weeks) control of hyperglycemia. It measures the percentage of glycohemoglobin in the blood. Glycohemoglobin, or HbA_{1c}, is the hemoglobin to which a glucose molecule is attached. Because glycosylation is a rather slow and essentially irreversible process, the test is not reliable for screening for gestational diabetes or for close daily control. However, in women with known pregestational DM, abnormal HbA_{1c} values correlate directly with the frequency of fetal congenital anomalies. A value greater than 10% is associated with a fetal anomaly rate of 20% to 25% (ACOG, 2005).

Antepartal Management of Diabetes Mellitus

The major goals of clinical care for all pregnant women with diabetes are (1) to maintain a physiologic equilibrium of insulin availability and glucose use during pregnancy and (2) to ensure an optimally healthy mother and newborn. To achieve these goals, good prenatal care using a team approach must be a top priority. The woman with gestational diabetes may find the diagnosis shocking and upsetting. She needs clear explanations and teaching to enlist her cooperation in ensuring a good outcome. The nurse educator plays a major role in this counseling.

The woman with pregestational diabetes needs to understand what changes she can expect during pregnancy; she should receive such teaching in preconception counseling. In addition to client education, preconception care focuses on stringent blood glucose control before conception and during the first trimester. Stringent glucose control during this period helps reduce the rate of infant malformations significantly (Slocum, 2007). A pregnant woman with preexisting diabetes may also require referral to specialists such as an ophthalmologist or nephrologist.

DIETARY REGULATION   The pregnant woman with diabetes needs to increase her caloric intake by about 300 kcal/day. During the first trimester the normal-weight woman generally requires about 30 kcal/kg of ideal body weight (IBW). During the second and third trimesters she needs about 35 kcal/kg IBW. Approximately 40% to 45% of the calories should come from complex carbohydrates, 12% to 20% from protein, and 35% to 40% from fats (Reece & Homko, 2008). The food is divided among three meals and three snacks. The bedtime snack is the most important and should include both protein and complex carbohydrates to prevent nighttime hypoglycemia. A nutritionist should work out meal plans with the woman based on the woman's lifestyle, culture, and food preferences. The woman needs to be familiar with the use of food exchanges so she can plan her own meals.

GLUCOSE MONITORING   Glucose monitoring is essential to determine the need for insulin and assess glucose control. Many physicians have the woman come in for weekly assessment of her fasting glucose levels and one or two postprandial levels. In addition, frequent self-monitoring of glucose levels is paramount in maintaining good glucose control. Self-monitoring is discussed on page 319.

INSULIN ADMINISTRATION   Many women with gestational diabetes require insulin to maintain normal glucose levels. Individuals with pregestational diabetes typically have type 1 diabetes and are already on insulin. In either case, human insulin should be used because it is the least likely to cause an allergic reaction. Insulin is given either in multiple injections or by continuous subcutaneous infusion. Multiple injections are more common and generally produce excellent results. Many women receive a combination of intermediate and regular insulin. Recently, clinicians have moved away from the use of regular human insulin, replacing it with an insulin analog (either lispro or aspart), which mimics physiologic insulin action. Research indicates that these analogs are more effective than regular insulin in achieving desired glucose levels and in reducing the risk of fetal macrosomia (Perkins et al., 2007). The analogs are convenient because they can be given closer to a meal than regular insulin (5 to 10 minutes vs 30 to 45 minutes). In addition, the analogs are associated with a lower incidence of hypoglycemia, and they do not cross the placenta (Scollan-Koliopoulos, Guadagno, & Walker, 2006). Often a four-dose approach is used, with regular insulin or an analog taken before each meal and NPH or Lente insulin added at bedtime (ACOG, 2005). Other clinicians vary the NPH and regular insulin patterns slightly but still prefer a four-dose approach.

Oral hypoglycemics are not generally used during pregnancy because they cross the placenta and have not been well studied. However, glyburide, a sulfonylurea taken orally, is now being used by clinicians as an alternative to insulin for women with GDM that is not controlled by diet and exercise alone. Glyburide enhances insulin secretion, but does not cross the placenta (Perkins et al., 2007).

EVALUATION OF FETAL STATUS   Information about the well-being, size, and maturation of the fetus is important for planning the course of pregnancy and the timing of birth. Because pregnancies complicated by diabetes are at increased risk of neural tube defects such as spina bifida in the fetus, maternal serum *alpha-fetoprotein (AFP)* screening is offered at 16 to 20 weeks' gestation (see Chapter 16 ∞).

Ultrasound is done at 18 weeks to establish gestational age and detect anomalies. It is then repeated at 28 weeks to monitor fetal growth for IUGR or macrosomia. Some agencies do *fetal biophysical profiles (BPP)* (ultrasound evaluation of fetal well-being in which fetal breathing movements, fetal activity, reactivity, muscle tone, and amniotic fluid volume are assessed) as part of an ongoing evaluation of fetal status.

Daily maternal evaluation of *fetal activity* is begun at about 28 weeks. Nonstress testing (NST) is usually begun weekly at 28 weeks and increased to twice weekly at 32 weeks' gestation. If the NST is nonreactive, a fetal biophysical profile or *contraction stress test* is performed. (For an explanation of these tests, see Chapter 16 ∞.) If the woman requires hospitalization for complications or to control blood sugar levels, NSTs may be done daily.

Intrapartal Management of Diabetes Mellitus

During the intrapartal period, medical therapy focuses on the following:

- *Timing of birth.* Most pregnant women with diabetes, regardless of the type, are allowed to go to term, with spontaneous labor. Some clinicians opt to induce labor in a woman at term to avoid problems related to an aging placenta. Cesarean birth may be indicated if evidence of nonreassuring fetal status exists. Birth before term may be indicated for diabetic women with vascular changes and worsening hypertension or if evidence of IUGR exists (ACOG, 2005). To determine fetal lung maturity, amniotic fluid (obtained by amniocentesis) is evaluated for lecithin/sphingomyelin (L/S) ratio and the presence of phosphatidylglycerol (PG) (see Chapter 16 ∞). Preterm birth, often by cesarean, must be considered if prenatal testing indicates that the fetal condition is deteriorating.
- *Labor management.* Frequently maternal insulin requirements decrease dramatically during labor. Consequently maternal glucose levels are measured hourly

to determine insulin need (Figure 15–1 ■). The primary goal in controlling maternal glucose levels intrapartally is to prevent neonatal hypoglycemia (ACOG, 2005). Often two intravenous lines are used, one with a 5% dextrose solution and one with a saline solution. The saline solution is then available for piggybacking insulin or if a bolus is needed. Because insulin clings to plastic IV bags and tubing, the tubing should be flushed with insulin before the prescribed amount is added. During the second stage of labor and the immediate postpartal period, the woman may not need additional insulin. The intravenous insulin is discontinued with the completion of the third stage of labor.

Postpartal Management of Diabetes Mellitus

Generally maternal insulin requirements fall significantly during the postpartal period for all diabetic women, regardless of the type of diabetes, because, with placental separation, hormone levels fall and the anti-insulin effect ceases. For the first 24 hours postpartum women with preexisting diabetes typically require very little insulin and are usually managed with a sliding scale. Afterward, a more regular insulin dosage pattern can be reestablished. Women with mild diabetes not requiring insulin often have sufficient glucose control and do not require any therapy while they are hospitalized.

Antihyperglycemics are contraindicated during breastfeeding. Consequently a nursing woman with diabetes that is not controlled by diet alone may need insulin for a time postpartally (ACOG, 2005).

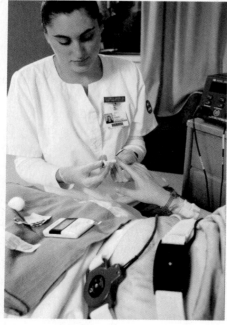

FIGURE 15–1 During labor the nurse closely monitors the blood glucose levels of the woman with diabetes mellitus.

Women with GDM seldom need insulin during the postpartum period. Clinicians routinely discontinue insulin for women with GDM following childbirth and then monitor blood glucose levels (Menato, Bo, Signorite et al., 2008). If elevated glucose levels develop, oral antihyperglycemic agents may be tried if the woman is not breastfeeding (ACOG, 2005). The woman should be reassessed 6 weeks postpartum to determine whether her glucose levels are normal. If the levels are normal, she should be reassessed at a minimum of 3-year intervals (ADA, 2006).

The establishment of parent-child relationships is a high priority during the postpartum period for all women with DM and their families. However that may become more challenging if the newborn requires a special-care nursery. In such cases, the parents need ongoing information, support, and encouragement to visit and be involved in the newborn's care.

Breastfeeding is encouraged as beneficial to both mother and baby. Maternal calorie needs increase during lactation to 500 to 800 kcal above prepregnant requirements, and insulin must be adjusted accordingly. Home blood glucose monitoring should continue for the insulin-dependent diabetic.

The woman and her partner, if he is involved, should also receive information on family planning. Barrier methods of contraception (diaphragm, cervical cap, condom) used with a spermicide are safe, effective, and economical and are the method of choice for insulin-dependent diabetic women. The use of combined oral contraceptives (COCs) by diabetic women is somewhat controversial. Many physicians who prescribe low-dose COCs to women with diabetes restrict them to women who have no vascular disease and do not smoke. The progesterone-only pill may also be used as may Depo-Provera. Many couples who have completed their families choose elective sterilization.

Nursing Care Management

The Nursing Care Plan for the Woman with Gestational Diabetes Mellitus addresses nursing management.

Nursing Assessment and Diagnosis

Whether diabetes has been diagnosed before pregnancy occurs or the diagnosis is made during pregnancy (GDM), careful assessment of the disease process and the woman's understanding of diabetes is important. A thorough physical examination—including assessment for vascular complications of the disease, any signs of infectious conditions, and urine and blood testing for glucose—is essential on the first prenatal visit. Follow-up visits are usually scheduled twice a month during the first two trimesters and once a week during the last trimester.

Assessment also yields vital information about the woman's ability to cope with the combined stress of pregnancy and diabetes and to follow a recommended regimen of care. It is necessary to determine the woman's knowledge about diabetes and self-care before formulating a teaching plan.

Nursing diagnoses that may apply to the pregnant woman with diabetes include the following:

- *Risk for Imbalanced Nutrition: More than Body Requirements* related to imbalance between intake and available insulin
- *Risk for Injury* related to possible complications secondary to hypoglycemia or hyperglycemia
- *Interrupted Family Processes* related to the need for hospitalization secondary to diabetes mellitus

Nursing Plan and Implementation

For the woman with preexisting diabetes, a nurse and a physician may provide prepregnancy counseling using a team approach. Ideally they see the couple before pregnancy so that the DM can be evaluated. The outlook for pregnancy is good if the diabetes is of recent onset without vascular complications, provided that glucose levels can be controlled.

For women with GDM, nursing care focuses heavily on client education about the condition, its implications, and its management.

CRITICAL THINKING

Patti Chang, a 35-year-old G3P2, is a well-educated, active Chinese American woman with no history of glucose intolerance. Her two children were born healthy at 36 weeks' gestation. She receives the usual 50 g glucose tolerance test at 26 weeks' gestation, and her plasma level is 160 mg/dL. She seems irritated and frustrated when her obstetrician tells her that it would be best to perform a 3-hour fasting glucose tolerance test. After the physician leaves the room, Patti asks the nurse the following questions: "Will the glucose hurt my baby? What will the treatment be?" How will the nurse answer the questions? Why does Patti seem so upset?

Answers can be found in Appendix F ∞.

Community-Based Nursing Care

In many cases, women with gestational diabetes mellitus are stabilized in the hospital and necessary teaching for self-care is begun. Women with preexisting diabetes may also require hospitalization for stabilization of their diabetes. In either case, the majority of ongoing teaching and supervision of pregnant women with diabetes is then carried out by nurses in clinics, community agencies, and the women's homes.

Effective Insulin Use

The nurse ensures that the woman and her partner understand the purpose of insulin, the types of insulin to be used, and the correct procedure for administering it. The woman's partner is also instructed about insulin administration in case it becomes necessary for the partner to give it. For some highly motivated women whose glucose levels are not well controlled with multiple injections, the continuous infusion pump may improve glucose control.

TEACHING TIP

It is essential to have a woman with GDM who is learning to test her blood glucose do a finger stick while you watch. For many women, actually sticking their finger can be a challenge to overcome. In addition, this observation enables you to verify that correct technique is used.

The nurse teaches the woman how and when to monitor her blood glucose level, the desired range of blood glucose levels, and the importance of good control (Figure 15–2 ■). Most women use a glucose meter to monitor blood sugar level because the meter provides a more accurate reading. The nurse teaches the woman to follow the manufacturer's directions exactly; to wash her hands thoroughly before puncturing her finger; and to touch the blood droplet, not her finger, to the test pad on the strip.

The nurse can provide the following tips about finger puncture: (1) Various spring-loaded devices are available that make puncturing easier; (2) letting the arm hang down for 30 seconds increases blood flow to the fingers; (3) warming the hands under warm running water increases the blood flow to them; and (4) the sides of fingers should be punctured instead of the ends because the ends contain more pain-sensitive nerves.

Clients with diabetes need to keep a record of each blood sugar reading as a guide for management. Specific record sheets are available for this purpose.

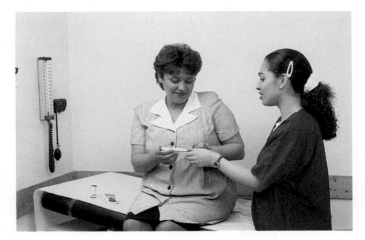

FIGURE 15–2 The nurse teaches the pregnant woman with gestational diabetes mellitus how to do home glucose monitoring.

Nursing Care Plan

For the Pregnant Woman with Gestational Diabetes Mellitus

CLIENT SCENARIO

Veronica Chavez, a 32-year-old primigravida of Latino descent, is 24 weeks' gestation. Although she began her pregnancy 30 lb overweight, she has not experienced complications until now. The 50 g glucose tolerance test Veronica took last week revealed a plasma level of 160 mg/dL. A subsequent 3-hour 100 g glucose tolerance test was positive for gestational diabetes mellitus (GDM). Veronica is now taking insulin injections twice a day. When she began the insulin, the nurse demonstrated how to monitor blood glucose levels and how to administer insulin injections correctly. The nurse also provided information about the condition and the importance of maintaining control of blood glucose levels.

Today, 1 week after beginning injections, Veronica has returned for a follow-up prenatal visit. She complains of urinary frequency and excessive thirst. She states that she has not monitored her blood glucose levels as often as directed, thereby affecting her insulin administration regimen. She also informs the nurse it is difficult to adhere to her new exercise program and diet plan. Veronica is frustrated and worried about the maternal risk factors associated with GDM and wonders how she will adapt.

ASSESSMENT

Subjective: Polydipsia, headache, general malaise, verbalizes concerns for maternal and fetal risk associated with GDM

Objective: Polyuria, BP 140/90, pulse 110, respirations 20, temperature 98.8°F, blood glucose level 200 mg/dL; glycosuria present, nonstress test is reactive

Nursing Diagnosis #1	Risk for Injury related to possible complications secondary to hypoglycemia or hyperglycemia*
Client Goal	The client will maintain appropriate blood glucose levels.
AEB:	• Verbalizes understanding of personal treatment regimen, to include diet, exercise, and insulin administration. • Establishes a daily routine for self-monitoring of blood glucose levels. • Maintains blood glucose levels within acceptable range. • Reports any signs or symptoms relating to hypoglycemia or hyperglycemia.

NURSING INTERVENTIONS

1. Educate the client about the procedure for using a glucose meter and when it should be used.

2. Encourage daily self-monitoring of blood glucose levels and reporting of any levels that are out of the normal range.

3. Educate client on proper insulin administration.

4. Monitor dipstick urine for ketones and protein and draw blood sample for hemoglobin A_{1c} (HbA$_{1c}$) during each prenatal visit.

RATIONALES

Rationale: Proper self-monitoring is an accurate method for determining insulin dosage. Self-monitoring of blood glucose levels should be performed four to six times a day. Insulin dosages are based on blood glucose levels and anticipated activity levels.

Rationale: Clients are encouraged to maintain blood sugar levels in the normal ranges as follows: fasting (before meals or taking insulin), 70 to 100 mg/dL; 2 hours after each meal, less than 120 mg/dL. Maintaining a normal blood glucose level during pregnancy helps prevent complications and promotes fetal and maternal well-being.

Rationale: Often women with GDM require insulin to maintain normal blood glucose levels. Insulin needs may increase with each trimester. Multiple injections of regular insulin or lispro may be required. Oral hypoglycemics cross the placenta and may have a teratogenic effect on the fetus; therefore they are never used during pregnancy.

Rationale: Increasing amounts of circulating maternal glucose and amino acids are diverted to the fetus, and maternal fat is metabolized more readily during fasting periods (during the night or after meal absorption). As a result of maternal metabolism of fat, ketones may be present in the urine. Hyperglycemia can lead to ketoacidosis. HbA$_{1c}$ lab results are helpful as an indicator of overall blood glucose control over the previous 4 to 8 weeks. Women with abnormal HbA$_{1c}$ values (greater than 10%) are at a higher risk for having a fetus with malformations.

Nursing Care Plan

For the Pregnant Woman with Gestational Diabetes Mellitus (Continued)

5. Educate client on the signs and symptoms of hyperglycemia.	**Rationale:** Early detection of signs and symptoms of hyperglycemia will prevent complications during pregnancy and promote positive pregnancy outcomes. Signs and symptoms of hyperglycemia include polyuria, polydipsia, dry mouth, fatigue, nausea, hot flushed skin, rapid deep breathing, abdominal cramps, acetone breath, headache, drowsiness, depressed reflexes, oliguria or anuria, and stupor or coma.
6. Educate client on the signs and symptoms of hypoglycemia.	**Rationale:** Hypoglycemia may develop rapidly. Early detection of signs and symptoms of hypoglycemia will prevent complications and allow for immediate action. Signs and symptoms include sweating, periodic tingling, disorientation, shakiness, pallor, clammy skin, irritability, hunger, headache, and blurred vision.
7. Educate client on proper dietary management.	**Rationale:** Caloric intake needs to increase by 300 calories per day for the pregnant diabetic woman. Complex carbohydrates should account for approximately 40–45% of the daily intake, whereas 12–20% should come from protein and 35–40% of calories per day should come from fat. Three meals and three snacks per day are recommended. To prevent nighttime hypoglycemia, the bedtime snack should include food sources high in protein and complex carbohydrates.

Evaluation of Client Goal	• Client verbalizes understanding of the importance of self-monitoring blood glucose levels. • Client maintains normal blood glucose levels. • Client follows diet and insulin administration routine as prescribed.
Nursing Diagnosis #2	Health-Seeking Behaviors related to an expressed desire to ensure healthy outcomes during pregnancy complicated by gestational diabetes mellitus
Client Goal	The client will participate in appropriate healthcare activities to improve overall health and wellness of pregnancy and prevent complications.
AEB:	• Schedules prenatal visits to monitor maternal and fetal well-being. • Reports signs of preeclampsia. • Uses various support services.

NURSING INTERVENTIONS

RATIONALES

1. Assess level of knowledge about the disease process.	**Rationale:** Provides information to formulate an individualized teaching plan to meet the client's learning needs. Provide written material about the disease process and lifestyle changes to help reinforce information discussed during prenatal visits.
2. Educate family members on various lifestyle changes needed during pregnancy.	**Rationale:** Care of the diabetic pregnant woman may involve the entire family. Family members may assist with alterations in meal preparations and help with insulin administration. Explain needed changes in diet, exercise, and insulin administration. In case the woman is unable to administer insulin, the partner or another family member is instructed how to give the insulin.
3. Schedule routine prenatal visits.	**Rationale:** During the first two trimesters follow-up visits are scheduled twice a month and once a week during the third trimester. Regular follow-up visits will provide for assessment of maternal and fetal well-being and allow for any adjustments or modifications to treatment plans to promote health and well-being.
4. Monitor for signs of preeclampsia.	**Rationale:** Preeclampsia occurs more frequently in diabetic pregnancies. Signs of preeclampsia include increased blood pressure and proteinuria.

(Continued on next page)

Nursing Care Plan

For the Pregnant Woman with Gestational Diabetes Mellitus *(Continued)*

NURSING INTERVENTIONS	RATIONALES
5. Perform routine nonstress test and assist with biophysical profile, ultrasound, alpha-fetoprotein, and amniocentesis.	**Rationale:** Nonstress test assesses fetal well-being and placental functioning. If the nonstress test is nonreactive a biophysical profile may be required. Ultrasounds may assess for fetal growth, size (macrosomia), and congenital anomalies. Alpha-fetoprotein screening assesses for neural tube defects. Amniocentesis can be used for a variety of tests, including alpha-fetoprotein and L/S ratio for assessment of lung maturity.
6. Assess fundal height every 2 weeks during first and second trimesters and once a week in the third trimester.	**Rationale:** A fundus that measures greater then expected for gestational age may be an indication of hydramnios, an increase in amniotic fluid volume. Excessive fetal diuresis may be a result of fetal hyperglycemia. Hydramnios puts the woman at risk for premature rupture of membranes.
7. Refer client to a diabetic nutritionist.	**Rationale:** A nutritionist can assist the client to individualize her diet and alter meal plans to reflect the client's lifestyle, culture, and food preferences.

Evaluation of Client Goal	• Client attends all prenatal visits. • Client displays no signs of complications. • Client enlists help from the nutritionists to assist with meal planning.

CRITICAL THINKING QUESTIONS

1. What data in Veronica's history might predispose her to GDM?

Answer: Veronica is over age 25, overweight prior to pregnancy, and Latino. These factors place her at average risk for developing GDM. Clients who present with these risk factors should be screened at 24 to 28 weeks' gestation using the 1-hour GTT.

2. Veronica states she is uncomfortable administering the insulin injections and asks if she could take oral medication instead of the insulin injections. What information would the nurse provide about the use of oral hypoglycemics?

Answer: Oral hypoglycemics may have a teratogenic effect on the fetus and have been associated with prolonged fetal hypoglycemia. Oral hypoglycemics are not used during pregnancy because women using them often break away from their control and become hyperglycemic.

3. Veronica has verbalized her concern about her condition and wonders how she will adapt. What nursing strategies might be implemented to help meet Veronica's psychosocial needs?

Answer: It is important to identify available support persons and to assess family perceptions of the change in Veronica's health status with this pregnancy. Include family in diabetic teaching. Explain purpose of scheduled tests and procedures.

*For your reference, this care plan provides an example of how two nursing diagnoses might be addressed.

Planned Exercise Program

Regardless of the type of diabetes, unless otherwise medically contraindicated, exercise is encouraged for the woman's overall well-being. If she is used to a regular exercise program, the nurse encourages her to continue. In addition, the nurse advises the woman to exercise after meals when blood sugar levels are high, to wear diabetic identification, to carry a simple sugar such as hard candy (because of the possibility of exercise-induced hypoglycemia), to monitor her blood glucose levels regularly, and to avoid injecting insulin into an extremity that will soon be used during exercise.

If the woman has not been following a regular exercise plan, the nurse can encourage her to begin gradually. Because of alterations in metabolism with exercise, the woman's blood glucose should be well controlled before she begins an exercise program.

Teaching for Self-Care

Using the information gained during the nursing assessment of the pregnant woman with diabetes, the nurse provides appropriate teaching to the woman and her family so that the woman can meet her own healthcare needs as much as possible.

- *Glucose monitoring.* Home monitoring of blood glucose levels is the most accurate and convenient method to determine insulin dose and assess control. Women are taught self-monitoring techniques according to a specified schedule. Women with GDM typically measure their blood glucose four times a day (fasting and 1 to 2 hours after meals), whereas women with preexisting diabetes monitor their blood five to seven times each day (Reece & Homko, 2008). They then regulate their insulin dosage based on blood glucose values and anticipated activity level. Women are encouraged to maintain blood glucose levels in normal ranges as follows: fasting (before eating or taking insulin), below 95 mg/dL; 2 hours after each meal, below 120 mg/dL (ADA, 2006).
- *Symptoms of hypoglycemia and ketoacidosis.* The pregnant diabetic woman must recognize symptoms of changing glucose levels and take appropriate action by immediately checking her capillary blood glucose level. Hypoglycemia may develop fairly rapidly. Symptoms include sweating, periodic tingling, disorientation, shakiness, pallor, clammy skin, irritability, hunger, headache, and blurred vision. If the woman's blood glucose is less than 60 mg/dL, she is advised to take 20 g of carbohydrate, which she can obtain by drinking 1 cup of skim milk, 1/2 cup orange or apple juice, or 1/2 cup regular soft drink or by eating four to six pieces of hard candy or 1 tablespoon honey, corn syrup, or brown sugar. She should then wait 15 minutes and retest her glucose level. If it remains under 60 mg/dL she should ingest another 20 g of carbohydrate (Cleveland Clinic, 2006). Many people overtreat their symptoms by continuing to eat, but doing so can cause rebound hyperglycemia. The woman should carry a snack at all times and should have other fast sources of glucose (simple carbohydrates such as hard candy) on hand to treat an insulin reaction when milk is not available. Family members are also taught how to inject glucagon in case food does not work or is not feasible (e.g., in the presence of severe morning sickness).
- *Smoking.* Smoking has harmful effects on both the maternal vascular system and the developing fetus and is contraindicated for both pregnancy and diabetes.
- *Travel.* Insulin can be kept at room temperature while traveling. Insulin supplies should be kept with the traveler and not packed in the baggage. Special meals can be arranged by notifying most airlines a few days before departure. The woman should wear a diabetic identification bracelet or necklace and should check with her physician for any instructions or advice before traveling.
- *Support groups.* Many communities have diabetes support groups or education classes that are helpful to women with newly diagnosed diabetes.
- *Cesarean birth.* Chances for a cesarean birth increase if the pregnant woman is diabetic. The possibility should

be anticipated and caregivers may suggest enrollment in cesarean birth preparation classes. Many hospitals offer classes, and information is available through state or national organizations. The couple may prefer simply to discuss cesarean birth with the nurse and their obstetrician and read some books on the topic.

Hospital-Based Nursing Care

Hospitalization may become necessary during the pregnancy to evaluate blood glucose levels and adjust insulin dosages. In such cases, the nurse monitors the woman's status and continues to provide teaching so that the woman is knowledgeable about her condition and its management.

During the intrapartal period, the nurse continues to monitor the woman's status, maintains her intravenous fluids, is alert for signs of hypoglycemia, and provides the care indicated for any woman in labor. If a cesarean birth becomes necessary, the nurse provides appropriate care, as described in Chapter 22 ∞.

Evaluation

Expected outcomes of nursing care include the following:

- The woman is able to discuss her condition and its possible impact on her pregnancy, labor and birth, and postpartal period.
- The woman participates in developing a healthcare regimen to meet her needs and follows it throughout her pregnancy.
- The woman avoids developing hypoglycemia or hyperglycemia.
- The woman gives birth to a healthy newborn.
- The woman is able to care for her newborn.

Care of the Woman with Anemia

Anemia indicates inadequate levels of hemoglobin (Hb) in the blood. During pregnancy, *anemia* is defined as hemoglobin less than 10 g/dL (Krakow, 2008). The common anemias of pregnancy are caused by either insufficient hemoglobin production related to nutritional deficiency in iron or folic acid during pregnancy or to hemoglobin destruction in an inherited disorder such as sickle cell anemia. Table 15–5 describes these common anemias.

Care of the Woman with HIV Infection

Infection with the **human immunodeficiency virus type 1 (HIV-1)** is one of today's major health concerns. It leads to a progressive disease that ultimately results in the

TABLE 15–5	Anemia and Pregnancy		
Condition	Brief Description	Maternal Implications	Fetal/Neonatal Implications
Iron deficiency anemia	Condition caused by inadequate iron intake resulting in hemoglobin levels below 11 g/dL. To prevent this, most women are advised to take supplemental iron during pregnancy.	Pregnant woman with this anemia tires easily, is more susceptible to infection, has increased chance of preeclampsia-eclampsia and postpartal hemorrhage, and cannot tolerate even minimal blood loss during birth. Healing of episiotomy or incision may be delayed.	Risk of low birth weight, prematurity, stillbirth, and neonatal death increases in women with severe iron deficiency anemia (maternal Hb less than 6 g/dL). Fetus may be hypoxic during labor because of impaired uteroplacental oxygenation.
Sickle cell anemia	Recessive autosomal disease in which normal adult hemoglobin, hemoglobin A, is abnormally formed. It occurs primarily in people of African descent and occasionally in people of Southeast Asian or Mediterranean descent (i.e., Greeks, Italians, Arabs, and Turks) (ACOG, 2000). The disease is characterized by sickling of the RBCs in the presence of decreased oxygenation. Condition may be marked by crisis with profound anemia, jaundice, high temperature, infarction, and acute pain. Crisis is treated by rehydration with intravenous fluids, administration of oxygen, antibiotics, and analgesics. The fetus is monitored throughout.	Pregnancy may aggravate sickle cell anemia and bring on a vaso-occlusive crisis. Maternal mortality is rare but there is a significant risk of maternal infection, often urinary tract infection or pulmonary infection, because of impaired immune functioning (Cunningham et al., 2005). Congestive heart failure or acute renal failure may also occur. The goal of treatment is to reduce anemia and maintain good health. Because the woman maintains her hemoglobin levels by intense erythropoiesis, additional folic acid supplements (1 mg/day) are necessary. Maternal infections are treated promptly because dehydration and fever can trigger sickling and crisis. Oxygen supplementation is used throughout labor and IV fluids are given to maintain hydration. Fetal heart rate is monitored closely. Antiembolism stockings are indicated postpartally.	Abortion, fetal death, and prematurity may occur. IUGR is also a characteristic finding in newborns of women with sickle cell anemia.
Folic acid deficiency anemia	Folic acid deficiency is the most common cause of megaloblastic anemia. In the absence of folic acid, immature RBCs fail to divide, become enlarged (megaloblastic), and are fewer in number. Increased folic acid metabolism during pregnancy and lactation can result in deficiency. Because the condition is difficult to diagnose, the best approach is prevention. All women who could become pregnant should take a multivitamin containing 400 mcg daily (generally found in prenatal vitamins) before conception and through at least the first trimester of pregnancy. The condition is treated with 1 mg folate daily (see Chapter 13 ∞).	Folate deficiency is the second most common cause of anemia in pregnancy. Severe deficiency increases the risk that the mother may need a blood transfusion following birth because of anemia. She also has an increased risk of hemorrhage caused by thrombocytopenia and is more susceptible to infection. Folic acid is readily available in foods such as fresh leafy green vegetables, red meat, fish, poultry, and legumes, but it is easily destroyed by overcooking or cooking with large quantities of water.	Maternal folic acid deficiency has been associated with an increased risk of neural tube defects (NTDs) such as spina bifida, meningomyelocele, and anencephaly in the newborn. Adequate folic acid intake can reduce the incidence of NTDs by 50% to 70% (CDC & Pan American Health Organization, 2003). Women who have already had one baby with a NTD are generally advised to take a larger dose of folic acid daily.

development of **acquired immunodeficiency syndrome (AIDS)**. The estimated number of diagnosed AIDS cases in the United States from 1981 to 2006 was 982,498. In 2006, 35,314 new cases of HIV/AIDS were diagnosed in the 33 states with long-term reporting data. Men still make up the majority of cases whereas women account for about 26% (CDC, 2008). The major transmission categories are identified in Figure 15–3 ■.

Among females 80% of the cases result from high-risk heterosexual contact, 19% from injection drug use, and 1% from other categories of transmission (CDC, 2008). Although about 24% of U.S. women are African American or Latino, these groups accounted for 82% of all female AIDS cases in 2005 (CDC, 2007).

CULTURAL PERSPECTIVES

The rate of HIV/AIDS-infected individuals varies significantly among races and ethnic groups. In 2006 it was 60.3 per 100,000 in the black population, 20.8 per 100,000 in the Hispanic population, and 6.4 per 100,000 in the white population (CDC, 2007).

Pathophysiology of HIV and AIDS

HIV-1, which causes AIDS, typically enters the body through blood, blood products, or other body fluids such as semen, vaginal fluid, and breast milk. HIV affects specific T cells, thereby decreasing the body's immune responses.

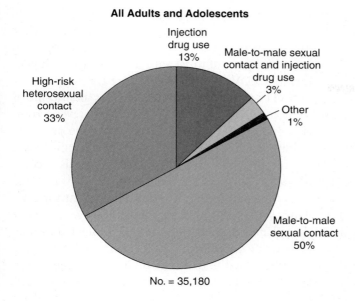

All Adults and Adolescents

Injection drug use 13%

Male-to-male sexual contact and injection drug use 3%

Other 1%

High-risk heterosexual contact 33%

Male-to-male sexual contact 50%

No. = 35,180

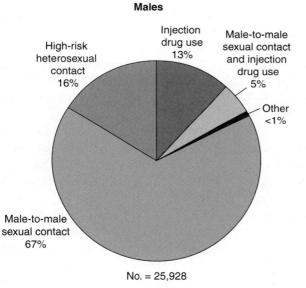

Males

Injection drug use 13%

Male-to-male sexual contact and injection drug use 5%

High-risk heterosexual contact 16%

Other <1%

Male-to-male sexual contact 67%

No. = 25,928

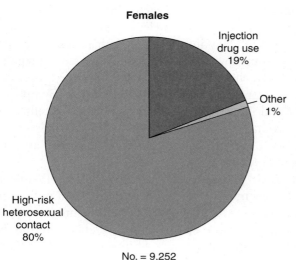

Females

Injection drug use 19%

Other 1%

High-risk heterosexual contact 80%

No. = 9,252

Figure 15–3 Transmission categories of adults and adolescents with HIV/AIDS diagnosed during 2006.
Source: Centers for Disease Control and Prevention. (March 2008). *HIV/AIDS in the United States.CDC/HIV AIDS Facts.* Retrieved April 29, 2008 from http://www.cdc.gov/hiv

This makes the affected person susceptible to opportunistic infections such as *Pneumocystis carinii*, which causes a severe pneumonia, candidiasis, cytomegalovirus, tuberculosis, and toxoplasmosis.

Once infected with the virus, the individual develops antibodies that can be detected with the enzyme-linked immunosorbent assay (ELISA) and confirmed with the Western blot test. Antibodies can be detected in most individuals within 6 months after exposure, but in rare circumstances the latent period is longer. An asymptomatic period lasting from a few months to as long as 17 years (with a median length of 10 years) follows seroconversion. The majority of infected pregnant women fall into this category.

The diagnosis of AIDS is made when an individual is HIV positive and is identified as having one of several specific opportunistic infections.

Maternal Risks

AIDS-defining diseases that are more common in women than in men include wasting syndrome, esophageal candidiasis, and herpes simplex virus disease. Non-AIDS-defining gynecologic disorders, such as candidiasis or cervical pathology, are prevalent among women in all stages of HIV infection.

Many women who are HIV positive choose to avoid pregnancy because of the risk of infecting the fetus and the increased risk of dying before the child is raised. Women who are asymptomatic and become pregnant should be advised that pregnancy is not believed to accelerate the progression of HIV/AIDS, that the use of antiretroviral therapy (ARV) during pregnancy significantly reduces the risk of transmitting the HIV-1 to the fetus, and that most medications used to treat HIV can be safely taken during the pregnancy.

Pregnant women who are HIV positive should receive information about known risk factors for perinatal transmission and ways of reducing the risk. Risk factors include cigarette smoking, illicit drug use, genital tract infections, and unprotected sexual intercourse with multiple partners (Public Health Service Task Force, 2007).

Fetal-Neonatal Risks

HIV/AIDS may develop in infants whose mothers are seropositive, usually because of perinatal transmission. Perinatal transmission occurs transplacentally, at birth when the infant is exposed to maternal blood and vaginal secretions, and via breast milk. In the United States, the rate of transmission has dropped dramatically and is now less than 2% because of the implementations of recommendations for universal prenatal HIV counseling and testing, the availability of antiretroviral prophylaxis, the use of scheduled cesarean birth, and the avoidance of breastfeeding (Public Health Service Task Force, 2007).

MyNursingKit | Aids in Pregnancy

Following birth, infants often have a positive antibody titer, which reflects the passive transfer of maternal antibodies and does not indicate HIV infection. For further discussion of the infant who is HIV positive, see Chapter 28 ∞.

Clinical Therapy

The goal for antenatal care is identification of the pregnant woman at risk for HIV infection. Thus the revised CDC HIV testing guidelines indicate that screening should be included in the routine panel of prenatal screening tests for all pregnant women with the understanding that the woman is notified that it is part of testing and that she can "opt out" of having the HIV portion of screening should she so choose (Branson, Handsfield, Lampe et al., 2006). Initial testing is done using enzyme-linked immunoabsorbent assay (ELISA). If the results are positive, the Western blot test is used to confirm the diagnosis. Women who test positive should be counseled about the implications of the diagnosis for themselves and their fetus to ensure an informed reproductive choice.

Two screening tests have been developed that are useful in assessing the HIV status of women who did not receive prenatal care before labor and for women in active labor who do not know their HIV status. These tests (OraQuick HIV-1 Antibody test and the SUDS HIV-1 test) require a small blood sample, can be read in 20 minutes, and are very sensitive and specific (Lachat, Scott, & Relf, 2006).

Antiretroviral prophylaxis or antiretroviral therapy should be recommended to all infected pregnant women regardless of CD4 count to reduce the rate of perinatal transmission. As more antiretroviral medications have been developed, a wide array of options exists. Highly active antiretroviral therapy (HAART) is a treatment approach that uses a minimum of three antiretroviral agents. It generally includes ZDV, a nucleoside reverse transcriptase inhibitor (NRTI), plus a second NRTI such as didanosine or lamivudine combined with a non-nucleoside reverse transcriptase inhibitor (NNRTI) such as nevirapine or a protease inhibitor such as indinavir, ritonavir, or saquinavir.

HIV antiretroviral drug resistance testing is recommended before beginning treatment in HIV-infected pregnant women who do not require treatment for their own health. When possible, treatment for these women is delayed until after the first trimester. HIV-infected women who are already receiving HAART when they become pregnant are advised to continue their current regimen if it is effective, but they should not receive drugs such as efavirenz (EFV), which have known teratogenic effects (Public Health Service Task Force, 2007).

Treatment recommendations have also been developed for the mother and infant for the intrapartum and postpartum periods. The decision about which regimen is most appropriate should be determined following discussion with the woman about the risks and benefits based on her individual HIV status.

HIV-infected women should be evaluated and treated for other sexually transmitted infections and for conditions occurring more commonly in women with HIV, such as tuberculosis, cytomegalovirus, toxoplasmosis, and cervical dysplasia. HIV-infected women with no history of hepatitis B should receive the hepatitis vaccine, which is not contraindicated prenatally, as well as the pneumococcal vaccine and an annual flu shot. In addition to routine prenatal laboratory tests, a platelet count and a complete blood count with differential should be obtained at the first prenatal visit and repeated each trimester to identify anemia, thrombocytopenia, and leukopenia, which are associated both with HIV infection and with antiviral therapy.

The woman with HIV also should be assessed regularly for serologic changes that indicate the disease is progressing. This is determined by the absolute CD4+ T-lymphocyte count, which provides the number of helper T4 cells. When CD4+ counts fall to 200/mm^3 or lower, opportunistic infections such as *Pneumocystis carinii* pneumonia are more likely to develop.

At each prenatal visit, asymptomatic HIV-infected women are monitored for early signs of complications, such as weight loss in the second or third trimester or fever. The woman is asked about signs of vaginal infection. Her mouth is inspected for signs of infections such as thrush (candidiasis) or hairy leukoplakia; her lungs are auscultated for signs of pneumonia; and her lymph nodes, liver, and spleen are palpated for signs of enlargement. Each trimester the woman should have a visual examination and

---

COMPLEMENTARY AND ALTERNATIVE THERAPIES

Effects of a Spiritual Mantram on HIV Outcomes

Bormann (2006) examined the effectiveness of the use of a psychosocial intervention—in this case a mantram repetition—on psychologic distress (anxiety, anger, depression, and so forth), quality of life enjoyment and satisfaction, and spiritual well-being in HIV-infected adults. In this study a mantram is defined as a word or phrase that has spiritual associations for the individual. Subjects were asked to repeat the mantram silently throughout the day. A wrist counter was used to track the number of times the mantram was repeated each day. Over time, the mantram group showed significantly more improvement than the control group in reducing anger and in increased quality of life, peace, spiritual connectedness, and faith.

Clearly further study is warranted but the authors suggest that mantram practice may contribute to managing psychologic distress and enhancing spiritual well-being in people living with HIV/AIDS.

Source: Bormann, J. E. (2006). Effects of spiritual mantram repetition on HIV outcomes: A randomized controlled trial. *Journal of Behavioral Medicine, 29*(4), 359–376.

a funduscopic examination to detect such complications as toxoplasmosis retinitis. Further discussion of therapy for the pregnant woman who is HIV positive or who has AIDS may be found in journal articles and specialty texts.

A pregnancy complicated by HIV infection, even if asymptomatic, is considered high risk, and the fetus is monitored closely. Weekly nonstress testing is begun at 32 weeks' gestation, and serial ultrasounds are done to detect intrauterine growth restriction. Biophysical profiles are also indicated (see Chapter 17 ∞). Invasive procedures such as amniocentesis are avoided when possible to prevent the contamination of a noninfected infant.

To reduce the risk of perinatal transmission, intrapartum intravenous ZDV is indicated for all pregnant women regardless of their prenatal therapy regimen. Scheduled cesarean birth at 38 weeks' gestation and before rupture of the membranes is recommended for women with elevated viral loads (Minkoff, 2008).

Women who are HIV positive are at increased risk for complications such as intrapartal or postpartal hemorrhage, postpartal infection, poor wound healing, and infections of the genitourinary tract. Thus they need careful monitoring and appropriate therapy as indicated.

Following childbirth, the HIV-positive woman should be referred to a physician knowledgeable about treating individuals with HIV infection. Because of the profound implications of HIV infection for the woman, her family, the fetus/newborn, and her healthcare providers, screening is recommended for all pregnant women, but especially those at increased risk, including the following: prostitutes; women with multiple sexual partners; women whose current or previous sex partners have been bisexual, have abused IV drugs, had hemophilia, or tested positive for HIV; women who are or have been IV drug users; and women from countries where heterosexual transmission is common. In addition, clinics located in areas with a large HIV-positive population may require routine HIV screening of all prenatal clients.

Nursing Care Management

Nursing Assessment and Diagnosis

A woman who tests positive for HIV may be asymptomatic or may present with any of the following signs or symptoms: fatigue, anemia, malaise, progressive weight loss, lymphadenopathy, diarrhea, fever, neurologic dysfunction, cell-mediated immunodeficiency, or evidence of Kaposi's sarcoma (purplish, reddish brown lesions either externally or internally).

If a woman tests positive for HIV or is involved in a relationship that places her at high risk, the nurse should assess the woman's knowledge level about the disease, its implications for her and her fetus, and self-care measures the woman can take.

Examples of nursing diagnoses that might apply for a pregnant woman who tests positive for HIV include the following:

- *Risk for Ineffective Health Maintenance* related to lack of information about HIV/AIDS and its long-term implications for the woman, her unborn child, and her family
- *Risk for Infection* related to altered immunity secondary to HIV infection
- *Compromised Family Coping* related to the implications of a positive HIV test in one of the family members

Nursing Plan and Implementation
Community-Based Nursing Care

Nurses need to help women understand that HIV/AIDS is a fatal disease. HIV infection can be avoided if women practice safe sex, including insisting that their partners wear a latex condom for each act of intercourse and avoid sharing IV drug needles.

Women at high risk for HIV/AIDS should be offered premarital and prepregnancy screening for HIV antibodies (ACOG, 2004). In many instances, the nurse will be responsible for counseling the woman about the test and its implications for her, her partner, and her child if she becomes pregnant.

In monitoring the asymptomatic pregnant woman who is HIV positive, the nurse needs to be alert for nonspecific symptoms such as fever, weight loss, fatigue, persistent candidiasis, diarrhea, cough, skin lesions, and behavior changes. These may be signs of developing symptomatic HIV infection. Laboratory findings such as increased viral load, decreased hemoglobin, hematocrit, and CD4 lymphocytes; elevated erythrocyte sedimentation rate (ESR); and abnormal complete blood count, differential, and platelets may indicate complications such as infection or progression of the disease.

Education about optimal nutrition and maintenance of wellness is important, and the information should be reviewed frequently with the woman. The woman should also receive information about her ZDV prophylaxis and the importance of following the established regimen for herself during pregnancy and for her newborn after birth.

HINTS FOR PRACTICE

Research indicates that prenatal care providers working in states with a low incidence of HIV/AIDS may not be as knowledgeable as they should be about follow-up when HIV testing is refused and about the disease itself as it relates to pregnancy and prenatal care (Ogles, Murphy, Caldwell, & Thornton, 2007). If you work with childbearing families it is crucial that you stay current on the diagnosis and treatment of pregnant women with HIV/AIDS, even if you live in an area where the incidence is low.

Nursing Care Plan For a Woman with HIV/AIDS

CLIENT SCENARIO

Janice Olsen, a 25-year-old gravida 1, para 0, is HIV positive. At 14 weeks' gestation she presents to the clinic with symptoms of a sore throat, chills, fatigue, diarrhea, and a weight loss of 2 lb since her last visit. She is unsure whether these symptoms are related to HIV or to the normal discomforts of pregnancy. Lab test reveals a decrease in CD4+ T lymphocyte count. Janice is placed on prophylactic HAART therapy. The nurse assesses Janice's emotional responses so that support and teaching can be planned accordingly. Janice is counseled on the signs and symptoms of infections, methods of disease transmission, and precautions that are necessary to prevent the spread of infection to her partner, fetus, and/or caregivers. The nurse also reinforces the importance of attending each prenatal visit.

ASSESSMENT

Subjective: myalgia, sore throat, chills

Objective: CD4+ T lymphocyte count is at a level of 182/mm³; candidiasis, temperature 101.4°F, diarrhea, and 2 lb weight loss in 1 week

Nursing Diagnosis	Risk for Infection related to inadequate secondary defenses (leukopenia, suppressed inflammatory response) secondary to HIV-positive status*
Client Goal	Client will remain free of opportunistic infection during course of pregnancy.
AEB:	• CD4+ T lymphocyte count within normal limits • No complaints of chills, fever, or sore throat • Normal weight gain during pregnancy

NURSING INTERVENTIONS

1. Obtain a complete health history during first prenatal visit.

2. Obtain a complete physical exam during first prenatal exam.

3. Educate the woman as to the signs and symptoms of infection.

4. Monitor the absolute CD4+ T lymphocyte count, ESR, CBC with differential, and hemoglobin and hematocrit (H & H) at each prenatal visit.

5. Obtain nutritional history and monitor weight gain at each prenatal visit.

RATIONALES

Rationale: A complete health history will help determine risk factors for the development of opportunistic infections during pregnancy. A comprehensive health history should include assessments for psychological well-being, social history, and habits, including risky behaviors such as recreational or illicit drug use involving the sharing of needles, multiple sexual partners, etc. Medical history should include data regarding previous episodes of illnesses such as pneumonias, persistent cough, herpes simplex types 1 and 2, lesions on retina, diarrhea, weight loss, gastroenteritis, abdominal pain, or any cognitive impairment.

Rationale: A complete physical exam will assist in identifying any underlying symptoms or illnesses that may compromise the pregnancy and/or complicate the treatment of HIV.

Rationale: Early recognition of signs and symptoms of infection will allow for immediate treatment, which may decrease the severity of the infection. Signs and symptoms of infections include fever, weight loss, fatigue, persistent candidiasis, diarrhea, cough, and skin lesions (Kaposi's sarcoma and hairy leukoplakia in the mouth).

Rationale: Lab results provide information about the woman's immune system and the potential for disease progression. Opportunistic infections are more likely to occur when the CD4+ T lymphocyte count drops below a level of 200/mm³. ESR can rise above 20 mm/hr with anemia and with acute and chronic inflammation. CBC with differential and platelet count helps identify anemia, thrombocytopenia, and leukopenia. H & H can also identify anemia.

Rationale: The HIV-infected woman needs to maintain optimal nutritional intake. A compromised nutritional status may affect maternal and fetal well-being. Depleted reserves of protein and iron may decrease the woman's ability to fight infection thereby making her more susceptible to opportunistic infections.

Nursing Care Plan For a Woman with HIV/AIDS *(Continued)*

Evaluation of Client Goal	• CD4+ T lymphocyte count is within normal limits. • Client reports no signs of opportunistic infections. • Client continues to gain appropriate amount of weight per week for the remainder of the pregnancy.

CRITICAL THINKING QUESTIONS

1. Janice agrees to follow the prescribed regimen for HAART therapy, which includes ZDV, but questions how long she will need to continue the medications. What will the nurse include in the discussion about her medications? Will Janice's newborn also have to take the medication?

Answer: To reduce the risk for perinatal transmission it is recommended that all HIV-infected women receive ZDV as part of therapy during pregnancy. Regardless of the therapy prescribed during pregnancy, ZDV is indicated for all pregnant women during the intrapartum period. Newborns of women with HIV also receive ZDV during the first 6 weeks of life.

2. Janice arrives at her next prenatal visit upset and stressed by all the testing and monitoring she needs to have during her pregnancy. What can the nurse do to help relieve some of Janice's stress and help her understand the basis for frequent monitoring of maternal and fetal well-being?

Answer: Counseling is imperative for the woman who is HIV positive. The nurse can provide the woman with up-to-

date, accurate information about the disease and its effect on the newborn. It is also helpful to explain that this disease puts the woman at a higher risk for opportunistic infections, which might complicate a pregnancy. Therefore monitoring the woman closely is essential so that complications are detected early, which will allow for immediate treatment and a better prognosis.

3. What measures will be taken to prevent the transmission of HIV to Janice's newborn during the birth process?

Answer: Care will be given to decrease the newborn's exposure to infected material. Certain procedures, such as internal fetal monitoring, forceps, vacuum extractors, and episiotomy will be avoided if possible. A scheduled cesarean before the onset of labor or rupture of membranes is recommended for women with high viral loads.

*For your reference, this care plan is an example of how one nursing diagnosis might be addressed.

Hospital-Based Nursing Care

The Nursing Care Plan for a Woman with HIV/AIDS summarizes essential nursing management.

In 1987, the CDC stated that the increasing prevalence of HIV/AIDS and the risk of exposure faced by healthcare workers is significant enough that *precautions should be taken with all clients* (not only those with known HIV infection), especially in dealing with blood and body fluids. These precautions are called *standard precautions.*

Nurses who deal with childbearing families are exposed frequently to blood and body fluids and need to pay careful attention to the CDC guidelines, which are addressed in introductory nursing courses as a preparation for clinical practice. See Key Facts to Remember: The Pregnant Woman with HIV Infection.

Protocols have been established for postexposure treatment of a caregiver who experiences a needlestick or exposure to body fluids of a person with HIV or a person whose HIV status is unknown. The effectiveness of the therapy, usually a combined drug approach, depends on

starting therapy rapidly. Thus such exposure should be reported immediately.

Teaching for Self-Care

The psychologic implications of HIV/AIDS for the childbearing family are staggering. The woman is faced with the knowledge that she and her newborn, if infected, have a decreased life expectancy. If her infant is not infected, she must face the possibility that others will raise her child. She must also face the reality that she can only hope to lengthen her life by carefully following an expensive, exacting medical regimen. The couple must deal with the impact of the illness on the partner, who may or may not be infected, and on other children. The woman and her family may have feelings of fear, helplessness, anger, and isolation.

The nonjudgmental, supportive nurse plays an essential role in preserving confidentiality and the client's right to privacy. The nurse can help ensure that the woman receives complete, accurate information about her condition and ways she might cope. The nurse also teaches transmission prevention using the specific language and

KEY FACTS TO REMEMBER

The Pregnant Woman with HIV Infection

- Following initial infection, antibodies usually become detectable within about 6 to 12 weeks, but it may take 6 months or longer. *Despite this, the woman is infected, and infectious.*
- HIV infection is spread primarily through sexual contact, exposure to contaminated blood, and (perinatally) from infected mother to child.
- Many women who are HIV positive are asymptomatic and may be unaware they have the infection. *Standard precautions are indicated in caring for all pregnant women.*
- A pregnant woman found to be HIV positive should receive prenatal counseling about the possible implications of HIV for the fetus so that she can make an informed choice about continuing her pregnancy. Her choice should be supported.
- During pregnancy, caregivers should be alert to nonspecific symptoms such as weight loss and fatigue, which may indicate progression of HIV disease.
- The incidence of vertical transmission of HIV infection from mother to baby has decreased significantly because of the administration of ZDV to the mother prenatally and during labor and to the newborn for a specified period following birth.
- Invasive procedures during the intrapartal period increase the risk of exposure to HIV for the fetus (who may be uninfected) and should be undertaken only after carefully weighing the advantages and risks.

The cardinal rule in caring for pregnant women is: If it's wet and it's not yours, use protection when handling it!

parlance of the woman and her partner. In addition the nurse ensures that the woman is referred to a comprehensive program that includes social services, psychologic support, and appropriate health care.

Evaluation

Expected outcomes of nursing care include the following:

- The woman discusses the implications of her HIV infection (or diagnosis of AIDS), its implications for her unborn child and for herself, the method of transmission, and the treatment options.
- The woman uses information about social services (or other agency referral) for follow-up assistance and counseling.
- The woman begins to verbalize her feelings about her condition and its implications for her and her family.

Care of the Woman with Heart Disease

Pregnancy results in increased cardiac output, heart rate, and blood volume. The normal heart is able to adapt to these changes without undue difficulty. The woman with

heart disease, however, has decreased cardiac reserve, making it more difficult for her heart to accommodate the higher workload of pregnancy.

Currently cardiac disease complicates about 1% of pregnancies (Cunningham, Leveno, Bloom et al., 2005). The pathology found in a pregnant woman with heart disease varies with the type of disorder. The more common conditions are discussed briefly here.

Congenital heart defects have become more common in pregnant women as improved surgical techniques enable females born with heart defects to live to childbearing age. Congenital heart defects most commonly seen in pregnant women include atrial septal defect, ventricular septal defect, patent ductus arteriosus, coarctation of the aorta, and tetralogy of Fallot.

For women with congenital heart disease, the implications of pregnancy depend on the specific defect. If the heart defect has been surgically repaired and no evidence of organic heart disease remains, pregnancy may be undertaken with confidence. Because many cardiac lesions are susceptible to subacute bacterial endocarditis, even in cases where the lesion was surgically repaired, antibiotic prophylaxis is often recommended at the time of birth. Women with congenital heart disease who experience cyanosis should be counseled to avoid pregnancy because the risk to mother and fetus is high.

Rheumatic fever, which may develop in untreated group A β-hemolytic streptococcal infections, is an inflammatory connective tissue disease that can involve the heart, joints, central nervous system, skin, and subcutaneous tissue. Once it occurs, rheumatic fever can recur; it is serious primarily because of the permanent damage it can do to the heart—rheumatic heart disease. Fortunately, rheumatic heart disease has declined rapidly in the past half century, primarily because of prompt identification of pharyngeal infections caused by streptococcus and the availability of antibiotics for treatment.

Rheumatic heart disease results when recurrent inflammation from bouts of rheumatic fever causes scar-tissue formation on the valves. The scarring results in stenosis (failure of the valve to open completely), regurgitation caused by failure of the valve to close completely, or a combination of both, thereby increasing the workload of the heart. Although mitral valve stenosis is the most commonly seen lesion, the aortic and tricuspid valves may also be affected.

The increased blood volume of pregnancy, coupled with the pregnant woman's need for increased cardiac output, stresses the heart of a woman with mitral stenosis and increases her risk of developing congestive heart failure. Even the woman who has no symptoms at the onset of her pregnancy is at risk.

Mitral valve prolapse (MVP) is usually an asymptomatic condition that is commonly found in women of childbearing age. The condition is more common in women than in men and seems to run in families. In MVP, the mitral valve leaflets tend to prolapse into the left atrium during ventricular systole because the chordae tendineae that support them are long, stretched, and thin. This produces a characteristic systolic click on auscultation. In more pronounced cases of MVP, mitral valve regurgitation occurs, producing a systolic murmur.

Women with MVP usually tolerate pregnancy well. Most women require assurance that they can continue with normal activities. A few women experience symptoms—primarily palpitations, chest pain, and dyspnea—which are often caused by arrhythmias. They are usually treated with propranolol hydrochloride (Inderal). Limiting caffeine intake also helps decrease palpitations. Antibiotic prophylaxis is no longer recommended (ACOG, 2003).

Peripartum cardiomyopathy is a relatively rare but serious dysfunction of the left ventricle that occurs in the last month of pregnancy or the first 5 months postpartum in a woman with no previous history of heart disease. The cause is unknown, but the mortality rate is as high as 18% to 56% (Klein & Galan, 2004). The symptoms are similar to those of congestive heart failure: dyspnea, orthopnea, fatigue, cough, chest pain, palpitations, and edema. The condition usually presents with anemia and infection; consequently, treatment focuses on underlying abnormalities. Digitalis, diuretics, vasodilators, anticoagulants, sodium restriction, and strict bed rest are often part of the treatment. Peripartum cardiomyopathy may resolve with bed rest as the heart gradually returns to normal size. Subsequent pregnancy is strongly discouraged because the disease tends to recur during pregnancy.

Eisenmenger syndrome is not a single congenital defect, but a complication that can develop as a result of other cardiac lesions causing left-to-right shunting (as with atrial septal defects or ventricular septal defects). This shunting can result in progressive pulmonary hypertension. As pulmonary vascular resistance increases, the shunting becomes bidirectional or reverses to right-to-left shunting. This condition cannot be corrected surgically and is associated with maternal mortality rates of 30% to 50% (Klein & Galan, 2004).

Clinical Therapy

The primary goal of clinical therapy is early diagnosis and ongoing management of the woman with cardiac disease. Echocardiogram, chest X-ray, auscultation of heart sounds, and sometimes cardiac catheterization are essential for establishing the type and severity of the heart disease. The severity of the disease can also be determined by the individual's ability to perform ordinary physical activity. The following classification of functional capacity has been standardized by the Criteria Committee of the New York Heart Association (1994).

- *Class I.* Asymptomatic. No limitation of physical activity.
- *Class II.* Slight limitation of physical activity. Asymptomatic at rest; symptoms occur with ordinary physical activity.
- *Class III.* Marked limitation of physical activity. Comfortable at rest but symptomatic during less-than-ordinary physical activity.
- *Class IV.* Inability to carry on any physical activity without discomfort. Even at rest the person experiences symptoms of cardiac insufficiency or anginal pain; discomfort increases with any physical activity.

Women in classes I and II usually experience a normal pregnancy and have few complications, whereas those in classes III and IV are at risk for more severe complications. Because anemia increases the work of the heart, it should be diagnosed early and treated if present. Infections, even if minor, also increase cardiac workload and should be treated. As pregnancy progresses, the woman's activity should be limited to minimize cardiac workload. Similarly, weight gain and sodium intake may also be restricted.

Drug Therapy

The pregnant woman with heart disease may need drug therapy in addition to the iron and vitamin supplements ordinarily prescribed to maintain health during pregnancy. Antibiotics, usually penicillin if not contraindicated by allergy, are used during pregnancy to prevent recurrent bouts of rheumatic fever and subsequent heart valve damage. Antibiotics may also be recommended during labor and the early postpartum period to prevent bacterial endocarditis in women with either acquired or congenital disease. If the woman develops coagulation problems, the anticoagulant heparin may be used. Heparin offers the greatest safety to the fetus because it does not cross the placenta. The thiazide diuretics and furosemide (Lasix) may be used to treat congestive heart failure if it develops. Digitalis glycosides and common antiarrhythmic drugs may be used to treat cardiac failure and arrhythmias. These agents cross the placenta but have no reported teratogenic effect. However, they have not been adequately studied to establish their safety in pregnancy (Klein & Galan, 2004).

Labor and Birth

Spontaneous natural labor with adequate pain relief is usually recommended for women in classes I and II. Special attention should be given to the prompt recognition and treatment of any signs of heart failure (Figure 15–4 ■). Those in classes III and IV may have labor induced and may need to be hospitalized before the onset of labor for cardiac stabilization. They also require invasive cardiac monitoring during labor.

Use of low forceps or vacuum assistance provides the safest method of birth, with lumbar epidural anesthesia to

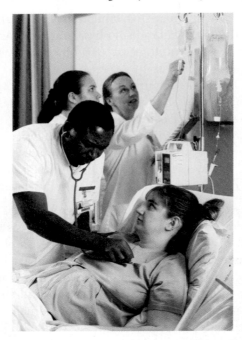

FIGURE 15–4 When a woman with heart disease begins labor, the nursing students and instructor caring for her monitor her closely for signs of congestive heart failure.

reduce the stress of pushing. Cesarean birth is used only if fetal or maternal indications exist, not on the basis of heart disease alone.

Nursing Care Management

Nursing Assessment and Diagnosis

The nurse assesses the stress of pregnancy on the functional capacity of the heart during every antepartal visit. The nurse notes the category of functional capacity assigned to the woman; takes the woman's pulse, respirations, and blood pressure; and compares the findings with the normal values expected during pregnancy. The nurse then determines the woman's activity level, including rest, and any changes in the pulse and respirations that have occurred since previous visits. The nurse also identifies and evaluates other factors that would increase strain on the heart. These factors might include anemia, infection, anxiety, lack of a support system, and household and career demands.

The following signs and symptoms, if they are progressive, are indicative of congestive heart failure:

- Cough (frequent, with or without blood-stained sputum [hemoptysis])
- Dyspnea (progressive, on exertion)
- Edema (progressive, generalized, including extremities, face, eyelids)
- Heart murmurs (heard on auscultation)
- Palpitations

- Rales (auscultated in lung bases)
- Weight gain (related to fluid retention)

Progressiveness of the cycle is the critical factor because some of these same behaviors are seen to a minor degree in a pregnancy without cardiac problems.

Nursing diagnoses that might apply to the pregnant woman with heart disease include the following:

- *Decreased Cardiac Output: Easy Fatigability*
- *Impaired Gas Exchange* related to pulmonary edema secondary to cardiac decompensation
- *Fear* related to the effects of the maternal cardiac condition on fetal well-being

Nursing Plan and Implementation

Nursing care is directed toward maintaining a balance between cardiac reserve and cardiac workload.

Antepartal Nursing Care

Nursing actions are designed to meet the physiologic and psychosocial needs of the pregnant woman with heart disease. The priority of nursing action varies based on the severity of the disease process and the individual needs of the woman determined by the nursing assessment.

The woman and her family should thoroughly understand her condition and its management and should recognize signs of potential complications; this level of understanding will decrease anxiety. When the nurse provides thorough explanations, uses printed material, and provides frequent opportunities to ask questions and discuss concerns, the woman is better able to meet her own healthcare needs and seek assistance appropriately.

As part of health teaching, the nurse explains the purposes of the dietary and activity changes that are required. A diet is instituted that is high in iron, protein, and essential nutrients but low in sodium, with adequate calories to ensure normal weight gain. Such a diet best meets the nutrition needs of the client with cardiac disease. To help preserve her cardiac reserves, the woman may need to restrict her activities. In addition, 8 to 10 hours of sleep, with frequent daily rest periods, are essential. Because upper respiratory infections may tax the heart and lead to decompensation, the woman must avoid contact with sources of infection.

During the first half of pregnancy, the woman is seen approximately every 2 weeks to assess cardiac status. During the second half of pregnancy, the woman is seen weekly. These assessments are especially important between weeks 28 and 30, when the blood volume reaches its maximum. If symptoms of cardiac decompensation occur, prompt medical intervention is indicated to correct the cardiac problem.

Intrapartum Period

Labor and birth exert tremendous stress on the woman and her fetus. This stress could be fatal to the fetus of a woman with cardiac disease because the fetus may be receiving a decreased oxygen and blood supply. Thus the intrapartal care of a woman with cardiac disease is aimed at reducing physical exertion and the accompanying fatigue.

The nurse evaluates maternal vital signs frequently to determine the woman's response to labor. A pulse rate greater than 100 beats per minute or respirations greater than 24 per minute may indicate the onset of cardiac decompensation and require further evaluation. The nurse also auscultates the woman's lungs frequently for evidence of rales and carefully observes for other signs that she is developing congestive heart failure.

To ensure cardiac emptying and adequate oxygenation, the nurse encourages the laboring woman to assume either a semi-Fowler's or side-lying position, with her head and shoulders elevated. Oxygen by mask, diuretics to reduce fluid retention, sedatives and analgesics, prophylactic antibiotics, and digitalis may also be used as indicated by the woman's status.

The nurse remains with the woman to support her. It is essential that the nurse keep the woman and her family informed of labor progress and management plans, collaborating with them to fulfill their wishes for the birth experience as much as possible. The nurse needs to maintain an atmosphere of calm to lessen the anxiety of the woman and her family.

Continuous electronic fetal monitoring is used to provide ongoing assessment of the fetal response to labor. To prevent overexertion and the accompanying fatigue, the nurse encourages the woman to sleep and relax between contractions and provides her with emotional support and encouragement. Epidural anesthesia is often used to decrease exertion. During pushing, the nurse encourages the woman to use shorter, more moderate pushing, with complete relaxation between pushes (Chapter 19 ∞). Forceps or vacuum extraction may be used if pushing is too difficult. Vital signs are monitored closely during the second stage.

Postpartum Period

The postpartum period is a significant time for the woman with cardiac disease. As extravascular fluid returns to the bloodstream for excretion, cardiac output and blood volume increase. This physiologic adaptation places great strain on the heart and may lead to decompensation, especially in the first 48 hours after birth.

So that the health team can detect any possible problems, the woman may remain in the hospital longer postpartally than the low-risk woman. Her vital signs are monitored frequently, and she is assessed for signs of decompensation. She stays in the semi-Fowler's or side-lying position, with her head and shoulders elevated, and begins a gradual, progressive activity program. Appropriate diet and stool softeners facilitate bowel movement without undue strain.

The postpartum nurse gives the woman opportunities to discuss her birth experience and helps her deal with any feelings or concerns that distress her. The nurse also encourages maternal-infant attachment by providing frequent opportunities for the mother to interact with her child.

No evidence exists that breastfeeding compromises cardiac output. Thus the only concern about breastfeeding for women with cardiovascular disease is related to medications the mother may be taking. These should be evaluated for the likelihood of passing into the milk or affecting lactation. The nurse can assist the breastfeeding mother to a comfortable side-lying position, with her head moderately elevated, or to a semi-Fowler's position. To conserve the mother's energy, the nurse should position the newborn at the breast and be available to burp the baby and reposition him or her at the other breast. The nurse can also encourage family members to assist the mother in this way.

In addition to providing the normal postpartum discharge teaching, the nurse should ensure that the woman and her family understand the signs of possible problems from her heart disease or other postpartal complications. The nurse also plans an activity schedule with the woman and her family. Visiting nurse referrals may be necessary, depending on the woman's health status.

Evaluation

Expected outcomes of nursing care include the following:

- The woman is able to discuss her condition and its possible impact on pregnancy, labor and birth, and the postpartal period.
- The woman participates in developing an appropriate healthcare regimen and follows it throughout her pregnancy.
- The woman gives birth to a healthy infant.
- The woman avoids congestive heart failure, thromboembolism, and infection.
- The woman is able to identify signs and symptoms of possible postpartum complications.
- The woman is able to care effectively for her newborn infant.

Other Medical Conditions and Pregnancy

A woman with a preexisting medical condition needs to be aware of the possible impact of pregnancy on her condition, as well as the impact of her condition on the successful outcome of her pregnancy. Table 15–6 discusses some of the less common medical conditions in relation to pregnancy.

TABLE 15–6	Less Common Medical Conditions and Pregnancy		
Condition	**Brief Description**	**Maternal Implications**	**Fetal/Neonatal Implications**
Asthma	Asthma, an obstructive lung condition, is the most common respiratory disease found in pregnancy, complicating 4% to 8% of all pregnancies (ACOG, 2008). Typical symptoms include wheezing, dyspnea, and episodic coughing. A severe asthmatic attack often requires hospitalization. It is managed by long-term comprehensive drug therapy to prevent airway inflammation, combined with drug treatment to manage attacks or exacerbations and client education about triggers (such as cold air, dust, smoke, exercise, food additives), methods of prevention, and treatment options.	The goal of therapy is to maintain adequate oxygenation of the fetus by preventing maternal hypoxia. Thus it is safer to treat symptoms with asthma medications than to let women have untreated symptoms and exacerbations. The effects of pregnancy on asthma symptoms varies with improvement in 23% and worsened symptoms in 30%. Thus all pregnant women with asthma should be monitored by assessing their symptoms and measuring their peak expiratory flow rate and forced expiratory volume. The use of medication is individualized using the lowest amount of medication necessary to maintain normal lung function. During pregnancy, Budesonide is the preferred inhaled corticosteroid for regular control. Asthma medications should be continued during labor and birth. To decrease the risk of bronchospasm, the woman should be well hydrated and receive adequate analgesia (ACOG, 2008).	Prematurity and low birth weight are more common among the infants of women who have asthma (Dombrowski, 2006). Asthma has also been linked with higher rates of hyperemesis gravidarum, preeclampsia, uterine hemorrhage, and perinatal mortality. The goal of therapy is to prevent maternal exacerbations because even a mild exacerbation can cause severe hypoxia-related complications in the fetus. If an exacerbation occurs, inhaled albuterol is recommended as rescue therapy if needed. If symptoms and pulmonary function levels do not improve, hospitalization may be necessary. Women are also taught to avoid or control their asthma triggers (allergens, irritants, tobacco smoke, and so forth) (ACOG, 2008).
Epilepsy	Chronic disorder characterized by seizures; may be idiopathic or secondary to other conditions, such as head injury, metabolic and nutritional disorders such as PKU or vitamin B_6 deficiency, encephalitis, neoplasms, or circulatory interferences. Treated with anticonvulsants.	Vast majority of pregnancies in women with seizure disorders are uneventful and have an excellent outcome. Women with more frequent seizures before pregnancy may have exacerbations during pregnancy, but this may be related to nausea and vomiting, lack of cooperation with drug regimen, or sleep deprivation. During pregnancy the woman should continue to be treated with the medication that best controls her seizures. Folic acid therapy should be started prior to conception if possible. Folic acid and vitamin D are indicated throughout pregnancy (AAFP, 2004).	Certain anticonvulsant medications are associated with increased incidence of congenital anomalies, especially cleft lip and heart defects, although the incidence has decreased in recent years. This may be due to the fact that the current ability to determine blood levels of medications has led to more accurate dosages and the resultant use of a single medication; consequently multiple medications are used less often (AAFP, 2004).
Hepatitis B	Hepatitis B, caused by the hepatitis B virus (HBV), is a major, growing health problem. Groups at risk include those from areas with a high incidence (primarily developing countries), illegal IV drug users, prostitutes, homosexuals, those with multiple sex partners, or occupational exposure to blood, although many infected people have no identifiable source of infection. HBV transmission is blood borne, primarily sexually and perinatally transmitted. Because of the dramatic increase and the difficulty of vaccinating high-risk individuals before they become infected, the CDC now recommends (1) testing all pregnant women for the presence of hepatitis B surface antigen and prophylactic treatment for all infants born to women who are HBsAG-positive or whose status is unknown; (2) routine infant vaccination; (3) vaccination of children and adolescents through age 18 years who have not been vaccinated; (4) vaccination of unvaccinated adults who are at risk for hepatitis B (CDC, 2006).	Hepatitis B does not usually affect the course of pregnancy. However, chronic HBV carriers have a great potential for infecting others when exposure to blood and body fluids occurs. In addition, chronic carriers may develop long-term sequelae, such as chronic liver disease and liver cancer. Approximately 4000 to 5000 deaths are caused annually by liver disease associated with chronic HBV infection. It is now recommended that all pregnant women be tested for the presence of hepatitis B surface antigen (HBsAg). A woman who is negative may be given the hepatitis vaccine.	Perinatal transmission most often occurs at or near the time of childbirth. More important, the risk of becoming a chronic carrier of the HBV is inversely related to the age of the individual at the time of initial infection. Therefore infants infected perinatally have the highest risk of becoming chronically infected if not treated. Recommendations now include routine vaccination of all newborns born to HBsAg-negative women and immunoprophylaxis to all newborns of HBsAg-positive women (CDC, 2006).

TABLE 15–6 Less Common Medical Conditions and Pregnancy *(Continued)*

Condition	Brief Description	Maternal Implications	Fetal/Neonatal Implications
Hyperthyroidism (thyrotoxicosis)	Enlarged, overactive thyroid gland; increased T_4: TBG ratio and increased BMR. Symptoms include muscle wasting, tachycardia, excessive sweating, and exophthalmos. Treatment by antithyroid drug propylthiouracil (PTU) while monitoring free T_4 levels. Surgery used only if drug intolerance exists.	Mild hyperthyroidism is not dangerous. Increased incidence of preeclampsia and postpartum hemorrhage if not well controlled. Serious risk related to thyroid storm characterized by high fever, tachycardia, sweating, and congestive heart failure. Now occurs rarely. When diagnosed during pregnancy, may be transient or permanent.	Neonatal thyrotoxicosis is rare. Even low doses of antithyroid drug in mother may produce a mild fetal/neonatal hypothyroidism; higher dose may produce a goiter or mental deficiencies. Fetal loss not increased in euthyroid women. If untreated, rates of abortion, intrauterine death, and stillbirth increase. Breast-feeding contraindicated for women on antithyroid medication because it is excreted in the milk (may be tried by woman on low dose if neonatal T_4 levels are monitored).
Hypothyroidism	Characterized by inadequate thyroid secretions (decreased T_4: TBG ratio), elevated TSH, lowered BMR, and enlarged thyroid gland (goiter). Symptoms include lack of energy, excessive weight gain, cold intolerance, dry skin, and constipation. Treated by thyroxine replacement therapy.	Long-term replacement therapy usually continues at same dosage during pregnancy as before. Weekly nonstress test (NST) after 35 weeks' gestation.	If mother untreated, fetal loss 50%; high risk of congenital goiter or true cretinism. Therefore newborns are screened for T_4 level. Mild TSH elevations present little risk because TSH does not cross the placenta.
Maternal phenylketonuria (PKU) (hyperphenylalaninemia)	Inherited recessive single gene anomaly causing a deficiency of the liver enzyme needed to convert the amino acid phenylalanine to tyrosine, resulting in high serum levels of phenylalanine. Brain damage and mental retardation occur if not treated early.	Low phenylalanine diet is mandatory before conception and during pregnancy. The woman should be counseled that her children will either inherit the disease or be carriers, depending on the zygosity of the father for the disease. Treatment at a PKU center is recommended.	Risk to fetus if maternal treatment not begun preconception. In untreated women increased incidence of fetal mental retardation, microcephaly, congenital heart defects, and growth retardation. Fetal phenylalanine levels are approximately 50% higher than maternal levels.
Multiple sclerosis	Neurologic disorder characterized by destruction of the myelin sheath of nerve fibers. The condition occurs primarily in young adults, more commonly in females, and is marked by periods of remission; progresses to marked physical disability in 10 to 20 years.	Associated with remission during pregnancy, but with slightly increased relapse rate postpartum (Haas, 2000). Rest is important; help with child care should be planned. Uterine contraction strength is not diminished, but because sensation is frequently lessened, labor may be almost painless.	Increased evidence of a genetic predisposition. Therefore reproductive counseling is recommended.
Rheumatoid arthritis	Chronic inflammatory disease believed to be caused by a genetically influenced antigen-antibody reaction. Symptoms include fatigue, low-grade fever, pain and swelling of joints, morning stiffness, pain on movement. Treated with salicylates, physical therapy, and rest. Corticosteroids used cautiously if not responsive to above.	Usually there is remission of rheumatoid arthritis symptoms during pregnancy, often with a relapse postpartum. Anemia may be present due to blood loss from salicylate therapy. Mother needs extra rest, particularly to relieve weight-bearing joints, but needs to continue range-of-motion exercises. If in remission, may stop medication during pregnancy.	Possibility of prolonged gestation and longer labor with heavy salicylate use. Possible teratogenic effects of salicylates.

(Continued)

TABLE 15–6	Less Common Medical Conditions and Pregnancy *(Continued)*		
Condition	Brief Description	Maternal Implications	Fetal/Neonatal Implications
Systemic lupus erythematosus (SLE)	Chronic autoimmune collagen disease, characterized by exacerbations and remissions; symptoms range from characteristic rash to inflammation and pain in joints, fever, nephritis, depression, cranial nerve disorders, and peripheral neuropathies.	Women who conceive when the disease is in remission appear to have little risk for adverse outcomes, whereas those with active disease have less favorable outcomes. Pregnancy does not appear to alter the long-term prognosis of women with SLE (Molad, Berkowski, Monselise, et al., 2005).	Increased incidence of spontaneous abortion, stillbirth, prematurity, and IUGR. Infants born to women with SLE may have characteristic skin rash, which usually disappears by 12 months. Infants are at increased risk for complete congenital heart block, a condition that can be diagnosed prenatally. Fetal echocardiography is then performed to rule out other cardiac defects (Buyon & Clancy, 2005). No known treatment exists although various therapies have been tried. The prognosis for the fetus varies but, because the heart damage is permanent, a pacemaker may be necessary if the newborn is to survive (Branch, Silver & Aagaard-Tillery, 2008).
Tuberculosis (TB)	Infection caused by *Mycobacterium tuberculosis;* inflammatory process causes destruction of lung tissue, increased sputum, and coughing. Associated primarily with poverty and malnutrition and may be found among refugees from countries where TB is prevalent. Treated with isoniazid and either ethambutol or rifampin, or both.	The incidence of tuberculosis has begun to increase significantly since the late 1980s, and it is increasingly associated with HIV infection (Laibl & Sheffield, 2005). If TB inactive due to prior treatment, relapse rate no greater than for nonpregnant women. When isoniazid is used during pregnancy, the woman should take supplemental pyridoxine (vitamin B$_6$). Extra rest and limited contact with others is required until disease becomes inactive.	If maternal TB is inactive, mother may breastfeed and care for her infant. If TB is active, newborn should not have direct contact with mother until she is noninfectious. Isoniazid crosses the placenta, but most studies show no teratogenic effects. Rifampin crosses the placenta. Possibility of harmful effects still being studied.

CHAPTER HIGHLIGHTS

- Almost any health problem that a person can have when not pregnant can coexist with pregnancy as well. Some problems, such as anemias, may be exacerbated by pregnancy. Others, such as collagen disease, may go into temporary remission with pregnancy. Regardless of the health problem, careful health care is needed throughout pregnancy to improve the outcome for mother and fetus.

- The diagnosis of high-risk pregnancy can shock an expectant couple. Providing emotional support, teaching about the condition and prognosis, and educating for self-care are important nursing measures that help clients cope.

- Substance abuse (either drugs or alcohol) not only is detrimental to the mother's health but also may have profound, lasting effects on the fetus. Nurses need to be alert to signs of substance abuse and be nonjudgmental in their care of women with substance abuse problems.

- The key point in the care of the pregnant diabetic is scrupulous maternal plasma glucose control. This is best achieved by home blood glucose monitoring, multiple daily insulin injections, and a careful diet.

- To reduce the incidence of congenital anomalies and other problems in the newborn, the woman should maintain a normal blood glucose level before conception and through-

out the pregnancy. Women with diabetes, even more than most other clients, need to be educated about their condition and involved with their own care.

- Anemia indicates inadequate levels of hemoglobin (Hb) in the blood. Anemia is defined as hemoglobin less than 12 g/dL in nonpregnant women and less than 11 g/dL in pregnant and postpartum women. Iron deficiency anemia is the most common form of anemia. Other anemias include folic acid deficiency, sickle cell anemia, and thalassemia.

- HIV infection, which is transmitted via blood and body fluids, may also be transmitted vertically from the mother to the fetus. Currently there is no definitive treatment for HIV/AIDS.

- Vertical transmission of HIV infection has been reduced dramatically with the administration of ZDV to the mother prenatally and during labor and to the newborn.

- Nurses should employ blood and body fluid precautions (standard precautions) in caring for all women to avoid potential spread of infection.

- Cardiac disease during pregnancy requires careful assessment, limitation of activity, and knowing and reporting signs of impending cardiac decompensation by both client and nurse.

CHAPTER REFERENCES

American Academy of Family Physicians. (AAFP). (2004). *Epilepsy and pregnancy: what you should know.* Retrieved December 11, 2005 from http://familydoctor.org/243.xml

American College of Obstetricians and Gynecologists (ACOG). (2000). *Genetic screening for hemoglobinopathesis* (ACOG Committed Opinion No. 238). Washington, DC: Author.

American College of Obstetricians and Gynecologists. (ACOG). (2003). *Prophylactic antibiotics in labor and delivery* (ACOG Practice Bulletin No. 47). Washington, DC: Author.

American College of Obstetricians and Gynecologists (ACOG). (2004). *Prenatal and perinatal human immunodeficiency virus testing: Expanded recommendations.* (ACOG Committed Opinion No. 304). Washington, DC: Author.

American College of Obstetricians and Gynecologists (ACOG). (2005). *Pregestational diabetes mellitus* (ACOG Practice Bulletin No. 60). Washington, DC: Author.

American College of Obstetricians and Gynecologists (ACOG). (2008). *Asthma in pregnancy* (ACOG Practice Bulletin No. 90). Washington, DC: Author.

American Diabetes Association (ADA). (2006). Position statement: Gestational diabetes mellitus. *Diabetes Care, 29*(Suppl. 1).

American Diabetes Association (ADA). (2007). Position statement: Diagnosis and classification of diabetes mellitus. *Diabetes Care, 30*(Suppl.), S42–S47.

Bormann, J. E. (2006). Effects of spiritual mantram repetition on HIV outcomes: A randomized controlled trial. *Journal of Behavioral Medicine, 29*(4), 359–376.

Branch, D. W., Silver, R. M., & Aagaard-Tillery, K. (2008). Immunologic disorders in pregnancy. In R. S. Gibbs, B. Y. Karlan, A. F. Haney, & I. E. Nygaard (Eds.), *Danforth's obstetrics and gynecology* (10th ed.). Philadelphia: Wolters Kluwer/Lippincott Williams & Wilkins.

Branson, B. M., Handsfield, H. H., Lampe, M. A., Janssen, R. S., Taylor, A. W., Lyss, S. B., & Clark, J. E. (2006). Revised recommendations for HIV testing of adults, adolescents, and pregnant women in health-care settings. *Morbidity and Mortality Weekly Report, 55*(RR-14), 1–36.

Byron, J. P., & Clancy, R. M. (2005). Neonatal lupus, basic research and clinical perspectives. *Rheumatic Diseases Clinics of North America, 31*(2), 299–313.

Centers for Disease Control and Prevention (CDC). (2006, August 4). Sexually transmitted disease guidelines, 2006. *Morbidity and Mortality Weekly Report, 55*: No. RR-11, 1–93.

Centers for Disease Control and Prevention (CDC). (2007). *HIV/AIDS among women.* Retrieved May 18, 2008, from www.cdc.gov/hiv/topics/women/resources/factsheets/print/women.htm

Centers for Disease Control and Prevention (CDC). (2008). *HIV/AIDS in the United States.* CDC HIV/AIDS Facts. Retrieved May 18, 2008, from www.cdc.gov

Centers for Disease Control and Prevention & the Pan American Health Organization. (2003). *The prevention of neural tube defects with folic acid.* Retrieved April 26, 2004, from www.cdc.gov/Images_-/_Video_and_Audio/Images/Birth_Defects/Folic_Acid/ntd_dave.pdf

Cleveland Clinic. (2006). *Gestational diabetes. Hypoglycemia.* Retrieved July 7, 2007, from http://www.clevelandclinic.org/health/health-info/docs/2300/2354.asp?index=9012

Criteria Committee of the New York Heart Association. (1994). *Nomenclature and criteria for diagnosis of diseases of the heart and great vessels* (9th ed.). Dallas: American Heart Association.

Cunningham, F. G., Leveno, K. J., Bloom, S. L., Hauth, J .C., Gilstrap III, L. C., & Wenstrom, K. D. (2005). *Williams obstetrics* (22nd ed.). New York: McGraw-Hill.

Dombrowski, M. P. (2006). Asthma and pregnancy. *Obstetrics and Gynecology, 108*, 667–681.

Food and Drug Administration (FDA). (2005). Alcohol warning for pregnant women. *FDA Consumer, 39*(3), 4.

Forsbach-Sanchez, G., Tamez-Perez, H. E., & Vazquez-Lara, J. (2005, May–June). Diabetes and pregnancy. *Archives of Medical Research, 36*(3), 291–299.

Gamma, A., Jerome, L., Liechti, M. E., & Sumnall, H. R. (2005). Is ecstasy perceived to be safe? A critical survey. *Drug & Alcohol Dependence, 77*(2), 185–193.

Haas, J. (2000). High dose IVIG in the postpartum period for prevention of exacerbations in MS. *Multiple Sclerosis, 6* (Suppl. 2), 518–520.

Jansson, L. M., Dipietro, J., & Elko, A. (2005). Fetal response to maternal methadone administration. *American Journal of Obstetrics & Gynecology, 193*(3 Pt 1), 611–617.

Klein, L. L., & Galan, H. L. (2004, June). Cardiac disease in pregnancy. *Obstetrics & Gynecology Clinics of North America, 31*(2), viii, 429–459.

Koprich, J. S., Chen, E. R., Kanaan, N. M., Campbell, N. C., Kordower, J. H., & Lipton, J. W. (2003). Prenatal 3,4-methylenedioxymethamphetamine (ecstasy) alters exploratory behavior, reduces monoamine metabolism, and increases forebrain tyrosine hydroxylase fiber density of juvenile rats. *Neurotoxicology and Teratology, 25*(5), 509–517.

Krakow, D. (2008). Medical and surgical complications of pregnancy. In R. S. Gibbs, B. Y. Karlan, A. F. Haney, & I. E. Nygaard (Eds.), *Danforth's obstetrics and gynecology* (10th ed.). Philadelphia: Wolters Kluwer/Lippincott Williams & Wilkins.

Lachat, M. F., Scott, C. A., & Relf, M. V. (2006). HIV and pregnancy: Considerations for nursing practice. *MCN, 31*(4), 233–240.

Laibl, V. R., & Sheffield, J. S. (2005). Tuberculosis in pregnancy. *Clinics in Perinatology, 32*(3), 739–747.

March of Dimes. (2007). Illicit drug use during pregnancy. *Fact Sheet.* Retrieved June 27, 2007, from www.marchofdimes.com

Menato, G., Bo, S., Signorite, A., Gallo, M., Cotrino, I., Poala, C. B., & Massobrioo, M. (2008). Current management of gestational diabetes. *Expert Review of Obstetrics and Gynecology, 3*(1), 73–91.

Minkoff, H. (2008). Human immunodeficiency virus. In R. S. Gibbs, B. Y. Karlan, A. F. Haney, & I. E. Nygaard (Eds.), *Danforth's obstetrics and gynecology* (10th ed.). Philadelphia: Wolters Kluwer/Lippincott Williams & Wilkins.

Molad, Y., Borkowski, T., Monselise, A., Ben-Haroush, A., Sulkes, J., Hod , M., et al. (2005). Maternal and fetal outcome of lupus pregnancy: A prospective study of 29 pregnancies. *Lupus 14*(2), 145–151.

Ogles, J. R., Murphy, B. S., Caldwell, G. G., & Thornton, A. C. (2007). Testing practices and knowledge of HIV among prenatal providers in a low seroprevalence state. *AIDS, Patient Care, and STDs, 21*(3), 187–194.

Perkins, J. M., Dunn, J. P., & Jagasia, S. (2007). Perspectives in gestational diabetes mellitus: A review of screening, diagnosis, and treatment. *Clinical Diabetes, 25*(2), 57–62.

Public Health Service Task Force. (2007, November 2). Recommendations for use of antiretroviral drugs in pregnant HIV-infected women for maternal health and interventions to reduce perinatal HIV transmission in the United States. Retrieved May 19, 2008, from http://aidsinfo.nih.gov/

Reece, E. A., & Homko, C. J. (2008). Diabetes mellitus and pregnancy. In R. S. Gibbs, B. Y. Karlan, A. F. Haney, & I. E. Nygaard (Eds.), *Danforth's obstetrics and gynecology* (10th ed.). Philadelphia: Wolters Kluwer/Lippincott Williams & Wilkins.

Scollan-Koliopoulos, M., Guadagno, S., & Walker, E. A. (2006). Gestational diabetes management: Guidelines to a healthy pregnancy. *The Nurse Practitioner, 31*(6), 14–23.

Slocum, J. M. (2007). Preconception counseling and type 2 diabetes. *Diabetes Spectrum, 20*, 117–123.

Substance Abuse and Mental Health Services Administration (SAMHSA). (2007). *Results from the 2006 National Survey on Drug Use and Health: National Findings.* Rockville MD: Office of Applied Studies (NSDUH Series H-32, DHHS Publication No. SMA 07-4293).

Wyatt, J. W., Frias, J. L., Hoyme, H. E., Jovanovic, L., Kaaja, R., Brown, F., et al. (2005). Congenital anomaly rate in offspring of mothers with diabetes treated with insulin lispro during pregnancy. *Diabetic Medicine, 22*(6), 803–807.

CHAPTER 16

Pregnancy at Risk: Gestational Onset

Working with women who are dealing with high-risk pregnancies has given me a much deeper appreciation of the stress a family faces when their unborn child is threatened or when the mother is ill. Some families seem so strong and resilient—they use me as a resource, and I am delighted to assist them in that way. Other families seem to crumble and have such needs. I do my best to help them gain the tools they need to cope. When I succeed, I am elated. When they can't seem to cope, no matter what any of us do, I feel such a sense of sadness for the family and their future.

—Maternity nurse working in a large medical center

LEARNING OUTCOMES

16-1. Relate the etiology, medical therapy, and cultural perspectives to community-based and hospital-based nursing care management of women with a bleeding problem associated with pregnancy.

16-2. Describe the maternal and fetal-neonatal risks and medical therapy in community-based and hospital-based nursing care management of the woman with hyperemesis gravidarum.

16-3. Describe the development and course of hypertensive disorders associated with pregnancy.

16-4. Describe the maternal and fetal-neonatal risks, clinical manifestations, and diagnosis in determining the community-based and hospital-based nursing care management of the pregnant woman with a hypertensive disorder in the antepartum, intrapartum, and postpartum periods.

16-5. Relate the cause, fetal-neonatal risks, prevention, and clinical therapy to the nursing care management of the woman at risk for Rh alloimmunization.

16-6. Explain the occurrence, cause, clinical treatment, and implications for the fetus or newborn in determining nursing care management of the woman at risk for ABO incompatibility.

16-7. Examine the effects of surgical procedures in the nursing care management of the pregnant woman requiring surgery.

16-8. Relate the impact of trauma caused by an accident to the nursing care management of the pregnant woman or her fetus.

16-9. Examine the needs and care of the pregnant woman who experiences abuse.

16-10. Explain the cause, fetal-neonatal risks, and clinical therapy in the nursing care management of the pregnant woman with a perinatal infection affecting the fetus.

Pregnancy is usually an uncomplicated experience. In some cases, however, problems arise that place the pregnant woman and her unborn child at risk. Regular prenatal care serves to detect these potential complications quickly so that effective care can be provided. This chapter focuses on problems that primarily occur during pregnancy; that is, problems with a *gestational onset*.

Care of the Woman with a Bleeding Disorder

Vaginal bleeding occurs in up to 25% of first trimester pregnancies (Harville, Wilcox, Bird, & Weinberg, 2004; Schauberger, Mathiason, & Rooney, 2005). During the first and second trimesters of pregnancy, the major cause of bleeding is abortion. **Abortion** is the expulsion of the fetus before viability, which is considered to be 20 weeks' gestation or weight of less than 500 g. Abortions are either *spontaneous* (occurring naturally) or *induced* (occurring as a result of artificial or mechanical interruption). Because the term *abortion* may carry a negative connotation, spontaneous abortion is often called **miscarriage**.

Other complications that can cause bleeding in the first half of pregnancy are ectopic pregnancy and gestational trophoblastic disease, discussed shortly. In the second half of pregnancy, particularly in the third trimester, the two major causes of bleeding are placenta previa and abruptio placentae. (These are discussed in detail in Chapter 21 ∞.) Regardless of the cause of bleeding, however, the nurse has certain general responsibilities in providing nursing care.

General Principles of Nursing Intervention

Spotting is relatively common during pregnancy and usually occurs following sexual intercourse or exercise because of trauma to the highly vascular cervix. However, the woman is advised to report any spotting or bleeding that occurs during pregnancy so that it can be evaluated.

It is often the nurse's responsibility to make the initial assessment of bleeding. In general, the following nursing measures should be implemented for pregnant women being treated for bleeding disorders.

- Monitor blood pressure and pulse frequently.
- Observe the woman for behaviors indicative of shock, such as pallor, clammy skin, perspiration, dyspnea, or restlessness.
- Count and weigh pads to assess amount of bleeding over a given time period; save any tissue or clots expelled.
- If pregnancy is of 12 weeks' gestation or beyond, assess fetal heart tones with a Doppler.
- Prepare for intravenous (IV) therapy. There may be standing orders to begin IV therapy on clients who are bleeding.
- Prepare equipment for examination.
- Have oxygen available.
- Collect and organize all data, including antepartal history, onset of bleeding episode, and laboratory studies (hemoglobin, hematocrit, Rh status, hormonal assays) for analysis.
- Obtain an order to type and crossmatch for blood if evidence of significant blood loss exists.
- Assess coping mechanisms of woman in crisis. Give emotional support to enhance her coping abilities by continuous, sustained presence; by clear explanation of procedures; and by communicating her status to her family. Prepare the woman for possible fetal loss. Assess her expressions of anger, denial, silence, guilt, depression, or self-blame.
- Assess the family's response to the situation.

Spontaneous Abortion (Miscarriage)

Many pregnancies end in the first trimester because of spontaneous abortion. Often the woman assumes she is having a heavy menstrual period when she is really having an early abortion; thus statistics regarding spontaneous abortions are inaccurate. The incidence is 10% to 15% for clinically recognized pregnancies; however, maternal age influences this significantly. A 40-year-old pregnant woman has twice the risk of a 20-year-old (Simpson & Jauniaux, 2007).

A majority of spontaneous abortions are related to chromosomal abnormalities. Other causes include teratogenic drugs, faulty implantation caused by abnormalities of the female reproductive tract, a weakened cervix, placental abnormalities, chronic maternal diseases, endocrine imbalances, and maternal infections. Women who use hot tubs or

Jacuzzis are twice as likely to have miscarriages as nonusers, probably because of the hyperthermia resulting from increased core body temperature (Li, Janevic, Odouli, & Liyan, 2004).

Classification

Spontaneous abortions are subdivided into the following categories.

- *Threatened abortion* (Figure 16–1A ■). The embryo or fetus is jeopardized by unexplained bleeding, cramping, and backache. The cervix is closed. Bleeding may persist for days. It may be followed by partial or complete expulsion of the embryo or fetus, placenta, and membranes (sometimes called the "products of conception").
- *Imminent abortion* (Figure 16–1B). Bleeding and cramping increase. The internal cervical os dilates. Membranes may rupture. The term *inevitable abortion* also applies.
- *Complete abortion.* All the products of conception are expelled.
- *Incomplete abortion* (Figure 16–1C). Some of the products of conception are retained, most often the placenta. The internal cervical os is dilated slightly.
- *Missed abortion.* The fetus dies in utero but is not expelled. Uterine growth ceases, breast changes regress, and the woman may report a brownish vaginal discharge. The cervix is closed. If the fetus is retained beyond 6 weeks, the breakdown of fetal tissues results in

the release of thromboplastin, and disseminated intravascular coagulation (DIC) may develop.
- *Recurrent pregnancy loss* (formerly called habitual abortion). Abortion occurs consecutively in three or more pregnancies.
- *Septic abortion.* Presence of infection. May occur with prolonged, unrecognized rupture of the membranes; pregnancy with an intrauterine device (IUD) in utero; or attempts by unqualified individuals to terminate a pregnancy.

Clinical Therapy

One of the more reliable indicators of potential spontaneous abortion is the presence of pelvic cramping and backache. These symptoms are usually absent in bleeding caused by polyps, ruptured cervical blood vessels, or cervical erosion.

Speculum examination is done to determine the presence of cervical polyps or cervical erosion. Ultrasound scanning may detect the presence of cardiac activity and a gestational sac, or reveal a crown-rump length that is small for gestational age. Laboratory determination of hCG level can confirm a pregnancy, but because the hCG level falls slowly after fetal death, it cannot confirm a live embryo/fetus. Serial hCG levels may be indicated to confirm a diagnosis. Hemoglobin and hematocrit levels are obtained to assess blood loss. Blood is typed and cross-matched for possible replacement needs.

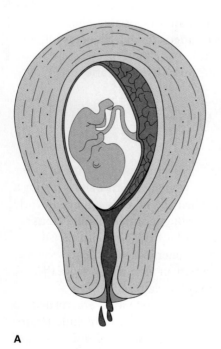
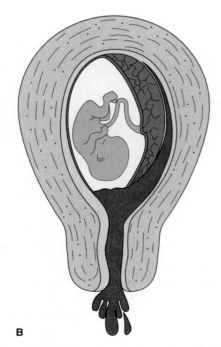
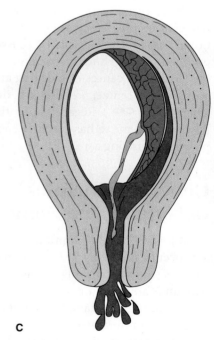

A   B   C

FIGURE 16–1 Types of spontaneous abortion. *A,* Threatened. The cervix is not dilated, and the placenta is still attached to the uterine wall, but some bleeding occurs. *B,* Imminent. The placenta has separated from the uterine wall, the cervix has dilated, and the amount of bleeding has increased. *C,* Incomplete. The embryo/fetus has passed out of the uterus; however, the placenta remains.

The therapy prescribed for the pregnant woman with bleeding is bed rest, abstinence from coitus, and emotional support. If bleeding persists and abortion is imminent or incomplete, the woman may be hospitalized, IV therapy or blood transfusions may be started to replace fluid, and dilatation and curettage (D&C) or suction evacuation is performed to remove the remainder of the products of conception. If the woman is Rh negative and not sensitized, Rh immune globulin (RhoGAM) is given within 72 hours (see discussion on Rh sensitization later in this chapter).

In missed abortions, the products of conception eventually are expelled spontaneously. If this does not occur within 4 to 6 weeks after embryo or fetal death, hospitalization is necessary. Dilatation and curettage or suction evacuation is done if the pregnancy is in the first trimester. In the second trimester, labor is induced or, alternatively, dilatation and evacuation (D&E) may be used.

Nursing Care Management

Nursing Assessment and Diagnosis

The nurse assesses the woman's vital signs, amount and appearance of any bleeding, level of comfort, and general physical health. The woman's blood type and antibody status should be identified to determine the need for Rh immune globulin (see page 362). If the pregnancy is 10 to 12 weeks or more, fetal heart rate should be assessed by Doppler. The nurse also assesses the responses of the woman and her family to this crisis and evaluates their coping mechanisms and ability to comfort each other.

Examples of nursing diagnoses that may apply include the following:

- *Fluid Volume Deficit* related to excessive bleeding secondary to spontaneous abortion
- *Acute Pain* related to abdominal cramping secondary to threatened abortion
- *Anticipatory Grieving* related to expected loss of unborn child

Nursing Plan and Implementation

Community-Based Nursing Care

If a woman in her first trimester of pregnancy begins cramping or spotting, she is often evaluated on an outpatient basis. The nurse provides analgesics for pain relief if the woman's cramps are severe and explains what is occurring throughout the process.

Feelings of shock or disbelief are normal. Couples who approached the pregnancy with feelings of joy and a sense of expectancy now also feel grief, sadness, and possibly anger.

Because many women, even with planned pregnancies, feel some ambivalence initially, guilt is also a common

emotion. These feelings may be even stronger for women who were negative about their pregnancies. The women may harbor negative feelings about themselves or even believe that the abortion may be a punishment for some wrongdoing.

The nurse can offer invaluable psychologic support to the woman and her family by encouraging them to talk about their feelings, allowing them the privacy to grieve, and listening sympathetically to their concerns about this pregnancy and future ones. The nurse may help decrease feelings of guilt or blame by informing the woman and her family about the causes of spontaneous abortion. The nurse can also refer them to other healthcare professionals for additional help as necessary. If the woman has older children, she may need guidance in how to help them understand and cope with what has occurred. Commemorating the pregnancy and baby is helpful in validating the significance of the loss (Easterwood, 2004). The grieving period following a spontaneous abortion usually lasts 6 to 24 months. Many couples can be helped during this period by an organization or support group established for parents who have lost a fetus or newborn.

Hospital-Based Nursing Care

A woman with an incomplete or missed abortion may need a D&C or other procedure, which is typically done on an outpatient basis. Barring any complications, the woman can return home a few hours after the procedure. The nurse monitors the woman's condition closely and administers Rh immune globulin if it is indicated. During discharge teaching, the nurse advises the woman to report heavy or bright red vaginal bleeding, to take the full course of antibiotics if they are prescribed, and to delay pregnancy for at least 2 months to allow sufficient time for healing. The nurse also

---

CULTURAL PERSPECTIVES

Remember that individual responses to fetal loss following miscarriage may vary greatly and may be influenced by ethnic or cultural norms.

- Miscarriage may be viewed in many ways. For example, it may be seen as a punishment from God, as the result of the evil eye or of a hex or curse by an enemy, or as a natural part of life.
- When grieving over a pregnancy loss, women from some cultures and ethnic groups may show their emotions freely, crying and wailing, whereas other women may hide their feelings behind a mask of stoicism.
- In some cultures the woman's partner is her primary source of support and comfort. In others, the woman turns to her mother or close female relatives for comfort.
- Avoid falling into the trap of stereotyping women according to culture. Individual responses are influenced by many factors including the degree of assimilation into the dominant culture.

shares information about the psychologic responses to the loss that the woman and her partner may experience.

Evaluation

Expected outcomes of nursing care include the following:

- The woman is able to explain spontaneous abortion and the treatment measures employed in her care.
- The woman suffers no complications.
- The woman and her partner begin verbalizing their grief and acknowledge that the grieving process lasts several months.

Ectopic Pregnancy

Ectopic pregnancy (EP) is the implantation of the fertilized ovum in a site other than the endometrial lining of the uterus. It has many associated risk factors including tubal damage caused by pelvic inflammatory disease (PID), previous tubal surgery, congenital anomalies of the tube, endometriosis, previous ectopic pregnancy, presence of an IUD, and in utero exposure to diethylstilbestrol (DES).

The incidence of EP has increased dramatically in the past several years from 4.5 per 1000 pregnancies in 1970 to 19.7 per 1000 pregnancies in 2000 (Van Den Eeden, Shan, Bruce, & Glasser, 2005). This increase is related to an increase in the associated risk factors, better diagnostic measures, and the increased use of assisted reproductive technology (Chapter 7 ∞), which carries a 5% risk of EP (Seeber & Barnhart, 2008). However, although the incidence has increased, the mortality rate has declined almost 90% because of better diagnostic techniques that allow detection before tubal rupture.

Ectopic pregnancy occurs when the fertilized ovum is prevented or slowed in its passage through the tube and thus implants before it reaches the uterus. The most common location for implantation is the ampulla of the fallopian tube. Figure 16–2 ■ illustrates this and other implantation sites.

Initially the normal symptoms of pregnancy may be present; specifically, amenorrhea, breast tenderness, and nausea. The hormone hCG is present in the blood and urine. As the pregnancy progresses, the chorionic villi grow into the wall of the tube or site of implantation and a blood supply is established. When the embryo outgrows this space, the tube ruptures and there is bleeding into the abdominal cavity. This bleeding irritates the peritoneum, causing the characteristic symptoms of sharp, one-sided pain, syncope, and referred shoulder pain. The woman may also experience lower abdominal pain. Vaginal bleeding occurs when the embryo dies and the decidua begins to slough.

Physical examination usually reveals adnexal tenderness. (The adnexae are the areas of the lower abdomen located over each ovary and fallopian tube.) An adnexal mass is palpable about half the time. Bleeding tends to be slow and chronic, and the abdomen gradually becomes rigid and very tender. With extensive bleeding into the abdominal cavity, pelvic examination causes extreme pain, and a mass of blood may be palpated in the cul-de-sac of Douglas. Laboratory tests may reveal low hemoglobin and hematocrit levels and rising leukocyte levels.

Clinical Therapy

Diagnosis of ectopic pregnancy begins with an assessment of menstrual history, including the last menstrual period (LMP), followed by a careful pelvic exam to identify any abnormal pelvic masses and tenderness. A serum progesterone level is drawn. A viable intrauterine pregnancy can be diagnosed with 97.5% sensitivity if the progesterone

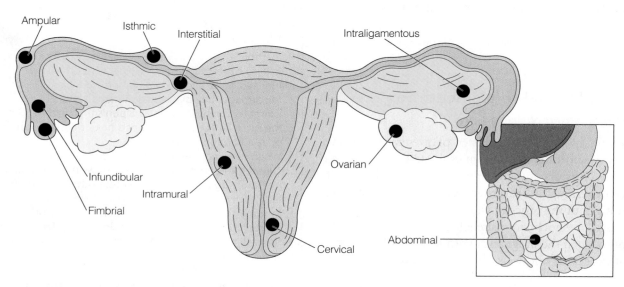

FIGURE 16–2 Various implantation sites in ectopic pregnancy. The most common site is within the fallopian tube, hence the name "tubal pregnancy."

level is 25 ng/mL or higher, whereas a serum progesterone level lower than 5 ng/mL indicates a dead fetus or an ectopic pregnancy. Levels from 5 to 25 ng/mL are inconclusive (Cunningham, Leveno, Bloom et al., 2005).

Serum β-hCG levels are drawn and reassessed in 48 hours if necessary. A woman with ectopic pregnancy tends to have abnormally low hCG levels. Moreover, in normal pregnancy, hCG levels double every 48 to 72 hours. Nondoubling hCG levels occur in ectopic pregnancy and in nonviable uterine pregnancies. If the β-hCG levels are above 1500 milli-international units per milliliter, transvaginal ultrasound is used to check for a uterine pregnancy or an adnexal mass. Confirming a uterine pregnancy nearly eliminates the diagnosis of ectopic pregnancy.

Treatment may be medical or surgical. Medical treatment using methotrexate is indicated for the woman who desires future pregnancy if her ectopic pregnancy is unruptured and of 3.5 cm size or less and if her condition is stable. In addition, there must be no fetal cardiac motion and the woman must have no evidence of acute intra-abdominal bleeding, a blood disorder, or kidney or liver disease. Methotrexate, a folic acid antagonist that interferes with DNA synthesis and cell multiplication, is administered intramuscularly. Although a single-dose approach requires fewer visits, a two-dose protocol has become increasingly popular because it has a lower failure rate. With the two-dose approach a second injection is given on day 4. A third dose can be given on day 7 if there has not been an appropriate drop in human chorionic gonadotropin (hCG) (Seeber & Barnhart, 2008). As an outpatient, the woman is monitored for increasing abdominal pain. β-hCG titers are monitored regularly. β-hCG titers typically increase for 1 to 4 days and then decrease (Lipscomb, Givens, Meyer, & Bran, 2005).

If surgery is indicated and the woman desires future pregnancies, treatment involves salpingostomy via a laparoscope. With this method, a linear incision is made and the products of conception are gently removed. The surgical incision is left open and allowed to close by secondary intention. If the tube is ruptured or if future childbearing is not an issue, laparoscopic salpingectomy (removal of the tube) is performed, leaving the ovary in place unless it is damaged.

With both medical and surgical therapies for ectopic pregnancy, the Rh-negative nonsensitized woman is given Rh immune globulin to prevent sensitization (discussed later in this chapter).

Nursing Care Management

Nursing Assessment and Diagnosis

When the woman with a suspected ectopic pregnancy is admitted to the hospital, the nurse assesses the appearance and amount of vaginal bleeding and monitors vital signs for evidence of developing shock.

The nurse assesses the woman's emotional state and coping abilities and determines the couple's informational needs. The woman may experience marked abdominal discomfort, so the nurse also determines the woman's level of pain. If surgery is necessary, the nurse performs the ongoing assessments that are appropriate postoperatively.

Nursing diagnoses that may apply for a woman with an ectopic pregnancy include the following:

- *Acute Pain* related to abdominal bleeding secondary to tubal rupture
- *Anticipatory Grieving* related to expected loss of unborn child

Nursing Plan and Implementation

Community-Based Nursing Care

Women with ectopic pregnancy are often seen initially in a clinic or office setting. Nurses need to be alert to the possibility of ectopic pregnancy if a woman presents with complaints of abdominal pain and lack of menses for 1 to 2 months. If a woman is to receive medical treatment using methotrexate, she is followed as an outpatient. The nurse advises the woman to avoid sun exposure because methotrexate causes photosensitivity. The nurse also stresses that some abdominal pain is common following the injection, but generally it is mild and lasts only 24 to 48 hours. More severe pain, which might indicate that the medical treatment was not successful and the ectopic pregnancy has ruptured, should be evaluated. The woman should also report heavy vaginal bleeding, dizziness, or tachycardia. The nurse stresses the need to return for follow-up β-hCG testing.

Hospital-Based Nursing Care

Once a diagnosis of ectopic pregnancy is made and surgery is scheduled, the nurse starts an IV as ordered and begins preoperative teaching. The nurse should immediately report signs of developing shock. If the woman is experiencing severe abdominal pain, the nurse can administer analgesics and evaluate their effectiveness.

Regardless of the treatment used, the woman and her family will need emotional support during this difficult time. Their feelings and responses to this crisis are generally similar to those that occur in cases of spontaneous abortion. As a result, similar nursing actions are required.

Evaluation

Expected outcomes of nursing care include the following:

- The woman is able to explain ectopic pregnancy, treatment alternatives, and implications for future childbearing.

- The woman and her caregivers detect possible complications early and manage them successfully.
- The woman and her partner are able to begin verbalizing their loss.

Gestational Trophoblastic Disease

Gestational trophoblastic disease (GTD) is the pathologic proliferation of trophoblastic cells (the trophoblast is the outermost layer of embryonic cells). In the United States the incidence is approximately 1 per 1500 live births (Copeland & Landon, 2007). Risk factors are largely unknown. GTD includes hydatidiform mole, invasive mole (chorioadenoma destruens), and choriocarcinoma.

Hydatidiform mole (molar pregnancy) is a disease in which (1) abnormal development of the placenta occurs, resulting in a fluid-filled, grapelike cluster; and (2) the trophoblastic tissue proliferates. The disease results in the loss of the pregnancy and the possibility, though remote, of developing choriocarcinoma, a form of cancer, from the trophoblastic tissue.

Molar pregnancies are classified into two types, complete and partial, both of which meet the previously mentioned criteria. A *complete mole* develops from an ovum containing no maternal genetic material, an "empty egg," which is fertilized by a normal sperm. The embryo dies very early, no circulation is established, the hydropic (fluid-filled) vesicles are avascular, and no embryonic tissue or membranes are found. Choriocarcinoma seems to be associated exclusively with the complete mole.

The *partial mole* usually has a triploid karyotype (69 chromosomes). Most often, a normal ovum with 23 chromosomes is fertilized by two sperm (dispermy) or by a sperm that has failed to undergo the first meiotic division and therefore contains 46 chromosomes. There may be a fetal sac or even a fetus with a heartbeat. The fetus has multiple anomalies because of the triploidy and little chance for survival. The villi are often vascularized and may be fluid-filled in only portions of the placenta. Often partial moles are recognized only after spontaneous abortion, and they may go unnoticed even then.

Invasive mole (chorioadenoma destruens) is similar to a complete mole, but it involves the uterine myometrium. Treatment is the same as for complete mole.

Clinical Therapy

Initially the clinical picture is similar to that of pregnancy; however, classic signs soon appear. Vaginal bleeding occurs almost universally. It is often brownish (like prune juice) because of liquefaction of the uterine clot, but it may be bright red. Uterine enlargement greater than expected for gestational age is a classic sign of a complete mole, which is present in about ⅓ to ½ of cases (Li, 2008).

In the remainder of cases, the uterus is appropriate or small for gestational age. Hydropic vesicles (grapelike clusters) may be passed; if so, they are diagnostic (Figure 16–3 ■). With a partial mole the vesicles are often smaller and may not be noticed. In addition, because serum hCG levels are higher with molar pregnancy than with normal pregnancy, the woman may experience hyperemesis gravidarum. Anemia occurs frequently and is caused by blood loss and poor nutrition secondary to hyperemesis. Symptoms of preeclampsia before 24 weeks' gestation strongly suggest a molar pregnancy. No fetal heart tones are auscultated, and no fetal movement is palpated. The advent of transvaginal ultrasound has led to earlier diagnosis of molar pregnancy, often in the first trimester.

Therapy begins with suction evacuation of the mole and curettage of the uterus to remove all fragments of the placenta. Early evacuation decreases the possibility of other complications. If the woman is older and has completed her childbearing, or if there is excessive bleeding, hysterectomy may be the treatment of choice to reduce the risk of choriocarcinoma.

Malignant GTD, usually choriocarcinoma, develops following evacuation of a mole in 20% of women (ACOG, 2004). To detect this serious problem early, the woman treated for hydatidiform mole should receive extensive follow-up therapy. Follow-up care includes a baseline chest X-ray to detect metastasis and a physical exam including pelvic exam. Serum β-hCG levels are monitored every 1 to 2 weeks until negative two consecutive times, then every 1 to 2 months for a year. During this time, the woman also has periodic pelvic exams. If hCG levels plateau for 3 to 6 consecutive weeks or rise more than 50%, evaluation for metastatic disease should be under-

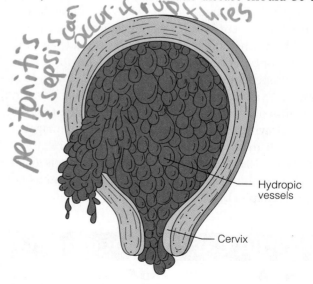

peritonitis & sepsis can occur if ruptures

Hydropic vessels

Cervix

FIGURE 16–3 Hydatidiform mole. A common sign is vaginal bleeding, often brownish (the characteristic "prune juice" appearance) but sometimes bright red. In this figure, some of the hydropic vessels are being passed. This occurrence is diagnostic for hydatidiform mole.

taken and prompt chemotherapy initiated (Berman et al., 2004). Effective contraception is needed during this time to prevent pregnancy and the resulting confusion about the cause of changes in hCG levels, which could mask an hCG rise associated with malignant GTD.

Continued high or rising hCG titers are abnormal. If they occur, D&C is performed and the tissue examined. If malignant cells are found, treatment at a center specializing in GTD is advised. Chemotherapy for choriocarcinoma is started using methotrexate alone or in combination with other chemotherapy agents. Persistent GTD is almost 100% curable if diagnosed early and treated appropriately.

If, after a year of monitoring, the hCG serum titers remain within normal limits, a couple may be assured that subsequent normal pregnancy can be anticipated, with a low probability of recurring hydatidiform mole.

Nursing Care Management

Nursing Assessment and Diagnosis

It is important for nurses involved in antepartal care to be aware of symptoms of hydatidiform mole and observe for them at each antepartal visit. The classic symptoms used to diagnose molar pregnancy are found more frequently with the complete than with the partial mole. Before evacuation, the partial mole may be difficult to distinguish from a missed abortion. If a molar pregnancy is diagnosed, the nurse should assess the woman's (or the couple's) understanding of the condition and its implications.

Nursing diagnoses that may apply to a woman with a hydatidiform mole include the following:

- *Fear* related to the possible development of choriocarcinoma
- *Anticipatory Grieving* related to the loss of the pregnancy secondary to GTD

Nursing Plan and Implementation

Community-Based Nursing Care

When a molar pregnancy is suspected, the woman needs emotional support. The nurse can relieve some of the woman's anxiety by answering questions about the condition and explaining what ultrasound and other diagnostic procedures will entail. Nurses also need to be alert to the psychologic impact of the diagnosis. The woman and her partner may experience feelings of powerlessness, anger, fear, self-blame, and guilt as well as altered perceptions about their sexuality and fertility (Bess & Wood, 2006). If a molar pregnancy is diagnosed, the nurse supports the parents as they deal with their grief about the lost pregnancy. Healthcare counselors, a member of the clergy, or a professional counselor may be able to help them deal with this loss.

Hospital-Based Nursing Care

When the woman is hospitalized for evacuation of the mole, the nurse must monitor vital signs and vaginal bleeding for evidence of hemorrhage. In addition, the nurse determines whether abdominal pain is present and evaluates the woman's emotional state and coping ability. Typed and crossmatched blood must be available for surgery because of previous blood loss and the potential for hemorrhage. Oxytocin is administered to keep the uterus contracted and prevent hemorrhage. If the woman is Rh negative and not sensitized, she is given Rh immune globulin to prevent antibody formation.

The woman needs to understand the importance of the follow-up visits. She is advised to delay becoming pregnant again until after the follow-up program is completed.

Evaluation

Expected outcomes of nursing care include the following:

- The woman has an uneventful recovery following successful evacuation of the mole.
- The woman is able to explain GTD and its treatment, follow-up, and long-term implications for pregnancy.
- The woman and her partner are able to begin verbalizing their grief at the loss of their anticipated child.
- The woman can discuss the importance of follow-up care and indicates her willingness to cooperate with the regimen.

Care of the Woman with Hyperemesis Gravidarum

Hyperemesis gravidarum, which is excessive vomiting during pregnancy, occurs in one-half of 1% of pregnancies (Cappell, 2007). It may be mild at first, but true hyperemesis may progress to a point at which the woman not only vomits everything she swallows but also retches between meals.

Although the exact cause of hyperemesis is unclear, increased levels of hCG may play a role. Higher levels of estradiol as well as lower levels of prolactin have been implicated as potential causes (Lagiou et al., 2003). Other variables that may relate to hyperemesis include transient hyperthyroidism, hypofunction of the anterior pituitary gland and adrenal cortex, abnormalities of the corpus luteum, *Helicobacter pylori* infection, and psychologic factors (Scott & Abu-Hamda, 2004). In severe cases, the pathology of hyperemesis begins with dehydration, which leads to fluid-electrolyte imbalance and alkalosis from loss of hydrochloric acid. Hypovolemia, hypotension, tachycardia, increased hematocrit and blood urea nitrogen (BUN), and decreased urine output can also occur. If untreated, metabolic acidosis may develop. Severe potassium loss may disrupt cardiac

MyNursingKit | Hyperemesis Education and Research Organization functioning. Starvation causes muscle wasting and severe protein and vitamin deficiencies. Fetal or embryonic death may result, and the woman may suffer irreversible metabolic changes or death.

The long-term impact of hyperemesis on a pregnancy depends on overall maternal weight gain. Infants of women with hyperemesis and low pregnancy weight gain have a higher incidence of low birth weight, preterm birth, and 5-minute Apgar scores below 7 (Note: An Apgar score of 7 to 10 indicates that the newborn is in good condition) (see Chapter 19 ∞). Infants born to women with hyperemesis and weight gains of 7 kg (15.4 lb) or more had no increased risk of these complications (Dodds, Fell, Joseph et al., 2006).

Clinical Therapy

The goals of treatment include control of vomiting, correction of dehydration, restoration of electrolyte balance, and maintenance of adequate nutrition. If the woman does not respond to standard approaches to the control of nausea and vomiting in pregnancy (see Chapter 11 ∞), she may require IV fluids on an outpatient basis. If her symptoms do not improve, hospitalization may be indicated. Initially the woman is given nothing by mouth (NPO), and IV fluids are administered. Potassium chloride is typically added to the IV infusion to prevent hypokalemia. Thiamine and pyroxidine (vitamin B_6) may also be replaced to correct deficiencies and prevent peripheral neuropathy. Antiemetics may also be administered. Typically the woman remains NPO for 48 hours. If her condition does not improve, total parenteral nutrition may be needed. She then begins controlled oral feedings.

Nursing Care Management

Nursing Assessment and Diagnosis

When a woman is hospitalized for control of vomiting, the nurse regularly assesses the amount and character of any emesis, intake and output, fetal heart rate, evidence of jaundice or bleeding, and the woman's emotional state.

Nursing diagnoses that may apply to a woman with hyperemesis gravidarum include the following:

- *Imbalanced Nutrition: Less than Body Requirements* related to persistent vomiting secondary to hyperemesis
- *Fear* related to the effects of hyperemesis on fetal well-being

Nursing Plan and Implementation

Community-Based Nursing Care

Total parenteral nutrition therapy provided at home in collaboration with a physician and a registered dietician is sometimes used to enable the woman to remain in her home. It also gives the nurse an opportunity to observe family interactions and evaluate the woman's environment. This assessment is often useful in determining the pregnant woman's level of support, any significant stressors in her life, and her understanding of nutrition and self-care measures.

Hospital-Based Nursing Care

Nursing care is supportive and directed at maintaining a relaxed, quiet environment away from food odors or offensive smells. Once oral feedings resume, food needs to be attractively served. Oral hygiene is important because the mouth is dry and may be irritated from vomitus. Weight is monitored regularly. In some cases emotional factors have appeared to play a role in this condition, although that remains controversial. Nevertheless, psychotherapy may sometimes be recommended. With proper treatment, prognosis is favorable.

Evaluation

Expected outcomes of nursing care include the following:

- The woman is able to explain hyperemesis gravidarum, its therapy, and its possible effects on her pregnancy.
- The woman's condition is corrected and complications are avoided.

Care of the Woman with a Hypertensive Disorder

Hypertensive disorders, which affect 5% to 10% of pregnant women, are the most common medical complications in pregnancies (Habli & Sibai, 2008). Various attempts have been made to classify these disorders. For clinical purposes, the following classification may be used (Sibai, 2007).

- Preeclampsia-eclampsia
- Chronic hypertension
- Chronic hypertension with superimposed preeclampsia or eclampsia
- Gestational (or transient) hypertension

Preeclampsia and Eclampsia

Preeclampsia, the most common hypertensive disorder in pregnancy, occurs in 2% to 7% of pregnancies although the incidence is significantly higher (14%) in women with a twin pregnancy (Habli & Sibai, 2008). In the United States, it is the second leading cause of maternal death (Baxter & Weinstein, 2004). Preeclampsia is defined as an increase in blood pressure after 20 weeks' gestation accompanied by proteinuria. Previously edema was included in the definition but was removed because it is such a common finding in pregnancy. However, sudden onset of severe edema warrants close evaluation to rule out preeclampsia or other pathologic processes such as renal disease.

Preeclampsia, typically categorized as mild or severe, is a progressive disorder. In its most severe form, **eclampsia**, generalized seizures, or coma develop. Most often preeclampsia is seen in the last 10 weeks of gestation, during labor, or in the first 48 hours after childbirth. Although birth of the fetus and removal of the placenta is the only known cure for preeclampsia, it can be controlled with early diagnosis and careful management. Preeclampsia is seen more often in teenagers and in women over age 35, especially if they are primigravidas. Women with a history of preeclampsia are at increased risk, as are women with a large placental mass associated with multiple gestation, GTD, Rh incompatibility, and diabetes mellitus.

Pathophysiology of Preeclampsia

The exact cause of preeclampsia-eclampsia remains unknown, despite decades of research. Preeclampsia affects all the major systems of the body. The following pathophysiologic changes are associated with the disease.

- In normal pregnancy, the lowered peripheral vascular resistance and the increased maternal resistance to the pressor effects of angiotensin II result in lowered blood pressure. In preeclampsia, blood pressure begins to rise after 20 weeks' gestation, probably in response to a gradual loss of resistance to angiotensin II. This response has been linked to the ratio between the prostaglandins prostacyclin and thromboxane. Prostacyclin is a potent vasodilator. It is decreased in preeclampsia, often several weeks before symptoms develop. This changes the ratio between the two prostaglandins, allowing the potent vasoconstriction and platelet-aggregating effects of thromboxane to dominate. These hormones are produced partially by the placenta, which would help explain the reversal of the condition when the placenta is removed and why the incidence is increased when there is a larger than normal placental mass.

- In addition, nitric oxide, a potent vasodilator, plays a role in the pregnant woman's resistance to vasopressors. Decreased nitric oxide production in women with preeclampsia may contribute to the development of hypertension.

- The loss of normal vasodilation of uterine arterioles and the concurrent maternal vasospasm result in decreased placental perfusion. The effect on the fetus may be growth restriction, decrease in fetal movement, and chronic hypoxia or nonreassuring fetal status.

↑ protein in urine

- In preeclampsia, normal renal perfusion is decreased. With a reduction of the glomerular filtration rate (GFR), serum levels of creatinine, BUN, and uric acid begin to rise from normal pregnant levels, whereas urine output decreases. Sodium is retained in increased amounts, which results in increased extracellular volume, increased sensitivity to angiotensin II, and edema. Stretching of the capillary walls of the glomerular endothelial cells allows the large protein molecules, primarily albumin, to escape in the urine, decreasing serum albumin levels. The decreased serum albumin concentration causes decreased plasma colloid osmotic pressure. This lowered pressure results in a further movement of fluid to the extracellular spaces, which also contributes to the development of edema.

- The decreased intravascular volume causes increased viscosity of the blood and a corresponding rise in hematocrit.

HELLP syndrome (*h*emolysis, *e*levated *l*iver enzymes, and *l*ow *p*latelet count) is sometimes associated with severe preeclampsia. Women who experience this multiple-organ-failure syndrome have high morbidity and mortality rates, as do their offspring.

The hemolysis that occurs is termed *microangiopathic hemolytic anemia*. It is thought that red blood cells are distorted or fragmented during passage through small, damaged blood vessels. Vascular damage is associated with vasospasm, and platelets aggregate at sites of damage, resulting in low platelet count (less than 100,000/mm^3) (Baxter & Weinstein, 2004). Elevated liver enzymes occur from blood flow that is obstructed by fibrin deposits. Hyperbilirubinemia and jaundice may also be seen. Liver distention causes epigastric pain and may ultimately result in liver rupture. Symptoms may include nausea, vomiting, flulike symptoms, or epigastric pain. HELLP syndrome is sometimes complicated by disseminated intravascular coagulation (DIC). See the discussion on DIC on page 358.

Women with HELLP syndrome are best cared for in a tertiary care center. Initially the mother's condition should be assessed and stabilized, especially if her platelet counts are very low. The fetus is also assessed, using a nonstress test and biophysical profile. Once HELLP syndrome is diagnosed and the woman's condition is stable, expeditious birth of the child is indicated regardless of gestational age.

Maternal Risks

Central nervous system changes associated with preeclampsia are hyperreflexia, headache, and seizures. Hyperreflexia may be caused by increased intracellular sodium and decreased intracellular potassium levels. Cerebral vasospasm causes headaches, and cerebral edema and vasoconstriction

due to constriction of vessel

are responsible for seizures. Thrombocytopenia (platelet count less than 100,000/mm^3) is a frequent finding in preeclampsia. It occurs when platelets aggregate at the sites of vascular damage associated with vasospasm.

Women with severe preeclampsia or eclampsia are at increased risk for renal failure, abruptio placentae, DIC, ruptured liver, and pulmonary embolism.

Fetal-Neonatal Risks

Infants of women with preeclampsia tend to be small for gestational age (SGA). The cause is related specifically to maternal vasospasm and hypovolemia, which result in fetal hypoxia and malnutrition. In addition, the newborn may be premature because of the necessity for early birth.

At birth, the newborn may be oversedated because of medications administered to the mother. The newborn may also have hypermagnesemia caused by treatment of

---

EVIDENCE IN ACTION
Preeclampsia is considered a risk factor of cardiovascular disease in women.
(meta-analysis and systematic review) (Bellamy, Casas, Hingorani, & Williams, 2007)

---

the woman with large doses of magnesium sulfate.

Clinical Therapy

The goals of medical management are prompt diagnosis of the disease; prevention of cerebral hemorrhage, seizures, hematologic complications, and renal and hepatic diseases; and birth of an uncompromised newborn as close to term as possible. Reduction of elevated blood pressure is essential in accomplishing these goals.

CLINICAL MANIFESTATIONS AND DIAGNOSIS

Mild Preeclampsia Women with mild preeclampsia may exhibit few if any symptoms. The blood pressure is elevated to 140/90 mm Hg or higher and the proteinuria is 1 g or less in 24 hours (2+ dipstick).

Although edema is no longer considered a diagnostic criterion, generalized edema, seen as puffy face or hands, and in dependent areas such as the ankles, may be present.

EVIDENCE-BASED PRACTICE

Anti-Platelet Agents to Prevent Preeclampsia and Its Complications

Clinical Question
Are anti-platelet agents—primarily low-dose aspirin—safe and effective in preventing preeclampsia and its complications?

The Evidence
The cause of preeclampsia is uncertain. However, it is known that preeclampsia results in an underperfused placenta, which leads, eventually, to placental damage. This damage is thought to activate platelets and blood clotting, and so it has been suggested that anti-platelet agents may be useful in preventing these problems. Multiple studies have been conducted on this subject with conflicting results, and so the Centre for Perinatal Health Services Research sponsored a meta-analysis of relevant research to determine if a clear answer emerged. Simultaneously, five experts conducted a review based on the Cochrane Pregnancy and Childbirth Group's trial register and a hand search of proceedings from professional research conferences focused on the study of hypertension in pregnancy. The meta-analysis represented 59 trials with more than 32,000 women as subjects, and the review included 31 trials with more than 37,000 subjects. These multiple-site, large sample reviews represent the strongest evidence for practice.

What Is Effective?
Anti-platelet agents, primarily low-dose aspirin, have moderate benefits in preventing preeclampsia and its complications. Preeclampsia was reduced by 10% to 17% in the treatment groups. The risk was reduced more for those women who were at high risk for preeclampsia as compared with women who were only moderately at risk. The risk of a

small-for-gestational-age infant was reduced by 10%, and aspirin was associated with an 8% reduction in the risk of a preterm birth. The risk of stillbirth or infant death before discharge was reduced by 9%. The agents did not reduce the risk of fetal death. There was no associated increase in bleeding events for either the mothers or their infants.

What Is Inconclusive?
No clear evidence emerged to determine which women are most likely to benefit from low-dose aspirin therapy. Further, no consensus was achieved on when treatment is best started and at what dosage. Doses up to 75 mg appear to be safe, but there is no evidence that benefits outweigh the risks with higher doses. More research is needed to determine the specifics of aspirin treatment efficacy.

Best Practice
Low doses of aspirin do help prevent preeclampsia and some of its complications, particularly in women who are at high risk. You can reassure the pregnant woman that taking prescribed low-dose aspirin will not result in bleeding complications for her or her baby, and may help her avoid the complications of preeclampsia.

References
Askie, L., Duley, L., Henderson-Smart, D., & Stewart, L. (2007). Antiplatelet agents for prevention of pre-eclampsia: A meta-analysis of individual patient data. *Obstetrical and Gynecological Survey, 62*(11), 697–699.

Duley, L., Henderson-Smart, D., Meher, S., & King, J. (2008). Antiplatelet agents for preventing pre-eclampsia and its complications. *Cochrane Database of Systematic Reviews*, Issue 2.

Edema is identified by a weight gain of more than 1.5 kg (3.3 lb) per month in the second trimester or more than 0.5 kg (1.1 lb) per week in the third trimester. Edema is assessed on a 1+ to 4+ scale.

Severe Preeclampsia Severe preeclampsia may develop suddenly. Blood pressure is 160/110 mm Hg or higher on two occasions at least 6 hours apart while the woman is on bed rest. Proteinuria equal to or greater than 5 g is found in a 24-hour urine collection while a dipstick urine protein measurement is 3+ to 4+ on two random samples obtained at least 4 hours apart. Oliguria is present with urine output equal to or less than 500 mL in 24 hours. Other characteristic symptoms include visual or cerebral disturbances (frontal headaches, blurred vision, scotomata [spots before the eyes]), cyanosis or pulmonary edema, epigastric or right upper quadrant pain, impaired liver function, thrombocytopenia or evidence of hemolysis or both, and intrauterine fetal growth restriction. Other signs or symptoms that may be present include nausea, vomiting, irritability, hyperreflexia, and retinal edema (retinas appear wet and glistening), with narrowed segments on the retinal arterioles when examined with an ophthalmoscope. Epigastric pain is often the sign of impending convulsion and is thought to be caused by increased vascular engorgement of the liver.

Eclampsia Eclampsia, characterized by a grand mal convulsion or coma, may occur before the onset of labor, during labor, or early in the postpartal period. Some women experience only one seizure; others have several. Unless they occur quite frequently, the woman often regains consciousness between seizures.

ANTEPARTAL MANAGEMENT The clinical therapy for preeclampsia depends on the severity of the disease.

Home Care of Mild Preeclampsia In general, women with preeclampsia are admitted to the hospital. However, for some women with mild preeclampsia, home care is now an option. The woman assesses her blood pressure, weight, and urine protein daily and does daily fetal movement monitoring. Weight gains of 1.4 kg (3 lb) in 24 hours or 1.8 kg (4 lb) in a 3-day period are generally cause for concern. Remote NSTs are performed twice per week or biophysical profiles are done weekly. Nursing contact varies from daily to weekly, depending on physician request. It is extremely important to advise the woman to report to the doctor if she develops signs of worsening preeclampsia.

Hospital Care of Mild Preeclampsia The woman is placed on bed rest, primarily on her left side, to decrease pressure on the vena cava, thereby increasing venous return, circulatory volume, and placental and renal perfusion. Improved renal blood flow helps decrease angiotensin II levels, promotes diuresis, and lowers blood pressure.

The woman is weighed daily and evaluated for worsening edema, persistent headache, visual changes, or epigastric pain. Urine dipstick is done daily to assess for protein; blood pressure is checked at least four times per day. Diet should be well balanced and moderate to high in protein (80 to 100 g/day, or 1.5 g/kg/day) to replace protein lost in the urine. Sodium intake should be moderate, not to exceed 6 g/day. Excessively salty foods should be avoided, but sodium restriction and diuretics are no longer used in treating preeclampsia.

To achieve a safe outcome for the fetus, tests to evaluate fetal status are done more frequently as preeclampsia progresses. The following tests are used:

- Fetal movement record
- Nonstress test
- Ultrasonography every 3 or 4 weeks for serial determination of growth
- Biophysical profile
- Amniocentesis to determine fetal lung maturity
- Doppler velocimetry beginning at 30 to 32 weeks gestation to screen for fetal compromise

Severe Preeclampsia If the uterine environment is considered detrimental to fetal well-being, birth may be the treatment of choice for both mother and fetus, even if the fetus is immature. Other medical therapies for severe preeclampsia include the following:

- *Bed rest.* Bed rest must be complete. Stimuli that may bring on a seizure should be reduced.
- *Diet.* A high-protein, moderate-sodium diet is given as long as the woman is alert and has no nausea or indication of impending seizure.
- *Anticonvulsants.* Magnesium sulfate is the treatment of choice for convulsions. Its depressant action on the central nervous system (CNS) reduces the possibility of seizure (see Drug Guide: Magnesium Sulfate in Chapter 21 ∞).
- *Fluid and electrolyte replacement.* The goal of fluid intake is to achieve a balance between correcting hypovolemia and preventing circulatory overload. Fluid intake may be oral or supplemented with intravenous therapy. Intravenous fluids may be started "to keep lines open" in case they are needed for drug therapy even when oral intake is adequate. Electrolytes are replaced as indicated by daily serum electrolyte levels.
- *Corticosteroids.* Betamethasone or dexamethasone is often administered to the woman whose fetus has an immature lung profile. Corticosteroids may also have a beneficial effect in women with HELLP syndrome.
- *Antihypertensives.* Antihypertensive therapy is generally given for sustained systolic blood pressure of at

least 160 to 180 mm Hg or diastolic blood pressures of 105 to 110 mm Hg or higher. Hydralazine (Apresoline) is the antihypertensive medication most commonly used. It is generally administered in IV boluses. Methyldopa is often used for long-term control of mild to moderate hypertension in pregnancy because it is effective and has a well-documented safety record. Recent studies indicate that intravenous labetalol and oral nifedipine are as effective as IV hydralazine and have fewer side effects (Sibai, 2007).

Eclampsia   An eclamptic seizure requires immediate, effective treatment. A bolus of 4 to 6 g magnesium sulfate is given intravenously over 5 minutes to control convulsions. Antihypertensive agents are used to keep the diastolic blood pressure between 90 to 100 mm Hg, thus avoiding a potential reduction in uteroplacental blood flow or cerebral perfusion. A sedative such as diazepam or amobarbital is used only if the seizures are not controlled by magnesium sulfate. Dilantin may be used for seizure prevention. The lungs are auscultated for pulmonary edema. The woman is observed for circulatory and renal failure and signs of cerebral hemorrhage. Furosemide (Lasix) may be given for pulmonary edema; digitalis may be given for circulatory failure. Intake and output are monitored hourly.

The woman is assessed for signs of labor. She is also checked every 15 minutes for evidence of vaginal bleeding and abdominal rigidity, which might indicate abruptio placentae. While she is comatose, she is positioned on her side with the side rails up.

Because of the severity of her condition, the woman is often cared for in an intensive care unit. Invasive hemodynamic monitoring of either central venous pressure (CVP) or pulmonary artery wedge pressure may be started using a Swan-Ganz catheter. Both these procedures carry risk to the woman, and the decision to use them should be made judiciously. When the condition of the woman and the fetus are stabilized, induction of labor is considered, because birth is the only known cure for preeclampsia. The woman and her partner should be given a careful explanation about her status and that of her unborn child and the treatment they are receiving. Plans for further treatment and for birth must be discussed with them.

INTRAPARTAL MANAGEMENT   Labor may be induced by IV oxytocin when there is evidence of fetal maturity and cervical readiness. In severe cases, cesarean birth may be necessary even if the fetus is immature.

Assessment for signs of worsening preeclampsia continues. The woman may receive intravenous oxytocin and magnesium sulfate simultaneously. Infusion pumps should be used, and bags and tubing must be carefully labeled. Magnesium levels are assessed regularly.

Meperidine (Demerol) or fentanyl may be given intravenously for pain relief in labor. A pudendal block is often used for vaginal birth. An epidural block may be used if it is administered by a skilled anesthesiologist who is knowledgeable about preeclampsia. However, spinal or epidural anesthesia is contraindicated in the presence of coagulopathy or a platelet count of 50,000/mm (Sibai, 2005).

Electronic fetal monitoring is used to assess fetal status continuously. Birth in the Sims' or semisitting position should be considered. If the lithotomy position is used, a wedge should be placed under the right buttock to displace the uterus. The wedge should also be used if birth is by cesarean. Oxygen is administered to the woman during labor if the need is indicated by fetal response to the contractions.

A pediatrician or neonatal nurse practitioner must be available to care for the newborn at birth. This caregiver must be informed of all amounts and times of medication the woman has received during labor.

POSTPARTUM MANAGEMENT   The woman with preeclampsia usually improves rapidly after giving birth, although seizures can still occur during the first 48 hours postpartum. When the hypertension is severe, the woman may continue to receive hydralazine or magnesium sulfate postpartally.

In general, the recurrence rate of preeclampsia is 18% to 25% in subsequent pregnancies. The rate is substantially higher in women with multiple gestations, early onset preeclampsia/eclampsia, previous HELLP syndrome, or underlying vascular disease (Sibai, 2005). Women who have had a normotensive previous pregnancy are at increased risk when they conceive with a new partner. Also, in vitro fertilization using donor eggs and/or donor sperm has a higher incidence of preeclampsia (Wiggins & Elliott, 2005).

Nursing Care Management

See Nursing Care Plan for a Woman with Preeclampsia for information on nursing care.

Nursing Assessment and Diagnosis

Blood pressure is taken and recorded during each antepartal visit. If the blood pressure rises, or if the normal slight decrease in blood pressure expected between 8 and 28 weeks of pregnancy does not occur, the woman should be followed closely. The woman's urine is checked for proteinuria at each visit.

If hospitalization becomes necessary, the nurse then assesses the following:

- *Blood pressure.* Blood pressure should be assessed every 1 to 4 hours, or more frequently if indicated by medication or other changes in the woman's status.

Nursing Care Plan   For a Woman with Preeclampsia

CLIENT SCENARIO

Ingrid Fruehoff, a 36-year-old primigravida, is 34 weeks' pregnant. Four days ago, during a routine prenatal visit, the nurse discovered that her blood pressure was elevated slightly, to 130/84. Normally, Ingrid's blood pressure readings had been 118/74. She had gained 4 lb since her previous monthly visit. A trace level of protein was found with a dipstick urine. In addition, Ingrid reported experiencing some headaches over the previous few days that had not been relieved by acetaminophen. The nurse explained to Ingrid the signs and symptoms of preeclampsia and encouraged her to call the clinic if her condition worsened over the next few days. She was sent home on bed rest and scheduled for a recheck in 4 days.

When Ingrid returns to the clinic today, she is admitted to the hospital with worsening preeclampsia. She is placed on complete bed rest. The nurse monitors her closely for signs of severe preeclampsia, which include hypertension, proteinuria, oliguria, cerebral or visual disturbances, pulmonary edema, epigastric pain, and sudden onset of severe edema. Ingrid is also observed for eclamptic seizure. Tests for fetal status, such as documentation of fetal movement, nonstress tests, serial ultrasounds, biophysical profile, amniocentesis, and Doppler flow studies, are performed. The nurse reassures Ingrid that everything will be done to make her comfortable and ensure the well-being of her baby.

ASSESSMENT

Subjective: Headache, irritability, scotomata

Objective: Blood pressure 148/90, deep tendon reflexes 3+, 600 cc of urine collected over the last 24 hours with a protein level of 5 g/L; weight gain of 3 lb over last 4 days; 2+ pitting edema on lower extremities

Nursing Diagnosis #1	Deficient Fluid Volume related to fluid shift from intravascular to extravascular space secondary to vasospasm*
Client Goal	The signs and symptoms of preeclampsia will decrease.
AEB:	• Decreased blood pressure • Decreased levels of protein in urine • Deep tendon reflexes return to normal (2+)

NURSING INTERVENTIONS

1. Encourage woman to lie in the left lateral recumbent position.

2. Assess blood pressure every 1 to 4 hours as necessary.

3. Monitor urine for volume and proteinuria every shift or every hour per agency protocol.

RATIONALES

Rationale: The left lateral recumbent position decreases pressure on the vena cava thereby increasing venous return, circulatory volume, and placental and renal perfusion. Angiotensin II levels are decreased when there is improved renal blood flow, which helps to promote diuresis and lower blood pressure.

Rationale: Frequent monitoring helps identify progression of the disorder and allows for early intervention to ensure maternal and fetal health and well-being.

Rationale: These measures help to assess renal perfusion. Urinary output decreases when there is a reduction of the glomerular filtration rate. Urinary output that falls below 30 mL per hour or less than 700 mL in a 24-hour period should be reported. Normally urine does not contain protein. As the disorder worsens, the capillary walls of the glomerular endothelial cells stretch, allowing protein molecules to pass into the urine. Readings of 3+ and 4+ indicate loss of 5 g or more protein in 24 hours.

(Continued on next page)

Nursing Care Plan   For a Woman with Preeclampsia *(Continued)*

NURSING INTERVENTIONS	RATIONALES
4. Assess deep tendon reflexes and clonus.	*Rationale:* Hyperreflexia indicates central nervous system (CNS) irritability and may develop as preeclampsia worsens. Eliciting deep tendon reflexes provides information about CNS status and is also used to assess for magnesium sulfate toxicity. Reflexes are graded on a scale of 0 to 4+ using the deep tendon reflex rating scale (refer to Clinical Skills: Assessing Deep Tendon Reflexes and Clonus). A rating of 0 or no response is abnormal and occurs with high maternal serum magnesium levels. Clonus, an abnormal finding, indicates a more pronounced hyperreflexia secondary to marked CNS irritability.
5. Assess for edema.	*Rationale:* Edema develops as fluid shifts from the intravascular to the extravascular spaces. Edema is assessed either by weight gain (more than 3.3 lb per month in the second trimester or more than 1.1 lb per week in the third trimester) or by assessing for pitting edema (assessed by using finger pressure to a swollen area, usually the lower extremities, and grading on a scale of 1+ to 4+).
6. Administer magnesium sulfate per infusion pump as ordered.	*Rationale:* As preeclampsia worsens, the risk of an eclamptic seizure increases. Magnesium sulfate is the treatment of choice for seizures because of its CNS depressant action. As a secondary effect, magnesium sulfate also relaxes smooth muscles and may therefore decrease the blood pressure.
7. Assess for magnesium sulfate toxicity.	*Rationale:* Side effects of magnesium sulfate are dose related. Therapeutic levels are in the range of 4.8 to 9.6 mg/dL. As maternal serum magnesium levels increase, toxicity may occur. Signs of toxicity include decreased or absent DTRs, urine output below 30 mL/hour, respirations below 12, and confusion.
8. Provide a balanced diet that includes 80 to 100 g/day or 1.5 g/kg/day of protein.	*Rationale:* A diet rich in protein is necessary to replace protein that is excreted in the urine. Sodium intake should be moderate but should not exceed 6 g/day.

Evaluation of Client Goal	• Blood pressure returns to client's normal level. • Urine protein levels are decreased to zero. • Deep tendon reflexes remain at 2+ with no beats of clonus.
Nursing Diagnosis #2	Risk for Injury to fetus related to uteroplacental insufficiency secondary to vasospasm.
Client Goal	• The fetus will have adequate supply of oxygen and nutrients.
AEB:	• No signs of fetal distress • Fetal diagnostic tests within normal limits

NURSING INTERVENTIONS	RATIONALES
1. Instruct woman to count fetal movements three times a day for 20 to 30 minutes, maintain a record of movement, and share the record with the nurse.	*Rationale:* Fetal activity provides reassurance of fetal well-being. Decrease in fetal movement or cessation of movement may indicate fetal compromise.
2. Encourage woman to rest in the left lateral recumbent position.	*Rationale:* Lying in the left lateral recumbent position decreases pressure on the vena cava, which increases venous return, circulatory volume, and placental and renal perfusion. Blood flow to the fetus is increased, thereby reducing the risk of fetal hypoxia and malnutrition.
3. Assist with serial ultrasounds.	*Rationale:* Maternal vasospasm and hypovolemia result from preeclampsia, which may lead to a small-for-gestational-age newborn. Ultrasound provides assessment of fetal growth by measuring the biparietal diameter of the fetal head or the fetal femur length.

Nursing Care Plan | For a Woman with Preeclampsia (Continued)

4. Perform nonstress tests as ordered.	**Rationale:** A nonstress test is performed to assess the fetal heart rate in response to fetal movement. Accelerations of fetal heart rate with fetal movement may indicate the fetus has adequate oxygenation and an intact central nervous system. (Refer to Chapter 14 ∞ for interpretation of NST results.)
5. Describe for the woman the purposes of a biophysical profile (BPP).	**Rationale:** Preeclampsia or eclampsia places the woman at risk for uteroplacental insufficiency because of the loss of normal vasodilation of uterine arterioles and maternal vasospasm. This results in decreased uteroplacental perfusion, which may lead to fetal hypoxia. A BPP is one assessment tool used to evaluate fetal well-being. Providing explanation of the diagnostic test helps relieve anxiety and ensures that the woman understands what the test evaluates and what the results mean. See discussion of BPP in Chapter 14 ∞.
6. Assist with amniocentesis to obtain lecithin/sphingomyelin (L/S) ratio.	**Rationale:** Women with preeclampsia may give birth before term. Amniotic fluid may be analyzed to determine the maturity of the fetal lungs. A lecithin/sphingomyelin ratio of 2:1 or greater indicates fetal lung maturity and is usually achieved by 35 weeks' gestation.
7. Explain the purpose of Doppler flow studies.	**Rationale:** Doppler flow studies (umbilical velocimetry) help to assess placental function and sufficiency. Uteroplacental insufficiency is a risk for a woman with preeclampsia (see Chapter 14 ∞).

Evaluation of Client Goal	• All diagnostic tests are within normal limits, which indicates that uteroplacental sufficiency is maintained. • No signs of fetal distress were documented during testing.

CRITICAL THINKING QUESTIONS

1. A woman gives birth at 39 weeks' gestation. The prenatal record reveals a history of preeclampsia with this pregnancy. Even though the newborn was full term, the birth weight falls below the 10th percentile. Describe how preeclampsia in the prenatal period can affect the growth of the fetus.

Answer: Maternal vasospasm and loss of normal vasodilation of uterine arterioles occur with preeclampsia. This results in decreased placental perfusion leading to fetal hypoxia and malnutrition. Therefore newborns tend to be small for gestational age.

2. The nurse is assisting a woman with preeclampsia to select a dinner menu. The choices include: menu #1: grilled chicken, broccoli with peanut sauce, brown rice, an oatmeal cookie, and a milkshake; menu #2: pasta with tomato sauce, fresh green salad, garlic bread, chocolate cake, and iced tea. Which menu plan is best for a woman with preeclampsia? Why?

Answer: Menu #1 is the better choice because it provides more protein. Each protein choice is a complete protein. Protein is excreted in the urine as a result of severe preeclampsia and replacement is needed. Recommended protein needs include 80 to 100 g/day or 1.5 g/kg/day of protein.

3. The nurse is admitting three women to the antepartum unit. Two rooms are available, one private room and one double occupancy room. One woman being admitted is in preterm labor, the second has preeclampsia, and the third has third-trimester bleeding. Which room assignment would be most appropriate for the woman with preeclampsia? Why?

Answer: The private room would be most appropriate for the woman with preeclampsia. Preeclampsia causes CNS irritability. If the disorder worsens, bright lights and loud noises may precipitate seizures. A private room allows the nurse to maintain a quiet, low-stimulus environment for the woman. Visitors and phone calls are also limited.

4. Your assessment of a client receiving magnesium sulfate for severe preeclampsia includes nausea and vomiting, blurred vision, absent deep tendon reflexes (previously DTRs were 3+), 70 mL total urine output over 4 hours. Are these findings normal? What, if any, actions would you take?

Answer: Nausea, vomiting, and blurred vision are common side effects of magnesium sulfate. Absent deep tendon reflexes and urine output less than 30 mL/hr are signs of magnesium toxicity. Actions include the following: Stop the infusion, notify the physician, and obtain a maternal serum magnesium level. Calcium gluconate should be available at the bedside.

*For your reference, this care plan provides an example of how two nursing diagnoses might be addressed.

The following factors may lead to errors in measuring blood pressure (BP):

Incorrect cuff size—a cuff that is too small results in a falsely elevated blood pressure, whereas one that is too large falsely lowers blood pressure.

Elevating the arm above the level of the heart, such as occurs when a woman lying on her left side raises her right arm for a blood pressure measurement, will falsely lower the blood pressure 10 to 20 mm Hg.

Korotkoff phase—when blood pressure is checked during pregnancy, the disappearance of the sound (phase V) is the preferred indicator rather than the muffling of the sound (phase IV).

Anxiety, exercise, and smoking can elevate blood pressure. Wait 10 minutes after the woman's arrival to check a resting blood pressure.

- *Temperature.* Temperature should be taken every 4 hours, or every 2 hours if elevated.
- *Pulse and respirations.* Pulse rate and respirations should be determined along with blood pressure.
- *Fetal heart rate.* The fetal heart rate should be checked with the blood pressure or monitored continuously with the electronic fetal monitor if the situation indicates.
- *Urinary output.* Every voiding should be measured. The woman frequently has an indwelling catheter. In this case, urine output can be assessed hourly. Output should be 700 mL or greater in 24 hours, or at least 30 mL/hr.
- *Urine protein.* Urinary protein is evaluated hourly if an indwelling catheter is in place or with each voiding. Readings of 3+ or 4+ indicate loss of 5 g or more of protein in 24 hours.
- *Urine specific gravity.* Specific gravity of the urine should be checked hourly or with each voiding. Readings over 1.040 correlate with oliguria and proteinuria.
- *Edema.* The face (especially eyelids and cheekbone area), fingers, hands, arms (ulnar surface and wrist), legs (tibial surface), ankles, feet, and sacral area are inspected and palpated for edema. The degree of pitting is determined by pressing over bony areas.
- *Weight.* The woman is weighed daily at the same time, wearing the same robe or gown and slippers. Weighing may be omitted if the woman is to maintain strict bed rest.
- *Pulmonary edema.* The woman is observed for coughing. The lungs are auscultated for moist respirations.
- *Deep tendon reflexes.* The woman is assessed for evidence of hyperreflexia in the brachial, wrist, patellar, or Achilles tendons. The patellar reflex is the easiest to assess (see Clinical Skills: Assessing Deep Tendon Reflexes and Clonus). Clonus should also be assessed by vigorously dorsiflexing the foot while the knee is held in a fixed position. Normally no clonus is present. If it is present, it is measured as beats and recorded as such.

- *Placental separation.* The woman should be assessed hourly for vaginal bleeding and/or uterine rigidity.
- *Headache.* The woman should be questioned about the existence and location of any headache.
- *Visual disturbance.* The woman should be questioned about any visual blurring or changes or scotomata. The results of the daily funduscopic exam should be recorded on the chart.
- *Epigastric pain.* The woman should be asked about any epigastric pain. It is important to differentiate it from simple heartburn, which tends to be familiar and less intense.
- *Laboratory blood tests.* Daily tests of hematocrit to measure hemoconcentration; BUN, creatinine, and uric acid levels to assess kidney function; clotting studies for any indication of thrombocytopenia or DIC; liver enzymes; and electrolyte levels for deficiencies are all indicated. Magnesium levels are monitored regularly in women receiving magnesium sulfate.

When caring for a woman with preeclampsia who is receiving IV magnesium sulfate, it is imperative that you follow protocols for monitoring blood levels of magnesium. You are probably already aware of the common signs of increasing magnesium levels, such as diminished reflexes and decreased respiratory rate. However, there are some subtle clues you can also watch for that may suggest either the therapeutic or toxic range. When a woman's magnesium level is in the therapeutic range, she usually has some slurring of speech, awkwardness of movement, and decreased appetite. If the woman begins to have difficulty swallowing and begins to drool, she may be approaching the toxic range.

- *Level of consciousness.* The woman is observed for alertness, mood changes, and any signs of impending convulsion or coma.
- *Emotional response and level of understanding.* The woman's emotional response should be carefully assessed so that support and teaching can be planned accordingly.

In addition, the nurse continues to assess the effects of any medications administered. Because the administration of prescribed medications is an important aspect of care, the nurse is, of course, familiar with the more commonly used medications and their purpose, implications, and associated untoward or toxic effects.

Examples of nursing diagnoses that might apply to the woman with preeclampsia include the following:

- Deficient Fluid Volume related to fluid shift from intravascular to extravascular space secondary to vasospasm
- Risk for Injury related to the possibility of seizure secondary to cerebral vasospasm or edema

Clinical Skill Assessing Deep Tendon Reflexes and Clonus

NURSING ACTION	RATIONALE

Preparation

1. Explain the procedure, indications for its use, and information that will be obtained.

2. Most nurses check the patellar reflex and one other such as the biceps, triceps, or brachioradialis.

DTRs are assessed to gain information about CNS irritability secondary to preeclampsia and to assess the effects of magnesium sulfate if the woman is receiving it.

Equipment and Supplies

• Percussion hammer

Procedure

1. Elicit reflexes.

   Patellar reflex. Position the woman with her legs hanging over the edge of the bed (feet should not be touching the floor) (see Figure 16–4 ■). Briskly strike the patellar tendon, which is located just below the patella. Normal response is extension or a thrusting forward of the foot.

   In an inpatient setting the patellar reflex is often assessed while the woman lies supine. Flex her knees slightly and support them.

   Biceps reflex. Flex the woman's arm 45 degrees at the elbow and place your thumb on the biceps tendon. Allow your fingers to hold the biceps muscle. Strike your thumb in a slightly downward motion and assess the response. Normal response is flexion of the arm.

   Triceps reflex. Flex the woman's arm up to 90 degrees and allow her hand to hang against the side of her body. Using the percussion hammer, strike the triceps tendon just above the elbow. Normal response is contraction of the muscle, which causes extension of the arm.

   Brachioradialis reflex. Flex the woman's arm slightly and lay it on your forearm with her hand slightly pronated. Using the percussion hammer, strike the brachioradialis tendon, which is found about 1 to 2 inches above the wrist. Normal response is pronation of the forearm and flexion of the elbow.

   The correct position causes the muscle to be slightly stretched. Then when the tendon is stretched, with a tap the muscle should contract. Correct positioning and technique are essential to elicit the reflex.

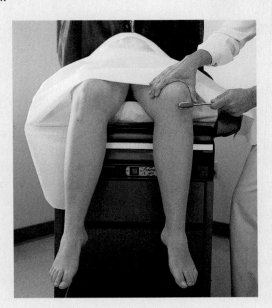

FIGURE 16–4 Correct position for eliciting patellar reflex: sitting.

(Continued on next page)

Clinical Skill Assessing Deep Tendon Reflexes and Clonus *(Continued)*

NURSING ACTION	RATIONALE
2. Grade reflexes. Reflexes are graded on a scale of 0 to 4+, as follows: 4+ Hyperactive; very brisk, jerky, or clonic response; abnormal 3+ Brisker than average; may not be abnormal 2+ Average response; normal 1+ Diminished response; low normal 0 No response; abnormal	*Normally reflexes are 1+ or 2+. With CNS irritation, hyperreflexia may be present; with high magnesium levels, reflexes may be diminished or absent.*
3. Assess for clonus. With the woman's knee flexed and the leg supported, vigorously dorsiflex the foot, maintain the dorsiflexion momentarily, and then release (Figure 16–5 ■). With a normal response, the foot returns to its normal position of plantar flexion. Clonus is present if the foot "jerks" or taps against the examiner's hand. If so, record the number of taps or beats of clonus.	*Clonus occurs with more pronounced hyperreflexia and indicates CNS irritability.*
4. Report and record findings. For example: DTRs 2+, no clonus or DTRs 4+, 2 beats clonus.	

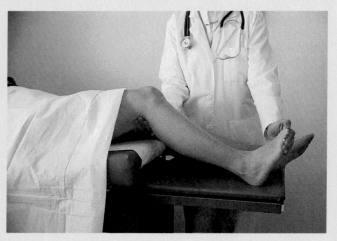

FIGURE 16–5 To elicit clonus, sharply dorsiflex the foot.

Nursing Plan and Implementation

Community-Based Nursing Care

A woman with preeclampsia has several major concerns. She may fear losing her fetus, she may worry about her personal relationship with her other children and her personal and sexual relationship with her partner, she may be concerned about finances, and she may also feel bored and a little resentful if she faces prolonged bed rest. If she has small children, she may have trouble providing for their care. The nurse should help the couple identify and discuss these concerns. The nurse can offer information and explanations if certain aspects of therapy cause difficulty. The nurse can also refer the woman and her family to community resources such as support groups or homemaker services as appropriate.

The woman needs to know which symptoms are significant and should be reported at once. Usually the woman with mild preeclampsia is seen once or twice a week, but she may need to come in earlier than her next scheduled appointment if symptoms indicate that her condition is progressing. She must understand her diet plan, which should reflect her culture, finances, and lifestyle (Figure 16–6 ■).

Hospital-Based Nursing Care

The development of severe preeclampsia is a cause for increased concern for the woman and her family. The most immediate concerns usually are about the prognosis for the woman and her fetus. The nurse can explain medical therapy and its purpose and offer honest, hopeful information. The nurse keeps the couple informed of fetal sta-

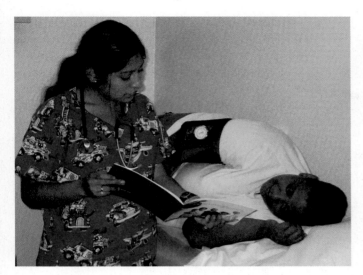

FIGURE 16–6 The nurse ensures that the woman with preeclampsia clearly understands her plan of care, especially with regard to the significance of her symptoms, her diet plan, and the importance of rest in a side-lying position.

tus and discusses other concerns the couple may express. The nurse provides as much information as possible and seeks other sources of information or aid for the family as needed. The nurse can also offer to contact a member of the clergy or hospital chaplain for additional support if the couple so chooses.

The nurse maintains a quiet, low-stimulus environment for the woman. The woman is generally placed in a private room in a quiet location where she can be watched closely. Visitors are limited to close family members or main support persons. The woman should maintain the left lateral recumbent position most of the time, with side rails up for her protection. Unlimited phone calls are avoided because the phone ringing unexpectedly may be too jarring. To avoid a sense of isolation, however, some women find it preferable to limit calls to a certain time of day. Bright lights and sudden loud noises may precipitate seizures in the woman with severe preeclampsia.

The occurrence of a convulsion is frightening to any family members who may be present, although the woman will not be able to recall it when she becomes conscious. Therefore, it is essential to offer explanations to the family members and the woman herself later.

A grand mal seizure has both a tonic phase, marked by pronounced muscular contraction and rigidity, and a clonic phase, marked by alternate contraction and relaxation of the muscles, which causes the woman to thrash about wildly. When the tonic phase of the contraction begins, the woman should be turned to her side (if she is not already in that position) to aid circulation to the placenta. Her head should be turned face down to allow saliva to drain from her mouth. The side rails should be padded or a pillow put between the woman and each side rail.

After 15 to 20 seconds the clonic phase starts. When the thrashing subsides, intensive monitoring and therapy begin. An oral airway is inserted, the woman's nasopharynx is suctioned, and oxygen is administered by nasal catheter. Fetal heart tones are monitored continuously. Maternal vital signs are monitored every 5 minutes until they are stable, then every 15 minutes.

Nursing Management During Labor and Birth

The laboring woman with preeclampsia must receive all the care and precautions necessary for normal labor, as well as those required for managing preeclampsia. The woman is kept positioned on her left side as much as possible. Both the woman and the fetus are monitored carefully throughout labor. The nurse notes the progress of labor and is alert to signs of worsening preeclampsia or its complications.

During the second stage of labor, the woman is encouraged to push in the side-lying position if possible. If she is unable to do so comfortably or effectively, she can be helped to a semisitting position for pushing and can then resume the lateral position between contractions. Birth is in the side-lying position or in the lithotomy position with a wedge placed under the woman's right hip.

A family member or other support person is encouraged to stay with the woman as much as possible. The woman in labor and the support person are kept informed of the progress and plan of care. In addition, their wishes concerning the birth experience are respected when possible. Preferably, the woman should be cared for by the same nurses throughout her stay.

Nursing Management During the Postpartal Period

Because the woman with preeclampsia is hypovolemic, even normal blood loss can be serious. The amount of vaginal bleeding must be assessed and the woman observed for signs of shock. Blood pressure and pulse are monitored every 4 hours for 48 hours. Hematocrit is checked daily. The woman is assessed for any further signs of preeclampsia. Intake and output are measured. Normal postpartum diuresis helps eliminate edema and is a favorable sign.

Postpartal depression can develop after such a difficult pregnancy. To help prevent it, the nurse provides opportunities for frequent maternal-infant contact and encourages family members to visit. The couple may have many questions, and the nurse should be available for discussion. The couple should be given family-planning information. Oral contraceptives may be used if the woman's blood pressure has returned to normal by the time they are prescribed (usually 4 to 6 weeks after birth). For a brief summary of preeclampsia, see Key Facts to Remember: Preeclampsia and Eclampsia.

KEY FACTS TO REMEMBER
Preeclampsia and Eclampsia

- Preeclampsia, which occurs after the 20th week of pregnancy, involves elevated BP and proteinuria. It may be mild or severe.
- A woman with preeclampsia who has a seizure is said to have eclampsia.
- The exact cause of preeclampsia is unknown.
- Vasospasm is responsible for most of the clinical manifestations, including the CNS signs of headache, hyperreflexia, and convulsion.
- Vasospasm also causes poor placental perfusion, which leads to IUGR.
- The only known cure for preeclampsia is birth of the infant, but symptoms may develop up to 48 hours postpartum.
- Management is supportive and includes anticonvulsant therapy, generally with magnesium sulfate; prevention of renal, hepatic, and hematologic complications; and careful assessment of fetal well-being.
- Nursing care focuses on implementing appropriate interventions based on the data gathered from regular assessment of vital signs, reflexes, degree of edema and proteinuria, response to therapy, fetal status, detection of developing complications, knowledge level, and psychologic state of the woman and her family.

Evaluation

Expected outcomes of nursing care include the following:

- The woman is able to explain preeclampsia, its implications for her pregnancy, the treatment regimen, and possible complications.
- The woman suffers no eclamptic seizures.
- The woman and her caregivers detect early evidence of increasing severity of the preeclampsia or possible complications so that appropriate treatment measures can be instituted.
- The woman gives birth to a healthy newborn.

Chronic Hypertensive Disease

Chronic hypertension exists when the blood pressure is 140/90 mm Hg or higher before pregnancy or before the 20th week of gestation or when hypertension persists 42 days following childbirth. If the diastolic blood pressure is greater than 80 mm Hg during the second trimester, chronic hypertension should be suspected. The cause of chronic hypertension has not been determined. In most women with chronic hypertension the disease is mild.

The goals of care are to prevent the development of preeclampsia and to ensure normal growth of the fetus. The woman is seen regularly for prenatal care (every 2 weeks until 28 weeks and then weekly until birth).

The woman is taught the importance of daily rest periods in the left lateral recumbent position and also learns to monitor her blood pressure at home. Sodium is limited to about 2.4 g/day. Antihypertensive medication is generally used only for women with blood pressure over 160/110. The drug of choice is methyldopa (Aldomet). Twenty-four-hour urines, serum creatinine, uric acid, hematocrit, and ultrasound examinations are repeated at least once in the second and third trimesters.

Nursing care is directed at providing sufficient information so that the woman can meet her healthcare needs. She is given information about her diet, the importance of regular rest, her medications, the need for blood pressure control, and any procedures used to monitor the well-being of her fetus.

Chronic Hypertension with Superimposed Preeclampsia

Preeclampsia develops in about 10% to 25% of women previously found to have chronic hypertension (Habli & Sibai, 2008). Close monitoring and careful management are indicated if the following signs develop: (1) elevations of systolic blood pressure 30 mm Hg above the baseline or diastolic blood pressure 15 to 20 mm Hg above the baseline, on two occasions at least 6 hours apart; (2) proteinuria; and (3) edema occurring in the upper half of the body. A woman with chronic hypertension who develops superimposed preeclampsia often progresses quickly to eclampsia, sometimes before 30 weeks of pregnancy.

Gestational or Transient Hypertension

Gestational hypertension occurs after 20 weeks, often during the last weeks of pregnancy. Its distinction from preeclampsia is the lack of proteinuria. Blood pressure is assessed 12 weeks after childbirth. If it remains elevated, the diagnosis is chronic hypertension. Women in whom gestational hypertension occurs are at increased risk of developing chronic hypertension later in life.

Disseminated Intravascular Coagulation

Disseminated intravascular coagulation (DIC) occurs more often in pregnancies complicated by preeclampsia, abruptio placentae, intrauterine fetal demise, amniotic fluid embolism, maternal liver disease, and septic abortion. Although DIC is not considered a component of severe preeclampsia, eclampsia, or HELLP syndrome, it can occur as a complication when any of these conditions exist. The incidence of DIC occurring when HELLP is the *only* risk factor is approximately 5% (Sibai, 2007).

DIC occurs when there is an overactivation of the normal clotting process. In most instances, tissue factor entering the circulation is the primary trigger for DIC. When this occurs, there is an imbalance between the coagulation and the fibrinolytic systems. This mechanism leads to hemorrhage and shock. During these events, clots are being formed and fibrin deposited into the microcirculation, resulting in cell or tissue damage. This triggers further coagulation, which eventually depletes the plasma clotting factors. These fibrin clots can lead to intravascular obstruction and infarctions. In addition, the fibrinolytic system is activated which results in the formation of fibrin-fibrinogen degradation products or fibrin split products. The release of these products decreases platelet functioning and further inhibits coagulation (Blackburn, 2007).

DIC is diagnosed when thrombocytopenia, low fibrinogen levels, and elevated fibrin split products are found in the laboratory findings. Serial platelet and serum fibrin degradation product counts are performed to monitor the mother's hematologic status. Supportive measures and reversing the causative factors are the primary interventions used to manage DIC.

Care of the Woman at Risk for Rh Alloimmunization

The Rh blood antigen, or Rh factor, is present on the surface of erythrocytes in a majority of the population. When it is present, a person is designated as Rh positive. Those without the factor are designated as Rh negative. If an Rh-negative individual is exposed to Rh-positive blood, an antigen-antibody response occurs, and the person forms anti-Rh agglutinin and is said to be sensitized. Subsequent exposure to Rh-positive blood can then cause a serious reaction that results in agglutination and hemolysis of red blood cells. In the United States about 85% of white Americans, 92% to 95% of African Americans, and 98% of Asian and Native Americans are Rh positive (ACOG, 2006).

Rh alloimmunization (sensitization) most commonly occurs when an Rh-negative woman carries an Rh-positive fetus, either to term or to termination by spontaneous or induced abortion. It can also occur if an Rh-negative non-pregnant woman receives an Rh-positive blood transfusion. The RBCs from the fetus invade the maternal circulation, thereby stimulating the production of Rh antibodies. Because this transfer of RBCs usually occurs at birth, the first offspring is not affected. In a subsequent pregnancy, however, Rh antibodies cross the placenta and enter the fetal circulation, causing severe hemolysis. The destruction of fetal RBCs, causing anemia in the fetus, is proportional to the extent of maternal sensitization (Figure 16–7 ■).

Fetal-Neonatal Risks

Although maternal sensitization can now be prevented by appropriate administration of Rh immune globulin (RhoGAM, or RhIgG), Rh alloimmunization still occurs in approximately 2.5 of 1000 births (McLean, Hedrianna, Lanouette, & Haesslein, 2004). If treatment is not initiated, the anemia resulting from this disorder can cause marked fetal edema, called **hydrops fetalis**.

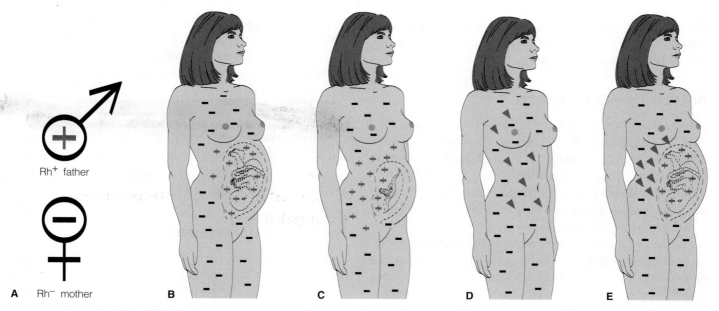

FIGURE 16–7 Rh alloimmunization sequence. *A,* Rh-positive father and Rh-negative mother. *B,* Pregnancy with Rh-positive fetus. Some Rh-positive blood enters the mother's blood. *C,* As the placenta separates, the mother is further exposed to the Rh-positive blood. *D,* The mother is sensitized to the Rh-positive blood; anti-Rh-positive anti-bodies (triangles) are formed. *E,* In subsequent pregnancies with an Rh-positive fetus, Rh-positive red blood cells are attacked by the anti-Rh-positive maternal antibodies, causing hemolysis of red blood cells in the fetus.

Congestive heart failure may result; marked jaundice (called *icterus gravis*), which can lead to neurologic damage (*kernicterus*), is also possible. This severe hemolytic syndrome is known as **erythroblastosis fetalis**.

Screening for Rh Incompatibility and Alloimmunization

At the first prenatal visit, caregivers (1) take a history of past pregnancies, previous sensitization, abortions, blood transfusions, or children who developed jaundice or anemia during the newborn period; (2) determine maternal blood type (ABO) and Rh factor and do a routine Rh antibody screening test; and (3) identify other medical complications such as diabetes, infections, or hypertension.

The antibody screening test (indirect Coombs' test) is important for the Rh-negative woman who may be pregnant with an Rh-positive fetus because it indicates whether the woman is sensitized to the Rh antigen. The test measures the number of antibodies in the maternal blood. If the pregnant woman is not sensitized, a second antibody screening test is done at 28 weeks' gestation. If the maternal antibody screen is positive, a maternal antibody titer is obtained. A woman with an elevated antibody titer should be considered sensitized and her pregnancy should be managed closely.

Clinical Therapy

The goals of clinical management are the early identification and treatment of maternal conditions that predispose to hemolytic disease, identification and evaluation of the Rh-sensitized woman, coordinated obstetric-pediatric treatment for the seriously affected newborn, and prevention of Rh sensitization if none is present.

Antepartal Management

If the antibody screen obtained at 28 weeks' gestation is negative, the woman is given 300 mcg of **Rh immune globulin (RhoGAM)** intramuscularly as a prophylactic (preventative) measure. RhoGAM provides passive antibody protection against Rh antigens. This "tricks" the body, which does not then produce antibodies of its own (active immunity).

When the woman is Rh negative and not sensitized and the father is Rh positive or unknown, Rh immune globulin is also given after each abortion (whether spontaneous or induced), ectopic pregnancy, chorionic villus sampling, multifetal pregnancy reduction, partial molar pregnancy, PUBS, antepartum hemorrhage, external version, or amniocentesis. It is also given if there has been maternal trauma such as injury resulting from a motor vehicle accident or from domestic violence. If abortion or ectopic pregnancy occurs in the first trimester, a smaller (50 mcg)

dose of Rh immune globulin (MICRhoGAM or Mini-Gamulin Rh) may be used although many hospitals do not stock this dose. Thus a full 300 mcg dose is generally given.

The fetus of a woman who is sensitized to the Rh factor is at risk. Two primary interventions can help the fetus whose blood cells are being destroyed by maternal antibodies: early birth and intrauterine transfusion; both carry risks. Ideally, birth should be delayed until fetal maturity is confirmed at about 36 to 37 weeks.

Ultrasound is an invaluable tool in managing the pregnancy of a woman with Rh alloimmunization. Ultrasound should be done at 14 to 16 weeks to determine gestational age. Then serial ultrasounds and amniotic fluid analysis can be used to follow fetal progress.

New technology enables clinicians to use a Doppler to measure peak systolic velocity in the middle cerebral artery (MCA) of the fetus. The increased fetal cardiac output and decreased blood viscosity seen in fetal anemia results in increased MCA blood flow velocity. MCA Dopplers can be done starting as early as 18 weeks' gestation but are unreliable after 34 to 35 weeks. The test is valuable because it reduces the need for invasive diagnostic procedures such as ultrasound (ACOG, 2006).

Ultrasound can also be used to detect ascites and subcutaneous edema, which are signs of severe fetal involvement. Other indicators of the fetal condition include an increase in fetal heart size and hydramnios.

As indicated previously, negative antibody titers can consistently identify the fetus not at risk. However, the titers cannot reliably point out the fetus in danger, because titer level does not always correlate with the severity of the disease. Thus, if the maternal antibody titer is 1:16 or greater, an optical density (OD) analysis of the amniotic fluid is performed. This optical density analysis measures the amount of pigment from the breakdown of red blood cells and can determine the severity of the hemolytic process.

If ΔOD indicates severe anemia or if fetal hydrops is present, percutaneous umbilical blood sampling (PUBS) (see Chapter 21 ∞) is performed to determine fetal hematocrit. If the hematocrit is low (generally less than 30%), the fetus is given an intrauterine blood transfusion. Severely sensitized fetuses may require birth at 32 to 34 weeks.

Postpartal Management

The Rh-negative mother who has no antibody titer (indirect Coombs' test negative, nonsensitized) and has given birth to an Rh-positive fetus (direct Coombs' test negative) is given an intramuscular injection of Rh immune globulin (RhoGAM). The woman must receive Rh immune globulin within 72 hours of childbirth so she does not have time to produce antibodies to fetal cells that entered her bloodstream when the placenta separated. A standard dose of RhoGAM (300 mcg) can prevent sensitization after exposure of up to 30 mL of Rh(D) positive blood. If there is a question about extent of fetal exposure, a Kleihauer-Betke test can be performed to determine the amount of Rh(D) positive blood that is present in the maternal circulation and to calculate the amount of RhoGAM needed. Up to five doses may be administered at one time. If additional doses are necessary, they are administered every 12 hours in alternating sites until the appropriate amount has been given (Shaver, 2004).

Rh immune globulin is not given to the newborn or the father. It is not effective for, and should not be given to, a previously sensitized woman. However, sometimes after birth or an abortion the results of the blood test do not clearly show whether the mother is already sensitized to the Rh antigen. In such cases, the Rh immune globulin should be given; it will cause no harm. For the major considerations in caring for an Rh-negative woman, see Key Facts to Remember: Rh Sensitization. (The treatment of the newborn with hemolytic disease is discussed in Chapter 27 ∞.)

KEY FACTS TO REMEMBER

Rh Sensitization

When trying to work through Rh problems, the nurse should remember the following:

- A potential problem exists when an Rh-negative mother and an Rh-positive father conceive a child who is Rh positive.
- In this situation, the mother may become sensitized or produce antibodies to her fetus's Rh-positive blood.

The following tests are used to detect sensitization:

- Indirect Coombs' test—done on the mother's blood to measure the number of Rh-positive antibodies.
- Direct Coombs' test—done on the infant's blood to detect antibody-coated Rh-positive RBCs.

Based on the results of these tests, the following may be done:

- If the mother's indirect Coombs' test is negative and the infant's direct Coombs' test is negative (confirming that sensitization has not occurred), the mother is given Rh immune globulin within 72 hours of birth.
- If the mother's indirect Coombs' test is positive and her Rh-positive infant has a positive direct Coombs' test, Rh immune globulin is *not* given; in this case, the infant is carefully monitored for hemolytic disease.
- It is recommended that Rh immune globulin be given antenatally at 28 weeks to decrease possible transplacental bleeding concerns.
- Rh immune globulin is also administered after each abortion (spontaneous or therapeutic), antepartum hemorrhage, mismatched blood transfusion, ectopic pregnancy, amniocentesis, chorionic villi sampling (CVS), percutaneous umbilical blood sampling (PUBS), fetal cephalic version, or maternal trauma.

Nursing Care Management

Nursing Assessment and Diagnosis

As part of the initial prenatal history, the nurse asks the mother if she knows her blood type and Rh factor. Many women are aware that they are Rh negative and that this status has implications for pregnancy. If the woman knows she is Rh negative, the nurse can assess the woman's knowledge of what that means. The nurse can also ask the woman if she has ever received Rh immune globulin, if she has had any previous pregnancies and what their outcome was, and if she knows her partner's Rh factor. If the partner is Rh negative, there is no risk to the fetus who will also be Rh negative.

If the woman does not know what Rh type she is, intervention cannot begin until the initial laboratory data are obtained. Once that is done, the nurse plans care based on the findings.

If the woman becomes sensitized during her pregnancy, nursing assessment focuses on the knowledge and coping skills of the woman and her family. The nurse also provides ongoing assessment during procedures to evaluate fetal well-being, such as ultrasound and amniocentesis.

After birth, the nurse reviews data about the Rh type of the fetus. If the newborn is Rh positive, the mother is Rh negative, and no sensitization has occurred, nursing assessment reveals the need to administer Rh immune globulin. If both the mother and her newborn are Rh negative, Rh immune globulin is not indicated.

Nursing diagnoses that might apply to the pregnant woman at risk for Rh sensitization include the following:

- *Health-Seeking Behaviors: Information about Rh Immune Globulin* related to an expressed need to understand the implications of being Rh negative and pregnant
- *Ineffective Individual Coping* related to depression secondary to the development of indications of the need for fetal exchange transfusion

Nursing Plan and Implementation

During the antepartal period the nurse explains the mechanisms involved in alloimmunization and answers any questions the woman and her partner have. It is imperative that the woman understand the importance of receiving Rh immune globulin after every spontaneous or therapeutic abortion or ectopic pregnancy. The nurse also explains the purpose of the Rh immune globulin administered at 28 weeks' gestation if the woman is not sensitized.

If the woman is sensitized to the Rh factor, it poses a threat to any Rh-positive fetus she carries. The nurse provides emotional support to the family to help the members deal with their grief and any feelings of guilt about the infant's condition. If an intrauterine transfusion becomes necessary, the

Clinical Skill Administration of Rh Immune Globulin (RhoGAM, HypRho-D)

NURSING ACTION	RATIONALE
Preparation	
1. Confirm that Rh immune globulin is indicated by checking the woman's prenatal or intrapartal record to verify that she is Rh negative. Then confirm that sensitization has not occurred—maternal indirect Coombs' negative. Postpartally, confirm that the baby is Rh positive but not sensitized (direct Coombs' negative) and that the mother's indirect Coombs' is negative. Rh immune globulin is *not* indicated if the infant is Rh negative, too.	*Rh immune globulin is only indicated for Rh-negative, unsensitized women.*
2. Confirm that the woman does not have a history of allergies to immune globulin preparations by checking entries on medication allergies in her chart and by asking her whether she has ever had any allergic reactions to medications, globulins, or blood products.	*Rh immune globulin is made from the plasma portion of blood. Allergic reactions are possible.*
3. Explain purpose and procedure. Have consent form signed if required by agency policy.	*Many agencies require separate consent for the administration of Rh immune globulin because it is a blood product.*
Equipment and Supplies	
• Rh immune globulin, which is obtained from the blood bank or pharmacy according to agency protocol. Lot numbers for the drug and the crossmatch should be the same.	*The woman should clearly understand the purpose of the Rh immune globulin, its rationale, the administration procedure, and any related risks. Generally the primary side effects are redness and tenderness at the injection site and allergic responses.*
• Syringe and IM needle	
Procedure	
1. Confirm the woman's identity and administer one vial of 300 mcg Rh immune globulin IM into the deltoid muscle.	
2. An immune globulin microdose is used after miscarriage, elective abortion, ectopic pregnancy, or molar pregnancy occurring within the first 12 weeks' gestation. Antepartally, the Rh immune globulin is generally given within 3 hours but not longer than 72 hours of the event.	
3. If a larger bleed is suspected at birth (as in cases of severe abruptio placentae), additional doses may be administered at one time using multiple sites or at regular intervals as long as all doses are given within 72 hours of childbirth.	*The normal 300 mcg dose provides passive immunity following exposure of up to 15 mL of transfused RBCs or 30 mL of fetal blood.*
4. Provide opportunities for the woman to ask questions and express concerns.	
5. Chart according to agency policy. Most agencies chart lot number, route, dose, and client education.	*Many women, especially primigravidas, are not aware of the risks for an Rh-positive fetus of a sensitized Rh-negative mother. They need to understand the importance of receiving Rh immune globulin for each pregnancy to ensure continued protection.*

nurse continues to provide emotional support while also assuming responsibility as part of the healthcare team.

During labor, the nurse caring for an Rh-negative woman who has not been sensitized ensures that the woman's blood is assessed for any antibodies and also has been crossmatched for Rh immune globulin. On the postpartum unit the nurse generally is responsible for administering the Rh immune globulin intramuscularly if the newborn is Rh positive (see Clinical Skill: Administration of Rh Immune Globulin).

Evaluation

Expected outcomes of nursing care include the following:

- The woman is able to explain the process of Rh sensitization and its implications for her unborn child and for subsequent pregnancies.
- If the woman has not been sensitized, she is able to discuss the importance of receiving Rh immune globulin when necessary and cooperates with the recommended dosage schedule.
- The woman gives birth to a healthy newborn.
- If complications develop for the fetus or newborn, they are detected quickly and therapy is instituted.

Care of the Woman at Risk Because of ABO Incompatibility

In addition to the Rh antigen, human red blood cells may present one or more antigens of the ABO group. People whose RBCs present the A antigen have type A blood. Those people whose RBCs present the B antigen have type B blood. People whose RBCs present both types of antigen have type AB blood, and those whose blood cells present neither A nor B have type O blood. ABO incompatibility occurs when a mother with one blood type is pregnant with a fetus of a different blood type. It is seen in about 20% to 25% of pregnancies, but it rarely causes significant hemolysis.

Group O infants, because they have no antigens on their red blood cells, are never affected regardless of the mother's blood type. In most cases ABO incompatibility is limited to type O mothers who become pregnant with a type A, B, or AB fetus. The incompatibility occurs as a result of the interaction of antibodies present in maternal serum and the antigen sites on the fetal red blood cells.

Anti-A and anti-B antibodies are naturally occurring; that is, women are naturally exposed to the A and B antigens through the foods they eat and through exposure to infection by gram-negative bacteria. As a result, some women have high serum anti-A and anti-B titers even before they become pregnant for the first time. Once they become pregnant, the maternal serum anti-A and anti-B antibodies cross the placenta and produce hemolysis of the fetal red blood cells. With ABO incompatibility, the first infant is frequently involved, and no relationship exists between the appearance of the disease and repeated sensitization from one pregnancy to the next.

Unlike Rh incompatibility, antepartal treatment is not warranted because it does not cause severe anemia. As part of the initial assessment, however, the nurse should note whether the potential for an ABO incompatibility exists (type O mother and type A or B father). This note alerts caregivers so that, following birth, the newborn can be assessed carefully for the development of hyperbilirubinemia (see Chapter 29 ∞).

Care of the Woman Requiring Surgery During Pregnancy

Although elective surgery should be delayed until the postpartal period, essential surgery can generally be undertaken during pregnancy. However, surgery poses some risks. The incidence of spontaneous abortion is increased for women who have surgery in the first trimester. Therefore, the early second trimester is the best time to operate because there is less risk of spontaneous abortion or early labor, and the uterus is not so large as to impinge on the abdominal field.

Although general preoperative and postoperative care is similar for gravid and nongravid women, special considerations must be kept in mind when the surgical client is pregnant. If a chest x-ray is done, the fetus should be shielded from the radiation. To prevent uterine compression of major blood vessels while the woman is supine, the caregiver must place a wedge under the woman's right hip to tilt the uterus during both surgery and recovery. The decreased intestinal motility and delayed gastric emptying that occur in pregnancy increase the risk of vomiting when anesthetics are given and during the postoperative period. Thus inserting a nasogastric tube is recommended before a pregnant woman has major surgery. An indwelling urinary catheter prevents bladder distention, decreases risk of injury to the bladder, and permits convenient monitoring of output.

Pregnancy causes increased secretions of the respiratory tract and engorgement of the nasal mucous membrane, often making breathing through the nose difficult. Consequently, pregnant women often need an endotracheal tube for respiratory support during surgery.

Caregivers must guard against maternal hypoxia. During surgery, uterine circulation decreases and fetal oxygenation may be reduced quickly. Fetal heart rate must be monitored electronically before, during, and after surgery. Blood loss is also closely monitored throughout the procedure and following it.

Postoperatively, the nurse encourages the woman to turn, breathe deeply, and cough regularly and to use any ventilation therapy, such as incentive spirometry, to avoid developing pneumonia. The pregnant woman is at increased risk for thrombophlebitis, so the nurse applies antiembolism stockings, encourages leg exercises while the woman is confined to bed, and introduces ambulation as soon as possible.

Discharge teaching is especially important. The woman and her family should clearly understand what to expect regarding activity level, discomfort, diet, medications, and any special considerations. In addition, they should know the warning signs they need to report to the physician immediately.

Care of the Woman Suffering Trauma from an Accident

Accidental injury complicates 6% to 7% of pregnancies (Gonik & Foley, 2004). Trauma from motor vehicle accidents is the leading cause of fetal and maternal death (Gonik & Foley, 2004). Falls and assault—including domestic violence—are the next most common causes of injury.

Late in pregnancy, when balance and coordination are adversely affected, the woman may fall. Her protruding abdomen is vulnerable to a variety of minor injuries. The fetus is usually well protected by the amniotic fluid, which distributes the force of a blow equally in all directions, and by the muscle layers of the uterus and abdominal wall. In early pregnancy, while the uterus is still in the pelvis, it is shielded from blows by the surrounding pelvic organs, muscles, and bony structures.

Trauma that causes concern includes blunt trauma (from an automobile accident, for example); penetrating abdominal injuries, such as knife and gunshot wounds; and the complications of maternal shock, premature labor, and spontaneous abortion. Maternal mortality most often occurs from head trauma or hemorrhage. Uterine rupture is a rare but life-threatening complication of trauma. It may result from strong deceleration forces in an automobile accident, with or without seat belts. Traumatic separation of the placenta can occur; it causes a high rate of fetal mortality. Premature labor, often following rupture of membranes during an accident, is another serious hazard to the fetus. Premature labor can ensue even if the woman is not injured. To help prevent trauma from automobile accidents, all pregnant women should wear both lap seat belts and shoulder harnesses.

Penetrating trauma includes gunshot wounds and stab wounds. The mother generally fares better than the fetus if the penetrating trauma involves the abdomen as the enlarged uterus is likely to protect the mother's bowel from injury. Unfortunately, the fetal injury rate is 59% to 80% (Gonik & Foley, 2004).

Treatment of major injuries during pregnancy focuses initially on life-saving measures for the woman. Such measures include establishing an airway, controlling external bleeding, and administering intravenous fluid to alleviate shock. The woman must be kept on her left side to prevent further hypotension. Fetal heart rate is monitored. Exploratory surgery may be necessary following abdominal trauma to determine the extent of injuries. If the fetus is late preterm and the uterus has been damaged, cesarean birth is indicated. If the fetus is still immature, the uterus can often be repaired, and the pregnancy continues until term. In all cases, emotional support and information about the woman's condition and its implications for her and for her fetus are essential components of care.

In cases of trauma in which the mother's life is not directly threatened, fetal monitoring for 4 hours should be sufficient if there are no contractions, vaginal bleeding, uterine tenderness, or leaking amniotic fluid. Abruptio placentae may occur following a blow to the abdomen. Increased uterine irritability in the first few hours after trauma helps identify women who may be at risk for this potentially catastrophic complication.

When cardiopulmonary resuscitation (CPR) is performed on the pregnant woman late in gestation, perimortem cesarean birth is advocated if CPR is unsuccessful in the first 4 minutes. Chest compressions are less effective in the third trimester because of compression of the inferior vena cava by the gravid uterus. Cesarean birth alleviates this compression and improves resuscitation efforts in both the fetus and the mother (Gonik & Foley, 2004; Katz, Balderston, & DeFreest, 2005).

Care of the Battered Pregnant Woman

Domestic violence, also called intimate partner abuse, may be defined as the intentional injury of a woman by her partner. Domestic violence often begins or increases during pregnancy. Estimates suggest that domestic violence impacts up to 20% of women although these estimates may be understated (AAP & ACOG, 2007; Kady, Gilbert, Xing, & Smith, 2005). Physical abuse may result in loss of pregnancy, preterm labor, low-birth-weight infants, and fetal death. Abused women have significantly higher rates of complications such as anemia, infection, low weight gain, and first- and second-trimester bleeding.

The first step toward helping the battered woman is to identify her. Asking every woman about abuse at various times during pregnancy is crucial because a woman may not disclose abuse until she knows her caregivers better. ACOG (1999a) recommends that all women be screened for abuse at the first prenatal visit, at least once each trimester, and then again during the postpartum period. Samples of questions the nurse can ask are provided in Chapter 5 ∞.

Chronic psychosomatic symptoms can also be an indicator of abuse. The woman may have nonspecific or vague complaints. It is important to assess old scars around the head, chest, arms, abdomen, and genitalia and to evaluate any bruising or evidence of pain. The nurse should be especially alert for signs of bruising or injury to the woman's breasts, abdomen, or genitalia because these areas are common targets of violence during pregnancy. Other indicators include a decrease in eye contact; silence when the partner is in the room; and a history of nervousness, insomnia, drug overdose, or alcohol problems. Frequent visits to the emergency room and a history of accidents without understandable causes are possible indicators of abuse.

The goals of treatment are to identify the woman at risk, increase her decision-making abilities to decrease the potential for further abuse, and provide a safe environment for the pregnant woman and her unborn child. An environment that is private, accepting, and nonjudgmental is necessary so the woman can express her concerns. She needs to be aware of community resources available to her, such as emergency shelters; police, legal, and social services; and counseling. Ultimately, it is the woman's decision to either seek assistance or return to old patterns.

Abuse may begin during pregnancy and may thus be a new, unexpected experience for the woman, one she believes is an isolated incident. She needs to know that battering may continue after childbirth and may extend to the child as well. This is an important time for the nurse to provide information and establish a trusted link for the woman with a health professional. (For further discussion see Chapter 5 ∞.)

Care of the Woman with a Perinatal Infection Affecting the Fetus

Fetal infection may develop at any time during pregnancy. In general, perinatal infections are most likely to cause harm when the embryo is exposed during the first trimester when organ development is occurring. Infections that occur later in pregnancy create other concerns such as growth restriction, preterm birth, and neurologic changes. This section addresses several of the most commonly occurring viral and parasitic infections that may have an impact on the fetus if acquired during pregnancy.

Toxoplasmosis

Toxoplasmosis is caused by the protozoan *Toxoplasma gondii*. It is innocuous in adults, but, when contracted in pregnancy, it can profoundly affect the fetus. The pregnant woman may contract the organism by eating raw or undercooked meat, by drinking unpasteurized goat's milk, or by contact with the feces of infected cats, either through the cat litter box or by gardening in areas frequented by cats.

Fetal-Neonatal Risks

The likelihood of fetal infection increases with each trimester of pregnancy, but the risk of serious impact on the fetus decreases. Thus maternal infection contracted during the first trimester is associated with the lowest incidence of fetal infection (15%) but the highest risk of se-

vere fetal disease or death (10%). The highest rate of fetal infection (60%) occurs when the mother contracts the infection in the third trimester, but most infants are born without clinical signs of infection (Davies & Gibbs, 2008). However, up to 85% of these infants will develop signs and symptoms if left untreated (Montoya & Rosso, 2005). The infection may vary from mild to severe. In mild cases, retinochoroiditis (inflammation of the retina and choroid of the eye) may be the only recognizable damage, and it and other manifestations may not appear until adolescence or young adulthood. Severe neonatal disorders associated with congenital infection include convulsions, coma, microcephaly, and hydrocephalus. The infant with a severe infection may die soon after birth. Survivors are often blind, deaf, and severely retarded. Treatment of the mother can reduce the incidence of fetal infection and decreases the late sequelae of the infection (Duff, 2007).

Clinical Therapy

The goal of therapy is to identify the woman at risk for toxoplasmosis and to treat the disease promptly if diagnosed. Diagnosis can be made by serologic testing of antibody titers, specifically the IgG and IgM fluorescent antibody (IFA) tests. If a pregnant woman is positive for IgG antibodies and negative for IgM in the third trimester, it indicates that she had a toxoplasmosis infection in the past and the baby is not at risk. If she has a positive IgM, it indicates a more recent infection and it should be followed by confirmatory testing at a toxoplasma reference lab (Montoya & Rosso, 2005). Toxoplasmosis polymerase chain reaction (PCR) test of amniotic fluid is useful in diagnosing congenital toxoplasmosis. Ultrasound may be useful in detecting signs of fetal infection such as ascites, microcephaly, intracranial calcifications, and fetal growth restriction (Duff, 2007).

Women in whom maternal infection is established should receive spiramycin to decrease the frequency of vertical transmission, particularly in the first trimester. Spiramycin is not commercially available in the United States, but it can be obtained for treatment through the CDC. Spiramycin does not reliably cross the placenta. Thus if fetal infection is suspected, spiramycin should be replaced with pyrimethamine, folinic acid, and a sulfonamide after the 18th week of pregnancy (Duff, 2007).

Nursing Care Management

Nursing Assessment and Diagnosis

The incubation period for the disease is 10 days. The woman with acute toxoplasmosis may be asymptomatic, or she may develop myalgia, malaise, rash, splenomegaly, and enlarged posterior cervical lymph nodes. Symptoms usually disappear in a few days or weeks.

Nursing diagnoses that might apply to the pregnant woman with toxoplasmosis include the following:

- *Risk for Ineffective Health Maintenance* related to lack of knowledge about ways in which a pregnant woman can contract toxoplasmosis
- *Anticipatory Grieving* related to potential effects on infant of maternal toxoplasmosis

Nursing Plan and Implementation

The nurse caring for women during the antepartal period has the primary opportunity to discuss methods of preventing toxoplasmosis. The woman must understand the importance of avoiding poorly cooked or raw meat, especially pork, beef, lamb, and, in the Arctic region, caribou. Fruits and vegetables should be washed. The woman should avoid contact with the cat litter box and have someone else clean it frequently, because it takes approximately 48 hours for a cat's feces to become infectious. The nurse should also discuss the importance of wearing gloves when gardening and of avoiding garden areas frequented by cats.

Evaluation

Expected outcomes of nursing care include the following:

- The woman is able to discuss toxoplasmosis, its methods of transmission, the implications for her fetus, and measures she can take to avoid contracting it.
- The woman implements health measures to avoid contracting toxoplasmosis.
- The woman gives birth to a healthy newborn.

Rubella

The effects of rubella (German measles) are no more severe, and there are no greater complications in pregnant women than in nonpregnant women of comparable age. However, the effects of this infection on the fetus and newborn are great because rubella causes a chronic infection that begins in the first trimester of pregnancy and may persist for months after birth.

Fetal-Neonatal Risks

Fortunately, the success of the rubella vaccination program in the United States has led to a dramatic decrease in the incidence of rubella. However, estimates suggest that approximately 20% of women are still susceptible to rubella and consequently their fetuses are at risk of congenital rubella syndrome should the mother become infected while pregnant (Gibbs et al., 2004).

The period of greatest risk for the teratogenic effects of rubella on the fetus is the first trimester. The most common clinical signs of congenital infection include congenital cataracts, sensorineural deafness, and congenital heart defects, particularly patent ductus arteriosus. Other abnormalities, such as mental retardation or cerebral palsy, may become evident in infancy. Diagnosis in the newborn can be conclusively made in the presence of these conditions and with an elevated rubella IgM antibody titer at birth.

Infants born with congenital rubella syndrome are infectious and should be isolated. These infants may continue to shed the virus for months.

The *expanded rubella syndrome* relates to effects that may develop for years after the infection. These include an increased incidence of insulin-dependent diabetes mellitus; sudden hearing loss; glaucoma; and a slow, progressive form of encephalitis.

Clinical Therapy

The best therapy for rubella is prevention. Live attenuated vaccine is available and should be given to all children. Women of childbearing age should be tested for immunity and vaccinated if susceptible and if it is established that they are not pregnant. Health counseling in high school and in premarital clinic visits can stress the importance of screening before planning a pregnancy. As part of the prenatal laboratory screen the woman is evaluated for rubella using hemagglutination inhibition (HAI), a serology test. The presence of a 1:18 titer or greater is evidence of immunity. A titer less than 1:8 indicates susceptibility to rubella. Because the vaccine is made with attenuated virus, pregnant women are not vaccinated. However, it is considered safe for newly vaccinated children to have contact with pregnant women.

If a woman who is pregnant becomes infected during the first trimester, therapeutic abortion may be an alternative.

Nursing Care Management

Nursing Assessment and Diagnosis

A woman who develops rubella during pregnancy may be asymptomatic or may show signs of a mild infection including a maculopapular rash, lymphadenopathy, muscular achiness, and joint pain. The presence of IgM antirubella antibody is diagnostic of a recent infection. These titers remain elevated for approximately 1 month after infection.

Nursing diagnoses that may apply to the woman who develops rubella early in her pregnancy include the following:

- *Ineffective Family Coping* due to an inability to accept the possibility of fetal anomalies secondary to maternal rubella exposure
- *Risk for Ineffective Health Maintenance* related to lack of knowledge about the importance of rubella immunization before becoming pregnant

Nursing Plan and Implementation

Nursing support and understanding are vital for the couple contemplating abortion because of a diagnosis of rubella. Such a decision may initiate a crisis for the couple who has planned the pregnancy. The parents need objective data to understand the possible effects on their unborn fetus and the prognosis for the offspring.

Evaluation

Expected outcomes of nursing care include the following:

- The woman is able to describe the implications of rubella exposure during the first trimester of pregnancy.
- If exposure occurs in a woman who is not immune, she is able to identify her options and make a decision about continuing her pregnancy that is acceptable to her and her partner.
- The nonimmune woman receives the rubella vaccine during the early postpartal period.
- The woman gives birth to a healthy infant.

Cytomegalovirus

Cytomegalovirus (CMV) belongs to the herpes virus group and causes both congenital and acquired infections referred to as cytomegalic inclusion disease (CID). The significance of this virus in pregnancy is related to its ability to be transmitted by asymptomatic women across the placenta to the fetus or by the cervical route during birth.

In the United States, over half of adults have antibodies for the CMV virus. The virus can be found in virtually all body fluids. It can be passed between humans by any close contact, such as kissing, breastfeeding, and sexual intercourse. Asymptomatic CMV infection is particularly common in children and gravid women. It is a chronic, persistent infection in that the individual may shed the virus continually over many years. The cervix can harbor the virus, and an ascending infection can develop after birth. Although the virus is usually innocuous in adults and children, it may be fatal to the fetus.

Accurate diagnosis in the pregnant woman is best documented by seroconversion. Shedding of the virus in urine and saliva can be intermittent and does not distinguish primary infection from recurrent infection (Landry, 2004). Identification of the virus in amniotic fluid by PCR or culture is the most specific way of diagnosing congenital infection (Davies & Gibbs, 2008). Ultrasound findings may include fetal hydrops, growth restriction, hydramnios, cardiomegaly, and fetal ascites. At present, no treatment exists for maternal CMV or for the congenital disease in the newborn.

CMV is the most frequent cause of viral infection in the human fetus, infecting 0.5% to 2% of all newborns. Of these, about 10% to 15% will have overt symptoms at birth and 20% to 30% of severely affected infants die; 90% of the survivors have significant neurologic complications (Hollier & Grissom, 2005). Subclinical infections in the newborn may produce mental retardation and hearing loss, sometimes not recognized for several months, or learning disabilities not seen until childhood. CMV may be the most common cause of mental retardation.

For the fetus, this infection can result in extensive intrauterine tissue damage that leads to fetal death; in survival with microcephaly, hydrocephaly, cerebral palsy, or mental retardation; or in survival with no damage at all. The infected newborn is often SGA. The principal tissues and organs affected are the blood, brain, and liver; however, virtually all organs are potentially at risk.

Herpes Simplex Virus

Herpes simplex virus (HSV-I or HSV-2) infection can cause painful lesions in the genital area. Lesions may also develop on the cervix. This condition and its implications for nonpregnant women are discussed in Chapter 6 ∞. However, because the presence of herpes lesions in the genital tract may profoundly affect the fetus, herpes infection as it relates to a pregnant woman is discussed here.

Fetal-Neonatal Risks

Primary infection poses the greatest risk to both the mother and her infant. Primary infection has been associated with spontaneous abortion, low birth weight, and preterm birth. Transmission to the fetus almost always occurs after the membranes rupture and the virus ascends or during birth through an infected birth canal. Transplacental infection is rare. Approximately 50% of all infants who are born vaginally to a mother who is experiencing a primary genital HSV infection develop some form of herpes infection. Exposure of the newborn to a *recurrent* infection drops the risk of transmission to between 1% and 5% (Hill & Roberts, 2005).

The infected infant is often asymptomatic at birth but after an incubation period of 2 to 12 days develops symptoms of fever (or hypothermia), jaundice, seizures, and poor feeding. Approximately one-half of infected infants develop the characteristic vesicular skin lesions. All infants who have neonatal herpes should be evaluated promptly and treated with acyclovir (CDC, 2006).

Clinical Therapy

The vesicular lesions of herpes have a characteristic appearance, and they rupture easily. Definitive diagnosis is made by culturing active lesions.

Oral antiviral therapies are available, including acyclovir (Zovirax), famciclovir, and valacyclovir. Famciclovir and

MyNursingKit | Herpes in Pregnancy

valacyclovir have an advantage of better absorption and a longer half-life than acyclovir (Gibbs et al., 2004). Currently, there is no evidence that there are any adverse fetal effects related to exposure to any of these drugs during any trimester (Hill & Roberts, 2005). The CDC (2006) does not recommend the routine use of acyclovir for recurrent infection during pregnancy but recognizes that the use of acyclovir late preterm may reduce the need for cesarean birth. The dosage is unchanged during pregnancy.

For a woman with either a primary or a secondary outbreak of genital herpes during labor, or symptoms that may indicate an impending outbreak, the preferred method of childbirth is cesarean birth. Although fetal transmission with recurrent outbreaks is low, a cesarean birth is warranted because of the serious nature of the disease in the newborn. An estimated 1500 to 2000 newborns contract herpes each year, with 85% of neonatal herpes resulting from viral transmission near the time of birth (Hill & Roberts, 2005). The risk of neonatal transmission is low in women with a history of HSV in the current pregnancy or in the past. Thus cost-benefit analysis suggests that oral acyclovir prophylaxis and vaginal birth are appropriate for women with a history of HSV but who have no evidence of active genital disease at the time of childbirth (Davies & Gibbs, 2008).

Nursing Care Management

Nursing Assessment and Diagnosis

During the initial prenatal visit it is important to learn whether the woman or her partner have had previous herpes infections. Ongoing assessment is indicated as pregnancy progresses.

Nursing diagnoses that may apply to the pregnant woman with HSV infection include the following:

- *Sexual Dysfunction* related to unwillingness to engage in sexual intercourse secondary to the presence of active herpes lesions
- *Ineffective Individual Coping* related to depression secondary to the risk to the fetus if herpes lesions are present at birth

Nursing Plan and Implementation

Nurses need to be particularly concerned with client education about this fast-spreading disease. Women should be informed of the association of HSV infection with spontaneous abortion, newborn mortality and morbidity, and the possibility of cesarean birth. A woman needs to inform all healthcare providers of her infection. She should also know of the possible association of genital herpes with cervical cancer and the importance of a yearly Pap smear.

The woman who acquired HSV infection as an adolescent may be devastated as a mature young adult who wants

to have a family. Clients may be helped by counseling that allows them to express the anger, shame, and depression often experienced by those with herpes. Literature may be helpful and is available from Planned Parenthood and many public health agencies. The American Social Health Association has established the HELP program to provide information and the latest research results on genital herpes. The association has a quarterly journal, *The Helper*, for clients with HSV infection and nurses.

Evaluation

Expected outcomes of nursing care include the following:

- The woman is able to describe her infection with regard to its method of spread, therapy and comfort measures, implications for her pregnancy, and long-term implications.
- The woman gives birth to a healthy infant.

Group B Streptococcal Infection

Group B streptococcus (GBS) infection is a bacterial infection found in the lower gastrointestinal or urogenital tracts of 20% to 25% of pregnant women (Duff, 2007). Women may transmit GBS infection to their fetus in utero or during childbirth. GBS is one of the major causes of early-onset neonatal infection. Newborns become infected in one of two ways: by vertical transmission from the mother during birth or by horizontal transmission from colonized nursing personnel or colonized infants.

GBS causes severe, invasive disease in infants. In newborns, the majority of cases occur within the first week of life and are designated as early-onset disease. Late-onset disease occurs 1 week or more after birth. Early-onset GBS is often characterized by signs of serious illness including pneumonia, apnea, and shock. Infants with late-onset GBS often develop meningitis. Long-term neurologic complications are common in both types of GBS. Fortunately, improved recognition and rapid treatment of infected infants has reduced mortality and morbidity rates significantly.

Risk factors for GBS neonatal sepsis include preterm labor, maternal intrapartum fever, prolonged rupture of the membranes, previous birth of an infected infant, and GBS bacteriuria in the current pregnancy. Guidelines for the detection and preventive treatment of newborns at risk include the following (Duff, 2007):

- All pregnant women should be screened for both vaginal and rectal GBS colonization at 35 to 37 weeks' gestation. Treatment should be based on these results, even if cultures were done earlier in pregnancy.
- Positive GBS screening culture should be done during current pregnancy.

- Women with GBS in their urine in any concentration should receive antibiotic prophylaxis intrapartally because such women typically have heavy colonization with GBS and thus have an increased risk of giving birth to a newborn with early-onset disease. These women do not need vaginal and rectal cultures at 35 to 37 weeks because therapy is already indicated.
- Women who have already given birth to a newborn with invasive GBS disease should receive intrapartum antibiotic prophylaxis. Culture-based screening is not necessary for them.
- If the results of GBS screening are not known when labor begins, prophylaxis is indicated for women with any of the following risk factors: gestation less than 37 weeks, membranes ruptured 18 hours or longer, temperature equal to or greater than 38.0°C (100.4°F).

Intrapartum antibiotic therapy is recommended as follows: initial dose of penicillin G 5 million units intravenously (IV) followed by 2.5 million units IV every 4 hours until childbirth. Alternately, ampicillin 2 g initial dose IV followed by 1 g IV every 4 hours until childbirth may be used. Women at high risk for an anaphylactic reaction to penicillin because of marked allergy may be treated with clindamycin or erythromycin.

Intrapartum prophylaxis is *not* indicated for women with intact membranes who have a planned cesarean birth before labor begins, for women who had positive GBS screening culture in a previous pregnancy (but have negative cultures in the current pregnancy), and women who have negative GBS cultures in late pregnancy regardless of risk factors (Davies & Gibbs, 2008).

Human B19 Parvovirus

Human B19 parvovirus causes erythema infectiosum or fifth disease in children. It is a mild disease in adults that produces a characteristic "slapped cheek" rash. Women with school-age children are more likely to acquire parvovirus, and serologic evaluation should be performed if the pregnant woman has been exposed to a child diagnosed with fifth disease.

CRITICAL THINKING

Your friend Jena Yoo, G1P0, is 6 months pregnant and mentions to you that she is developing symptoms of a bladder infection. She has had several bladder infections over the past few years and feels she has warded off others by increasing her fluid intake and drinking acidic juices. Jena tells you that she plans to use the same approach this time because she just had her prenatal appointment last week. She assures you that if symptoms persist, she will discuss it with her caregiver at her next prenatal visit. What advice would you give her?

Answer can be found in Appendix F ∞.

Although there is a low risk of fetal morbidity, transplacental transmission is reported to be as high as 33% with a fetal loss rate of 9% (Wilkins, 2004). Fetal infection is associated with spontaneous abortion, fetal hydrops, and stillbirth (Landry, 2004). Severe effects occur most frequently with maternal infection before 20 weeks' gestation. The major fetal concern is fetal anemia, which, if left untreated, may result in death (Ramirez & Mastrobattista, 2005). Weekly measurements of peak systolic velocity of the MCA are indicated to assess for anemia. Fetal transfusion may be required to treat severe anemia.

Other Infections in Pregnancy

Table 16–1 summarizes other urinary tract, vaginal, and sexually transmitted infections that contribute to risk during pregnancy. (These are described in more detail in Chapter 6 ∞.) Spontaneous abortion is frequently the result of a severe maternal infection. Some evidence links infection and prematurity. In addition, if the pregnancy is carried to term in the presence of infection, the risk of maternal and fetal morbidity and mortality increases. Thus it is essential to maternal and fetal health that infection be diagnosed and treated promptly.

TABLE 16–1   Infections That Put Pregnancy at Risk

Condition and Causative Organism	Signs and Symptoms	Treatment	Implications for Pregnancy
Urinary Tract Infections (UTI)			
Asymptomatic bacteriuria (ASB): *Escherichia, Klebsiella, Proteus* most common	Bacteria present in urine on culture with no accompanying symptoms.	Oral sulfonamides early in pregnancy, ampicillin and nitrofurantoin (Furadantin) in late pregnancy. Antibody sensitivity results will guide the selection of an appropriate antibiotic.	Women with ASB in early pregnancy may go on to develop cystitis or acute pyelonephritis by third trimester if not treated. Oral sulfon-amides taken in the last few weeks of pregnancy may lead to neonatal hyperbilirubinemia and kernicterus.
Cystitis (lower UTI): Causative organisms same as for ASB	Dysuria, urgency, frequency; low-grade fever and hematuria may occur. Urine culture (clean catch) shows ↑ leukocytes. Presence of 10^5 (100,000) or more colonies bacteria per mL urine.	Same	If not treated, infection may ascend and lead to acute pyelonephritis.
Acute pyelonephritis: Causative organisms same as for ASB	Sudden onset. Chills, high fever, flank pain. Nausea, vomiting, malaise. May have decreased urine output, severe colicky pain, dehydration. Increased diastolic BP, positive fluorescent antibody (FA) test, low creatinine clearance. Marked bacteremia in urine culture, pyuria, WBC casts.	Hospitalization; IV antibiotic therapy. Other antibiotics safe during pregnancy include carbenicillin, methenamine, cephalosporins. Catheterization if output is ↓. Supportive therapy for comfort. Follow-up urine cultures are necessary.	Increased risk of premature birth and intrauterine growth restriction (IUGR). These antibiotics interfere with urinary estriol levels and can cause false interpretations of estriol levels during pregnancy.
Vaginal Infections			
Vulvovaginal candidiasis (yeast infection): *Candida albicans*	Often thick, white, curdy discharge, severe itching, dysuria, dyspareunia. Diagnosis based on presence of hyphae and spores in a wet-mount preparation of vaginal secretions.	Intravaginal insertion of miconazole, butoconazole, or other topical azole preparation, or clotrimazole suppositories at bedtime for 1 week. Cream may be prescribed for topical application to the vulva if necessary (CDC, 2006).	If the infection is present at birth and the fetus is born vaginally, the fetus may contract thrush.
Bacterial vaginosis: *Gardnerella vaginalis*	Thin, watery, yellow-gray discharge with foul odor often described as "fishy." Wet-mount preparation reveals "clue cells." Application of potassium hydroxide (KOH) to a specimen of vaginal secretions produces a pronounced fishy odor.	Metronidazole 250 mg PO TID × 7 days or metronidazole 500 mg PO BID × 7 days or clindamycin 300 mg PO BID × 7 days (CDC, 2006).	CDC (2006) reports that multiple studies have failed to demonstrate a teratogenic effect from metronidazole.
Trichomoniasis: *Trichomonas vaginalis*	Occasionally asymptomatic. May have frothy greenish gray vaginal discharge, pruritus, urinary symptoms. Strawberry patches may be visible on vaginal walls or cervix. Wet-mount preparation of vaginal secretions shows motile flagellated trichomonas.	Single 2 g dose of metronidazole orally (CDC, 2006).	Increased risk for PROM, preterm birth, and low birth weight.
Sexually Transmitted Infections			
Chlamydial infection: *Chlamydia trachomatis*	Women are often asymptomatic. Symptoms may include thin or purulent discharge, urinary burning and frequency, or lower abdominal pain. Lab test available to detect monoclonal antibodies specific for *Chlamydia*.	Although nonpregnant women are treated with tetracycline, it may permanently discolor fetal teeth. Thus, pregnant women are treated with azithromycin or amoxicillin followed by repeat culture in 3 weeks (CDC, 2006).	Infant of woman with untreated chlamydial infection may develop newborn conjunctivitis, which can be treated with erythromycin eye ointment (but not silver nitrate). Infant may also develop chlamydial pneumonia. May be responsible for premature labor and fetal death.
Syphilis: *Treponema pallidum*, a spirochete	Primary stage: chancre, slight fever, malaise. Chancre lasts about 4 weeks, then disappears. Secondary stage: occurs 6 weeks to 6 months after infection. Skin eruptions (condyloma lata) are also symptoms of acute arthritis, liver enlargement, iritis, chronic sore throat with hoarseness. Diagnosed by blood tests such as VDRL, RPR, FTA, ABS. Dark-field examination or spirochetes may also be done.	Treatment of pregnant woman follows the regimen recommended for the general population and is based on the stage of syphilis. For syphilis less than 1 year in duration: 2.4 million units benzathine penicillin G IM. For syphilis of more than 1 year's duration or latent syphilis of unknown duration: 2.4 million units benzathine penicillin G once a week for 3 weeks. Sexual partners should also be screened and treated (CDC, 2006).	Syphilis can be passed transplacentally to the fetus. If untreated, one of the following can occur: second trimester abortion, stillborn infant at term, congenitally infected infant, uninfected live infant.

Gonorrhea: *Neisseria gonorrhoeae*	Majority of women asymptomatic; disease often diagnosed during routine prenatal cervical culture. If symptoms are present they may include purulent vaginal discharge, dysuria, urinary frequency, inflammation, and swelling of the vulva. Cervix may appear eroded.	Nonpregnant women are treated with a single dose of ceftriaxone IM or a single dose of cefixime, ciprofloxacin, ofloxacin, or levofloxacin orally. They are also treated for chlamydia using azithromycin or doxycycline. Quinolones (ofloxacin, levofloxacin) and tetracyclines are not used to treat pregnant women. Pregnant women are treated with a cephalosporin (ceftriaxone, cefixime); if they cannot tolerate a cephalosporin, they should receive spectinomycin. The chlamydia is treated with azithromycin or amoxicillin (CDC, 2006). All sexual partners are also treated.	Infection at time of birth may cause ophthalmia neonatorum in the newborn.
Condyloma acuminata: caused by a papovavirus	Soft, grayish pink lesions on the vulva, vagina, cervix, or anus.	Podophyllin, podofilox, and imiquimod are contraindicated during pregnancy. Some caregivers recommend removing warts by surgical methods or laser because the warts can proliferate and become friable (bleed easily) during pregnancy (CDC, 2006).	Possible teratogenic effect of podophyllin. Large doses have been associated with fetal death.

CHAPTER HIGHLIGHTS

- Several health problems associated with bleeding arise from the pregnancy itself, such as spontaneous abortion, ectopic pregnancy, and gestational trophoblastic disease. The nurse needs to be alert to early signs of these situations, to guard the woman against heavy bleeding and shock, to facilitate the medical treatment, and to provide educational and emotional support.

- Ectopic pregnancy is the implantation of a fertilized ovum in a site other than the uterus. Treatment may be medical, using IM methotrexate, or surgical.

- Hyperemesis gravidarum, excessive vomiting during pregnancy, may cause fluid and electrolyte imbalance, dehydration, and signs of starvation in the mother and, if severe enough, death of the fetus. Treatment is aimed at controlling the vomiting, correcting fluid and electrolyte imbalance, correcting dehydration, and improving nutritional status.

- Hypertension may exist before pregnancy or, more often, may develop during pregnancy. Preeclampsia can lead to growth retardation for the fetus, and if untreated it may lead to convulsions (eclampsia) and even death for the mother and fetus. A woman's understanding of the disease process helps motivate her to maintain the required rest periods in the left lateral recumbent position. Antihypertensive or anticonvulsive drugs may be part of the therapy.

- Rh incompatibility can exist when an Rh-negative woman and an Rh-positive partner conceive a child who is Rh positive. The use of Rh immune globulin has greatly decreased the incidence of severe sequelae caused by Rh because the drug "tricks" the body into thinking antibodies have been produced in response to the Rh antigen.

- The impact of surgery, trauma, or battering on the pregnant woman and her fetus is related to timing in the pregnancy, seriousness of the situation, and other factors influencing the situation.

- Physical violence often begins or continues during pregnancy. The nurse needs to be alert for signs of abuse, including bruising or injury to the breasts, abdomen, or genitalia. The woman should be given information about domestic violence and about community resources available to assist her.

- Toxoplasmosis, rubella, cytomegalovirus, herpes, GBS, and other perinatal infections pose a grave threat to the fetus. Prevention is the best therapy. There is no known treatment for rubella or CMV, but antimicrobial drugs are available for toxoplasmosis, herpes, and GBS.

- Universal screening for GBS is now recommended for all pregnant women at 35 to 37 weeks' gestation.

CHAPTER REFERENCES

American Academy of Pediatrics (AAP) & American College of Obstetricians and Gynecologists (ACOG). (2007). *Guidelines for perinatal care* (6th ed.). Elk Grove Village, IL: Author.

American College of Obstetricians and Gynecologists (ACOG). (1999a). *Domestic violence* (ACOG Educational Bulletin No. 257). Washington, DC: Author.

American College of Obstetricians and Gynecologists (ACOG). (2004). *Diagnosis and treatment of gestational trophoblastic disease* (ACOG Practice Bulletin No. 53). Washington, DC: Author.

American College of Obstetricians and Gynecologists (ACOG). (2006). *Management of alloimmunization during pregnancy* (ACOG Practice Bulletin No. 75). Washington, DC: Author.

Baxter, J. K., & Weinstein, L. (2004). HELLP syndrome: The state of the art. *Obstetrical & Gynecological Survey, 59*(12), 838–845.

Bellamy, L., Casas, J. P., Hingorani, A. D., & Williams, D. J. (2007). Pre-eclampsia and risk of cardiovascular disease and cancer in later life: Systematic review and meta-analysis. *BMJ, 335,* 974–986.

Berman, M. L., Di Saia, M. J., & Tewari, K. S. (2004). Pelvic malignancies, gestational trophoblastic neoplasia, and nonpelvic malignancies. In R. K. Creasy, R. Resnik, & J. Iams (Eds.), *Maternal fetal medicine* (5th ed.). Philadelphia: W.B. Saunders.

Bess, K. A., & Wood, T. L. (2006). Understanding gestational trophoblastic disease: How nurses can help those dealing with a diagnosis. *AWHONN Lifelines, 10*(4), 321–326.

Blackburn, S. T. (2007). *Maternal, fetal, and neonatal physiology: A clinical perspective* (3rd ed.). St. Louis: Saunders.

Cappell, M. S. (2007). Hepatic and gastrointestinal diseases. In S. G. Gabbe, J. R. Niebyl, & J. L. Simpson (Eds.), *Obstetrics: Normal and problem pregnancies* (5th ed.). Philadelphia: Churchill Livingstone.

Centers for Disease Control and Prevention (CDC). (2006). Sexually transmitted diseases treatment guidelines, 2006. *Morbidity and Mortality Weekly Report, 55*(RR-11), 1–93.

Copeland, L. J., & Landon, M. B. (2007). Malignant diseases and pregnancy. In S. G. Gabbe, J. R. Niebyl, & J. L. Simpson (Eds.), *Obstetrics: Normal and problem pregnancies* (5th ed.). Philadelphia: Churchill Livingstone.

Cunningham, F. G., Leveno, K. J., Bloom, S. L., Hauth, J. C., Gilstrap III, L. C., & Wenstrom, K. D. (2005). *Williams obstetrics* (22nd ed.). New York: McGraw-Hill.

Davies, J. K., & Gibbs, R. S. (2008). Obstetric and perinatal infections. In R. S. Gibbs, B. Y. Karlan, A. F. Haney, & I. E. Nygaard (Eds.), *Danforth's obstetrics and gynecology* (10th ed.). Philadelphia: Wolters Kluwer/Lippincott Williams & Wilkins.

Dodds, L., Fell, D. B., Joseph, K. S., Allen, V. M., & Butler, B. (2006). Outcomes of pregnancy complicated by hyperemesis gravidarum. *Obstetrics and Gynecology, 107,* 285–292.

Duff, P. (2007). Maternal and perinatal infection–bacterial. In S. G. Gabbe, J. R. Niebyl, & J. L. Simpson (Eds.), *Obstetrics: Normal and problem pregnancies* (5th ed.). Philadelphia: Churchill Livingstone.

Easterwood, B. (2004). Silent lullabies: Helping parents cope with early pregnancy loss. *AWHONN Lifelines, 8*(4), 356–360.

Gibbs, R. S., Sweet, R. L., & Duff, W. P. (2004). Maternal and fetal infectious disorders. In R. K. Creasy, R. Resnik, & J. Iams (Eds.), *Maternal fetal medicine* (5th ed.). Philadelphia: W.B. Saunders.

Gonik, B., & Foley, M. R. (2004). Intensive care monitoring of the critically ill pregnant patient. In R. K. Creasy, R. Resnik, & J. Iams (Eds.), *Maternal fetal medicine* (5th ed.). Philadelphia: W.B. Saunders.

Habli, M., & Sibai, B. M. (2008). Hypertensive disorders of pregnancy. In R. S. Gibbs, B. Y. Karlan, A. F. Haney, & I. E. Nygaard (Eds.), *Danforth's obstetrics and gynecology* (10th ed.). Philadelphia: Wolters Kluwer/Lippincott Williams & Wilkins.

Harville, E. W., Wilcox, A. J., Bird, D. D., & Weinberg, C. R. (2004). Vaginal bleeding in very early pregnancy. *Obstetrical & Gynecological Survey, 59*(3), 172–173.

Hill, J., & Roberts, S. (2005). Herpes simplex virus in pregnancy: New concepts in prevention and management. *Clinics in Perinatology, 32*(3), 657–670.

Hollier, L. M., & Grissom, H. (2005). Human herpes viruses in pregnancy: Cytomegalovirus, Epstein-Barr virus, and varicella zoster virus. *Clinics in Perinatology, 32*(3), 671–696.

Kady, D. E., Gilbert, W. M., Xing, G., & Smith, L. H. (2005). Maternal and neonatal outcomes of assaults during pregnancy. *Obstetrics & Gynecology, 105*(2), 357–363.

Katz, V., Balderston, K., & DeFreest, M. (2005). Perimortem cesarean delivery: Were our assumptions correct? *American Journal of Obstetrics & Gynecology, 192*(6), 1916–1921.

Lagiou, P., Tamimi, R., Mucci, L. A., Trichopoulos, D., Adami, H-O., & Shieh, C-C. (2003). Nausea and vomiting in pregnancy in relation to prolactin, estrogen, and progesterone: A prospective study. *Obstetrics & Gynecology, 101*(4), 639–644.

Landry, M. L. (2004). Viral infections. In G. N. Burrow, T. P. Duffy, & J.A. Copel (Eds.), *Medical complications during pregnancy* (6th ed.). Philadelphia, PA: Elsevier Saunders.

Li, A. J. (2008). Gestational trophoblastic neoplasms. In R. S. Gibbs, B. Y. Karlan, A. F. Haney, & I. E. Nygaard (Eds.), *Danforth's obstetrics and gynecology* (10th ed.). Philadelphia: Wolters Kluwer/Lippincott Williams & Wilkins.

Li, D., Janevic, T., Odouli, R., & Liyan, L. (2003). Hot tub use during pregnancy and the risk of miscarriage. *American Journal of Epidemiology, 158,* 931–937.

Lipscomb, G. H., Givens, V. M., Meyer, N. L., & Bran, D. (2005). Comparison of multidose and single-dose methotrexate protocols for the treatment of ectopic pregnancy. *American Journal of Obstetrics & Gynecology, 192*(6), 1844–1848.

McLean, L. K., Hedrianna, H. L., Lanouette, J. M., & Haesslein, H. C. (2004). A retrospective review of isoimmunized pregnancies managed by middle cerebral artery peak systolic velocity. *American Journal of Obstetrics & Gynecology, 190*(6), 1732–1738.

Montoya, J. G., & Rosso, F. (2005). Diagnosis and management of toxoplasmosis. *Clinics in Perinatology, 32*(3), 705–726.

Ramirez, M. M., & Mastrobattista, J. M. (2005). Diagnosis and management of human parvovirus B19 infection. *Clinics in Perinatology, 32*(3), 697–704.

Schauberger, C. W., Mathiason, M. A., & Rooney, B. L. (2005). Ultrasound assessment of first-trimester bleeding. *Obstetrics & Gynecology, 105*(2), 333–338.

Scott, L. D., & Abu-Hamda, E. (2004). Gastrointestinal disease in pregnancy. In R. K. Creasy, R. Resnik, & J. Iams (Eds.), *Maternal fetal medicine* (5th ed.). Philadelphia: W.B. Saunders.

Seeber, B. E., & Barnhart, K. T. (2008). Ectopic pregnancy. In R. S. Gibbs, B. Y. Karlan, A. F. Haney, & I. E. Nygaard (Eds.), *Danforth's obstetrics and gynecology* (10th ed.). Philadelphia: Wolters Kluwer/Lippincott Williams & Wilkins.

Shaver, S. M. (2004). Isoimmunization in pregnancy. *Critical Care Nursing Clinics of North America, 16,* 205–209.

Sibai, B. M. (2005). Diagnosis, prevention, and management of eclampsia. *Obstetrics and Gynecology, 105*(2), 402–410.

Sibai, B. M. (2007). Hypertension. In S. G. Gabbe, J. R. Niebyl, & J. L. Simpson (Eds.), *Obstetrics: Normal and problem pregnancies* (5th ed.). Philadelphia: Churchill Livingstone.

Simpson, J. L., & Jauniaux, R. M. (2007). Pregnancy loss. In S. G. Gabbe, J. R. Niebyl, & J. L. Simpson (Eds.), *Obstetrics: Normal and problem pregnancies* (5th ed.). Philadelphia: Churchill Livingstone.

Van Den Eeden, S. K., Shan, J., Bruce, C., & Glasser, M. (2005). Ectopic pregnancy rate and treatment utilization in a large managed care organization. *Obstetrics & Gynecology, 105*(5), pt. 1, 1052–1057.

Wiggens, D. A., & Elliott, M. (2005). Outcomes of pregnancies achieved by donor egg in vitro fertilization—A comparison with standard in vitro fertilization pregnancies. *American Journal of Obstetrics and Gynecology, 192*(6), 2002–2008.

Wilkins, I. (2004). Nonimmune hydrops. In R. K. Creasy, R. Resnik, & J. Iams (Eds.), *Maternal fetal medicine* (5th ed.). Philadelphia: W.B. Saunders.

PART FOUR

Birth and the Family

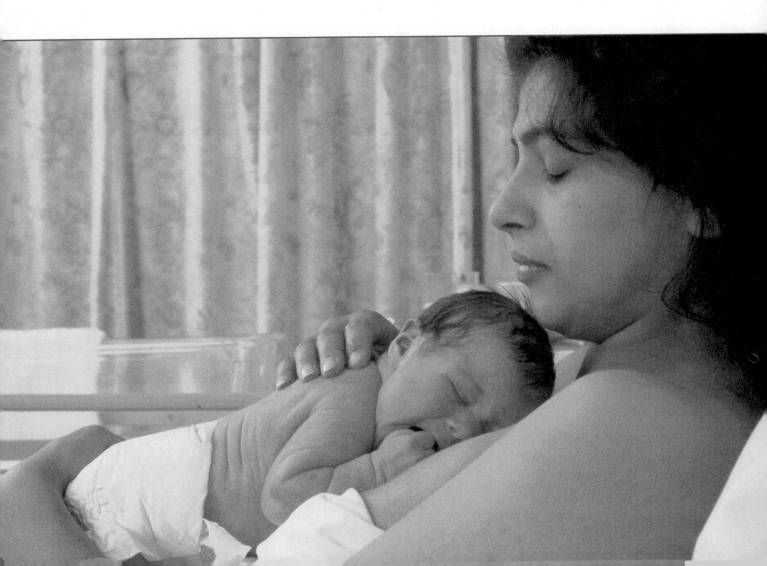

CHAPTER 17

Processes and Stages of Labor and Birth

There is no doubt in my mind that I have the most wonderful job in nursing! What an enormous privilege to be allowed to share in the birth of a new life, in the birth of a new family. The sheer miracle of it never ceases to amaze and humble me. I only hope that I am able to demonstrate that sense of awe and respect even when things don't go as we would expect or like to see them.

—A Labor and Delivery Nurse

LEARNING OUTCOMES

17-1. Describe the five critical factors that influence labor in the assessment of an expectant woman's and fetus's progress in labor and birth.

17-2. Summarize the implications of abnormalities present in each of the five critical factors on the outcome of labor and the health of the expectant woman and the fetus.

17-3. Examine an expectant woman's and fetus's response to labor based on the physiological processes that occur during labor.

17-4. Assess for the premonitory signs of labor when caring for the expectant woman.

17-5. Differentiate between false and true labor in an expectant woman.

17-6. Describe the physiologic and psychologic changes occurring in an expectant woman during each stage of labor in the nursing care management of the expectant woman.

17-7. Predict an expectant mother's progression through the various stages of labor based on assessment data.

17-8. Explain the maternal systemic response to labor in the nursing care of an expectant woman.

17-9. Examine fetal responses to labor.

KEY TERMS

Artificial rupture of membranes (AROM) **388**
Asynclitism **379**
Bloody show **386**
Braxton Hicks contractions **386**
Cardinal movements **390**
Crowning **389**
Duration **381**
Effacement **385**
Engagement **379**

In the final weeks of pregnancy, both mother and baby begin to prepare for birth. The fetus develops and grows in readiness for life outside of the womb. At the same time, the expectant woman undergoes various physiologic and psychologic changes that prepare her for childbirth and for the role of mother.

During labor, a woman instinctively knows she is engaging in one of the most important tasks she will ever do. A precious life is about to emerge. In those hours and moments the birth process may seem to carry all the power in the universe. The mother-to-be and her partner may be stretched beyond all of their normal limits of concentration, purpose, endurance, and pain. The dynamic nature of this experience is what makes the birth of a baby both a physiologic and a psychologic transition into parenthood.

Critical Factors in Labor

Five factors are important in the process of labor and birth: the passage, the fetus, the relationship between the passage and the fetus, the physiologic forces of labor, and the psychosocial considerations. The progress of labor is critically dependent on the complementary relationship of these five factors, which are described in this section and are summarized in the accompanying Key Facts to Remember: Critical Factors in Labor. Abnormalities affecting any one of these factors can alter the outcome of labor and jeopardize both the expectant woman and her baby. Complications of labor and birth are discussed in Chapter 22 ∞.

The Birth Passage

The true pelvis, which forms the bony canal through which the fetus must pass, is divided into three sections: the inlet, the pelvic cavity (midpelvis), and the outlet. (See Chapter 3 ∞ for a discussion of the pelvis and Chapter 10 ∞ for assessment techniques.)

The Caldwell-Moloy classification of pelvises is widely used to differentiate bony pelvis types. The four classic types of pelvis are *gynecoid, android, anthropoid,* and *platypelloid* (Figure 17–1 ■). The gynecoid, or female, pelvis is most common, and all of its diameters are adequate for childbirth. Implications of each type of pelvis for childbirth are summarized in Table 17–1.

KEY FACTS TO REMEMBER
Critical Factors in Labor

1. Birth passage
   a. Size of the maternal pelvis (diameters of the pelvic inlet, midpelvis, and outlet)
   b. Type of maternal pelvis (gynecoid, android, anthropoid, platypelloid, or a combination)
   c. Ability of the cervix to dilate and efface and ability of the vaginal canal and the external opening of the vagina (the introitus) to distend
2. Fetus
   a. Fetal head (size and presence of molding)
   b. Fetal attitude (flexion or extension of the fetal body and extremities)
   c. Fetal lie
   d. Fetal presentation (the body part of the fetus entering the pelvis in a single or multiple pregnancy)
3. The relationship between the passage and the fetus
   a. Engagement of the fetal presenting part
   b. Station (location of fetal presenting part in the maternal pelvis)
   c. Fetal position (relationship of the presenting part to one of the four quadrants of the maternal pelvis)
4. Physiologic forces of labor
   a. Frequency, duration, and intensity of uterine contractions as the fetus moves through the passage
   b. Effectiveness of the maternal pushing effort
5. Psychosocial considerations
   a. Mental and physical preparation for childbirth
   b. Sociocultural values and beliefs
   c. Previous childbirth experience
   d. Support from significant others
   e. Emotional status

The Fetus

Several aspects of the fetal body and position are critical to the outcome of labor. Primary among these are the size and the orientation of the fetal head.

Fetal Head

The fetal head is the least compressible and largest part of the fetus. Once it has been born, the birth of the rest of the body is rarely delayed. The fetal skull (cranium) has three major parts: the face, the base of the skull, and the vault of the cranium (roof). The bones of the face and cranial base are well fused and essentially fixed. The base of the cranium

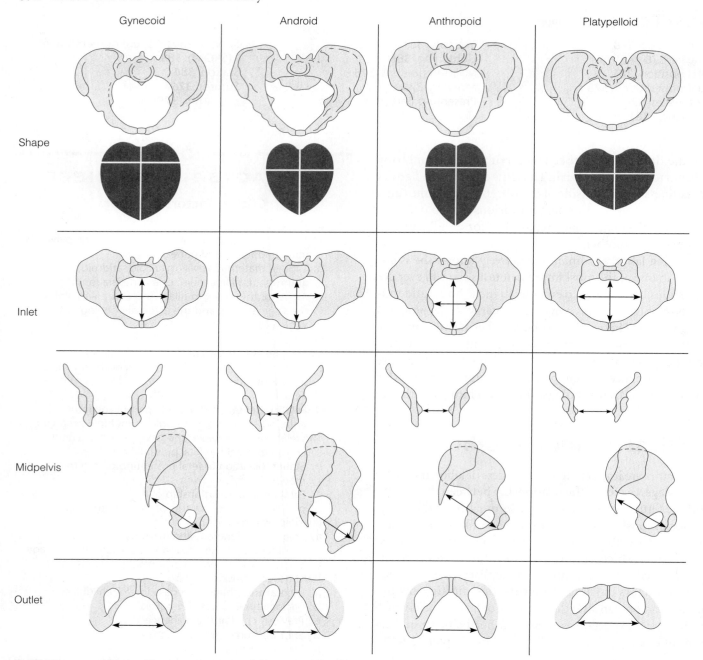

FIGURE 17–1 Comparison of Caldwell-Moloy pelvic types.

is composed of the two temporal bones, each with a sphenoid and ethmoid bone. The bones composing the vault are the two frontal bones, the two parietal bones, and the occipital bone (Figure 17–2 ■). These bones are not fused, allowing this portion of the head to adjust in shape as the presenting part passes through the narrow portions of the pelvis. The cranial bones overlap under pressure of the powers of labor and the demands of the unyielding pelvis. This overlapping is called **molding**.

The **sutures** of the fetal skull are membranous spaces between the cranial bones. The intersections of these sutures are called **fontanelles**. Cranial sutures allow for molding of the fetal head and help the clinician to identify the position of the fetal head during vaginal examination. The important sutures of the cranial vault are as follows (see Figure 17–2):

- *Frontal (mitotic) suture.* Located between the two frontal bones, this becomes the anterior continuation of the sagittal suture.
- *Sagittal suture.* Located between the parietal bones, this divides the skull into left and right halves; it runs anteroposteriorly, connecting the two fontanelles.
- *Coronal suture.* Located between the frontal and parietal bones, this extends transversely left and right from the anterior fontanelle.

TABLE 17–1	Implications of Pelvic Type for Labor and Birth	
Pelvic Type	**Pertinent Characteristics**	**Implications for Birth**
Gynecoid	Inlet rounded with all inlet diameters adequate Midpelvis diameters adequate with parallel side walls Outlet adequate	Favorable for vaginal birth
Android	Inlet heart-shaped with short posterior sagittal diameter Midpelvis diameters reduced Outlet capacity reduced	Not favorable for vaginal birth Descent into pelvis is slow
Anthropoid	Inlet oval in shape, with long anteroposterior diameter Midpelvis diameters adequate Outlet adequate	Favorable for vaginal birth
Platypelloid	Inlet oval in shape, with long transverse diameters Midpelvis diameters reduced Outlet capacity inadequate	Not favorable for vaginal birth Fetal head engages in transverse position Difficult descent through midpelvis Frequent delay of progress at outlet of pelvis

Note: Description of pelvic shape is exaggerated for easier comprehension.

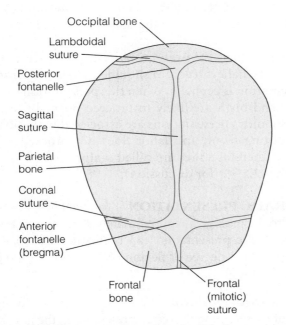

FIGURE 17–2 Superior view of the fetal skull.

- *Lambdoidal suture.* Located between the two parietal bones and the occipital bone, this extends transversely left and right from the posterior fontanelle.

The anterior and posterior fontanelles are clinically useful (along with the sutures) in identifying the position of the fetal head in the pelvis and in assessing the status of the newborn after birth. The anterior fontanelle is diamond shaped and measures about 2 by 3 cm (0.8 to 1.2 in.). It permits growth of the brain by remaining unossified for as long as 18 months. The posterior fontanelle is much smaller and closes within 8 to 12 weeks after birth. It is shaped like a small triangle and marks the meeting point of the sagittal suture and the lambdoidal suture (Blackburn, 2007).

Following are several important landmarks of the fetal skull (Figure 17–3 ■):

- *Mentum.* This is the fetal chin.
- *Sinciput.* This anterior area is known as the brow.
- *Bregma.* This is a large diamond-shaped anterior fontanelle.
- *Vertex.* This is the area between the anterior and posterior fontanelles.
- *Posterior fontanelle.* This is the intersection between posterior cranial sutures.
- *Occiput.* This is the area of the fetal skull occupied by the occipital bone, beneath the posterior fontanelle.

The diameters of the fetal skull vary considerably within normal limits. Some diameters shorten and others lengthen as the head is molded during labor. Fetal head diameters are measured between the various landmarks on the skull. For example, the suboccipitobregmatic diameter

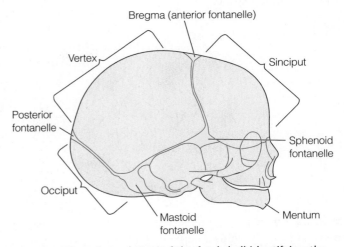

FIGURE 17–3 Lateral view of the fetal skull identifying the landmarks that have significance during birth.

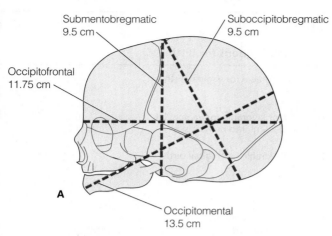

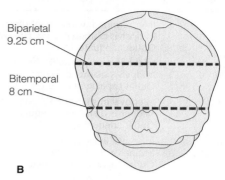

FIGURE 17–4 *A,* Anteroposterior diameters of the fetal skull. When the vertex of the fetus presents and the fetal head is flexed with the chin to the chest, the smallest anteroposterior diameter (suboccipitobregmatic) enters the birth canal. *B,* Transverse diameters of the fetal skull.

is the distance from the undersurface of the occiput to the center of the bregma, or anterior fontanelle. Typical fetal skull measurements are given in Figure 17–4 ■.

Fetal Attitude

Fetal attitude refers to the relation of the fetal parts to one another. The normal attitude of the fetus is one of moderate flexion of the head, flexion of the arms onto the chest, and flexion of the legs onto the abdomen (Figure 17–5 ■).

Fetal Lie

Fetal lie refers to the relationship of the cephalocaudal (spinal column) axis of the fetus to the cephalocaudal axis of the woman. The fetus may assume either a longitudinal (in an up-and-down position or vertical position) or a transverse lie (horizontal or side-to-side position). A longitudinal lie occurs when the cephalocaudal axis of the fetus is parallel to the woman's spine. A transverse lie occurs when the cephalocaudal axis of the fetus is at a right angle to the woman's spine.

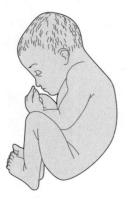

FIGURE 17–5 Fetal attitude. The attitude (or relationship of body parts) of this fetus is normal. The head is flexed forward with the chin almost resting on the chest. The arms and legs are flexed.

FETAL PRESENTATION **Fetal presentation** is determined by fetal lie and by the body part of the fetus that enters the pelvic passage first. This portion of the fetus is referred to as the **presenting part**. Fetal presentation may be cephalic, breech, or shoulder. The most common presentation is cephalic. When this presentation occurs, labor and birth are likely to proceed normally. Breech and shoulder presentations are associated with difficulties during labor, and labor does not proceed as expected; therefore, they are called **malpresentations** (see Chapter 22 ∞ for discussion).

CEPHALIC PRESENTATION The fetal head presents itself to the passage in approximately 97% of term births. The cephalic presentation can be further classified according to the degree of flexion or extension of the fetal head (attitude).

Vertex presentation Vertex is the most common type of presentation. In vertex presentation, the fetal head is completely flexed onto the chest, and the smallest diameter of the fetal head (suboccipitobregmatic) presents to the maternal pelvis (Figure 17–6A ■). The occiput is the presenting part.

Military presentation In military presentation, the fetal head is neither flexed nor extended. The occipitofrontal diameter presents to the maternal pelvis (Figure 17–6B); the top of the head is the presenting part.

Brow presentation In brow presentation, the fetal head is partially extended. The occipitomental diameter, the largest anteroposterior diameter, is presented to the maternal pelvis (Figure 17–6C); the sinciput is the presenting part (refer to Figure 17–3).

Face presentation In face presentation, the fetal head is hyperextended (complete extension). The sub-

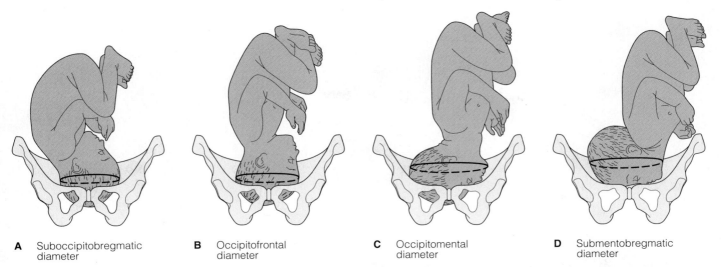

A Suboccipitobregmatic diameter   **B** Occipitofrontal diameter   **C** Occipitomental diameter   **D** Submentobregmatic diameter

FIGURE 17–6 Cephalic presentation. *A*, Vertex presentation. Complete flexion of the head allows the suboccipitobregmatic diameter to present to the pelvis. *B*, Military (median vertex) presentation with no flexion or extension. The occipitofrontal diameter presents to the pelvis. *C*, Brow presentation. The fetal head is in partial (halfway) extension. The occipitomental diameter, which is the largest diameter of the fetal head, presents to the pelvis. *D*, Face presentation. The fetal head is in complete extension, and the submentobregmatic diameter presents to the pelvis.

mentobregmatic diameter presents to the maternal pelvis (Figure 17–6D); the face is the presenting part.

BREECH PRESENTATION Breech presentations occur in 3% to 4% of all births (Royal College of Obstetricians & Gynaecologists, 2006). These presentations are classified according to the attitude of the fetus's hips and knees. In all variations of the breech presentation, the sacrum is the landmark to be noted.

Complete breech In complete breech, the fetal knees and hips are both flexed; the thighs are on the abdomen, and the calves are on the posterior aspect of the thighs. The buttocks and feet of the fetus present to the maternal pelvis (refer to Chapter 22, Figure 22–7 ∞).

Frank breech In frank breech, the fetal hips are flexed, and the knees are extended. The buttocks of the fetus present to the maternal pelvis.

Footling breech In footling breech, the fetal hips and legs are extended, and the feet of the fetus present to the maternal pelvis. In a single footling, one foot presents; in a double footling, both feet present.

SHOULDER PRESENTATION A shoulder presentation is also called a transverse lie. Most frequently, the shoulder is the presenting part and the acromion process of the scapula is the landmark to be noted. However, the fetal arm, back, abdomen, or side may present in a transverse lie. The incidence of shoulder presentation is 0.3% of all births (Family Practice Notebook, 2008). (See Chapter 22 ∞ for further discussion of transverse lie.)

Relationship of Maternal Pelvis and Presenting Part

We have discussed the birth passage and the fetus, but the third critical factor is the relationship between these two. When assessing the relationship of the maternal pelvis and the presenting part of the fetal body, the nurse considers engagement, station, and fetal position.

Engagement

Engagement of the presenting part occurs when the largest diameter of the presenting part reaches or passes through the pelvic inlet (Figure 17–7 ■). Whereas engagement confirms the adequacy of the pelvic inlet, it does not indicate whether the midpelvis and outlet are also adequate.

Engagement can be determined by vaginal examinations and leopold's maneuvers. (See Chapter 18 ∞ for assessment techniques.) In primigravidas, engagement occurs approximately 2 weeks before term. Multiparas, however, may experience engagement several weeks before the onset of labor or during the process of labor.

Another variable of engagement is the relationship of the fetal sagittal suture to the mother's symphysis pubis and sacrum. The terms *synclitism* and *asynclitism* describe this relationship. **Synclitism** occurs when the sagittal suture is midway between the symphysis pubis and the sacral promontory. Upon vaginal examination, the suture feels midline between these two maternal landmarks and feels as though it is in alignment. **Asynclitism** occurs when the sagittal suture is directed toward either the symphysis pubis or the sacral promontory and feels misaligned. Upon vaginal examination,

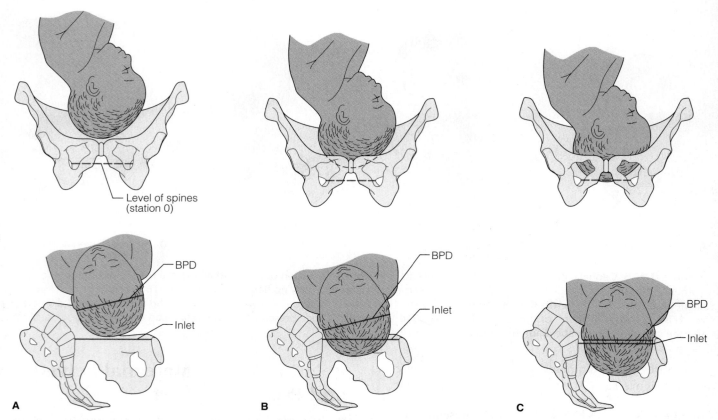

FIGURE 17–7 Process of engagement in cephalic presentation. *A,* Floating. The fetal head is directed down toward the pelvis but can still easily move away from the inlet. *B,* Dipping. The fetal head dips into the inlet but can be moved away by exerting pressure on the fetus. *C,* Engaged. The biparietal diameter (BPD) of the fetal head is in the inlet of the pelvis. In most instances, the presenting part (occiput) will be at the level of the ischial spines (0 station).

the suture feels somewhat turned to one side within the pelvis, making it asymmetrical. Asynclitism can be either anterior or posterior. It is important to identify asynclitism, because it can lengthen the time of descent or interfere with the descent process. Sometimes, this can lead to the inability of the fetal head to fit through the birth canal and can result in the need for a cesarean birth.

Station

Station refers to the relationship of the presenting part to an imaginary line drawn between the ischial spines of the maternal pelvis. In a normal pelvis, the ischial spines mark the narrowest diameter through which the fetus must pass. These spines are not sharp protrusions that harm the fetus, but blunted prominences at the midpelvis. As a landmark, the ischial spines have been designated as zero (0) station (Figure 17–8 ■). If the presenting part is higher than the ischial spines, a negative number is assigned, noting centimeters above zero (0) station. Engagement is represented when the fetal head reaches the 0 station. Positive numbers indicate that the presenting part has passed the ischial spines. Station −5 is at the pelvic inlet, and station +5 is at the outlet.

During labor, the presenting part should move progressively from the negative stations to the midpelvis at zero (0)

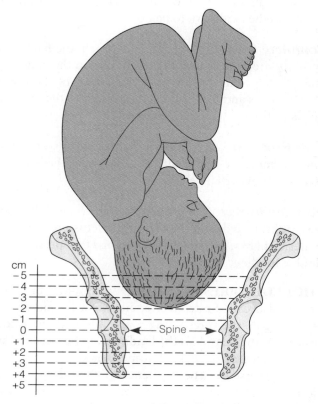

FIGURE 17–8 Measuring the station of the fetal head while it is descending. In this view the station is −2/−3.

station and into the positive stations. If the presenting part can be seen at the woman's perineum, birth is imminent. Failure of the presenting part to descend in the presence of strong contractions may be caused by disproportion between the maternal pelvis and fetal presenting part, malpresentation, asynclitism, or multiple fetuses. Station is determined by vaginal examination. (See Chapter 18 ∞ for assessment techniques.)

Fetal Position

Fetal position refers to the relationship between a designated landmark on the presenting fetal part and the front, sides, or back of the maternal pelvis. The chosen landmarks differ according to presentation:

- The landmark for vertex presentations is the occiput.
- The landmark for face presentations is the mentum.
- The landmark for breech presentations is the sacrum.
- The landmark for shoulder presentations is the acromion process on the scapula.

To determine position, the nurse notes which quadrant of the maternal pelvis the appropriate landmark is directed toward: the left anterior, right anterior, left posterior, or right posterior. If the landmark is directed toward the side of the pelvis, fetal position is designated as *transverse*, rather than anterior or posterior. In documentation, the following abbreviations are used:

1. Right (R) or left (L) side of the maternal pelvis
2. The landmark of the fetal presenting part: occiput (O), mentum (M), sacrum (S), or acromion process (A)
3. Anterior (A), posterior (P), or transverse (T), depending on whether the landmark is in the front, back, or side of the pelvis

These abbreviations help the healthcare team communicate the fetal position. Thus when the fetal occiput is directed toward the back and to the left of the birth passage, the abbreviation used is LOP (left-occiput-posterior). The term *dorsal* (D) is used when denoting the fetal position in a transverse lie; it refers to the fetal back. Thus RADA indicates that the acromion process of the scapula is directed toward the woman's right and the fetus's back is anterior.

The most common fetal position is occiput anterior. When this position occurs, labor and birth are likely to proceed normally. Positions other than occiput anterior are more frequently associated with problems during labor; therefore they are called malpositions (see Chapter 22 ∞). The most commonly occurring positions and malpositions are illustrated in Figure 17–9 ■.

Assessment techniques to determine fetal position include inspection and palpation of the maternal abdomen and vaginal examination. They are discussed in Chapter 18 ∞.

Physiologic Forces of Labor

Primary and secondary forces work together to achieve birth of the fetus, the fetal membranes, and the placenta. The *primary force* is uterine muscular contractions, which cause the changes of the first stage of labor—complete effacement and dilatation of the cervix. The *secondary force* is the use of abdominal muscles to push during the second stage of labor. The pushing adds to the primary force after full dilatation.

Contractions

In labor, uterine contractions are rhythmic but intermittent. Between contractions there is a period of relaxation. This allows uterine muscles to rest and provides respite for the laboring woman. It also restores uteroplacental circulation, which is important to fetal oxygenation and adequate circulation in the uterine blood vessels.

Each contraction has three phases. These are (1) *increment,* the building up of the contraction (the longest phase); (2) *acme,* or the peak of the contraction; and (3) *decrement,* or the letting up of the contraction.

When describing uterine contractions during labor, caregivers use the terms *frequency, duration, and intensity* (Figure 17–10 ■). **Frequency** refers to the time between the beginning of one contraction and the beginning of the next contraction. **Duration** is measured from the beginning of a contraction to the completion of that same contraction. **Intensity** refers to the strength of the contraction during acme. In most instances intensity is estimated by palpating the uterine fundus during a contraction, but it may be measured directly with an intrauterine catheter. When estimating intensity by palpation, the nurse determines whether it is mild, moderate, or strong by judging how indentable the uterine wall is during the acme of a contraction. If the uterine wall can be indented easily, the contraction is considered mild. Strong intensity exists when the uterine wall cannot be indented. Moderate intensity falls between these two ranges. When intensity is measured with an intrauterine catheter, the normal resting pressure in the uterus (between contractions) averages 10 to 12 mm Hg. During acme the intensity ranges from 25 to 40 mm Hg in early labor, 50 to 70 mm Hg in active labor, 70 to 90 mm Hg during transition, and 70 to 100 mm Hg while the woman is pushing in the second stage (Funai, Evans, & Lockwood, 2008). (See Chapter 18 ∞ for further discussion of assessment techniques.)

At the beginning of labor, the contractions are usually mild. As labor progresses, the duration of the contractions, intensity, and frequency increase. Because the contractions are involuntary, the laboring woman cannot control their duration, frequency, or intensity.

MyNursingKit | First and Second Stages of Labor

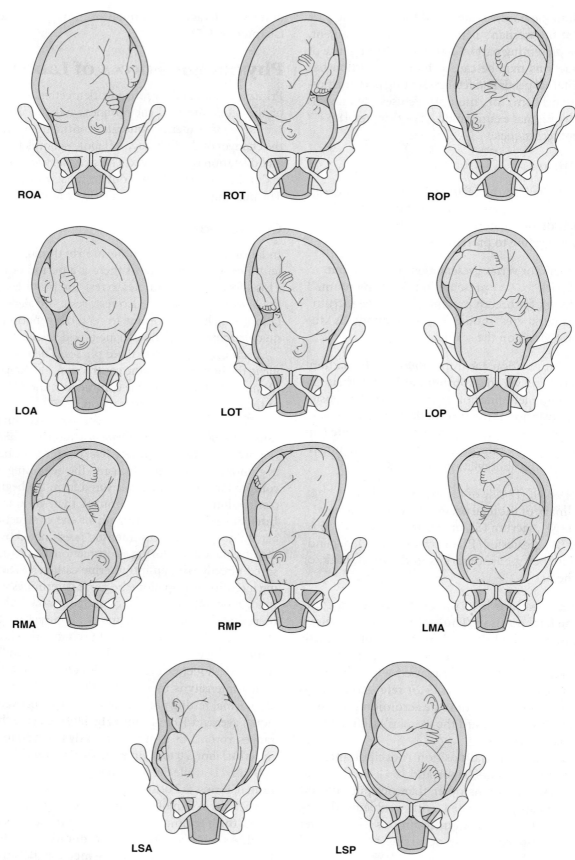

FIGURE 17–9 Categories of presentation.
Source: Ross Laboratories, Columbus, OH.

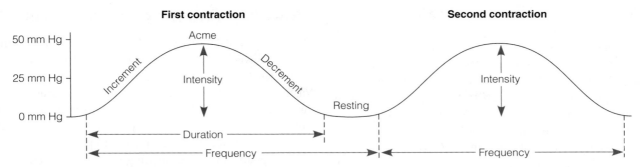

FIGURE 17–10 Characteristics of uterine contractions.

Bearing Down

After the cervix is completely dilated, the maternal abdominal muscles contract as the woman pushes. This pushing action (called *bearing down*) aids in expulsion of the fetus and placenta. If the cervix is not completely dilated, however, bearing down can cause cervical edema (which retards dilatation), possible tearing and bruising of the cervix, and maternal exhaustion.

Psychosocial Considerations

Thus far, the discussion has focused on physical influences on labor outcomes. However the final critical factor is the parents' psychosocial readiness, including their fears, anxieties, birth fantasies, excitement level, feelings of joy and anticipation, and level of social support. Similar psychosocial factors affect the mother and the father. Both are making a transition into a new role, and both have expectations of themselves during the labor and birth experience, as caregivers for their child and their new family. Psychosocial factors affecting labor and birth include the couple's accomplishment of the tasks of pregnancy, usual coping mechanisms in response to stressful life events, support system, preparation for childbirth, and cultural influences. Even mothers and fathers who attend childbirth preparation classes and have a solid support system can be concerned about what labor will be like. Many couples, even in the intense happiness and excitement of the event, may be concerned about whether they will be able to perform the way they expect, whether the pain will be more than the mother expects or can cope with, and whether the father can provide helpful support. Although birth is usually a happy and joyful event, it is a physical and emotional stress. Whether stress is positive or negative, it still can impact a couple's responses to the labor itself.

A woman approaching her first labor faces a totally new experience, and the woman who has given birth before knows that this labor might be very different from her past experience. Most women wonder if they will live up to their expectations for themselves; whether they will be physically injured through laceration, episiotomy, or cesarean inci-

sion; and whether significant others will be supportive. Many women are excited and happy that labor has occurred, even if they have concerns about the labor process itself.

Expectant women mentally prepare for labor through meaningful action and imaginary rehearsal. The actions frequently consist of "nesting behavior" (housecleaning, decorating the nursery) and a "psyching up" for the labor, which varies depending on the woman's self-confidence, self-esteem, and previous experiences with stress. Specific actions to prepare for labor may focus on becoming better informed and prepared. In addition, just as a woman tries on the maternal role during pregnancy, fantasizing about labor seems to help her understand and become better prepared for it. Fantasies about the excitement of the baby's birth and the sharing of the experience involve the woman in constructive preparation. Many pregnant women have dreams about their infant, labor, birth, and parenting. These dreams may result from sleep deprivation, rapid eye movement sleep deprivation, and altered hormone levels (Nielson & Paquette, 2007).

Some women may fear the pain of contractions, whereas others welcome the opportunity to feel the birth process. Some women view the pain as threatening and associate it with a loss of control over their bodies and emotions. Other women see pain as a rite of passage into motherhood and a necessary means to an end. It is helpful for women to realize that the pain of labor is natural. Assurances that labor is progressing normally can go a long way toward reducing anxiety and thereby reducing pain, and providing positive reinforcement that the mother is doing "a good job." Empowerment and having control over one's body plays a key role in determining whether the woman views her labor and birth positively (Hardin & Buckner, 2005). Women who viewed their births as a positive experience were also more likely to have a sense of well-being about themselves after the experience (Hardin & Buckner, 2005). Some women view the birth experience as a challenge in which they will have the opportunity to succeed and provide their baby with joyful reception into the world. A wide variety of coping techniques to assist both the laboring woman and her partner are discussed in Chapters 19 and 20 ∞.

The laboring woman's support system also influences the course of labor and birth. Some women prefer not to have a support person or family member with them. For some, the birth process is a private moment that the woman may wish to reserve for herself. However, most women choose to have significant persons (family members, father, and friend) with them during labor and birth. Social support tends to have a positive effect. For some families, the birth event is a celebration in which they may want as many significant others present as possible. Some women may want to create a joyful festive atmosphere that includes the grandparents, friends, and other children. A labor partner's presence at the bedside provides a means to enhance communication and to demonstrate feelings of love. Communication needs may include talking and the use of affectionate and reassuring words from the partner. Affection may take the form of holding hands, hugging, or touching or gentle reassurance for the woman.

How the woman views the birth experience in hindsight may affect her mothering behaviors. It appears that any activities by the expectant woman or by healthcare providers that enhance the birth experience will be beneficial to the mother-baby connection. Some studies have shown that when some women are disappointed with their birth experience, they may have some initial difficulties and be more prone to postpartum mood disorders (Bryant, Porter, Tracy et al., 2007; Lobel & DeLuca, 2007). The father's experience of the birth and his opportunities for bonding may have important implications for fathering as well (Goodman, 2005). Psychosocial factors associated with a positive birth experience are summarized in Table 17–2.

The Physiology of Labor

In addition to considering the five critical factors affecting the progress of labor and birth, it is essential to explore the physiology of the normal birth experience.

TABLE 17–2	Factors Associated with a Positive Birth Experience

Motivation for the pregnancy

Attendance at childbirth education classes

A sense of competence or mastery

Self-confidence and self-esteem

Feelings of empowerment

Positive relationship with mate

Maintaining control during labor

Support from mate or other person during labor

Not being left alone in labor

Trust in the medical/nursing staff

Having personal control of breathing patterns, comfort measures

Choosing a physician/certified nurse-midwife who has a similar philosophy of care

Receiving clear information regarding procedures

Possible Causes of Labor Onset

The process of labor usually begins between the 38th and the 42nd week of gestation, when the fetus is mature and ready for birth. Despite research, the exact cause of labor onset is not clearly understood. However, some important aspects have been identified: progesterone relaxes smooth muscle tissue, estrogen stimulates uterine muscle contractions, and connective tissue loosens to permit the softening, thinning, and eventual opening of the cervix (Blackburn, 2007). Currently, researchers are focusing on the role of fetal membranes (chorion and amnion), the decidua, and the effect of progesterone withdrawal, of prostaglandin, and of corticotropin-releasing hormone in relation to labor onset (Blackburn, 2007).

Progesterone Withdrawal Hypothesis

Progesterone, produced by the placenta, relaxes uterine smooth muscle by interfering with the conduction of impulses from one cell to the next. Therefore during pregnancy, progesterone exerts a quieting effect and the uterus generally is without coordinated contractions. Toward the end of gestation, biochemical changes decrease the availability of progesterone to myometrial cells and may be associated with an antiprogestin that inhibits the relaxant effect but allows other progesterone actions such as lactogenesis. With the decreased availability of progesterone, estrogen is better able to stimulate contractions (Blackburn, 2007). Progesterone administration is now used as a mechanism to prevent preterm labor and childbirth (Szekeres-Bartho, Wilczynski, Basta et al., 2008).

Prostaglandin Hypothesis

Although the exact relationship between prostaglandin and the onset of labor is not yet known, the effect is clinically demonstrated by the successful induction of labor after vaginal application of prostaglandin E. In addition, preterm labor may be stopped by using an inhibitor of prostaglandin synthesis (Challis, 2004).

The amnion and decidua are the focus of research on the source of prostaglandins. Once prostaglandin is produced, stimuli for its synthesis may include rising levels of estrogen, decreased availability of progesterone, and increased levels of oxytocin, platelet-activating factor, and endothelin-1 (Challis, 2004).

Corticotropin-Releasing Hormone Hypothesis

Corticotropin-releasing hormone (CRH) increases throughout pregnancy, with a sharp increase at term, and has a possible role in labor onset. There also is an increase in plasma CRH before preterm labor, and CRH levels are elevated in multiple gestation. CRH also is known to stimulate the synthesis of prostaglandin F and prostaglandin E by amnion cells (Vogel, Thorsen, Currey et al., 2005).

Myometrial Activity

In true labor, with each contraction, the muscles of the upper uterine segment shorten and exert a longitudinal traction on the cervix, causing effacement. **Effacement** is the drawing up of the internal os and the cervical canal into the uterine side walls. The cervix changes progressively from a long, thick structure to a structure that is tissue-paper thin (Figure 17–11 ■). In primigravidas, effacement usually precedes dilatation.

Contractions are stimulated by the hormone oxytocin. Oxytocin is a potent uterine stimulant (Arthur, Taggart, & Mitchell, 2007). Oxytocin is frequently used as an agent to induce or augment labor in term fetuses or when delivery is necessitated. Uterine sensitivity to oxytocin is increased during pregnancy (Blackburn, 2007). Oxytocin is produced in the hypothalamus and secreted into the bloodstream but is also produced in uterine tissues during late gestation, with concentrations increasing at the onset of labor (Arthur, Taggart, & Mitchell, 2007). The oxytocin receptors are most likely formed in the gestational tissues which when stimulated produce myometrial activity (Blackburn, 2007).

The uterus elongates with each contraction, decreasing the horizontal diameter. This elongation causes a straightening of the fetal body, pressing the upper portion against the fundus and thrusting the presenting part down toward the lower uterine segment and the cervix. The pressure exerted by the fetus is called the *fetal axis pressure.* As the uterus elongates, the longitudinal muscle fibers are pulled upward over the presenting part. This action and the hydrostatic pressure of the fetal membranes cause cervical dilatation. The cervical os and cervical canal widen from less than 1 cm (0.4 in.) to approximately 10 cm (3.9 in.), allowing birth of the fetus. When the cervix is completely dilated and retracted up into the lower uterine segment, it can no longer be palpated. At the same time the round ligament pulls the fundus forward, aligning the fetus with the bony pelvis.

Musculature Changes in the Pelvic Floor

The levator ani muscle and fascia of the pelvic floor draw the rectum and vagina upward and forward with each contraction, along the curve of the pelvic floor. As the fetal head descends to the pelvic floor, the pressure of the presenting part causes the perineal structure, which was once 5 cm (2 in.) in thickness, to change to a structure less than 1 cm (0.4 in.) thick. A normal physiologic anesthesia

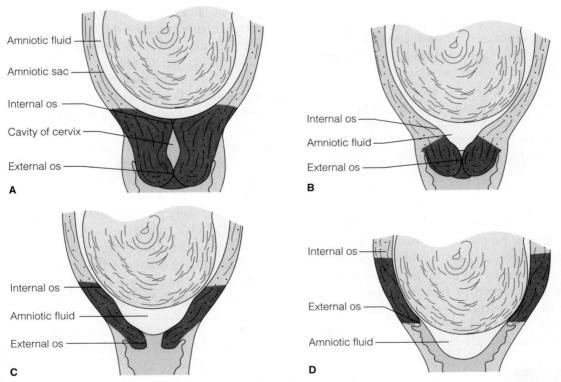

FIGURE 17–11 Effacement of the cervix in the primigravida. *A,* Beginning of labor. There is no cervical effacement or dilatation. The fetal head is cushioned by amniotic fluid. *B,* Beginning cervical effacement. As the cervix begins to efface, more amniotic fluid collects below the fetal head. *C,* Cervix is about one-half (50%) effaced and slightly dilated. The increasing amount of amniotic fluid below the fetal head exerts hydrostatic pressure on the cervix. *D,* Complete effacement and dilatation.

is produced as a result of the decreased blood supply to the area. The anus everts, exposing the interior rectal wall as the fetal head descends forward (Blackburn, 2007).

Premonitory Signs of Labor

Most primigravidas and many multiparas experience the following signs and symptoms of impending labor.

Lightening

Lightening describes the effects that occur when the fetus begins to settle into the pelvic inlet (engagement). With fetal descent, the uterus moves downward, and the fundus no longer presses on the diaphragm, which eases breathing. However, with increased downward pressure of the presenting part, the woman may notice the following:

- Leg cramps or pains caused by pressure on the nerves that course through the obturator foramen in the pelvis
- Increased pelvic pressure
- Increased urinary frequency
- Increased venous stasis, leading to edema in the lower extremities
- Increased vaginal secretions resulting from congestion of the vaginal mucous membranes

Braxton Hicks Contractions

Before the onset of labor, **Braxton Hicks contractions** (the irregular, intermittent contractions that have been occurring throughout the pregnancy) may become uncomfortable. The pain seems to be focused in the abdomen and groin but may feel like the "drawing" sensations experienced by some women with dysmenorrhea. When these contractions are strong enough for the woman to believe she is in labor, she is said to be in false labor. False labor is uncomfortable and may be exhausting. Because the contractions can be fairly regular, the woman has no way of knowing if they are the beginning of true labor. She may come to the hospital or birthing center for a vaginal examination to determine if cervical dilatation is occurring. Frequent episodes of false labor, as well as trips back and forth to the certified nurse-midwife or physician's office or hospital, may frustrate or embarrass the woman who feels that she should know when she is really in labor. Reassurance by nursing staff can ease embarrassment. It is important to remember that women with contractions that occur on a regular basis before 38 weeks should be assessed to determine if they are experiencing preterm labor (see Chapter 21 ∞).

Cervical Changes

Considerable change occurs in the cervix during the prenatal and intrapartal period. At the beginning of pregnancy the cervix is rigid and firm, and it must soften so that it can stretch and dilate to allow the fetus passage. This softening of the cervix is called *ripening*.

As term approaches, collagen fibers in the cervix are broken down by the action of enzymes such as collagenase and elastase. As the collagen fibers change, their ability to bind together decreases because of increasing amounts of hyaluronic acid (which loosely binds collagen fibrils) and decreasing amounts of dermatan sulfate (which tightly binds collagen fibrils). The water content of the cervix also increases. All these changes result in a weakening and softening of the cervix.

Bloody Show

During pregnancy, cervical secretions accumulate in the cervical canal to form a barrier called a *mucous plug*. With softening and effacement of the cervix, the mucous plug is often expelled, resulting in a small amount of blood loss from the exposed cervical capillaries. The resulting pink-tinged secretions are called **bloody show**. Bloody show is considered a sign that labor will begin within 24 to 48 hours. Vaginal examination that includes manipulation of the cervix may also result in a blood-tinged discharge, which is sometimes confused with bloody show.

Rupture of Membranes

Approximately 8% of women at term (38 through 41 weeks' gestation) experience rupture of the amniotic membranes (ROM) before the onset of labor. After the membranes rupture, 50% of these women gave birth within 5 hours and 95% gave birth within 28 hours (ACOG, 2007). ACOG recommends that women who present with ruptured membranes without contractions should be started on an oxytocin infusion at the time of presentation to decrease the incidence of chorioamnionitis. Women with group beta streptococcus (GBS) or those with no documented GBS culture should begin antibiotic therapy immediately (ACOG, 2007). Labor is induced only if the pregnancy is beyond 34 weeks. Women with preterm gestations of less than 34 weeks are managed conservatively provided both the mother and fetus are stable (ACOG, 2007).

When the membranes rupture, the amniotic fluid may be expelled in large amounts. If engagement has not occurred, there is danger of the umbilical cord washing out with the fluid (prolapsed cord). In addition, the open pathway into the uterus increases the risk of infection. Because of these threats, when the membranes rupture, the woman is advised to notify her certified nurse-midwife or physician and proceed to the hospital or birthing center. In some instances, the fluid is expelled in small amounts and may be confused with episodes of urinary incontinence associated with urinary urgency, coughing, or sneezing. The discharge should be checked to determine its source and the appropriate action. (See Chapter 18 ∞ for assessment techniques.)

Sudden Burst of Energy

Some women report a sudden burst of energy approximately 24 to 48 hours before labor. The cause of the energy spurt is unknown. In prenatal teaching the nurse should warn prospective mothers not to overexert themselves during this energy burst to avoid being overtired when labor begins.

TEACHING TIP

Encourage mothers who experience a sudden burst of energy to eat small, frequent nutritious meals during this period, and to rest. Encourage the pregnant woman to have her significant other or a friend do chores and activities that she feels are essential to complete before the baby arrives.

Other Signs

Additional premonitory signs include the following:

- Weight loss of 1 to 3 lb resulting from fluid loss and electrolyte shifts produced by changes in estrogen and progesterone levels.
- Diarrhea, indigestion, or nausea and vomiting just before onset of labor. The cause of these signs is unknown.

Differences Between True and False Labor

The contractions of true labor produce progressive dilatation and effacement of the cervix. They occur regularly and increase in frequency, duration, and intensity. The discomfort of true labor contractions usually starts in the back and radiates around to the abdomen. The pain is not relieved by ambulation (in fact, walking may intensify the pain).

The contractions of false labor do not produce progressive cervical effacement and dilatation. Classically, they are irregular and do not increase in frequency, duration, and intensity. The contractions may be perceived as a hardening or "balling up" without discomfort, or discomfort may occur mainly in the lower abdomen and groin. The discomfort may be relieved by ambulation, changes of position, drinking a large amount of water, or a warm shower or tub bath (Edwards & Byrom, 2007).

The woman will find it helpful to know the characteristics of true labor contractions as well as the premonitory signs of ensuing labor. However, at times the only way to differentiate accurately between true and false labor is to assess dilatation. The woman must feel free to come in for accurate assessment of labor and should be counseled not to feel foolish if the labor is false. The nurse must reassure the woman that false labor is common and that it often cannot be distinguished from true labor except by vaginal

---

KEY FACTS TO REMEMBER

Comparison of True and False Labor

TRUE LABOR	FALSE LABOR
Contractions are at regular intervals.	Contractions are irregular.
Intervals between contractions gradually shorten.	Usually no change.
Contractions increase in duration and intensity.	Usually no change.
Discomfort begins in back and radiates around to abdomen.	Discomfort is usually in abdomen.
Intensity usually increases with change in activity.	Change of activity has no effect on contractions.
Cervical dilatation and effacement are progressive.	No change.
Contractions do not decrease with rest or warm tub bath.	Rest and warm tub lessen contractions.

---

examination. (See Key Facts to Remember: Comparison of True and False Labor.)

Stages of Labor and Birth

To assist caregivers, common terms have been developed as benchmarks to subdivide the labor process into phases and stages of labor. It is important to note, however, that these represent theoretical separations in the process. A laboring woman will not usually experience distinct differences from one stage to another.

The first stage begins with the onset of true labor and ends when the cervix is completely dilated at 10 cm (3.9 in.). The second stage begins with complete dilatation and ends with the birth of the newborn. The third stage begins with the birth of the newborn and ends with the delivery of the placenta.

Some clinicians identify a fourth stage. During this stage, which lasts 1 to 4 hours after delivery of the placenta, the uterus effectively contracts to control bleeding at the placental site (Edwards & Byrom, 2007).

First Stage

The first stage of labor is divided into the latent, active, and transition phases. Each phase of labor is characterized by physical and psychologic changes and is summarized in Table 17–3.

Latent Phase

The *latent phase* starts with the beginning of regular contractions, which are usually mild. The woman feels able to cope with the discomfort. She may be relieved that labor

MyNursingKit | Video: Labor 1st Stage—Part 1

TABLE 17–3	Characteristics of Labor			
		First Stage		**Second Stage**
	Latent Phase	**Active Phase**	**Transition Phase**	
Nullipara	8.6 hr	4.6 hr	3 hr	Up to 3 hr
Multipara	5.3 hr	2.4 hr	less than 1 hr	less than 1 hr, averages 15 min
Cervical dilatation	0 to 3 cm	4 to 7 cm	8 to 10 cm	
Contractions				
Frequency	Every 10 to 30 min	Every 2 to 5 min	Every 1½ to 2 min	Every 1½ to 2 min
Duration	30 sec	40 to 60 sec	60 to 90 sec	60 to 90 sec
Intensity	Begin as mild and progress to moderate; 25 to 40 mm Hg by intrauterine pressure catheter (IUPC)	Begin as moderate and progress to strong; 50 to 70 mm Hg by IUPC	Strong by palpation; 70 to 90 mm Hg by IUPC	Strong by palpation; 70 to 100 mm Hg by IUPC

has finally started and that the end of pregnancy has come. Although she may be anxious, she is able to recognize and express those feelings of anxiety. The woman is often smiling and eager to talk about herself and answer questions. Excitement is high, and her partner or other support person is often equally elated.

Uterine contractions become established during the latent phase and increase in frequency, duration, and intensity. They may start as mild contractions lasting 30 seconds with a frequency of 10 to 30 minutes and progress to moderate ones lasting 30 to 40 seconds with a frequency of 5 to 7 minutes. As the cervix begins to dilate, it also effaces, although little or no fetal descent is evident. For a woman in her first labor (nullipara), the latent (or early) phase of the first stage of labor averages 8.6 hours but should not exceed 20 hours. The latent phase in multiparas averages 5.3 hours but should not exceed 14 hours.

At the beginning of labor, the amniotic membranes bulge through the cervix in the shape of a cone. **Spontaneous rupture of membranes (SROM)** generally occurs at the height of an intense contraction with a gush of fluid out of the vagina. In many instances, the membranes are ruptured by the certified nurse-midwife or physician, using an instrument called an amnihook. This procedure is called *amniotomy*, or **artificial rupture of membranes (AROM)**, and is discussed in Chapter 23 ∞.

Active Phase

When the woman enters the early *active phase*, her anxiety and her sense of the need for energy and focus tends to increase as she senses the intensification of contractions and pain. She may begin to fear a loss of control or may feel the need to "really work and focus" on the contractions. Women will use a variety of coping mechanisms. Some

women exhibit a sense of purpose and the need for regrouping whereas others may feel a decreased ability to cope and a sense of helplessness. Women who have support persons and family available often experience greater satisfaction and have less anxiety than those without support.

During this phase, the cervix dilates from about 4 cm to 7 cm (1.6 to 2.8 in.). Fetal descent is progressive. The cervical dilatation averages 1.2 cm/hr in nulliparas and 1.5 cm/hr (0.5 in./hr) in multiparas (Edwards & Byrom 2007). During the active and transition phases, contractions become more frequent and longer in duration, and they increase in intensity. By the end of the active phase, contractions have a frequency of 2 to 3 minutes, a duration of 60 seconds, and strong intensity.

> **EVIDENCE IN ACTION**
> *Twelve contractions an hour is considered a meaningful signal that spontaneous birth is beginning or is imminent.*
> (Prospective observational cohort study)
> (Pates, McIntire & Leveno, 2007)

Transition Phase

The *transition phase* is the last part of the first stage of labor. When the woman enters the transition phase, she may demonstrate an acute awareness of the need for her energy and attention to be completely focused to the task at hand. She may experience significant anxiety or feel out of control. She becomes acutely aware of the increasing force and intensity of the contractions. She may become restless, frequently changing position in an attempt to get comfortable. By the time the woman enters the transition phase, she is inner directed and often tired. She may not want to be left alone at the same time the support person may be feeling the need for a break. The nurse should reassure the woman that she will not be left alone. It is crucial that the nurse be available as relief support at this time and keep the woman informed about where her labor support people are, if they leave the room. Some women have the intuition that the end of labor is occurring and know that birth is nearing, so an instinct to have support people remain with her often occurs.

During transition, contractions have a frequency of about every 1½ to 2 minutes, a duration of 60 to 90 seconds, and strong intensity (Edwards & Byrom, 2007). Cervical dilatation slows as it progresses from 8 to 10 cm (3.1 to 3.9 cm) and the rate of fetal descent dramatically increases. The average rate of descent is 1.6 cm/hr (0.6 in./hr) and at least 1 cm/hr (0.4 in./hr) in nulliparas. In addition, the average rate of descent is 5.4 cm/hr (2.1 in./hr) and at least 2.1 cm/hr (0.8 in./hr) in multiparas. The transition phase does not usually last longer than 3 hours for nulliparas or longer than 1 hour for multiparas (Edwards & Byrom, 2007). The total duration of the first stage may be increased by approximately 1 hour if epidural anesthesia is used.

As dilatation approaches 10 cm (3.9 in.), there may be increased rectal pressure and an uncontrollable desire to bear down, increased amount of bloody show, and rupture of membranes (if it has not already occurred). With the peak of a contraction, she may experience a sensation of pressure so great that she may fear that she will be "torn open" or "split apart." She may also fear that the sensations indicate that something is wrong. Thus, the nurse should inform the woman that what she is feeling is normal in this stage of labor. Even with assurance, the woman may increasingly doubt her ability to cope with labor and may become apprehensive, irritable, and withdrawn. She may be terrified of being left alone, though she does not want anyone to talk to or touch her. However, with the next contraction she may ask for verbal and physical support.

Other characteristics of this phase may include the following:

- Increasing bloody show
- Hyperventilation, as the woman increases her breathing rate
- Generalized discomfort, including low backache, shaking and cramping in legs, and increased sensitivity to touch
- Increased need for partner's and/or nurse's presence and support
- Restlessness
- Increased apprehension and irritability
- An inner focusing on her contractions
- A sense of bewilderment, frustration, and anger at the contractions
- Requests for medication
- Hiccupping, belching, nausea, or vomiting
- Beads of perspiration on the upper lip or brow
- Increasing rectal pressure and feeling the urge to bear down

The woman in this phase is anxious to "get it over with." She may be amnesic and sleep between her now-frequent contractions. Her support persons may start to feel fatigue and may feel helpless. They may turn to the nurse for increased participation as their efforts to alleviate her discomfort seem less effective.

Second Stage

The second stage of labor begins with complete cervical dilatation and ends with birth of the infant. Traditional thought suggests that the second stage should be completed within 3 hours after the cervix becomes fully dilated for primigravidas; the stage averages 15 minutes for multiparas (see Table 17–3). Contractions continue with a frequency of about every 1½ to 2 minutes, a duration of 60 to 90 seconds, and strong intensity (Edwards & Byrom, 2007). Descent of the fetal presenting part continues until it reaches the perineal floor.

As the fetal head descends, the woman usually has the urge to push because of pressure of the fetal head on the sacral and obturator nerves. As she pushes, intra-abdominal pressure is exerted from contraction of the maternal abdominal muscles. As the fetal head continues its descent, the perineum begins to bulge, flatten, and move anteriorly. Most women feel acute, increasingly severe pain and a burning sensation as the perineum distends. The amount of bloody show may increase. The labia begin to part with each contraction. Between contractions the fetal head appears to recede. With succeeding contractions and maternal pushing effort, the fetal head descends farther. **Crowning** occurs when the fetal head is encircled by the external opening of the vagina (introitus), and it means birth is imminent.

The woman may feel some relief that the transition phase is over, the birth is near, and she can push. Some women feel a sense of purpose now that they can be actively involved. The woman may be focused and should be encouraged to center all her energy into pushing. Resting between contractions should be encouraged. There are often many opportunities for the support person to assist the woman. The support person can provide support to the legs, offer ice chips, fan the woman who is often overheated and fatigued, and offer verbal encouragement. For women without childbirth preparation, this stage can become frightening; the woman should be encouraged to work with her contractions and not fight them. A support person who has never seen a labor may become disconcerted during this time. The nurse can assist the support person in performing activities and offering encouragement that assists the woman during the birth process. The woman may feel she has lost her ability to cope and become embarrassed, or she may demonstrate extreme irritability toward the staff or her supporters as she attempts to regain control over her body. Some women feel a great sense of purpose and are unrelenting in their efforts to work with each and every contraction. Some women will be very forceful and directive with staff and support persons. Again, all of these reactions and emotions are common and should be supported as the woman works toward the birth.

Spontaneous Birth (Vertex Presentation)

As the fetal head distends the vulva with each contraction, the perineum becomes extremely thin and the anus stretches and protrudes. With time, the head extends under the symphysis pubis and is born. When the anterior shoulder meets the underside of the symphysis pubis, a gentle push by the mother aids in the birth of the shoulders. The body then follows (Figure 17–12 ■). (Birth of a fetus in other than a vertex presentation is discussed in Chapter 22 ∞.)

Positional Changes of the Fetus

For the fetus to pass through the birth canal, the fetal head and body must adjust to the passage by certain positional changes. These changes, called **cardinal movements** or

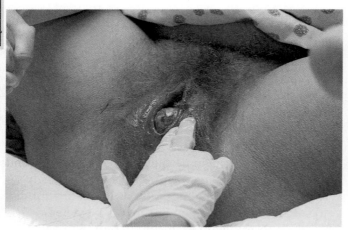

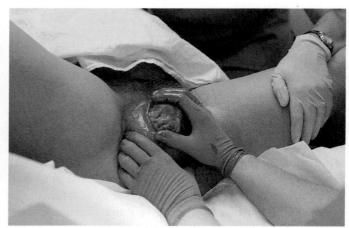

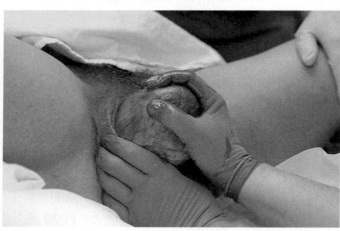

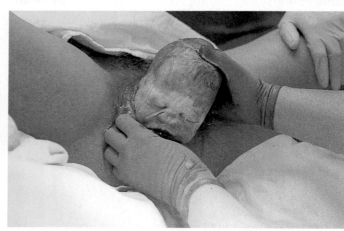

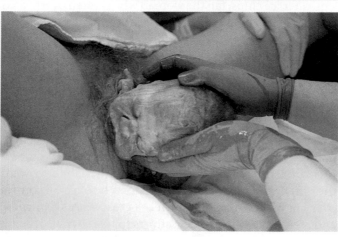

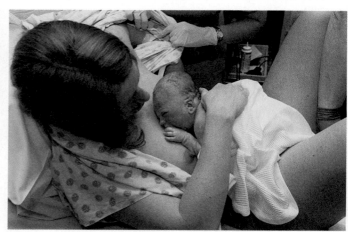

FIGURE 17–12 The birth sequence.
Source: © Stella Johnson (www.stellajohnson.com).

mechanisms of labor, are described in the order in which they occur (Figure 17–13 ■).

DESCENT *Descent* occurs because of four forces: (1) pressure of the amniotic fluid, (2) direct pressure of the uterine fundus on the breech, (3) contraction of the abdominal muscles, and (4) extension and straightening of the fetal body. The head enters the inlet in the occiput transverse or oblique position because the pelvic inlet is widest from side to side. The sagittal suture is an equal distance from the maternal symphysis pubis and sacral promontory.

FLEXION *Flexion* occurs as the fetal head descends and meets resistance from the soft tissues of the pelvis, the muscles of the pelvic floor, and the cervix. As a result of the resistance, the fetal chin flexes downward onto the chest.

INTERNAL ROTATION The fetal head must rotate to fit the diameter of the pelvic cavity, which is widest in the anteroposterior diameter. As the occiput of the fetal head meets resistance from the levator ani muscles and their fascia, the occiput rotates—usually from left to right—and the sagittal suture aligns in the anteroposterior pelvic diameter.

EXTENSION The resistance of the pelvic floor and the mechanical movement of the vulva opening anteriorly and forward assist with extension of the fetal head as it passes under the symphysis pubis. With this positional change, the occiput, then brow and face, emerge from the vagina.

RESTITUTION The shoulders of the fetus enter the pelvis inlet obliquely and remain oblique when the head rotates to the anteroposterior diameter through internal rotation. Because of this rotation, the neck becomes twisted. Once the head is born and is free of pelvic resistance, the neck untwists, turning the head to one side (restitution), and aligns with the position of the back in the birth canal.

EXTERNAL ROTATION As the shoulders rotate to the anteroposterior position in the pelvis, the head turns farther to one side (external rotation).

EXPULSION After the external rotation, and through the pushing efforts of the laboring woman, the anterior shoulder meets the undersurface of the symphysis pubis and slips under it. As lateral flexion of the shoulder and head occurs, the anterior shoulder is born before the posterior shoulder. The body follows quickly.

Third Stage

The third stage of labor is defined as the period of time from the birth of the infant until the completed delivery of the placenta. The third stage should be completed within 30 minutes of the birth of the infant. If the time of placenta delivery is delayed, the cervix begins to close as the uterus contracts and the risk of hemorrhage and placenta retention (retained placenta) occurs.

Placental Separation

After the infant is born, the uterus contracts firmly, diminishing its capacity and the surface area of placental attachment. The placenta begins to separate because of this decrease in surface area. As this separation occurs, bleeding

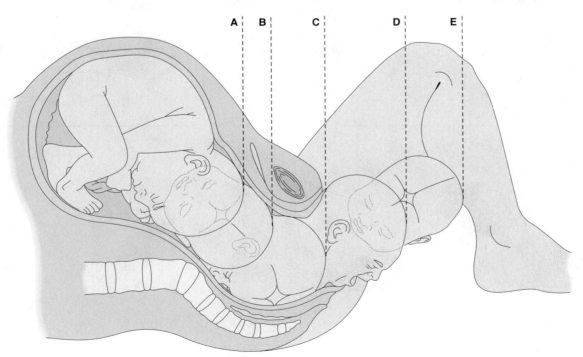

FIGURE 17–13 Mechanisms of labor. *A,* Descent. *B,* Flexion. *C,* Internal rotation. *D,* Extension. *E,* External rotation.

results in the formation of a hematoma between the placental tissue and the remaining decidua. This hematoma accelerates the separation process. The membranes are the last to separate. They are peeled off the uterine wall as the placenta descends into the vagina.

Signs of placental separation usually appear about 5 minutes after the birth of the newborn. These signs are (1) a globular-shaped uterus, (2) a rise of the fundus in the abdomen, (3) a sudden gush or trickle of blood, and (4) further protrusion of the umbilical cord out of the vagina.

Placental Delivery

When the signs of placental separation appear, the woman may bear down to aid in placental expulsion. If this fails and the certified nurse-midwife or physician has ascertained that the fundus is firm, gentle traction may be applied to the cord while pressure is exerted on the fundus. The weight of the placenta as it is guided into the placental collection pan aids in the removal of the membranes from the uterine wall. A placenta is considered to be retained if 30 minutes have elapsed from completion of the second stage of labor.

If the placenta separates from the inside to the outer margins, it is delivered with the fetal (shiny) side presenting (Figure 17–14 ■). This is known as the Schultze mechanism of placental delivery or, more commonly, "shiny Schultze." If the placenta separates from the outer margins inward, it will roll up and present sideways with the maternal surface delivering first. This is known as the Duncan mechanism of placental delivery and is commonly called "dirty Duncan" because the placental surface is rough.

Fourth Stage

The fourth stage of labor is the time, from 1 to 4 hours after birth, during which physiologic readjustment of the mother's body begins. With the birth, hemodynamic changes occur. Blood loss ranges from 250 to 500 mL. With this blood loss and removal of the weight of the pregnant uterus from the surrounding vessels, blood is redistributed into venous beds. This results in a moderate drop in both systolic and diastolic blood pressure, increased pulse pressure, and moderate tachycardia (Cunningham, Leveno, Bloom et al., 2005).

The uterus remains contracted in the midline of the abdomen. The fundus is usually midway between the symphysis pubis and umbilicus. Its contracted state constricts the vessels at the site of placental implantation. Immediately after birth of the placenta, the cervix is widely spread and thick.

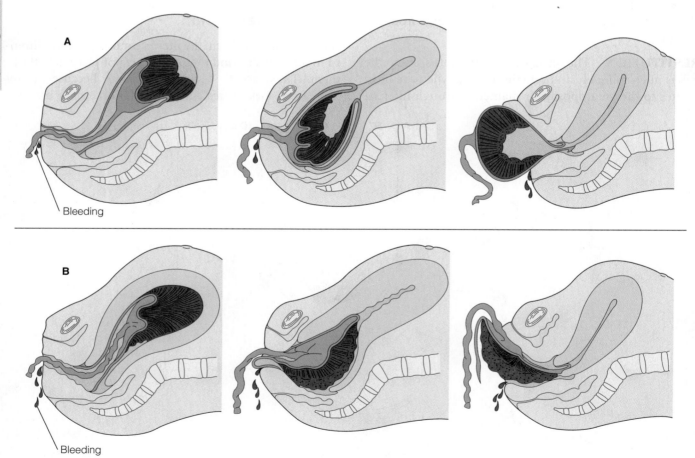

FIGURE 17–14 Placental separation and expulsion. *A,* Schultze mechanism. *B,* Duncan mechanism.

Nausea and vomiting usually cease. The woman may be thirsty and hungry. She may experience a shaking chill, which is thought to be associated with the ending of the physical exertion of labor. The bladder is often hypotonic because of trauma during the second stage and/or the administration of anesthetics that decrease sensations. Hypotonic bladder can lead to urinary retention.

Maternal Systemic Response to Labor

The labor and birth process affects nearly all of the maternal physiological systems.

Cardiovascular System

The woman's cardiovascular system is stressed both by the uterine contractions and by the pain, anxiety, and apprehension she experiences. During pregnancy, there is a 50% increase in circulating blood volume. The increase in cardiac output peaks between the second and third trimester although during labor there is a significant increase in cardiac output. With each contraction, 300 to 500 mL of blood volume is forced back into the maternal circulation, which results in an increase in cardiac output of as much as 10% to 15% over the typical third trimester levels (Blackburn, 2007; Sharma, 2006). Further increases in cardiac output occur as the laboring woman experiences pain with uterine contractions and her anxiety and apprehension increase.

Maternal position also affects cardiac output. In the supine position, cardiac output lowers as a result of the gravid uterus, heart rate increases, and stroke volume decreases. When the woman turns to a lateral (side-lying) position, cardiac output increases (ACC & AHA, 2006; Blackburn, 2007). Women with preexisting heart disease have higher rates of arrhythmias in labor (Flores & Marquez, 2007).

Blood Pressure

As a result of increased cardiac output, blood pressure (both systolic and diastolic) rises during uterine contractions. In the first stage, systolic pressure increases by 35 mm Hg and diastolic pressure increases by about 25 mm Hg. There may be further increases in the second stage during pushing (Blackburn, 2007).

Respiratory System

Oxygen demand and consumption increase at the onset of labor because of the presence of uterine contractions. As anxiety and pain from contractions increase, hyperventilation frequently occurs. With hyperventilation there is a fall in $PaCO_2$, and respiratory alkalosis results (Tomimatsu, Peña, & Longo, 2007).

By the end of the first stage, most women have developed a mild metabolic acidosis compensated by respiratory alkalosis. As they push in the second stage of labor, the women's $PaCO_2$ levels may rise along with blood lactate levels (because of muscular activity), leading to mild respiratory acidosis. By the time the baby is born (end of second stage), there is metabolic acidosis uncompensated for by respiratory alkalosis (Blackburn, 2007).

The changes in acid-base status that occur in labor are quickly reversed in the fourth stage because of changes in women's respiratory rates. Acid-base levels return to pregnancy levels by 24 hours after birth, and nonpregnant values are attained a few weeks after birth (Blackburn, 2007).

Renal System

During labor there is an increase in maternal renin, plasma renin activity, and angiotensinogen. This elevation is thought to be important in the control of uteroplacental blood flow during birth and the early postpartal period (Blackburn, 2007).

Structurally, the base of the bladder is pushed forward and upward when engagement occurs. The pressure from the presenting part may impair blood and lymph drainage from the base of the bladder, leading to edema.

Gastrointestinal System

During labor, gastric motility and absorption of solid food are reduced. Gastric emptying time is prolonged, and gastric volume (amount of contents that remain in the stomach) remains increased, regardless of the time the last meal was taken (Blackburn, 2007). Some narcotics also delay gastric emptying time and add to the risk of aspiration if general anesthesia is used.

Immune System and Other Blood Values

The white blood cell (WBC) count increases to 25,000 to 30,000/mm³ during labor and the early postpartum period. The change in WBCs is mostly because of increased neutrophils resulting from a physiologic response to stress. The increased WBC count makes it difficult to identify the presence of an infection.

Maternal blood glucose levels decrease because glucose is used as an energy source during uterine contractions. The decreased blood glucose levels lead to a decrease in insulin requirements (Blackburn, 2007).

Pain

Pain during labor comes from a complexity of physical causes. Each woman will experience and cope with pain differently. Multiple factors affect a woman's reaction to labor pain.

Causes of Pain During Labor

The pain associated with the first stage of labor is unique in that it accompanies a normal physiologic process. Even though perception of the pain of childbirth varies among women, there is a physiologic basis for discomfort during labor. Pain during the first stage of labor arises from (1) dilatation of the cervix, which is the primary source of pain; (2) stretching of the lower uterine segment; (3) pressure on adjacent structures; and (4) hypoxia of the uterine muscle cells during contraction (Blackburn, 2007). The areas of pain include the lower abdominal wall and the areas over the lower lumbar region and the upper sacrum (Figure 17–15 ■).

During the second stage of labor, pain is caused by (1) hypoxia of the contracting uterine muscle cells, (2) distention of the vagina and perineum, and (3) pressure on adjacent structures. The area of pain increases as shown in Figures 17–16 ■ and 17–17 ■.

Pain during the third stage results from uterine contractions and cervical dilatation as the placenta is expelled. This stage of labor is short, and after it anesthesia is needed primarily for episiotomy repair.

Factors Affecting Response to Pain

Many factors affect the individual's perception and response to pain. For example, childbirth preparation classes may reduce the need for analgesia during labor.

Preparing for labor and birth through reading, talking with others, or attending a childbirth preparation class frequently has positive effects for the laboring woman and her partner. The woman who knows what to expect and what techniques she may use to increase comfort tends to be less anxious during the labor. A tour of the birthing center and an opportunity to see and feel the environment also help reduce anxiety because during admission (especially with the first child) many new things are happening and they seem to occur all at once.

In addition, individuals tend to respond to painful stimuli in the way that is acceptable in their culture. In some cultures, it is natural to communicate pain, no matter how mild, whereas members of other cultures stoically accept pain out of fear or because it is expected. Nurses need to be aware of cultural norms and demonstrate culturally sensitive care to women and their families in the intrapartum setting (Khademian & Vizeshfar, 2008.).

Response to pain may also be influenced by fatigue and sleep deprivation. The fatigued woman has less energy and ability to use such strategies as distraction or imagination to deal with pain. As a result, she may lose her ability to cope with labor and choose analgesics or other medications to relieve the discomfort.

The woman's previous experience with pain and anxiety level also affects her ability to manage current and future pain. Those who have had experience with pain seem more sensitive to painful stimuli than those who have not. Unfamiliar surroundings and events can increase anxiety, as does separation from family and loved ones. Anticipation of discomfort and questions about whether she can cope with the contractions may also increase anxiety.

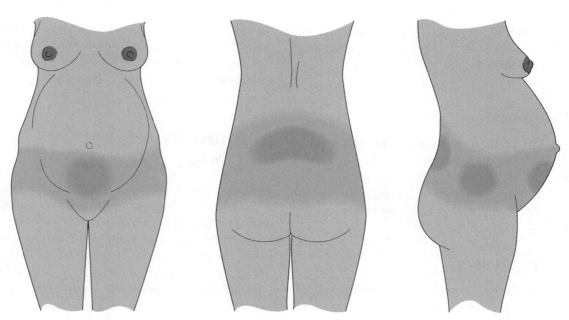

FIGURE 17–15 Area of reference of labor pain during the first stage. Pain is most intense in the darkened areas.
Source: Bonica, J. J. (1972). *Principles and practice of obstetric analgesia and anesthesia* (p. 108). Philadelphia: Davis.

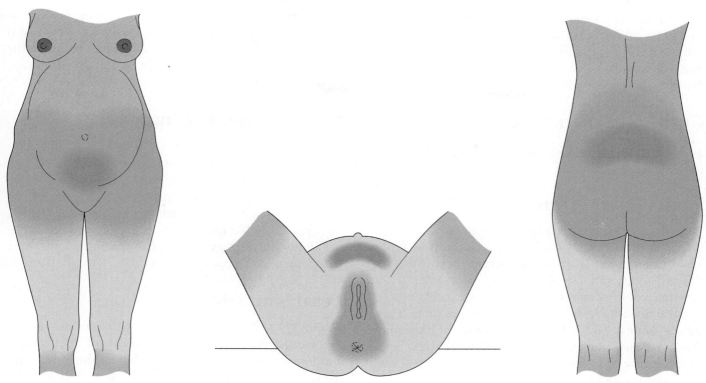

FIGURE 17–16 Distribution of labor pain during the later phase of the first stage and early phase of the second stage. The darkest colored areas indicate the location of the most intense pain; moderate color, moderate pain; and light color, mild pain. The uterine contractions, which at this stage are very strong, produce intense pain.
Source: Bonica, J. J. (1972). *Principles and practice of obstetric analgesia and anesthesia* (p. 109). Philadelphia: Davis.

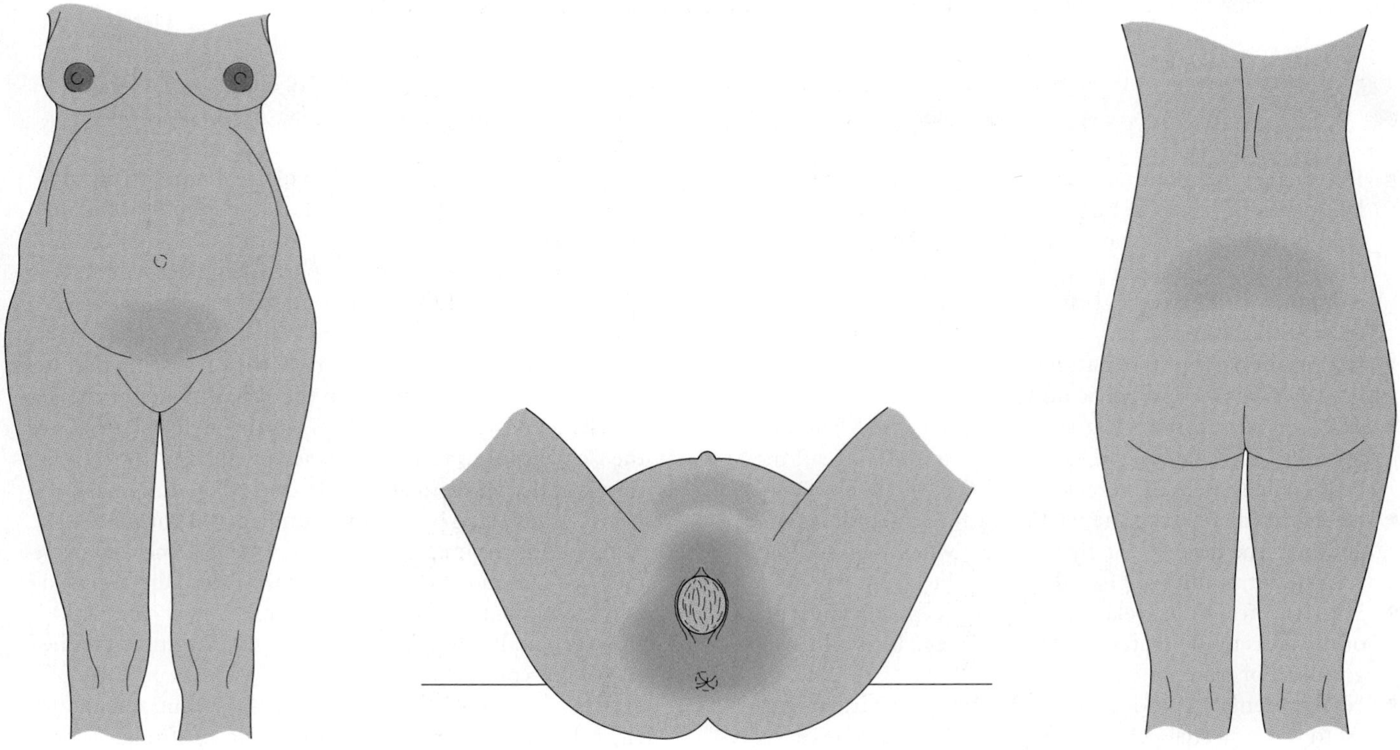

FIGURE 17–17 Distribution of labor pain during the later phase of the second stage and actual birth. The perineal component is the primary cause of discomfort. Uterine contractions contribute much less to the level of pain.
Source: Bonica, J. J. (1972). *Principles and practice of obstetric analgesia and anesthesia* (p. 109). Philadelphia: Davis.

Both attention and distraction influence the perception of pain. When pain sensation is the focus of attention, the perceived intensity is greater. A sensory stimulus such as a back rub can be a distraction that focuses the woman's attention on the stimulus rather than the pain.

Fetal Response to Labor

When the fetus is healthy, the mechanical and hemodynamic changes of normal labor have no adverse effects.

Heart Rate Changes

Early fetal heart rate decelerations can occur with intracranial pressures of 40 to 55 mm Hg, as the head pushes against the cervix. The currently accepted explanation of this early deceleration is hypoxic depression of the central nervous system, which is under vagal control. The absence of these head-compression decelerations in some fetuses during labor is explained by the existence of a threshold that is reached more gradually in the presence of intact membranes and lack of maternal resistance. These early decelerations are harmless in a normal fetus.

Acid-Base Status in Labor

Blood flow is decreased to the fetus at the peak of each contraction, which leads to a slow decrease in pH status. During the second stage of labor, as uterine contractions become longer and stronger and the woman often holds her breath to push, the fetal pH decreases more rapidly. Although women are encouraged to maintain slow paced breathing, holding of the breath does often occur. As the base deficit increases, fetal oxygen saturation drops approximately 10% (Blackburn, 2007).

Hemodynamic Changes

The adequate exchange of nutrients and gases in the fetal capillaries and intervillous spaces depends in part on the fetal blood pressure. Fetal blood pressure is a protective mechanism for the normal fetus during the anoxic periods caused by the contracting uterus during labor. The fetal and placental reserve is usually enough to see the fetus through these anoxic periods unharmed (Blackburn, 2007).

Fetal Sensation

Beginning at about 37 or 38 weeks' gestation (full term), the fetus is able to experience sensations of light, sound, and touch. The full-term fetus is able to hear music and the maternal voice. Even in utero, the fetus is sensitive to light and will move away from a bright light source. Additionally, the term baby is aware of pressure sensations during labor such as the touch of the caregiver during a vaginal exam or pressure on the head as a contraction occurs. Although the fetus may not be able to process this input, it is important to note that as the woman labors, the fetus is experiencing the labor as well.

CHAPTER HIGHLIGHTS

- Five factors that continuously interact during the process of labor and birth are the birth passage, the fetus, the relationship between the passage and the fetus, the forces of labor (contractions and pushing efforts), and the emotional components the woman brings to the birth setting (psychosocial status).
- Important parts of the maternal pelvis include the pelvic inlet, pelvic cavity, and pelvic outlet.
- The fetal head contains bones that are not fused. This allows for some overlapping and for a change in the shape of the head, called molding, to facilitate birth.
- Fetal attitude refers to the relation of the fetal parts to one another. The head is usually moderately flexed at midline, and the extremities are flexed close to the body.
- Fetal lie refers to the relationship of the cephalocaudal axis of the fetus to the maternal spine. The fetal lie is either longitudinal or transverse.
- Fetal presentation is determined by the body part lying closest to the maternal pelvis. Fetal presentation can be cephalic (head down), breech (buttocks or one or both feet), or shoulder.

- Fetal position is the relationship of the landmark on the presenting fetal part to the front, sides, or back of the maternal pelvis.
- Engagement of the presenting part takes place when the largest diameter of the presenting part reaches or passes through the pelvic inlet.
- Station refers to the relationship of the presenting part to an imaginary line drawn between the ischial spines of the maternal pelvis. Negative numbers (−5 through −1) are above the ischial spines, and the fetus is not engaged. Zero (0) station is at the pelvic inlet, and descent below the ischial spines is indicated by positive numbers (+1 through +4).
- Each uterine contraction has an increment, acme, and decrement. Contraction frequency is the time from the beginning of one contraction to the beginning of the next contraction.
- Contraction duration is the time from the beginning to the end of one contraction.
- Contraction intensity is the strength of the contraction during acme. Intensity is termed mild, moderate, or strong.
- Factors that affect the woman's response to labor pain include education, cultural beliefs, fatigue, personal significance of

pain, previous experience, anxiety, and availability of coping techniques and support.

- Possible causes of labor include progesterone withdrawal, prostaglandin release, or increased concentrations of CRH.

- Premonitory signs of labor include lightening, Braxton Hicks contractions, cervical softening and effacement, bloody show, sudden burst of energy, weight loss, and sometimes rupture of membranes.

- True labor contractions occur regularly, with an increase in frequency, duration, and intensity over time. The contractions usually start in the back and radiate around the abdomen. The discomfort is not relieved by ambulation or rest. False labor contractions do not produce progressive cervical effacement and dilatation. They are usually irregular and do not increase in intensity. The discomfort may be relieved by changes in activity.

- There are four stages of labor and birth: the first stage is from the beginning of true labor to complete dilatation of the cervix, the second stage is from complete dilatation of the cervix to birth, the third stage is from birth to expulsion of the placenta, and the fourth stage is from expulsion of the placenta to a period of 1 to 4 hours after.

- The fetus accommodates itself to the maternal pelvis in a series of movements called the cardinal movements of labor, which include descent, flexion, internal rotation, extension, restitution, external rotation, and expulsion.

- Placental separation is indicated by lengthening of the umbilical cord, a small spurt of blood, change in uterine shape, and a rise of the fundus in the abdomen.

- The placenta is delivered by the Schultze or Duncan mechanism, which is determined by the way it separates from the uterine wall.

- Maternal systemic responses to labor involve the cardiovascular, respiratory, renal, gastrointestinal, and immune systems.

- The fetus is usually able to tolerate the labor process with no untoward changes.

EXPLORE PEARSON **mynursingkit**™

MyNursingKit is your one stop for online chapter review materials and resources. Prepare for success with additional NCLEX®-style practice questions, interactive assignments and activities, web links, animations and videos, and more!

Register your access code from the front of your book at
www.mynursingkit.com

CHAPTER REFERENCES

American College of Cardiology (ACC) & American Heart Association (AHA). (2006). ACC/AHA guidelines for the management of patients with valvular heart disease. *Journal of the American College of Cardiology, 48*(3), 1–148.

American College of Obstetricians & Gynecologists. [ACOG]. (2007). Premature rupture of membranes (ACOG Practice Bulletin No. 80). Washington, DC: ACOG.

Arthur, P., Taggart, M. J., & Mitchell, B. F. (2007). Oxytocin and parturition: A role for increased myometrial calcium and calcium sensitization? *Front Biosciences, 1*(12), 619–633.

Blackburn, S. T. (2007). *Maternal, fetal, and neonatal physiology: A clinical perspective* (3rd ed.). Philadelphia: Saunders.

Bryant, J., Porter, M., Tracy, S. K., & Sullivan, E. A. (2007). Caesarean birth: Consumption, safety, order, and good mothering. *Social Science & Medicine, 65*(6), 1192–1201.

Challis, J. R. G. (2004). Characteristics of parturition. In R. Creasy, R. Resnik, & J. Iams (Eds.). *Maternal-fetal medicine* (5th ed., pp. 484–497). Philadelphia: Saunders.

Cunningham, F. G., Leveno, K. J., Bloom, S. L., Hauth, J. C., & Wenstrom, K. D. (2005). *William's obstetrics* (22nd ed.). New York: McGraw Hill.

Edwards, G., & Byrom, S. (2007). *Essential midwifery practice: Public health.* Hoboken, NJ: Wiley-Blackwell.

Family Practice Notebook. (2008). Shoulder presentation. Retrieved April 11, 2008, from http://www.fpnotebook.com/OB/LD/ShldrPrsntn.htm

Flores, J. R., & Marquez, M. F. (2007). Arrhythmias in pregnancy: How and when to treat? *Archives of Mexican Cardiology, 77*(Suppl. 2), S2-24, S2-31.

Funai, E. F., Evans, M., & Lockwood, C. J. (2008). *High risk obstetrics: The requisites in obstetrics & gynecology.* Mosby: St. Louis.

Goodman, J. H. (2005). Becoming an involved father of an infant. *Journal of Obstetric, Gynecologic, & Neonatal Nursing 34*(2), 190–200.

Hardin, A. M., & Buckner, E. B. (2005). Characteristics of a positive experience for women who have an unmedicated birth. *Journal of Perinatal Education, 13*(4), 10–16.

Khademian, Z., & Vizeshfar, F. (2008). Nursing students' perceptions of the importance of caring behaviors. *Journal of Advanced Nursing, 61*(4), 456–462.

Lobel, M., & DeLuca, R. S. (2007). Psychosocial sequelae of cesarean delivery: Review and analysis of their causes and implications. *Social Science & Medicine, 64*(11), 2272–2284.

Nielson, T., & Paquette, T. (2007). Dream-associated behaviors affecting pregnant and postpartum women. *Sleep, 30*(9), 1162–1169.

Pates, J. A., McIntire, D. D. & Leveno, K. J. (2007). Uterine contractions preceding labor. *Obstetrics & Gynecology, 110* (3), 566–569.

Royal College of Obstetricians & Gynaecologists (RCOG). (2006). External cephalic version and reducing the incidence of breech presentation (Guideline No. 20A). Edinburgh: Author.

Sharma, S. (2006). Pulmonary disease in pregnancy. e-Medicine. Retrieved February 12, 2008, from http://www.emedicine.com/med/topic3252.htm

Szekeres-Bartho, J., Wilczynski, J. R., Basta, P., & Kalinka. J. (2008). Role of progesterone and progestin therapy in threatened abortion and preterm labour. *Front Bioscience, 1*(13), 1981–1990.

Tomimatsu, T., Peña, J. P., & Longo, L. D. (2007). Fetal cerebral oxygenation: The role of maternal hyperoxia with supplemental CO_2 in sheep. *American Journal of Obstetrics & Gynecology, 196*(4), 359. e1-5.

Vogel, I., Thorsen, P., Curry, A., Sandager, P., & Uldbjerg, N. (2005). Biomarkers for the prediction of preterm delivery. *Acta obstetrician et Gynecologica Scandinavica, 84*(6), 516–525.

CHAPTER 18

Intrapartal Nursing Assessment

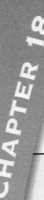

As charge nurse on a busy birthing unit, sometimes I feel like I'm meeting myself coming and going. At any one time I may be called upon to do a great number of things, seemingly all at once: maintain a safe and adequate staffing, be the extra pair of hands at a high-risk delivery, consult with members of the hospital's support services team, arrange for the smooth transfer of a labor patient to the operating room for a cesarean, help a mom who is having difficulty breastfeeding, or simply cuddle a newborn whose parents (and nurse) need a few minutes of rest. Would I trade this bustle for anything else? Not on your life!

—Birth Center Charge Nurse

LEARNING OUTCOMES

18-1. Describe a maternal assessment of the laboring woman that includes the client history, high-risk screening, and physical and psychosociocultural factors.

18-2. Evaluate the progress of labor by assessing the laboring woman's contractions, cervical dilatation, and effacement.

18-3. Describe an intrapartal fetal assessment to determine fetal position and presentation, fetal heart rate, and fetal status.

18-4. Describe the steps and frequency for performing auscultation of fetal heart rate.

18-5. Delineate the procedure for performing Leopold's maneuvers and the information that can be obtained.

18-6. Describe the indications, methods, and steps for performing and recording electronic fetal monitoring.

18-7. Distinguish between baseline and periodic changes in fetal heart rate monitoring, and the appearance and significance of each.

18-8. Evaluate fetal heart rate tracings using a systematic approach.

18-9. Compare nonreassuring fetal heart rate patterns to appropriate nursing responses.

18-10. Explain the family's responses to electronic fetal monitoring in nursing care management.

18-11. Describe how fetal arterial oxygen saturation (FSpO2) monitoring uses pulse oximetry to monitor oxygenation of the fetal blood to determine if hypoxia is occurring.

The physiologic and psychologic events that occur during labor call for continual and rapid adaptations by the mother and fetus. Frequent and accurate assessments are crucial to the progress of these adaptations. In current nursing practice, the traditional assessment techniques of observation, palpation, and auscultation are augmented by the judicious use of technology such as ultrasound and electronic monitoring. These tools may provide more detailed information for assessment; however, it is important for the nurse to remember that the technology only provides data. It is the nurse who monitors the mother and her baby.

Maternal Assessment

Assessment of the mother begins with a client history and screening for intrapartal risk factors.

History

The nurse obtains a brief oral history when the woman is admitted to the birthing area. Typically the maternal and fetal vital signs are immediately assessed. If the vital signs are within normal limits, the interview continues. If there is an identified problem, nursing care is then prioritized.

It is common for the provider to send the prenatal records to the labor and birthing unit before the woman's due date. The information should be reviewed in a nonjudgmental manner to ensure changes have not occurred since the information was documented. During the initial interview, the nurse is building a trusting relationship. It is often helpful if the nurse sits down and appears unrushed, makes direct eye contact (if culturally appropriate), and begins the interview with a statement such as, "I am going to be asking you some very personal and specific questions so that we can provide the best care for both you and your baby." This conveys a nonjudgmental approach, shows respect, and makes the woman feel more at ease. Each agency has its own admission forms, but they usually include the following information.

- Woman's name and age
- Last menstrual period (LMP) and estimated date of birth (EDB)
- Attending physician or certified nurse-midwife (CNM)
- Personal data: blood type; Rh factor; results of serology testing; prepregnant and present weight; allergies to medications, foods, or other substances; prescribed

and over-the-counter medications taken during pregnancy; and history of drug and alcohol use and smoking during the pregnancy
- History of previous illness, such as tuberculosis, heart disease, diabetes, convulsive disorders, and thyroid disorders; asthma; sickle cell/Tay Sachs and other inherited disorders; pregnancy-related complications (such as preterm labor, gestational diabetes, preeclampsia, low platelets)
- Problems in the prenatal period, such as elevated blood pressure, bleeding problems, recurrent urinary tract infections, other infections, abnormal laboratory findings (such as abnormal glucose screen indicating gestational diabetes or low hemoglobin or hematocrit indicating anemia), or sexually transmitted infections
- Pregnancy data: gravida, para, abortions, and neonatal deaths
- The method chosen for infant feeding
- Type of childbirth education or infant care classes
- Previous infant care experience
- Woman's preferences regarding labor and birth, such as no episiotomy, no analgesics or anesthetics, or the presence of the father or others at the birth
- Pediatrician, family practice physician, or nurse practitioner
- Additional data: history of special tests such as non-stress test (NST), biophysical profile (BPP), or ultrasound; history of any preterm labor; onset of labor; amniotic fluid membrane status; and brief description of any previous labor and birth
- Onset of labor, status of amniotic membranes (intact, ruptured, time of rupture, color, and odor)

Assessment of psychosocial history is a critical component of intrapartal nursing assessment. More than 500,000 pregnancies annually are affected by some type of mental illness that is either present before or emerges with pregnancy (ACOG, 2008). An estimated one-third of all pregnant women are exposed to some type of psychotropic medication during their pregnancies. In addition, an estimated 17% of pregnant women have diagnosed depression during pregnancy; up to 70% report depressive symptoms while pregnant (ACOG, 2008). Other mental illnesses include bipolar disorder, anxiety disorders, and schizophrenia. It is also not uncommon for adults to be diagnosed with eating disorders, autism, learning disabilities, and attention deficit or attention deficit hyperactivity disorder. All of these diagnoses can play a role in how the woman copes with the labor and birth experience and should be assessed by the admitting nurse. Women with identified disorders will need ongoing assessment during the labor and birth.

Because of the prevalence of domestic violence in our society (see Chapter 5 ∞), the nurse needs to consider the possibility that the woman may have experienced abuse at some point in her life. Although the incidence of rape in the United States is declining, sexual assault affects 0.8 per 1000 individuals over the age of 12 in the United States (U.S. Department of Justice, 2006). In addition, it is estimated that one out of every three women has been victimized by the age of 18 (Siegfried, 2007). Many victims of domestic violence, sexual assault, or childhood abuse may be anxious about the labor process, or anxiety may arise during labor. Therefore, it is essential to review the woman's prenatal record and any other available records for information that may indicate abuse or a history of victimization of violence. Antepartal assessment for domestic violence is discussed in Chapter 10 ∞.

HINTS FOR PRACTICE

Many nurses have difficulty asking questions about domestic violence, sexual abuse, and drug or alcohol use during pregnancy. However, this information is necessary to provide the best nursing care possible. To create a relationship of trust in which the woman feels safe answering uncomfortable questions, the following tips may be helpful:

- Explore your own beliefs and values.
- Use open-ended questions.
- Be receptive of the answers.
- Be accepting of others' life experiences.

CRITICAL THINKING

You are the birthing center nurse and you have reason to suspect that Lynn Ling, who has just been admitted in labor, may be in an abusive relationship. How could you set up an interview so that the partner would leave the room (and take any accompanying children) without feeling that you are possibly increasing the risk to the woman? What communication techniques would you use to encourage Lynn to reveal if her partner is abusive?

Answers can be found in Appendix F ∞.

Intrapartal High-Risk Screening

Screening for intrapartal high-risk factors is an integral part of assessing the normal laboring woman. As the history is obtained, the nurse notes the presence of any potential risk factors that may be considered high-risk conditions. For example, the woman who reports a physical symptom such as intermittent bleeding needs further assessment to rule out abruptio placentae or placenta previa before the admission process continues. It is important

to determine the difference between vaginal bleeding and bloody show. Bloody show is usually brown to reddish brown in color with a tinged vaginal discharge that is mucousy in consistency, whereas vaginal bleeding is bright red in color and is more like the type of bleeding encountered from a cut or laceration. In addition to identifying the presence of a high-risk condition, the nurse must recognize the implications of the condition for the laboring woman and her fetus. For example, if there is an abnormal fetal presentation, the nurse understands that the labor may be prolonged, prolapse of the umbilical cord is more likely, and the possibility of a cesarean birth is increased.

Although physical conditions are frequently listed as the major factors that increase risk in the intrapartal period, socioeconomic and cultural variables such as poverty, nutrition, the amount of prenatal care, crowded living conditions, cultural beliefs regarding pregnancy, and communication patterns may also precipitate a high-risk situation. Mental illness is also a risk factor because it can result in episodic prenatal care or the need to take psychotropic medications during the pregnancy (ACOG, 2008). In addition, recent research indicates that women who suffer from post-traumatic stress disorder (PTSD) may be at increased risk for some pregnancy complications (Griebenow, 2006). Other risk factors include smoking, drug use, and consumption of alcohol during pregnancy. The nurse can quickly review the prenatal record for number of prenatal visits; weight gain during pregnancy; progression of fundal height; assistance such as Medicaid and the Special Supplemental Food Program for Women, Infants, and Children (WIC); exposure to environmental agents; and history of traumatic life events, including abuse.

The nurse can begin gathering data about sociocultural factors as the woman enters the birthing area. The nurse observes the communication pattern between the woman and her support person(s) and their responses to admission questions and initial teaching. If the woman and her support person(s) do not speak English and translators are not available among the birthing unit staff, the course of labor and the nurse's ability to interact and provide support and education are affected. The couple must receive information in their primary language to make informed decisions. Communication may also be affected by cultural practices such as beliefs about when to speak, who should ask questions, or whether it is acceptable to let others know about discomfort. People from certain cultures may want to experience birth naturally and may decline pain medications. In some cultures, the father is not expected to be present in the birthing area. Nurses need to be culturally sensitive so that this is not interpreted as being disinterested in the birth, the mother, or the infant (Spector, 2009).

A partial list of intrapartal risk factors appears in Table 18–1. The factors precede the Intrapartal Assessment Guide because they must be kept in mind during the assessment.

TABLE 18-1 Intrapartal High-Risk Factors

Factor	Maternal Implication	Fetal-Neonatal Implication
Abnormal presentation	↑ Incidence of cesarean birth ↑ Incidence of prolonged labor ↑ Incidence of fibroids	↑ Incidence of placenta previa Prematurity ↑ Risk of congenital abnormality Neonatal physical trauma ↑ Risk of intrauterine growth restriction
Multiple gestation	↑ Uterine distention → ↑ risk of postpartum hemorrhage ↑ Risk of cesarean birth ↑ Risk of preterm labor	Low birth weight Prematurity ↑ Risk of congenital anomalies Feto-fetal transfusion
Hydramnios	↑ Discomfort ↑ Dyspnea ↑ Risk of preterm labor Edema of lower extremities/varicosities	↑ Risk of esophageal or other high alimentary tract atresias ↑ Risk of CNS anomalies (myelocele) ↑ Risk of prolapsed cord
Oligohydramnios	Maternal fear of "dry birth"	↑ Incidence of congenital anomalies ↑ Incidence of renal lesions ↑ Risk of intrauterine growth restriction ↑ Risk of fetal acidosis ↑ Risk of cord compression Postmaturity
Meconium staining of amniotic fluid	↑ Psychologic stress caused by fear for baby	↑ Risk of fetal asphyxia ↑ Risk of meconium aspiration ↑ Risk of pneumonia caused by aspiration of meconium
Premature rupture of membranes	↑ Risk of infection (chorioamnionitis) ↑ Risk of preterm labor ↑ Anxiety/fear for the baby Prolonged hospitalization ↑ Incidence of tocolytic therapy	↑ Perinatal morbidity Prematurity ↓ Birth weight ↑ Risk of respiratory distress syndrome Prolonged hospitalization
Induction of labor	↑ Risk of hypercontractility of uterus ↑ Risk of uterine rupture ↑ Length of labor if cervix not ready ↑ Anxiety	Prematurity if gestational age not assessed correctly Hypoxia if hyperstimulation occurs
Abruptio placentae/placenta previa	Hemorrhage Uterine atony ↑ Incidence of cesarean birth ↑ Maternal morbidity	Fetal hypoxia/acidosis Fetal exsanguination ↑ Perinatal mortality
Failure to progress in labor	Maternal exhaustion ↑ Incidence of augmentation of labor ↑ Incidence of cesarean birth	Fetal hypoxia/acidosis Intracranial birth injury
Precipitous labor (less than 3 hours)	Perineal, vaginal, cervical lacerations ↑ Risk of postpartum hemorrhage	Tentorial tears
Prolapse of umbilical cord	↑ Fear for baby Cesarean birth → emergent	Acute fetal hypoxia/acidosis
Fetal heart aberrations	↑ Fear for baby ↑ Risk of cesarean birth, forceps, vacuum Continuous electronic monitoring and intervention in labor	Tachycardia or bradycardia Acute or chronic asphyxic insult Chronic hypoxia Congenital heart block
Uterine rupture	Hemorrhage Cesarean birth/hysterectomy ↑ Risk of morbidity/mortality	Fetal anoxia Fetal hemorrhage ↑ Neonatal morbidity and mortality
Postdates (greater than 42 weeks)	↑ Anxiety ↑ Incidence of induction of labor ↑ Incidence of cesarean birth ↑ Use of technology to monitor fetus ↑ Risk of shoulder dystocia	Postmaturity syndrome ↑ Risk of fetal-neonatal mortality and morbidity ↑ Risk of antepartum fetal death ↑ Incidence/risk of large baby
Diabetes	↑ Risk of hydramnios ↑ Risk of hypoglycemia or hyperglycemia ↑ Risk of preeclampsia	↑ Risk of malpresentation ↑ Risk of macrosomia ↑ Risk of intrauterine growth restriction ↑ Risk of respiratory distress syndrome ↑ Risk of congenital anomalies
Preeclampsia	↑ Abruptio placentae ↑ Risk of seizures ↑ Risk of stroke ↑ Risk of HELLP	↑ Risk of small-for-gestational-age baby ↑ Risk of preterm birth ↑ Risk of mortality
AIDS/STI	↑ Risk of additional infections	↑ Risk of transplacental transmission

EVIDENCE-BASED PRACTICE

Third Trimester Antiviral Prophylaxis for Genital Herpes Simplex Virus

Clinical Question

How effective is antenatal antiviral prophylaxis for recurrent genital herpes in preventing maternal recurrence and transmission of the infection to the newborn?

The Evidence

Infection with genital herpes simplex virus (HSV) is one of the most common sexually transmitted infections. Three out of four women with HSV infection before pregnancy will have a recurrence during the prenatal period or will demonstrate clinical presence at birth. Transmission of the virus to the newborn typically occurs by direct contact with the virus in the genital tract during birth. The traditional approach has been to recommend a cesarean birth to any woman with active genital lesions or prodromal symptoms when labor begins. Several antiviral agents are available for use both for therapy and for preventing a flare-up. Seven studies that compared the use of antiviral agents to placebo were systematically appraised and the findings were aggregated in the Cochrane Database of Systematic Reviews. This type of unbiased review of multiple trials that meets the rigorous standards of the Cochrane review represents the strongest level of evidence for practice.

What Is Effective?

Women who received antiviral prophylaxis were significantly less likely to have an active recurrence of genital herpes at the time of birth. They were also less likely to need cesarean birth specifically for genital herpes. The women receiving the antiviral drugs were also less likely to have active disease detected in the vagina at birth, limiting neonatal exposure to viral shed.

What Is Inconclusive?

The effect of antiviral prophylaxis before the onset of labor could not be assessed, as women in neither the experimental nor control groups had active disease during the intrapartum period. Little evidence exists about the effects of antiviral usage on neonatal outcomes, including the rate of neonatal herpes infection.

Best Practice

Antenatal antiviral prophylaxis reduces viral shedding and prenatal recurrence, and so reduces the need for cesarean birth specifically for genital herpes. The risks, benefits, and alternatives should be explained to women who have a history of HSV, but you can also reassure the mother that the risk of the baby getting herpes during birth is low regardless of preventive treatment.

Reference

Hollier, L., & Wendel, G. (2008). Third trimester antiviral prophylaxis for preventing maternal genital herpes simplex virus (HSV) recurrences and neonatal infection. *Cochrane Database of Systematic Reviews.* Issue 2.

Intrapartal Physical and Psychosociocultural Assessment

A physical examination is part of the admission procedure and part of the ongoing care of the client. Although the intrapartal physical assessment is not as complete and thorough as the initial prenatal physical examination (Chapter 10 ∞), it does involve assessment of some body systems and the actual labor process. The Intrapartal Assessment Guide provides a framework the maternity nurse can use when examining the laboring woman.

The physical assessment portion includes assessments performed immediately on admission as well as ongoing assessments. Nurses should conduct ongoing assessments in all clinical situations. For example, when the woman is changing into her gown, the nurse can assess the skin for bruises, needlemarks, burns, or other abnormalities. The nurse can also determine if the woman appears under- or overnourished. When labor is progressing rapidly, the nurse may not have time for a complete assessment. In that case, the critical physical assessments include maternal vital signs, labor status, fetal status, and laboratory findings.

The cultural assessment portion provides a starting point for this important aspect of assessment. Individual-ized nursing care can best be planned and implemented when the values and beliefs of the laboring woman are known and honored (Spector, 2009). To avoid stereotyping clients the nurse always asks the woman and her family about individual beliefs and preferences. Nurses who feel uncertain about what to ask or consider need to explore the varying cultural values and beliefs of the people residing in their community. Some communities have a prominent culture that may follow certain rituals but it is still important for the nurse to ask each woman about her own beliefs and preferences.

The final section of the assessment guide addresses psychosocial factors, including ideas, knowledge, fantasies, and fears about childbearing. In addition, women with a previous history of psychologic disorders, such as anxiety or depression, may have unique needs during labor. The nurse should specifically ask the woman if she has any special needs in which she anticipates knowing that some women may not know what needs will arise. This makes ongoing assessments imperative. It is important that the nurse pay specific attention to body language, eye contact, and other nonverbal cues which may indicate that the woman is experiencing anxiety or other feelings. By assessing her psychosocial status, the nurse can meet the

ASSESSMENT GUIDE   INTRAPARTAL—FIRST STAGE OF LABOR

Physical Assessment/ Normal Findings	Alterations and Possible Causes*	Nursing Responses to Data†
Vital Signs		
Blood pressure (BP): Less than or equal to 135 systolic and 85 diastolic in adult 18 years of age or older or no more than 15 to 20 mm Hg use in systolic pressure over baseline BP during early pregnancy	High blood pressure (essential hypertension, preeclampsia, renal disease, apprehension, anxiety, or pain) Low blood pressure (supine hypotension) Hemorrhage/hypovolemia Shock Drugs	Evaluate history of preexisting disorders and check for presence of other signs of preeclampsia. Do not assess during contractions; implement measures to decrease anxiety and reassess. Turn woman on her side and recheck BP. Provide quiet environment. Have O_2 available.
Pulse: 60 to 90 bpm	Increased pulse rate (excitement or anxiety, cardiac disorders, early shock, drug use)	Evaluate cause, reassess to see if rate continues; report to physician/CNM.
Respirations: 16 to 24/min (or pulse rate divided by 4)	Marked tachypnea (respiratory disease), hyperventilation in transition phase Decreased respirations (narcotics)	Assess between contractions; if marked tachypnea continues, assess for signs of respiratory disease or respiratory distress.
	Hyperventilation (anxiety/pain)	Encourage slow breaths if woman is hyperventilating.
Pulse oximetry 95% or greater	Less than 90%: hypoxia, hypotension, hemorrhage	Apply O_2; notify physician/CNM.
Temperature: 36.2°C to 37.6°C (97°F to 99.6°F)	Elevated temperature (infection, dehydration, prolonged rupture of membranes, epidural regional block)	Assess for other signs of infection or dehydration.
Weight		
25 to 35 lb greater than prepregnant weight	Weight gain greater than 35 lb (fluid retention, obesity, large infant, diabetes mellitus, preeclampsia), weight gain less than 15 lb (SGA, substance abuse, psychosocial problems)	Assess for signs of edema. Evaluate, OATA from prenatal record.
Lungs		
Normal breath sounds, clear and equal	Rales, rhonchi, friction rub (infection), pulmonary edema, asthma	Reassess; refer to physician/CNM.
Fundus		
At 40 weeks' gestation located just below xiphoid process	Uterine size not compatible with estimated date of birth (SGA, large for gestational age [LGA], hydramnios, multiple pregnancy, placental/fetal anomalies, malpresentation)	Reevaluate history regarding pregnancy dating. Refer to physician/CNM for additional assessment.
Edema		
Slight amount of dependent edema	Pitting edema of face, hands, legs, abdomen, sacral area (preeclampsia)	Check deep tendon reflexes for hyperactivity; check for clonus; refer to physician/CNM.
Hydration		
Normal skin turgor, elastic	Poor skin turgor (dehydration)	Assess skin turgor; refer to physician for deviations. Provide fluids per physician/CNM orders.
	*Possible causes of alterations are identified in parentheses.	†This column provides guidelines for further assessment and initial nursing intervention.

(Continued)

ASSESSMENT GUIDE   INTRAPARTAL—FIRST STAGE OF LABOR (Continued)

Physical Assessment/ Normal Findings	Alterations and Possible Causes*	Nursing Responses to Data†
Perineum		
Tissues smooth, pink color (see Initial Prenatal Assessment Guide, Chapter 10 ∞)	Varicose veins of vulva, herpes lesions/genital warts	Note on client record need for follow-up in postpartal period; reassess after birth, refer to physician/CNM.
Clear mucus; may be blood tinged with earthy or human odor	Profuse, purulent, foul-smelling drainage	Suspected gonorrhea or chorioamnionitis; report to physician/CNM; initiate care to newborn's eyes; notify neonatal nursing staff and pediatrician.
Presence of small amount of bloody show that gradually increases with further cervical dilatation	Hemorrhage	Assess BP and pulse, pallor, diaphoresis, report any marked changes. Standard precautions.
Labor Status		
Uterine contractions: Regular pattern	Failure to establish a regular pattern, prolonged latent phase Hypertonicity Hypotonicity Dehydration	Evaluate whether woman is in true labor. Ambulate if in early labor. Evaluate client status and contractile pattern. Obtain a 20-minute EFM strip. Notify physician/CNM. Provide hydration.
Cervical dilatation: Progressive cervical dilatation from size of fingertip to 10 cm (Clinical Skill: Performing an Intrapartal Vaginal Examination)	Rigidity of cervix (frequent cervical infections, scar tissue, failure of presenting part to descend)	Evaluate contractions, fetal engagement, position, and cervical dilatation. Inform client of progress.
Cervical effacement: Progressive thinning of cervix (Clinical Skill: Performing an Intrapartal Vaginal Examination)	Failure to efface (rigidity of cervix, failure of presenting part to engage); cervical edema (pushing effort by woman before cervix is fully dilated and effaced, trapped cervix)	Evaluate contractions, fetal engagement, and position. Notify physician/CNM if cervix is becoming edematous; work with woman to prevent pushing until cervix is completely dilated. Keep vaginal exams to a minimum.
Fetal descent: Progressive descent of fetal presenting part from station −5 to + 4 (Figure 18–4 in Clinical Skill: Performing an Intrapartal Vaginal Examination)	Failure of descent (abnormal fetal position or presentation, macrosomic fetus, inadequate pelvic measurements)	Evaluate fetal position, presentation, and size.
Membranes: May rupture before or during labor	Rupture of membranes more than 12 to 24 hours before onset of labor	Assess for ruptured membranes using Nitrazine test tape before doing vaginal exam. Follow standard precautions. Instruct woman with ruptured membranes to remain on bed rest if presenting part is not engaged and firmly down against the cervix. Keep vaginal exams to a minimum to prevent infection. When membranes rupture in the birth setting *immediately assess FHR* to detect changes associated with prolapse of umbilical cord (FHR slows).
Findings on **Nitrazine test tape:** Membranes probably intact Yellow pH 5.0 Olive pH 5.5 Olive green pH 6.0	False-positive results may be obtained if large amount of bloody show is present, previous vaginal examination has been done using lubricant, or tape is touched by nurse's fingers	Assess fluid for consistency, amount, odor; assess FHR frequently. Assess fluid at regular intervals for presence of meconium staining. Follow standard precautions while assessing amniotic fluid.
	*Possible causes of alterations are identified in parentheses.	†This column provides guidelines for further assessment and initial nursing intervention.

ASSESSMENT GUIDE   INTRAPARTAL—FIRST STAGE OF LABOR (Continued)

Physical Assessment/ Normal Findings	Alterations and Possible Causes*	Nursing Responses to Data†
Membranes probably ruptured Blue-green pH 6.5 Blue-gray pH 7.0 Deep blue pH 7.5		Teach woman that amniotic fluid is continually produced (to allay fear of "dry birth"). Teach woman that she may feel amniotic fluid trickle or gush with contractions. Change chux pads often.
Amniotic fluid clear, with earthy or human odor, no foul-smelling odor	Greenish amniotic fluid (fetal stress) Bloody fluid (vasoprevia abruptio placentae)	Assess FHR; do vaginal exam to evaluate for prolapsed cord; apply fetal monitor for continuous data; report to physician/CNM.
	Strong or foul odor (amnionitis)	Take woman's temperature and report to physician/CNM.
Fetal Status		
FHR: 110 to 160 bpm	Less than 110 or greater than 160 bpm (nonreassuring fetal status); abnormal patterns on fetal monitor: decreased variability, late decelerations, variable decelerations, absence of accelerations with fetal movement	Initiate interventions based on particular FHR pattern.
Presentation: Cephalic, 97% Breech, 3%	Face, brow, breech, or shoulder presentation	Report to physician/CNM; after presentation is confirmed as face, brow, breech, or shoulder, woman may be prepared for cesarean birth.
Position: Left-occiput-anterior (LOA) most common	Persistent occipital-posterior (OP) position; transverse arrest	Carefully monitor maternal and fetal status. Reposition mother side-lying or hands/knee to promote rotation of fetal head.
Activity: Fetal movement	Hyperactivity (may precede fetal hypoxia)	Carefully evaluate FHR; apply fetal monitor.
	Complete lack of movement (nonreassuring fetal status or fetal demise)	Carefully evaluate FHR; apply fetal monitor. Report to physician/CNM.
Laboratory Evaluation		
Hematologic tests **Hemoglobin:** 12 to 16 g/dL	Less than 11 g/dL (anemia, hemorrhage, sickle cell disorders, pernicious anemia)	Evaluate woman for problems associated with decreased oxygen-carrying capacity caused by lowered hemoglobin.
CBC **Hematocrit:** 38% to 47% **RBC:** 4.2 to 5.4 million/mm³ **WBC:** 4500 to 11,000/mm³, although leukocytosis to 20,000/mm³ is not unusual **Platelets:** 150,000 to 400,000/mm³	Presence of infection or blood dyscrasias, loss of blood (hemorrhage, disseminated intravascular coagulation [DIC])	Evaluate for other signs of infections, petechiae, bruising, or unusual bleeding.
Serologic testing STS or VDRL test: nonreactive Rh	Positive reaction (Chapter 10 ∞, Initial Prenatal Assessment Guide)	For reactive test notify newborn nursery and pediatrician.
	Rh-positive fetus in Rh-negative woman	Assess prenatal record for titer levels during pregnancy.
		Obtain cord blood for direct Coombs' at birth.
	*Possible causes of alterations are identified in parentheses.	†This column provides guidelines for further assessment and initial nursing intervention.

(Continued)

ASSESSMENT GUIDE   INTRAPARTAL—FIRST STAGE OF LABOR (Continued)

Physical Assessment/ Normal Findings	Alterations and Possible Causes*	Nursing Responses to Data†
Urinalysis		
Glucose: negative	Glycosuria (low renal threshold for glucose, diabetes mellitus)	Assess blood glucose; test urine for ketones; ketonuria and glycosuria require further assessment of blood sugars.†
Ketones: negative	Ketonuria (starvation ketosis)	
Proteins: negative	Proteinuria (urine specimen contaminated with vaginal secretions, fever, kidney disease); proteinuria of 2+ or greater found in uncontaminated urine may be a sign of ensuing preeclampsia	Instruct woman in collection technique; incidence of contamination from vaginal discharge is common. Report any increase in proteinuria to physician/CNM.
Red blood cells: negative	Blood in urine (calculi, cystitis, glomerulonephritis, neoplasm)	Assess collection technique (may be bloody show).
White blood cells: negative	Presence of white blood cells (infection in genitourinary tract)	Assess for signs of urinary tract infections.
Casts: none	Presence of casts (nephrotic syndrome)	

Cultural Assessment§	Variations to Consider	Nursing Responses to Data†
Cultural influences determine customs and practices regarding intrapartal care.	Individual preferences may vary.	
Ask the following questions: Who would you like to remain with you during your labor and birth?	She may prefer only her partner/significant other to remain or may also want family and/or friends.	Provide support for her wishes by encouraging desired people to stay. Provide information to others (with the woman's permission) who are not in the room.
What would you like to wear during labor?	She may be more comfortable in her own clothes.	Offer supportive materials such as chux if needed to protect her own clothing. Avoid subtle signals to the woman that she should not have chosen to remain in her own clothes. Have other clothing available if the woman desires. If her clothing becomes contaminated, it will be simple to place it in a plastic bag.
What activity would you like during labor?	She may want to ambulate most of the time, stand in the shower, sit in the jacuzzi, sit on a chair/stool/birthing ball, remain on the bed, and so forth.	Support the woman's wishes; provide encouragement and complete assessments in a manner so her activity and positional wishes are disturbed as little as possible.
What position would you like for the birth?	She may feel more comfortable in lithotomy with stirrups and her upper body elevated, or side-lying or sitting in a birthing bed, or standing, or squatting, or on hands and knees.	Collect any supplies and equipment needed to support her in her chosen birthing position. Provide information to the coach regarding any changes that may be needed based on the chosen position.

§These are only a few suggestions. We do not mean to imply that this is a comprehensive cultural assessment; rather, it is a tool to encourage cultural sensitivity.

*Possible causes of alterations are identified in parentheses.

†This column provides guidelines for further assessment and initial nursing intervention.

ASSESSMENT GUIDE INTRAPARTAL—FIRST STAGE OF LABOR *(Continued)*

Cultural Assessment[§]	Variations to Consider	Nursing Responses to Data[†]
Is there anything special you would like?	She may want the room darkened or to have curtains and windows open, music playing, a Leboyer birth, her coach to cut the umbilical cord, to save a portion of the umbilical cord, to save the placenta, to videotape the birth, and so forth.	Support requests, and communicate requests to any other nursing or medical personnel (so requests can continue to be supported and not questioned). If another nurse or physician does not honor the request, act as advocate for the woman by continuing to support her unless her desire is truly unsafe.
Ask the woman if she would like fluids, and ask what temperature she prefers.	She may prefer clear fluids other than water (tea, clear juice). She may prefer iced, room-temperature, or warmed fluids.	Provide fluids as desired.
Observe the woman's response when privacy is difficult to maintain and her body is exposed.	Some women do not seem to mind being exposed during an exam or procedure; others feel acute discomfort.	Maintain privacy and respect the woman's sense of privacy. If the woman is unable to provide specific information, the nurse may draw from general information regarding cultural variation: Southeast Asian women may not want any family member in the room during exam or procedures. Her partner may not be involved with coaching activities during labor or birth. Muslim women may need to remain covered during the labor and birth and avoid exposure of any body part. The husband may need to be in the room but remain behind a curtain or screen so he does not view his wife at this time.
If the woman is to breastfeed, ask if she would like to feed her baby immediately after birth.	She may want to feed her baby right away or may want to wait a little while.	

Psychosocial Assessment	Variations to Consider	Nursing Responses to Data[†]
Preparation for Childbirth		
Woman has some information regarding process of normal labor and birth.	Some women do not have any information regarding childbirth.	Add to present information base.
Woman has breathing and/or relaxation techniques to use during labor.	Some women do not have any method of relaxation or breathing to use, and some do not desire them.	Support breathing and relaxation techniques that client is using; provide information if needed.
Woman and support person have done extensive preparation for childbirth (Bradley classes, Lamaze).	Some women have strong opinions regarding labor and birth preparation.	Support woman's wishes to participate in her birth experience; support birthplan.
Response to Labor		
Latent phase: Relaxed, excited, anxious for labor to be well established	May feel unable to cope with contractions because of fear, anxiety, or lack of information	Provide support and encouragement, establish trusting relationship.

[§]These are only a few suggestions. We do not mean to imply that this is a comprehensive cultural assessment; rather, it is a tool to encourage cultural sensitivity.

[†]This column provides guidelines for further assessment and initial nursing intervention.

(Continued)

ASSESSMENT GUIDE INTRAPARTAL—FIRST STAGE OF LABOR (Continued)

Psychosocial Assessment	Variations to Consider	Nursing Responses to Data[†]
Active phase: Becomes more intense, begins to tire	May remain quiet and without any sign of discomfort or anxiety, may insist that she is unable to continue with the birthing process	Provide support and coaching if needed.
Transitional phase: Feels tired, may feel unable to cope, needs frequent coaching to maintain breathing patterns		
Coping mechanisms: Ability to cope with labor through use of support system, breathing, relaxation techniques, and comfort measures including frequent position changes in labor, warm water immersion, and massage	May feel marked anxiety and apprehension, may not have coping mechanisms that can be brought into this experience, or may be unable to use them at this time	Support coping mechanisms if they are working for the woman; provide information and support if she exhibits anxiety or needs alternative to present coping methods.
	Survivors of sexual abuse may demonstrate fear of IVs or needles, may recoil when touched, may insist on a female caregiver, may be very sensitive to body fluids and cleanliness, and may be unable to labor lying down	Encourage participation of coach/significant other if a supportive relationship seems apparent. Establish rapport and a trusting relationship. Provide information that is true and offer your presence.
Anxiety		
Some anxiety and apprehension is within normal limits	May show anxiety through rapid breathing, nervous tremors, frowning, grimacing, clenching of teeth, thrashing movements, crying, increased pulse and blood pressure	Provide support, encouragement, and information. Teach relaxation technique. Support controlled breathing efforts. May need to provide a paper bag to breathe into if woman says her lips are tingling. Note FHR.
Sounds During Labor		
	Some women are very quiet; others moan or make a variety of noises.	Provide a supportive environment. Encourage woman to do what feels right for her.
Support System		
Physical intimacy between mother and father (or mother and support person/doula) caretaking activities such as soothing conversation, touching	Some women would prefer no contact, others may show clinging behaviors.	Encourage caretaking activities that appear to comfort the woman; encourage support for the woman; if support is limited, the nurse may take a more active role.
Support person stays in close proximity	Limited interaction may come from a desire for quiet.	Encourage support person to stay close (if this seems appropriate).
Relationship between mother and father or support person: involved interaction	The support person may seem to be detached and maintain little support, attention, or conversation.	Support interactions; if interaction is limited, the nurse may provide more information and support. Ensure that partner/significant other has short breaks, especially before transition.

[†]This column provides guidelines for further assessment and initial nursing intervention.

woman's needs for information and support. The nurse can then assist the woman and her partner; in the absence of a partner, the nurse may become the support person.

While performing the intrapartal assessment, it is imperative that the nurse follow Centers for Disease Control and Prevention (CDC) guidelines to prevent exposure to body substances. Gloves should be worn at all times when performing vaginal assessments or providing pericare. A waterproof apron and mask or eye protection should be worn if fluid exposure is likely.

Methods of Evaluating Labor Progress

The nurse assesses the woman's contractions and cervical dilatation and effacement to evaluate labor progress.

Contraction Assessment

Uterine contractions may be assessed by palpation or continuous electronic monitoring.

PALPATION The nurse assesses contractions for frequency, duration, and intensity by placing one hand on the uterine fundus. The hand is kept relatively still because excessive movement may stimulate contractions or cause discomfort. The nurse determines the frequency of the contractions by noting the time from the beginning of one contraction to the beginning of the next. If contractions begin at 7:00, 7:04, and 7:08, for example, their frequency is every 4 minutes. To determine contraction duration, the nurse notes the time when tensing of the fundus is first felt (beginning of contraction) and again as relaxation occurs (end of contraction). During the peak or acme of the contraction, intensity can be evaluated by estimating the indentability of the fundus. The nurse should assess at least three successive contractions to provide enough data to determine the contraction pattern. See Key Facts to Remember: Contraction and Labor Progress Characteristics for review of characteristics in different phases of labor.

HINTS FOR PRACTICE

Many experienced nurses note that mild contractions are similar in consistency to the tip of the nose, moderate contractions feel more like the chin, and with strong contractions, there is little indentability, much like the forehead. When palpating a woman's uterus during a contraction, compare the consistency to your nose, chin, and forehead to determine the intensity.

This is also a good time to assess the laboring woman's perception of pain. How does she describe the pain? What is her affect? Is this contraction more uncomfortable than the last one? Is the nurse's palpation of intensity congruent with the woman's perception? (For instance, the nurse

KEY FACTS TO REMEMBER
Contraction and Labor Progress Characteristics

CONTRACTION CHARACTERISTICS

Latent phase:	Every 10 to 30 min × 30 sec; mild, progressing to Every 5 to 7 min × 30 to 40 sec; moderate
Active phase:	Every 2 to 5 min × 40 to 60 sec; moderate to strong
Transition phase:	Every 1½ to 2 min × 60 to 90 sec; strong

LABOR PROGRESS CHARACTERISTICS

Primipara:	At least 1.2 cm/hr dilatation At least 1 cm/hr descent Less than 2 hr in second stage
Multipara:	At least 1.5 cm/hr dilatation At least 2.1 cm/hr descent Less than 1 hr in second stage

might evaluate a contraction as mild in intensity whereas the laboring woman evaluates it as very strong.) A nurse's assessment is not complete unless the laboring woman's affect and response to the contractions are also noted and charted.

ELECTRONIC MONITORING OF CONTRACTIONS Electronic monitoring of uterine contractions provides continuous data. In many birth settings electronic monitoring is routine for high-risk clients and women who are having oxytocin-induced labor; other facilities monitor all laboring women. Although electronic monitoring offers many advantages, it is useless unless it is coupled with careful nursing assessment.

Electronic monitoring may be done externally, with a device that is placed against the maternal abdomen, or internally, with an **intrauterine pressure catheter (IUPC)**. When monitoring by external means, the portion of the monitoring equipment called a *tocodynamometer*, or "toco," is positioned against the fundus of the uterus and held in place with an elastic belt (Figure 18–1 ■). The toco contains a flexible disk that responds to pressure. When the uterus contracts, the fundus tightens and the change in pressure against the toco is amplified and transmitted to the electronic fetal monitor. The monitor displays the uterine contraction as a pattern on graph paper.

External monitoring offers several advantages including providing a continuous recording of the frequency and duration of uterine contractions and is noninvasive. However, it does not accurately record the intensity of the uterine contraction, and it is difficult to obtain an accurate fetal heart rate in some women, such as those who are

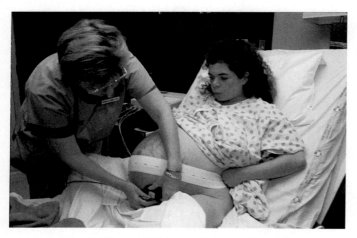

FIGURE 18–1 Woman in labor with external monitor applied. The tocodynamometer placed on the uterine fundus is recording uterine contractions. The lower belt holds the ultrasonic device that monitors the fetal heart rate. The belts can be adjusted for comfort.
Source: © Stella Johnson (www.stellajohnson.com).

very obese, those who have hydramnios (an abnormally large amount of amniotic fluid), or those whose fetus is very active. In addition, the woman may be bothered by the belt if it requires frequent readjustment when she changes position. It allows the nurse to continually monitor the fetus if there are concerns in the FHR. Continuous monitoring also enables the nurse and physician/CNM to observe the pattern of the fetal heart rate over a period of time, enabling them to examine the electronic fetal monitoring strip.

Internal intrauterine monitoring provides the same data and also provides accurate measurement of uterine contraction intensity (the strength of the contraction and the actual pressure within the uterus). After membranes have ruptured, the certified nurse-midwife (or the nurse in some facilities) or the physician inserts the IUPC into the uterine cavity and connects it by a cable to the electronic fetal monitor. It is importnat to first assess the fetal position and to review a past ultrasound to determine placenta placement. The internal monitor should be placed away from the placenta. If one has not been previously obtained, the physician/CNM may wish to do one on the unit or have the radiologist perform such an exam.

The pressure within the uterus in the resting state and during each contraction is measured by a small micropressure device located in the tip of the catheter. Internal electronic monitoring is used when it is imperative to have accurate intrauterine pressure readings to evaluate the stress on the uterus or to determine the adequacy of contractions. The advantage of the intrauterine pressure monitor is that it can directly measure the intensity of the contraction. It can be used in cases where the external monitor may not be accurately assessing the contraction strength, such as in cases of maternal obesity. It can also be used when oxytocin is being administered to ensure that uterine contractions are adequate.

It is important that the nurse also evaluate the woman's labor status by palpating the intensity and resting tone of the uterine fundus during contractions. Technology is a useful tool if used as an adjunct to good assessment skills.

Internal monitoring has both risks and benefits. It provides a more accurate fetal tracing and is more effective in monitoring the fetal status. Placement of an intrauterine pressure catheter can cause vaginal bleeding. In rare cases, the scalp electrode can be placed on the fetal fontanelle or on an eye if the fetus is in a face presentation, thus causing fetal injury. Women with certain medical conditions, such as HIV, should not be monitored with internal monitoring because it can increase the risk of viral transmission.

CERVICAL ASSESSMENT Cervical dilatation and effacement are evaluated directly by vaginal examination (see Clinical Skill: Performing an Intrapartal Vaginal Examination). The vaginal examination can provide information about the adequacy of the maternal pelvis, membrane status, characteristics of amniotic fluid, and fetal position and station.

Fetal Assessment

A complete intrapartal fetal assessment requires determination of the fetal position and presentation, and evaluation of the fetal status.

Fetal Position

Fetal position is determined in several ways:

- Inspection of the woman's abdomen
- Palpation of the woman's abdomen
- Vaginal examination to determine the presenting part
- Ultrasound
- Auscultation of fetal heart rate

Inspection

The nurse should observe the woman's abdomen for size and shape. The lie of the fetus should be assessed by noting whether the uterus projects up and down (longitudinal lie) or left to right (transverse lie).

Palpation: Leopold's Maneuvers

Leopold's maneuvers are a systematic way to evaluate the maternal abdomen. Frequent practice increases the examiner's skill in determining fetal position by palpation. Leopold's maneuvers may be difficult to perform on an obese woman or on a woman who has excessive amniotic

Clinical Skill Performing an Intrapartal Vaginal Examination

NURSING ACTION	RATIONALE

Preparation

1. Explain the procedure, the indications for the exam, what the exam may feel like, and that it may cause discomfort.

2. Assess for latex allergies.

3. Position the woman with her thighs flexed and abducted. Instruct her to put the heels of her feet together. Drape the woman with a sheet, leaving a flap to access the perineum.

   This position provides access to the woman's perineum. The drape ensures privacy.

4. Encourage the woman to relax her muscles and legs.

   Relaxation decreases muscle tension and increases comfort.

5. Inform the woman before touching her. Be gentle.

Equipment and Supplies

- Clean disposable gloves if membranes are not ruptured
- Sterile gloves if membranes are ruptured
- Lubricant
- Nitrazine test tape
- Slide
- Sterile cotton-tipped swab (Q-tip)

Before the Procedure: *Test for Fluid Leakage*

If fluid leakage has been reported or noted, use Nitrazine test tape and Q-tip with slide for fern test before performing the exam.

As long as lubricant has not been used, Nitrazine tape registers a change in pH if amniotic fluid is present.

Procedure (Sterile if membranes ruptured)

1. Pull glove onto dominant hand.

   Single glove is worn when membranes are intact. If a sterile exam is needed, both hands will be gloved with sterile gloves.

2. Using your gloved hand, position the hand with the wrist straight and the elbow tilted downward. Insert your well-lubricated second and index fingers of the gloved hand gently into the vagina until they touch the cervix. Use care when positioning your hand.

   This position allows the fingertips to point toward the umbilicus and find the cervix.

3. If the woman verbalizes discomfort, acknowledge it and apologize. Pause for a moment and allow her to relax before progressing.

   This validates the woman's discomfort and helps her feel more in control.

4. To determine the status of labor progress, perform the vaginal examination during and between contractions.

   Cervical effacement, dilatation, and fetal station are affected by the presence of a contraction.

5. Palpate for the opening, or a depression, in the cervix. Estimate the diameter of the depression to identify the amount of dilatation (see Figure 18–2 ■).

   Allows determination of effacement and dilatation.

6. Determine the status of the fetal membranes by observing for leakage of amniotic fluid. If fluid is expressed, test for amniotic fluid.

7. Palpate the presenting part (see Figure 18–3 ■).

   Determination of the presenting part is necessary to assess the position of the fetus and to evaluate fetal descent.

8. Assess the fetal descent (see Figure 18–4 ■) and station by identifying the position of the posterior fontanelle.

9. Record findings on woman's chart and on fetal monitor strip if fetal monitor is being used.

(Continued on next page)

Clinical Skill Performing an Intrapartal Vaginal Examination *(Continued)*

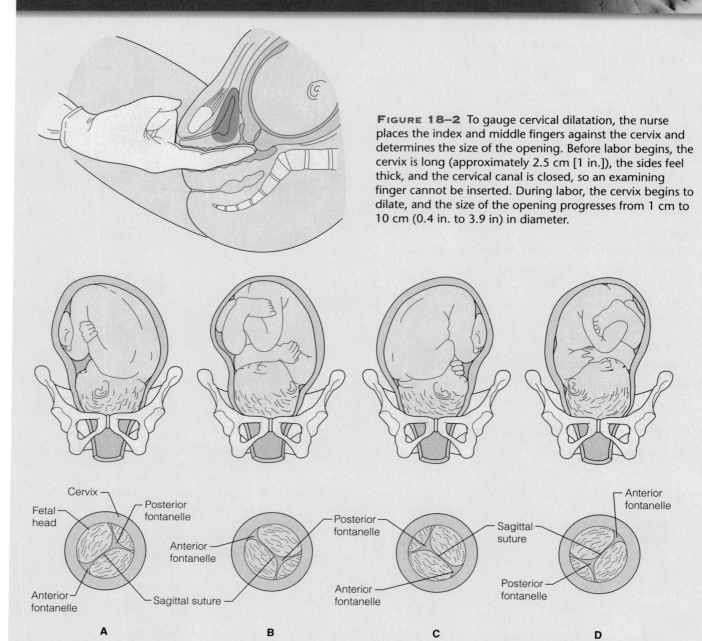

FIGURE 18–2 To gauge cervical dilatation, the nurse places the index and middle fingers against the cervix and determines the size of the opening. Before labor begins, the cervix is long (approximately 2.5 cm [1 in.]), the sides feel thick, and the cervical canal is closed, so an examining finger cannot be inserted. During labor, the cervix begins to dilate, and the size of the opening progresses from 1 cm to 10 cm (0.4 in. to 3.9 in) in diameter.

FIGURE 18–3 Palpation of the presenting part (the portion of the fetus that enters the pelvis first). *A,* Left occiput anterior (LOA). The occiput (area over the occipital bone on the posterior part of the fetal head) is in the left anterior quadrant of the woman's pelvis. When the fetus is in LOA, the posterior fontanelle (located just above the occipital bone and triangular in shape) is in the upper left quadrant of the maternal pelvis. *B,* Left occiput posterior (LOP). The posterior fontanelle is in the lower left quadrant of the maternal pelvis. *C,* Right occiput anterior (ROA). The posterior fontanelle is in the upper right quadrant of the maternal pelvis. *D,* Right occiput posterior (ROP). The posterior fontanelle is in the lower right quadrant of the maternal pelvis.
Note: The anterior fontanelle is diamond shaped. Because of the roundness of the fetal head, only a portion of the anterior fontanelle can be seen in each of the views, so it appears to be triangular in shape.

Clinical Skill Performing an Intrapartal Vaginal Examination *(Continued)*

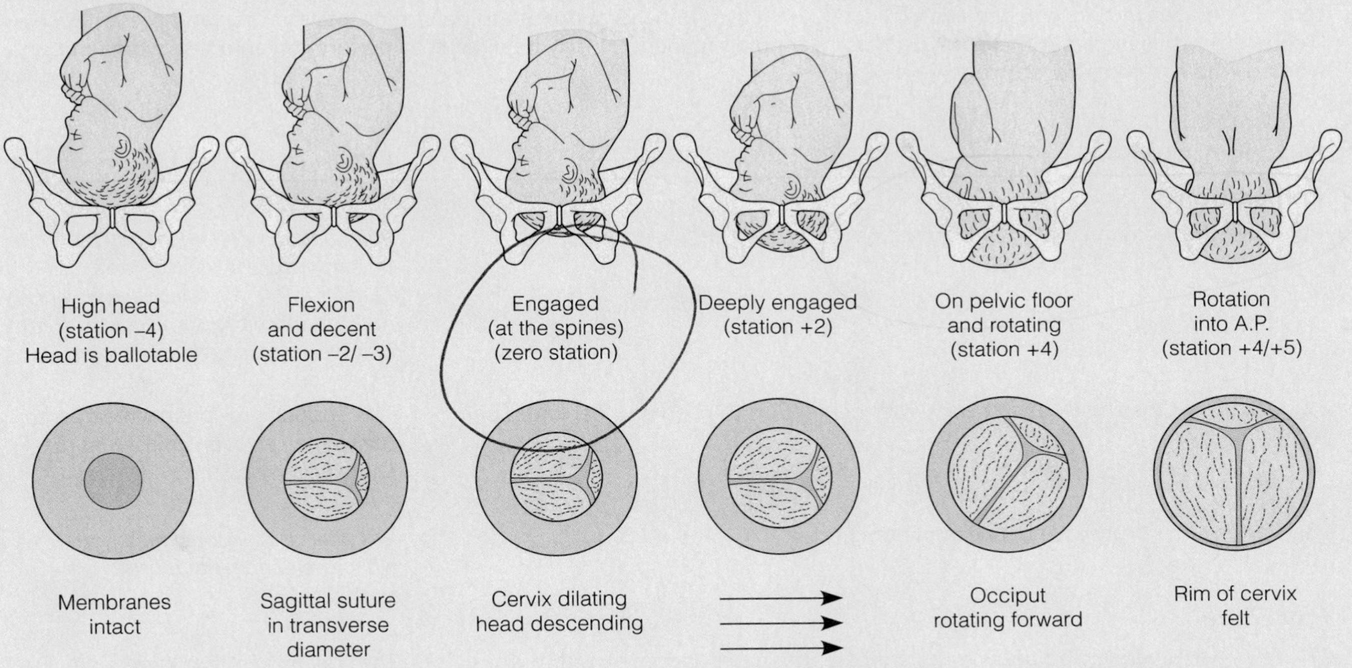

High head
(station –4)
Head is ballotable

Flexion
and decent
(station –2/ –3)

Engaged
(at the spines)
(zero station)

Deeply engaged
(station +2)

On pelvic floor
and rotating
(station +4)

Rotation
into A.P.
(station +4/+5)

Membranes
intact

Sagittal suture
in transverse
diameter

Cervix dilating
head descending

Occiput
rotating forward

Rim of cervix
felt

FIGURE 18–4 Top: The fetal head progressing through the pelvis. Bottom: The changes that the nurse will detect on palpation of the occiput through the cervix while doing a vaginal examination.
Source: Myles, M. F. (1975). *Textbook for midwives* (p. 246). Edinburgh, Scotland: Churchill-Livingstone.

fluid (hydramnios). Before performing Leopold's maneuvers, have the woman (1) empty her bladder and (2) lie on her back with her feet on the bed and her knees bent (see Clinical Skill: Performing Leopold's Maneuvers).

Vaginal Examination and Ultrasound

Other assessment techniques to determine fetal position and presentation include vaginal examination and the use of ultrasound to visualize the fetus. During the vaginal examination, the examiner can palpate the presenting part if the cervix is dilated. Information about the position of the fetus and the degree of flexion of its head (in cephalic presentations) can also be obtained (see the Clinical Skill: Performing an Intrapartal Vaginal Examination). Visualization by ultrasound is used when the fetal position cannot be determined by abdominal palpation (see Chapter 16 ∞).

Auscultation of Fetal Heart Rate

The handheld Doppler ultrasound is used to auscultate the fetal heart rate (FHR) between, during, and immediately after uterine contractions. A fetoscope can also be used. Instead of listening haphazardly over the client's

abdomen for the FHR, the nurse may choose to perform Leopold's maneuvers first. Leopold's maneuvers not only indicate the probable location of the FHR but also help determine the presence of multiple fetuses, fetal lie, and fetal presentation.

The FHR is heard most clearly at the fetal back (Figure 18–6 ■). Thus in a cephalic presentation, the FHR is best heard in the lower quadrants of the maternal abdomen. In a breech presentation, it is heard at or above the level of the maternal umbilicus. In a transverse lie, FHR may be heard best just above or just below the umbilicus. As the presenting part descends and rotates through the pelvic structure during labor, the location of the FHR tends to descend and move toward the midline.

After the FHR is located, it is usually counted for 30 seconds and multiplied by 2 to obtain the number of beats per minute. The nurse should occasionally listen for a full minute, through and just after a contraction, to detect any abnormal heart rate, especially if the FHR is over 160 bpm (tachycardia), under 110 bpm (bradycardia), or irregular. If the FHR is irregular or has changed markedly from the last assessment or if the nurse hears an audible deceleration, the nurse should listen for a full minute through and immediately after a contraction. In these situations, continuous

Clinical Skill Performing Leopold's Maneuvers

Leopold's maneuvers are a systematic way to evaluate the woman's abdomen to determine fetal position and presentation. Frequent practice increases the examiner's skill. Leopold's maneuvers may be difficult to perform on an obese woman or on a woman who has excessive amniotic fluid.

NURSING ACTION	RATIONALE
Preparation	
1. Have the woman empty her bladder.	*Palpating the abdomen may be uncomfortable if the woman's bladder is full. A full bladder may also make it difficult to complete the third and fourth maneuvers. See later discussion.*
2. Ask the woman to lie on her back with her feet on the bed and her knees bent.	*This position provides good access to the woman's abdomen. Flexing the knees helps relax the abdominal muscles.*
3. Perform the procedure between contractions.	*It is difficult to identify fetal parts when the abdominal muscles are contracted.*
Procedure	
1. First maneuver: Facing the woman, palpate the upper abdomen with both hands. Note the shape, consistency, and mobility of the palpated part (see Figure 18–5A ■).	*The fetal head is firm, hard, and round and moves independently of the trunk. The breech (fetal buttocks) feels softer and symmetric and has small bony prominences; it moves with the trunk.*
2. Second maneuver: After determining whether the head or buttocks occupies the fundus, try to determine the location of the fetal back. Still facing the woman, palpate the abdomen with gentle but deep pressure, using the palms. Hold the right hand steady while the left hand explores the right side of the uterus. Then repeat the maneuver, holding the left hand steady while exploring the left side of the woman's abdomen with your right hand (see Figure 18–5B).	*The fetal back, on one side of the abdomen, feels firm and smooth and should connect what was found in the fundus with a mass in the outlet. The fetal extremities, which feel small and knobby, should be found on the other side.*

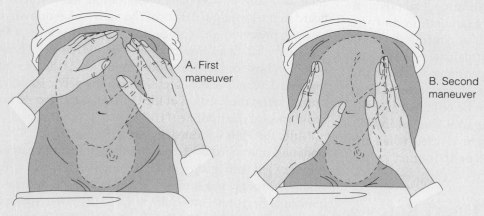

A. First maneuver

B. Second maneuver

FIGURE 18–5 Leopold's maneuvers for determining fetal position, presentation, and lie. *Note:* Many nurses do the fourth maneuver first to identify the part of the fetus in the pelvic inlet.

Clinical Skill Performing Leopold's Maneuvers *(Continued)*

NURSING ACTION	RATIONALE
3. Third maneuver: Determine what fetal part is lying just above the pelvic outlet. To do this, gently grasp the abdomen with the thumb and fingers just above the symphysis pubis. Note whether the presenting part feels like the fetal head or buttocks and whether it is engaged (see Figure 18–5C).	*This maneuver yields the opposite information from that gained with the first maneuver and validates the presenting part. If the head is presenting and is not engaged, it may be gently pushed back and forth.*
4. Fourth maneuver: Facing the woman's feet, place both hands on the lower abdomen and move the hands gently down the sides of the uterus toward the pubis. Attempt to locate the cephalic prominence or brow (see Figure 18–5D).	*The brow is located on the side where there is the greatest resistance to the descent of the fingers toward the pubis. It is located on the side opposite the fetal back if the head is well flexed. However, when the fetal head is extended, the occiput is the first cephalic prominence felt, and it is located on the same side as the fetal back. Thus when completing the fourth maneuver, if the first cephalic prominence palpated is on the same side as the back, the head is not flexed. If the cephalic prominence is found opposite the back, the head is well flexed.*

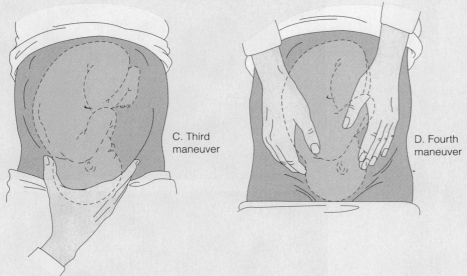

C. Third maneuver

D. Fourth maneuver

FIGURE 18–5 (continued) Leopold's maneuvers for determining fetal position, presentation, and lie. *Note:* Many nurses do the fourth maneuver first to identify the part of the fetus in the pelvic inlet.

electronic fetal monitoring is warranted (American College of Obstetricians & Gynecologists, 2005). (For guidelines about how often to auscultate the FHR, see Clinical Skill: Auscultation of Fetal Heart Rate.)

It is important to note that intermittent auscultation has been found to be as effective as the electronic method for fetal surveillance. A growing number of healthcare professionals, doctors and nurses alike, are beginning to question the widespread usage of this technology. Although fetuses who are monitored continuously have a reduction in seizures, there is no reduction in cerebral palsy, infant mortality, or adverse neonatal outcomes. Women who receive continuous fetal monitoring are more likely to undergo a cesarean birth or an instrument-assisted birth (Alfirevic, Devane, & Gyte, 2006). Figure 18–7 ■ shows three methods for auscultating the FHR.

Electronic Monitoring of Fetal Heart Rate

Electronic fetal monitoring (EFM) produces a continuous tracing of the FHR, which allows visual assessment of many characteristics of the FHR (see Clinical Skill: Electronic Fetal Monitoring).

Indications for Electronic Monitoring

If one or more of the following factors are present, the fetal heart rate and contractions are monitored by EFM.

1. Previous history of a stillbirth at 38 or more weeks' gestation
2. Presence of a complication of pregnancy (e.g., preeclampsia, placenta previa, abruptio placentae,

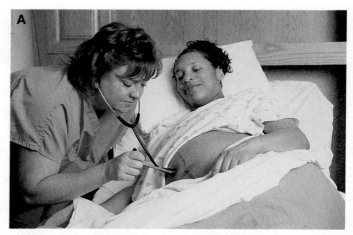

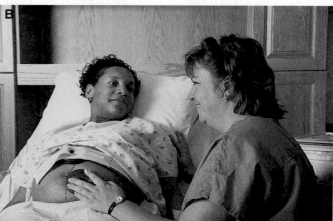

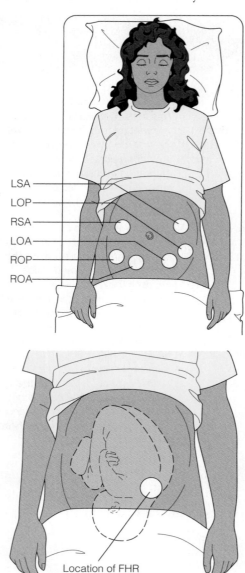

LSA

LOP

RSA

LOA

ROP

ROA

Location of FHR
in LOA position

FIGURE 18–6 Location of FHR in relation to the more commonly seen fetal positions. The fetal heart rate is heard more clearly over the fetal back.

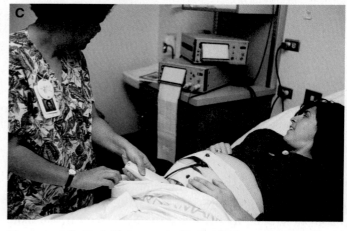

FIGURE 18–7 *A,* The nurse holds the fetoscope as she places it against the maternal abdomen. *B,* The nurse uses a Doppler to assess the fetal heart rate. Doppler monitors can be used for intermittent labor monitoring or in the outpatient or community setting. *C,* When the fetal heart rate is picked up by the electronic monitor, the sound of the heartbeat can be heard by all persons in the room.
Source: A & B, Photographer: Elena Dorfman, C, Michael Newman/PhotoEdit.

multiple gestation, prolonged or premature rupture of membranes)

3. Induction of labor (labor that is begun as a result of some type of intervention such as an intravenous infusion of pitocin)

4. Preterm labor

5. Decreased fetal movement

6. Nonreassuring fetal status

7. Meconium staining of amniotic fluid (meconium has been released into the amniotic fluid by the fetus, which may indicate a problem)

8. Trial of labor following a previous cesarean birth (ACOG, 2004)

9. Maternal fever

10. Placental problems

Methods of Electronic Monitoring of FHR

External monitoring of the fetus is usually accomplished by ultrasound. A transducer, which emits continuous sound waves, is placed on the maternal abdomen. When

Clinical Skill Auscultation of Fetal Heart Rate

NURSING ACTION	RATIONALE

Preparation

1. Explain the procedure, the indications for it, and the information that will be obtained.

2. Uncover the woman's abdomen.

Equipment and Supplies

- Doppler device
- Ultrasonic gel

Procedure

1. To use the Doppler:
   - Place ultrasonic gel on the diaphragm of the Doppler. Gel is used to maintain contact with the maternal abdomen and enhances conduction of sound.
   - Place the Doppler diaphragm on the woman's abdomen halfway between the umbilicus and symphysis and in the midline. You are most likely to hear the FHR in this area. Listen carefully for the sound of the fetal heartbeat.

2. Check the woman's pulse against the fetal sounds you hear. If the rates are the same, reposition the Doppler and try again.

   If the rates are the same, you are probably hearing the maternal pulse and not the FHR.

3. If the rates are not similar, count the FHR for 1 full minute. Note that the FHR has a double rhythm and only one sound is counted.

4. If you do not locate the FHR, move the Doppler laterally.

5. Auscultate the FHR between, during, and for 30 seconds following a uterine contraction (UC).

6. Frequency recommendations:

   This evaluation provides the opportunity to assess the fetal status and response to labor.

   - *Low-risk women:* Every 1 hour in the latent phase, every 30 minutes in the active phase, and every 15 minutes in the second stage.
   - *High-risk women:* Every 30 minutes in the latent phase, every 15 minutes in the active phase, and every 5 minutes in the second stage.

7. Document FHR data (rate and rhythm), characteristics of uterine activity, and any actions taken as a result of the FHR.

Auscultation with the Fetoscope

The fetoscope is an older assessment tool; however, some clinicians prefer it because it is "natural" and does not rely on ultrasound.
To use the fetoscope:

- Place the fetoscope earpieces in your ears; use the handpiece to position the bell of the fetoscope on the mother's abdomen.
- Place the diaphragm halfway between the umbilicus and symphysis and in the midline. *You are most likely to hear the FHR in this area.*
- Without touching the fetoscope, listen carefully for the FHR.

placed correctly, the sound waves bounce off the fetal heart and are picked up by the electronic monitor. The actual moment-by-moment FHR is displayed graphically on a screen (Figure 18–8 ■). In some instances, the monitor may track the maternal heart rate instead of the fetal heart rate. However, the nurse can avoid this error by comparing the maternal pulse to the FHR.

Recent advances in technology have led to the development of new ambulatory methods of external monitoring. Using a telemetry system, a small, battery-operated transducer transmits signals to a receiver connected to the monitor. This system, which is held in place with a shoulder strap, allows the woman to ambulate, helping her to feel more comfortable and less confined during labor. Many of the newer models can also be worn in the tub and can be completely submerged in water, making a more natural birthing expereince possible even for women who require continuous monitoring for medical indications. In contrast, the system depicted in Figure 18–8 requires the woman to remain close to the electrical power source for the monitor.

Internal monitoring requires an internal spiral electrode. Women who require internal monitoring are typically confined to bed and cannot ambulate. To place the spiral electrode on the fetal occiput, the amniotic membranes must be ruptured, the cervix must be dilated at least 2 cm, the presenting part must be down against the cervix, and the presenting part must be known (i.e., the nurse must be able to detect the actual part of the fetus that is down against the cervix). In cases of a breech presentation, the electrode can be placed on the fetal buttocks. The exact position should be identified because the electrode should not be placed on the external genitalia. If all these factors are present, the labor and birth nurse (if specialty training has been completed) or the physician or CNM inserts a sterile internal spiral electrode into the vagina and places it against the fetal presenting part. The spiral electrode is rotated clockwise until it is attached to the presenting part. It is essential that the electrode not be placed over the eye or a fontanelle, so the fetal position should be determined before a scalp electrode is applied. Wires that extend from the spiral electrode are attached to a leg plate (which is placed on the woman's thigh) and then attached to the electronic fetal monitor. This method of monitoring the FHR provides more accurate continuous data than external monitoring, because the signal is clearer and movement of the fetus or the woman does not interrupt it (Figure 18–9 ■).

The FHR tracing at the top of Figure 18–10 ■ was obtained by internal monitoring with a spiral electrode; the uterine contraction tracing at the bottom of the figure was obtained by external monitoring with a toco. Note that the FHR is variable (the tracing moves up and down instead of in a straight line). In this figure each dark vertical line represents 1 minute; therefore, contractions are occurring about every 2½ to 3 minutes. The FHR is evaluated by assessing an electronic monitor tracing for baseline rate, baseline variability, and periodic changes.

Baseline Fetal Heart Rate

The **baseline rate** refers to the average FHR rounded to increments of 5 bpm observed during a 10-minute period of monitoring. This excludes periodic or episodic changes, periods of marked variability, and segments of the baseline that differ by more than 25 bpm. The duration should be at least 2 minutes (Macones, Hankins, Spong et al., 2008). Normal FHR (baseline rate) ranges from 110 to 160 bpm. There are two abnormal variations of the baseline rate—those above 160 bpm (tachycardia) and those below 110 bpm (bradycardia). Another change affecting the baseline is called **variability**, which is a change in FHR over a few seconds to a few minutes.

A **wandering baseline** is a smooth meandering unsteady baseline in the normal range without variability

Clinical Skill Electronic Fetal Monitoring

NURSING ACTION	RATIONALE
Preparation	
Explain the procedure, the indications for it, and the information that will be obtained.	
Equipment and Supplies	
• Monitor	
• Two elastic monitor belts	
• Tocodynamometer ("toco")	
• Ultrasound transducer	
• Ultrasound gel	
Procedure	
1. Turn on the monitor.	
2. Place the two elastic belts around the woman's abdomen.	
3. Place the "toco" over the uterine fundus off the midline on the area palpated to be most firm during contractions. Secure it with one of the elastic belts.	*The uterine fundus is the area of greatest contractility.*
4. Note the UC tracing. The resting tone tracing (that is, without a UC) should be recording on the 10 or 15 mm Hg pressure line. Adjust the line to reflect that reading.	*If the resting tone is set on the zero line, there often is a constant grinding noise.*
5. Apply the ultrasonic gel to the diaphragm of the ultrasound transducer.	*Ultrasonic gel is used to maintain contact with the maternal abdomen. The ultrasonic beam is directed toward the fetal heart.*
6. Place the diaphragm on the maternal abdomen in the midline between the umbilicus and the symphysis pubis.	
7. Listen for the FHR, which will have a whiplike sound. Move the diaphragm laterally if necessary to obtain a stronger sound.	
8. When the FHR is located, attach the second elastic belt snugly to the transducer.	*Firm contact is necessary to maintain a steady tracing.*
9. Place the following information on the beginning of the fetal monitor paper: date, time, woman's name, gravida, para, membrane status, and name of physician or certified nurse-midwife.	
10. Ongoing documentation should provide information about FHR including baseline rate in beats per minute (bpm), long-term variability (LTV), short-term variability (STV), response to uterine contractions (accelerations or decelerations), procedures performed, changes in position and the like, as well as any therapy initiated.	

Note: Each birthing unit may have specific guidelines about additional information to include. A full description of fetal monitoring analysis is beyond the scope of this text.

MyNursingKit | Association of Women's Health, Obstetric and Neonatal Nurses

(Cunningham et al., 2005). Possible causes for this pattern include congenital defects or metabolic acidosis. Immediate interventions should be taken to enhance fetal oxygenation. Birth should be anticipated (AWHONN, 2006).

Fetal tachycardia is a sustained rate of 161 bpm or above. *Marked tachycardia is* 180 bpm or above. Causes of tachycardia include the following (Cunningham et al., 2005):

1. Early fetal hypoxia, which leads to stimulation of the sympathetic system as the fetus compensates for reduced blood flow
2. Maternal fever, which accelerates the metabolism of the fetus
3. Maternal dehydration
4. Beta-sympathomimetic drugs such as ritodrine, terbutaline, atropine, and isoxsuprine, which have a cardiac stimulant effect

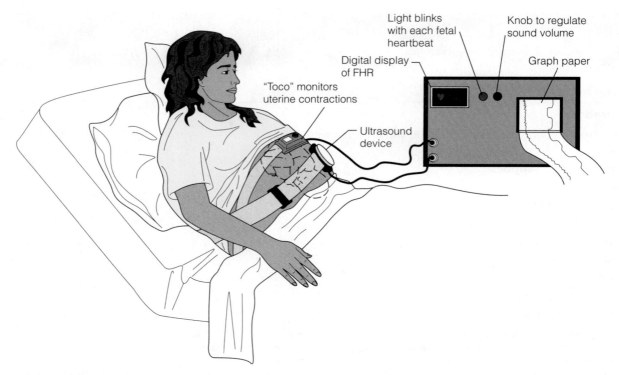

FIGURE 18–8 Electronic fetal monitoring by external technique. The ultrasound device, placed over the fetal back, transmits information on the fetal heart rate. Information from both the tocodynamometer and ultrasound device is transmitted to the electronic fetal monitor. The fetal heart rate is indicated four ways: on the digital display, as a blinking light, by sound, and on special monitor paper. The uterine contractions are displayed on the graph paper.

5. Amnionitis (fetal tachycardia may be the first sign of developing intrauterine infection)
6. Maternal hyperthyroidism (thyroid-stimulating hormones may cross the placenta and stimulate fetal heart rate)
7. Fetal anemia (the heart rate is increased as a compensatory mechanism to improve tissue perfusion)
8. Tachydysrhythmias (fetal dysrhythmias occur in less than 1% of all pregnancies)

Tachycardia is considered an ominous sign if it is accompanied by late decelerations, severe variable decelerations, or decreased variability. If tachycardia is associated with maternal fever, treatment may consist of antipyretics and/or antibiotics.

Fetal bradycardia is a rate less than 110 bpm during a 10-minute period or longer. Causes of fetal bradycardia include the following (Cunningham et al., 2005):

1. Late (profound) fetal hypoxia (depression of myocardial activity)
2. Maternal hypotension, which results in decreased blood flow to the fetus
3. Prolonged umbilical cord compression; fetal baroreceptors are activated by cord compression and this produces vagal stimulation, which results in decreased FHR
4. Fetal arrhythmia, which is associated with complete heart block in the fetus

5. Uterine hyperstimulation
6. Abruptio placentae
7. Uterine rupture
8. Vagal stimulation in the second stage (because this does not involve hypoxia, the fetus can recover)
9. Congenital heart block
10. Maternal hypothermia

Bradycardia may be a benign or an ominous (preterminal) sign. If there is variability, the bradycardia is considered benign. Bradycardia accompanied by decreased variability and late decelerations is considered ominous and a sign of nonreassuring fetal status (Cunningham et al., 2005).

Arrythmias and Dysrhythmias

Arrythmias, a term often used interchangeably with *dysrhythmias,* are disturbances in the FHR pattern that are not associated with abnormal electrical impulse formation or conduction in the fetal cardiac tissue, but are related to a structural abnormality or congenital heart disease (Iaizzio, 2005). Fetal arrythmias may be detected when listening to the FHR on a fetal monitor. It is important to rule out artifacts or electrical interference because this sometimes occurs. Most true arrhythmias are accompanied by baseline bradycardia, baseline tachycardia, or an abrupt baseline spiking (Cunningham et al., 2005). Ninety

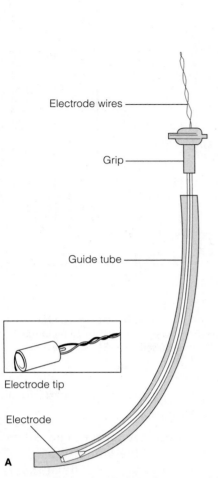

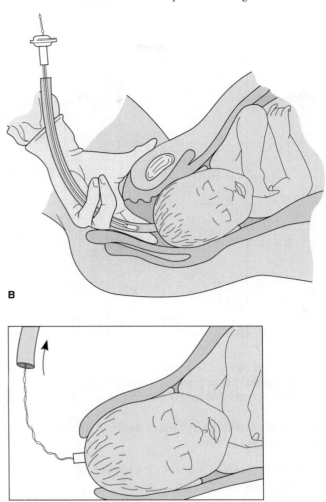

FIGURE 18–9 Technique for internal, direct fetal monitoring. *A,* Spiral electrode. *B,* Attaching the spiral electrode to the scalp. *C,* Attached spiral electrode with the guide tube removed.

percent of fetal cardiac arrhythmias are benign. The most common serious arrhythmias are superventricular tachycardia and complete heart block (Iaizzio, 2005).

Variability

Baseline variability is a measure of the interplay (the push-pull effect) between the sympathetic and parasympathetic nervous systems. Baseline variability is the fluctuations in the FHR of two cycles per minute or greater. Figure 18–11 ■ depicts the different ranges of variability. The amplitude of peak and trough in beats per minute are defined as follows (Macones, 2008):

- *Absent:* amplitude undetectable
- *Minimal:* amplitude detectable but less than 5 bpm
- *Moderate:* amplitude 6 to 25 bpm
- *Marked:* amplitude greater than 25 bpm

Reduced variability is the best single predictor for determining fetal compromise (Cunningham et al., 2005). Fetal acidosis and subsequent hypoxia is highest in fetuses

that have absent or minimial variability (Siira, Ojala, Ekholm et al., 2007).

Causes of decreased variability include the following (Cunningham et al., 2005):

1. Hypoxia and acidosis (decreased blood flow to the fetus)
2. Administration of drugs such as meperidine hydrochloride (Demerol), diazepam (Valium), or hydroxyzine (Vistaril), which depress the fetal central nervous system
3. Fetal sleep cycle (during fetal sleep, variability is decreased; fetal sleep cycles usually last for 20 to 40 minutes each hour)
4. Fetus of less than 32 weeks' gestation (fetal neurologic control of heart rate is immature)
5. Fetal dysrhythmias
6. Fetal anomalies affecting the heart, central nervous system, or autonomic nervous system
7. Previous neurological insult
8. Tachycardia

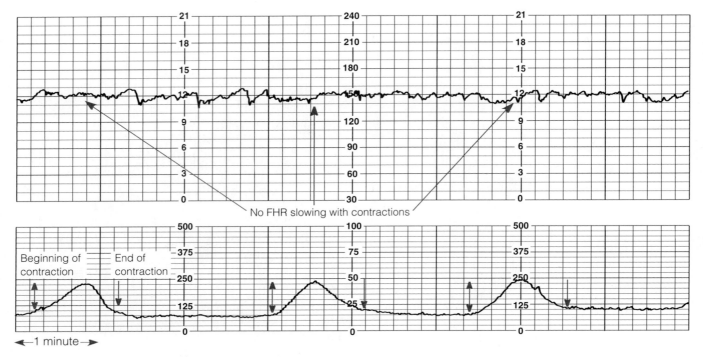

FIGURE 18-10 Normal FHR range is from 110 to 160 bpm. The FHR tracing in the upper portion of the graph indicates an FHR range of 140 to 155 bpm. The bottom portion depicts uterine contractions. Each dark vertical line marks 1 minute, and each small rectangle represents 10 seconds. The contraction frequency is about every 2½ minutes, and the duration of the contractions is 50 to 60 seconds.

Causes of marked variability include the following (Cunningham et al., 2005):

1. Early mild hypoxia (variability increases as a result of compensatory mechanism)
2. Fetal stimulation or activity (stimulation of autonomic nervous system because of abdominal palpation, maternal vaginal examination, application of spiral electrode on fetal head, or acoustic stimulation)
3. Fetal breathing movements
4. Advancing gestational age (greater than 30 gestational weeks)

Absent variability that does not appear to be associated with a fetal sleep cycle or the administration of drugs is a warning sign of nonreassuring fetal status. It is especially ominous if absent or minimal variability is accompanied by late decelerations, explained shortly. If

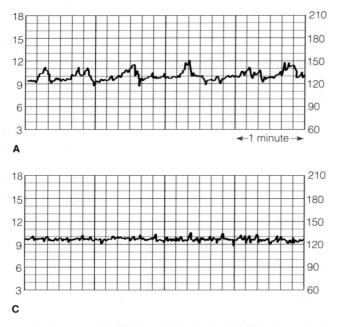

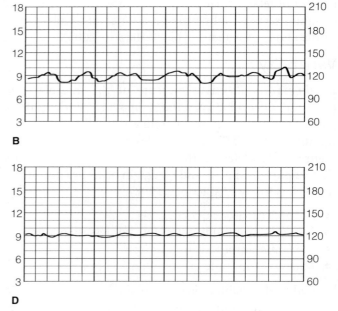

FIGURE 18-11 Variability. *A,* Marked variability. *B,* Moderate variability. *C,* Minimal variability. *D,* Absent variability.

decreased variability is noted on monitoring, application of a spiral electrode should be considered to obtain more accurate information.

Accelerations

Accelerations are transient increases in the FHR normally caused by fetal movement. When the fetus moves, its heart rate increases, just as the heart rates of adults increase during exercise. Often accelerations accompany uterine contractions, usually because the fetus moves in response to the pressure of the contractions. Accelerations of this type are thought to be a sign of fetal well-being and adequate oxygen reserve. They indicate a mature autonomic nervous system and the absence of acidosis (Blackburn, 2007). The accelera-

tions with fetal movement are the basis for nonstress tests (see Chapter 16 ∞).

Decelerations

Decelerations are periodic decreases in FHR from the normal baseline. They are categorized as early, late, and variable according to the time of their occurrence in the contraction cycle and their waveform (Figure 18–12 ■). When the fetal head is compressed, cerebral blood flow is decreased, which leads to central vagal stimulation and results in early deceleration. The onset of early deceleration is associated with the onset of the uterine contraction. This type of deceleration is of uniform shape, is usually considered benign, and does not require intervention.

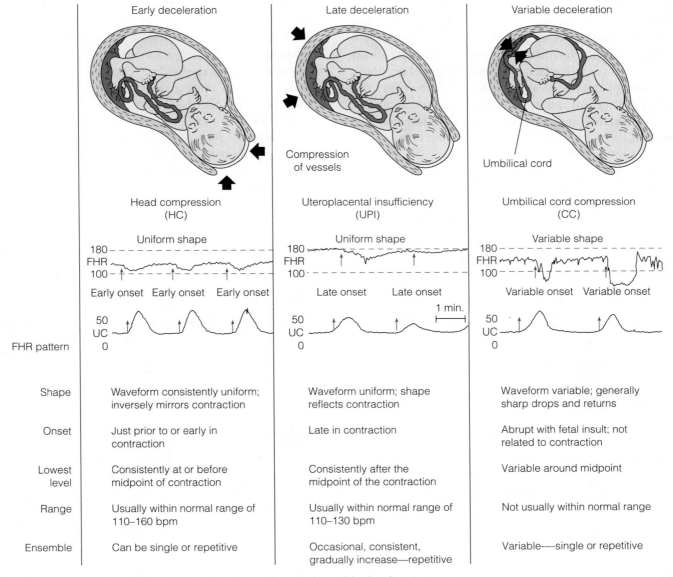

FHR pattern	Early deceleration	Late deceleration	Variable deceleration
Shape	Waveform consistently uniform; inversely mirrors contraction	Waveform uniform; shape reflects contraction	Waveform variable; generally sharp drops and returns
Onset	Just prior to or early in contraction	Late in contraction	Abrupt with fetal insult; not related to contraction
Lowest level	Consistently at or before midpoint of contraction	Consistently after the midpoint of the contraction	Variable around midpoint
Range	Usually within normal range of 110–160 bpm	Usually within normal range of 110–130 bpm	Not usually within normal range
Ensemble	Can be single or repetitive	Occasional, consistent, gradually increase—repetitive	Variable——single or repetitive

FIGURE 18–12 Types and characteristics of early, late, and variable decelerations.
Source: Hon, E. (1976). *An introduction to fetal heart rate monitoring* (2nd ed., p. 29). Los Angeles: University of Southern California School of Medicine.

HINTS FOR PRACTICE

The presence of repetitive early decelerations may be a sign of advanced dilatation or the beginning of the second stage of labor. If the monitoring strip shows reoccurring early decelerations, ask the laboring woman if she is experiencing any pressure. Pressure that occurs only with the contractions typically indicates advanced dilatation. Intense pressure that does not change or ease up when the contractions cease may indicate the beginning of the second stage. A vaginal examination may be performed to establish the dilatation.

Late deceleration is caused by uteroplacental insufficiency resulting from decreased blood flow and oxygen transfer to the fetus through the intervillous spaces during uterine contractions. The most common causes of late decelerations are maternal hypotension resulting from the administration of epidural anesthesia and uterine hyperstimulation associated with oxytocin infusion (Caracostea, Stamatian, Lerintiu et al., 2007). Maternal hypertension, diabetes, collagen-vascular disorders, and placenta abruption are also causative factors (Cunningham et al., 2005). The onset of the deceleration occurs after the onset of a uterine contraction and is of a uniform shape that tends to reflect associated uterine contractions. The late deceleration pattern is considered a nonreassuring sign and requires continuous assessment. If late decelerations continue, and the time until birth is not imminent, a cesarean birth may be indicated.

Variable decelerations occur if the umbilical cord becomes compressed, thus reducing blood flow between the placenta and fetus. The resulting increase in peripheral resistance in the fetal circulation causes fetal hypertension. The fetal hypertension stimulates the baroreceptors in the aortic arch and carotid sinuses, which slow the FHR. The onset of variable decelerations varies in timing with the onset of the contraction, and the decelerations are variable in shape. This pattern requires further assessment. Nursing interventions for late and variable decelerations in the FHR are presented in Table 18–2.

A *sinusoidal pattern* appears similar to a waveform. The characteristics of this pattern include absence of variability and the presence of a smooth wavelike shape (Figure 18–13 ■). The pattern resembles a perfect letter "S" lying on its side. These patterns can be benign (pseudosinusoidal) or true sinusoidal. The true pattern is associated with Rh alloimmunization, fetal anemia, severe fetal hypoxia, umbilical cord occlusion, twin-to-twin transfusion, or a chronic fetal bleed. Pseudosinusoidal patterns are usually temporary and commonly occur with the administration of medications such as meperidine (Demerol) or butorphanol tartrate (Stadol) (Cunningham et al., 2005).

Decelerations are also classified based on the rate in which the FHR leaves the baseline FHR. *Abrupt decelerations* occur in less than 30 seconds (Macones et al., 2008). Variable decelerations descend abruptly. *Gradual decelerations* require 30 seconds or more to descend. Both early and late decelerations descend gradually. Decelerations can also be episodic

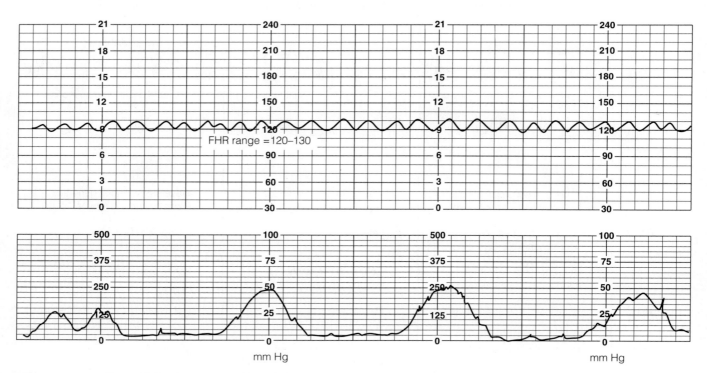

FIGURE 18–13 Sinusoidal pattern. Note the undulating waveform evenly distributed between the 120 and 130 bpm baseline. There is no STV; accelerations or decelerations are not present.

Pattern	Nursing Interventions

TABLE 18–2 Guidelines for Management of Variable, Late, and Prolonged Deceleration Patterns

Pattern	Nursing Interventions
Variable decelerations	Report findings to physician/CNM and document in chart. Provide explanation to woman and partner.
Isolated or occasional	Change maternal position to one in which FHR pattern is most improved.
Moderate	Discontinue oxytocin if it is being administered and other interventions are unsuccessful. Perform vaginal examination to assess for prolapsed cord or change in labor progress. Monitor FHR continuously to assess current status and for further changes in FHR pattern.
Variable decelerations Severe and uncorrectable	Administer oxygen by face mask at 7 to 10 L/min. Report findings to physician/CNM and document in chart. Provide explanation to woman and partner. Prepare for probable cesarean birth. Follow interventions listed above. Prepare for vaginal birth unless baseline variability is decreasing or FHR is progressively rising—then cesarean, forceps, or vacuum birth is indicated. Assist physician with fetal scalp sampling if ordered. Prepare for cesarean birth if scalp pH shows acidosis or downward trend.
Late decelerations	Administer oxygen by face mask at 7 to 10 L/min. Report findings to physician/CNM and document in chart. Provide explanation to woman and partner. Monitor for further FHR changes. Maintain maternal position on left side. Maintain good hydration with IV fluids (normal saline or lactated Ringer's). Discontinue oxytocin if it is being administered and late decelerations persist despite other interventions. Monitor maternal blood pressure and pulse for signs of hypotension; possibly increase flow rate of IV fluids to treat hypotension. Follow physician's orders for treatment for hypotension if present. Increase IV fluids to maintain volume and hydration (normal saline or lactated Ringer's). Assess labor progress (dilatation and station). Assist physician with fetal blood sampling: If pH stays above 7.25, physician will continue monitoring and resample; if pH shows downward trend (between 7.25 and 7.20) or is below 7.20, prepare for birth by most expeditious means.
Late decelerations with tachycardia or decreasing variability	Report findings to physician/CNM and document in chart. Maintain maternal position on left side. Administer oxygen by face mask at 7 to 10 L/min. Discontinue oxytocin if it is being administered. Assess maternal blood pressure and pulse. Increase IV fluids (normal saline or lactated Ringer's). Assess labor progress (dilatation and station). Prepare for immediate cesarean birth. Explain plan of treatment to woman and partner. Assist physician with fetal blood sampling (FBS) (if ordered).
Prolonged decelerations	Perform vaginal examination to rule out prolapsed cord or to determine progress in labor status. Change maternal position as needed to try to alleviate decelerations. Discontinue oxytocin if it is being administered. Notify physician/CNM of findings/initial interventions and document in chart. Provide explanation to woman and partner. Increase IV fluids (normal saline or lactated Ringer's). Administer tocolytic if hypertonus noted and ordered by physician/CNM. Anticipate normal FHR recovery following deceleration if FHR previously normal. Anticipate intervention if FHR previously abnormal or deceleration lasts more than 3 minutes.

or periodic. *Episodic decelerations* occur independently of the uterine contractions and are frequently the result of external stimulations, such as vaginal exams. *Periodic decelerations* refer to decelerations that occur with the contractions and are considered repetitive if they occur with 50% of the contractions (ACOG, 2005, AWHONN, 2006). Decelerations that leave the baseline for more than 2 minutes but less than 10 minutes are known as *prolonged decelerations*.

Evaluation of FHR Tracings

With a systematic approach to evaluating FHR tracings, the nurse can make a more accurate and rapid assessment,

avoid interpreting findings on the basis of inadequate or erroneous data, and easily communicate data to the woman, physician or CNM, and staff. A universal language for documentation should be used consistently within the facility to avoid errors.

Evaluation of the electronic monitor tracing begins by looking at the uterine contraction pattern. To evaluate the contraction pattern, the nurse should do the following:

1. Determine the uterine resting tone.
2. Assess the contractions: What is the frequency? What is the duration? What is the intensity?

After evaluating the FHR tracing for the contraction pattern, the nurse may categorize the tracing according to the Three Tier FHR Interpretation System below. The three-tier system for the categorization of FHR patterns is recommended by ACOG, AWHONN, and NICHD (Macones et al., 2008). Categorization of the FHR tracing evaluates the fetus at that point in time; tracing patterns can and will change. A FHR tracing may move back and forth between categories depending on the clinical situation and management strategies employed.

The Three-Tier Fetal Heart Rate Interpretation System (Macones et al., 2008).

Category I

Category I FHR tracings include <u>all</u> of the following:

- Baseline rate: 110-160 bpm
- Baseline FHR variability: moderate
- Late or variable de3celerations: absent
- Early decelerations: present or absent
- Accelerations: present or absent

Category II

Category II FHR tracings include all FHR tracings not categorized as Category I or Category III. Category II tracings may represent an appreciable fraction of those encountered in clinical care. Examples of Category II FHR tracings include any of the following:

- Baseline rate –
  - Bradycardia not accompanied by absent baseline variability
  - Tachycardia
- Baseline FHR variability
  - Minimal baseline variability
  - Absent baseline variability not accompanied by recurrent decelerations
  - Marked baseline variability
- Accelerations
  - Absence of induced accelerations after fetal stimulation

- Periodic or episodic decelerations
  - Recurrent variable decelerations accompanied by minimal or moderate baseline variability
  - Prolonged deceleration of 2 minutes or more but less than 10 minutes
  - Recurrent late decelerations with moderate baseline variability
  - Variable decelerations with other characteristics, such as slow return to baseline, "overshoots", or "shoulders"

Category III

Category III FHR tracings include either:
- Absent baseline FHR variability and any of the following:
  - Recurrent late decelerations
  - Recurrent variable decelerations
  - Bradycardia
- Sinusoidal pattern

Category I FHR tracings are normal. They are strongly predictive of normal fetal acid-base status at the time of observation. The FHR tracings may be followed in a routine manner, and no specific action is required. *Category II FHR tracings are indeterminate.* They are not predictive of abnormal fetal acid-base status, yet we do not have adequate evidence at present to classify these as Category I or Category III. Category II tracings require evaluation and continued surveillance and reevaluation, taking into account the entire associated clinical circumstances.

Category III FHR tracings are abnormal. They are predictive of abnormal fetal acid-base status at the time of observation. They require prompt evaluation. Depending on the clinical situation, efforts to expeditiously resolve the abnormal FHR pattern may include, but are not limited to, provision of maternal oxygen, change in maternal position, discontinuation of labor stimulation, and treatment of maternal hypotension.

Nursing Care Management

Technology has been advancing at a rapid rate in the labor and birthing arena, and each new development challenges nurses to understand, include, and balance technology with holistic nursing practice. A key strength of technology is its potential to explain and predict health patterns or problems with precision. It can also save time and reduce the risk of more invasive procedures. However, technology also has the potential to dehumanize the nurse-client relationship. This can happen when nurses focus on a device instead of the client; or in other words, on data that are objectively measurable, tangible, and visible rather than cues that may arise from intuition or from observations of or interactions with the client and family. In addition, the technical language of EFM and other procedures may act as a barrier, isolating the client and deemphasizing her experience.

For these reasons, it is important to recognize that every encounter with the childbearing family offers the nurse an opportunity to provide education and empowerment. These encounters include times when technology is utilized. By helping to provide information when needed, answering questions, and encouraging the family to make decisions, a trusting relationship can be established. Within this bond of trust resides an awareness of the client's whole being and the healing power of each moment.

Before using the electronic fetal monitor, the nurse needs to fully explain the reason for its use and the information that it can provide. After the monitor is applied, basic information can be recorded on the monitor strip. These data should include the date, client's name, physician's or CNM's name, hospital identification number, age, gravida, para, estimated date of birth (EDB), membrane status, and maternal vital signs.

It is important for the laboring woman to feel that what is happening to her is the central focus. The nurse can acknowledge this need by always speaking to and looking at the woman when entering the room, before looking at the monitor.

As the monitor strip runs and care is provided, the following occurrences should be recorded not only in the medical record but also on the monitoring strip. This information helps the healthcare team assess current status and evaluate the tracing (American Academy of Pediatrics [AAP] & ACOG, 2007).

1. Vaginal examination (dilatation, effacement, station, position)
2. Amniotomy or spontaneous rupture of membranes, color of amniotic fluid, amount of fluid, and any presence of odor
3. Maternal vital signs
4. Maternal position in bed and changes of position
5. Application of spiral electrode or intrauterine pressure catheter
6. Medications given
7. Oxygen administration
8. Maternal behaviors (emesis, coughing, hiccups)
9. Fetal scalp stimulation or fetal scalp blood sampling
10. Vomiting
11. Pushing
12. Administration of anesthesia blocks

Most electronic fetal monitors automatically post the time at periodic intervals on the monitoring strip; however, if the monitor does not automatically add the time, the time should be included when recording any information. When adding information to the monitoring strip, it is essential to initial each note. The tracing is considered a legal part of the woman's medical record and is submissible as evidence in court.

Fetal Scalp Stimulation Test

When there is a question regarding fetal status, a scalp stimulation test can be used before the more invasive fetal blood sampling (FBS). In this test, the examiner applies pressure to the fetal scalp while doing a vaginal examination. The fetus who is not in any stress responds with an acceleration of the FHR (Gabbe, Simpson, Niebyl et al., 2007).

Fetal Arterial Oxygen Saturation Monitoring

Fetal arterial oxygen saturation (FSpO$_2$) monitoring was approved by the Food and Drug Administration (FDA) in 2000 as a direct, real-time method to determine fetal oxygenation levels (Bloom, Spong, Thom et al., 2006). An intrauterine device is placed adjacent to the fetal cheek or temple maintaining constant contact with the fetal skin. Using pulse oximetry, the monitor displays fetal oxygenation saturation as a percentage of oxygen within the fetal blood. Levels of 40% to 70% are considered reassuring. Levels less than 30% indicate hypoxia and require immediate birth. Levels between 30% and 40% indicate mild acidosis and require continuous monitoring and assessment (Bloom et al., 2006).

FSpO$_2$ monitoring can be used when the fetus is in a vertex presentation, the membranes are ruptured, the cervix is at least 2 cm (0.8 in.) dilated, the station is −1 or lower, and the pregnancy is at least 36 weeks' gestation or more. Use of FSpO$_2$ monitoring allows labor to continue despite a nonreassuring tracing if fetal oxygen levels are within normal range.

Cord Blood Analysis at Birth

In cases where significant abnormal FHR patterns have been noted, meconium-stained amniotic fluid is present, or the infant is depressed at birth, umbilical cord blood may be analyzed immediately following the birth to determine if acidosis is present. AAP and ACOG (2007) recommend performing cord blood analyses in cases where the Apgar score is below 7 at 5 minutes of age (Normal Apgar score is 7 to 10).

The cord is clamped before the infant takes the first breath. Using a third hemostat, the practitioner clamps an 8- to 10-inch portion of the umbilical cord. A small amount of blood (1.0 mL is required for a full panel) is aspirated with a syringe from one of the umbilical arteries. An artery is selected because it gives a more reliable blood gas reading and fetal tissue pH level. If the cord blood will not be analyzed immediately, a heparinized syringe should be used. Normal fetal blood pH should be above 7.25 (AAP & ACOG, 2007). Lower levels indicate acidosis and hypoxia. Many practitioners obtain cord blood analysis to minimize medicolegal exposure.

CHAPTER HIGHLIGHTS

- Intrapartal assessment includes attention to both the physical and the psychosociocultural parameters of the laboring woman, assessment of the fetus, and ongoing assessment for conditions that place the woman and her fetus at increased risk.

- A vaginal examination determines the status of fetal membranes; cervical dilatation and effacement; and fetal presentation, position, and station.

- Uterine contractions may be assessed by palpation or by an electronic monitor.

- Leopold's maneuvers provide a systematic evaluation of fetal presentation and position.

- Fetal presentation and position may also be assessed by vaginal examination or ultrasound.

- The fetal heart rate may be assessed by auscultation (with a fetoscope or Doppler) or by electronic monitoring.

- Electronic fetal monitoring is accomplished by indirect ultrasound or by direct methods that require the placement of a spiral electrode on the fetal presenting part.

- Indications for electronic monitoring include fetal, maternal, and uterine factors; presence of pregnancy complications; regional anesthesia; and elective monitoring.

- Variability is the single most important indictor of fetal compromise.

- Baseline FHR refers to the range of FHR observed between contractions, during a 10-minute period of monitoring.

- The normal range of FHR is 110 to 160 bpm.

- Baseline changes of the FHR include tachycardia, bradycardia, and variability.

- Fetal tachycardia is defined as a rate of 161 bpm or more for a 10-minute period.

- Fetal bradycardia is defined as a rate of less than 110 bpm for a 10-minute period.

- Baseline variability is an important parameter of fetal well-being.

- Periodic changes are transient decelerations or accelerations of the FHR from the baseline. Accelerations are normally caused by fetal movement; decelerations may be termed early, late, variable, or sinusoidal.

- Early decelerations are caused by compression of the fetal head during contractions and are considered reassuring.

- Late decelerations are associated with uteroplacental insufficiency and are considered ominous.

- Variable decelerations are associated with compression of the umbilical cord and require further assessment.

- Sinusoidal patterns are characterized by an undulant sine wave.

- Psychologic reactions to monitoring vary between feelings of relief and feelings of being tied down.

- Birthing room nurses have responsibilities in recognizing and interpreting fetal monitoring patterns, notifying the physician or CNM of problems, and initiating corrective and supportive measures when needed.

- Fetal scalp stimulation can be used when fetal status is in question.

- Fetal oxygenation can be assessed by fetal arterial oxygen saturation ($FSpO_2$) monitoring.

- Cord blood analysis can be obtained from the umbilical artery immediately after birth to determine the acid-base status.

CHAPTER REFERENCES

Alfirevic, Z., Devane, D., & Gyte, G. M. L. (2006). Continuous cardiotocography (CTG) as a form of electronic fetal monitoring (EFM) for fetal assessment during labour. *Cochrane Database of Systematic Reviews* 2006, Issue 3. Art. No.: CD006066. DOI: 10.1002/14651858.CD006066.

American Academy of Pediatrics (AAP) & American College of Obstetricians and Gynecologists (ACOG). (2007). *Guidelines for perinatal care* (6th ed.). Washington, DC: Author.

American College of Obstetricians and Gynecologists [ACOG]. (2004). *Vaginal birth after previous cesarean delivery.* ACOG Practice Bulletin No. 54. Washington, DC: Author.

American College of Obstetricians and Gynecologists [ACOG]. (2005). *Intrapartum fetal heart rate monitoring.* ACOG Practice Bulletin No. 70. Washington, DC: Author.

American College of Obstetricians and Gynecologists [ACOG]. (2008). *Use of psychiatric medications during pregnancy and lactation.* ACOG Practice Bulletin No. 92. Washington, DC: Author.

Association of Women's Health, Obstetric, and Neonatal Nurses (AWHONN). (2006). In J. Poole (Ed.). *Foundations of fetal heart rate monitoring: An introduction to AWHONN's fetal heart rate monitoring principles and practices program.* Baltimore: Williams & Wilkins.

Blackburn, S. (2007). Maternal, fetal, & neonatal physiology: A clinical perspective (3rd ed.). St. Louis: Saunders.

Bloom, S. L., Spong, C. Y., Thom, E., Varner, M. W., Rouse, D. J., Weininger, S., et al. (2006). Fetal pulse oximetry and cesarean delivery. *New England Journal of Medicine, 355,* 2195–2202.

Caracostea, G., Stamatian, F., Lerintiu, M., & Herghea, D. (2007). The influence of maternal epidural anesthesia upon intrapartum fetal oxygenation. *Journal of Maternal Fetal Neonatal Medicine, 20*(2), 161–165.

Cunningham, F. G., Leveno, K. J., Bloom, S. L., Hauth, J. C., Gilstrap, L. C., & Wenstrom, K. D. (2005). *Williams obstetrics* (22nd ed.). New York: McGraw-Hill.

Gabbe, S. G., Simpson, J. L., Niebyl, J. R., Galan, H., Goetzl, L., Jauniaux, E. R. M., & Landan, M. (2007). *Obstetrics: Normal and problem pregnancies* (5th ed.). CITY: Churchill Livingstone.

Griebenow, J. J. (2006). Healing the trauma: Entering motherhood with posttraumatic stress disorder (PTSD). *Midwifery Today International Midwife, 80,* 28–31, 68.

Iaizzio, P. A. (2005). *Handbook of cardiac anatomy, physiology, and devices.* Totowa, NJ: Humana Press.

Macones, G. A., Hankins, G. D. V., Spong, C. Y., Hauth, J., & Moore, T. (2008). The 2008 National Institute of Child Health and Human Development Workshop Report on Electronic Monitoring: Update on Definitions, Interpretation, and Research Guidelines. *JOGNN: The Journal of Obstetrics, Gynecology and Neonatal Nursing, 37*(5) 510–515.

Siegfried, C. (2007). Victimization and youth. *The Prevention Researcher, 17*(1),14–16.

Siira, S., Ojala, T., Ekholm, E., Vahlberg, T., Blad S., & Rosen, K. G. (2007). Change in heart rate variability in relation to a significant ST-event associates with newborn metabolic acidosis. *British Journal of Obstetrics & Gynecology, 114*(7), 819–823. Epub 2007 May 16.

Spector, R. E. (2009). *Cultural diversity in health and illness* (7th ed.). Upper Saddle River, NJ: Prentice Hall Health.

U.S. Department of Justice. (2006). National crime victimization survey: Criminal victimization, 2005. Retrieved July 23, 2007, from http://www.ojp.gov/bjs/pub/pdf/cv05.pdf

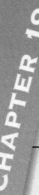

CHAPTER 19

The Family in Childbirth: Needs and Care

For as long as I can remember I have been fascinated with birth. I began as a hospital volunteer, then taught childbirth preparation, and then became a labor nurse before going back to school to become a certified nurse-midwife. It has been a challenge, and sometimes I wondered if I would make it. But here I am, practicing in the same hospital that I used to volunteer in. I'm still fascinated with birth.

—A Certified Nurse-Midwife

LEARNING OUTCOMES

19-1. Identify admission data of a woman admitted to the birthing area.

19-2. Describe the nursing care of a woman and her partner/family upon admission to the birthing area.

19-3. Use assessment data to determine the nursing interventions to meet the psychologic, social, physiologic, and spiritual assessment of the woman and her partner/family during each stage of labor.

19-4. Compare methods of promoting comfort during the first and second stages of labor.

19-5. Explain the immediate needs and physical assessment of the newborn following birth in the provision of nursing care.

19-6. Examine the unique needs of the adolescent during birth in the provision of nursing care.

19-7. Describe the role and responsibility of the nurse in management of a precipitous birth.

KEY TERMS

Apgar score 453
Birthing room 431
Doula 447
Family-centered care 431
Hyperventilation 446
Precipitous birth 461

It is time for a child to be born. The waiting is over; labor has begun. The dreams and wishes of the past months fade as the mother-to-be or the expectant parents face the reality of the childbearing and childrearing tasks that lie ahead.

The parents are about to undergo one of the most meaningful and stressful events of their lives. The adequacy of their preparation for childbirth, including the coping mechanisms, communication, and support systems that they have established, will be put to the test. In particular, the childbearing woman may feel that her psychologic and physical limits are about to be challenged. Social and peer relationships may dramatically change after the birth of a child. These events may be even more challenging for a single woman or an adolescent, especially if she lacks a strong support system.

Family-centered care is a model of care based on the philosophy that physical, sociocultural, spiritual, and economic needs of the family are combined and considered collectively when planning care for the childbearing family (Chai-Chen, 2007). To reflect the consumer demand for family-centered care, most birthing centers now have **birthing rooms**, single rooms where the woman and her partner or other family members will stay for the labor, birth, recovery, and possibly the postpartum period. These rooms may be called *labor, delivery, recovery, and postpartum (LDRP) rooms* or *single-room maternity care (SRMC)*.

The atmosphere of a birthing room is more relaxed than a traditional hospital room and families seem to feel more comfortable in them. Another benefit to a birthing room is that the woman does not have to be transferred from one area to another for the actual birth. A birthing room setting helps the laboring woman create her own space to labor in and enhances the family's comfort and involvement. Birthing rooms usually have beds that can be adapted for birth by removing a small section near the foot. The decor is designed to produce a homelike atmosphere in which families can feel both safe and at ease.

Maternal-newborn nursing has kept pace with the changing philosophy of childbirth. Nurses who choose positions in a birthing area are presented with opportunities to interact with clients in a wide variety of situations, from a family who wants maximum interaction to one that wants to be left alone as much as possible. In addition, despite the increasing focus on family-centered care, the nurse must always be ready to meet the needs and concerns of the single woman who is laboring alone. In every case, nurses strive to provide high-quality, individualized care.

The previous two chapters provided a database about physiologic and psychologic changes during labor and birth and needed nursing assessments. This chapter presents nursing care during labor and birth and includes a Clinical Pathway for Intrapartal Stages on pages 432 to 434. A brief summary of the responsibilities of the birthing room nurse is provided on the Teaching Card on Nursing Care During Labor inserted in the center of this text.

Nursing Diagnosis During Labor and Birth

When a plan of care is devised for the intrapartal period, the nurse can develop a general plan that encompasses the total process, from the beginning of labor through the fourth stage, or a plan can be developed for each stage of labor and birth. A general plan presents an overview of the whole process, whereas a plan of care that identifies nursing diagnoses for each stage provides an opportunity to identify more specific nursing care.

In the first stage, examples of appropriate nursing diagnoses may include the following:

- *Fear/Anxiety* related to discomfort of labor and unknown labor outcome
- *Acute Pain* related to uterine contractions, cervical dilatation, and fetal descent
- *Health-Seeking Behaviors* related to the normal labor process and comfort measures

Examples of nursing diagnoses for the second and third stages may include the following:

- *Acute Pain* related to uterine contractions, the birth process, and/or perineal trauma from birth
- *Health-Seeking Behaviors* related to pushing methods to assist in the birth
- *Fear/Anxiety* related to the outcome of the birth process
- *Readiness for enhanced cognition* related to birth process

In the fourth stage, possible nursing diagnoses include the following:

- *Acute Pain* related to perineal trauma
- *Health-Seeking Behaviors* related to the involution process and self-care needs
- *Readiness for Enhanced Family Processes* related to incorporation of the newborn into the family

Nursing Care During Admission

During her prenatal visits the woman is instructed to call her healthcare provider and come to the birthing unit if any of the following occur:

- Rupture of membranes (ROM)
- Regular, frequent uterine contractions (nulliparas, 5 minutes apart for 1 hour; multiparas, 6 to 8 minutes apart for 1 hour)
- Any vaginal bleeding
- Decreased fetal movement

Clinical Pathway FOR INTRAPARTAL STAGES

FIRST STAGE	SECOND AND THIRD STAGE	FOURTH STAGE BIRTH TO 1 HOUR PAST BIRTH
REFERRAL		
Review prenatal record Advise physician/CNM of admission	Labor record for first stage	Report to recovery room nurse **Expected Outcomes** Appropriate resources identified and utilized

ASSESSMENTS

FIRST STAGE	SECOND AND THIRD STAGE	FOURTH STAGE BIRTH TO 1 HOUR PAST BIRTH
Admission assessments: Ask about problems since last prenatal visit; labor status (contraction frequency and duration), membrane status (intact or ruptured); coping level; support; woman's desires during labor and birth; ability to verbalize needs; laboratory testing (blood and UA) Intrapartal assessments: Cervical assessment: from 1 to 10 cm dilatation; nullipara (1.2 cm/h), multipara (1.5 cm/h) Cervical effacement: from 0% to 100% Fetal descent: progressive descent from −4 to +4 Membrane assessment: intact or ruptured; when ruptured, nitrazine positive, fluid clear, no foul odor Comfort level: woman states is able to cope with contractions Behavioral characteristics: facial expressions, tone of voice, and verbal expressions are consistent with comfort level and ability to cope Latent Phase: • BP, P, R q1h if in normal range (BP less than or equal to 135/85 or not greater than 30 mm Hg systolic or 15 mm Hg diastolic over baseline; pulse 60 to 90; respirations 16 to 24/min, quiet, easy) • Temp q4h unless greater than 37.6°C (99.6°F) or membranes ruptured then q2h • Uterine contractions q30min (contractions q5–10min, 15–40 sec, mild intensity) • FHR q60min (for low-risk women) and q30min (for high-risk women) if reassuring (reassuring FHR has: baseline 110 to 160, STV and LTV present, accelerations with fetal movement, no late decelerations); if nonreassuring, position on side, start O$_2$, assess for hypotension, monitor continuously, notify physician/CNM Active Phase: • BP, P, R, q1h if WNL • Temp as above • Uterine contractions q15–30min: contractions q2–5min, 40–60 sec, moderate to strong • FHR q30min (for low-risk women) and q15min (for high-risk women) if reassuring; if nonreassuring institute interventions and continuous electronic monitoring Transition: • BP, P, R, q30min • Uterine contractions q15min: contractions q1½–2min, 60–90 sec, strong • FHR q15min if reassuring; if nonreassuring, see above	Second stage assessments: • BP, P, R q5–15min • Uterine contractions palpated continuously • FHR q15min (for low-risk women) and q5min (for high-risk women) if reassuring; if nonreassuring, monitor continuously Fetal descent: descent continues to birth Comfort level: woman states is able to cope with contractions and pushing Behavioral characteristics: response to pushing, facial expressions, verbalization Third stage assessments: • BP, P, R q5min • Uterine contractions, palpate occasionally until placenta is delivered, fundus maintains tone and contraction pattern continues to birth of placenta Newborn assessments: • Assess Apgar score of newborn • Respirations: 30 to 60, irregular • Apical pulse: 110 to 160 and somewhat irregular • Temperature: Skin temp above 36.5°C (97.8°F) • Umbilical cord: two arteries, one vein (if one artery, assess for anomalies and urine output) • Gestational age: 38 to 42 weeks	Immediate postbirth assessments of mother q15min for 1h: • BP: /135/85; should return to pre-labor level • Pulse: slightly lower than in labor; range is 60 to 90 • Respirations: 16 to 24/min; easy; quiet • Temperature: 36.2°C to 37.6°C (97°F to 99.6°F) • Fundus firm, in midline, at the umbilicus • Lochia rubra; moderate amount; not more than 2 pad/hr; no free flow or passage of clots with massage • Perineum: sutures intact; no bulging or marked swelling; minimal bruising may be present; no c/o severe pain or rectal pain • Bladder nondistended; spontaneous void of at least 100 mL clear, straw-colored urine; bladder nondistended following voiding • If hemorrhoids present, no tenseness or marked engorgement; less than 2 cm diameter Comfort level: equal to or less than 3 on scale of 1 to 10 Energy level: awake and able to hold newborn Newborn assessments if newborn remains with parents: • Respirations: 30 to 60; irregular • Apical pulse: 110 to 160 and somewhat irregular • Temperature: skin temp above 36.5°C (97.8°F); skin feels warm to touch • Skin color noncyanotic • Mucus: small amount, clear, easily suctioned with bulb syringe without skin color change • Behavioral: newborn opens eyes widely if room is slightly darkened • Movements rhythmic; no hand tremors present **Expected Outcomes** Findings indicate normal progression with absence of complications

	FIRST STAGE	**SECOND AND THIRD STAGE**	**FOURTH STAGE BIRTH TO 1 HOUR PAST BIRTH**
TEACHING/PSYCHOSOCIAL	Establish rapport Orient to environment, expected assessments, and procedures Answer questions and provide information Orient to EFM if used Teach relaxation, visualization, and breathing pattern if needed Explain comfort measures available Assume advocacy role for woman/family during labor and birth	Orient to expected assessments and procedures Answer questions and provide information Explain comfort measures available Continue advocacy role	Explain immediate assessments and care after this first hour Teach self-massage of fundus and expected findings Instruct to call for assistance if mother desires to get OB Begin newborn teaching; bulb syringe, positioning; maintaining warmth Assist parents in exploring their newborn Assist with first breastfeeding experience **Expected Outcomes** Client and partner verbalize/demonstrate understanding of teaching
NURSING CARE MANAGEMENT AND REPORT	Straight cath PRN if bladder distended If regional block administered monitor BP, FHR, sensation per protocol Provide continuing status reports to physician/CNM Perform sterile vaginal examination as indicated	Straight cath PRN if bladder distended Continue monitoring VS, FHR, and sensation if regional block has been given	Straight cath if bladder distended and woman unable to void Monitor return of motor ability and sensation if regional block has been given Weigh perineal pads if lochia flow greater than or equal to 1 saturated pad in 15 min, presence of boggy uterus and clots; ↓ BP, ↑ P **Expected Outcomes** • Maternal/fetal well-being maintained and supported • Mother and newborn experience safe labor and birth • Family participates in process as desired
ACTIVITY	Encourage ambulation unless contraindicated Maintain bed rest immediately after administration of IV pain medication, or following regional block Woman rests comfortably between contractions	Position comfortably for birth Woman rests comfortably between pushing efforts and while awaiting birth of placenta	Position of comfort **Expected Outcomes** • Activity maintained as desired unless contraindicated • Comfort enhanced by positioning/movement
COMFORT	Institute comfort measures: ambulation, frequent position change, effleurage, focal point, patterned paced breathing, visualization, therapeutic touch, backrub, moist cloths to face, holding hand, words of encouragement, changing underpad, shower, whirlpool, staying with the woman/family, warmed blanket at back, sacral pressure Offer pain medication or administer if requested Assist with administration of regional block	Institute comfort measures: • Second stage: cool cloth to forehead, encouragement, coaching, help support legs while pushing, position of comfort for pushing and birth • Third stage: cool cloth to forehead, assist parents to see newborn, position mother to hold newborn, provide encouragement	Institute comfort measures: • Perineal discomfort: gently cleanse and apply ice pack; position to decrease pressure on perineum • Uterine discomfort: palpate fundus gently • Hemorrhoids: ice pack • General fatigue: position of comfort, encourage rest • Administer pain medication PRN **Expected Outcomes** • Optimal comfort level maintained • Active reduction of pain/discomfort achieved

(Continued)

Clinical Pathway FOR INTRAPARTAL STAGES *(Continued)*

FIRST STAGE	SECOND AND THIRD STAGE	FOURTH STAGE BIRTH TO 1 HOUR PAST BIRTH
NUTRITION		
Ice chips and clear fluids Evaluate for signs of dehydration	Ice chips and clear fluids	Regular diet if assessments are WNL Encourage fluids **Expected Outcomes** Nutritional needs met
ELIMINATION		
Voids at least q2h; urine clear, straw-colored, negative for protein Bladder nondistended May have bowel movement Monitor I&O with IVs	May void spontaneously with pushing May pass stool with pushing	Voids spontaneously **Expected Outcomes** Urinary bladder and bowel function unimpaired
MEDICATIONS		
Administer pain medication per woman's request	Local infiltration of anesthetic agent for birth by physician/CNM Pitocin 10 to 20 units IM, IVP per IV tubing, or added to IV fluids	Continue Pitocin infusion Administer pain medication PRN **Expected Outcomes** Comfort enhanced by pain-relieving techniques, administration of analgesia agent or an analgesic or anesthetic block
DISCHARGE PLANNING		
Evaluate knowledge of labor and birth process Evaluate support system and need for referral after birth		Provide information if mother is to be moved from LDR room Provide opportunity for parents to ask questions regarding newborn Evaluate knowledge of normal postpartum, newborn care **Expected Outcomes** Mother and newborn transferred to low-risk postpartal and newborn care
FAMILY INVOLVEMENT		
Identify available support person(s) Recognize possible impact of culture on responses Observe interaction between woman and partner Create moment alone with woman to identify possible abuse Assess current parenting skills	Provide opportunities for woman and support person(s) to watch newborn assessments Perform newborn assessment on mother's abdomen/chest if possible	Provide opportunity for parents to be with baby Encourage skin-to-skin contact Darken room to encourage eye-to-eye contact Provide quiet time for new family Parenting: demonstrates early culturally expected parenting behaviors **Expected Outcomes** • Incorporation of newborn into family • Family verbalizes comfort with newborn care
DATE		

The woman in labor and her partner or support person(s) tend to be concerned about arriving at the birth center in time for the birth. Sometimes the labor is advanced and birth is imminent, but usually the woman is in early labor at admission. If time permits and the family is not familiar with what will occur during labor, the nurse can provide necessary information. (See Client Teaching: What to Expect During Labor.)

The manner in which the maternity nurse greets the woman and her partner influences the course of the woman's hospital stay. The arrival into the healthcare setting and the sometimes impersonal and technical aspects of admission can produce profound stress, fear, and anxiety. If women and their families are greeted in a brusque, harried manner, they are less likely to look to the nurse for support. A calm, pleasant manner indicates to the woman that she is important. It helps to instill in the couple a sense of confidence in the staff's ability to provide quality care during this critical time.

Following the initial greeting, the nurse escorts the woman to the birthing room and provides a quick yet thorough orientation to the facility including the location of the restrooms, public phones, and nurse-call or emergency call system. These simple steps can go a long way toward helping the couple feel more at ease. The nurse also explains the monitoring equipment or other unfamiliar technology. Every effort needs to be made to demystify the environment for the laboring woman and her support person(s). Some women prefer that their partner remain with them during the admission process, although others prefer to have the partner wait outside.

As the nurse helps the woman undress and get into a hospital gown, he or she can start to develop rapport and begin the assessment process. The experienced labor and birth nurse can obtain essential information about the woman and her pregnancy within a few minutes after admission, initiate any immediate interventions needed, and

Client Teaching WHAT TO EXPECT DURING LABOR

Content	**Teaching Method**
Describe aspects of the admission process, including: • Taking an abbreviated history. • Physical assessment (maternal vital signs [VS], fetal heart rate [FHR], contraction status, status of membranes). • Assessment of uterine contractions (frequency, duration, intensity). • Orientation to surroundings. • Introductions to other support staff. • Determination of woman's and family support person's expectations of the nurse.	Provide information on the basic assessment and care activities. Allow time for questions and discussion as labor progress permits.
Present aspects of ongoing physical care, such as when to expect assessment of maternal VS, FHR, and contractions.	
If the electronic fetal monitor is used, describe how it works and the information it provides. Orient the woman to the sights and sounds of the monitor. Explain what "normal" data will look like and what characteristics are being watched for.	Demonstrate the fetal monitor.
Be sure to note that assessments will increase as the labor progresses, especially during the transition phase (usually the time the woman would like to be left alone) to help keep the mother and baby safe by noting deviations from normal course.	
Describe the vaginal examination and the information it elicits.	Use a cervical dilatation chart to illustrate the amount of dilatation. Focus on open discussion.
Review comfort techniques that may be used in labor and ascertain what the woman thinks will promote comfort.	
Review the breathing techniques the woman has learned so that you will be able to support her technique.	Ask the woman to demonstrate the techniques she has learned. Focus on open discussion.
Review comfort and support measures, such as positioning, backrub, effleurage, touch, distraction techniques, and ambulation.	
If the woman is in early labor, offer her a tour of the birthing area.	Provide a tour of the birthing area, explaining equipment and routines. Include the woman's partner.

establish individualized priorities and preferences. A major challenge for nurses is the formulation of realistic objectives for laboring women, because each woman has different coping mechanisms and support systems.

The woman may be facing a number of unfamiliar procedures that may seem routine for healthcare providers. It is important to remember that all women have the right to accept or reject care measures. The woman's informed consent should be obtained before any procedure that involves touching her body. The admission process therefore includes signing an informed consent for treatment and providing information regarding advanced directives. Typically, an identification bracelet and an allergy band are attached to the expectant woman's wrist.

If indicated, the woman is assisted into bed. A side-lying or semi-Fowler's position rather than a supine position is most comfortable and avoids supine hypotensive syndrome (vena caval syndrome). After obtaining the essential information from the woman and her records, the nurse begins the intrapartal assessment. (Chapter 18 ∞ considers intrapartal maternal assessment in depth.) Once the assessment is complete, the nurse can make effective nursing decisions about intrapartal care, such as the following:

- Should ambulation, bed rest, or a combination of both be encouraged?
- Is more frequent or continuous electronic fetal monitoring needed?
- What preferences does the woman have for her labor and birth?
- Is a support person available?
- What special needs do this woman and her partner have?

The nurse auscultates the fetal heart rate (FHR) as described in Chapter 18 ∞. The nurse determines the woman's blood pressure, pulse, respirations, oral temperature, and level of pain or discomfort, and assesses contraction frequency, duration, and intensity (possibly while gathering other data). Before the vaginal examination, the nurse informs the woman about the procedure and its purpose and obtains her consent; afterward, the nurse conveys the findings. If there are signs of advanced labor (frequent contractions, an urge to bear down, and so on), a vaginal examination must be done immediately upon admission. If the woman shows signs of excessive bleeding or reports episodes of painless bleeding in the last trimester, the nurse should not perform a vaginal examination. Instead, he or she should notify the physician or certified nurse-midwife immediately.

Results of FHR assessment, uterine contraction evaluation, and the vaginal examination help determine whether the rest of the admission process can proceed at a leisurely pace or whether additional interventions are required. For example, a FHR of less than 110 beats per minute on auscultation indicates that a fetal monitor should be applied immediately to obtain additional data and continuous fetal monitoring should be performed. The woman's vital signs can be assessed once the monitor is in place. (See the Teaching Card on Fetal Heart Rate Monitoring in the center of this book.)

HINTS FOR PRACTICE

If the fetal monitor is no longer recording the fetal heart tracing, check for adequate gel under the transducer and reposition it before you assume there is a problem with the fetus. Maternal and fetal movement are the most common causes of an inability to trace the fetal heart rate.

The admission process includes collecting a clean voided midstream urine specimen. The woman with intact membranes may collect her specimen in the bathroom. If the membranes are ruptured and the presenting part is not well applied to the cervix, the woman generally remains in bed to avoid prolapse of the umbilical cord. The appropriateness of ambulation when membranes are ruptured varies. The decision is generally based on physical findings, clinician orders, the woman's desires, agency policy, and safety concerns.

The nurse may test the woman's urine for the presence of protein, ketones, and glucose by using a dipstick before sending the sample to the laboratory. This procedure is especially important if edema or elevated blood pressure is noted on admission. Proteinuria of +1 or more may be a sign of impending preeclampsia. Glycosuria is found frequently in pregnant women because of the increased glomerular filtration rate in the proximal tubules and the inability of these tubules to increase reabsorption of glucose. However, it may also be associated with gestational diabetes and should not be discounted. While the woman is collecting the urine specimen, the nurse can gather the equipment for any preparation procedures ordered by the physician/CNM. Laboratory tests are done during early admission. Hemoglobin and hematocrit values help determine the oxygen-carrying capacity of the circulatory system and the woman's ability to withstand blood loss at birth. Elevation of the hematocrit indicates hemoconcentration of blood, which occurs with edema or dehydration. A low hemoglobin, in the absence of other evidence of bleeding, suggests anemia. Blood may be typed and crossmatched if the woman is in a high-risk category. Platelets are evaluated as well because low platelets can lead to bleeding problems. Low platelets are also a contraindication for epidural anesthesia. In addition, a type and screen is performed in case an obstetrical emergency arises and the woman needs to get blood products. Additional serological testing may be performed as indicated. HIV testing should be offered to all women who have not been previously screened (Perinatal HIV Guidelines Working Group, 2006).

Depending on how rapidly labor is progressing, the nurse notifies the physician/CNM before or after completing the admission procedures. The report should include the following information: parity, cervical dilatation and effacement, station, presenting part, status of the membranes, contraction pattern, FHR, vital signs that are not in the normal range, any significant prenatal history, the woman's birth preferences, her reaction to labor, and her preferences for pain relief.

A nursing admission note is entered into the computer or the charting system. The admission note should include the reason for admission, the date and time of the woman's arrival and notification of the physician/CNM, the condition of the woman and her baby, and labor and membrane status.

Nursing Care During the First Stage of Labor

After completing the nursing assessment and diagnosis steps, the nurse creates a plan of care to achieve identified nursing goals. For instance, if the woman and her support person did not have the opportunity to attend childbirth education classes, the nursing goal is to provide desired information. To accomplish this goal, the nurse assesses the current level of the couple's understanding and then plans to provide brief explanations as labor progresses.

Integration of Family Expectations

Laboring families have specific expectations of the labor and birth experience, of themselves, of the nurse, and of the physician/CNM. Sometimes families have unrealistic expectations, which can increase anxiety, create stress, and end in disappointment if expectations are not met. All families should be encouraged to discuss their preferences and special requests with the nurse. Some families may present to the birthing center with a birth plan (discussed in Chapter 8 ∞). Reviewing the plan provides the nurse with the opportunity to explore the family's wishes. Requests that cannot be met should be explained thoroughly. All members of the healthcare team should be informed of the family's requests.

Some families may want the nurse present at all times, whereas others will desire privacy and want to spend time alone. Couples may want a great deal of support if they have not attended childbirth education classes or if they are anxious. Others may want to enjoy the experience as a couple, with as few outside interruptions as possible. In this case, the nurse informs the couple of her or his availability and of the need to make intermittent assessments.

Integration of Cultural Beliefs

Knowledge of values, customs, and practices of different cultures is as important during labor as it is in the prenatal period. Without this knowledge, a nurse is less likely to understand a family's behavior and may attempt to im-

pose personal values and beliefs on them. As cultural sensitivity increases, so does the likelihood of providing high-quality care (Spector, 2009).

The following sections briefly present a few possible responses to labor. General examples about any culture or belief system need to be viewed as background information only. The nurse must always remain aware that an individual example of a birthing practice will never be pertinent to all women in a given group. Within every culture, each person develops his or her own beliefs, values, and behaviors. Culture is also discussed in Chapter 2 ∞.

Modesty

Modesty is an important consideration for most women regardless of culture. Many women are uncomfortable with the degree of exposure needed for certain procedures during labor and the birth. Some women may be particularly uncomfortable when men are present and feel more comfortable with women; others may be uncomfortable with exposure regardless of the gender of the caregivers. The nurse needs to be alert to the woman's responses to examinations and procedures and provide appropriate draping and privacy. It is more prudent to assume that embarrassment will occur with exposure and take measures to provide privacy than to assume that it will not matter to the woman if she is exposed. In particular, some Middle Eastern women are not accustomed to male physicians and attendants.

Orthodox Jewish women may follow several Jewish laws during the childbearing period. The law of *Tznuit* requires the woman to maintain modesty in order to preserve dignity. The woman may prefer a gown that covers her elbows and knees. She may also wish to wear a hair covering such as a wig, scarf, or other form of head covering. The men typically do not observe the woman while she is changing and should be given the opportunity to leave the room to maintain the woman's dignity (Lutwak, Ney, & White, 2004).

CRITICAL THINKING

Fatima Al Ahala is a 22-year-old, G1 who presents in labor. Fatima and her husband Samir are from Pakistan. The couple has stated that they can accept care only from female providers. The couple is being attended to by a female nurse-midwife and the backup physician is also a female. When her labor intensifies, Fatima requests an epidural. The only anesthesiologist available is a male physician. What actions can you take to help this family meet their cultural preferences?

Answer can be found in Appendix F ∞.

Expression and Meaning of Pain

The manner in which a woman chooses to deal with the discomfort of labor varies widely. Some women seem to turn inward and remain very quiet during the whole process. They speak only to ask others to leave the room or cease conversation. Others may be very vocal, with behaviors such as counting out loud, moaning, crying, or shouting. They may also turn from side to side or change positions frequently, often appearing restless.

In many Asian cultures, it is important for individuals to act in a way that will not bring shame on the family. Therefore, the Korean woman may not express pain outwardly for fear of shaming herself or her family, and a Filipina woman may say it is best to lie quietly. Silence is valued in Chinese society, so a Chinese client may be quiet and stoic to avoid dishonoring herself or her family. Japanese women often prefer natural childbirth and prefer to eat during labor. The male partner is often present for the birth. Mexican women often chant the phrase "Aye yie yie" while in labor, which is actually a form of "folk lamaze." Repeating the phrase in succession several times necessitates taking long, slow, deep breaths. Thus, it is a cultural method for alleviating pain (St. Elizabeth's Medical Center, 2007). Many Mexican women will want their partners and female relatives present during the birthing process. European Americans demonstrate a wide variety of behaviors in response to pain, from silence to shouting. The nurse supports a woman's individual expression, as long as it is not harmful, in order to enhance the birthing experience for mother, baby, and family.

Different cultures also have differing beliefs about the meaning and value of labor pain. Because childbearing is considered a woman's "career" by ancient Chinese custom, elders advise the pregnant woman not to fear childbirth. South or Central American women may view pain during labor as a symbol of love toward the baby—the more intense the pain, the more intense the love. Native American women typically view labor pain as natural, and may use meditation, self-control, or indigenous plants or herbs, such as black cohosh, throughout their labor as well as to aid them during birth (Spector, 2009). European American women may value pain as aiding in the birth of their baby and signaling that all is well, or they may find themselves feeling angry about the intensity of the pain and fearful of losing control.

Examples of Cultural Beliefs

Although it is important to avoid stereotyping, descriptions of a few women's responses to labor may be helpful. The following are "snapshots" from Hmong, Vietnamese, Hispanic, Muslim, and Orthodox Judaism cultures.

Hmong women from Laos report that squatting during childbirth is common in their culture. During labor they may want to be active and move about. The husband is frequently present and actively involved in providing comfort. Traditionally, the woman prefers that the amniotic membranes not be ruptured until just before birth. It is thought that the escape of fluid at this time makes the birth easier. During labor the woman usually prefers only

---

CULTURAL PERSPECTIVES

In the Muslim culture, male healthcare providers are usually not allowed to care for female clients. In the hospital setting, if a male provider such as an anesthesiologist or neonatologist will be needed, it is best to speak to the husband first and obtain his permission. Because modesty is of great concern for Muslim women, care should be taken to cover the woman as much as possible. She may want to put her *khimar* (head covering) on before the male enters the room.

"hot" foods and warm water to drink (Spector, 2009). As soon as the baby is born the family may request that the mother be given a soft-boiled egg to restore her energy.

Vietnamese women usually maintain self-control and may even smile throughout labor. They may prefer to walk about during labor and to give birth in a squatting position. In labor, the mother often prefers cold beverages because pregnancy is viewed as a "hot" condition. However, during the postpartum period, which is viewed as a "cold" condition, she will prefer warm liquids (Ethnomed, 2007). The newborn is protected from praise and the "evil eye" to prevent jealousy (Spector, 2009).

Latina women have identified expectations of their partners during labor and birth such as wanting their partners to stay with them and to reassure them that everything will be alright. As they labor, the women want their partners to show their love and to speak using affectionate words. Latina women also typically want their mothers present during the birth process.

Muslim women may have their husband or a female friend or relative with them during childbirth. However, the father may take a very passive, hands-off approach, speaking up only as an advocate as needed. Family support may be particularly important but does not preclude the importance of the nurse's presence. The woman may want to retain her head covering (*khimar*), and the nurse can offer two long-sleeved gowns. It is important for a female nurse, physician, or CNM to perform examinations when possible. If a male physician or nurse is involved, the woman may wish for her husband to remain in the room. After the birth Muslim fathers may call praise to Allah (*adhan*) in the newborn's right ear and clean the newborn.

Orthodox Jews observe the law of *niddah*, which begins with the onset of regular uterine contractions or the appearance of bloody show or membrane rupture. Once this occurs, the *niddah law* mandates a physical separation of husband and wife. Usually, husbands will not touch their wives during this time, but may remain in the room, or just outside of the curtain. The nurse can encourage the father to offer verbal support, prayer, and eye contact if the couple feels comfortable with these interventions. Once the father stops providing physical care, the nurse will need to assist the woman and serve as the primary caretaker and coach. Sometimes, the laboring woman's mother or another female friend or relative may be present. It is common for the father to read prayers during this time. It is also usual practice that the husband does not observe the birth and reenters the room only after the woman is draped (Lutwak Ney, & White, 2004).

Maternity nurses can provide culturally sensitive care by first becoming acquainted with the beliefs and practices of the various subcultures in their communities. In the birthing situation, the truly effective nurse supports the family's cultural practices as long as it is safe to do so. Nurses should not assume that because a woman is from a certain ethnic group that her preferences will always follow cultural norms. Instead, the nurse should assess her individualized preferences and wishes.

HINTS FOR PRACTICE

When providing care for a culturally diverse woman and her family, ask yourself what your assumptions are regarding their expectations. Ask direct questions to ensure that you are not making false assumptions based on her cultural identity alone. Consider how these factors will affect her behavior during the labor and birth and incorporate these into your plan of care.

Provision of Care in the First Stage

As discussed in Chapter 18 ∞, the nurse needs to evaluate physical parameters of the woman and her fetus. Maternal temperature is monitored every 4 hours unless the temperature is over 37.5°C (99.6°F); in such cases it is taken every hour. When the amniotic membranes have ruptured, maternal temperature is assessed every 1 to 2 hours depending on the policy of the institution. Blood pressure, pulse, respirations, and response to pain are monitored every hour. If the woman's blood pressure is over 135/85 mm Hg or her pulse is more than 100, the nurse must notify the physician/CNM and reevaluate the blood pressure and pulse more frequently. The woman's pain level should be monitored continually because this can elevate the blood pressure and pulse, especially during contractions.

The nurse palpates uterine contractions for frequency, intensity, and duration every 30 minutes. The nurse also auscultates the FHR every 30 minutes for low-risk women and every 15 minutes for high-risk women as long as it remains between 110 and 160 beats per minute and is reassuring (American College of Obstetricians & Gynecologists, 2005). The FHR should be auscultated throughout one contraction and for about 15 seconds after the contraction to ensure that there are no decelerations. If the FHR baseline is not in the 110 to 160 range or decelerations are heard, continuous electronic monitoring is recommended (Table 19–1).

Latent Phase

The nurse should offer fluids in the form of clear liquids or ice chips at frequent intervals, unless complications exist that may necessitate general anesthesia. Some certified childbirth educators advise the woman to bring lollipops to help combat the dryness that occurs with some of the labor breathing patterns. Avoiding both liquids and solids during labor, which was once standard practice, is no longer so as evidence-based practice research and new guidelines indicate that clear fluids can be consumed throughout labor and up to 2 hours before an elective cesarean birth. Research shows that the volume of liquid consumed is less important than the presence of particulate matter ingested because this increases the risk of aspiration. Certain women with specific risk factors for aspiration should be evaluated on a case-by-case basis to assess their specific risk factors and determine the most appropriate recommendation. Current guidelines suggest avoiding solids for 6 to 8 hours before an elective cesarean birth (American Society of Anesthesiologists [ASA], 2006). Eating during labor has not been associated with an increase in aspiration and is therefore no longer contraindicated, although some institutions may continue to limit oral intake in labor (Gennaro, Mayberry, & Kafulafula, 2007). Previously, it was believed that drinking fluids should be avoided because it can lead to

TABLE 19–1	Nursing Assessments in the First Stage	
Phase	Mother	Fetus
Latent	Blood pressure, respirations each hour if in normal range. Temperature every 4 hours unless over 37.5°C (99.6°F) or membranes ruptured, then every 2 hours. Uterine contractions every 30 minutes.	FHR every 60 minutes for low-risk women and every 30 minutes for high-risk women if normal characteristics present (average variability, baseline in the 110 to 160 bpm range, without late or variable decelerations). Note fetal activity. If electronic fetal monitor is in place, assess for reactive NST.
Active Transition	Blood pressure, pulse, respirations every hour if in normal range. Uterine contractions palpated every 15 to 30 minutes. Blood pressure, pulse, respirations every 30 minutes. Contractions palpated at least every 15 minutes.	FHR every 30 minutes for low-risk women and every 15 minutes for high-risk women if normal characteristics are present. FHR every 15 minutes if normal characteristics are present.

vomiting caused by the decreased gastric emptying time. Although vomiting is common during the first stage of labor, many women have more energy and tolerate labor better with oral intake and have higher satisfaction with their labor and birth experience (ASA, 2006). If vomiting does occur, the nurse provides reassurance and oral care.

Active Phase

During the active phase, the contractions have a frequency of 2 to 5 minutes, a duration of 40 to 60 seconds, and a moderate to strong intensity. As the contractions become more frequent and intense, a woman who has been ambulatory may choose to sit in a chair or lie down. (Laboring positions are discussed shortly.) Contractions need to be palpated every 15 to 30 minutes.

Vaginal exams may be performed to assess cervical dilatation and effacement as well as fetal station and position. Vaginal examinations should be limited because they introduce bacteria which can lead to maternal infection. During the active phase, the cervix dilates from 4 to 7 cm, and vaginal discharge and bloody show increase; thus, the nurse needs to change the perineal pads more frequently.

The FHR is auscultated and evaluated every 30 minutes for low-risk women and every 15 minutes for high-risk women (ACOG, 2005). Maternal blood pressure, pulse, and respirations are monitored during the FHR assessment or more frequently if indicated. The woman's level of pain and coping mechanisms are assessed continuously.

The woman is encouraged to void because a full bladder can interfere with fetal descent. If the woman is unable to void, catheterization or an indwelling Foley catheter may be necessary.

If the amniotic membranes have not ruptured previously, they may do so during this phase. When the membranes rupture, the nurse notes the amount, color, odor, and consistency of the amniotic fluid and the time of rupture and immediately auscultates the FHR. The fluid should be clear, with no odor. Nonreassuring fetal status may lead to intestinal and anal sphincter relaxation, and meconium may be released into the amniotic fluid, which turns the fluid greenish brown. When the nurse notes meconium-stained fluid, an electronic monitor is applied to assess the FHR continuously. The time of rupture is noted. Current management of rupture of membranes without labor varies. The group beta streptococcus status should be evaluated and intrapartum antibiotics should be administered as indicated. Labor induction may be initiated on a case-by-case basis (ACOG, 2007).

An additional concern is prolapse of the umbilical cord, which may occur when membranes rupture and the fetal presenting part is not well applied to the cervix. The concern is that the amniotic fluid coming through the cervix will propel the umbilical cord through the cervix (prolapsed cord). The FHR is auscultated because a drop in the rate might indicate an undetected prolapsed cord. Immediate intervention is necessary to remove pressure on a prolapsed umbilical cord (see Chapter 21 ∞). (See Table 19–2 for additional deviations from normal.)

Transition

During transition, the contraction frequency is every 1½ to 2 minutes, duration is 60 to 90 seconds, and intensity is strong. Cervical dilatation increases from 8 to 10 cm, effacement is complete (100%), and there is usually a heavy amount of bloody show. Contractions are palpated at least every 15 minutes. Sterile vaginal examinations may be done more frequently because this stage of labor usually is accompanied by rapid change. Maternal blood pressure, pulse, and respirations are monitored when the FHR is assessed, the woman's pain level is monitored continuously, and the FHR is auscultated every 30 minutes for low-risk women and every 15 minutes for high-risk women. It should be noted that women may receive more frequent assessments based on individualized needs. Women may also shake uncontrollably, feel nausea, or vomit during this stage.

Comfort measures become very important in this phase of labor, but continual assessment is required to intervene appropriately. The woman may rapidly change from wanting a back rub and other hands-on care to wanting to be left completely alone. The support person and the nurse need to follow her cues and change interventions as needed. Because the woman is breathing more rapidly, the nurse can increase her comfort by offering small spoons of ice chips to moisten her mouth or by applying an emollient to dry lips. The nurse can encourage the woman to rest between contractions. If analgesics have been administered, a quiet environment enhances the quality of rest between contractions.

Some women have difficulty coping during this time and need help with their breathing. Either the support person or the nurse can breathe along with the woman during each contraction to help her maintain her pattern. A gentle reminder to "slow down your breathing" can help prevent hyperventilation (discussed shortly). It is helpful to encourage the woman and to assure her that she is doing a good job. The woman will begin to feel increased rectal pressure as the fetal presenting part moves down the birth canal. The nurse encourages the woman to refrain from pushing until the cervix is completely dilated. To help the woman avoid involuntary pushing during contractions, the nurse can encourage *pant-blow breathing*, suggesting that the woman "pant like a puppy" or "blow in short breaths as if you were blowing out a candle." This measure helps prevent cervical edema.

The end of transition and the beginning of the second stage may be indicated by a change in the woman's voice or the sounds she is making. As the fetus moves down and

TABLE 19–2	Deviations from Normal Labor Process Requiring Immediate Intervention
Problem	Immediate Action
Woman admitted with vaginal bleeding or history of painless vaginal bleeding	Do not perform vaginal examination. Assess FHR. Evaluate amount of blood loss. Evaluate labor pattern. Notify physician/CNM immediately.
Presence of greenish or brownish amniotic fluid	Continuously monitor FHR. Evaluate dilatation of cervix and determine if umbilical cord is prolapsed. Evaluate presentation (vertex or breech). Maintain woman on complete bed rest on left side. Notify physician/CNM immediately.
Absence of FHR and fetal movement	Notify physician/CNM. Provide truthful information and emotional support to laboring couple. Remain with the couple.
Prolapse of umbilical cord	Relieve pressure on cord manually. Continuously monitor FHR; watch for changes in FHR pattern. Notify physician/CNM. Assist woman into knee-chest position or place in Trendelenburg position. Administer oxygen.
Woman admitted in advanced labor; birth imminent	Prepare for immediate birth. Obtain critical information: • Estimated date of birth (EDB), history of bleeding problems, history of medical or obstetric problems • Past and/or present use/abuse of prescription/OTC/illicit drugs. Problems with this pregnancy. FHR and maternal vital signs. Whether membranes are ruptured and how long since rupture. Blood type and Rh. Direct another person to contact physician/CNM. Do not leave woman alone. Provide support to couple. Put on gloves.

she feels increased pressure and a bearing-down sensation, her voice tends to deepen. If she moans during a contraction, it takes on a more guttural quality. Expert nurses recognize this sound as a sign of changes in the woman.

Promotion of Comfort in the First Stage

The first step in planning care is to talk with the woman and her partner or support person to identify their goals. Usually the woman or the couple is concerned with discomfort, so it is helpful to identify factors that may contribute to discomfort. These factors include uncomfortable positions or infrequent position changes, diaphoresis, continual leaking of amniotic fluid, a full bladder, a dry mouth, anxiety, and fear. Nursing interventions can minimize the effects of these factors. These interventions are described later in this section.

There are many types of responses to pain. As the intensity of the contractions increase with the progress of labor, the woman becomes less aware of the environment and may have difficulty hearing and understanding verbal instructions. Some women may become irritable during this time. The pattern of coping with labor contractions varies from the use of highly structured breathing techniques to turning inward. Low moaning that begins deep in the throat, rocking or swaying, counting, facial grimacing, and using loud vocalizations are all effective means of dealing with the discomfort of labor and birth. Some women feel that making sounds helps them cope and do the work of labor, whereas others make loud sounds only as they lose their perception of control.

The most frequent physiologic manifestations of pain are increased pulse and respiratory rates, dilated pupils, increased blood pressure, and muscle tension. In labor, these reactions are transitory because the pain is intermittent. Increased muscle tension is most significant because it may impede the labor process. Women in labor frequently tighten skeletal muscles voluntarily during a contraction and remain motionless. This method of dealing with the contractions may actually increase her discomfort, but the woman may believe it is the only acceptable way to cope with the pain.

A woman generally wants touching, massage, effleurage, and other forms of physical contact during the first part of labor, but when she moves into the transition phase, she may pull away. Alternatively, the woman may beseech her partner or nurse to hold her hand or rub her back, or may even reach out and grasp the support person. Some women are uncomfortable with being touched at all, regardless of the phase of labor, whereas others do not welcome touch from a nonfamily member. It is important to validate the unique strengths and coping techniques of the individual

COMPLEMENTARY AND ALTERNATIVE THERAPIES

Acupressure During Labor

Acupressure is an ancient Chinese medical treatment that involves using the fingers to press key pressure points on the surface of the skin. This pressure ultimately stimulates the immune system to promote healing by triggering the release of endorphins, reducing stress through muscle relaxation, and promoting circulation. The specific acupressure point used in laboring women is the San Yin-Jiao (SP-6) acupressure point. The SP-6 acupressure point is located on the medial side of the leg, in the calf region, approximately 3 cm (1.2 in.) superior to the prominence of the inner malleus. The use of acupressure in labor has been associated with shorter labors and lower subjective and objective pain scores. Women who receive acupressure typically use less pain medication than those who do not receive acupressure (Smith, Collins, Cyna, & Crowther, 2006).

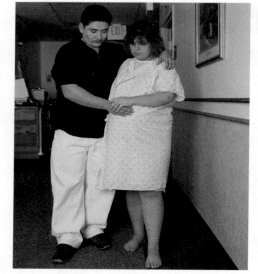

FIGURE 19–1 Woman and her partner walking in the hospital during labor.

and to meet each family on their own terms, always keeping in mind that this is *their* experience. Cultural influences can also affect how a woman will react to support and touch in labor. The nurse should take cues from the woman and make adjustments in her care to meet her specific needs.

HINTS FOR PRACTICE

The nurse can introduce and facilitate the following nonpharmacologic pain relief techniques in labor to encourage maternal comfort and facilitate coping: massage, effleurage, hydrotherapy, position changes, hypnosis, aromatherapy, sitting in a rocking chair or glider, or on a birthing ball, walking, leaning against the bed or her partner, using TENs unit, visualization, relaxation techniques, the use of prayer or meditation, and breathing techniques.

Most nurses like to incorporate comfort measures into their nursing care, and they readily respond to the woman's needs. As the nurse and woman or couple work together to increase comfort during contractions, a ritual of supportive measures begins to develop. The nurse watches for cues and nonverbal behaviors and asks for feedback from the woman. As labor progresses, the nurse and couple will use their prior experience and growing rapport to change comfort measures as needed.

A decrease in the intensity of discomfort is one of the goals of nursing support during labor. Nursing measures used to decrease pain include the following:

- Ensuring general comfort
- Providing information to decrease anxiety
- Using specific supportive relaxation techniques
- Encouraging controlled breathing
- Administering pharmacologic agents as ordered by the physician/CNM

EVIDENCE IN ACTION
The hands and knees posture to relieve persistent back pain during labor is supported by a review of the research.
(Cochrane Review) (Hunter, Hofmeyr, & Kulier 2007)

General Comfort

General comfort measures are of great importance during labor. By relieving minor discomforts, the nurse helps the woman optimize her coping abilities to deal with pain.

The woman is encouraged to ambulate as long as there are no contraindications, such as vaginal bleeding or rupture of membranes (ROM) before the fetus is engaged in the pelvis. Ambulation can increase comfort and aid in fetal descent (Figure 19–1 ■).

Even if the woman prefers not to walk around, upright positions such as sitting in a rocker or leaning against a wall or bed can enhance comfort. If she stays in bed, the nurse can encourage the woman to assume positions that she finds comfortable (Figure 19–2 ■).

A side-lying position is generally the most advantageous for the laboring woman, although frequent position changes seem to achieve more efficient contractions. In one facility where evidence-based practice was embraced, changes were implemented to benefit the care of laboring women. Lithotomic position was once the position of choice (100%) in this facility; however, after reviewing the evidence, the use of the lithotomic position fell to 30% (Bardzulin, Bochoriashvili, Abashhidze, & Konaia, 2006). Care should be taken to support all body parts, with the joints kept slightly flexed. For instance, when the woman is in a side-lying position, pillows may be placed against her chest and under the uppermost arm. The nurse should place a pillow or folded bath blanket between her knees to support the uppermost leg and relieve tension or muscle strain. Placing a pillow at the woman's midback and placing one to support the uterus also help provide support.

If the woman is more comfortable on her back, the head of the bed

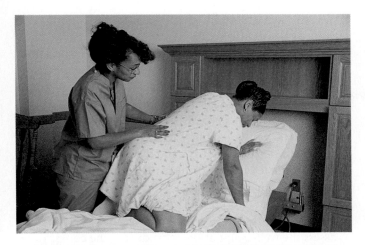

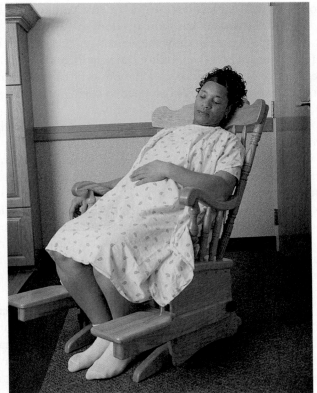

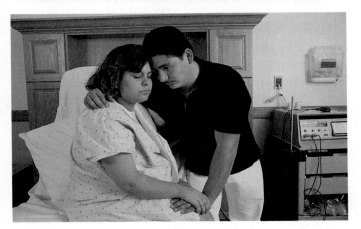

FIGURE 19–2 The laboring woman is encouraged to choose a position of comfort. The nurse modifies assessments and interventions as necessary.

should be elevated to relieve the pressure of the uterus on the vena cava. Pillows may be placed under each arm and under the knees to provide support. Because a pregnant woman is at increased risk for thrombophlebitis, excessive pressure behind the knee and calf should be avoided. The nurse needs to assess pressure points frequently. Frequent changes of position contribute to comfort and relaxation.

Wearing socks or slippers may alleviate cold feet, just as adjusting the room's thermostat can offset excessive warmth. Attention to such details allows the woman to focus on the more important issues of giving birth. The woman may be offered a warmed or cooled facial cloth, which is placed on her forehead or across or behind her neck. Providing a toothbrush and toothpaste for oral care can also increase comfort.

Diaphoresis and the constant leaking of amniotic fluid can dampen the woman's gown and bed linen. Offering fresh, smooth, dry bed linen promotes comfort. To avoid having to change the bottom sheet following rupture of the membranes, the nurse may replace absorbent underpads at frequent intervals (following standard precautions). The perineal area should be kept as clean and dry as possible to promote comfort and to prevent infection. A full bladder adds to discomfort during a contraction and may prolong labor by interfering with the descent of the fetus. The bladder should be kept as empty as possible. Even if the woman is voiding, urine may be retained because of the pressure of the fetal presenting part. The nurse can detect a full bladder by palpating directly over the symphysis pubis. Some of the regional procedures for analgesia and anesthesia during labor contribute to the inability to void, and catheterization may be necessary. The woman should be encouraged to empty her bladder every 1 to 2 hours.

Family members also need to be encouraged to maintain their own comfort. Because their attention is directed toward the laboring woman, they may forget their own needs. The nurse may have to encourage them to take breaks, to maintain food and fluid intake, and to rest.

HINTS FOR PRACTICE

Many support persons and family members are reluctant to leave the woman unattended while they meet their own personal needs. Offer to stay with the woman during their absence. This provides reassurance to the support person or family member that the woman will be well cared for in his or her absence.

Handling Anxiety

The anxiety experienced by women beginning labor is related to a combination of factors inherent to the process. A moderate amount of anxiety about pain enhances the woman's ability to deal with it. In contrast, an excessive degree of anxiety decreases her ability to cope with the pain.

Women in the latent phase of labor who are experiencing increased levels of anxiety about their ability to cope and their own personal safety are much more likely to describe their pain as unbearable. Women at risk for greater anxiety during labor include women who are young, poor, minority, and unmarried. Women with preexisting mental illness, such as depression and anxiety, are at a greater risk for developing post-traumatic stress disorder (PTSD) related to their labor and birth experience (Maggioni, Margola, & Filipi, 2006). Women with mental illness issues may need additional support to assist them with identifying effective coping mechanisms during the labor and birth.

Ways to decrease anxiety not related to pain are to give information (which eases fear of the unknown), establish rapport with the couple (which helps them preserve their personal integrity), and express confidence in the couple's ability to work with the labor process. In addition to being a good listener, the nurse must demonstrate genuine concern for the laboring woman. Remaining with the woman as much as possible conveys a caring attitude and dispels fears of abandonment. Praise for breathing, relaxation, and pushing efforts not only encourages repetition of the behavior but also decreases anxiety about the ability to cope with labor.

Client Teaching

Providing truthful information about the nature of the discomfort that will occur during labor is important. Stressing the intermittent nature and maximum duration of the contractions can be helpful. The woman can cope with pain better when she knows that a period of relief will follow. Describing the type of discomfort and specific sensations that will occur as labor progresses helps the woman recognize these sensations as normal and expected when she does experience them.

TEACHING TIP

Advise women that the strength and intensity of contractions are different for each person, but they may feel like a tightening sensation or a menstrual cramp initially. Over time as the labor progresses, the contractions become more intense and more uncomfortable with the uterus tightening and becoming very hard with the pain radiating from the back around to the front. For some women, the pain takes their breath away or they may feel anxiety and fear. As the contractions become more painful, they also occur closer together. The sensation of having to push occurs as the head progresses into the pelvis and feels like the woman has to have a bowel movement. Once the contraction goes away, this intense feeling of having to have a bowel movement usually lets up some.

Descriptions of sensations are best accompanied by information on specific comfort measures. As previously noted, some women experience the urge to push during transition, when the cervix is not fully dilated and effaced. This sensation can be controlled by pant-blow breathing (it is difficult to pant or blow and bear down at the same time); the nurse should provide instructions about this technique before it is required.

Thorough orientation and explanation of surroundings, procedures, and equipment being used also decreases anxiety, thereby reducing pain. Attachment to an electronic monitor can produce fear because the woman may associate equipment of this type with critically ill people. It can also limit the woman's ability to move about and comfort herself with position changes and ambulation. If continuous electronic fetal monitoring is needed, the nurse can explain beeps, clicks, and other strange noises and give a simplified explanation of the monitor strip. The nurse can emphasize that the use of the fetal monitor provides a way to assess the well-being of the fetus during the course of labor. If available, a less intrusive telemetry monitor can be applied so the woman has more freedom to move about. In addition, the nurse can show the woman and her partner or support person how the monitor can help them identify the beginnings of contractions. At the onset of each contraction, the woman can be encouraged to begin her breathing technique to lessen her perception of pain.

Labor and childbirth may be a critical time for the woman with a history of childhood sexual abuse or rape. It is estimated that of the 872,000 children abused in some way annually, 9.3% have experienced sexual abuse (United States Department of Health & Human Services, 2007). Between 2004 to 2005, there were approximately 200,780 victims of sexual assault (National Sexual Assault Hotline, 2007). Women with a history of sexual abuse experiencing current life stressors, such as pregnancy, are more apt to have medical complications than those with no history of abuse (Cromer & Sachs-Ericsson, 2006).

To develop a competent plan of care, all women entering the healthcare arena should be evaluated for a history of sexual abuse or rape. Culturally diverse women may need specific examples of abuse to determine if they have had these types of experiences because some behaviors that are considered abusive in our society may be considered normal patterns of behavior in other cultures (Thombs, Bennett, Ziegelstein et al., 2007). Women may or may not be able to address this issue with the nurse, because sharing such personal information is difficult and may stir up painful memories. It is therefore especially important for the nurse to be alert for nonverbal cues, such as excessive unexplained anxiety, unrelenting pain, and/or intense fear during vaginal exams, and to be prepared to offer additional teaching to help offset the woman's anxiety.

TEACHING TIP

If a woman is experiencing severe fear or anxiety about a vaginal examination, advise her to slowly count to 10 during the examination while continually wiggling her toes. This source of distraction may lessen her fear and anxiety. It also enables the woman to have a sense of control.

Supportive Relaxation Techniques

Tense muscles increase resistance to the descent of the fetus and contribute to maternal fatigue. This fatigue increases pain perception and decreases the woman's ability to cope with the pain. Comfort measures, massage, techniques for decreasing anxiety, and client teaching can contribute to relaxation. Adequate sleep and rest are also important. The laboring woman needs to be encouraged to use the period between contractions for rest and relaxation. A prolonged prodromal phase of labor may interfere with sleep. An aura of excitement naturally accompanies the onset of labor, making it difficult for the woman to sleep even though the contractions are mild and infrequent. The nurse may have to act as an advocate for the woman to limit the number of her visitors, interruptions, and phone calls.

Distraction is another method of increasing relaxation and coping with discomfort. During early labor, conversation or activities such as watching television, light reading, or playing cards or other games can serve as distractions. One technique that is effective for relieving moderate pain is to have the woman concentrate on a pleasant experience she has had in the past. Other techniques include the use of a specific visual or mental focal point (such as a picture of a loved one), breathing techniques, counting or humming, or visualization.

Touch—discussed earlier—is another type of distraction (Figure 19–3 ■). Although some women regard touching as an invasion of privacy or threat to their independence, many want to touch and be touched during a painful experience. To determine whether the woman desires touch, the nurse can place a hand on the side of the bed within the woman's reach. The woman who needs touch will reach out for contact, and the nurse can follow through with this behavioral cue.

Specific touch techniques useful for relaxation include effleurage and massage. Mild to moderate abdominal discomfort during contractions may be relieved or lessened by effleurage. Back pain associated with labor may be relieved by firm pressure on the lower back or sacral area. To apply

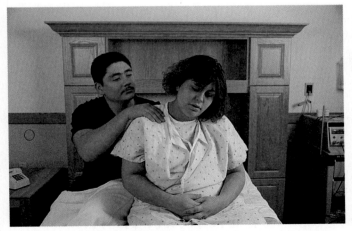

FIGURE 19–3 The woman's partner provides support and encouragement during labor.

firm pressure, the nurse can either place her or his hand or a rolled, warmed towel or blanket in the small of the woman's back, or instruct the woman's support person to do so.

In some instances, analgesics or regional anesthetic blocks may be used to enhance comfort and relaxation during labor. (See Chapter 20 ∞ for a discussion of analgesia and anesthesia.) In addition to the measures just described, the nurse can enhance the woman's relaxation by providing encouragement and support for her controlled breathing techniques, discussed next.

Breathing Techniques

Breathing techniques may help the laboring woman. Used correctly, they increase the woman's pain threshold, permit relaxation, enhance the woman's ability to cope with contractions, provide a sense of control, and allow the uterus to function more efficiently.

Various types of breathing techniques can be used in labor. Many women learn patterned-paced breathing during prenatal education classes. This type of controlled breathing often has three levels. The woman tends to begin with the first level and then proceed to the next when she feels the need. Regardless of the level of breathing used, a cleansing breath (involving only the chest) begins and ends each pattern. The cleansing breath consists of inhaling through the nose slowly until a sense of fullness in the lungs occurs, holding the breath for a few seconds, and then exhaling slowly through pursed lips (Table 19–3).

The first pattern may also be called slow, deep breathing or slow-paced breathing. During the breathing movements only the chest moves. The woman inhales slowly through her nose, moves her chest up and out during the inhalation, and exhales through pursed lips. The breathing rate is six to nine breaths a minute.

The second pattern may be called shallow or modified-paced breathing. The woman begins with a cleansing breath. At the end of the cleansing breath she pushes out a short breath. She then inhales and exhales through the mouth at a rate of about four breaths every 5 seconds. This pattern can be altered into a more rapid rate that does not exceed two to two-and-a-half breaths every second.

The third pattern, introduced earlier, is called pant-blow or patterned-paced breathing. It is similar to modified-paced breathing except the breathing is punctuated every few breaths by a forceful exhalation through pursed lips. A pattern of four breaths may be used to begin. All breaths are kept equal and rhythmic. As the contraction becomes more intense, the woman may adjust the pattern as needed to 3:1, 2:1, and finally 1:1. (Instructions for the three patterns of breathing are summarized on the Teaching Card on Breathing Techniques for Labor inserted in the center of this text.)

Abdominal breathing is another technique that can be effective in labor. In abdominal breathing, the woman moves the abdominal wall outward as she inhales and inward as she exhales. This method tends to lift the abdominal wall off the contracting uterus and thus helps to provide pain relief. The breathing is deep and rhythmic, and typically relaxing. As transition approaches, the woman using abdominal breathing may feel the urge to breathe more rapidly. The pant-blow pattern discussed earlier can be suggested to slow the breathing and help the woman avoid the urge to bear down (see Table 19–3).

Hyperventilation is the result of an imbalance of oxygen and carbon dioxide (i.e., too much carbon dioxide is exhaled, and too much oxygen remains in the body). Hyperventilation may occur when a woman breathes very rapidly over a prolonged period. The signs and symptoms of hyperventilation are tingling or numbness in the tip of the nose, lips, fingers, or toes; dizziness; spots before the eyes; or spasms of the hands or feet (carpal-pedal spasms). If hyperventilation occurs, the woman should be encouraged to slow her breathing rate and take shallow breaths. With instruction and encouragement, many women are able to change their breathing to correct the problem. Encouraging the woman to relax and counting out loud for her so she can pace her breathing during contractions are also helpful actions. If the signs and symptoms continue or become more severe (they progress from numbness to spasms), the woman can breathe into a paper surgical mask or a paper bag until symptoms abate. Breathing into a mask or bag causes rebreathing of carbon dioxide. The nurse should remain with the woman to reassure her because a great deal of anxiety often occurs.

Role of the Doula

Throughout the first stage of labor, the nurse assesses and supports the interaction between the woman and her partner. In the absence of a partner, or when the partner

---

TABLE 19–3 Nursing Support of Patterned-Paced Breathing

Determine which breathing method the woman (couple) has learned.
Provide encouragement as needed in maintaining breathing pattern.
Provide support to the labor coach and assist as needed.

Lamaze Breathing Pattern Level

First level (slow paced)

Pattern begins and ends with a cleansing breath (in through the nose and out through pursed lips as if cooling a spoonful of hot food). While inhaling through the nose and exhaling through pursed lips, slow breaths are taken, moving only the chest. The rate should be approximately 6–9/minute or 2 breaths/15 seconds. The coach or nurse may assist by reminding the woman to take a cleansing breath, and then the breaths could be counted out if needed to maintain pacing. The woman inhales as someone counts "one one thousand, two one thousand, three one thousand, four one thousand." Exhalation begins and continues through the same count.

First level for use during uterine contractions (the level begins and ends with a cleansing breath [CB]).

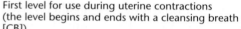

Second level (modified paced)

Pattern begins and ends with a cleansing breath. Breaths are then taken in and out silently through the mouth at approximately 4 breaths/5 seconds. The jaw and entire body need to be relaxed. The rate can be accelerated to 2 to 2¹⁄₂ breaths/second. The rhythm for the breaths can be counted out as "one and two and one and two and . . ." with the woman exhaling on the numbers and inhaling on "and."

Second level

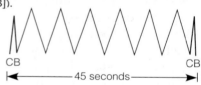

Third level (pattern paced)

Pattern begins and ends with a cleansing breath. All breaths are rhythmical, in and out through the mouth. Exhalations are accompanied by a "hee" or "hoo" sound in a varying pattern, 2:1, which begins as 3:1 (hee hee hee hoo) and can change to 2:1 (hee hee hoo) or 1:1 (hee hoo) as the intensity of the contraction changes. The rate should not be more rapid than 2 to 2¹⁄₂ breaths/second. The rhythm of the breaths would match a "one and two and" count.

Third level (Darkened spike represents "hoo.")

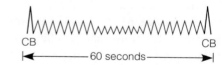

Abdominal Breathing Pattern Cues

The abdomen moves outward during inhalation and inward during exhalation. The rate remains slow with approximately 6 to 9 breaths/minute.

Breathing sequence for abdominal breathing

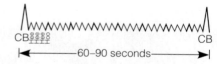

Quick Method

When the woman has not learned a particular method and is in active phase of labor, the nurse may teach her a combination of two patterns. Abdominal breathing may be used until labor is more advanced. Then a more rapid pattern consisting of two short blows from the mouth followed by a longer blow can be used. (This pattern is called "pant-pant-blow" even though all exhalations are a blowing motion.)

Pant-pant-blow breathing pattern

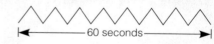
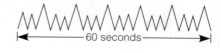

TABLE 19–4	Psychologic Characteristics and Nursing Support During First and Second Stages of Labor	
Phase	**Woman's Response**	**Support Measures**
Stage 1 Latent phase	Usually happy, talkative, and eager to be in labor Exhibits need for independence by taking care of own bodily needs and seeking information	Establish rapport on admission and continue to build during care. Assess information base and learning needs. Be available to consult regarding breathing technique if needed; teach breathing technique if needed and in early labor. Orient family to room, equipment, monitors, and procedures. Encourage woman and partner to participate in care as desired. Provide needed information. Assist woman into position of comfort; encourage frequent change of position; encourage ambulation during early labor. Offer fluids/ice chips. Keep couple informed of progress. Encourage woman to void every 1 to 2 hours. Assess need for and interest in using visualization to enhance relaxation and teach if appropriate.
Active phase	May experience feelings of helplessness Exhibits increased fatigue and may begin to feel restless and anxious as contractions become stronger Expresses fear of abandonment Becomes more dependent as she is less able to meet her needs	Encourage woman to maintain breathing patterns. Provide quiet environment to reduce external stimuli. Provide reassurance, encouragement, support; keep couple informed of progress. Promote comfort by giving back rubs, sacral pressure, cool cloth on forehead, assistance with position changes, support with pillows, effleurage. Provide ice chips, ointment for dry mouth and lips. Encourage to void every 1 to 2 hours. Offer shower/whirlpool/warm bath if available.
Transition phase	Tires and may exhibit increased restlessness and irritability May feel she cannot keep up with labor process and is out of control Physical discomforts Fear of being left alone May fear tearing open or splitting apart with contractions	Encourage woman to rest between contractions. If she sleeps between contractions, wake her at beginning of contraction so she can begin breathing pattern (increases feeling of control). Provide support, encouragement, and praise for efforts. Keep couple informed of progress; encourage continued participation of support persons. Promote comfort as previously listed but recognize many women do not want to be touched when in transition. Provide privacy. Provide ice chips, ointment for lips. Encourage to void every 1 to 2 hours.
Stage 2	May feel out of control, helpless, panicky, or may be happy that she can take a more active role in pushing	Assist woman in pushing efforts. Encourage woman to assume position of comfort. Provide encouragement and praise for efforts. Keep couple informed of progress. Provide ice chips. Maintain privacy as woman desires.

desires a less active role, it is becoming more common for women to employ a paid caregiver who has experience in caring for laboring women. The caregiver, often called a **doula**, has typically received special training and may even be certified. The doula's role is to enhance the laboring woman's comfort and decrease her anxiety. A doula can be a valuable advocate to the laboring woman and her family, as well as an asset to the labor nurse. For example, the doula might support the woman by helping to identify the beginning of each contraction and encouraging her as she breathes through it. A constant presence offering continued encouragement and support with each contraction throughout labor has immeasurable benefits.

Table 19–4 summarizes labor progress, possible responses of the laboring woman, and support measures.

Nursing Care During the Second Stage of Labor

Nursing care during the second stage focuses on providing care, promoting comfort, and assisting during the birth.

Provision of Care in the Second Stage

The second stage is reached when the cervix is completely dilated (10 cm [3.9 in.]). The uterine contractions continue as in the transition phase. Maternal pulse is assessed at the onset of the second stage. The blood pressure is assessed every 30 minutes, but may be done more frequently if fetal decelerations or bradycardia occur. The FHR is assessed every 15 minutes in low-risk women and every 5 minutes in women with high-risk complications (ACOG, 2005). Once the second stage is reached, the nurse remains with the woman continually and does not generally leave the room.

As the woman pushes during the second stage, she may make a variety of sounds. A low-pitched, grunting sound ("uhhh") usually indicates that the woman is working with the pushing. The nurse who feels comfortable with maternal sounds and stays sensitive to changes in the sounds may be able to detect if the woman is losing her ability to cope. For instance, if the woman feels afraid of the sensations produced by her pushing effort, her sound may change to a high-pitched cry or whimper.

MyNursingKit | Video: Labor 2nd Stage—Part 1

It is not uncommon for the woman to be afraid to push. In these situations, the woman may talk or cry out during the contraction instead of actively pushing. During this time, the nurse should provide support, reassurance, and clear directions for the woman to follow. Often it is helpful to direct the woman to concentrate on a single voice, listen for suggestions, and let her body do the work. Many women find this type of interaction comforting as it allows them to focus on one person.

TEACHING TIP

When teaching the woman the effective technique for pushing, instruct her to bear down and push into her bottom as if she is having a bowel movement. Watch the woman's perineum and rectum while she is pushing and give verbal praise and encouragement when change in the perineum or rectum is seen, indicating she is successfully pushing.

During the second stage, the woman may feel intense rectal pressure. The instinctive response is to resist and to tighten muscles rather than bear down (push). A sensation of splitting apart or burning also occurs in the latter part of the second stage when the woman is pushing. The woman who expects these sensations and understands that bearing down contributes to progress at this stage is more likely to do so.

When the urge to bear down becomes uncontrollable and pushing begins, the nurse can help by encouraging her and by supporting her efforts (Figure 19–4 ■). Birthing positions are discussed shortly.

Most women push spontaneously and effectively in response to messages from their body. This more natural approach that lets the mother wait to bear down until she feels an urge to push may shorten the pushing phase, reducing the incidence of physiological stress in the mother and acidosis in the newborn. This technique decreases the incidence of instrument births and damage to maternal perineal tissue (Gennaro et al., 2007; Roberts, Gonzalez, & Sampselle, 2007). In some settings, however, sustained, forceful pushing is still advocated. In that case, when the contraction begins, the nurse tells the woman to take a cleansing breath or two, then to take a third large breath and hold it while pushing down with her abdominal muscles (called the *Valsalva maneuver*).

EVIDENCE-BASED PRACTICE

Passive Descent versus Active Pushing

Clinical Question
Which method of pushing—passive descent or active pushing as soon as full cervical dilation is achieved—provides the most benefit for mothers with epidural anesthesia?

The Evidence
Epidural analgesia is a common method of pain management during active labor, but one of the negative effects is that it often decreases the mother's sensation of the urge to push. Women have traditionally been directed to push immediately at 10-cm cervical dilatation, but there exists little evidence for the efficacy of this practice. The second stage of labor includes a period of time in which the fetus descends, and the literature refers to this as "passive descent." Passive descent allows the woman to delay pushing until she feels the urge to push or until the head is visible. A meta-analysis published by the professional association for obstetrical nurses (AWOHNN) and a large, multisite randomized trial provides evidence from eight studies that included more than 2800 women. These studies were all randomized controlled trials, and so this systematic review of multiple experiments represents the strongest level of evidence for practice.

What Is Effective?
Passive descent increases the chance that a mother will have a spontaneous vaginal birth, decreases the risk of having instrument-assisted birth procedures, and reduces the amount of time women need to push before the baby is born. Concerns about lengthening the second stage of labor appear unwarranted, as these studies found that it is the length of time pushing—not the length of the second stage—that is associated with complications. There was no difference between passive descent and active pushing in the rate of cesarean birth, perineal lacerations, or episiotomy. Women who were directed to push actively had increased rates of fetal oxygen desaturation during the second stage, and so the baby may have fewer complications with passive descent. Thus, delayed pushing is more supportive of favorable fetal well-being than active pushing.

What Is Inconclusive?
The actual method of coaching mothers was not consistent among studies, and so you cannot specify to the mother the best way to push when she has the urge. These studies allowed only 2 hours for passive descent to occur, so it is unknown whether these superior outcomes are achieved when more than 2 hours are allowed to pass before pushing.

Best Practice
Passive descent appears to be superior to active pushing in women with epidural anesthesia with respect to improving the chance of a spontaneous vaginal birth and reducing birth-related procedures. You can reassure mothers that passive descent is better for the fetus as well, even if the second stage of labor seems longer.

References
Brancato, R., Church, S., & Stone, P. (2008). A meta-analysis of passive descent versus immediate pushing in nulliparous women with epidural analgesia in the second stage of labor. *JOGNN: The Journal of Obstetrical, Gynecological, and Neonatal Nursing, 37*(1), 4–12.

Simpson, K., & James, D. (2005). Effects of immediate versus delayed pushing during second-stage labor on fetal well-being: A randomized clinical trial. *Nursing Research, 54*(3), 149–157.

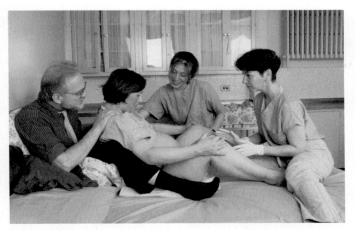

FIGURE 19–4 The nurse provides encouragement and support during pushing efforts.
Source: Margaret Miller/Photo Researchers, Inc.

A nullipara is usually prepared for birth when perineal bulging is noted. A multipara usually progresses much more quickly, so she may be prepared for the birth when the cervix is dilated 7 to 8 cm. As the birth approaches, the woman's partner or support person also prepares for the birth. (See Key Facts to Remember: Indications of Imminent Birth.)

The woman's blood pressure and the FHR are monitored between contractions, and the contractions are palpated at least every 5 minutes until the birth (Table 19–5). The nurse continually assesses the woman's level of pain or her ability to cope with the discomfort of labor. The nurse continues to assist the woman in her pushing efforts, to keep both the woman and the coach informed of procedures and progress, and to support them both throughout the birth.

Promotion of Comfort in the Second Stage

Most of the comfort measures that have been used during the first stage remain appropriate at this time. Applying cool cloths to the face and forehead may help cool the woman involved in the intense physical exertion of pushing. The woman may feel hot and want to remove some of her clothing or bed linens. Care still needs to be taken to provide privacy even though covers are removed. The woman can be encouraged to rest and relax all muscles during the periods between contractions. The nurse and support person(s) can

TABLE 19–5	Nursing Assessments in the Second Stage	
Mother	**Fetus**
Blood pressure, pulse, respirations every 5 to 15 minutes.	FHR every 15 minutes for low-risk women and every 5 minutes for high-risk women.
Uterine contractions palpated continuously.	

KEY FACTS TO REMEMBER

Indications of Imminent Birth

Birth is imminent if the woman shows the following changes:
- Bulging of the perineum
- Uncontrollable urge to bear down
- Increased bloody show

---

assist the woman into a pushing position with each contraction to further conserve energy. Between contractions, the woman should be assisted into a comfortable position. Sips of fluids or ice chips may be used to provide moisture and relieve dryness of the mouth. Positive reinforcement and encouragement should be continually provided.

Assisting During Birth

In addition to assisting the woman and her partner, the nurse also assists the physician/CNM in preparing for the birth. The physician/CNM dons a sterile gown and gloves and may place sterile drapes over the woman's abdomen and legs. An episiotomy may be performed just before the actual birth. (See the discussion of episiotomy in Chapter 23 ∞.)

Shortly before the birth, the birthing room or delivery room is prepared with the equipment and materials that may be needed. These materials typically come in a prepackaged kit and contain the instruments and disposable drapes, gowns, and containers that will be used during the birth. The nurse ensures that all supplies and a pair of sterile gloves are placed on the instrument table. This table can be prepared before the birth and covered with a sterile drape. Family members do not need to change into other clothing if the birth occurs in a birthing room; they don a disposable scrub suit or scrubs provided by the facility if the birth is to occur in a delivery room or surgery suite. Thorough handwashing is required of the nurses and physician/CNM. Nurses who will be in direct contact with the mother at the time of birth need to wear protective clothing such as an apron or gown with a splash apron, disposable gloves, and eye covering. The physician/CNM also needs to wear a plastic apron or a gown with a splash apron, eye covering, and sterile gloves.

HINTS FOR PRACTICE

Some physicians/CNMs may routinely use other equipment or supplies during the birth. Examples of equipment include mineral oil, warm water, and clean washcloths for perineal massage. Gathering these supplies early can save time and enable the nurse to stay with the woman during pushing.

If for any reason the laboring woman is to give birth in a location other than the birthing room (such as in the case of a cesarean birth), she is moved on her bed or a cart shortly before birth. It is important that the woman move from one bed to another *between contractions*. During the contraction, the woman feels increased discomfort and may be involved in pushing efforts. Perineal bulging may be occurring, which adds to the discomfort and difficulty in moving. Care should be taken to preserve her privacy during the transfer, and safety must be provided by raising the side rails. The bed itself should be placed in a locked position. The labor bed or transfer cart must be carefully braced against the delivery table to ensure the woman's safety during the transfer.

Even though there are differences in the delivery room setting, the family can still be together during the birth. It is important to provide encouragement for family members to participate, because the delivery room environment may be unfamiliar and seem intimidating. The family member may hesitate to continue providing support because of fear of interfering or being in the way. The nurse provides clear simple directions that help the support person participate throughout the birth process. The nurse can ensure the support person is sitting as close as possible to the woman. The nurse can also encourage hand holding and touching or stroking of the woman's face.

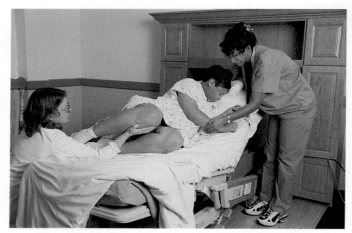

Maternal Birthing Positions

The upright posture for birth was considered normal in most societies until modern times. Women variously selected squatting, kneeling, standing, and sitting positions for birth (Figure 19–5 ■). During the mid-twentieth century, the recumbent position (lithotomy) became common in North American hospitals because of the convenience it offered in applying new technology. In recent years, however, consumers and healthcare professionals have begun searching for alternative positions, refocusing on the comfort of the laboring woman rather than on the convenience of the physician/CNM (Table 19–6). Evidence-based practice research has shown that the squatting position results in fewer instrumental deliveries, fewer episiotomy extensions, and less perineal tears than lithotomic positions (Nasir, Korejo, & Noorani, 2007). An upright position, which has been found to be the most effective birthing position, is possible even for women who have epidural anesthesia (Gennaro et al., 2007).

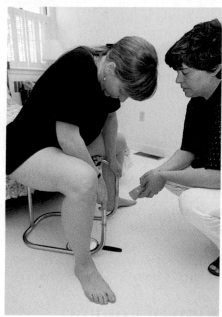

The woman may be positioned for birth on a bed with use of leg supports, in a squatting position, or perhaps on her hands and knees. If a birthing bed is used, the back is elevated 30 to 60 degrees to help the woman bear down. Stirrups, if needed and used, are padded to alleviate pressure. If assisting the woman to place her legs in the stirrups, both legs should be lifted simultaneously to avoid strain on abdominal, back, and perineal muscles. Stirrups are sometimes needed if the woman is unable to control her legs following epidural anesthesia, if forceps or a vacuum extractor is being used, or if a difficult birth is anticipated. The stirrups should be adjusted to fit the woman's

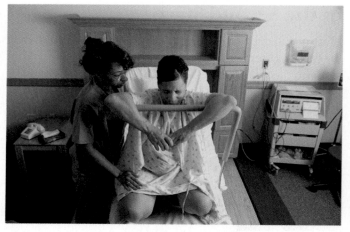

FIGURE 19–5 Birthing positions. *A,* Side-lying (also known as left lateral Sims') position. *B,* Using a birthing stool. *C,* Using a birthing bar.
Source: B © Stella Johnson (www.stellajohnson.com).

legs. The feet are supported in the stirrup holders. The height and angle of the stirrups are adjusted so there is no pressure on the back of the knees or the calves, which

TABLE 19–6	Comparison of Birthing Positions		
Position	**Advantages**	**Disadvantages**	**Nursing Actions**
Recumbent	Enhances ability to maintain sterile field. May be easier to monitor FHR. Easier to perform episiotomy or laceration repair.	May decrease blood pressure. It is difficult for the woman to breathe because of pressure on the diaphragm. There is an increased risk of aspiration. May increase perineal pressure making laceration more likely. May interfere with uterine contractions.	Ensure that stirrups do not cause excess pressure on the legs. Assess legs for adequate circulation and support.
Left lateral Sims'	Does not compromise venous return from lower extremities. Increases perineal relaxation and decreases need for episiotomy. Appears to prevent rapid descent.	It is difficult for the woman to see the birth.	Adjust position so that the upper leg lies on the bed (scissor fashion) or is supported by the partner or on pillows.
Squatting	Size of pelvic outlet is increased. Gravity aids descent and expulsion of newborn. Second stage may be shortened.	It may be difficult to maintain balance while squatting.	Help woman maintain balance. Use a birthing bar if available.
Semi-Fowler's	Does not compromise venous return from lower extremities. Woman can view birth process.	If legs are positioned wide apart, relaxation of perineal tissues is decreased.	Assess that upper torso is evenly supported. Increase support of body by changing position of bed or using pillows as props.
Sitting in birthing bed	Gravity aids descent and expulsion of the fetus. Does not compromise venous return from lower extremities. Woman can view the birth process. Leg position may be changed at will.		Ensure that legs and feet have adequate support.
Sitting on birthing stool	Gravity aids descent and expulsion of infant. Does not compromise venous return from lower extremities. Woman can view birth process.	It is difficult to provide support for the woman's back.	Encourage woman to sit in a position that increases her comfort.
Hands and knees	Increases perineal relaxation and decreases need for episiotomy. Increases placental and umbilical blood flow and decreases fetal distress. Improves fetal rotation. Better able to assess perineum. Better access to fetal nose and mouth for suctioning at birth. Facilitates birth of infant with shoulder dystocia.	Woman cannot view birth. There is decreased contact with birth attendant. Caregivers cannot use instruments. There may be increased maternal fatigue.	Adjust birthing bed by dropping the foot down. Supply extra pillows for increased support.

might cause discomfort and postpartal vascular problems. Some practitioners may opt to leave the bed assembled and instead lower the foot of the bed into a lower position. Many times, women are more comfortable with this position. When stirrups are not used for the birth, the woman's legs may be placed in stirrups after the birth if a repair of the perineum is needed.

Cleansing the Perineum

After the woman has been positioned for the birth, her vulvar and perineal area are cleansed to increase her com-

fort, to remove the bloody discharge that is present before the actual birth, and to prevent infection. Perineal cleansing methods range from use of warm soapy water to aseptic technique depending on the agency protocol or on physician/CNM orders. Once the cleansing is completed, the woman returns to the desired birthing position.

Supporting the Couple

Both the woman's partner and the nurse who has been with the woman during the labor continue to provide support during contractions. The woman is encouraged to

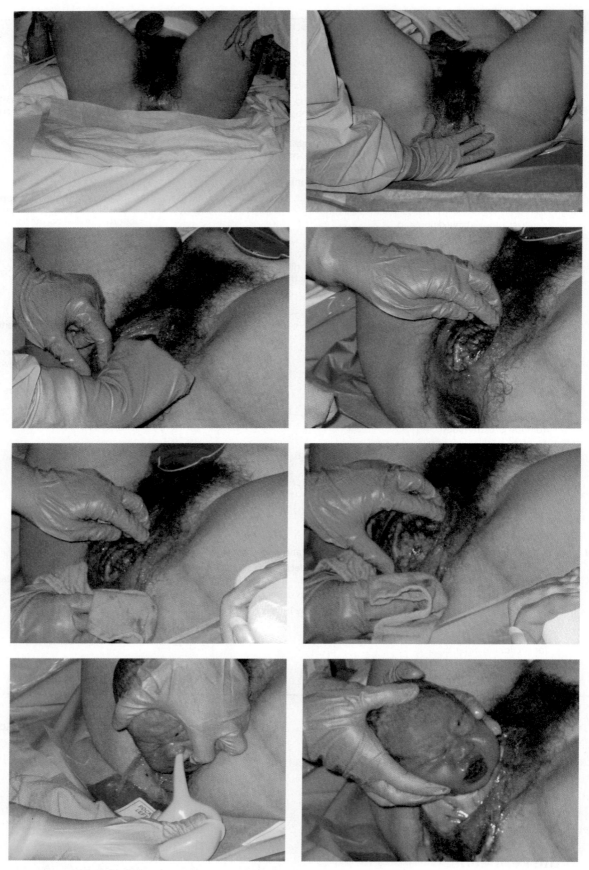

FIGURE 19–6 A birthing sequence.

push with each contraction and, as the fetal head emerges, is asked to take shallow breaths or to pant to prevent pushing. The physician/CNM may instruct her to "push and breathe, push and breathe" in an effort to ease the fetal head out to prevent perineal trauma and tearing. While supporting the head, the physician/CNM assesses whether the umbilical cord is around the fetal neck and removes it if it is, then suctions the mouth and nose with a bulb syringe. The mouth is suctioned first to prevent reflex inhalation of mucus when the sensitive nares are touched with the bulb syringe tip. The woman is encouraged to push again as the rest of the newborn's body is born. Figure 19–6 ■ depicts an entire birthing experience.

Nursing Care During the Third and Fourth Stages of Labor

Nursing care during the third and fourth stages focuses on initial care of the newborn, enhancing attachment, assisting with placenta delivery, and providing care for the mother.

Initial Care of the Newborn

The physician/CNM places the newborn on the mother's abdomen or under the radiant-heated unit. Placing the newborn on the maternal abdomen promotes attachment and bonding and gives the mother the opportunity to immediately interact with her baby. Placing the baby on the mother's chest also promotes early breastfeeding opportunities. Even though the baby may not breastfeed immediately, placement on the mother's chest enables the baby to smell, touch, and lick the mother's nipples. The newborn is maintained in a modified Trendelenburg position which aids drainage of mucus from the nasopharynx and trachea by gravity. The newborn is dried immediately and wet blankets are removed. The nurse helps maintain infant warmth by placing warmed blankets over the newborn or by placing the newborn in skin-to-skin contact with the mother. If the newborn is under a radiant-heated unit, he or she is dried, placed on a dry blanket, and left uncovered under the radiant heat. Because radiant heat warms the outer surface of objects, a newborn wrapped in blankets will receive no benefit from radiant heat.

The newborn's nose and mouth are suctioned with a bulb syringe as needed. Most immediate care of the newborn can be accomplished while the newborn is in the parent's arms or under the radiant-heated unit. Many women request that their infant be left on their abdomen or chest while initial care is given. Unless a medical complication exists, the nurse should complete assessments in this position because it promotes parental attachment.

Apgar Scoring System

The Apgar scoring system (Table 19–7) is used to evaluate the physical condition of the newborn at birth. The newborn is rated 1 minute after birth and again at 5 minutes and receives a total score (**Apgar score**) ranging from 0 to 10 based on the following assessments. If the Apgar score is less than 7 at 5 minutes, the scoring should be repeated every 5 minutes up to 20 minutes (ACOG, 2006a).

1. *Heart rate* is auscultated or palpated at the junction of the umbilical cord and skin. This is the most important assessment. A newborn heart rate of less than 100 beats per minute indicates the need for immediate resuscitation.
2. *Respiratory effort* is the second most important Apgar assessment. Complete absence of respirations is termed apnea. A vigorous cry indicates adequate respirations.
3. *Muscle tone* is determined by evaluating the degree of flexion and resistance to straightening of the extremities. A normal newborn's elbows and hips are flexed, with the knees positioned up toward the abdomen.
4. *Reflex irritability* is evaluated by stroking the baby's back along the spine or by flicking the soles of the feet. A cry merits a full score of 2. A grimace is 1 point, and no response is 0.
5. *Skin color* is inspected for cyanosis and pallor. Generally, newborns have blue extremities, with a pink body, which merits a score of 1. This condition is termed *acrocyanosis* and is present in 85% of normal newborns at 1 minute after birth. A completely pink newborn scores a 2, and a totally cyanotic, pale infant scores 0. Newborns with darker skin pigmentation will not be pink in color. Their skin color is assessed for pallor and acrocyanosis, and a score is selected based on the assessment.

TABLE 19–7 The Apgar Scoring System			
	Score		
Sign	**0**	**1**	**2**
Heart rate	Absent	Slow—below 100	Above 100
Respiratory effort	Absent	Slow—irregular	Good crying
Muscle tone	Flaccid	Some flexion of extremities	Active motion
Reflex irritability	None	Grimace	Vigorous cry
Color	Pale blue	Body pink, blue extremities	Completely pink

Source: Apgar, V. (1966, August). The newborn (Apgar) scoring system, reflections and advice. *Pediatric Clinics of North America, 13,* 645.

A score of 7 to 10 indicates a newborn in good condition who requires only nasopharyngeal suctioning and perhaps some oxygen near the face (called "blow-by" oxygen). If the Apgar score is below 7, resuscitative measures may need to be instituted. (See the discussion in Chapter 28 ∞.) Apgar scores of less than 3 at 5 minutes post-birth may correlate with neonatal mortality (ACOG, 2006a).

Assisting with Clamping the Cord

If the physician/CNM has not placed some type of cord clamp on the newborn's umbilical cord, the nurse must do so. Before applying the cord clamp, the nurse examines the cut end of the cord for the presence of two arteries and one vein. The umbilical vein is the largest vessel, and the arteries are seen as smaller vessels. The number of vessels is recorded on the birth and newborn records. The cord is clamped approximately ½ to 1 in. from the abdomen to allow room between the abdomen and clamp as the cord dries. Abdominal skin must not be clamped, because this will cause necrosis of the tissue. The most common type of cord clamp is the plastic Hollister cord clamp (Figure 19–7 ■). The Hollister clamp is removed in the newborn nursery approximately 24 hours after the cord has dried.

In recent years, the timing of umbilical cord clamping has been the focus of discussion and research. In one study of preterm infants (equal to and less than 32 gestational weeks), infants in the group with delayed cord clamping had fewer intraventricular hemorrhages and less late-onset sepsis. Evidence-based practice therefore suggests that delayed clamping in premature infants may yield more benefits than immediate cord clamping (Mercer, Vohr, McGrath et al., 2006). In full-term infants, delayed cord clamping can result in polycythemia; however, this appears to be benign.

These infants were more likely to have improved hematocrit, ferritin, and iron levels resulting in a reduction in anemia (Hutton & Hassan, 2007). Early cord clamping was previously advocated for as a preventive treatment for postpartum hemorrhage, but it has also been associated with an increase in alloimmunization. Based on these findings, delayed cord clamping is now the treatment of choice (Levy & Blickstein, 2006).

Cord Blood Collection for Banking

A growing number of parents are arranging for cord blood banking (see discussion in Chapter 1 ∞). Immediately after the newborn's umbilical cord is clamped and cut, the CNM or physician withdraws blood from the remaining umbilical cord by inserting a large gauge needle into the umbilical vein. The needle allows the blood to be collected into a special container that parents receive from the Cord Blood Registry and bring with them for the birth. The nurse labels the specimen immediately and follows the directions required for storage and pickup. The collected cord blood can then be used to treat childhood cancers, rare genetic disorders, and cerebral palsy. The main drawback of cord blood banking remains the cost. Although cord blood can be donated, much like blood donations at some hospital facilities, most hospitals do not have these services available.

Newborn Physical Assessment by the Nurse

The nurse performs an abbreviated systematic physical assessment in the birthing area to detect any abnormalities (Table 19–8). First, the nurse notes the size of the newborn and the contour and size of the head in relationship to the rest of the body. The newborn's posture and movements indicate tone and neurologic functioning.

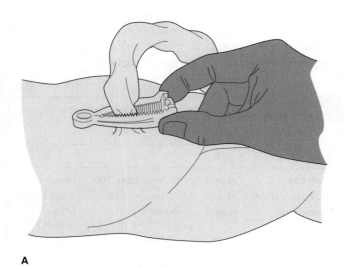

A

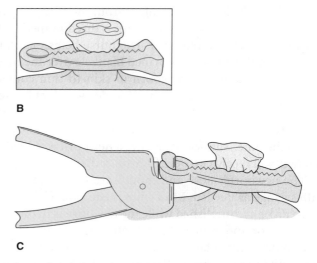

B

C

FIGURE 19–7 Hollister cord clamp. A, Clamp is positioned $^{1}/_{2}$ to 1 in. from the abdomen and then secured. B, Cut cord. The one vein and two arteries can be seen. C, Plastic device for removing clamp after the cord has dried. After the cord is cut, the nurse grasps the Hollister clamp on either side of the cut area and gently separates it.

TABLE 19–8	Initial Newborn Evaluation
Assess	Normal Findings
Respirations	Rate 30 to 60, irregular
	No retractions, no grunting
Apical pulse	Rate 110 to 160 and somewhat irregular
Temperature	Skin temp above 36.5°C (97.8°F)
Skin color	Body pink with bluish extremities
Umbilical cord	Two arteries and one vein
Gestational age	Should be 38 to 42 weeks to remain with parents for extended time
Sole creases	Sole creases that involve the heel

In general, expect scant amount of vernix on upper back, axilla, groin; lanugo only on upper back; ears with incurving of upper ⅔ of pinnae and thin cartilage that springs back from folding; male genitals—testes palpated in upper or lower scrotum; female genitals—labia majora larger; clitoris nearly covered.

In the following situations, newborns should generally be stabilized rather than remaining with parents in the birth area for an extended period of time:

- Apgar less than 8 at 1 minute and less than 9 at 5 minutes or baby requires resuscitation measures (other than whiffs of oxygen)
- Respirations below 30 or above 60, with retractions and/or grunting
- Apical pulse below 110 or above 160 with marked irregularities
- Skin temperature below 36.5°C (97.8°F)
- Skin color pale blue or circumoral pallor
- Baby less than 38 weeks' or more than 42 weeks' gestation
- Baby very small or very large for gestational age
- Congenital anomalies involving open areas in the skin (meningomyelocele)

The nurse inspects the skin for discoloration, presence of vernix caseosa and lanugo, and evidence of trauma and desquamation (peeling of skin). Vernix caseosa is a white, cheesy substance found normally on newborns. It is absorbed within 24 hours after birth. Vernix is abundant on preterm infants and absent on postterm newborns. A large quantity of fine hair (lanugo) is often seen on preterm newborns, especially on the shoulders, foreheads, backs, and cheeks. Desquamation of the skin is seen in postterm newborns.

The nurse observes the nares for flaring and, as the newborn cries, inspects the palate for cleft palate. The nurse looks for mucus in the nose and mouth and removes it with a bulb syringe as needed. The nurse inspects the chest for respiratory rate and the presence of retractions. If retractions are present, the nurse assesses the newborn for grunting or stridor. A normal respiratory rate is 30 to 60 per minute. The nurse auscultates the lungs bilaterally for breath sounds. Absence of breath sounds on one side could indicate a pneumothorax. Rales may be heard immediately after birth because a small amount of fluid may remain in the lungs; this fluid will be absorbed. Rhonchi indicate aspiration of oral secretions. If there is excessive mucus or respiratory distress, the nurse suctions the newborn with a

mucus trap. (See Clinical Skill: Performing Nasal Pharyngeal Suctioning.) The nurse notes and records elimination of urine or meconium on the newborn record.

Newborn Identification and Security Measures

Identification bands typically come in a set of four, all preprinted with identical numbers. The nurse places two bands on the newborn—one on the wrist and one on the ankle. The newborn bands must fit snugly to prevent their loss. The nurse then gives the mother and partner each a band. The band number is recorded in both the maternal and infant chart. The bands allow access to the infant care areas and must not be removed until the infant is discharged. In most facilities, as a security measure, only individuals with a band are given unlimited access to the newborn. Some facilities also include an umbilical clamp with a preprinted number identical to the number printed on the bands.

Although some institutions rely on an umbilical band system to ensure the safety of newborns, others attach an alarm to the band (Figure 19–8 ■). The alarm is triggered if the device is tampered with or if the infant is removed from the parameters of the security field.

Additional hospital security measures are now commonplace in maternity settings. This includes mandating that all staff wear appropriate identification at all times. Parents are instructed that individuals without appropriate identification should not be allowed to remove their infant under any circumstances. The nurse also advises the parents to place the infant on the side of the bed away from the window, and to have the baby return to the nursery whenever the mother naps or showers and no other family member is present.

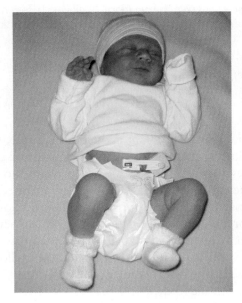

FIGURE 19–8 Umbilical alarm in place on a newborn infant.

Clinical Skill Performing Nasal Pharyngeal Suctioning

NURSING ACTION	RATIONALE

Preparation

1. Suction equipment is always available in the birthing area to clear secretions from the newborn's nose or oropharynx if respirations are depressed or if amniotic fluid was meconium stained.

2. Tighten the lid on the DeLee mucus trap or other suction device collection bottle.

This avoids spillage of secretions and prevents air from leaking out of the lid.

3. Connect one end of the DeLee tubing to low suction.

Equipment and Supplies

- DeLee mucus trap or other suction device

Procedure

1. Don gloves.

2. Without applying suction, insert the free end of the DeLee tubing 3 to 5 in. into the newborn's nose or mouth (Figure 19–9 ■).

Applying suction while passing the tube would interfere with smooth passage of the tube.

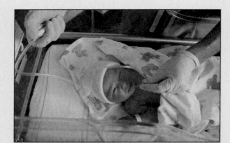

FIGURE 19–9 DeLee mucous trap being used to suction a newborn's mouth to remove excess secretions.

3. Place your thumb over the suction control and begin to apply suction. Continue to suction as you slowly remove the tube, rotating it slightly.

Suctioning during withdrawal removes fluid and avoids redepositing secretions in the newborn's nasopharynx.

4. Continue to reinsert the tube and provide suction for as long as fluid is aspirated.

Excessive suctioning can cause vagal stimulation, which decreases the heart rate.

5. If it is necessary to pass the tube into the newborn's stomach to remove meconium secretions that the newborn swallowed before birth, insert the tube through the newborn's mouth into the stomach. Apply suction and continue to suction as you withdraw the tube.

Because the newborn's nares are small and delicate, it is easier and faster to pass the suction tube through the mouth.

6. Document the completion of the procedure and the amount and type of secretions.

This documentation provides a record of the intervention and the status of the infant at birth.

Although hospital infant abductions are rare, they are catastrophic in nature to the family, hospital, and community. Many abductors pose as medical personnel to gain access to the mother and infant. Women should be advised to ask all hospital personnel for proper identification. If the mother or family feels unsure of the individual, they should immediately call on the call bell to alert the nurse and ask for other verification. If a woman is reluctant to allow a student nurse to transport her infant, the staff nurse should be asked to assist the student.

Delivery of the Placenta

After birth, the physician/CNM prepares for the delivery of the placenta (see Chapter 17 ∞). The following signs suggest placental separation:

1. The uterus rises upward in the abdomen.
2. As the placenta moves downward, the umbilical cord lengthens.
3. A sudden trickle or spurt of blood appears.
4. The shape of the uterus changes from a disk to a globe.

Drug Guide Carboprost Tromethamine (Hemabate)

Overview of Action Carboprost tromethamine (Hemabate) is used to reduce blood loss secondary to uterine atony. It stimulates myometrial contractions to control postpartum hemorrhaging that is unresponsive to usual techniques. Carboprost tromethamine can also be used to induce labor in women desiring an elective termination of a pregnancy. The drug is also used to induce labor in cases of intrauterine fetal death and hydatidiform mole (Wilson, Shannon, & Shields, 2009).

Pregnancy Risk Category: D

Route, Dosage, Frequency In cases of immediate postpartum hemorrhage the usual intramuscular dose is 250 mcg (1 mL) which can be repeated every 1½ to 3½ hours if uterine atony persists. The dosage can be increased to 500 mcg (2 mL) if uterine contractility is inadequate after several doses of 250 mcg. The total dosage should not exceed 12 mg. The maximum duration of use is 48 hours (Wilson et al., 2009).

Contraindications The drug is contraindicated in women with active cardiac, pulmonary, or renal disease. It should not be administered during pregnancy or in women with acute pelvic inflammatory disease. It should be used with caution in women with asthma, adrenal disease, hypotension, hypertension, diabetes mellitus, epilepsy, fibroids, cervical stenosis, or previous uterine surgery (Wilson et al., 2009).

Side Effects The most common side effects are nausea and diarrhea. Fever, chills, and flushing can occur. Headache, muscle, joint, abdominal, or eye pain can also occur (Wilson et al., 2009).

Nursing Considerations

- The injection should be given in a large muscle. Aspiration should be performed to avoid injection into a blood vessel which can result in bronchospasm, tetanic contractions, and shock.
- After administration, monitor uterine status and bleeding carefully.
- Report excess bleeding to the physician/CNM.
- Check vital signs routinely, observing for an increase in temperature, elevated pulse, and decreased blood pressure.
- Breastfeeding should be delayed for 24 hours after administration (Wilson et al., 2009).

While waiting for these signs, the nurse palpates the uterus to check for bogginess and fullness caused by uterine relaxation and subsequent bleeding into the uterine cavity. After the placenta has separated, the woman may be asked to bear down to aid delivery of the placenta.

Oxytocics are frequently given at the time of the delivery of the placenta, so the uterus will contract and bleeding will be minimized. Oxytocin (Pitocin), 10 to 20 units, may be added to an intravenous (IV) infusion or 10 units may be given intramuscularly. In the presence of hemorrhage caused by uterine atony, some physicians/ CNMs may order up to 40 units to a liter of intravenous fluid, methylergonovine maleate (Methergine), 0.2 mg, administered intramuscularly, or carboprost tromethamine (Hemabate), 250 mcg/mL, administered intramuscularly. Cytotec has been commonly used when other pharmacologic interventions have failed. Cytotec is administered rectally in dosages of 800 to 1000 mcg (ACOG, 2006b; Bradley, Prata, Young-Lin et al., 2007). In addition to administering the ordered medications, the nurse assesses and records maternal blood pressure before and after administration of oxytocics and assesses the amount of bleeding. For further information, refer to the Drug Guide: Oxytocin (in Chapter 23 ∞), the Drug Guide: Methylergonovine Maleate (in Chapter 31 ∞), and the Drug Guide: Carboprost Tromethamine in this chapter.

After the delivery of the placenta, the physician/CNM inspects the placental membranes to make sure they are intact and that all cotyledons are present. If there is a defect or a part missing from the placenta, a manual uterine examination or *uterine exploration* is done. The nurse notes on the birth record the time of delivery of the placenta.

Enhancing Attachment

Dramatic evidence indicates that the first few hours and even minutes after birth are an important period for the attachment of mother and infant.

If contact can occur during the first hour after birth, the newborn will be in the quiet state and able to interact with parents by looking at them. Newborns also turn their heads in response to a spoken voice. (See Chapter 23 ∞ for further discussion of newborn states.) If possible and desired by the mother, the newborn should be placed on the woman's chest so she can directly see her infant. This early interaction promotes attachment, early breastfeeding, and family interaction.

The first parent-newborn contact may be brief (a few minutes), and may be followed by a more extended contact after the mother completes other uncomfortable procedures (delivery of the placenta and suturing of the episiotomy or laceration). When the newborn is returned to the mother, the nurse can assist her to begin breastfeeding if she so desires. The baby may seek out the mother's breast, and early contact between the two can

EVIDENCE IN ACTION
Infant to mother skin-to-skin care immediately following birth supports breastfeeding and bonding.
(Meta-analysis) (Moore, Anderson, & Bergman, 2007)

MyNursingKit | Video: Inspection of the Placenta ∞

greatly affect breastfeeding success. Even if the newborn does not actively nurse, he or she can lick, taste, and smell the mother's skin. This activity by the newborn stimulates the maternal release of prolactin, which promotes the onset of lactation. These early interactions are associated with greater breastfeeding success.

Darkening the birthing room by turning out most of the lights causes newborns to open their eyes and gaze around. This in turn enhances eye-to-eye contact with the parents.

(Note: If the physician/CNM needs a light source, the spotlight can be left on.) Treatment of the newborn's eyes with antibiotic eye ointment may also be delayed up to an hour after birth. Many parents who establish eye contact with the newborn are content to quietly gaze at their infant. Others may show more active involvement by touching or inspecting the newborn. Some mothers talk to their babies in a high-pitched voice, which seems to be soothing to newborns. Some couples verbally express amazement and pride when they see they have produced a beautiful, healthy baby. Their verbalization enhances feelings of accomplishment and ecstasy.

Both parents need to be encouraged to do whatever they feel most comfortable doing. Some parents prefer only limited contact with the newborn immediately after birth and instead desire private time together in a quiet environment. In spite of the current zeal for providing immediate attachment opportunities, nursing personnel need to be aware of parents' wishes. The desire to delay interaction with the newborn does not necessarily imply a decreased ability of the parents to bond with their newborn. (See Chapter 28 ∞ for further discussion of parent-infant attachment.)

Provision of Care in the Fourth Stage

The physician/CNM inspects the vagina, cervix, and perineum for lacerations and makes any necessary repairs. The episiotomy may be repaired now if it has not been done previously (see Chapter 23 ∞).

The nurse assesses the uterus for firmness by palpating the fundus. The normal position is at the midline and below the umbilicus. A displaced fundus may be caused by a full bladder or blood collected in the uterus. The clots or blood accumulation in the uterus may be expelled by grasping it with one hand anteriorly and posteriorly and squeezing. The nurse continues to palpate the uterine fundus at frequent intervals for at least 4 hours to ensure that it remains firmly contracted (Figure 19–10 ■). It is palpated but not massaged unless it is soft (boggy). If it becomes boggy or appears to rise in the abdomen, the fundus is massaged until firm; then the nurse exerts firm pressure on the fundus in an attempt to express retained clots. During all aspects of fundal massage, the nurse uses one hand to provide support for the lower portion of the uterus and

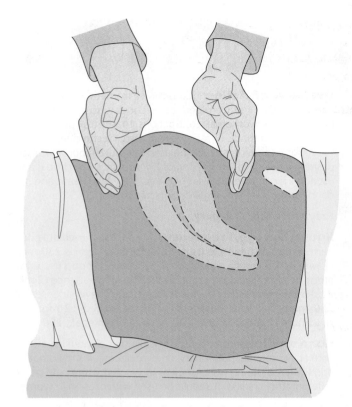

FIGURE 19–10 Suggested method of palpating the fundus of the uterus during the fourth stage. The left hand is placed just above the symphysis pubis, and gentle downward pressure is exerted. The right hand is cupped around the uterine fundus.

prevent damage to the round ligaments. The uterus is very tender at this time; all palpation and massage should be done as gently as possible.

The nurse washes the woman's perineum with gauze squares and warmed solution and dries the area well with a towel before placing the sanitary pad. Many times, an ice pack is also placed against the perineum to promote comfort and decrease swelling. If stirrups have been used, the woman's legs are removed from the stirrups at the same time to avoid muscle strain. The woman is encouraged to move her legs gently up and down in a bicycle motion. The woman remains in the same bed or is transferred to a recovery room bed, and the nurse helps her don a clean gown. Soiled linens are removed and the woman is typically offered something to drink.

During the recovery period (1 to 4 hours) the woman is monitored closely. Frequent checking for deviations from normal in vital signs is required. The maternal blood pressure is monitored at 5- to 15-minute intervals to detect any changes. Blood pressure should return to the prelabor level because an increased volume of blood is returning to the maternal circulation from the uteroplacental shunt. Pulse rate should be slightly lower than it was during labor. Baroreceptors cause a vagal response, which slows the pulse. A rise in blood pressure may be a response to oxytocic drugs or may be caused by preeclampsia. Blood loss may be reflected by a lowered blood pressure and a rising pulse rate (Table 19–9).

TABLE 19–9	Maternal Adaptations Following Birth
Characteristic	**Normal Finding**
Blood pressure	Returns to prelabor level
Pulse	Slightly lower than in labor
Uterine fundus	In the midline at the umbilicus or 1 to 2 finger breadths below the umbilicus
Lochia	Red (rubra), small to moderate amount (from spotting on pads to ¼ to ½ of pad covered in 15 minutes) Doesn't exceed saturation of one pad in first hour
Bladder	Nonpalpable
Perineum	Smooth, pink, without bruising or edema
Emotional state	Wide variation, including excited, exhilarated, smiling, crying, fatigued, verbal, quiet, pensive, and sleepy

The nurse also monitors the woman's temperature. Frequently women have tremors or uncontrollable shaking in the immediate postpartum period that may be caused by a difference in internal and external body temperatures (higher temperature inside the body than outside). Another theory is that the woman is reacting to the fetal cells that have entered the maternal circulation at the placental site. A heated blanket may be placed next to the woman's skin to alleviate the problem and can be replaced as often as the mother desires.

The woman's pain level should also be assessed. If the woman is experiencing any type of discomfort, pain medications can be administered as ordered. The nurse can also assist the woman with comfort measures, such as position changes, frequent ice pack changes, and administration of topical medications that are often ordered to reduce perineal edema and discomfort.

The nurse inspects the bloody vaginal discharge for amount and charts it as minimal, moderate, or heavy and with or without clots. This discharge, lochia rubra, should be bright red. A soaked perineal pad contains approximately 100 mL of blood. If the perineal pad becomes soaked in a 15-minute period or if blood pools under the buttocks, continuous observation is necessary. When the fundus is firm, a continuous trickle of blood may signal laceration of the vagina or cervix or an unligated vessel in the episiotomy. (See Key Facts to Remember: Immediate Postbirth Danger Signs.)

If the fundus rises and displaces to the right, the nurse must be concerned about two factors:

1. As the uterus rises, the uterine contractions become less effective and increased bleeding may occur.
2. The most common cause of uterine displacement is bladder distention.

The nurse palpates the bladder to determine whether it is distended. The bladder fills rapidly with the extra fluid volume returned from the uteroplacental circulation (and with any fluid received intravenously during labor and birth). The postpartal woman may not realize that her

KEY FACTS TO REMEMBER

Immediate Postbirth Danger Signs

In the immediate postbirth recovery period the following conditions should be reported to the physician/CNM:

- Hypotension
- Tachycardia
- Uterine atony
- Excessive bleeding
- Hematoma

bladder is full because trauma to the bladder and urethra during childbirth and the use of regional anesthesia decrease bladder tone and the urge to void.

All measures should be taken to enable the mother to void. The nurse may place a warm towel across the lower abdomen or pour warm water over the perineum to relax the urinary sphincter and facilitate voiding. The woman may also try running warm water over her hand. If the woman is unable to void, catheterization is necessary. The perineum is inspected for edema and hematoma formation.

The couple may be tired, hungry, and thirsty. Some agencies serve the couple a meal. Most women are very hungry after birth. The tired mother will probably drift off into a welcome sleep. The partner can also be encouraged to rest, because his supporting role is physically and mentally tiring. If the mother is not in a birthing room, she is usually transferred from the birthing unit to the postpartal or mother-baby area after 2 hours or more, depending on agency policy and whether the following criteria are met:

- Stable vital signs
- Stable bleeding
- Undistended bladder
- Firm fundus
- Sensations fully recovered from any anesthetic agent received during birth

For some women, the childbirth experience has been extremely painful, filled with hours of feeling powerless or out of control. In this circumstance, the woman is at higher risk for developing post-traumatic stress disorder (Ayers, Eagle, & Waring, 2006). (See Chapter 21 ∞ for further discussion.)

Support of the Adolescent During Birth

As with all women, each adolescent in labor is different. The nurse must assess what each teen brings to the experience by asking the following questions:

- Has the young woman received prenatal care?
- What are her attitudes and feelings about the pregnancy?
- Who will attend the birth and what is the person's relationship to her?

- What preparation has she had for the experience?
- What are her expectations and fears regarding labor and birth?
- How has her culture influenced her?
- What are her usual coping mechanisms?
- Does she plan to keep the newborn?

Any adolescent who has not had prenatal care requires close observation during labor. Fetal well-being is established by fetal monitoring. Adolescent women are at risk for pregnancy and labor complications and must be assessed carefully. The nurse should be especially alert for any physiologic complications of labor. The young woman's prenatal record is carefully reviewed for risks, and the adolescent is screened for preeclampsia, cephalopelvic disproportion (CPD), anemia, cigarette smoking, alcohol and drugs ingested during pregnancy, sexually transmitted infections, and size-date discrepancies.

The support role of the nurse depends on the young woman's support system during labor. The adolescent may not be accompanied by someone who will stay with her during childbirth, or she may have her mother, the father of the baby, or a close friend as her labor partner. Regardless of whether the teen has a support person, it is important for the nurse to establish a trusting relationship with her. In this way, the nurse can help the teen understand what is happening to her. Establishing a nurturing rapport is essential. Some nurses may view adolescent pregnancy as a negative event; however, it is important to treat the young woman with respect. The adolescent who is given positive reinforcement for "work well done" will leave the experience with increased self-esteem, despite the emotional problems that may accompany her situation.

If a support person accompanies the adolescent, that person also needs the nurse's encouragement and support. The nurse must explain changes in the young woman's behavior and substantiate her wishes. The nursing staff should reinforce the adolescent's feelings that she is wanted and important.

The adolescent who has taken childbirth education classes is generally better prepared for labor than the adolescent who has not. However, the nurse must keep in mind that the younger the adolescent, the less she may be able to participate actively in the process, even if she has taken prenatal classes.

The very young adolescent (age 14 and under) has fewer coping mechanisms and less experience to draw on than her older counterparts. Because her cognitive development is incomplete, the younger adolescent may have fewer problem-solving capabilities. Her ego integrity may be more threatened by the experience, and she may be more vulnerable to stress and discomfort. Thus, she needs someone to rely on at all times during labor. She may be more childlike and dependent than older teens. The nurse must be sure that

instructions and explanations are simple and concrete. During the transition phase, she may become withdrawn and unable to express her need to be nurtured. Touch, soothing encouragement, and measures to provide comfort help her maintain control and meet her needs for dependence. During the second stage of labor, the young adolescent may feel as if she is losing control and may reach out to those around her. By remaining calm and giving directions, the nurse helps her cope with feelings of helplessness.

The middle adolescent (age 15 to 17 years) often attempts to remain calm and unflinching during labor. The experienced nurse realizes that a caring attitude will still help the young woman. Many older adolescents believe that they "know it all," but they may be no more prepared for childbirth than their younger counterparts. The nurse's reinforcement and nonjudgmental manner will help them save face. If the adolescent has not taken childbirth preparation classes, she may require preparation and explanations. The older teenager's (age 18 to 19) response to the stresses of labor, however, is similar to that of the adult woman.

Adolescents, regardless of their age, need ongoing education throughout labor and in the early postpartal period (Figure 19–11 ■). Clear explanations should be provided. They should be encouraged to ask questions and seek out information.

Even if the adolescent is planning to relinquish her newborn, she should be given the option of seeing and holding the infant. She may be reluctant to do this at first, but the grieving process is facilitated if the mother sees the infant. However, seeing or holding the newborn should be the young woman's choice. (See Chapter 30 ∞ for further discussion of the relinquishing mother and the adolescent parent.)

Adolescents need individualized care for the issues that they face in the postpartum period. They may experience additional psychosocial issues unique to their age group and their developmental level. Adolescents are also at an increased risk for unintended subsequent pregnancies and abortions. Proper discharge teaching should include contraceptive options (Falk, Ostlund, Magnuson et al., 2006).

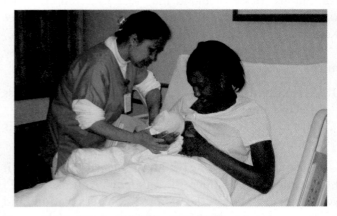

FIGURE 19–11 An adolescent mother receives breastfeeding assistance in the immediate postpartum period.

Nursing Care During Precipitous Birth

Occasionally labor progresses so rapidly that the nurse is faced with the task of managing the actual birth of the baby. A **precipitous birth** occurs when the labor and birth occur in 3 hours or less. If this happens, the attending nurse has the primary responsibility for providing a physically and psychologically safe experience for the woman and her baby. A woman whose physician/CNM is not present may feel disappointed, frightened, abandoned, angry, and cheated. She may fear what is going to happen and feel that everything is out of her control. In working with the woman, the nurse provides support by keeping her informed about the labor progress and assuring her that the nurse will stay with her. If birth is imminent, the nurse must not leave the mother alone. Auxiliary personnel can be directed to contact the physician/CNM and retrieve the emergency birth pack ("precip pack"), which should be readily accessible to birthing rooms. A typical pack contains the following items:

1. Small drape that can be placed under the woman's buttocks to provide a sterile field
2. Bulb syringe to clear mucus from the newborn's mouth
3. Two sterile clamps (Kelly or Rochester) to clamp the umbilical cord before applying a cord clamp
4. Sterile scissors to cut the umbilical cord
5. Sterile umbilical cord clamp, either Hesseltine or Hollister
6. Baby blanket to wrap the newborn in after birth
7. Package of sterile gloves

At all times during the birth, the nurse remains calm; the woman is reassured by the composure of the nurse and feels that the nurse is competent.

The nurse attends the precipitous birth as follows: The woman is encouraged to assume a comfortable position. Women who give birth in the lateral positions are less prone to perineal lacerations (Hastings-Tolsma, Vincent, Emeis et al., 2007). If time permits, the nurse scrubs his or her hands with soap and water and puts on sterile gloves. Sterile drapes may be placed under the woman's buttocks if time allows. The bed should be left in an intact position without the use of the stirrups. The nurse may place an index finger inside the lower portion of the vagina and the thumb on the outer portion of the perineum and gently massage the area to help stretch perineal tissues and prevent perineal lacerations. Warm compresses also protect against lacerations, although there may not be time to implement them (Hastings-Tolsma et al., 2007).

As the infant's head crowns, the nurse should support the perineum with her thumb on one side and four fingers on the other side providing manual support while instructing the woman to pant, which decreases her urge to push. The nurse checks whether the amniotic sac is intact. If it is, the

nurse tears the sac, usually with a Kelly clamp, so the newborn will not breathe in amniotic fluid with the first breath.

With one hand, the nurse applies gentle pressure in a downward motion against the fetal head to prevent it from popping out rapidly. The nurse does not hold the head back forcibly. Rapid birth of the head may result in tears in the woman's perineal tissues. In the fetus, the rapid change in pressure within the fetal head may cause subdural or dural tears. The nurse supports the perineum with the other hand and allows the head to be born between contractions.

As the woman continues to pant, the nurse inserts one or two fingers along the back of the fetal head to check for the umbilical cord. If there is a nuchal cord (umbilical cord around the neck), the nurse bends her or his fingers like a fish hook, grasps the cord, and pulls it over the baby's head. It is important to check that the cord is not wrapped around the neck more than one time. If the cord is tightly looped and cannot be slipped over the baby's head, two clamps are placed on the cord, the cord is cut between the clamps, and the cord is unwound.

Immediately after birth of the head, the nurse suctions the baby's mouth and nasal passages. The head will then rotate to one side or the other. The head will move in one direction; the nurse does not attempt to rotate the head to one side or another. The nurse then places one hand on each side of the head, over the fetal ears. Care should be taken to ensure that the hands are not exerting pressure on the fetal neck. The nurse then exerts gentle downward traction until the anterior shoulder passes under the symphysis pubis. After the anterior shoulder is seen, gentle upward traction is used to aid the birth of the posterior shoulder. The nurse then instructs the woman to push gently so that the rest of the body can be born quickly. The newborn must be supported as she or he emerges.

The newborn is held at the level of the uterus to facilitate blood flow through the umbilical cord. The combination of amniotic fluid and vernix makes the newborn very slippery, so the nurse must be careful to avoid dropping the baby. Leaving the birthing bed in an intact position provides the nurse with an area to place the newborn immediately after the birth. The nose and mouth of the newborn are suctioned again, using a bulb syringe. The nurse then dries the newborn and removes the wet blankets to prevent heat loss.

The umbilical cord may now be cut. The nurse places two sterile Kelly clamps approximately 1 to 3 in. from the newborn's abdomen. The cord is cut between the Kelly clamps with sterile scissors. The nurse places a sterile umbilical cord clamp adjacent to the Kelly clamp on the newborn's cord, between the clamp and the newborn's abdomen. The clamp must not be placed snugly against the abdomen, because the cord will dry and shrink. As soon as the nurse determines that the newborn's respirations are adequate, the infant can be placed on the mother's abdomen. The newborn's head should be slightly lower than the body to aid drainage of fluid and mucus. The weight of the newborn on the mother's abdomen stimulates uterine contractions, which aid in placental separation. The umbilical cord should not be pulled.

The nurse is alert for signs of placental separation (slight gush of dark blood from the vagina, lengthening of the cord, or a change in uterine shape from discoid to globular). The nurse can also place a hand in the vagina to see if the placenta is present. When these signs are present, the mother is instructed to push so that the placenta can be delivered. The nurse inspects the placenta to determine whether it is intact. Cord blood can be obtained from the placenta after delivery.

The nurse checks the firmness of the uterus. The fundus may be gently massaged to stimulate contractions and decrease bleeding. Putting the newborn to breast also stimulates uterine contractions through release of oxytocin from the pituitary gland.

The nurse cleanses the area under the mother's buttocks and inspects her perineum for lacerations. Bleeding from lacerations may be controlled by pressing sterile gauze or a clean perineal pad against the perineum and instructing the woman to keep her thighs together.

If the physician/CNM's arrival is delayed or if the newborn is having respiratory distress, the newborn should be transported immediately to the nursery. The newborn must be properly identified before he or she leaves the birth area. The nurse notes and places on a birth record the following information:

- Position of fetus at birth
- Presence of cord around neck or shoulder (nuchal cord)
- Time of birth
- Apgar scores at 1 and 5 minutes after birth
- Gender of newborn
- Time of expulsion of placenta
- Method of placental expulsion
- Appearance and intactness of placenta
- Mother's condition
- Any medications that were given to mother or newborn (per agency protocol)

Evaluation

Evaluation provides an opportunity to determine the effectiveness of nursing care. As a result of comprehensive nursing care during the intrapartal period, the following outcomes may be anticipated:

- The mother's physical and psychologic well-being has been maintained and supported.
- The baby's physical and psychologic well-being has been protected and supported.
- The woman and her family members have had input into the birth process and have participated as much as they desired.
- The mother and her baby have had a safe birth.

CHAPTER HIGHLIGHTS

- Nursing diagnoses in the intrapartum period typically include a general plan that includes the beginning of labor through the fourth stage.
- During labor, before procedures are begun, it is important to explain what will be done, the reasons, potential benefits and risks, and possible alternatives. These explanations help the woman determine what happens to her body.
- Behavioral responses to labor vary with the phase of labor, the preparation the woman has had, and her previous experience, cultural beliefs, and developmental level.
- The childbearing family may have a variety of expectations of the nurse during labor and birth. Some families want to make all decisions themselves with limited nursing contact, whereas others want a moderate amount of contact and see the relationship as a cooperative venture. Still other families want a lot of involvement and look to the nurse to instill confidence in them that everything will be alright.
- Each woman's cultural beliefs affect her need for privacy, expression of discomfort, and expectations for the birth and the role she wishes the father to play in the birth event.
- The phases of the first stage of labor include the latent phase (dilatation up to 3 cm [1.2 cm]), the active phase

(dilatation from 4 to 7 cm [1.6 to 2.8 in.]), and the transition phase (dilatation from 8 to 10 cm [3.1 to 3.9 in.]).
- The laboring woman's comfort may be increased by general comfort measures, methods of handling anxiety, client teaching, supportive relaxation techniques, controlled breathing, and support by a caring person.
- During the second stage of labor the nurse assists the woman with establishing an effective pattern for pushing, finding a comfortable pushing position, and providing continuous encouragement for her efforts.
- Maternal birthing positions include a wide variety of possibilities, from side-lying (lateral) to sitting, squatting, and semi-Fowler's.
- Immediate assessments of the newborn include evaluation of the Apgar score and an abbreviated physical assessment. These early assessments help determine the need for resuscitation and whether the newborn's adaptation to extrauterine life is progressing normally. The newborn who is not experiencing problems may remain with the parents for an extended period after birth.
- Immediate care of the newborn includes maintenance of respirations, promotion of warmth, prevention of infection, and accurate identification.

- The placenta separates from the uterine wall and is expelled with either the maternal or fetal side emerging from the vagina. The maternal side contains the cotyledons, appears rough in texture, and may be associated with retention of placental fragments.
- The fourth stage includes the first 1 to 4 hours following birth. Many physiologic and psychologic changes occur during this period.

- The adolescent mother has special needs in the birth setting. Her developmental needs require specialized nursing care.
- At times a baby is born rapidly, in less than 3 hours, without the physician/CNM present. This event is referred to as a precipitous birth. The nurse in the birthing area remains with the woman and attends to her needs during the birth until the physician/CNM arrives.

EXPLORE PEARSON **mynursingkit**™

MyNursingKit is your one stop for online chapter review materials and resources. Prepare for success with additional NCLEX®-style practice questions, interactive assignments and activities, web links, animations and videos, and more!

Register your access code from the front of your book at
www.mynursingkit.com

CHAPTER REFERENCES

American College of Obstetricians & Gynecologists (ACOG). (2005). Intrapartum fetal heart rate monitoring (ACOG Practice Bulletin No. 70). Washington, DC: Author.

American College of Obstetricians & Gynecologists (ACOG). (2006a). Apgar score (Committee Opinion No. 333). Washington, DC: Author.

American College of Obstetricians & Gynecologists (ACOG). (2006b). Postpartum hemorrhage (ACOG Practice Bulletin No. 76). Washington, DC: Author.

American College of Obstetricians & Gynecologists (ACOG). (2007). Premature rupture of membranes (ACOG Practice Bulletin No. 80). Washington, DC: Author.

American Society of Anesthesiologists (ASA). (2006). *Practice guidelines for obstetric anesthesia.* Park Ridge, IL: Author.

Ayers, S., Eagle, A., & Waring, H. (2006). The effects of childbirth-related post-traumatic stress disorder on women and their relationships: A qualitative study. *Psychological Health Medicine, 11*(4), 389–398.

Bardzulin, N. T., Bochoriashvili, K. A., Abashhidze, T. T., & Konaia, N. A. (2006). Early results of evidence-based perinatal care technologies implemented by Zestafoni Maternity Hospital. *Georgian Medical News, 138,* 45–48.

Bradley, S. E., Prata, N., Young-Lin, N., & Bishai, D. M. (2007). Cost-effectiveness of misoprostol to control postpartum hemorrhage in low-resource settings. *International Journal of Gynaecology & Obstetrics, 97*(1), 52–56.

Chai-Chen, A. (2007). Family-centered care. *Journal for Specialists in Pediatric Nursing, 12*(2), 119–122.

Cromer, K. R., & Sachs-Ericsson, N. (2006). The association between childhood abuse, PTSD, and the occurrence of adult health problems: Moderation via current life stress. *Journal of Trauma and Stress, 19*(6), 967–971.

Ethnomed. (2007). Peripartum and infant care issues and practices among refugee groups. Retrieved April 15, 2007, at http://ethnomed. org/ethnomed/clin_topics/peri.html

Falk, G., Ostlund, I., Magnuson, A., Scholin, J., & Nilsson, K. (2006). Teenage mothers—a high-risk group for new unintended pregnancies. *Contraception, 74*(6), 471–475. Epub.

Gennaro, S., Mayberry, L. J., & Kafulafula, U. (2007). The evidence supporting nursing management of labor. *JOGNN, 36*(6), 598–604.

Hastings-Tolsma, M., Vincent, D., Emeis, C., & Francisco, T. (2007). Getting through birth in one piece: protecting the perineum. *MCN. The American Journal of Maternal-Child Nursing, 32*(3), 158–164.

Hunter, S., Hofmeyr, G. J., & Kulier, R. (2007). Hands and knees posture in late pregnancy of labour for fetal malposition (lateral or posterior). [Cochrane Review]. In *Cochrane Database of Systematic Reviews.* 2007. Retrieved May 19, 2008, from The Cochrane Library, Wiley Interscience.

Hutton, E. K., & Hassan, E. S. (2007). Late versus early clamping of the umbilical cord in full-term neonates: Systematic review and meta-analysis of controlled trials. *JAMA, 297*(11), 1257–1258.

Levy, T., & Blickstein, I. (2006). Timing of cord clamping revisited. *Journal of Perinatal Medicine, 34*(4), 293–297.

Lutwak, R. A., Ney, A. M., & White, J. A. (2004). Jewish perspectives on the birthing experience. Retrieved May 28, 2008, from http://mikvah. org/inside.asp?id=146

Maggioni, C., Margola, D., & Filipi, F. (2006). PTSD, risk factors, and expectations among women having a baby: A two-wave longitudinal study. *Journal of Psychosomatic Obstetrics & Gynaecology, 27*(2), 81–90.

Mercer, J. S., Vohr, B. R., McGrath, M. M., Padbury, J. F., Wallace, M., & Oh, W. (2006). Delayed cord clamping in very premature infants reduces the risk of intraventricular hemorrhage and late-onset sepsis: A randomized controlled trial. *Pediatrics, 117,* 1235–1242.

Moore, E. R., Anderson, G. C., Bergman, N. (2007). Early skin-to-skin contact for mothers and their healthy newborn infants. [Cochrane Review]. In *Cochrane Database of Systematic Reviews.* 2007. Retrieved April 10, 2008, from The Cochrane Library, Wiley Interscience.

Nasir, A., Korejo, R., & Noorani, K. J. (2007). Childbirth in squatting position. *Journal of Pakistanian Medical Association, 57*(1), 19–22.

National Sexual Assault Hotline. (2007). Statistics and key facts. Retrieved April 20, 2007, from http://www.rainn.org/statistics/index.html

Perinatal HIV Guidelines Working Group. (2006). Public Health Service Task Force recommendations for use of antiretroviral drugs in pregnant HIV-1 infected women for maternal health and interventions to reduce perinatal HIV-1 transmission in the United States. October 12, 2006 1-65. Retrieved April 17, 2007, at http:// aidsinfo.nih.gov/ContentFiles/PerinatalGL.pdf

Roberts, J. M., Gonzalez, C. B., & Sampselle, C. (2007). Why do supportive birth attendants become directive of maternal bearing-down efforts in second-stage labor? *Journal of Nurse Midwifery & Women's Health, 52*(2), 134–141.

Smith, C. A., Collins, C. T., Cyna, A. M., & Crowther, C. A. (2006). Complementary and alternative therapies for pain management in labour. *Cochrane Database Systematic Review, 18*(4), CD003521.

Spector, R. E. (2009). *Cultural diversity in health and illness* (7th ed.). Upper Saddle River, NJ: Prentice Hall Health.

St. Elizabeth's Medical Center. (2007). Cultural diversity: Latinos. Retrieved April 17, 2007, from http://www.stemc.org/about_stemc/cultural_ diversity/latinos.php?id=294

Thombs, B. D., Bennett, W., Ziegelstein, R. C., Bernstein, D. P., Scher, C. D., & Forde, D. R. (2007). Cultural sensitivity in screening adults for a history of childhood abuse: Evidence from a community sample. *Journal of General Internal Medicine, 22*(3), 368–373.

U.S. Department of Health and Human Services, Administration on Children, Youth and Families (2007). *Child Maltreatment 2005.* Washington, DC: U.S. Government Printing Office.

Wilson, B. A., Shannon, M. T., & Shields, K. M. (2009). *Nurse's drug guide 2009.* Upper Saddle River, NJ: Pearson Education.

CHAPTER 20

Pharmacologic Management of Pain

I had the unique opportunity to join the staff of a brand-new women's hospital as it was opening. The team I work with is very tight knit, and we really support each other. Our schedule rotates so that I cover the regular (daytime) surgical cases for 2 days a week and then I have a 24-hour call shift on the birthing unit. I may do 10 to 12 epidurals during that call period, so I really have to be efficient. Still, it's important to me (and the others on my team) to spend as much time as that laboring woman needs, to explain things, and help her feel comfortable with her choice of pain relief.

—Certified Registered Nurse Anesthetist

LEARNING OUTCOMES

20-1. Describe the use, administration, dose, onset of action, adverse effects, and contraindications of systemic drugs that promote pain relief during labor in determining the nursing care management of the woman in labor and her fetus.

20-2. Compare the major types of regional analgesia and anesthesia, including area affected, advantages, disadvantages, contraindications, techniques, and nursing care management of the laboring woman and her fetus.

20-3. Explain the possible complications of regional anesthesia in nursing care management of the laboring woman and her fetus.

20-4. Explain the use and major complications of general anesthesia during labor in nursing care management of the woman in labor and her fetus.

KEY TERMS

Analgesic potentiators **468**
Epidural block **471**
General anesthesia **478**
Local infiltration anesthesia **477**
Pudendal block **477**
Regional analgesia **469**
Regional anesthesia **468**
Spinal block **475**

Childbearing women experience varying levels of pain and other demanding sensations during labor and birth. As discussed in Chapter 19 ∞, nursing interventions directed toward pain relief begin with psychologic measures such as providing information, support, and encouragement. Measures to promote physical comfort include back rubs, showers, whirlpools (Jacuzzi), and the application of cool cloths. Some laboring women need no further interventions.

For other women, the progression of labor brings increasing pain that interferes with their ability to cope. These women may elect to use pharmacologic agents such as systemic medications, regional nerve blocks (epidural, spinal, or combined epidural-spinal), and local anesthetic blocks (pudendal and perineal) to decrease discomfort, increase relaxation, and reestablish their ability to participate more effectively in the labor and birth experience. The methods are not all mutually exclusive, and any of them may be used in combination with nonpharmacologic comfort measures. The use of general anesthesia has very limited use in modern obstetrics. It is occassionally used during emergency cesarean births although this trend continues to decrease because of the adverse maternal and fetal effects associated with its use.

Although systemic analgesics and regional anesthetic blocks may affect the fetus, so do the pain and stress experienced by the laboring woman. During labor there is an increase in maternal respirations and oxygen consumption, which decreases the amount of oxygen available to the fetus. In addition, the pain and stress can lead to metabolic acidosis and the release of catecholamines, which causes maternal blood vessels to constrict, lessening oxygen and nutrient supply to the fetus (Hawkins, Goetzl & Chestnut, 2007).

There is a good deal of peer pressure on expectant parents to have the "ideal" birth experience. They may plan a natural childbirth, in which case the need for analgesia may make them feel inadequate and guilty. The nurse has a special role in helping a woman and her partner accept alterations in their original plan and recognize the unique qualities of their birth experience. Reassurance that accepting analgesia for discomfort is not a fail-ure can help maintain the woman's self-esteem. The emphasis should be on achieving a healthy, satisfying outcome for the family.

Systemic Medications

The goal of pharmacologic analgesia during labor is to provide maximum pain relief at minimum risk for the mother and fetus. To reach this goal, clinicians must consider a number of factors, including the following:

- All systemic medications used for pain relief during labor cross the placental barrier by simple diffusion, but some medications cross more readily than others.
- Medication action in the body depends on the rate at which the substance is metabolized by liver enzymes and excreted by the kidneys.
- High medication doses may remain in the fetus for long periods because fetal liver enzymes and kidney excretion are inadequate for metabolizing analgesic agents.

Nursing Care Management

Analgesic medications provide pain relief for the laboring woman but also affect the fetus and the labor process. Pain medication given too early may prolong labor and depress the fetus; if given too late it is of minimal use to the woman and may lead to respiratory depression in the newborn. The nurse assesses the mother and fetus and also evaluates the contraction pattern before administering prescribed systemic medications.

Maternal assessment parameters include:

- The woman is willing to receive medication after being advised about the risks and benefits of the medication.
- Maternal vital signs are stable.
- Contraindications (such as specific medication allergy, respiratory compromise, or current medication dependence) are not present.

Fetal assessment parameters include:

- The fetal heart rate (FHR) baseline is between 110 and 160 beats per minute, and no late decelerations or non-reassuring FHR patterns are present.
- Variability is present.
- The fetus exhibits normal movement, and accelerations are present with fetal movement.
- The fetus is term.

Assessment of labor includes:

- Documentation of the contraction pattern
- The cervical status including cervical position, consistency, effacement, dilatation, and station.

CRITICAL THINKING

Luisa Silva, a 33-year-old G1P0, is 32 weeks pregnant. She is trying to decide whether she should accept any analgesia during her labor. She has finished childbirth education classes and wants an unmedicated labor and birth. She says, "I want to do this on my own, but I'm afraid it may be too much. Will it be OK if I need to take something?" What will you tell her?

Answers can be found in Appendix F ∞.

Before administering the medication, the nurse once again ascertains whether the woman has a history of any medication reactions or allergies and provides information about the medication. (See Key Facts to Remember: What Women Need to Know About Pain Relief Medications.) Maternal vital signs, FHR, contraction pattern, and pain level should be assessed and documented before the administration of any pain medication. After giving the medication, the nurse records the medication name, dose, route, and site, as well as the woman's blood pressure (BP) and pulse, on the FHR monitor strip and on the woman's medical record. If the woman is alone, side rails should be raised to provide safety. The nurse assesses the FHR for possible adverse effects of the medication. After the medication has been administered, the nurse should document the woman's pain level, the effectiveness of the medication, and any adverse effects if they occurred.

When an analgesic medication is administered by intramuscular or subcutaneous route, it takes a few minutes for the effect to be felt. The nurse can continue with other supportive measures to enhance comfort, such as ensuring a quiet environment, providing a back rub or cool cloth, assisting with relaxation and visualization exercises, or providing therapeutic touch until the woman feels the effect of the medication. Often, continued reassurance and verbal praise have a calming effect. When the medication begins to take effect, the woman may sleep between contractions. This short period of rest helps her relax and can restore her energy. When an intravenous route is ordered by the physician/CNM, the effect of the medication will be felt within a few minutes, so if any change of position is necessary or if the woman needs to void, the nurse may suggest that these activities be completed before the medication administration. Some women may be so uncomfortable that they do not want anything except the medication. In this case, administering the medication first would be more helpful for the woman.

◈

KEY FACTS TO REMEMBER

What Women Need to Know About Pain Relief Medications

Before receiving medications, the woman should understand the following:
- Type of medication administered
- Route of administration
- Expected effects of medication
- Implications for fetus or newborn
- Safety measures needed (e.g., remain in bed with side rails up)

Opioid Analgesics

Opioid analgesic agents that are injected into the circulation have their primary action at sites in the brain, activating the neurons that descend to the spinal cord. The opioid analgesics used in early labor are given in either intermittent doses or, less commonly, by patient-controlled administration. These medications work by providing some analgesic effect and by inducing sedation (Hawkins, 2008).

Butorphanol Tartrate (Stadol)

Butorphanol tartrate (Stadol) is a synthetic agonist-antagonist opioid analgesic agent that can be given via the intramuscular or intravenous (IV) route. The medication has been proven effective in reducing pain intensity in laboring women. A study that compared butorphanol (Stadol) with meperidine (Demerol) found that both medications relieved pain intensity although the magnitude of pain following the administration of butorphanol (Stadol) was less (Nelson & Eisenach, 2005). Its onset of action is rapid after IV injection, peak analgesia occurs in 30 to 60 minutes, and the duration is from 3 to 4 hours (Wilson, Shannon, & Shields, 2009). The recommended initial dose is 1 to 2 mg administered intramuscularly (IM) or intravenously every 4 hours. These medications can have a "ceiling effect" where providing additional medication will not result in more analgesic effects but will result in increased side effects. Respiratory depression of both the mother and fetus or newborn can occur. The effects of butorphanol can be reversed with naloxone (Narcan). Butorphanol should not be used for women with a known opiate dependency and should be used with caution if medication dependence is suspected because it may precipitate withdrawal (Medscape, 2007c). Butorphanol tartrate (Stadol) can increase maternal blood pressure and should not be used in women with chronic hypertension or preeclampsia (Medscape, 2007c).

The most common side effect associated with butorphanol (Stadol) is drowsiness. Dizziness, fainting, and hypotension can also occur (Medscape, 2007c). If these symptoms do occur, the woman should remain in bed with the side rails up to prevent injury. Urinary retention following administration of butorphanol is not common but does occur. Therefore, the nurse should be alert for bladder distention when a woman has received butorphanol for analgesia during labor, has IV fluids infusing, and receives regional anesthesia for the birth. Butorphanol needs to be protected from light and stored at room temperature (Medscape, 2007c).

Nalbuphine Hydrochloride (Nubain)

Like butorphanol, nalbuphine hydrochloride (Nubain) is a synthetic agonist-antagonist opioid analgesic and may precipitate medication withdrawal if the woman is physically dependent on opioids. It also crosses the placenta to the fetus and can cause a nonreassuring fetal heart rate and neonatal respiratory depression (Medscape, 2007b). Nalbuphine may be given via the intramuscular, subcutaneous, or intravenous route, although it is most frequently given by the intravenous route in the birth setting. The usual dose for adults is 10 to 20 mg (Medscape, 2007b). If given intravenously, onset of action occurs in 2 to 3 minutes, peak of action occurs in 15 to 20 minutes, and duration is 3 to 6 hours. When given through the intramuscular or subcutaneous route, the onset of action occurs in less than 15 minutes, peak of action occurs in 30 to 60 minutes, and duration is 3 to 6 hours (Wilson et al., 2009). When given via the IV route, nalbuphine may be given directly into the tubing of a running IV infusion; 10 mg should be administered over 3 to 5 minutes (Wilson et al., 2009). Like butorphanol tartrate (Stadol), nalbuphine can also have a ceiling effect where the pain reduction qualities do not increase, but the side effects increase. Adverse effects in the woman include respiratory depression, drowsiness, flushing, dizziness, blurred vision, bradycardia, nausea, diaphoresis, and urinary urgency (Medscape, 2007b). Nalbuphine is often the medication of choice because it is associated with less nausea and vomiting, and a lower incidence of respiratory depression. Nalbuphine is also associated with increased maternal sedation, which allows the mother an opportunity to rest between contractions (ACOG, 2002). See Drug Guide: Nalbuphine Hydrochloride (Nubain).

Meperidine (Demerol)

Meperidine was once the most commonly used synthetic agonist-antagonist opioid analgesic in obstetrical practice. Meperidine is used less commonly because of the associated prolonged neonatal neurobehavioral depression when compared with fentanyl or Nubain (ACOG, 2002). Meperidine should not be used in women who are opioid dependent. It can be administered IM or IV in labor; the typical dose is 50 to 100 mg IM every 1 to 2 hours as needed. Meperidine administered intravenously should be given slowly and diluted. The typical dosage is 25 to 50 mg IV (Medscape, 2007a). The continuous IV dosage is 15 mg/h to 35 mg/h as needed for pain (Medscape, 2007a). The most serious adverse effect is respiratory depression. Other adverse maternal effects include constipation, dizziness, itching, drowsiness, fainting,

Drug Guide Nalbuphine Hydrochloride (Nubain)

Overview of Action Nubain is a synthetic opioid analgesic with agonist and weak antagonist properties. Analgesic properties are equal to those produced by morphine. Nubain's potency is three to four times greater than pentazocine. The incidence of respiratory depression that occurs is equivalent to morphine.

Dosage Route Nubain is indicated for moderate to severe pain. Adults: 10 to 20 mg every 3 to 6 hours PRN subcutaneous/IM/IV.

Maternal Contraindications Hypersensitivity or allergy to nalbuphine hydrochloride, respiratory depression, acute asthma attack, bradycardia, inflammatory bowel disease, and substance abuse.

Maternal Side Effects Abdominal pain with cramps, allergic dermatitis, allergic reactions, angioedema, anorexia, atelectasis, biliary spasm, blurred vision, bradycardia, bronchial asthma, bronchospastic pulmonary disease, depression, diplopia, dizziness, drowsiness, dysgeusia, dyspnea, fainting, false sense of well-being, flushing, gastrointestinal irritation, general weakness, hallucinations, headache disorder, hypertension, hypotension, impaired cognition, insomnia, laryngeal edema, laryngismus, malaise, nausea, nervousness, nightmares, oliguria, pruritus of skin, pulse changes, respiratory depression, skin rash, tachyarrhythmia, ureteral spasm, urticaria, vertigo, visual changes, vomiting, xerostomia.

Nursing Considerations

- Assess client's allergy, sensitivity, or dependence to opioids on admission.
- Inform woman of potential side effects.
- Monitor and evaluate analgesic effect. Ask client about comfort level and notify analgesia provider of inadequate pain relief.
- Observe for symptoms of hypersensitivity: pruritus, urticaria, and/or burning sensation.
- May produce an allergic response in clients with sulfite sensitivity.
- If allergic reaction (urticaria, edema, or respiratory difficulties) occurs, administer naloxone or diphenhydramine per physician order.
- Assess respiratory rate before administration. Notify healthcare provider if respirations are less than 12 per minute.
- Monitor urinary output and assess bladder for distention. Assist client to void.
- Maintain bedrest or assist client with ambulation after administration.
- Counsel client that use with alcohol or other central nervous system depressants may increase medication effects.
- Prolonged use with abrupt discontinuation can result in symptoms consistent with opioid withdrawal in both the mother and infant.

flushing, general weakness, sedation, hypotension, malaise, nausea, urinary retention, and vomiting (Medscape, 2007a).

Meperidine has fetal side effects including alterations in the electroencephalogram, decreased or absent respiratory movements, a decrease in fetal movement, and a decrease in variability with the FHR tracing (Braveman, 2006). Newborns who receive meperidine take longer to sustain respirations after birth and have lower Apgar scores, lower oxygen saturation rates, more respiratory acidosis, and a higher incidence of abnormal neurological examiniations at birth (Braveman, 2006). The use of meperidine has also been associated with delays and difficulties with breastfeeding, including lack of sucking, and incorrect sucking technique (Braveman, 2006).

Fentanyl (Sublimaze)

Fentanyl is a short-acting opiate that has been used during labor to relieve pain and induce sedation. Fentanyl should not be administered to women with an opioid dependency. The typical dosage is 50 to 100 mcg every 2 hours intravenously or intramuscularly (Ryan-Haddad, 2006). The intravenous dosage is given over a period of 1 to 2 minutes. The onset of relief is almost immediate and the peak effect occurs in 30 to 60 minutes. Although the onset is fast, the duration of effectiveness is limited to 30 to 60 minutes. The onset of the intramuscular dose is 7 to 15 minutes (Ryan-Haddad, 2006). Fentanyl is 50 to 100 times more potent than morphine. Fentanyl has less neonatal neurobehavioral depression than Demerol because it does not cross the placenta. However, neonatal depression can still occur, although at much lower rates when compared with Demerol. Adverse effects to fentanyl include bradycardia, hypotension, nausea, vomiting, and respiratory depression. Fentanyl results in less sedation, nausea, vomiting, and pruritis compared with Demerol. Fentanyl can also cause muscle rigidity, especially in the respiratory muscles.

Analgesic Potentiators

The use of **analgesic potentiators**, also known as *ataractics,* can decrease anxiety and increase the effectiveness of analgesics when given simultaneously. These medications, which are classified as tranquilizers, have no specific properties that decrease pain; however, they do work well to potentiate the effects of opioid analgesics without increasing unwanted side effects. This enhancement enables the woman to receive a smaller dose of the opioid being administered. These medications can also be used to manage unpleasant side effects, such as nausea or vomiting, associated with the administration of opioid analgesics.

Commonly used analgesic potentiators include promethazine (Phenergan), hydroxyzine (Vistaril), propiomazine (Largon), and promazine (Sparine). The main side effect associated with these medications is sedation.

Sedation may be helpful in promoting rest in women who have had a prolonged labor or who have had little sleep; however, the effect may be undesirable to other women.

Opiate Antagonist: Naloxone (Narcan)

Because naloxone is an antagonist with little or no agonistic effect, it exhibits little pharmacologic activity in the absence of opioids. Naloxone can be used to reverse the mild respiratory depression that follows administration of small doses of opiates. The medication is useful for respiratory depression caused by fentanyl and meperidine, as well as butorphanol tartrate and nalbuphine hydrochloride. Naloxone is the medication of choice when the depressant is unknown because it will cause no further depression (Wilson et al., 2009). An initial dose of 0.4 to 2 mg may be administered intravenously to the laboring woman. If the woman is nonresponsive, the medication can be readministered every 2 to 3 minutes. Knowledge of basic airway management is imperative in cases where the woman or infant is not immediately responsive and respiratory depression is occurring. The nurse should be prepared to provide basic airway management, including chin lift, jaw thrust maneuver, and initiation of respirations through a bag valve mask device. Naloxone may be given to the newborn if needed after birth. The newborn dose is 0.1 mg/kg and may need to be repeated. It is typically administered to mothers who have received opioids within 4 hours of the birth (Wilson et al., 2009). (See Drug Guide: Naloxone Hydrochloride (Narcan), in Chapter 29 ∞ .)

When naloxone is given, other resuscitative measures may be indicated, and trained personnel should be readily available. The duration of the medication's effect is shorter than that of the analgesic medication for which it is acting as an antagonist, so the nurse must be alert to the return of respiratory depression and the need for repeated doses. Naloxone should not be given in women with known or suspected opiate dependency because it may precipitate severe withdrawal (Wilson et al., 2009).

Regional Anesthesia and Analgesia

Regional anesthesia is the temporary loss of sensation produced by injecting an anesthetic agent (called a *local*) into direct contact with nervous tissue. Loss of sensation happens because the local agents stabilize the cell membrane, which prevents initiation and transmission of nerve impulses. The regional anesthetic blocks most commonly used in childbirth include the epidural, spinal, and combined epidural-spinal blocks. Epidural blocks may be used for analgesia during labor and vaginal birth and for anesthesia during cesarean birth.

An epidural relieves pain associated with the first stage of labor by blocking the sensory nerves supplying the uterus. Pain associated with the second stage of labor and with birth can be alleviated with epidural, combined epidural-spinal, and pudendal blocks (see Figure 20–1 ■).

Until the past few years, the same anesthetic agents used for regional epidurals were also used to produce **regional analgesia** (pain relief to a body region) during labor. This practice was problematic because the anesthetic agents used alter the transmission of impulses to the bladder, making voiding difficult. The agents also interfere with blood pressure stability and leg movement. The descent of the fetus is slowed and an increased risk of perineal lacerations occurs more commonly in women with epidural anesthesia (Fitzgerald, Weber, Howden et al., 2007; Sheiner, Walfisch, Hallak et al., 2006). To address these difficulties, regional analgesia is now obtained by injecting an opioid such as fentanyl along with only a small amount of anesthetic agent. New medication combinations relieve the woman's pain while minimizing the side effects just mentioned (Hawkins, Goetzl & Chestnut, 2007).

The intrathecal injection of opioids results in another type of regional analgesia. In this case, the opioid is injected into the subarachnoid space. It is important for the anesthesia provider to provide a test dose before giving the entire dose to determine that the catheter is correctly placed. Fentanyl citrate and preservative-free morphine are the most commonly used medications. This typically results in more effective pain relief over the subsequent 24 hours after birth although the incidence of nausea may be increased in some women (Vasudevan, Snowman, Sundar et al., 2007).

Nursing care during administration of regional analgesia is directed toward helping the woman void before administration, assisting her with positioning during and after the procedure, monitoring and assessing vital signs and respiratory status, monitoring analgesic effect, and determining fetal well-being. Reassurance and thorough explanations help decrease anxiety and fear. Additional measures may be needed to address pruritus, nausea and vomiting, and urinary retention.

As with other procedures, the woman needs to know how the block is given, the expected effect on her and the fetus, advantages and disadvantages, and possible complications (Datta, 2006). Many women discuss possible anesthetic blocks with their care provider at some point in the pregnancy. If they have not, it is important to give them an opportunity to ask questions and obtain information before receiving the block while in labor.

Anesthetic Agents for Regional Blocks

Local anesthetic agents block the conduction of nerve impulses from the periphery to the central nervous system by preventing the propagation of an action potential from the source of pain (Datta, 2006). The types of nerve fibers are differentially sensitive to the various anesthetic agents. In general, the smaller the fiber, the more sensitive it is to local agents. For example, it is possible to block the small C and A delta fibers, which transmit pain and temperature, without blocking the larger A alpha, A beta, and A gamma fibers, which continue to maintain a sense of pressure, muscle tone, position sense, and motor function.

Absorption of local anesthetics depends primarily on the vascularity of the area of injection. The agents themselves contribute to increased blood flow by causing vasodilation. High concentrations of medications cause greater vasodilation. Good maternal physical condition or a high

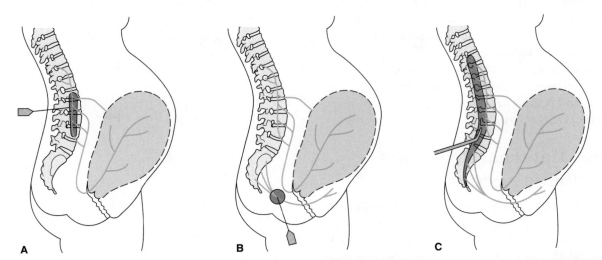

FIGURE 20–1 Schematic diagram showing pain pathways and sites of interruption. *A,* Lumbar sympathetic (spinal) block: Relief of uterine pain only. *B,* Pudendal block: Relief of perineal pain. *C,* Lumbar epidural block: Dark area demonstrates peridural (epidural) space and nerves affected, and the gray tube represents a continuous plastic catheter.
Source: Bonica, J. J. (1972). *Principles and practice of obstetric analgesia and anesthesia* (pp. 492, 512, 521, 614). Philadelphia: F. A. Davis.

metabolic rate aids absorption. Malnutrition, dehydration, electrolyte imbalance, and cardiovascular and pulmonary problems increase the potential for toxic effects. The pH of tissues affects the rate of absorption, which has implications for fetal complications such as acidosis. The addition of vasoconstrictors such as epinephrine delays absorption and prolongs the anesthetic effect. Epinephrine decreases uteroplacental blood flow, making it an undesirable additive in many situations. The breakdown of local anesthetics in the body is accomplished by the liver and plasma esterase, and the resulting substance is eliminated by the kidneys. It is important to use the weakest concentration and the smallest amount necessary to produce the desired results.

Types of Local Anesthetic Agents

Two types of local anesthetic agents are currently available: esters and amides. The ester type includes procaine hydrochloride (Novocain), chloroprocaine hydrochloride (Nesacaine), and tetracaine hydrochloride (Pontocaine). Esters are rapidly metabolized; therefore, toxic maternal levels are not as likely to be reached, and placental transfer to the fetus is prevented. Ester-linked agents have a higher incidence of allergic reactions when compared with amides. However, they do not appear to have a higher incidence of fetal effects (Datta, 2006).

Amide types include lidocaine hydrochloride (Xylocaine), mepivacaine hydrochloride (Carbocaine), and bupivacaine hydrochloride (Marcaine). Amide types are more powerful and longer-acting agents. They readily cross the placenta, can be measured in the fetal circulation, and affect the fetus for a prolonged period. Lidocaine (Xylocaine) has been associated with major neurological and minor neurological toxicity; therefore, the dose of lidocaine should not exceed 75 mg.

Ropivacaine (Naropin) is a new generation amide that is now being used in labor. The pain relief effects are similar to other amides. However, the blockade effect is slightly lower than other amides, thus increasing the rates of vaginal births and decreasing instrument-assisted births.

Levobupivacaine (Chirocaine) has less toxicity than ropivacaine and is safer in longer surgical procedures because it has decreased toxicity.

Adverse Maternal Reactions to Anesthetic Agents

Reactions to local anesthetic agents range from mild symptoms to cardiovascular collapse. Mild reactions include palpitations, tinnitus, apprehension, confusion, and a metallic taste in the mouth. Moderate reactions include more severe degrees of mild symptoms plus nausea and vomiting, hypotension, and muscle twitching, which may progress to convulsions. Severe reactions are sudden loss of consciousness, coma, severe hypotension, bradycardia, respiratory depression, and cardiac arrest. Anesthetic agents should not be used unless an intravenous line is in place.

The preferred treatment for a mild toxic reaction is administration of oxygen and IV injection of a short-acting barbiturate to diminish anxiety. Nursing interventions for adverse reactions are included in the Nursing Care Plan for Epidural Anesthesia (see pages 474–475).

Neonatal Neurobehavioral Effects of Anesthesia and Analgesia

Many studies have focused on the neurobehavioral effects on the newborn of pharmacologic agents used during labor and birth. Although analgesic and anesthetic agents may alter the behavioral and adaptive function of the newborn,

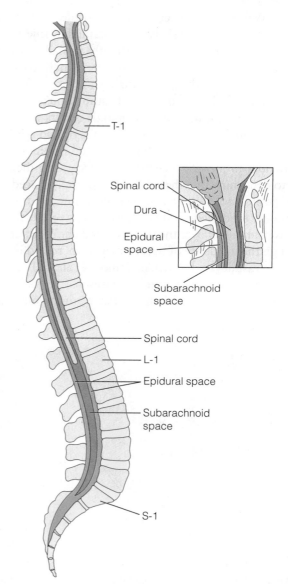

T-1

Spinal cord

Dura

Epidural space

Subarachnoid space

Spinal cord

L-1

Epidural space

Subarachnoid space

S-1

FIGURE 20–2 The epidural space lies between the dura mater and the ligamentum flavum, extending from the base of the skull to the end of the sacral canal.

physiologic factors such as hunger, degree of hydration, and time within the sleep-wake cycle may also exert an influence (Datta, 2006). It should be noted that more neurological impairment occurs in the newborn resulting from normal birth process than from epidural complications.

Epidural Block

A lumbar **epidural block** involves injection of an anesthetic agent into the epidural space to provide pain relief throughout labor. The epidural space, a potential space between the dura mater and the ligamentum flavum, is accessed through the lumbar area (Figure 20–2 ■). The epidural is most frequently used as a continuous block to provide analgesia and anesthesia from active labor through episiotomy repair (Figure 20–3 ■).

Epidurals have become a relatively common method of analgesia and anesthesia during labor and birth in the United States. It is estimated that 68% of all women in the United States receive an epidural during their labor. Non-Hispanic white women had the highest rates of epidural use (70.2%), followed by non-Hispanic black women (65.6%). Hispanic women used epidural anesthesia the least (57.8%). Epidural use did not differ among age groups (Martin & Menacker, 2007). An epidural can be given as soon as active labor is established (Datta, 2006).

Advantages

The epidural block relieves discomfort during labor and birth, and the woman is fully awake and a part of the birth process. Epidural anesthesia results in less adverse fetal effects when compared with intravenous analgesia or general anesthesia. It can also allow the woman to rest and regain strength before the woman needs to push during the second stage. The continuous epidural allows different blocking for each stage of labor, so that the fetus is able to descend and rotate in the maternal pelvis; many times the woman's urge to bear down is preserved. Epidurals that combine anesthesia and an opioid agent are often effective in providing postoperative pain relief for longer periods of time.

Opioids are used with epidural blocks for labor. Some of the agents used include morphine, fentanyl, butorphanol, and meperidine (Datta, 2006). When only opioids are used epidurally, rather than in combination with another type of agent, the amount of pain relief is not as effective, especially

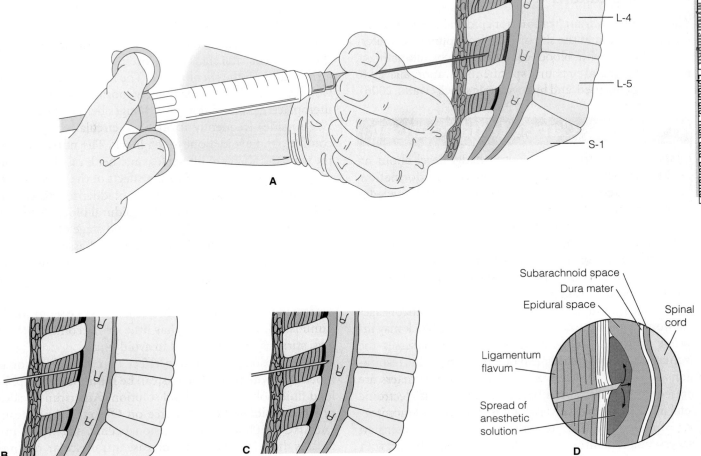

FIGURE 20–3 Technique for lumbar epidural block. *A*, Proper position for insertion. *B*, Needle in the ligamentum flavum. *C*, Tip of needle in epidural space. *D*, Force of injection pushing dura away from tip of needle.
Source: Bonica, J. J. (1972). *Principles and practice of obstetric analgesia and anesthesia* (p. 631). Philadelphia: F. A. Davis.

toward the end of labor; therefore, a combination of opioids and a low dose of local are given (Datta, 2006).

Disadvantages

The most common complication of an epidural block is maternal hypotension, which is generally prevented by administering intravenous fluid before epidural placement, left uterine displacement, and maternal positioning on her side. In some instances, labor progress and fetal descent may be slowed, and pushing efforts in the second stage may be less effective because of a decrease in sensation. The average increase in the length of labor is approximately 25 minutes. There does not appear to be an increase in forceps or vacuum use or in cesarean section births related to epidural anesthesia (ACOG, 2006). Delay in return of bladder sensation may result in urinary retention and the need for catheterization during labor and in the fourth stage (Musselwhite, Faris, Moore et al., 2007). Low back pain can also occur after an epidural and is usually more common in women who underwent vaginal deliveries. Typically, epidurals do not cause chronic low back pain, although the woman can have soreness at the insertion site for a few days.

Contraindications

The absolute contraindications for epidural block are client refusal, infection at the site of the needle puncture, maternal problems with blood coagulation (coagulopathies), raised intracranial pressure, specific medication allergy to the agent being used, and hypovolemic shock (Datta, 2006).

Nursing Care Management

Assessment of the woman's knowledge level about an epidural block is essential. Before providing information, the nurse determines the woman's current knowledge and evaluates factors related to learning, such as primary language spoken, ability to hear and interpret information, and the presence of anxiety. Although the nurse is an integral person in providing information, the anesthesia provider is the essential person to provide information and to obtain written informed consent.

In preparation for the epidural, the nurse encourages the woman to empty her bladder, because the block may interfere with her ability to void. The nurse assesses the woman's pain level, maternal blood pressure, pulse, respirations, and FHR to determine that normal parameters are present and to establish a baseline. Continuous electronic fetal monitoring to assess fetal status and frequent monitoring of maternal blood pressure and pulse for hypotension are essential. An intravenous infusion is usually begun with an 18 gauge plastic indwelling catheter. A large gauge catheter is used so that IV fluids can be administered quickly if hypotension occurs. A bolus of 500 to 1000 mL of

IV fluid is given before beginning the epidural block to decrease the incidence of hypotension.

Either of two positions can be used to achieve epidural placement: side-lying or sitting. If the side-lying position is used, the nurse assists the woman to move to the edge of the bed, where the mattress is firmer and provides more support. The woman's head is supported with a small pillow so it remains in alignment with the spine. A pillow may also be placed in front of her chest to provide support for her upper arm. Her back needs to remain straight, with the shoulders square. Her legs are bent and her knees kept together so that the upper hip does not roll forward and cause the spine to twist.

The block may also be given with the woman in a sitting position, with her back flexed and her feet supported on a stool. The woman should be advised to push her back toward the anesthesia provider. The nurse typically stands directly in front of the woman with hands placed on the woman's shoulders. The woman is encouraged to arch her back and push back toward the analgesia provider. After positioning, the nurse continues to provide support and tries to ensure that the woman does not move during the procedure. After the needle and catheter are placed, the woman is assisted into a reclining position.

Maternal vital signs are assessed frequently per protocol until the block wears off. The blood pressure can be monitored by a mechanical blood pressure device or directly by the nurse. The vital signs are recorded on the fetal monitor strip and/or on the client record. The nurse encourages the woman to maintain a side-lying position to maximize uteroplacental blood flow and changes her position (from side to side) frequently to increase circulation, promote comfort, and avoid a one-sided block. The nurse assesses the woman's ability to lift her legs and her level of sensation every 30 minutes to monitor the effects of the nerve block.

The nurse assesses the woman's bladder for distention at frequent intervals because the epidural block decreases the urge to urinate. During the second stage of labor, the woman with an epidural block may need assistance with pushing. The nurse may need to tell the woman when contractions begin and give extra assistance by holding her legs during pushing efforts. The woman's legs need to be protected from pressure applied to them while sensation is diminished. If the woman has little or no control of her legs, stirrups may be needed to avoid injury.

The most common side effect of epidural regional block is hypotension. The risk can be minimized by a preload fluid bolus of crystalloid solution (American Society of Anesthesiologists Task Force on Obstetric Anesthesia [ASAHQ], 2006). If hypotension occurs, the nurse increases the IV flow rate (to increase intravascular volume and raise the blood pressure), ensures or verifies left uterine displacement (to increase circulation), and administers oxygen (to improve oxygenation). If blood pressure is not restored in 1 to 2 minutes, ephedrine, 5 to 10 mg IV, is administered (ASAHQ, 2006). After ephedrine is administered, the blood pressure is continually monitored and the maternal and fetal responses are recorded.

The epidural may cause elevation of maternal temperature (pyrexia). Pyrexia may be confused with maternal infection and frequently results in additional testing of the newborn to rule out infection (Hughes et al., 2002).

Headache (which may occur with spinal blocks) is not a side effect of epidural anesthesia because the dura mater of the spinal canal has not been penetrated and there is no leakage of spinal fluid. Motor control of the legs is weak but not totally absent after birth. Return of complete sensation and the ability to control the legs are essential before ambulation is attempted. Recovery may take several hours, depending on the anesthetic agent and the dose given.

To assess sensation the nurse can touch various parts of the woman's legs and abdomen bilaterally to determine if the touch can be felt. The nurse can evaluate motor control by asking the woman to raise her knees, to lift her feet (one at a time) off the bed, or to dorsiflex her foot. Even though assessments may indicate that sensation and motor control have returned, the nurse needs to be ready to support the woman's weight as she stands and quickly return her to bed if motor control is inadequate. In addition, blood pressure assessments help the nurse determine the safety of ambulation. The nurse assesses blood pressure while the woman is lying down, then sitting in the bed. As long as blood pressure values remain stable (no evidence of orthostatic hypotension), a standing blood pressure is assessed. It is advisable to have additional assistance when the woman stands for the first time, to maintain safety.

Continuous Epidural Infusion

Epidural anesthesia may be given with a continuous infusion pump. Some of the benefits include good to excellent analgesia, infrequent nausea, minimal sedation, decreased anxiety, earlier mobilization, retained cough reflex, decreased risk of deep vein thrombosis, decreased myocardial oxygen demand, and ease of administration. A continuous infusion reduces the use of bolus dosages which may provide intermittent pain control.

Obviously, ease of administration does not imply lack of need for close observation. Malfunctioning equipment with subsequent overdose is always a possibility. Fortunately, infusion pumps designed specifically for use in epidural anesthesia have safety factors incorporated. Continuous epidural infusions should be administered with the same precautions used for intermittent injections.

Some of the potential problems of epidural infusions include breakthrough pain, sedation, nausea and vomiting, pruritus, and hypotension. Breakthrough pain may occur at any time during the epidural infusion but usually occurs when the infusion rate of the agent is below the recommended therapeutic rate. It may also occur when the infusion pump rate is altered or the integrity of the epidural line is broken. When breakthrough pain occurs, the nurse checks the integrity of the epidural infusion line and notifies the analgesia provider. There may be standing orders for treatment of breakthrough pain, but it is best to inform the analgesia provider of any problems that occur. Often, breakthrough pain can be corrected with a bolus dose of medication. In rare circumstances, the epidural itself may need to be replaced.

Some women may experience *hot spots* or areas of incomplete anesthesia coverage. Nursing interventions include position changes. If the hot spot becomes too uncomfortable, an anesthesia provider can administer additional medication. In some cases, the epidural will need to be replaced.

General sedation and resulting respiratory depression may occur from the systemic effect of the epidural agents as they are absorbed into the circulation. The respiratory rate, along with the quality of respirations, should be assessed no less frequently than every 15 to 30 minutes. The nurse should notify the anesthetist of any significant decreases in respiratory rate or respiratory pattern change. If respiratory rate decreases below 14 respirations per minute, naloxone may be given to counteract the effect of the anesthetic agent; typically respirations then return to a normal rate.

Nausea and vomiting can occur at any time during or after epidural infusion. The nurse should give an antiemetic if one is ordered and notify the analgesia provider. The nausea and vomiting can make the woman very uncomfortable, and the infusion rate of the epidural may need to be decreased or terminated to alleviate this discomfort. Nausea and vomiting can sometimes occur as a result of transition rather than as a direct side effect of the epidural infusion.

Pruritus (itching and rash) may occur at any time during the epidural infusion. It usually appears first on the face, neck, or torso and is usually the result of the agent in the epidural infusion. Treatment generally involves administration of diphenhydramine hydrochloride (Benadryl). If no standing order exists, the nurse notifies the anesthetist and identifies the problem. The epidural infusion may need to be decreased or terminated.

Hypotension may occur from hypovolemia or from the effect of the epidural. Treatment involves administering oxygen by mask, administering a bolus of crystalloid fluid, and notifying the anesthetist. Usually standing orders for treatment of hypotension are graded in terms of the degree of hypotension. The epidural infusion may have to be terminated and the woman placed in the Trendelenburg position. See the Nursing Care Plan for Epidural Anesthesia for further nursing assessment and interventions.

Nursing Care Plan For Epidural Anesthesia

CLIENT SCENARIO

Barbara, a 25-year-old G1P0, at 40 weeks is accompanied to the labor and birthing room by her husband and the nurse. After 3 hours the contractions are every 4 min, lasting 60 sec with moderate intensity. She is now requesting an epidural.

The analgesia provider arrives and provides Barbara with information in order to obtain written informed consent for the procedure. Barbara is placed on continuous epidural infusion. The nurse answers Barbara's questions concerning comfort and labor progress once the epidural takes effect. She is reassured that every precaution will be taken to ensure the health and well-being of her and her baby.

ASSESSMENT

Subjective: Facial grimace, rates pain level of 7 on a scale of 10, crying, reports fatigue.

Objective: Cervix is anterior, 100% effaced, 5 cm dilated, and the fetal head is at 0 station. Blood pressure is 90/60, pulse 70, respirations 16, lungs clear. Fetal heart rate between 136 and 152 bpm, with good long-term variability. Abdomen is soft between contractions. No edema noted in hands and feet.

Nursing Diagnosis	Risk for Injury related to maternal hypotension associated with epidural anesthesia secondary to vasodilation and venous pooling*
Client Goal	Maternal and fetal effects associated with hypotension will be minimized.
AEB:	• Decrease in blood pressure identified and treated successfully • Blood pressure within normal limits • Fetal heart rate within normal limits with good long-term variability

NURSING INTERVENTIONS

1. Obtain baseline maternal vital signs and fetal heart rate.

2. Insert IV with large gauge catheter.

3. Provide hydration with 500 to 1000 mL of intravenous solution (e.g., lactated Ringer's) 15 to 30 min before procedure. Dextrose-free solution is recommended.

4. Educate the client about treatment measures to expect if unwanted side effects from the epidural occur.

5. Assist the client into position for the procedure.

6. Monitor blood pressure every 1 to 2 min for the first 10 min then every 5 to 15 min until the block wears off.

7. Observe, record, and report symptoms of hypotension, including systolic pressure <100 mm Hg or a 20% to 30% fall in systolic pressure, apprehension, restlessness, dizziness, tinnitus, and headache.

RATIONALES

Rationale: Normal ranges include temperature 98°F to 99.6°F/36.6°C to 37.5°C, pulse 60 to 90, respirations 14 to 22/min, blood pressure 90–140/60–90, fetal heart rate 110 to 160 bpm. A baseline assessment allows for a comparison over the course of care to assess for any fluctuations.

Rationale: Allows for IV fluids to be administered quickly if hypotension occurs.

Rationale: Increases intravascular volume and maintains cardiac output by preloading the client before epidural anesthesia. Rapid infusion of dextrose solutions can cause fetal hyperglycemia and rebound neonatal hypoglycemia.

Rationale: Advance preparation will decrease anxiety and the client will be more compliant. Treatment measures include oxygen administration, increase of IV fluids, possible administration of a vasopressor such as ephedrine, and repositioning of the client. For discussion of other possible side effects such as loss of bladder function or motor control and their management, see text discussion.

Rationale: Place client in a supine position for 5 to 10 min following administration of block to allow medication to diffuse bilaterally. After 5 to 10 min, position client on side.

Rationale: Hypotension is the most common side effect of epidural anesthesia. Close monitoring will allow for quick assessment and treatment of any changes from baseline blood pressures before the procedure.

Rationale: These signs are related to hypotension and must be treated immediately to avoid health risk to mother and fetus.

Nursing Care Plan | For Epidural Anesthesia *(Continued)*

NURSING INTERVENTIONS

8. Initiate treatment measures to reverse hypotension.

9. Observe, record, and report fetal bradycardia (FHR less than 110 bpm) and loss of beat-to-beat variability.

RATIONALES

Rationale: Treatment measures include placing client in left lateral position as directed, increase IV rate, administer oxygen by face mask at 7 to 10 L/min as needed, administer vasopressors as ordered (usually ephedrine 5 to 10 mg IV), manually displace uterus laterally to left using a wedge or pillow. Notify analgesia provider or certified registered nurse anesthesist immediately.

Rationale: Maternal hypotension results in decreased blood flow to the fetus. Normal fetal heart rate ranges between 110 and 160 bpm. Fetal bradycardia occurs when the fetal heart rate falls below 110 bpm during a 10-min period of continuous monitoring. When fetal bradycardia is accompanied by decreased beat-to-beat variability it is considered ominous and could be a sign of advanced fetal compromise.

Evaluation of Client Goal

- Hypotension was identified and treated successfully.
- Blood pressure remained within normal limits.
- No signs of fetal bradycardia identified.
- Fetal heart rate within normal limits with good beat-to-beat variability.

CRITICAL THINKING QUESTIONS

1. It has been 5 hours since the epidural began and your assessment reveals the client is fully dilated and at 0 station. You tell the client she can push but she states she can't feel anything. How will you assist her in pushing?

Answer: Have client place her hand on her abdomen to let her know when a contraction begins. She may also feel some rectal pressure. At this point help her to get into pushing position and give extra assistance by holding her legs up and apart. Instruct her to bear down. Inform her when the contraction is over and to lay back and rest until the next contraction begins.

2. For which of the following clients would an epidural seem most appropriate?

   A. Cervix 2 cm, 50% effaced, contractions every 20 min lasting 30 sec, mild intensity, client relaxed
   B. Cervix 4 cm, 100% effaced, contractions every 4 min with decreased beat-to-beat variability. Client uncomfortable but breathing well with contractions.
   C. Cervix 6 cm, 100% effaced, contractions every 2 minutes, moderate intensity, FHR 140 with good

beat-to-beat variability. Client unable to relax between contractions

Answer: The client who is 6 cm dilated, 100% effaced, contractions every 2 min, moderate intensity, FHR 140 with good beat-to-beat variability but unable to relax between contractions is the most appropriate candidate for an epidural. An epidural can be given once a regular pattern of labor is established and the woman requests pharmacologic relief. Because everyone's pain is different, a woman's request alone is an adequate indication that pain medication is warranted. Epidurals that are placed before a normal contraction pattern is established can slow the labor process and lead to additional interventions. This client is in active labor with an established contraction pattern and appears to need something to help with relaxation and decrease the pain of contractions. Epidural anesthesia may cause maternal hypotension thereby causing fetal bradycardia and a loss of beat-to-beat variability. If a client's fetal heart rate is showing decreased beat-to-beat variability she may not be a candidate for an epidural at this time.

*For your reference, this care plan is an example of how one nursing diagnosis might be addressed.

Epidural Opioid Analgesia After Birth

To provide analgesia for approximately 24 hours after the birth, the analgesia provider may inject an opioid, such as morphine sulfate (Duramorph) or fentanyl (Sublimaze), into the epidural space immediately after the birth. The analgesic effect begins approximately 30 to 60 minutes after the injection. The side effects include pruritus, nausea and vomiting, and urinary retention (Wilson et al., 2009). The onset seems to occur early, and it resolves within 14 to 16 hours after the birth. (See Drug Guide: Postpartum Epidural Morphine in Chapter 31 ∞.)

Spinal Block

In a **spinal block,** a local anesthetic agent is injected directly into the spinal fluid in the spinal canal to provide anesthesia for cesarean birth and occasionally for vaginal birth. This technique involves passing through the epidural space and dura mater and injecting the medication directly into the cerebral spinal fluid. The technique of administration varies depending on whether the spinal block is being given for a cesarean or vaginal birth (Figure 20–4 ■).

Advantages

The advantages of spinal block are immediate onset of anesthesia, relative ease of administration, a need for smaller medication volume, and maternal compartmentalization of the medication.

Disadvantages

The primary disadvantage of spinal block is blockade of sympathetic nerve fibers, resulting in a high incidence of hypotension; maternal hypotension may lead to alterations in the fetal heart rate and fetal hypoxia. In addition, uterine tone is maintained, which makes intrauterine manipulation difficult.

Contraindications

Contraindications for spinal block include severe hypovolemia, regardless of the cause; central nervous system disease; infection over the puncture site; allergy to local anesthetic agents; coagulation problems; and client refusal (Datta, 2006).

Nursing Care Management

If an intravenous infusion is not already in place, it is started with a 16 to 18 gauge plastic catheter. A bolus of 500 to 1000 mL is infused rapidly. The nurse assesses maternal vital signs, pain level, and the FHR to establish a baseline and then positions the woman in a sitting (or a side-lying) position. The woman sits on the side of the bed or operating room table and places her feet on a stool. The woman places her arms between her knees or up around the nurse's shoulders, places her head to her chest, and arches her back to widen the intervertebral spaces. The nurse supports the woman in this position and palpates the uterus to identify the beginning of uterine contractions (if labor is present). The analgesia provider injects the anesthetic agent between contractions. If the anesthetic agent is injected during a contraction, the level of anesthesia obtained is higher and may compromise respirations.

The woman remains in a sitting position for 30 seconds and then returns to a lying position, with a rolled towel or blanket under her right hip to displace the uterus from the vena cava. The nurse monitors maternal blood pressure and pulse frequently per protocol or physician's order. The blood pressure is also reassessed when the woman is moved after birth, because movement may lower blood pressure.

If the spinal block is being used during vaginal birth, the nurse monitors uterine contractions and instructs the woman to bear down during a contraction. The block may reduce the woman's ability to push, although the new combinations of medications tend to decrease this side effect. Sometimes, the birth may be assisted with forceps or vacuum extractor (see Chapter 22 ∞).

After birth, the temporary motor paralysis of the woman's legs continues. The nurse needs to exercise caution when moving the woman from the birthing bed (or operating room table) to protect her from injury. The woman remains in bed for 6 to 12 hours following the block; she may not regain sensation and control of her bladder for 8 to 12 hours and may need to be catheterized. An indwelling bladder catheter is usually inserted before surgery for women undergoing cesarean birth.

The epidural or spinal catheter is removed by either an analgesia provider or the nurse. The tape used to se-

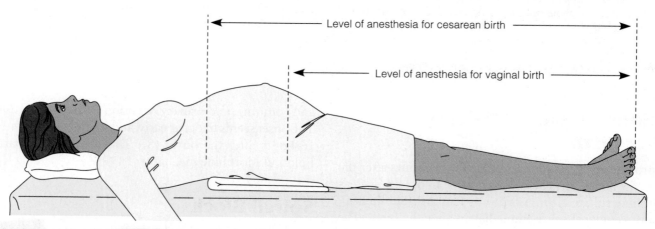

FIGURE 20–4 Levels of spinal anesthesia for vaginal and cesarean births.
Source: Reprinted with permission of Ross Laboratories, Columbus, OH. From Clinical Education Aid No. 17.

cure the block is removed. The catheter is then grasped between the fingers and slowly removed with gentle traction. The catheter should be inspected to ensure the tip did not break off. A band-aid or gauze and tape is placed over the site. It is not unusual for a small amount of bleeding to occur initially upon removal. Continuous bleeding warrants a call to the anesthesia provider. The nurse documents removal of the catheter and any adverse effects.

Combined Spinal-Epidural Block

Spinal anesthesia may be combined with an epidural block. The combined spinal-epidural (CSE) block can be used for labor analgesia and for cesarean birth. The anesthetic and analgesic agents used differ according to the purpose of the CSE block. A CSE is accomplished by inserting an epidural needle into the epidural space. A narrow gauge atraumatic (24 to 27 gauge pencil-point) needle is inserted through the epidural needle, through the dura, and into the cerebral spinal fluid. A small amount of local anesthetic agent, opioid, or both is injected, and the atraumatic needle is withdrawn. An epidural catheter is then threaded through the epidural needle and into the epidural space. The epidural needle is removed, and the epidural catheter is secured.

An advantage of CSE block is that the spinal (intrathecal) anesthetic and/or analgesic agent has a faster onset than medications that are injected into the epidural space. Most medications are used in low dose, so spinal analgesia may be given in early labor to assist in alleviating labor pain. The epidural is activated when active labor begins. Another advantage of a CSE block is that laboring women can ambulate after the CSE is placed.

TEACHING TIP

Advise women with a CSE in place always to have assistance during ambulation to prevent falls.

Pudendal Block

A **pudendal block,** administered by a transvaginal method, intercepts signals to the pudendal nerve (Figure 20–5 ■). The pudendal block provides perineal anesthesia for the latter part of the first stage of labor, the second stage, birth, and episiotomy repair. The pudendal block relieves the pain of perineal distention and typically relieves pain in the lower vagina, vulva, and perineum but not the discomfort of uterine contractions (Datta, 2006).

Advantages of the pudendal block are ease of administration and absence of maternal hypotension. It also may be used to decrease the discomfort of low forceps or vacuum-assisted birth. Because a pudendal block does not alter maternal vital signs or FHR, additional assessments are not necessary. The nurse explains the procedure and answers any questions.

The disadvantages of the pudendal block include possible broad ligament hematoma, perforation of the rectum, and trauma to the sciatic nerve. A moderate dose of anesthetic agent has minimal ill effects on the course of labor, but the urge to push may decrease.

Local Infiltration Anesthesia

Local infiltration anesthesia is accomplished by injecting an anesthetic agent into the intracutaneous, subcutaneous, and intramuscular areas of the perineum (Figure 20–6 ■). It is generally used at the time of birth, both in preparation for an episiotomy if one is needed and for the episiotomy repair. Women who have followed some type of prepared childbirth method and want minimal analgesia and anesthesia usually do not object to local anesthesia for the episiotomy or laceration repair. The administration procedure is technically uncomplicated and is practically free from complications.

A disadvantage of local infiltration is that large amounts of local anesthetic must be used to infuse the tissues. Although any local anesthetic may be used, chloroprocaine hydrochloride (Nesacaine), lidocaine

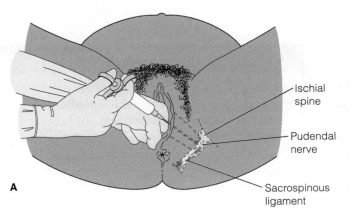

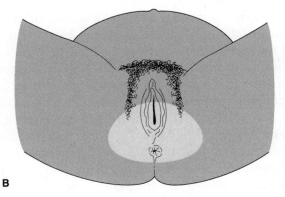

Ischial spine

Pudendal nerve

Sacrospinous ligament

A

B

FIGURE 20–5 *A,* Pudendal block by the transvaginal approach. *B,* Area of perineum affected by pudendal block.

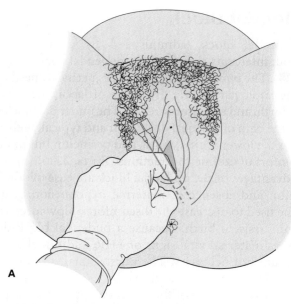

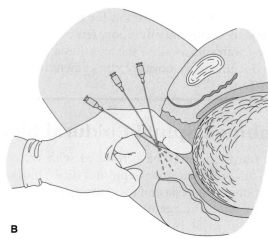

Figure 20–6 Local infiltration anesthesia. *A,* Technique of local infiltration for episiotomy and repair. *B,* Technique of local infiltration showing fan pattern for the fascial planes.
Source: Bonica, J. J. (1972). *Principles and practice of obstetric analgesia and anesthesia* (p. 505). Philadelphia: F. A. Davis.

hydrochloride (Xylocaine), tetracaine hydrochloride (Pontocaine), and mepivacaine hydrochloride (Carbocaine) are the agents of choice because of their capacity for diffusion. Because local anesthetic agents have no effect on maternal vital signs or FHR, additional assessments are unnecessary.

General Anesthesia

Occasionally, **general anesthesia** (induced unconsciousness) may be needed for cesarean birth and for surgical intervention with some complications. The method used to achieve general anesthesia is usually a combination of intravenous injection and inhalation of anesthetic agents.

Complications of General Anesthesia

A primary danger of general anesthesia is fetal depression. Another significant risk is difficulty with maternal intubation. Pregnant women are more difficult to intubate than non-pregnant individuals. Most general anesthetic agents reach the fetus in about 2 minutes. The depression in the fetus is directly proportional to the depth and duration of the anesthesia. The poor fetal metabolism of general anesthetic agents is similar to that of analgesic agents administered during labor. General anesthesia is not advocated when the fetus is considered to be at high risk, particularly in preterm birth. Infants whose mothers receive general anesthesia suffer more respiratory depression than those whose mothers have received epidural anesthesia. Infants

born to mothers who have received general anesthesia have lower 1 minute Apgar scores than those who are given regional anesthesia for an emergency cesarean birth (Gori, Pasqualucci, Corradetti et al., 2007).

General anesthesia is associated with greater blood loss (Afolabi, Lesi, & Merah, 2006). The majority of general anesthetic agents cause some degree of uterine relaxation. They may also cause vomiting and aspiration. Because pregnancy results in decreased gastric motility, and the onset of labor halts the process almost entirely, food eaten hours earlier may remain undigested in the stomach. The nurse must find out when the laboring woman last ate and record this information on the client's chart and on her anesthesia record. Even when food and fluids have been withheld, the gastric juice produced during fasting is highly acidic and can cause chemical pneumonitis if aspirated. Women who receive general anesthesia may experience difficulty remembering events in the early postpartum period or may have some recall of the events during the birth.

Nursing Care Management

Prophylactic antacid therapy to reduce the acidic content of the stomach before general anesthesia is common practice. A nonparticulate antacid (such as bicitra) is often used. Cimetidine (Tagamet) has also been suggested by some analgesia providers (Cunningham et al., 2005). Famotidine is also commonly used. The use of prokinetic medications, such as metoclopramide, may also help empty gastric contents.

Before induction of anesthesia, the nurse places a wedge under the woman's right hip to displace the uterus and prevent vena caval compression in the supine position. The woman should also be preoxygenated with 3 to 5 minutes of 100% oxygen. Intravenous fluids are started so that access to the intravascular system is immediately available. During the preparation, the woman should be counseled on what to expect and should be told that the baby will have limited exposure to the anesthesia agents.

During the process of rapid induction of anesthesia, the nurse applies cricoid pressure to occlude the esophagus and prevent possible aspiration; the esophagus is oc-cluded by applying 1 to 2 kg before the loss of consciousness and increase that to 2 to 4 kg after the induction of anesthesia. The amount of pressure applied is critical because too much pressure can result in difficulty in performing a successful intubation. Too little pressure can result in aspiration. Cricoid pressure is maintained until the anesthesia provider has placed the endotracheal tube and indicates that the pressure can be released. Figure 20–7 ■ shows the appropriate technique.

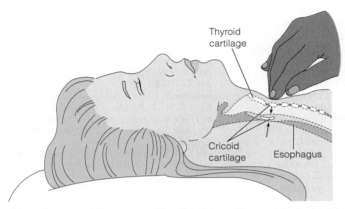

FIGURE 20–7 Proper position for fingers in applying cricoid pressure until a cuffed endotracheal tube is placed by the analgesia provider or certified nurse-anesthetist. The cricoid cartilage is depressed 2 to 3 cm posteriorly so that the esophagus is occluded.

Thyroid cartilage
Cricoid cartilage
Esophagus

HINTS FOR PRACTICE

Some women may wake from general anesthesia with an awareness of events that occurred during a cesarean birth. A small number of women experience unpleasant thoughts or nightmares as a result. If a woman expresses anxiety or states she has unpleasant memories of the birth, the nurse should encourage her to discuss her feelings and the experiences she remembers. The analgesia provider and physician should be notified so they can establish a therapeutic dialogue with the woman. Some women may have to be referred for counseling to prevent or treat post-traumatic stress disorder.

It should be noted that this discussion of obstetric analgesia and anesthesia applies only to a healthy woman and fetus. Pain relief during labor and birth for women with high-risk conditions, such as preterm labor, preeclampsia, blood disorders, or diabetes mellitus, requires skilled decision making, close observation, and awareness of all the potential threats to both the woman and her baby.

CHAPTER HIGHLIGHTS

- Pain relief during labor may be enhanced by childbirth preparation methods and by the administration of analgesics and/or regional anesthesia blocks.
- The goal of pharmacologic pain relief during labor is to provide maximum analgesia with minimal risk for the mother and fetus.
- The best time for administering analgesia is determined after a complete assessment. An analgesic agent is generally administered when cervical change has occurred.
- Analgesic agents include a variety of medications, such as butorphanol tartrate (Stadol), nalbuphine hydrochloride (Nubain), meperidine (Demerol), and fentanyl (Sublimaze).
- Opioid antagonists (such as naloxone) counteract the respiratory depressant effect of the opiate opioids by acting at specific receptor sites in the CNS.

- Regional analgesia and anesthesia are achieved by injecting local anesthetic agents into an area that will bring the agent into direct contact with nerve tissue. Methods most commonly used in childbearing include epidural block, spinal block, pudendal block, and local infiltration.
- Three types of local anesthetic agents used in regional blocks are the amides, esters, and opiates.
- Adverse reactions of the woman to local anesthetic agents range from mild symptoms such as palpitations to cardiovascular collapse.
- Complications of general anesthesia include fetal depression, uterine relaxation, vomiting, and aspiration.
- The choice of analgesia and anesthesia for the high-risk woman and fetus requires careful evaluation.

CHAPTER REFERENCES

Afolabi, B. B., Lesi, F. E., & Merah, N. A.(2006). Regional versus general anesthesia for caesarean section. *Cochrane Database Systematic Review, 18*(4), CD004350.

American College of Obstetricians and Gynecologists [ACOG]. (2002). Obstetrics analgesia and anesthesia (ACOG) Practice Bulletin No. 36.) Washington, DC: Author.

American College of Obstetricians and Gynecologists [ACOG]. (2006). ACOG committee opinion. No. 339: Analgesia and cesarean delivery rates. *Obstetrics & Gynecology, 107*(6), 1487–1488.

American Society of Anesthesiologists Task Force on Obstetric Anesthesia [ASAHQ]. (2006). Practice guidelines for obstetric anesthesia. Retrieved June 7, 2007, at http://www.asahq.org/publicationsAndServices/OBguide.pdf

Braveman, F. R. (2006). Obstetric and gynecologic anesthesia: The requisites. St. Louis, MO: Mosby.

Cunningham, F. G., MacDonald, P. C., Gant, N. F., Leveno, K. J., Gilstrap, L. C., Hankins, D. V., & Clark, S. L. (2005). *Williams obstetrics* (22nd ed.). Stamford, CT: Appleton & Lange.

Datta, S. (2006). *Obstetric anesthesia handbook* (4th ed.). New York: Springer Publishing Company.

Fitzgerald, M. P., Weber, A. M., Howden, N., Cundiff, G. W., Brown, M. B., & Pelvic Floor Disorders Network. (2007). Risk factors for anal sphincter tear during vaginal delivery. *Obstetrics & Gynecology, 109*(1), 29–34.

Gori, F., Pasqualucci, A., Corradetti, F., Milli, M., & Peduto, V. A. (2007). Maternal and neonatal

outcome after cesarean section: The impact of anesthesia. *Journal of Maternal Fetal Neonatal Medicine, 20*(1), 53–57.

Hawkins, J. L. (2008). Obstetric analgesia and anesthesia. In R. S. Gibbs, B. Y. Karlan, A. F. Haney & I. E. Nygaard (Eds.). Dansforth's obstetrics and gynecology. (10th ed., pp. 43–60). Philadelphia, PA: Lippincott Williams & Wilkins.

Hawkins, J. L., Goetzl, L., & Chestnut, D. H. (2007). Obstetric anesthesia. In S. G. Gabbe, J. R. Niebyl, & J. L. Simpson (Eds.), *Obstetrics: Normal and problem pregnancies* (5th ed., pp. 396–427). Philadelphia, PA: Churchill Livingstone.

Hughes, S. C., Levinson, G., Rosen, M. A., & Shnider, S. M. (2002). *Shnider and Levinson's anesthesia for obstetrics* (4th ed.). Phildelphia: Lippincott, Williams & Wilkins.

Martin, J. A., & Menacker, F. (2007). Expanded health data from the new birth certificate, 2004. *National Vital Statistics Report, 55*(12), 1–23.

Medscape. (2007a). Medscape drug guide: Demeral. Retrieved July 22, 2008, at http://www.medscape.com/druginfo/dosage?drugid=3914&drugname=Demeral+Inj&monotype=default

Medscape. (2007b). Medscape drug guide: Nubain. Retrieved July 12, 2008, at http://www.medscape.com/druginfo/dosage?drugid=11255&drugname=Nubain+Inj&monotype=default&cid=med.

Medscape. (2007c). Medscape drug guide: Stadol. Retrieved July 12, 2008, at http://www.medscape.com/druginfo/dosage?drugid=982&drguname=Stadol+Inj&monotype=default

Musselwhite, K. L., Faris, P., Moore, K., Berci, D., & King, K. M. (2007). Use of epidural anesthesia and the risk of acute postpartum urinary retention. *American Journal of Obstetrics & Gynecology, 196*(5), 472.e1–5.

Nelson, K. E., & Eisenach, J. C. (2005). Intravenous butorphanol, meperidine, and their combination relieve pain and distress in women in labor. *Anesthesiology, 102*(5), 1008–1013.

Ryan-Haddad, A. (2006). Options in analgesia in labor. *U.S. Pharmacist, 31*, 11. Retrieved June 6, 2007, at http://www.uspharmacist.com/index.asp?show=article&page=8_1893.htm

Sheiner, E., Walfisch, A., Hallak, M., Harlev, S., Mazor, M., & Shoham-Vardi, I. (2006). Length of the second stage of labor as a predictor of perineal outcome after vaginal delivery. *Journal of Reproductive Medicine, 51*(2), 115–119.

Vasudevan, A., Snowman, C. E., Sundar, S., Sarge, T. W., & Hess, P. E. (2007). Intrathecal morphine reduces breakthrough pain during labour epidural analgesia. *British Journal of Anaesthia, 98*(2), 241–245. Epub 2007 Jan 8.

Wilson, B. A., Shannon, M. T., & Shields, K. L., (Eds.). (2009). *Nurse's drug guide: 2009.* Upper Saddle River, NJ: Prentice Hall.

CHAPTER 21

Childbirth at Risk: Pre-Labor Complications

As a nurse midwife who has worked with high-risk pregnant women for over a decade, I have gained some insight into the challenges high-risk women face in trying to follow medical advice and in dealing with the realities of that advice. It was not until I spent nearly 6 months on bedrest with my 4th child, however, that I truly understood the hardships and difficulties they endure. As I found myself unable to care for my other children or to work as a nurse midwife, as I faced a variety of physical, emotional, and financial strains, I gained a new appreciation for all that a high-risk mother sacrifices for the well-being of her unborn child. These women need a great deal of support, education, and reassurance to deal with the daily struggles of a high-risk pregnancy.

—A Certified Nurse-Midwife and Former High-Risk Maternity Client

LEARNING OUTCOMES

21-1. Explain the possible causes, risk factors, and clinical therapy for premature rupture of the membranes or preterm labor in determining the hospital-based and community-based nursing care management of the woman and her fetus-newborn.

21-2. Compare placenta previa and abruptio placenta, including implications for the mother and fetus, as well as nursing care.

21-3. Explain the maternal and fetal-neonatal implications and the clinical therapy in determining the community-based and hospital-based nursing care management of the woman with multiple gestation.

21-4. Compare the identification, maternal and fetal-neonatal implications, clinical therapy, and nursing care management of women with hydramnios and oligohydramnios.

KEY TERMS

Abruptio placentae **491**
Hydramnios **498**
Oligohydramnios **499**
Placenta previa **489**
Premature rupture of membranes (PROM) **482**
Preterm labor (PTL) **484**
Tocolysis **485**

After the first trimester, the majority of pregnancies progress smoothly to term. In some cases, however, complications can occur before the onset of labor that significantly impact the outcome of pregnancy. This chapter presents content related to the most common of these conditions. It also serves as a prelude to the complications discussed in Chapter 22 ∞.

Care of the Woman with Premature Rupture of Membranes

Premature rupture of membranes (PROM) is spontaneous rupture of the membranes before the onset of labor. PROM affects approximately 5% to 10% of all pregnancies. *Preterm PROM (PPROM),* which affects approximately 3% of all pregnancies, is the rupture of membranes occurring before 37 weeks' gestation (Mercer, 2007). PPROM is associated with infection, previous history of PPROM, hydramnios, multiple pregnancy, urinary tract infection (UTI), amniocentesis, placenta previa, abruptio placentae, trauma, incompetent cervix, history of laser conization or LEEP procedure, bleeding during pregnancy, and maternal genital tract anomalies.

Maternal risk is related to infection, specifically *chorioamnionitis* and *endometritis* (postpartal infection of the endometrium). In addition, abruptio placentae occurs more frequently in women with PROM. Other rare complications include retained placenta and hemorrhage, maternal sepsis, and maternal death.

Fetal-newborn implications include risk of respiratory distress syndrome (with PPROM), fetal sepsis, malpresentation, prolapse of the umbilical cord, nonreassuring fetal heart rate tracings, compression of the umbilical cord, premature birth, and increased perinatal morbidity and mortality. Gestations from 32 to 36 weeks generally have favorable outcomes although there may be some complications. In general, infants born before 32 weeks have some complications, including respiratory distress syndrome (RDS), necrotizing enterocolitis, intraventricular hemorrhage, and sepsis. The earlier the gestational age, the greater the likelihood of infant complications (Mercer, 2007).

Cervical insufficiency or cervical incompetence is painless dilatation of the cervix without contractions because of a structural or functional defect of the cervix. The woman is usually unaware of contractions and presents with advanced effacement and dilatation and, possibly, bulging membranes. (ACOG, 2008).

Factors that may contribute to the tendency for the cervix to dilate prematurely can be divided into three categories: congenital factors, acquired factors, and biochemical (hormonal) factors. Endovaginal ultrasound

measurements of cervical length between 15 and 28 weeks' gestation identify groups at risk for preterm birth. Medical therapies used are serial cervical ultrasound assessments, bed rest, progesterone supplementation, antibiotics, and anti-inflammatory drugs (Berghella, et al., 2007; Mancuso & Owen, 2009). Surgical options include cervical and abdominal cerclage procedures.

Clinical Therapy

A sterile speculum examination is done to detect the presence of amniotic fluid in the vagina. If fluid is not obviously pooling, the diagnosis can be supported with nitrazine paper (which turns deep blue). Because certain bacterial pathogens can also result in a positive nitrazine test, a microscopic examination (ferning test) should be used as a confirmation of rupture because it is considered a definitive test. Digital examination increases the risk and is not recommended.

Fetal well-being is assessed through a fetal heart rate tracing or biophysical profile. The gestational age of the fetus is calculated in order to decide. If maternal signs and symptoms of infection are evident, antibiotic therapy (usually by intravenous infusion) is begun immediately, and the fetus is born vaginally or by cesarean regardless of the gestational age. Prophylactic antibiotics are often administered for the first 48 hours while awaiting culture results. Upon admission to the nursery, the newborn is assessed for sepsis and placed on antibiotics. (Chapter 29 ∞ provides further information about the newborn with sepsis.)

Management of PROM in the absence of infection and gestation of less than 37 weeks is usually conservative. On admission, complete blood cell count (CBC), C-reactive protein, and urinalysis are obtained. Cultures, including chlamydia, gonorrhea, and group B streptococcus, should be obtained. An ultrasound is obtained to determine gestational age, amniotic fluid level, and fetal well-being. Regular nonstress tests (NSTs) or biophysical profiles are used to monitor fetal well-being. (These tests are discussed in Chapter 16 ∞.) Maternal blood pressure, pulse, temperature, and fetal heart rate (FHR) are assessed every 4 hours. (see Chapter 16 ∞).

Maternal corticosteroid administration promotes fetal lung maturity and helps to prevent respiratory distress syndrome, intraventricular hemorrhage, necrotizing enterocolitis, perinatal death, and long-term neurological morbidity. Currently a single course of corticosteroids is recommended (see Drug Guide: Betamethasone).

Nursing Care Management

Nursing Assessment and Diagnosis

Determining the duration of the rupture of the membranes is a significant component of the intrapartal as-

MyNursingKit | Placenta Problems
MyNursingKit | Fetal Distress

Drug Guide   Betamethasone (Celestone Soluspan)

Overview of Maternal-Fetal Action   Studies have provided ample evidence that glucocorticoids such as betamethasone are capable of inducing pulmonary maturation and decreasing the incidence of respiratory distress syndrome in preterm infants. The mechanism by which corticosteroids accelerate fetal lung maturity is unclear, but it is related to the stimulation of enzyme activity by the drug. The enzyme is required for biosynthesis of surfactant by the type II pneumocytes. Surfactant is of major importance to the proper functioning of the lung in that it decreases the surface tension of the alveoli. Glucocorticoids also increase the rate of glycogen depletion, which leads to thinning of the interalveolar septa and increases the size of the alveoli. The thinning of the epithelium brings the capillaries into closer proximity with the air spaces and improves oxygen exchange.

Route, Dosage, Frequency   Prenatal maternal intramuscular injections of 12 mg of betamethasone are given once a day for 2 days. Dexamethasone has also been given in doses of 6 mg every 12 hours for four doses (Iams & Romero, 2007). To obtain maximum results, birth should be delayed for at least 24 hours after completing the first round of treatment. The effect of corticosteroids may be transient. Repeat courses of cortico-steroids should not be used routinely (Gibbs, 2008).

Contraindications

Inability to delay birth

Adequate L/S ratio

Presence of a condition that necessitates immediate birth (e.g., maternal bleeding)

Presence of maternal infection, diabetes mellitus (relative contraindication)

Gestational age greater than 34 completed weeks

Maternal Side Effects   Increased risk for infection has not been supported in large studies. There may, however, be some increase in the incidence of infection in women with premature rupture of the membranes. Maternal hyperglycemia may occur during corticosteroid administration. Insulin-dependent diabetics may require insulin infusions for several days to prevent ketoacidosis. Corticosteroids may possibly increase the risk of pulmonary edema, especially when used concurrently with tocolytics (Briggs, Freeman, & Yaffee, 2005).

Effects on Fetus/Newborn

Lowered cortisol levels at birth, but rebound occurs by 2 hours of age

Hypoglycemia

Increased risk of neonatal sepsis

Animal studies have shown serious fetal side effects such as reduced head circumference and decreased placental weight. Human studies have not shown these effects, however (Briggs et al., 2005).

Nursing Considerations

- Assess for presence of contraindications.
- Provide education regarding possible side effects.
- Administer betamethasone deep into gluteal muscle, avoiding injection into deltoid (high incidence of local atrophy). (Dexamethasone may be administered IM or IV.)
- Periodically evaluate BP, pulse, weight, and edema.
- Assess lab data for electrolytes and blood glucose.
- Although concomitant use of betamethasone and tocolytic agents has been implicated in increased risk of pulmonary edema, the betamethasone has little mineral corticoid activity; therefore, it probably doesn't add significantly to the salt and water retention effects of beta-adrenergic agonists. Other causes of noncardiogenic pulmonary edema should also be investigated if pulmonary edema develops during administration of betamethasone to a woman in preterm labor.

---

sessment. The nurse asks the woman when her membranes ruptured and when labor began. Gestational age is determined to prepare for the possibility of a preterm birth. The nurse observes the mother for signs and symptoms of infection, especially by reviewing her white blood cell (WBC) count, temperature, pulse rate, and the character of her amniotic fluid. When a preterm or cesarean birth is anticipated, the nurse evaluates the childbirth preparation and coping abilities of the woman and her partner.

Nursing diagnoses that may apply to a woman with PROM include the following:

- *Risk for Infection* related to premature rupture of membranes
- *Impaired Gas Exchange* in the fetus related to compression of the umbilical cord secondary to prolapse of the cord
- *Risk for Ineffective Individual Coping* related to unknown outcome of the pregnancy

Nursing Plan and Implementation

Uterine activity and fetal response to the labor are evaluated, but vaginal exams are not done unless absolutely

MyNursingKit | Guidelines for Managing the Second Stage of Labor

necessary because this increases the risk of infection. The woman is encouraged to rest on her left side to promote optimal uteroplacental perfusion. Comfort measures may help promote rest and relaxation. The nurse must also ensure that hydration is maintained, particularly if the woman's temperature is elevated.

Education is another important aspect of nursing care. The woman and her partner, if he is involved, need to understand the implications of PROM and all treatment methods. It is important to address side effects and alternative treatments. The couple needs to know that although the membranes are ruptured, amniotic fluid continues to be produced.

TEACHING TIP

To help a laboring woman and her family understand how the amniotic membranes provide protection, use a color chart that shows a side view of the fetus in the uterus with the membranes intact. Ask the couple to visualize what would happen if the membranes rupture. They will be able to see that pathogens have direct access to the uterus, increasing the risk of infection. They will also see that, when the membranes rupture and the fluid escapes, the cord could "wash out" with the fluid and become trapped between the pelvis and fetal head, causing cord compression.

Providing psychologic support for the couple is critical. The nurse may reduce anxiety by listening empathetically, relaying accurate information, and providing explanations of procedures. Preparing the couple for a cesarean birth, a preterm newborn, and the possibility of fetal or newborn demise may be necessary. Consultation with the neonatologist or pediatric provider can give the woman and her partner an opportunity to ask questions if a preterm birth is anticipated.

Evaluation

Expected outcomes of nursing care include the following:

- The woman's risk of infection and of cord prolapse decrease.
- The couple is able to discuss the implications of PROM and all treatments and alternative treatments.
- The couple verbalizes understanding that they did not cause the event.
- The pregnancy is maintained without trauma to the mother or fetus.

MyNursingKit | Premature Rupture of Membranes

Care of the Woman at Risk Because of Preterm Labor

Labor that occurs between 20 and 36 completed weeks of pregnancy is called **preterm labor (PTL)**. Prematurity continues to be the number one perinatal and neonatal

problem in the United States, with 12.7% of all live births occurring prematurely. In fact, the incidence of premature birth has risen by more than 20% since 1990 (March of Dimes, 2007). Often PTL is related to multiple risk factors; only rarely is there a single cause. Table 21–1 presents a list of risk factors for spontaneous preterm labor.

Maternal implications of PTL include psychologic stress related to the baby's condition and physiologic stress related to medical treatment for preterm labor.

Fetal-neonatal implications include increased morbidity and mortality, especially caused by respiratory distress syndrome (RDS), increased risk of trauma during birth, and maturational deficiencies (fat storage, heat regulation, immaturity of organ systems).

Clinical Therapy

Women who are at risk for PTL are taught to recognize the symptoms associated with preterm labor and, if any symptoms are present, to notify their certified nurse-midwife or physician immediately. Prompt diagnosis is necessary to

TABLE 21–1 Risk Factors for Spontaneous Preterm Labor	
Multiple gestation	Cervical shortening / 1 cm
DES exposure	Uterine irritability
Known cervical incompetence	Age (less than 17 or over 35)
Polyhydramnios	Low socioeconomic status
Uterine anomaly	Cigarettes—more than 10/day
Cervix dilated / 1 cm at 32 weeks	Substance abuse
Second-trimester abortion	Low maternal weight
Fetal abnormality	Poor weight gain
Febrile illness	More than two first-trimester abortions
Bleeding after 12 weeks	Non-white race
History of pyelonephritis or other maternal infection	Cervical cerclage in situ
Diabetes	In vitro fertilization (singleton or multiple gestation)
Previous preterm birth	STI (trichomoniasis, chlamydia)
Previous preterm labor with term birth	Anemia
Abdominal surgery during second or third trimester	Abdominal trauma
History of cone biopsy	Foreign body (e.g. IUD)
Uteroplacental ischemia	Bacterial vaginosis, E. coli (ascending intrauterine infection)
Stress	Periodontal disease
Inadequate or no prenatal care	Domestic violence
Lack of social support	Long work hours with prolonged standing
Hypertension (preeclampsia, gestational hypertension, chronic hypertension)	Clotting disorders
Obesity	Interval of less than 6 to 9 months between pregnancies

stop preterm labor before it progresses to the point at which intervention will be ineffective.

Prompt diagnosis of PTL is often difficult because many of the symptoms are common in normal pregnancy. Research suggests that the strongest predictors of preterm birth include the following: cervicovaginal fibronectin, abnormal cervical length on ultrasound, history of previous preterm birth, and the presence of infection (discussed later in this chapter) (Iams & Romero, 2007).

Fetal fibronectin (fFN) is a protein normally found in the fetal membranes and decidua. It is in the cervicovaginal fluid in early pregnancy but is not usually present in significant quantities between 22 and 37 weeks' gestation (Ness, Visintine, Ricci et al., 2007). A positive fFN test (fFN found in the cervicovaginal fluid) during this time puts the woman at increased risk for preterm birth. Conversely, a negative fFN in a woman with preterm contractions is associated with a very low risk of birth within 7 to 14 days (Ness et al., 2007). The test is over 99% accurate for predicting no preterm birth within 7 days. The procedure for collecting a sample is similar to that of the Pap smear; results can be available within 1 hour.

The length of the cervix can be measured fairly reliably after 16 weeks' gestation using an ultrasound probe inserted into the vagina. A cervix that is shorter than expected may be useful in assisting physician to identify the need for a cerclage to prevent preterm birth because of incompetent cervix. In general, cervical length less than 25 mm before term is abnormal (Iams & Romero, 2007).

Diagnosis of preterm labor is confirmed if the pregnancy is between 20 and 37 weeks, there are documented uterine contractions (four in 20 minutes or eight in 1 hour), and documented cervical change or cervical dilatation of greater than 1 cm (0.4 in.) or cervical effacement of 80% or more.

Labor is not interrupted if one or more of the following conditions are present: severe preeclampsia or eclampsia, chorioamnionitis, hemorrhage, maternal cardiac disease, poorly controlled diabetes mellitus or thyrotoxicosis, severe abruptio placentae, fetal anomalies incompatible with life, fetal death, nonreassuring fetal status, or fetal maturity.

The goal of clinical therapy is to prevent preterm labor from advancing to the point that it no longer responds to medical treatment. The initial management of preterm labor is directed toward maintaining good uterine blood flow, detecting uterine contractions, and ensuring that the fetus is stable. The mother is asked to lie on her side to increase placental profusion, an IV infusion is started to promote maternal hydration, and maternal laboratory studies including CBC, C-reactive protein, vaginal cultures, fetal fibronectin (fFN), and urine culture are completed. An ultrasound may be obtained to determine cervical shortening or funneling, as well as assess fetal well-being.

Tocolysis is the use of medications in an attempt to stop labor. Drugs currently used as tocolytics include the β-adrenergic agonists (also called β-mimetics), magnesium sulfate, cyclooxygenase (prostaglandin synthetase) inhibitors, and calcium channel blockers. The β-mimetics terbutaline sulfate (Brethine) and magnesium sulfate are the most widely used tocolytics.

Although tocolytic drugs suppress uterine contractions and allow pregnancy to continue, they may cause maternal side effects; the most serious is maternal pulmonary edema. Reducing the dose and duration of therapy sometimes reduces the side effects.

Recent research has indicated that outcomes are similar between magnesium sulfate and nifedipine (Procardia); however, nifedipine (Procardia) has significantly fewer maternal side effects and is becoming a first-line treatment in managing preterm labor (Lyell, Pullen, Campbell et al., 2007). The selection of magnesium sulfate, calcium channel blockers, or β-mimetics also depends on the experience of the healthcare providers. For magnesium sulfate, the recommended loading dose is 4 g IV in 100 mL of IV fluid using an infusion pump over 30 minutes, followed by a maintenance dose of 1 to 4 g/hr titrated to response and side effects (Iams & Romero, 2007). The therapy is continued for 12 hours after uterine contractions have stopped.

Side effects with the loading dose may include flushing, a feeling of warmth, headache, nystagmus, nausea, and dizziness. Other side effects include lethargy, sluggishness, and pulmonary edema (see Drug Guide: Magnesium Sulfate). Fetal side effects may include hypotonia and lethargy that persists for 1 or 2 days following birth. Respiratory depression in the newborn can also occur (Iams & Romero, 2007).

One calcium channel blocker, nifedipine (Procardia), is becoming increasingly popular in treating preterm labor because it is easily administered orally or sublingually and has few serious maternal side effects. It decreases smooth muscle contractions by blocking the slow calcium channels at the cell surface. The most common side effects are related to arterial vasodilation and include hypotension, tachycardia, facial flushing, and headache. Nifedipine may be coadministered with the β-mimetics. However, it should *not* be used with magnesium because both drugs block calcium and simultaneous administration has been implicated in serious maternal side effects related to low calcium levels.

Prostaglandin synthesis inhibitors (PSIs) such as indomethacin (Indocin) have been used for tocolysis in selected instances. Although this medication has been highly effective in delaying birth, potential fetal side effects, such as constriction of the ductus arteriosus, necrotizing enterocolitis (NEC), and intraventricular hemorrhage (IVH), have made it an uncommon treatment modality (Gill, 2004).

Drug Guide Magnesium Sulfate

Pregnancy Risk Category: B

Overview of Obstetric Action Magnesium sulfate acts as a CNS depressant by decreasing the quantity of acetylcholine released by motor nerve impulses and thereby blocking neuromuscular transmission. This action reduces the possibility of convulsion, which is why magnesium sulfate is used in the treatment of preeclampsia. Because magnesium sulfate secondarily relaxes smooth muscle, it may decrease the blood pressure, although it is not considered an antihypertensive. Magnesium sulfate may also decrease the frequency and intensity of uterine contractions; as a result it is also used as a tocolytic in the treatment of preterm labor.

Route, Dosage, Frequency Magnesium sulfate is generally given intravenously to control dosage more accurately and prevent overdosage. The intravenous route allows for immediate onset of action. It must be given by infusion pump for accurate dosage.

For Treatment of Preterm Labor

Loading dose: 4 to 8 g magnesium sulfate in a 10% to 20% solution administered over a 20 to 60 minute period.
Maintenance dose: 2 to 4 g/hr via infusion pump (Carey & Gibbs, 2008).

For Treatment of Preeclampsia

Loading dose: 4 to 6 g magnesium sulfate administered over a 20- to 30-minute period.
Maintenance dose: 2 to 3 g/hr via infusion pump (Habli & Sibai, 2008).

Note: Magnesium sulfate is excreted via the kidneys. Because women in preterm labor typically have normal renal function, they generally require higher levels of magnesium to achieve a therapeutic range than women who have preeclampsia and may have compromised renal function. Maintenance dose may need to be adjusted based on serum magnesium levels.

Maternal Contraindications Diagnosed maternal myasthenia gravis is the only absolute contraindication to the administration of magnesium sulfate. A history of myocardial damage or heart block is a relative contraindication to use of the drug because of the effects on nerve transmission and muscle contractility. Extreme care is necessary in administration to women with impaired renal function because the drug is eliminated by the kidneys, and toxic magnesium levels may develop quickly.

Maternal Side Effects Most maternal side effects are dose related. Lethargy and weakness related to neuromuscular blockade are common. Sweating, a feeling of warmth, flushing, and nasal congestion may be related to peripheral vasodilation. Other common side effects include nausea and vomiting, constipation, visual blurring, headache, and slurred speech. Signs of developing toxicity include depression or absence of reflexes, oliguria, confusion, respiratory depression, circulatory collapse, and respiratory paralysis. Rapid administration of large doses may cause cardiac arrest. If any of these occur, the drip should be stopped immediately.

Effects on Fetus/Newborn The drug readily crosses the placenta. Some authorities suggest that transient decrease in FHR variability may occur; others report that no change occurred. In general, magnesium sulfate therapy does not pose a risk to the fetus. Occasionally, the newborn may demonstrate neurologic depression or respiratory depression, loss of reflexes, and muscle weakness. Ill effects in the newborn may actually be related to fetal growth retardation, prematurity, or perinatal asphyxia.

Nursing Considerations

- Monitor the blood pressure every 10 to 15 minutes during administration.
- Monitor maternal serum magnesium levels as ordered (usually every 6 to 8 hours). Therapeutic levels are in the range of 4 to 8 mg/dL. Reflexes often disappear at serum magnesium levels of 9 to 13 mg/dL; respiratory depression occurs at levels of 14 mg/dL; cardiac arrest occurs at levels above 30 mg/L (Rideout, 2005).
- Monitor respirations closely. If the rate is less than 12/minute, magnesium toxicity may be developing, and further assessments are indicated. Many protocols require stopping the medication if the respiratory rate falls below 12/minute.
- Assess knee jerk (patellar tendon reflex) for evidence of diminished or absent reflexes. Loss of reflexes is often the first sign of developing toxicity. Also note marked lethargy or decreased level of consciousness and hypotension.
- Determine urinary output. Output less than 30 mL/hr may result in the accumulation of toxic levels of magnesium.
- If the respirations or urinary output fall below specified levels or if the reflexes are diminished or absent, no further magnesium should be administered until these factors return to normal.
- The antagonist of magnesium sulfate is calcium. Consequently, an ampule of calcium gluconate should be available at the bedside. The usual dose is 1 g given IV over a period of about 3 minutes.
- Monitor fetal heart tones continuously with IV administration.
- Continue magnesium sulfate infusion for approximately 24 hours after birth as prophylaxis against postpartum seizures if given for preeclampsia.
- If the mother has received magnesium sulfate close to birth, the newborn should be closely observed for signs of magnesium toxicity for 24 to 48 hours.
- The antidote for magnesium sulfate is calcium gluconate. Calcium gluconate should always be on hand in case the magnesium levels get too high.

Note: Protocols for magnesium sulfate administration may vary somewhat according to agency policy. Consequently, individuals are referred to their own agency protocols for specific guidelines.

(ACOG) (2003a) recommends that corticosteroids (typically betamethasone or dexamethasone) be administered antenatally to women at risk for preterm birth because of their beneficial effect on the prevention of neonatal respiratory distress syndrome (RDS), intraventricular hemorrhage (IVH), necrotizing enterocolitis (NEC), and neonatal mortality (ACOG, 2003a). Women who are candidates for tocolysis are candidates for antenatal corticosteroids, regardless of fetal gender, race, or availability of surfactant therapy for the newborn, especially between 24 and 34 weeks' gestation (see Drug Guide: Betamethasone). Betamethasone is primarily used and should be administered in two intramuscular doses. When dexamethasone is used, four doses are given.

Recent research trials have shown that progesterone therapy is effective in reducing the incidence of preterm birth, at least in certain high-risk populations (Fonseca, Celik, Parra et al., 2007; How, Barton, Istwan et al., 2007). Currently experts are evaluating whether this therapy should become an accepted part of clinical practice. Further research is indicated to determine if progesterone can prevent preterm births in woman with multiple gestations and shortened cervical lengths.

Nursing Care Management

Nursing Assessment and Diagnosis

During the antepartal period, the nurse identifies the woman at risk for preterm labor by noting the presence of risk factors. During the intrapartal period, the nurse assesses the progress of labor and the physiologic impact of labor on the mother and fetus.

Nursing diagnoses that may apply to the woman with preterm labor include the following:

- *Fear* related to risk of early labor and birth
- *Ineffective Individual Coping* related to need for constant attention to pregnancy
- *Acute Pain* related to uterine contractions

Nursing Plan and Implementation

Community-Based Nursing Care

Once the woman at risk for preterm labor has been identified, she needs to be taught about the importance of recognizing the onset of labor (see Client Teaching: Preterm Labor). This teaching is often provided by clinic nurses or home care nurses.

Home uterine activity monitoring transmitted by telemetry to review stations, combined with daily telephone calls from a nurse to offer support and advice, remains a common approach to care following discharge. Research indicates that when women are monitored at home, there is a lower incidence of preterm births when compared with women who receive standard obstetric care in an outpatient setting (Morrison & Chauhan, 2003; Newman, 2005). Periodic home visits by a home care nurse are also a common part of care. During these visits the nurse completes physical assessments similar to those done in the hospital and assesses the woman's emotional state. The nurse can also provide information about support groups and other community resources for women at risk for preterm birth. Referrals for in-home services, such as assistance with child care, cleaning, and cooking, are also essential to ensure that women who have been placed on bed rest are able to maintain medically indicated restrictions.

Increasing the woman's awareness of the signs and symptoms of preterm labor is one of the nurse's most important teaching objectives. These include the following:

- Uterine contractions that occur every 10 minutes or less, with or without pain
- Mild menstrual-like cramps felt low in the abdomen
- Constant or intermittent feelings of pelvic pressure that feel like the baby pressing down
- Rupture of membranes
- Constant or intermittent low, dull backache
- A change in the vaginal discharge (an increase in amount, a change to more clear and watery, or a pinkish tinge)
- Abdominal cramping with or without diarrhea

The woman is also taught to evaluate contraction activity once or twice a day. She does so by lying down tilted to one side with a pillow behind her back for support. The woman places her fingertips on the fundus of the uterus, which is above the umbilicus (navel). She checks for contractions (hardening or tightening in the uterus) for about 1 hour. It is important for the pregnant woman to know that uterine contractions occur occasionally throughout the pregnancy. If they occur every 10 minutes for 1 hour, however, the cervix could begin to dilate, and labor could ensue.

The nurse ensures that the woman knows when to report signs and symptoms. If contractions occur every 10 minutes (or more frequently) for 1 hour, if any of the other signs and symptoms are present for 1 hour, or if clear fluid begins leaking from the vagina, the woman should telephone her physician or certified nurse-midwife, clinic, or hospital birthing unit and make arrangements to be checked for ongoing labor. Caregivers need to be aware that the woman's call must be taken seriously. When a woman is at risk for preterm labor, she may have many episodes of contractions and other signs or symptoms. If she is treated positively, she will feel freer to report problems as they arise.

Preventive self-care measures are also important. The nurse has a vital role in communicating the self-care measures described in Table 21–2.

Client Teaching PRETERM LABOR

Content	**Teaching Method**
• Describe the dangers of preterm labor, especially the risk of prematurity in the infant, and all the potential problems.	Discuss the risks specifically. Many people understand in a general way that prematurity can be dangerous, but they fail to understand how the baby is affected.
• Although decreased because of insurance reimbursements, stress the value of home monitoring in evaluating uterine activity on a regular basis if ordered. Emphasize that many of the early symptoms of labor, such as backache and increased vaginal discharge, may be subtle initially. Home monitoring can often detect increased uterine activity in the early stages before cervical changes progress to the point where it is impossible to stop labor.	Use handouts during the discussion. Help the woman clearly understand the value of the program because, to be successful, it requires a real commitment on her part.
If the woman is to be part of a home monitoring program, the monitoring nurse will usually do the initial teaching. Be prepared to reinforce the information provided and answer questions that may arise.	Teach the woman how to palpate for uterine contractions. Do a demonstration and ask for a return demonstration.
• Summarize self-care measures, such as maintaining generous fluid intake (2 to 3 quarts daily), voiding every 2 hours, avoiding lifting and overexertion, avoiding nipple stimulation or orgasm, limiting sexual activity, and cooperating with activity restrictions and bed rest requirements.	Use a handout during the discussion. Provide opportunities for discussion. If the woman has concerns about certain recommendations, try to modify the approach to best meet her needs.

TABLE 21–2 Self-Care Measures to Prevent Preterm Labor

• Rest two or three times a day lying on your left side.

• Drink 2 to 3 quarts of water or fluid each day. Avoid caffeine drinks. Filling a quart container and drinking from it will eliminate the need to keep track of numerous glasses of fluid.

• Empty your bladder at least every 2 hours during waking hours.

• Avoid lifting heavy objects. If small children are in the home, work out alternatives for picking them up, such as sitting on a chair and having them climb on your lap.

• Avoid prenatal breast preparation such as nipple rolling or rubbing nipples with a towel. This is not meant to discourage breastfeeding but to avoid the potential increase in uterine irritability.

• Pace necessary activities to avoid overexertion.

• Curtail or eliminate sexual activity, if necessary.

• Find pleasurable ways to help compensate for limitations of activities and boost the spirits.

• Try to focus on 1 day or 1 week at a time rather than on longer periods of time.

• If on bed rest, get dressed each day and rest on a couch rather than becoming isolated in the bedroom.

Source: Prepared in consultation with Susan Bennett, RN, ACCE, Coordinator of the Prematurity Prevention Program.

Hospital-Based Nursing Care

Supportive nursing care is important to the woman in preterm labor during hospitalization. This care consists of promoting bed rest, monitoring vital signs (especially blood pressure and respirations), measuring intake and output, and continuous monitoring of FHR and uterine contractions. Placing the woman on her left side facilitates maternal-fetal circulation. Vaginal examinations are kept to a minimum. If medications are being used, the nurse administers them and closely monitors the mother and fetus for any adverse effects.

Whether preterm labor is arrested or proceeds, the woman and her partner, if involved, experience intense psychologic stress. Decreasing the anxiety associated with the risk of a preterm newborn by providing emotional support is a primary aim of the nurse. The nurse also recognizes the stress of prolonged bed rest and of lack of sexual contact and helps the couple find satisfactory ways of dealing with those stresses. With empathetic communication, the nurse can assist the couple to express their feelings, which commonly include guilt and anxiety, thereby helping the couple identify and implement coping mechanisms. The nurse also keeps the couple informed about the labor progress, the treatment regimen, and the status of the fetus. In the event of imminent vaginal or cesarean birth, the couple should be offered brief but ongoing explanations to prepare them for the actual birth process and the events following the birth. The nurse can also arrange for consultations for the neonatologist or pediatrician to assist the couple in anticipating potential neonatal complications and risks for the newborn.

Evaluation

Expected outcomes of nursing care include the following:

- The woman is able to discuss the cause, identification, and treatment of preterm labor.
- The woman states that she feels comfortable in her ability to cope with her situation and has resources available to her.
- The woman can describe appropriate self-care measures and can identify characteristics that need to be reported to her caregiver.
- The woman successfully gives birth to a healthy infant.
- Both premature rupture of the membranes and preterm labor place the fetus at risk. Women with PROM and no signs of infection are managed conservatively with bed rest and careful monitoring of fetal well-being. If preterm labor develops, tocolytics are often effective in stopping labor, but they have associated side effects.

Care of the Woman at Risk Because of Bleeding During Pregnancy

Bleeding during pregnancy always requires assessment. The most common causes of bleeding during the first and second trimesters, namely spontaneous abortion, ectopic pregnancy, gestational trophoblastic disease, and incompetent cervix, are addressed in Chapter 16 ∞. The two most clinically significant causes of bleeding in the second half of pregnancy, placenta previa and abruption placentae, are discussed here. Other placental problems are addressed in Chapter 22 ∞.

Placenta Previa

In **placenta previa,** the placenta is implanted in the lower uterine segment rather than the upper portion of the uterus. This implantation may be on a portion of the lower segment or over the internal cervical os. As the lower uterine segment contracts and dilates in the later weeks of pregnancy, the placental villi are torn from the uterine wall, thus exposing the uterine sinuses at the placental site. Bleeding begins, but because its amount depends on the number of sinuses exposed, initially it may be either scanty or profuse (Figure 21–1 ■). Placenta previa is categorized as being *complete* (the internal os is completely covered), *partial* (the internal os is partially covered), *marginal* (the edge of the placenta is covered), or *low-lying* (the placenta is implanted in the lower uterine segment in close proximity to but not covering the os) (Cunningham et al., 2005).

The cause of placenta previa is unknown. Statistically it occurs in about 4 per 1000 births (Francois & Foley, 2007). Women who are black or minorities and women who have undergone a prior cesarean birth are at higher risk of placenta previa. Other risk factors include high gravidity, high parity, advanced maternal age, previous miscarriage, previous induced abortion, cigarette smoking, and male fetus (Kay, 2008).

Fetal-Neonatal Implications

The prognosis for the fetus depends on the extent of placenta previa. In cases of a marginal previa or a low-lying placenta, the woman may be allowed to labor. Changes in the FHR and meconium staining of the amniotic fluid may be apparent. In a profuse bleeding episode, the fetus is compromised and suffers some hypoxia. FHR monitoring is imperative when the woman is admitted, particularly if a vaginal birth is anticipated, because the presenting part of the fetus may obstruct the flow of blood from the placenta or umbilical cord. If nonreassuring fetal status occurs,

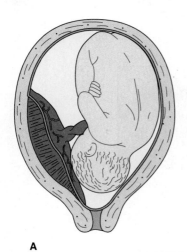 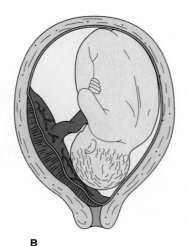 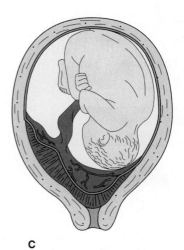

A   B   C

Figure 21–1 Placenta previa. *A,* Low placental implantation. *B,* Partial placenta previa. *C,* Total placenta previa.

cesarean birth is indicated. Women who are diagnosed with a complete or partial previa will undergo a cesarean birth because the risk of intrapartum hemorrhage is high. After birth, blood sampling should be done to determine whether the intrauterine bleeding episodes of the woman have caused anemia in the newborn.

Clinical Therapy

The goal of medical care is to identify the cause of bleeding and to provide treatment that will ensure birth of a mature newborn. Indirect diagnosis is made by localizing the placenta through tests that require no vaginal examination, such as a transabdominal ultrasound scan. Until placenta previa is ruled out, vaginal examinations should never be performed on a woman with bleeding because the examiner's fingers could perforate the placenta if cervical dilatation has occurred. Once placenta previa is ruled out, a vaginal examination can be performed with a speculum to determine the cause of bleeding (such as cervical lesions).

The differential diagnosis of placental or cervical bleeding takes careful consideration. Partial separation of the placenta may also present with painless bleeding, and true placenta previa may not demonstrate overt bleeding until labor begins, thus confusing the diagnosis.

Care of the woman with painless late-gestational bleeding depends on (1) the week of gestation during which the first bleeding episode occurs and (2) the amount of bleeding (Figure 21–2 ■). If the pregnancy is less than 37 weeks' gestation, expectant management is employed to delay birth until about 37 weeks' gestation to allow the fetus to mature. Expectant management involves stringent regulation of the following:

1. Providing bed rest with bathroom privileges as long as the woman is not bleeding
2. Performing no vaginal exams
3. Monitoring blood loss, pain, and uterine contractility
4. Evaluating FHR with an external fetal monitor
5. Monitoring maternal vital signs
6. Performing a complete laboratory evaluation: hemoglobin, hematocrit, Rh factor, and urinalysis
7. Providing intravenous fluid (lactated Ringer's solution)
8. Having two units of crossmatched blood available for transfusion

If frequent, recurrent, or profuse bleeding persists, or if fetal well-being appears threatened, a cesarean birth may be required.

Nursing Care Management

Nursing Assessment and Diagnosis

Assessment of the woman with placenta previa must be ongoing to prevent or treat complications that are potentially lethal to the mother and fetus. Painless, bright-red vaginal bleeding is the most accurate diagnostic sign of placenta previa. If this sign develops during the last

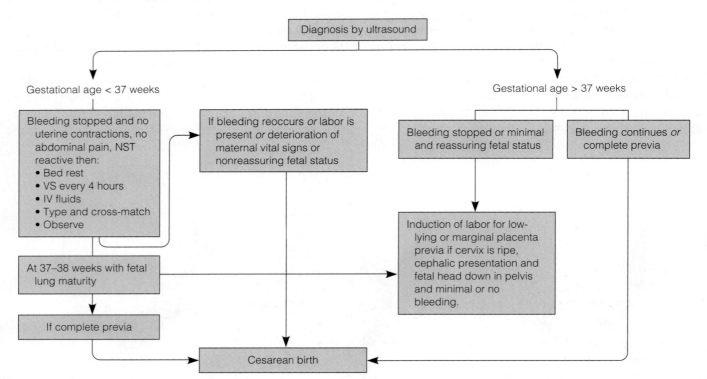

FIGURE 21–2 Management of placenta previa.
Source: Zuspan, F. P., & Quilligan, E. J. (1998). *Handbook of obstetrics, gynecology, and primary care.* Copyright 1998, with permission from Elsevier Science.

3 months of pregnancy, placenta previa should always be considered until ruled out by ultrasound examination. The first bleeding episode is generally scanty. If no vaginal examinations are performed, it often subsides spontaneously. However, each subsequent hemorrhage is more profuse.

The uterus remains soft; if labor begins, it relaxes fully between contractions. The FHR usually remains stable unless profuse hemorrhage and maternal shock occur. As a result of the placement of the placenta, the fetal presenting part is often unengaged, and transverse lie is common.

The nurse assesses blood loss, pain, and uterine contractility both subjectively and objectively. Maternal vital signs and the results of blood and urine tests provide the nurse with additional data about the woman's condition. The FHR is evaluated with continuous external fetal monitoring. Another pressing nursing responsibility is to observe and verify the family's ability to cope with the anxiety associated with an unknown outcome.

Nursing diagnoses that may apply include the following:

- *Fluid Volume Deficit* related to hypovolemia secondary to excessive blood loss
- *Risk for Impaired Gas Exchange* of the fetus related to decreased blood volume and maternal hypotension
- *Anxiety* related to concern for own personal status and the baby's safety

Nursing Plan and Implementation

The nurse monitors the woman and her fetus to determine the status of the bleeding and the responses of the mother and baby. Vital signs, intake and output, and other pertinent assessments must be made frequently. The nurse uses the electronic monitor tracing to evaluate fetal status. A whole-blood setup should be ready for intravenous infusion and a patent intravenous line established before caregivers undertake any invasive procedures. Maternal vital signs should be monitored every 15 minutes in the absence of hemorrhage and every 5 minutes with active hemorrhage. The external tocodynamometer should be connected to the maternal abdomen to continuously monitor uterine activity.

Provision of emotional support for the family is an important nursing care goal. During active bleeding, the assessments and management must be directed toward physical support. However, emotional aspects need to be addressed simultaneously. The nurse can explain the assessments and treatment measures needed. Time can be provided for questions, and the nurse can act as an advocate in obtaining information for the family. Emotional support can also be offered by staying with the family and using touch.

Promotion of neonatal physiologic adaptation is another important nursing responsibility. The newborn's hemoglobin, cell volume, and erythrocyte count should be checked immediately and then monitored closely. The newborn may require oxygen, administration of blood, and admission into a special-care nursery.

Evaluation

Anticipated outcomes of nursing care include the following:

- The cause of hemorrhage is recognized promptly and corrective measures are taken.
- The woman's vital signs remain in the normal range.
- Any other complications are recognized and treated early.
- The family understands what has happened and the implications and associated problems of placenta previa.
- The woman and her baby have a safe labor and birth.

Abruptio Placentae

Abruptio placentae is the premature separation of a normally implanted placenta from the uterine wall. Premature separation, the leading cause of perinatal mortality, is considered a catastrophic event because of the severity of the resulting hemorrhage. The incidence of abruptio placentae is 0.5% to 1.0% of all pregnancies but it accounts for 10% to 15% of all perinatal deaths (Kay, 2008).

The cause of abruptio placentae is largely unknown. Risk factors associated with placental abruption include increased maternal age, increased parity, cigarette smoking, cocaine abuse, trauma, maternal hypertension, rapid uterine decompression associated with hydramnios and multiple gestation, PPROM, uterine malformations or fibroids, placental anomalies, previous abruption, and inherited thrombophilia (Francois & Foley, 2007).

Abruptio placentae is subdivided into three types (Figure 21–3 ■):

- *Marginal.* In this case the placenta separates at its edges, the blood passes between the fetal membranes and the uterine wall, and the blood escapes vaginally (also called marginal sinus rupture).
- *Central.* In this situation, the placenta separates centrally, and the blood is trapped between the placenta and the uterine wall. Entrapment of the blood results in concealed bleeding.
- *Complete.* Massive vaginal bleeding is seen in the presence of total separation.

Abruptio placentae may also be graded according to the severity of clinical and laboratory findings as follows (Francois & Foley, 2007):

- *Grade 1.* Mild separation with slight vaginal bleeding. Fetal heart rate (FHR) pattern and maternal blood pressure unaffected. Accounts for 40% of abruptions.

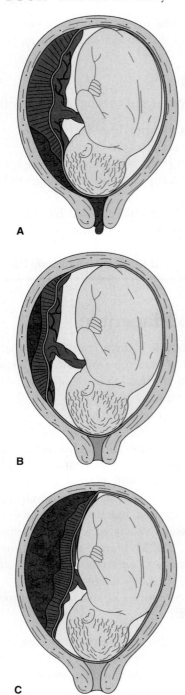

FIGURE 21–3 Abruptio placentae. *A*, Marginal abruption with external hemorrhage. *B*, Central abruption with concealed hemorrhage. *C*, Complete separation.

- *Grade 2.* Partial abruption with moderate bleeding. Significant uterine irritability is present. Maternal pulse may be elevated although blood pressure is stable. Signs of fetal compromise evident in FHR. Accounts for 45% of abruptions.
- *Grade 3.* Large or complete separation with moderate to severe bleeding. Maternal shock and painful uterine contractions present. Fetal death common. Accounts for about 15% of abruptions.

The signs and symptoms of placental abruption are listed in Table 21–3. In severe cases of central abruptio placentae, the blood invades the myometrial tissues between the muscle fibers. This occurrence accounts for the uterine irritability that is a significant sign of abruptio placentae. If hemorrhage continues, eventually the uterus turns entirely blue because the muscle fibers are filled with blood. After birth the uterus contracts poorly. This condition is known as a *Couvelaire uterus* and frequently necessitates hysterectomy.

Maternal Implications

As a result of the damage to the uterine wall and the retroplacental clotting with central abruption, large amounts of thromboplastin are released into the maternal blood supply. This thromboplastin in turn triggers the development of DIC and resultant hypofibrinogenemia. Fibrinogen levels, which are ordinarily elevated in pregnancy, may drop in minutes to the point at which blood will no longer coagulate.

Maternal mortality is now uncommon, although maternal morbidity still occurs (Cunningham et al., 2005). Postpartal problems depend in large part on the severity of the intrapartal bleeding, coagulation defects (DIC), hypofibrinogenemia, and time between separation and birth. Moderate to severe hemorrhage results in hemorrhagic shock, which may prove fatal to the mother if it is not rapidly reversed. In the postpartal period, women with this disorder are at risk for hemorrhage and renal failure

TABLE 21–3	Differential Signs and Symptoms of Placenta Previa and Abruptio Placentae	
	Placenta Previa	Abruptio Placentae
Onset	Quiet and sneaky	Sudden and stormy
Bleeding	External	External or concealed
Color of blood	Bright red	Dark venous
Anemia	= to blood loss	Greater than apparent blood loss
Shock	= to blood loss	Greater than apparent blood loss
Toxemia	Absent	May be present
Pain	Only labor	Severe and steady
Uterine tenderness	Absent	Present
Uterine tone	Soft and relaxed	Firm to stony hard
Uterine contour	Normal	May enlarge and change shape
Fetal heart tones	Usually present	Present or absent
Engagement	Absent	May be present
Presentation	May be abnormal	*No relationship*

Source: Oxorn, H. (1986). *Human labor and birth* (5th ed., p. 507). Norwalk, CT: Appleton & Lange.

caused by shock, vascular spasm, intravascular clotting, or a combination of these factors.

Fetal-Neonatal Implications

Perinatal mortality associated with abruptio placentae is about 25% (Cunningham et al., 2005). In severe cases, in which most of the placenta has separated, the infant mortality rate is near 100%. In less severe separation, fetal outcome depends on the level of maturity and the length of time to birth. The most serious complications in the newborn arise from preterm labor, anemia, and hypoxia. If fetal hypoxia progresses unchecked, irreversible brain damage or fetal demise may result. Thorough assessment and prompt action on the part of the healthcare team can improve both fetal and maternal outcomes.

Clinical Therapy

Because of the risk of DIC, evaluating the results of coagulation tests is imperative. In DIC, fibrinogen levels and platelet counts usually decrease; prothrombin times and partial thromboplastin times are normal to prolonged. If the values are not markedly abnormal, serial testing may be helpful in establishing an abnormal trend indicative of coagulopathy. Another test determines levels of fibrin-degradation products; these values rise with DIC.

After establishing the diagnosis, immediate priorities are maintaining the cardiovascular status of the mother and developing a plan for the birth of the fetus. The birth method selected depends on the condition of the woman and fetus and the speed in which the birth will occur; in many circumstances, cesarean birth will be the safest option.

If the separation is mild and the pregnancy is late preterm, labor may be induced and the fetus born vaginally with as little trauma as possible. If rupture of membranes and oxytocin infusion by pump do not initiate labor, a cesarean birth is required. A long delay would raise the risk of increased hemorrhage, with resulting hypofibrinogenemia. Supportive actions to decrease the risk of DIC include typing and crossmatching for blood transfusions (at least three units), evaluating the clotting mechanism, and providing intravenous fluids.

In cases of moderate to severe placental separation, a cesarean birth is done after treatment of hypofibrinogenemia by intravenous infusion of cryoprecipitate or fresh frozen plasma. Vaginal birth is impossible with a Couvelaire uterus, because the uterus would not contract properly in labor, and a hysterectomy is often needed.

The hypovolemia that accompanies severe abruptio placentae is life threatening and must be combated with whole blood. If the fetus is alive but experiencing stress, emergency cesarean birth is the method of choice. With a stillborn fetus, vaginal birth is preferable if bleeding has stabilized, unless maternal shock from hemorrhage is un-

controllable. Intravenous fluids are administered. Central venous pressure (CVP) monitoring may be needed to evaluate intravascular fluid replacement. An absolute level is not as important as the response to fluid replacement. CVP is evaluated hourly, and the results are communicated to the physician. Elevations of CVP may indicate fluid overload and pulmonary edema. Laboratory testing is ordered to provide ongoing data regarding hemoglobin, hematocrit, and coagulation status. The hematocrit is maintained at 30% through the administration of packed red blood cells or whole blood (Cunningham et al., 2005). Measures are taken to stimulate labor to effect a vaginal birth, if possible. An amniotomy may be performed, and oxytocin is given. Progressive dilatation and effacement usually occur.

Nursing Care Management

Electronic monitoring of the uterine contractions and resting tone between contractions provides information about the labor pattern and effectiveness of the oxytocin induction. Because uterine resting tone is frequently increased with abruptio placentae, it must be evaluated frequently for further increase. Abdominal girth measurements may be ordered hourly and are obtained by placing a tape measure around the maternal abdomen at the level of the umbilicus. Another method of evaluating uterine size, which increases as more bleeding occurs at the site of abruption, involves placing a mark at the top of the uterine fundus; the distance from the symphysis pubis to the mark may be measured hourly. Overdistention of the uterus can lead to a ruptured uterus, another life-threatening complication. See the Nursing Care Plan for a Woman with Hemorrhage in the Third Trimester and at Birth.

Care of the Woman with Multiple Gestation

In part because of advances in infertility treatments, the incidence of twins in the United States has increased by 65% since 1980 (ACOG, 2004). In 2004, the rate of twins was 32.2 per 1000 births. Although the number of twins rose by 2%, triplet and higher-order multiple births decreased by 6% to 176.9 per 100,000 for triplets and 187.4 per 100,000 for higher-order multiple births (Martin, Hamilton, Sutton et al., 2006). The reduction in triplet and higher-order multiple births has been driven by recommendations to transfer fewer embryos during in-vitro fertilization (IVF) procedures in an attempt to decrease neonatal mortality and morbidity that is common in triplet and higher-order multiple births. Multifetal births account for only 3% of all births in the United States (ACOG, 2004). The incidence of spontaneous twins varies but is highest among African Americans, women of greater age and parity, women with

Nursing Care Plan   For a Woman with Hemorrhage in Third Trimester and at Birth

CLIENT SCENARIO

Manuela Suarez is 34 years old, G5P4, and at term (38 weeks) when she is transported to the labor and birthing unit via stretcher. She is experiencing sharp pain on the left side of her abdomen and has been bleeding heavily over the last hour. Manuela states that the contractions have been lasting 45 to 60 seconds every 8 to 10 minutes over the last 3 hours. The nurse assesses dark red venous bleeding and palpates Manuela's abdomen, which is rigid. The nurse places Manuela on an external fetal monitor, starts an IV, and draws blood to evaluate platelet, hemoglobin, and fibrinogen levels. Partial thromboplastin time (PTT) levels are also evaluated.

The nurse provides emotional care to Manuela as well as factual information and reassurance about her care. The nurse also explains the procedures while including Manuela in the plan of care.

ASSESSMENT

Subjective: Sharp pain in abdomen and tender upon palpation

Objective: Dark red bleeding with saturation of a pad in 1 hour, rigid abdomen, BP 100/70, urine output over last 2 hours 80 mL

Nursing Diagnosis #1	Deficient Fluid Volume related to hypovolemia secondary to excessive blood loss from placental abruption*
Client Goal	Client will remain hemodynamically stable.
AEB:	• Vital signs within normal limits • Lab values within normal range • Urinary output greater than 30 mL per hour with specific gravity within normal range • Central venous pressure within normal range • No signs of DIC

NURSING INTERVENTIONS

1. In active hemorrhage, monitor vital signs every 5 minutes and compare to maternal baseline measurements.

2. Evaluate pulse pressure and quality of pulse, and determine pulse deficit hourly.

3. Inspect skin color, temperature, and capillary refill.

4. Count and weigh pads hourly. Record pad saturation amount using a specific amount of time (50 mL dark red blood on pad in 20 minutes).

5. Administer whole blood or packed red blood cells via IV with a large gauge cannula.

RATIONALES

Rationale: Vital signs indicate maternal systemic responses to blood loss. For example, hypotension (BP less than 90/60) indicates loss of large amounts of circulatory fluid or lack of compensation in circulatory system and the need for whole blood administration.

Rationale: Pulse is used to evaluate maternal effects of blood loss. Pulse pressure can be assessed by evaluating the difference between the systolic and diastolic pressure (normally 30 to 40 mm Hg). As cardiac output decreases, there is usually a fall in pulse pressure. Quality of pulse should be even in rhythm and normal (+2) in strength. A thready pulse may indicate vasoconstriction and reflects decreased cardiac output; peripheral pulses may be absent if vasoconstriction is intense. Pulse deficit occurs when the peripheral pulse is less than the apical pulse, which may indicate a lack of peripheral perfusion.

Rationale: To assess for tissue perfusion and oxygenation. Skin should not exhibit signs of pallor or cyanosis and should not be cold or clammy. Normal capillary refill is less than 3 seconds.

Rationale: To monitor blood loss (1 g = 1 mL of blood).

Rationale: A large gauge cannula is needed to allow IV fluids to be administered quickly and can be used for the administration of blood products such as whole blood or packed red blood cells. Blood products may be needed to replace blood loss and maintain hematocrit levels at 30% (see text for normal levels). While waiting for whole blood to be available, infuse isotonic fluids, plasma, plasma expanders, or serum albumin per physician orders.

Nursing Care Plan	For a Woman with Hemorrhage in Third Trimester and at Birth (Continued)

NURSING INTERVENTIONS

6. Review and evaluate diagnostic tests.

7. Measure central venous pressure hourly.

8. Evaluate level of consciousness frequently.

9. Monitor urinary output via urinary catheter and urine-specific gravities.

10. Monitor for signs of DIC.

11. Assess uterine resting tone every 15 minutes and abdominal girth hourly in suspected placental abruption.

12. Prepare client for possible cesarean section.

RATIONALES

Rationale: To assess for the maternal effects of blood loss and the possibility of DIC. Diagnostic tests should include hemoglobin levels (normal range 10 to 14 g/dL), hematocrit (normal range 32% to 42%), partial thromboplastin time (normal levels for nonpregnant woman are 12 to 14 seconds but in normal pregnancy it will be slightly decreased), fibrinogen levels (normal is 400 mg/dL), platelets are decreased (nonpregnant values = 150,000 to 350,000/mm^3). If admission lab values are not markedly abnormal then serial testing may be helpful in establishing a trend indicative of coagulopathy.

Rationale: Monitoring CVP hourly will guide intravenous fluid replacement. Normal CVP is 5 to 10 cm H_2O. Low CVP indicates a decrease in circulating blood volume (hypovolemia).

Rationale: Moderate to severe hemorrhage from abruptio placentae may lead to hypovolemia resulting in cerebral hypoxia. Changes in consciousness may indicate a decrease in blood flow to the brain.

Rationale: Indwelling urinary catheter provides continual assessment of urine output that evaluates renal perfusion and fluid loss. If urine output is decreased below 30 mL per hour this may indicate a sign of shock. Inability to concentrate urine may indicate renal damage from vasoconstriction and decreased blood perfusion.

Rationale: Signs and symptoms of DIC include bleeding from unusual places (i.e., from IV and IM injection site, nose, and mouth), petechiae around blood pressure cuff site, maternal tachycardia, and diaphoresis. Platelets and fibrinogen levels may be decreased although PTT may be normal to prolonged. (Refer to text for normal levels.) When large amounts of thromboplastin are released into the maternal blood supply, the thromboplastin in turn triggers the development of DIC resulting in hypofibrinogenemia.

Rationale: There is an increase in uterine resting tone with abruptio placentae which may decrease oxygen to the fetus. Resting tone should be measured every 15 minutes. Uterine size increases as bleeding occurs at the separation site. Measure abdominal girth hourly by placing a tape measure around the maternal abdomen at the level of the umbilicus or place a mark at the top of the uterine fundus.

Rationale: To promote maternal and fetal well-being. A cesarean section may be necessary after the treatment of hypofibrinogenemia if the separation is moderate to severe.

Evaluation of Client Goal	• No signs of hypovolemia or DIC are present. • Skin is warm and not clammy. • Vital signs are within normal limits. • Urine output is greater than 30 mL per hour and specific gravity is 1.010 to 1.025.
Nursing Diagnosis #2	Ineffective Tissue Perfusion related to decreased blood flow to fetus secondary to partial separation of placenta from uterine wall
Client Goal	The fetus will receive adequate uteroplacental perfusion.
AEB:	• Fetal heart rate and pattern within normal limits • Reactive nonstress test • Score of 8 or above on biophysical profile

(Continued on next page)

Nursing Care Plan

For a Woman with Hemorrhage in Third Trimester and at Birth (Continued)

NURSING INTERVENTIONS	RATIONALES
1. Monitor fetal heart rate by continuous fetal monitoring.	**Rationale:** When the placenta separates from the uterine wall fetal oxygenation is compromised and fetal hypoxia (FHR below 110 bpm) may develop. Continuous fetal monitoring will identify any changes in fetal heart rate that might indicate inadequate uteroplacental perfusion.
2. Assess fetal heart rate pattern every 15 minutes.	**Rationale:** A fetal heart rate pattern that shows late decelerations and a decrease in FHR variability are signs of nonreassuring fetal status. Immediate birth may be indicated to ensure fetal well-being.
3. Monitor uterine contractions and resting tone every 15 minutes.	**Rationale:** Increase in the strength and frequency of contractions places greater stress on the fetus. This is compounded by the decrease in uteroplacental blood flow caused by placental separation. Resting tone may also increase, placing greater demand on the fetus and limiting the fetus's ability to rest or compensate between contractions.
4. Encourage client to rest in the left lateral recumbent position.	**Rationale:** Placing a client in the left lateral recumbent position will decrease pressure on the vena cava which will increase venous return, circulatory volume, and placental and renal perfusion. Blood flow will be increased to the fetus, therefore reducing the risk of fetal hypoxia.
5. Evaluate nonstress test results.	**Rationale:** A nonstress test is performed to assess the fetal heart rate in response to fetal movement. Accelerations of fetal heart rate with fetal movement may indicate the fetus has adequate oxygenation and an intact central nervous system. A good outcome for a nonstress test is documented as reactive: This indicates there were at least two accelerations of 15 bpm above baseline, lasting 15 seconds in a 20-minute period.
6. Evaluate biophysical profile results.	**Rationale:** A biophysical profile evaluates fetal breathing, fetal movement of body or limbs, fetal tone, amniotic fluid volume, and reactive FHR with activity. A score of 8 to 10 is considered normal. A score less than 8 may indicate a fetus at risk for fetal death.

CRITICAL THINKING QUESTIONS

1. The nurse assesses a 40-year-old client at 16 weeks' gestation. The prenatal history for this client includes BP 140/90, presence of uterine fibroids, cocaine use, vegetarian diet, short umbilical cord, a spontaneous abortion 10 months ago, and a 7 lb weight gain. Which data in the prenatal history puts this client at risk for abruptio placentae? For placenta previa?

Answer: The client's prenatal history of uterine fibroids, cocaine use, and short umbilical cord puts her at risk for abruptio placentae. A spontaneous abortion 10 months ago puts her at risk for placenta previa.

2. A client at 38 weeks' gestation is admitted with mild abruptio placentae. She has been contracting for the past 6 hours but contractions are mild and infrequent. If her labor pattern does not progress, is the client at risk for possible complications? What might be done to avoid complications?

Answer: Rupture of membranes and Pitocin infusion by pump may help labor progress. If labor does not progress or an increase in bleeding occurs, a cesarean birth may be done to avoid the risk of increased hemorrhage which could result in hypofibrinogenemia.

*For your reference, this care plan provides an example of how two nursing diagnoses might be addressed.

---

a family history of fraternal twins, and women who are tall and overweight. The incidence is low in the Asian and Hispanic populations (Martin et al., 2006). The physiology of multiple gestation is discussed in Chapter 4 ∞.

Twins that occur from two separate ova are called dizygotic (two zygotes) or fraternal twins. The fetuses may be the same sex or different sexes and are no more closely related genetically than any other siblngs. In contrast, 33%

of twins are monozygotic or identical twins; they develop from one fertilized ovum. They are genetically identical and always the same sex (Blackburn, 2007).

During the prenatal period, visualization of two gestational sacs at 5 to 6 weeks, fundal height greater than expected for the length of gestation, and auscultation of heart rates that differ by at least 10 beats per minute are the most likely clues to multiple-gestation pregnancies. In addition, the alpha-fetoprotein level on the quadruple screen is usually elevated and many women experience severe nausea and vomiting (caused by elevated levels of the human chorionic gonadotropin [hCG] hormone) (Blackburn, 2007).

Maternal Implications

During her pregnancy, the woman may experience physical discomfort such as shortness of breath, dyspnea on exertion, backaches and musculoskeletal disorders, and pedal edema. Other associated problems include urinary tract infections, threatened abortion, anemia, gestational hypertension, preeclampsia, preterm labor and birth, premature rupture of membranes, thromboembolism, and placenta previa, placenta abruption, and other types of placenta disorders (Blackburn, 2007; Cleary-Goldman, Chitkara, & Berkowitz, 2007). Complications during labor include abnormal fetal presentations, uterine dysfunction, prolapsed cord, and hemorrhage at birth or shortly after (Blackburn, 2007; Cleary-Goldman et al., 2007).

Fetal-Neonatal Implications

The perinatal mortality rate is approximately three times greater for twins than for a single fetus, although the mortality rate for triplets and higher-order multiple births is four times higher (MacDorman, Hoyert, Martin et al., 2007). The perinatal mortality rate for monoamniotic siblings has been estimated to be as high as 10% to 32% (Cleary-Goldman et al., 2007). Fetal problems include decreased intrauterine growth rate for each fetus, increased incidence of fetal anomalies, increased risk of prematurity and its associated problems, abnormal presentations, increase in cord accidents, and an increase in cerebral palsy (Blackburn, 2007; Cleary-Goldman et al., 2007). Twins are more likely to have long-term disabilities when compared with children who were singleton births. Recent research has shown that primiparous women who are pregnant with twins have higher rates of complications and prematurity than multiparous women (Erez, Mayer, Shoham-Vardi et al., 2007). Multifetal pregnancies that are conceived spontaneously have better outcomes than those achieved with assisted reproductive technology (Koranantakul, Suwanrath, Suntharasaj et al., 2007).

Clinical Therapy

Once the presence of twins has been detected, preventing and treating problems that infringe on the development and birth of normal fetuses is the most significant clinical goal. Prenatal visits are more frequent for women with twins than for those with one fetus. Women with multiple-gestation pregnancies need to understand the nutritional implications of multiple fetuses, the assess-

ment of fetal activity, the signs of preterm labor, and the danger signs of pregnancy.

If the initial ultrasound scan performed at 18 to 20 weeks' gestation is normal and no risk factors are identified, serial ultrasounds performed every 3 to 4 weeks are used to assess the growth of each fetus. If the pregnancy has identified risks, including monochorionic diamniotic placentation, ultrasounds are performed every 2 to 3 weeks to detect possible twin-to-twin transfusion syndrome (Cleary-Goldman et al., 2007).

A systematic review of studies of hospitalization and bed rest for multiple pregnancy showed insufficient evidence to support routine bed rest (ACOG, 2004). More recent strategies include work leave, lifestyle modifications, and pelvic rest, although well-designed controlled studies supporting the use of these interventions is lacking in the current literature.

Third trimester testing usually begins at 32 to 34 weeks' gestation and may include NST or BPP. A reactive NST is associated with good fetal outcome if birth occurs within 1 week of the testing. The NST is done every 3 to 7 days until birth or until results become nonreactive. The BPP is also accurate in assessing fetal status with twin pregnancies. A biophysical profile of 8 or better for each fetus is considered reassuring, and weekly or biweekly BPPs and NSTs continue until birth.

Intrapartal management requires careful attention to maternal and fetal status. The mother should have an IV with a large bore needle in place. Anesthesia and cross-matched blood should be readily available. The twins are monitored by continuous dual electronic fetal monitoring.

The decision about method of birth, which depends on a variety of factors, may not be made until labor occurs. The presence of maternal complications such as placenta previa, abruptio placentae, or severe preeclampsia usually indicates the need for cesarean birth. Fetal factors such as severe IUGR, preterm birth, fetal anomalies, nonreassuring fetal status, and unfavorable fetal position or presentation also require cesarean birth.

Any combination of presentations and positions can occur with multiple births. Figure 21–4 ■ shows some possible presentations of twins. When the presenting fetus is in a nonvertex position, cesarean birth is indicated.

Nursing Care Management

Community-Based Nursing Care

During pregnancy the woman may need counseling about diet and daily activities. The nurse can help her plan meals to meet her increased needs. Nutritional requirements vary somewhat based on the mother's prepregnancy weight and the estimated weight of the twins. A daily intake of 3500 kcal (minimum) and 175 g protein is recommended

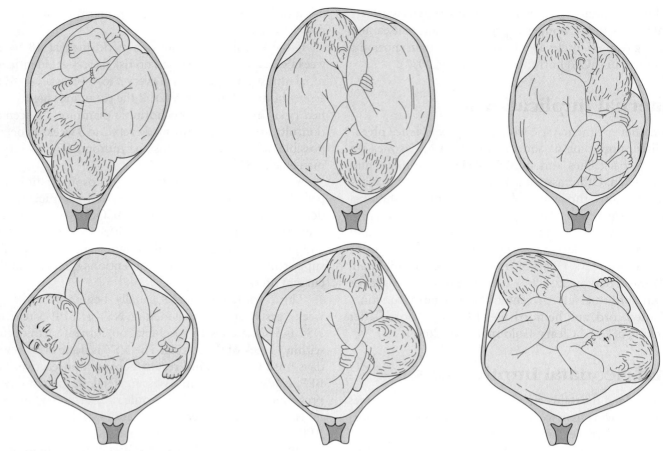

Figure 21–4 Twins may be in any of these presentations while in utero.

for a woman with normal-weight twins although an intake of 4000 kcal and 200 g of protein is recommended if the twins are underweight. A prenatal vitamin and 1 mg of folic acid should also be taken daily. A total weight gain of 40 to 45 lb, with a 24-lb gain by 24 weeks, is recommended for women with multiple-gestation pregnancy (Newman & Rittenberg, 2008).

Counseling about daily activities may include encouraging the woman to plan frequent rest periods during the day. The rest period is most effective if the woman rests in a side-lying position (which increases uteroplacental blood flow) and elevates her lower legs and feet to reduce edema. Back discomfort may be relieved by pelvic rocking, maintaining good posture, consistent use of a pregnancy belt to support the abdomen and lower back, and using good body mechanics when lifting objects and moving about.

Hospital-Based Nursing Care

During labor, the FHRs of the siblings are monitored continuously by an electronic fetal monitor (EFM). Electronic monitoring equipment now makes it possible to monitor the fetuses simultaneously. They are monitored throughout labor and vaginal birth or up to the time of abdominal incision if a cesarean is done. Most multiple gestations are now delivered via cesarean birth.

After birth the nurse must prepare to receive two or more newborns instead of one. This means duplicating everything, including resuscitation equipment, radiant warmers, and newborn identification papers and bracelets. Additional staff members should be available for newborn resuscitation, monitoring, and newborn care. Special precautions should be taken to ensure correct identification of the newborns. The first born is usually tagged Baby A; the second, Baby B; and so on.

Care of the Woman with Abnormal Amniotic Fluid Volume

Amniotic fluid serves many important functions during pregnancy. However, some pregnancies are complicated by either an excessive amount of amniotic fluid or a reduced amount of fluid.

Hydramnios

Hydramnios (also called *polyhydramnios*), a situation in which there is more than 2000 mL of amniotic fluid, occurs in about 1% of all pregnancies (Cunningham et al., 2005).

The exact cause of hydramnios is unknown; however, it often occurs in cases of major congenital anomalies.

During the second half of a normal pregnancy, the fetus begins to swallow and inspire amniotic fluid and to urinate, which contributes to the amount of amniotic fluid present. In cases of hydramnios, no pathology has been found in the amniotic epithelium. However, hydramnios is associated with fetal malformations that affect the fetal swallowing mechanism and neurologic disorders in which the fetal meninges are exposed in the amniotic cavity. This condition is also found in cases of anencephaly, in which the fetus is thought to urinate excessively because of overstimulation of the cerebrospinal centers. When monozygotic twins manifest hydramnios, it is because the twin with the increased blood volume urinates excessively. Because the weight of the placenta has been found to be increased in some cases of hydramnios, increased functioning of the placental tissue may be a factor.

There are two types of hydramnios: chronic and acute. In the chronic type, the fluid volume gradually increases and is a problem of the third trimester. Most cases are of this variety. In acute cases, the volume increases rapidly over a period of a few days. The acute type is usually diagnosed between 20 and 24 weeks' gestation.

Maternal Implications

When the amount of amniotic fluid is over 3000 mL, the woman experiences shortness of breath and edema in the lower extremities from compression of the vena cava. Milder forms of hydramnios occur more frequently and are associated with minimal symptoms. Hydramnios is associated with maternal disorders such as diabetes and Rh sensitization and with multiple-gestation pregnancies. It can also occur as a result of infections such as syphilis, toxoplasmosis, cytomegalovirus, herpes, and rubella.

If the amniotic fluid is removed rapidly before birth, abruptio placentae can result from too sudden a change in the size of the uterus. Because of overdistention of uterine muscles, uterine dysfunction can occur in the intrapartal period, and the incidence of postpartal hemorrhage increases.

Fetal-Neonatal Implications

Fetal malformations and preterm birth are common with hydramnios; thus the perinatal mortality rate is fairly high. Prolapsed cord can occur when the membranes rupture, creating a further complication for the fetus. The incidence of malpresentations also increases. In addition, the incidence of preterm labor and cesarean birth is significantly increased in pregnancies complicated by hydramnios.

Clinical Therapy

Hydramnios is managed with supportive treatment unless the intensity of the woman's distress and symptoms dictates otherwise. If the accumulation of amniotic fluid is severe enough to cause maternal dyspnea and pain, hospitalization and removal of the excessive fluid are required. Fluid can be removed vaginally or by amniocentesis. The dangers of performing the technique vaginally are prolapsed cord and the inability to remove the fluid slowly. If amniocentesis is performed, it should be done with the aid of sonography to prevent inadvertent damage to the fetus and placenta. In addition, the fluid should be removed slowly to prevent abruption.

MyNursingKit | Amniotic Fluid Problems

Nursing Care Management

Hydramnios should be suspected when the fundal height increases out of proportion to the gestational age. As the amount of fluid increases, the nurse may have difficulty palpating the fetus and auscultating the FHR. In more severe cases, the maternal abdomen appears extremely tense and tight on inspection. On sonography, large spaces can be identified between the fetus and the uterine wall.

When amniocentesis is performed, it is vital to maintain sterile technique to prevent infection. The nurse can offer support to the couple by explaining the procedure to them.

If the fetus has been diagnosed with a congenital defect in utero or is born with a defect, the family needs psychologic support. Often the nurse collaborates with social services to offer the family this additional help.

Oligohydramnios

Oligohydramnios is defined as a less-than-normal amount of amniotic fluid (approximately 500 mL is considered normal). This condition affects 1% to 3% of all pregnancies (Gilbert, 2007). Oligohydramnios is diagnosed when the largest vertical pocket of amniotic fluid visible on ultrasound examination is 5 cm (2 in.) or less (Cunningham et al., 2005).

The exact cause of this condition is unknown. It is found in cases of postmaturity; maternal hypertensive disorders, with IUGR secondary to placental insufficiency; and in fetal conditions associated with major renal malformations, including renal aplasia with dysplastic kidneys and obstructive lesions of the lower urinary tract. If oligohydramnios occurs in the first part of pregnancy, there is a danger of fetal adhesions (one part of the fetus may adhere to another part).

Maternal Implications

When oligohydramnios exists, labor can be dysfunctional, and progress is slow. The woman should be monitored for hypertensive disorders.

Fetal-Neonatal Implications

During the gestational period, fetal skin and skeletal abnormalities may occur because fetal movement is impaired as a result of reduced amniotic fluid volume. Because there is less fluid available for the fetus to use during fetal breathing movements, pulmonary hypoplasia may develop. During the labor and birth, oligohydramnios reduces the cushioning effect for the umbilical cord, and cord compression is more likely to occur. Decreased amniotic fluid also contributes to fetal head compression.

Clinical Therapy

During the antepartum period oligohydramnios may be suspected when the uterus does not increase in size according to the dates, the fetus is easily palpated and outlined by the examiner, and the fetus is not ballottable. The fetus can be assessed by biophysical profiles, nonstress tests, and serial ultrasounds. As soon as the fetus is term, induction is typically scheduled because the fetus is at an increased risk for intrauterine fetal demise. During labor, the fetus is monitored by continuous EFM to detect cord compression, which is indicated by variable decelerations. Some clinicians advocate the use of an *amnioinfusion* (a transcervical instillation of 250 mL of warmed sterile saline, followed by a continuous infusion rate of 100 to 200 mL/hr) after membranes have ruptured to decrease the frequency and severity of variable decelerations in the FHR during labor. The fluid is administered in a blood warmer to maintain a constant temperature. It is imperative to monitor for expulsion of the fluid to prevent overdistention of the uterus. The infusion of saline provides more fluid for the umbilical cord to float in and thereby lessens or prevents cord compression. Amnioinfusions are also used in cases of thick meconium to decrease the consistency and decrease the incidence of meconium below the infant's vocal cords (Gilbert, 2007).

Nursing Care Management

Continuous electronic fetal monitoring is an important part of the assessment during the labor and birth. The nurse evaluates the EFM tracing for the presence of variable decelerations or other nonreassuring signs (such as increasing or decreasing baseline, decreased variability, presence of late decelerations). If variable decelerations are noted, the woman's position can be changed (to relieve pressure on the umbilical cord), and the physician/CNM is notified. If the tracing is not reassuring, a cesarean birth is performed. After the birth, the newborn is evaluated for signs of congenital anomalies, pulmonary hypoplasia, and postmaturity.

CHAPTER HIGHLIGHTS

- Both premature rupture of the membranes and preterm labor place the fetus at risk. Women with preterm PROM and no signs of infection are managed conservatively with bed rest and careful monitoring of fetal well-being. If preterm labor develops, tocolytics are often effective in stopping labor, but they have associated side effects.

- Placenta previa occurs when the placenta implants low in the uterus near or over the cervix. A low-lying or marginal placenta is one that lies near the cervix. In partial placenta previa, part of the placenta lies over the cervix; in complete placenta previa, the cervix is completely covered.

- Abruptio placentae is the separation of the placenta from the side of the uterus before the birth of the infant. Abruptio placentae may be central, marginal, or complete.

- Hydramnios, also known as polyhydramnios, occurs when there is more than 2000 mL of amniotic fluid contained within the amniotic membranes. Hydramnios is associated with fetal malformations that affect fetal swallowing and with maternal diabetes mellitus, Rh sensitization, and multiple gestation pregnancies.

- Oligohydramnios occurs when there is a severely reduced volume of amniotic fluid. Oligohydramnios is associated with IUGR, postmaturity, and fetal renal or urinary malformations. The fetus is more likely to experience variable decelerations because the amniotic fluid is insufficient to keep pressure off the umbilical cord.

American College of Obstetricians & Gynecologists (ACOG). (2003a). Management of preterm labor. ACOG Practice Bulletin No. 43. Washington, DC: Author.

American College of Obstetricians and Gynecologists (ACOG). (2003. Reaffirmed 2008). *Cervical insufficiency* (ACOG Practice Bulletin No. 48). Washington, DC: Author.

American College of Obstetricians & Gynecologists (ACOG). (2004). Multiple gestation: Complicated twin, triplet, and higher-order multifetal pregnancy. ACOG Practice Bulletin No. 56. Washington, DC: Author.

Berghella, V, Roman, A., Daskalakis, C., Ness, A., Baxter, J.K. (2007). Gestational age at cervical length measurement and incidence of preterm birth. *Obstetrics & Gynecology*, (110)2, Part 1, 311–317.

Blackburn, S. T. (2007). *Maternal, fetal, and neonatal physiology: A clinical perspective* (3rd ed.). Philadelphia: Saunders.

Briggs, G. G., Freeman, R. K., & Yaffee, S. J. (2005). *Drugs in pregnancy and lactation* (7th ed.). Philadelphia: Lippincott, Williams, & Wilkins.

Carey, J. C., & Gibbs, R. S. (2008). Preterm labor and postterm delivery. In R. S. Gibbs, B. Y. Karlan, A. F. Haney, & I. E. Nygaard (Eds.), *Danforth's obstetrics and gynecology* (10th ed.). Philadelphia: Wolters Kluwer/Lippincott Williams & Wilkins.

Cleary-Goldman, J., Chitkara, U., & Berkowitz, R. L. (2007). Multiple gestations. In S. G. Gabbe, J. R. Niebyl, & J. L. Simpson (Eds.), *Obstetrics: Normal and problem pregnancies* (5th ed.). Philadelphia: Churchill Livingstone.

Cunningham, F. G., Leveno, K. J., Bloom, S. L., Hauth, J. C., Gilstrap III, L. C., & Wenstrom, K. D. (2005). *Williams obstetrics* (22nd ed.). New York: McGraw-Hill.

Erez, O., Mayer, A., Shoham-Vardi, I., Dukler, D., & Mazor, M. (2007). Primiparity, assisted reproduction, and preterm birth in twin pregnancies: A population based study. *Archives of Gynecology & Obstetrics* (2007 Oct 31) [Epub ahead of print].

Fonseca, E. B., Celik, E., Parra, M., Singh, M., Nicolaides, K. H., & Fetal Medicine Foundation Second Trimester Screening Group. (2007). Progesterone and the risk of preterm birth among women with a short cervix. *New England Journal of Medicine, 2, 357*(5), 462–469.

Francois, K. E., & Foley, M. R. (2007). Antepartum and postpartum hemorrhage. In S. G. Gabbe, J. R. Niebyl, & J. L. Simpson (Eds.), *Obstetrics: Normal and problem pregnancies* (5th ed.). Philadelphia: Churchill Livingstone.

Gibbs, R. S. (2008). Premature rupture of the membranes. In R. S. Gibbs, B. Y. Karlan, A. F. Haney, & I. E. Nygaard (Eds.), *Danforth's obstetrics and gynecology* (10th ed.). Philadelphia: Wolters Kluwer/Lippincott Williams & Wilkins.

Gilbert, W. M. (2007). Amniotic fluid disorders. In S. G. Gabbe, J. R. Niebyl, & J. L. Simpson (Eds.), *Obstetrics: Normal and problem pregnancies* (5th ed.). Philadelphia: Churchill Livingstone.

Gill, G. (2004). Etiology and prevention of preterm labor. Retrieved November 4, 2007, from www.acog.org/acog_sections/download/EtiologyandPreventionofPretermLabor.pdf-2004-05-17

Habli, M., & Sibai, B. (2008). Hypertensive disorders of pregnancy. In R. S. Gibbs, B. Y. Karlan, A. F. Haney, & I. E. Nygaard (Eds.), *Danforth's obstetrics and gynecology* (10th ed.). Philadelphia: Wolters Kluwer/Lippincott Williams & Wilkins.

How, H. Y., Barton, J. R., Istwan, N. B., Rhea, D. J., & Stanziano, G. J. (2007). Prophylaxis with 17 alpha-hydroxyprogesterone caproate for prevention of recurrent preterm delivery: Does gestational age at initiation of treatment matter? *American Journal of Obstetrics & Gynecology, 197*(3), 260.e1–4.

Iams, J. D., & Romero, R. (2007). Preterm birth. In S. G. Gabbe, J. R. Niebyl, & J. L. Simpson (Eds.), *Obstetrics: Normal and problem pregnancies* (5th ed.). Philadelphia: Churchill Livingstone.

Johnson, J.R., & Iams, J.D. (2009). Cervical insufficiency. Retrieved 9/23/2009 at www.UpToDate.com.

Kay, H. H. (2008). Placenta previa and abruption. In R. S. Gibbs, B. Y. Karlan, A. F. Haney, & I. E. Nygaard (Eds.), *Danforth's obstetrics and gynecology* (10th ed.). Philadelphia: Wolters Kluwer/Lippincott Williams & Wilkins.

Koranantakul, O., Suwanrath, C., Suntharasaj, T., Getpook, C., & Leetanaporn, R. (2007). Outcomes of multifetal pregnancies. *Journal of Obstetric & Gynaecology Research, 33*(1), 49–55.

Lyell, D. J., Pullen, K., Campbell, L., Ching, S., Druzin, M. L., Chitkara, U., Burrs, D., Caughey, A. B., & El-Sayed, Y. Y. (2007). Magnesium sulfate compared with nifedipine for acute tocolysis of preterm labor: A randomized controlled trial. *Obstetrics & Gynecology, 110*(1), 61–67.

MacDorman, M. F., Hoyert, D. L., Martin, J. A., Munson, M. L., & Hamilton, B. E. (2007). Fetal and perinatal mortality, United States, 2003. *National Vital Statistics Reports, 55*(6), 1–18.

Mancuso, M.S. & Owen, J. (2009). Prevention of preterm birth based on a short cervix: Cerclage. *Seminars in Perinatology*(33), 325–333.

March of Dimes (MOD). (2007). March of Dimes Peristats: More babies born prematurely, new report shows. Retrieved August 20, 2008 from www.marchofdomes.com

Martin, J. A., Hamilton, B. E., Sutton, P. D., Ventura, S. J., Menacker, F., & Kirmeyer, S. (2006). Births: Final data for 2004. *National Vital Statistics Reports, 55*(1), 1–102.

Mercer, B. M. (2007). Premature rupture of the membranes. In S. G. Gabbe, J. R. Niebyl, & J. L. Simpson (Eds.), *Obstetrics: Normal and problem pregnancies* (5th ed.). Philadelphia: Churchill Livingstone.

Morrison, J. C., & Chauhan, S. P. (2003). Current status of home uterine activity monitoring. *Clinical Perinatology, 30*(4), 757–801.

Ness, A., Visintine, J., Ricci, E., & Berghella, V. (2007). Does knowledge of cervical length and fetal fibronectin affect management of women with threatened preterm labor? A randomized trial. *American Journal of Obstetricians & Gynecologists, 197*(4), 426.e1–7.

Newman, R. B. (2005). Uterine contraction assessment. *Obstetrics & Gynecology Clinics in North America, 32*(3), 341–367.

Newman, R. B., & Rittenberg, C. (2008). Multiple gestation. In R. S. Gibbs, B. Y. Karlan, A. F. Haney, & I. E. Nygaard (Eds.), *Danforth's obstetrics and gynecology* (10th ed.). Philadelphia: Wolters Kluwer/Lippincott Williams & Wilkins.

Noehr, B, Jensen, A, Frederiksen, K, Tabor, A, Kjaer, S.K. (2009). Loop electrosurgical excision of the cervix and subsequent risk for spontaneous preterm delivery: A population-based study of singleton deliveries during a 9-year period. *American Journal of Obstetrics & Gynecology*, (201)1, 33.e1–33.e6. Retrieved 10/24/2009 at www.sciencedirect.com.

Rideout, S. L. (2005). Tocolytics for pre-term labor: What nurses need to know. *AWHONN Lifelines, 9*(1), 56–61.

CHAPTER 22

Childbirth at Risk: Labor-Related Complications

I am very conscientious about making sure that I cover "unexpected outcomes" in my childbirth preparation classes. Although everyone hopes and anticipates that labor and birth will proceed normally, unfortunately it sometimes doesn't. At those times, when the family is anxious or afraid, maybe somewhere in the back of their minds is a little seed of reassurance because we have already talked about problems a little.

—Labor/Delivery Nurse and Childbirth Educator (CBE)

LEARNING OUTCOMES

22-1. Explain the psychologic factors that may contribute to complications during labor and birth in determining the nursing care management of the woman during labor and birth.

22-2. Compare hypertonic and hypotonic labor patterns, including risks, clinical therapy, and nursing care management.

22-3. Describe the risks and clinical therapy in determining the community-based and hospital-based nursing care management of postterm pregnancy on the childbearing family.

22-4. Relate the various types of fetal malposition and malpresentation, risks, and clinical therapy to the nursing care management for each.

22-5. Explain the identification, risks, and clinical therapy in determining the nursing care management of the woman and fetus at risk for macrosomia.

22-6. Relate the maternal implications, clinical therapy, prenatal history, and conditions that may be associated with nonreassuring fetal status to the nursing care of the mother and fetus.

22-7. Describe the nursing care for the mother and fetus with a prolapsed umbilical cord.

22-8. Summarize the identification, maternal and fetal-neonatal implications, clinical therapy, and nursing care management of women with amniotic fluid embolus.

22-9. Explain the types, maternal and fetal-neonatal implications, and clinical therapy in determining the nursing care management of the woman with cephalopelvic disproportion.

22-10. Identify common complications of the third and fourth stages of labor.

22-11. Explain the etiology, diagnosis, and phases of grief in determining the nursing care management of the family experiencing perinatal loss.

KEY TERMS

Successful completion of a pregnancy requires the harmonious functioning of the five critical factors discussed in Chapter 17 ∞: the birth passage, the fetus, the relationship between the passage and the fetus, the forces of labor, and psychosocial considerations. Disruptions in any of these components may cause **dystocia**, which is abnormal or difficult labor. This chapter discusses the most common of these disruptions.

Care of the Woman with a Psychologic Disorder

The onset of labor is a time of mixed emotions. Joy, excitement, happiness, fear of the unknown, and anxiety related to pain may all occur. These reactions are expected, and pose no health risk in women with adequate coping mechanisms. In contrast, laboring women with psychologic disorders face additional emotional challenges and require additional nursing support in the intrapartum period.

The prevalence of psychologic disorders among adults in the United States is 26.2% or roughly 1 in 4 adults (National Institute of Mental Health, 2008). **Psychologic disorders** are characterized by alterations in thinking, mood, or behavior. Although many such disorders can affect labor and birth, only the most common are discussed here. Because an in-depth discussion of psychologic disorders is beyond the scope of this text, students are encouraged to consult a mental-health nursing textbook for further reference. Postpartum psychologic disorders are discussed in Chapter 33 ∞.

The psychologic disorders which most commonly affect pregnant women are depression, bipolar disorder, anxiety, phobias, obsessive-compulsive disorder, posttraumatic stress disorder, and schizophrenia. These disorders may manifest themselves in different ways during the birth process; however, all require the nurse to provide compassionate and consistent nursing care.

Maternal Implications

Depression can reduce the woman's ability to concentrate or process information being provided by healthcare team members. The labor process may feel overwhelming to her, and she may feel hopelessness about the outcome of her labor. Women with bipolar disorder experience the symptoms of depression during the depressive phase; however, if labor occurs during a manic phase, the woman may be hyperexcitable. Anxiety disorders may cause the laboring woman to experience physical symptoms such as chest pain, shortness of breath, faintness, fear, or even terror. In general, laboring women with psychologic disorders tend to exhibit the behaviors characteristic of their disorder, but these behaviors may be somewhat exaggerated because of the intense emotions that are evoked in the woman's memory. Women with a past history of abuse, including physical and sexual abuse, are often fearful of losing control.

Clinical Therapy

The goal of clinical therapy is to provide strategies that will help decrease the woman's anxiety (as well as that of her partner), keep her oriented to reality, and promote optimal functioning while in labor. The woman should be oriented to her new environment. All questions and concerns should be addressed promptly. When needed, pharmacologic measures such as sedatives, analgesics, or antianxiety medications may be ordered. Women who are on psychologic medications during pregnancy often continue these during labor, birth, and the postpartum period. The woman should have an extensive assessment. The partner or family should be asked to leave the room at this time in case the assessment reveals domestic violence, a past history of violence, or current violence.

Nursing Care Management

The nurse uses therapeutic communication and sharing of information to allay anxiety for both the woman and her support person. Consistency in her care enables the woman to adjust to a new environment and begin to establish a relationship with her nurse.

Nursing Assessment and Diagnosis

Unless birth is imminent or severe complications exist, the nurse begins the assessment by reviewing the woman's background. Factors such as age, marital and socioeconomic status, culture, methods of coping, support system, and understanding of the labor process contribute to the woman's psychologic response to labor. It is important to ask all women if they have ever been diagnosed with a psychologic disorder. If the woman has, the nurse needs to ask her if she is currently receiving any treatment, including medications or psychotherapy. The nurse should also ask if she has ever had a psychiatric hospitalization or if she has ever had thoughts of hurting herself or others. The prenatal record should be reviewed for additional information regarding any psychiatric illnesses.

The nurse also assesses the woman for objective cues indicating a psychologic disorder. Monotone replies and/or a flat affect may indicate depression. Women with schizophrenia may lack orientation to person, time, and place. Objective cues indicating acute anxiety or signs of a panic attack include tachycardia and hyperventilation.

As labor progresses, the nurse remains alert to the woman's verbal and nonverbal behavioral responses to the pain and anxiety. The woman who is too quiet and compliant, is disoriented, is agitated and seems uncooperative, or is experiencing acute anxiety symptoms may require further appraisal for psychologic disorders. These rare circumstances require one-on-one nursing care. A consult with a psychiatrist is often warranted.

Nursing diagnoses that may apply to the woman with a psychologic disorder include the following:

- Anxiety related to stress of the labor process, unfamiliar environment, and unknown caregivers
- Fear related to unknown outcome of labor and invasive medical procedures
- Acute Pain related to increased anxiety and stress
- Ineffective Individual Coping related to increased anxiety and stress

Nursing Plan and Implementation

The primary nursing interventions center on providing support to the laboring woman and her partner or family. Families that have had the opportunity to attend prenatal classes may benefit from encouragement as they employ some of the coping techniques they have learned (see Chapter 8 ∞). If the woman begins to lose her ability to cope or her orientation to reality, the nurse can assist her in regaining control and orientation by explaining where she is, why she is there, and what is currently happening; providing reassurance; decreasing stimuli; and acknowledging her fears, concerns, and symptoms.

The nurse's ability to help the woman and her partner cope with the stress of labor is directly related to the rapport they have established. By employing a calm, caring, confident, nonjudgmental approach, the nurse may be able not only to acknowledge the anxiety or other emotions the woman is feeling but also to identify the source of the distress.

Once the causative factors are known, the nurse can implement appropriate interventions such as offering information, comfort measures, touch, or therapeutic communication. Some women with severe psychologic disorders may have excessive symptoms during their labor and birth. Although providing emotional support is imperative, care of these women should focus on maintaining a safe environment and ensuring maternal and fetal well-being. Pharmacologic interventions may be necessary for excessive symptoms.

Evaluation

Anticipated outcomes of nursing care include the following:

- The woman experiences a decrease in physiologic and psychologic stress and an increase in physical and psychologic comfort.
- The woman remains oriented to person, time, and place.
- The woman uses effective coping mechanisms to manage her stress and anxiety in labor.
- The woman is able to verbalize feelings about her labor.
- The woman's and her family's fear is decreased.

Care of the Woman with Dystocia Related to Dysfunctional Uterine Contractions

Dystocia, or difficult labor, may be caused by a wide variety of problems, the most common of which is dysfunctional (or uncoordinated) uterine contractions. These uncoordinated contractions result in a prolonged labor. Contractions that result in a more normal progression of labor tend to be moderate to strong when palpated and occur regularly (two to four contractions in 10 minutes in early labor and four to five per 10 minutes in later phases). Dysfunctional contractions are typically irregular in strength, timing, or both. These irregular uterine contractions are not effective in producing dilatation or effacement.

Hypertonic Labor Patterns

A normal contraction pattern is shown in Figure 22–1A ■. In hypertonic labor patterns, ineffective uterine contractions of poor quality occur in the latent phase of labor, and the resting tone of the myometrium (uterine muscle) increases. Contractions usually become more frequent, but their intensity may decrease (see Figure 22–1B). The contractions are painful but ineffective in dilating and effacing the cervix, and a prolonged latent phase may result. These prolonged contractions can result in fetal hypoxia.

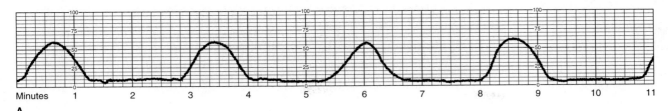

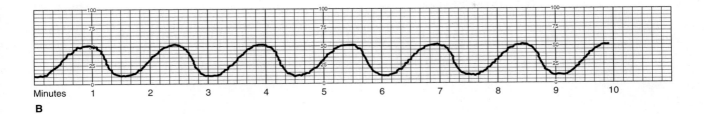

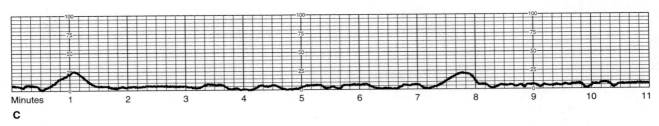

FIGURE 22-1 Comparison of labor patterns. *A,* Normal uterine contraction pattern. Note that the contraction frequency is every 3 minutes; duration is 60 seconds. The baseline resting tone is below 10 mm Hg. *B,* Hypertonic uterine contraction pattern. Note that the contraction frequency is every 1 to 2 minutes, duration is 90 seconds. The baseline resting tone is 10 mm Hg. *C,* Hypotonic uterine contraction pattern. Note in this example that the contraction frequency is every 7 minutes with some uterine activity between contractions, duration is 50 seconds, and intensity increases approximately 25 mm Hg during contractions.

Risks of Hypertonic Labor

Maternal risks of hypertonic labor include:

- Increased discomfort caused by uterine muscle cell anoxia
- Fatigue as the pattern continues and no labor progress results
- Frustration and stress on coping abilities
- Dehydration and increased incidence of infection if labor is prolonged

Fetal-neonatal risks include:

- Nonreassuring fetal status caused by contractions and increased resting tone interfering with the uteroplacental exchange of gases and nutrients.
- Prolonged pressure on the fetal head, which may result in cephalohematoma, caput succedaneum, or excessive molding (Figure 22–2 ■).

Clinical Therapy

Management of hypertonic labor may include bed rest and sedation to promote relaxation and reduce pain. Of-ten pharmacologic intervention to promote sedation will stop these contractions. If the hypertonic pattern continues and develops into a prolonged latent phase, Pitocin (oxytocin) infusion or amniotomy may be considered. An amniotomy can help a normal labor progress because of pressure on the cervix. Pitocin can be used to strengthen existing contractions and lead to a more productive pattern (see Chapter 23 ∞). These methods are instituted only after cephalopelvic dispro-portion (CPD) and fetal malpresentation have been ruled out. If the maternal pelvic diameters are less than average, if the fetus is particularly large, or if the fetus is in a malpresentation or malposition, CPD is said to be present. In such cases, labor is not stimulated because vaginal birth is not possible. Instead, a cesarean birth will be performed.

HINTS FOR PRACTICE

To determine if the fetal heart rate (FHR) is reassuring, the following components should be present: a baseline FHR of 110 to 160 bpm, presence of variability, and spontaneous accelerations.

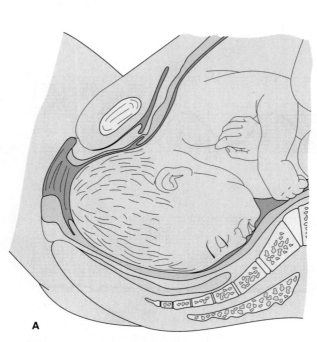

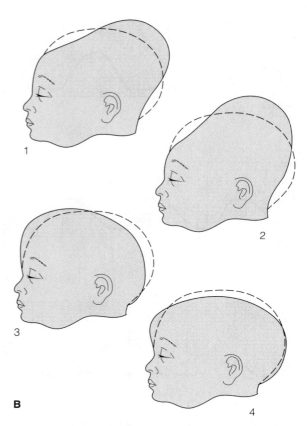

FIGURE 22–2 Effects of labor on the fetal head. *A,* Caput succedaneum formation. The presenting portion of the scalp area is encircled by the cervix during labor, causing swelling of the soft tissue. *B,* Molding of the fetal head in cephalic presentations: (1) occiput anterior, (2) occiput posterior, (3) brow, (4) face.

Nursing Care Management

Nursing Assessment and Diagnosis

As part of the labor assessment, the nurse should evaluate the intensity of the uterine contractions, the woman's perception of discomfort experienced, and the degree of cervical change. The nurse should also note whether anxiety is negatively affecting labor progress. Evidence of increasing frustration and discouragement on the part of the mother and her partner may indicate that the nurse needs to provide some additional information or reassurance.

Nursing diagnoses that may apply to the woman in a hypertonic labor pattern include the following:

- Fatigue related to inability to relax and rest secondary to a hypertonic labor pattern
- Increased discomfort related to the woman's inability to relax secondary to hypertonic uterine contractions
- Ineffective Individual Coping related to ineffectiveness of breathing techniques to relieve discomfort
- Anxiety related to slow labor progress

Nursing Plan and Implementation

A key nursing responsibility is to provide comfort and support to the laboring woman and her partner. The woman experiencing a hypertonic labor pattern will probably be very uncomfortable because of the increased frequency of contractions. Her anxiety level and that of her partner may be high. The nurse attempts to reduce the woman's discomfort and promote a more effective labor pattern.

The nurse may suggest supportive measures such as a change of position: left lateral side-lying, high Fowler's, on her knees in the bed with her arms up around the top of the bed while it is in high Fowler's, rocking in a rocking chair, sitting up, and walking. Soothing measures, such as a quiet environment, use of music the woman finds calming, back rub, therapeutic touch, and visualization, and comfort measures, such as mouth care, change of linens, effleurage, and relaxation exercises, may also be helpful. The use of tub baths or a warm shower can help promote comfort and uterine relaxation. If sedation is ordered, the nurse ensures that the environment is conducive to relaxation. The labor partner may also need assistance in helping the woman cope. A calm, understanding approach by the nurse offers the woman and her partner further support. Providing information about the cause of the hypertonic labor pattern and assuring the woman that she is not overreacting to the situation are important nursing actions.

Some women may request pain medication during this time period. For many women, the administration of a pain medication can assist with relaxation, promote rest, and allow them to reestablish coping mechanisms. For a complete guide to pain medication during labor, see Chapter 20 ∞.

Client education is key for the woman experiencing hypertonic labor. She needs information about the dysfunctional labor pattern and the possible implications for her and her baby. Information will help relieve anxiety and thereby increase relaxation and comfort. The nurse needs to explain treatment options and offer opportunities to ask questions.

Evaluation

Anticipated outcomes of nursing care include the following:

- The woman states she has increased comfort and decreased anxiety.
- The woman and her partner verbalize they are able to cope with the labor.
- The woman experiences a more effective labor pattern.
- The woman rates her pain as less than 3 on a 1 to 10 pain scale.

Hypotonic Labor Patterns

A hypotonic labor pattern usually develops in the active phase of labor, after labor has been well established. Hypotonic labor is characterized by fewer than two to three contractions in a 10-minute period (see Figure 22–1C). The contractions may be of low intensity and are characterized as causing minimal discomfort. Hypotonic labor may occur when the uterus is overstretched from a twin gestation, or in the presence of a large fetus, hydramnios, fetal malposition, prematurity, or grand multiparity. Bladder or bowel distention and CPD may also be associated with this pattern.

Risks of Hypotonic Labor

Maternal implications of hypotonic labor patterns include the following risks:

- Maternal exhaustion
- Stress on coping abilities
- Postpartal hemorrhage from insufficient uterine contractions following birth
- Intrauterine infection if labor is prolonged

Fetal-neonatal implications include the following risks.

- Nonreassuring fetal status caused by prolonged labor pattern
- Fetal sepsis from pathogens that ascend from the birth canal

Clinical Therapy

The goals of therapy are to improve the quality of the uterine contractions while ensuring a safe outcome for the woman and her baby. Uterine contractions can be stimulated in several ways including the use of Pitocin, amniotomy, or stimulation of the nipples which causes the release of endogenous oxytocin. Before initiating treatment for hypotonic labor, the physician/CNM validates the adequacy of pelvic measurements and establishes gestational age to ensure the fetus has reached maturity. After CPD, fetal malpresentation, and fetal immaturity have been ruled out, Pitocin may be given intravenously via an infusion pump to improve the quality of uterine contractions. Intravenous fluid is useful to maintain adequate hydration and prevent maternal exhaustion. Amniotomy may be used to stimulate the labor process. An amniotomy is used to allow the presenting part to directly apply pressure on the cervix and promote effacement and dilatation. The application of an electric breast pump or manual stimulation of the nipples may help strengthen uterine contractions, and is an excellent starting point for women who want an unmedicated birth.

Some physicians support the use of **active management of labor (AMOL)**, a process whereby labor is managed from the beginning with client education, identifying true labor by strict definition, amniotomy, timed cervical exams to determine abnormal labor patterns, and augmentation of labor with high-dose intravenous (IV) administration of Pitocin if a specified level of progress is not met. Supporters of AMOL contend that it is a preventative treatment that reduces the chance for protracted labor and decreases the cesarean birth rate (ACOG, 2003). Other components of AMOL include strict identification of fetal compromise, one-to-one nursing care, and peer review of operative births. Often, the individualized nursing care and peer review are not carried out as strictly as the other components. Opponents argue that the use of AMOL increases the incidence of infection (because of frequent vaginal examinations), necessitates the use of additional interventions, and increases the incidence of instrument-assisted births (Albers, 2007).

An improvement in the quality of uterine contractions is demonstrated by changes in the cervical exam

KEY FACTS TO REMEMBER

When an amniotomy is used to augment labor, women who are GBS positive, who have not had a culture, or whose culture results are unknown should have already been given antibiotic treatment to ensure that the fetus does not become infected. Some practitioners may prefer to wait to ensure that two doses have been administered before rupturing the membranes.

and a more active labor pattern. If the labor pattern does not become effective or if other complications develop, further interventions, including cesarean birth, may be necessary.

Nursing Care Management

Nursing Assessment and Diagnosis

Assessment of contractions (for frequency, intensity, and duration), maternal vital signs, and fetal heart rate provides the nurse with data to evaluate maternal-fetal status. The nurse is also alert for signs and symptoms of infection and dehydration. Because of the stress associated with a prolonged labor, observing the woman and her partner's success in implementing coping mechanisms is important, too.

Nursing diagnoses that may apply to the woman in hypotonic labor include the following:

- Acute Pain related to uterine contractions secondary to dysfunctional labor
- Ineffective Individual Coping related to unanticipated discomfort and slow progress in labor
- Fatigue related to prolonged labor and discomfort

Nursing Plan and Implementation

Nursing measures to promote maternal-fetal physical well-being include frequent monitoring of contractions, maternal vital signs, and FHR. If amniotic membranes are ruptured, the nurse assesses for the presence of meconium (dark green or black stool expelled from the fetal large intestine). The presence of meconium in the amniotic fluid makes close observation of fetal status more critical because it often indicates that the fetus is experiencing some form of stress. An intake and output record provides a way of determining maternal hydration or dehydration. The woman should be encouraged to void every 2 hours, and her bladder should be checked for distention. Because labor may be prolonged, the nurse must continue to monitor the woman and the fetus for signs of infection (elevated temperature, chills, foul-smelling amniotic fluid, and fetal tachycardia). Vaginal examinations should be kept to a minimum to decrease the risk of introducing an infection.

Women experiencing a hypotonic labor pattern require emotional support. The nurse assists the woman and her partner to cope with the frustration of a lengthy labor process. A warm, caring approach is coupled with techniques to reduce anxiety and discomfort.

The teaching plan needs to include information regarding the dysfunctional labor process and implications for the mother and baby. Disadvantages of and alternatives to treatment also need to be discussed and understood.

Evaluation

Anticipated outcomes of nursing care include the following:

- The woman maintains comfort during labor.
- The woman states that she understands the type of labor pattern that is occurring and the treatment plan.

Care of the Woman Experiencing Precipitous Labor

Precipitous labor is labor that lasts less than 3 hours and results in rapid birth. Contributing factors in precipitous labor are multiparity, large pelvis, previous precipitous labor, and a small fetus in a favorable position. One or more of these factors, plus strong contractions, result in a rapid descent of the infant through the birth canal. The incidence of precipitous birth in the United States is about 2% (Battista & Wing, 2007). A significant risk factor for precipitous labor is a previous rapid labor. Women with a history of rapid labor and birth can be monitored antepartally with cervical exams. Once the woman is 38 weeks, the healthcare provider may wish to schedule an induction. A careful review of the woman's past history should alert the physician or certified nurse-midwife of the risk of subsequent precipitous labors.

Precipitous labor and precipitous birth are not the same. A precipitous birth is an unexpected, sudden, and often unattended birth (see Chapter 19 ∞).

Risks of Precipitous Labor

Maternal risks of precipitous labor include:

- Loss of coping abilities
- Lacerations of the cervix, vagina, and perineum caused by rapid descent and birth of the fetus
- Postpartal hemorrhage caused by undetected lacerations or inadequate uterine contractions after birth

Fetal-neonatal implications include:

- Nonreassuring fetal status or hypoxia from decreased uteroplacental circulation caused by intense uterine contractions
- Brachial plexus injuries caused by rapid descent and uncontrolled birth

Clinical Therapy

Any woman with a history of precipitous labor requires close monitoring in the last few weeks of pregnancy. If the cervix softens and begins to dilate, the woman may be scheduled for immediate induction of labor. Women who are GBS positive may also be scheduled for an induction to reduce the likelihood of giving birth without appropriate antibiotic therapy.

Nursing Care Management

Nursing Assessment and Diagnosis

During the intrapartal nursing assessment, the nurse can identify a woman at increased risk of precipitous labor (e.g., a previous history of precipitous or short labor places a woman at risk). During labor the presence of one or both of the following factors may indicate potential problems:

- Accelerated cervical dilatation (more than 2 cm/hr in multigravidas and more than 1.2 cm/hr in primigravidas) and fetal descent
- Intense uterine contractions with little uterine relaxation between contractions

Nursing diagnoses that may apply to the woman with precipitous labor include the following:

- *Risk for Injury* related to rapid labor and birth
- *Acute Pain* related to rapid labor process
- *Fear* related to uncontrolled environment and potential absence of medical provider

Nursing Plan and Implementation

If the woman has a history of precipitous labor, she is closely monitored, and an emergency birth pack is kept at hand. The nurse stays in constant attendance if possible and promotes comfort and rest by assisting the woman to a comfortable position and providing a quiet environment. The nurse provides information and support before and after the birth.

To avoid possible precipitous labor and hyperstimulation of the uterus during Pitocin administration, the nurse should be alert to the dangers of Pitocin overdosage (see Drug Guide: Oxytocin in Chapter 23 ∞). If the woman who is receiving Pitocin develops an accelerated labor pattern, discontinue the Pitocin immediately, and turn the woman on her left side to improve uterine perfusion. Oxygen may be administered to increase the available oxygen in the maternal circulating blood, which in turn increases the amount available for exchange at the placental site. The fetus is continually monitored for signs of hypoxia and other indications of nonreassuring fetal status, such as late decelerations, loss of variability, or a change in the FHR baseline rate.

Evaluation

Anticipated outcomes of nursing care include the following:

- The woman and her baby are closely monitored during labor, and a safe birth occurs.
- The woman maintains optimal comfort.

Care of the Woman with Postterm Pregnancy

A **postterm pregnancy** is one that extends more than 294 days or 42 weeks past the first day of the last menstrual period. It is important to distinguish between the term *postdate,* which means that the pregnancy has gone beyond the estimated date of birth (EDB), and *postterm,* which indicates that the pregnancy has gone at least 1 day beyond 42 complete weeks from the last menstrual period. The actual incidence of postterm pregnancies is small, approximately 7% (ACOG, 2004). The majority of postterm pregnancies are actually incorrectly dated pregnancies. The cause of true postterm pregnancy is unknown, but it seems to occur more frequently in primigravidas, women with a past history of postterm pregnancies, and less commonly with fetal anencephaly or placental sulfatase deficiency. Research also indicates that postterm pregnancy is more common in male fetuses and may have a genetic disposition (ACOG, 2004).

Risks of Postterm Pregnancy

Maternal risks associated with postterm pregnancy include the following (ACOG, 2004; Blackburn, 2007):

- Probable labor induction
- Increased risk of dystocia
- Increased risk for large-for-gestational-age (LGA) infant
- Increased incidence of forceps-assisted or vacuum-assisted birth
- Increased psychologic stress as the due date passes and concern for the baby increases
- Increased risk of infection
- Increased risk of severe perineal trauma related to macrosomia
- Double the risk of cesarean birth

Fetal risks include the following (ACOG, 2004; Blackburn, 2007):

- Decreased perfusion from the placenta
- Fetal demise
- Oligohydramnios (decreased amount of amniotic fluid), which increases the risk of cord compression
- Meconium aspiration (aspiration of meconium-stained amniotic fluid by the fetus at the time of birth), which is more likely if oligohydramnios and thick meconium are present
- Low 5-minute Apgar score
- Risk for death of the infant in the first year of life

Some fetuses continue to grow beyond the 42nd week of pregnancy and can be excessively large at birth (macrosomia). The macrosomic fetus is at risk for birth trauma associated with shoulder dystocia. In other cases, the intrauterine environment becomes unfavorable for growth, and at birth the infant has lost muscle mass and subcutaneous fat resulting in an intrauterine growth restriction that occurs as a result of uteroplacental insufficiency. This is known as *dysmaturity syndrome,* which occurs in 20% of all postterm pregnancies and is frequently associated with oligohydramnios, meconium aspiration, and short-term neonatal complications (ACOG, 2004). The small-for-gestational-age (SGA) fetus is at risk for nonreassuring fetal status during labor because there is frequently associated oligohydramnios (Blackburn, 2007).

Clinical Therapy

When the 40th week of gestation is completed and birth has not occurred, most practitioners begin using the nonstress test (NST) and biophysical profile (BPP), modified BPP (especially the amniotic fluid volume portion of the BPP), or contraction stress test (CST) as assessment tools. These tests may be done two times a week to help evaluate fetal well-being (ACOG, 2004). Research has not demonstrated a clear benefit in performing postdate pregnancy monitoring; however, because the practice is in no way harmful to the fetus, the practice of fetal surveillance will likely continue. If at any time the fetal assessment tests indicate a problem, interventions are initiated to accomplish the birth.

Nursing Care Management

Nursing Assessment and Diagnosis

When the woman is admitted into the birthing area, ongoing assessments of fetal well-being begin as soon as the postterm condition has been verified. The nurse needs to identify reassuring FHR characteristics and evaluate for the presence of nonreassuring patterns, such as nonperiodic variable decelerations (which are associated with cord compression or oligohydramnios), so that corrective actions can be taken. When the amniotic membranes rupture, the nurse assesses the fluid for meconium. In addition, the nurse assesses the woman's knowledge about the condition, implications for her baby, risks, and possible interventions.

Nursing diagnoses that may apply to the woman with postterm pregnancy include the following:

- *Deficient Knowledge* related to lack of information about postterm pregnancy
- *Fear* related to the unknown outcome for the baby
- *Ineffective Individual Coping* related to anxiety about the status of the baby

Nursing Plan and Implementation

If the woman has not been assessing fetal movement every day, the nurse teaches her how to do so. It is vital to stress the importance of identifying inadequate fetal movement and immediately contacting her healthcare provider. (See Chapter 11 ∞ for further discussion of techniques to detect fetal movement.)

Client education about the postterm pregnancy is another important nursing responsibility. The nurse should address the implications and associated risks for the baby, as well as possible treatment plans. The woman and her partner need opportunities to ask questions and clarify information.

Hospital-Based Nursing Care

Promotion of fetal well-being requires careful assessment of the response of the fetus during labor. If oligohydramnios exists, a continuous FHR tracing is obtained and evaluated frequently. Some facilities may choose to use continuous monitoring on any fetus who is postterm because of the increased incidence of oligohydramnios. Variable decelerations are often associated with oligohydramnios, because the decreased amount of fluid allows compression of the umbilical cord. If the fetus is macrosomic, careful assessment of labor progress (contraction characteristics, progressive cervical dilatation, and fetal descent) is also needed.

Emotional support is a key nursing intervention for women with pregnancies that extend past the due date. Women experiencing postterm pregnancy frequently feel increased stress and anxiety and have difficulty coping. Women are also uncomfortable and have difficulty sleeping, resting, or obtaining a comfortable position. Many women are emotionally prepared for the duration of 40 weeks; however, after that period women may become discouraged, anxious, and irritable. Encouragement, support, and recognition of the woman's anxiety are helpful strategies.

Evaluation

Anticipated outcomes of nursing care include the following:

- The woman has knowledge about the postterm pregnancy.
- The woman and her partner feel supported and able to cope with the postterm pregnancy.
- Fetal status is maintained, any abnormalities are quickly identified, and supportive measures are initiated.

Care of the Woman and Fetus at Risk Because of Fetal Malposition

The *occiput-posterior (OP) position* is the most common fetal malposition. **Malposition** refers to any position that is not ROA, OA, or LOA. When the fetus is OP, the occiput of the fetal head is directed toward the back of the maternal pelvis. During labor, 90% to 95% of OP fetuses rotate to an occiput-anterior (OA) position.

A variation of OP called the **persistent occiput-posterior (POP) position** occurs in less than 10% of unmedicated labors. In this case the fetus enters the birth canal, descends, and is born in the OP position. Lack of rotation can be caused by poor contractions, abnormal flexion of the head, incomplete rotation, inadequate maternal pushing efforts usually related to epidural anesthesia, or a large fetus. Labor may be prolonged; however, most POP fetuses are born without the aid of forceps or a vacuum.

Risks of Fetal Malposition

Maternal risks related to the persistent occiput-posterior position include the following:

- Risk of third- or fourth-degree perineal lacerations during birth
- Risk of extension of a midline episiotomy

Fetal implications do not include an increased mortality risk unless labor is prolonged or additional interventions such as forceps-assisted, vacuum-assisted, or cesarean birth are required.

Clinical Therapy

Clinical treatment focuses on close monitoring of maternal and fetal status and labor progress to determine whether vaginal or cesarean birth is the safer birth method. A cesarean birth is chosen if maternal or fetal problems make a vaginal birth unwise or if CPD is present. Although the majority of persistent occiput-posterior fetuses are born vaginally, in some cases forceps-assisted or vacuum-assisted births may be necessary. The forceps can be used to deliver the fetus while it is still in the occiput-posterior position or to rotate the occiput to an anterior position (called Scanzoni's maneuver). A rotation from the left occiput-posterior (LOP) or right occiput-posterior (ROP) position to an anterior position may also be accomplished with a vacuum-assistance

---

EVIDENCE-BASED PRACTICE

Assessment and Intervention for Occiput-Posterior Malposition

Clinical Question
How is occiput-posterior (OP) malposition most accurately detected? What nursing interventions are effective in enhancing rotation from OP to occiput anterior?

The Evidence
The cause of occiput-posterior (OP) malposition is unclear, but the condition has well-documented risks for both maternal and neonatal morbidity. Many complications can be avoided if the fetus is successfully rotated to occiput anterior before birth, but doing so requires confidence in the detection of OP. AWOHNN, the professional organization for obstetric and neonatal nurses, requested a systematic review of research that focused on the diagnosis and treatment of OP malposition. Eight studies focused on diagnosis and five studies focused on fetal rotation were systematically reviewed by a clinical expert. The findings from multiple studies that have undergone rigorous review provide the strongest evidence for nursing practice.

What Is Effective?
A common diagnostic method, Leopold's maneuver, was only 60% effective in correctly identifying OP malposition. Digital vaginal examination was inaccurate the majority of the time in the first stage of labor, and in the second stage of labor was only slightly better than Leopold's maneuver. Transabdominal sonography was accurate more than 90% of the time, and it was as accurate as transvaginal sonography, which is more invasive and may be uncomfortable for the laboring mother. Interventions to rotate the fetus focused on maternal posturing. There was no support for maternal positioning before labor begins. The hands-and-knees position

has traditionally been advanced as a mechanism for antepartal fetal rotation, but these studies did not provide evidence supporting this intervention. For women presenting in labor with a fetus in the OP position, maternal posturing using Sims' position on the same side as the fetal spine is recommended during labor. Women in these studies who used this position throughout labor had better rotation to the occiput-anterior position, a lower cesarean birth rate, and shorter labors than women using other positions.

What Is Inconclusive?
The studies that investigated diagnostic use of sonography correlated the diagnosed position with the birth position. Because the fetus can rotate during birth, this method of study may be flawed. None of these studies conducted a cost-benefit analysis of sonography as a means of determining fetal position.

Best Practice
Leopold's maneuver and digital vaginal examination are not sufficiently accurate to detect occiput-posterior malposition of the fetus, particularly in early labor. Ultrasound evaluation is the most sensitive in identifying this position. Maternal positions before labor are not helpful, as is the case with most intrapartum positions. Sims' position on the same side as the fetal spine after OP fetal position is the most effective in achieving rotation. This position should be maintained as much as possible during latent and active phases of labor in order to enhance rotation.

References
Ridley, R. (2007). Diagnosis and intervention for occiput posterior malposition. *JOGNN: The Journal of Obstetric, Gynecologic, and Neonatal Nursing, 36*(2), 135–143.

device. (See Chapter 23 ∞ for further discussion of forceps and vacuum.)

Nursing Care Management

Nursing Assessment and Diagnosis

Signs and symptoms of a persistent occiput-posterior position include complaints of intense back pain by the laboring woman, a dysfunctional labor pattern, hypotonic labor (the fetal head does not put adequate pressure on the cervix), arrest of dilatation, or arrest of fetal descent. The back pain is caused by the fetal occiput compressing the sacral nerves. Further assessment may reveal a depression in the maternal abdomen above the symphysis. FHR is typically heard far laterally on the abdomen, and on vaginal examination the physician/CNM finds the wide, diamond-shaped anterior fontanelle in the anterior portion of the pelvis. This fontanelle may be difficult to feel because of molding of the fetal head.

Nursing diagnoses that may apply to women with persistent occiput-posterior position include the following:

- *Acute Pain* related to back discomfort secondary to the OP position
- *Ineffective Individual Coping* related to unanticipated discomfort and slow progress in labor

Nursing Plan and Implementation

Changing maternal posture has been used for many years to enhance rotation of OP or occiput-transverse (OT) to OA. A number of position changes may be tried. For instance, the woman may be asked to lie on one side and then asked to move to the other side as the fetus begins to rotate. This side-lying position may promote rotation; it also enables the support person to apply counterpressure on the sacral area to decrease discomfort. A knee-chest position provides a downward slant to the vaginal canal, directing the fetal head downward on descent. A hands-and-knees position is often effective in rotating the fetus. In addition to maintaining a hands-and-knees position on the bed, the woman may try pelvic rocking, and the support person may firmly stroke the abdomen. The stroking begins over the fetal back and swings around to the other side of the abdomen. After the fetus has rotated, the woman lies in a Sims' position on the side opposite the fetal back.

Some studies have shown success with the physician/CNM manually rotating the head during labor. Manual rotation done before complete dilatation was associated with a higher failure rate. When the occiput-posterior position resulted in an arrest of labor, the incidence of failure quadrupled. Inability to manually rotate the fetus was associated with a higher cesarean birth rate (Le Ray, Serres, Schmitz et al., 2007).

Evaluation

Anticipated outcomes of nursing care include the following:

- The woman's discomfort is decreased.
- The coping abilities of the woman and her partner are strengthened.

Care of the Woman and Fetus at Risk Because of Fetal Malpresentation

In a normal presentation, the occiput is the presenting part (Figure 22–3A ■). Fetal malpresentations include brow, face, breech, shoulder (transverse lie), and compound presentation. With a face or chin presentation, an internal scalp electrode should not be used.

Brow Presentation

In a brow presentation, the forehead of the fetus becomes the presenting part. In the military presentation, the fetal head is between flexion and extension (Figure 22–3B), whereas in the occipitomental presentation, the fetal head enters the birth canal with the widest diameter of the head (approximately 13.5 cm [5.3 in.]) foremost (Figure 22–3c).

The brow presentation occurs more often in multiparas than in nulliparas and is thought to be caused by lax abdominal and pelvic musculature. Grand multiparous women have a greater risk. Brow presentations can also occur in cases of CPD or pelvic contracture and in premature fetuses. Premature rupture of membranes precedes 27% of brow presentations (Parker & Napolitano, 2005). Many brow presentations spontaneously convert to face or occipital presentations. Brow presentations are the least common types of abnormal presentations and occur in about 1 in 1500 births (Lanni & Seeds, 2007).

Risks of Brow Presentation

Maternal implications of brow presentation include increased risk of the following:

- Longer labor caused by ineffective contractions and slow or arrested fetal descent
- Cesarean birth if brow presentation persists or if the fetus is large

Fetal-neonatal risks include increased mortality because of cerebral and neck compression and damage to the trachea and larynx. In addition, facial edema, bruising, and exaggerated molding of the newborn's head may be observed.

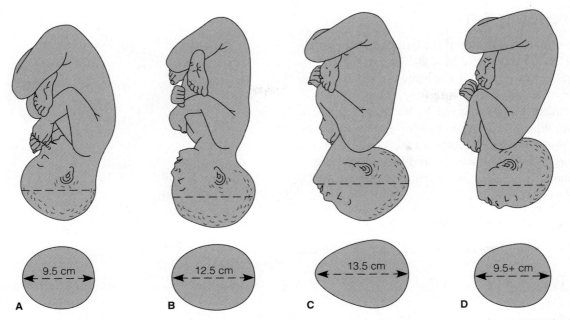

FIGURE 22–3 Types of cephalic presentations. *A,* The occiput is the presenting part because the head is flexed and the fetal chin is against the chest. The largest anteroposterior (AP) diameter that presents and passes through the pelvis is approximately 9.5 cm. *B,* Military (sinciput) presentation. The head is neither flexed nor extended. The presenting AP diameter is approximately 12.5 cm. *C,* Brow presentation. The largest diameter of the fetal head (approximately 13.5 cm) presents in this situation. *D,* Face presentation. The AP diameter is 9.5 cm.
Source: Danforth, D. N., & Scott, J. R. (Eds.). (1990). *Obstetrics and gynecology* (5th ed., p. 170, fig. 8–9). New York: Lippincott.

Clinical Therapy

If a brow presentation fails to convert to occipital or face presentation, cesarean birth is indicated in most cases (Lanni & Seeds, 2007). If a vaginal birth is attempted, the woman is closely monitored for CPD, caput succedaneum, facial edema, and nonreassuring fetal status. Attempts to convert brow presentations via manual attempt, forceps, or vacuum are contraindicated, as is the use of oxytocin. Scalp electrodes should not be placed when the fetus is in a brow presentation (FP Notebook, 2007). Attempts to facilitate birth using oxytocin can result in a dystocia.

Nursing Care Management

Nursing Assessment and Diagnosis

A brow presentation can be detected on vaginal examination by palpation of the diamond-shaped anterior fontanelle on one side and orbital ridges and root of the nose on the other side.

Nursing diagnoses that may apply to a woman with a brow presentation include the following:

- *Deficient Knowledge* related to lack of information about the possible maternal-fetal effects of brow presentation
- *Risk for Injury* to the fetus related to pressure on fetal structures secondary to brow presentation
- *Fear* related to sudden need for cesarean birth if conversion does not occur

Nursing Plan and Implementation

The nurse closely observes the woman for labor problems and the fetus for signs of hypoxia as evidenced by late decelerations and bradycardia.

The nurse also provides emotional support to the family. In this role the nurse explains the fetal position to the woman and her support person or interprets what the physician/CNM has told them. The nurse should stay close at hand to reassure the couple, inform them of any changes, and assist them with labor-coping techniques. In face and brow presentations, the newborn's face may be edematous. The couple may need help in beginning the attachment process because of the newborn's facial appearance. After the infant is inspected for any abnormalities, the pediatrician and nurse can assure the couple that the facial edema is only temporary and will subside in 3 or 4 days and that the molding will be much less visible in a few days (even though completion of the process takes several weeks).

Evaluation

Anticipated outcomes of nursing care include the following:

- The woman and her partner understand the implications and associated problems of brow presentation.
- The mother and her baby have a safe labor and birth.

Face Presentation

In a face presentation, the face of the fetus is the presenting part (Figure 22–3D and Figure 22–4 ■). The fetal head is hyperextended even more than in the brow presentation. Face presentation occurs most frequently in grand multiparity, in preterm birth, in fetuses affected by anencephaly or trisomies, in multiple gestations, in hydramnios, in macrosomia, in hydrocephaly, or in mothers with placenta previa, pelvic tumors, pelvic contractures, and uterine malformations. The incidence of face presentation is about 1 in 500 live births (Lanni & Seeds, 2007).

Risks of Face Presentation

Maternal risks related to face presentation include the following:

- Increased risk of CPD
- Prolonged labor
- Increased risk of infection (with prolonged labor)
- Cesarean birth if fetal chin is posterior (mentum posterior)

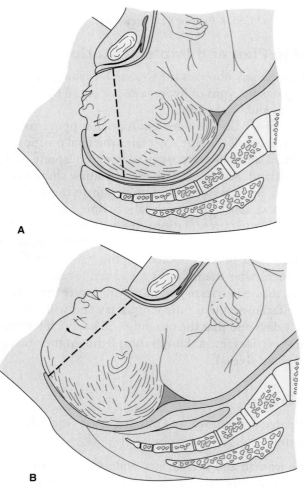

A

B

FIGURE 22–4 Face presentation. Mechanism of birth in mentoanterior position. *A*, The submentobregmatic diameter at the outlet. *B*, The fetal head is born by movement of flexion.

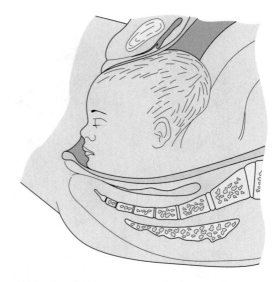

FIGURE 22–5 Face presentation. Mechanism of birth in mentoposterior position. Fetal head is unable to extend farther. The face becomes impacted.

Fetal-neonatal risks include the following (Lanni & Seeds, 2007):

- Cephalohematoma of the face
- Facial edema
- Laryngeal and tracheal edema
- Pronounced molding of the head
- Increased intrapartum deaths
- Nonreassuring fetal status

Clinical Therapy

A vaginal birth may be anticipated if no CPD is present, the chin (mentum) is anterior, the labor pattern is effective, and the fetal status is reassuring. Many mentum posterior presentations spontaneously convert to anterior in the late stages of labor. If the mentum remains posterior, a vaginal birth is not possible and a cesarean birth is necessary (Figure 22–5 ■). Attempts to rotate the fetus often result in higher maternal and fetal morbidity rates and should not be performed (Lanni & Seeds, 2007).

Nursing Care Management

Nursing Assessment and Diagnosis

When performing Leopold's maneuvers, the nurse finds that the back of the fetus is difficult to outline, and a deep furrow can be palpated between the hard occiput and the fetal back (Figure 22–6 ■). Fetal heart tones are audible on the side where the fetal feet are palpated. It may be difficult to determine by vaginal examination whether a breech or face is presenting, especially if facial edema is already present. During the vaginal examination, palpation of the saddle of the nose and the gums should be attempted. When assessing engagement, the nurse must

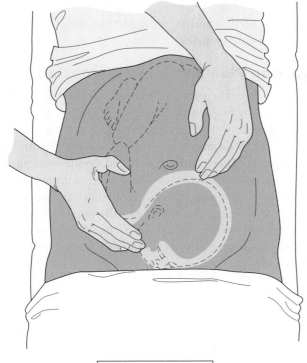

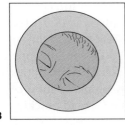

FIGURE 22–6 Face presentation. *A,* Palpation of the maternal abdomen with the fetus in right mentum posterior (RMP). *B,* Vaginal examination may permit palpation of facial features of the fetus.

remember that the face has to be deep within the pelvis before the biparietal diameters have entered the inlet.

Nursing diagnoses that may apply to the woman with a fetus in face presentation include the following:

- *Fear* related to unknown outcome of the labor and a possible instrument-assisted or cesarean birth
- *Risk for Injury* to the newborn's face related to edema secondary to the birth process

Nursing Plan and Implementation

Nursing interventions are the same as those indicated for the brow presentation.

Evaluation

Anticipated outcomes of nursing care include the following:

- The woman and her partner understand the implications and associated problems of face presentation.
- The mother and her baby have a safe labor and birth.

Breech Presentation

The exact cause of breech presentation (Figure 22–7 ■) is unknown. This malpresentation occurs in about 3% to 4% of labors and is frequently associated with preterm birth, placenta previa, hydramnios, multiple gestation, uterine anomalies (such as bicornuate uterus), and fetal anomalies (especially anencephaly and hydrocephaly) (Cunningham et al., 2005).

Risks of Breech Presentation

The maternal implication of breech presentation is a likelihood of cesarean birth. Fetal-neonatal implications include the following (Lanni & Seeds, 2007):

- Higher perinatal morbidity and mortality rates
- Increased risk of prolapsed cord, especially in incomplete breeches, because space is available between the cervix and presenting part
- Increased risk of cervical spinal cord injuries caused by hyperextension of the fetal head during vaginal birth
- Increased brachial plexus injuries
- Increased risk of asphyxia and nonreassuring fetal status

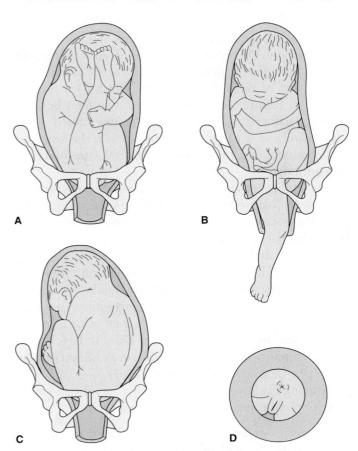

FIGURE 22–7 Breech presentation. *A,* Frank breech. *B,* Incomplete (footling) breech. *C,* Complete breech in left sacral anterior (LSA) position. *D,* On vaginal examination, the nurse may feel the anal sphincter. The tissue of the fetal buttocks feels soft.

- Increased risk of dystocia
- Increased risk of birth trauma (especially of the head) during either vaginal or cesarean breech birth
- Nulliparous women had increases in neonatal morbidity and mortality (Gilbert, Hicks, Boe, & Danielson, 2003)

Clinical Therapy

Current clinical therapy is directed toward converting the breech presentation to a cephalic presentation before the beginning of labor. Breech presentations are 16 times more likely to result in intrapartum fetal death (Lanni & Seeds, 2007). Some physicians attempt an *external cephalic version (ECV)* at 36 to 38 weeks' gestation as long as the woman is not in labor. ACOG currently recommends that breech presentations be born via planned cesarean because of the significant increase in complications associated with breech vaginal births (ACOG, 2006). (See Chapter 23 ∞ for discussion of external version.)

Nursing Care Management

Nursing Assessment and Diagnosis

Frequently it is the nurse who first recognizes a breech presentation. On palpation the nurse feels the firm fetal head in the uterine fundus and the wider sacrum in the lower part of the abdomen. If the sacrum has not descended, ballottement causes the entire fetal body to move. Furthermore, FHR is usually auscultated above the umbilicus. Passage of meconium into the amniotic fluid caused by compression of the fetal intestinal tract is common.

If membranes are ruptured, the nurse is particularly alert for a prolapsed umbilical cord, especially in footling breeches, because there is space between the cervix and presenting part through which the cord can slip. If the infant is small and the membranes rupture, the danger is even greater. The risk of a prolapsed umbilical cord is one reason why any woman with ruptured membranes should not ambulate until a full assessment, including vaginal examination, has been performed. Women with a breech presentation are 5 to 20 times more likely to have a prolapsed umbilical cord than women whose infants are in vertex presentation (Lanni & Seeds, 2007).

Nursing diagnoses that may apply to a woman with a breech presentation include the following:

- *Impaired Gas Exchange* in the fetus related to interruption in umbilical blood flow secondary to compression of the cord
- *Deficient Knowledge* related to lack of information about the implications and associated complications of breech presentation for the mother and fetus

- *Risk for Injury* related to possible prolapsed umbilical cord, birth trauma, intrapartum asphyxia, or fetal spinal cord injuries

Nursing Plan and Implementation

During labor, the nurse promotes maternal-fetal physical well-being by frequently assessing fetal and maternal status. Because the fetus is at increased risk for prolapse of the cord, agency protocols may call for continuous fetal monitoring. If the head is not completely engaged, continuous monitoring is warranted and the woman should maintain complete bed rest. The nurse provides teaching and information about the breech presentation and the nursing care needed.

As many as 86.9% of infants in breech presentations are born by cesarean birth (ACOG, 2006). Most breech vaginal births are performed on multiparous women with a proven pelvis (prior birth of a normal or large size fetus without difficulty) that presents in active labor with an unknown breech presentation. The nurse assists with the vaginal birth by including Piper forceps (used to guide the after-coming fetal head) in the birth table setup. The nurse may assist the physician if forceps are needed for the birth. If the family and physician/CNM decide on a cesarean birth, the nurse assists as with any cesarean birth. Breech births commonly occur in the operating room with a "double setup" in place. If difficulties arise with the birth, the room is already prepared for a cesarean birth and the procedure can be performed quickly.

Evaluation

Anticipated outcomes of nursing care include the following:

- The woman and her partner understand the implications and associated problems of breech presentation.

COMPLEMENTARY AND ALTERNATIVE THERAPIES

Moxibustion to Promote Version in Breech Presentation

Traditional Chinese medicine (TCM) uses the herb mugwort in the form of moxa to promote version in a breech presentation. *Moxa* is a system of treatment, often combined with acupuncture, in which an herb is dried, rolled into cones (like incense cones), and placed on certain meridian parts of the body. The moxa is then lit and allowed to burn close to the skin, hence the *-bustion* component of the name. The heat and pungency of mugwort stimulates the point, and energy moves through. It is believed that the effect of moxibustion increases fetal activity.

The meridian point used in moxibustion to promote version in breech presentations is acupoint BL67, located beside the outer corner of the fifth toenail. Treatment may take from 7 days to 2 weeks. There is limited evidence that suggests that moxibustion is an effective modality in the management of breech presentations (Coyle, Smith, & Peat, 2005).

- Major complications are recognized early and corrective measures are instituted.
- The mother and baby have a safe labor and birth.

Transverse Lie (Shoulder Presentation) of a Single Fetus

A transverse lie occurs in approximately 1 in 300 term births (Lanni & Seeds, 2007). An abnormal presentation that is identified in the early third trimester has a 22% risk of persisting at term (Fox & Chapman, 2006). Maternal conditions associated with a transverse lie are grand multiparity with relaxed uterine muscles, preterm fetus, abnormal uterus, excessive amniotic fluid, placenta previa, and contracted pelvis (Figure 22–8 ■).

The management of shoulder presentation depends on the gestational age. If discovered before term, the management is expectant (watchful), because some fetuses change presentation without intervention. When a shoulder presentation is still evident at 37 completed weeks of gestation, an external cephalic version (ECV) attempt (followed, if successful, by induction of labor) is recommended, because the associated risk of prolapsed cord is 20 times higher if the fetus is in an abnormal axis (Lanni & Seeds, 2007). If the ECV is unsuccessful, a cesarean birth should be performed before the onset of spontaneous labor.

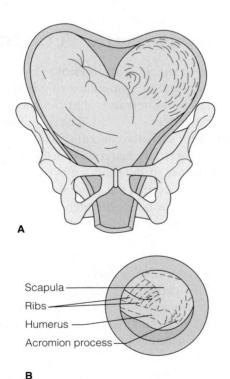

A

Scapula
Ribs
Humerus
Acromion process

B

FIGURE 22–8 Transverse lie. *A,* Shoulder presentation. *B,* On vaginal examination, the nurse may feel the acromion process as the fetal presenting part.

Nursing Care Management

The nurse can identify a transverse lie by inspection and palpation of the abdomen, by auscultation of FHR, and by vaginal examination. On inspection the woman's abdomen appears widest from side to side as a result of the long axis of the infant's body lying parallel to the ground and across the mother's uterus.

On palpation no fetal part is felt in the fundal portion of the uterus or above the symphysis. The head may be palpated on one side and the breech on the other. Fetal heart rate is usually auscultated just below the midline of the umbilicus. On vaginal examination, if a presenting part is palpated, it is the ridged thorax or possibly an arm that is compressed against the chest.

The nurse assists in the interpretation of the fetal presentation and provides information and support to the couple. The nurse also assesses maternal and fetal status frequently and prepares the woman for a cesarean birth. (See Chapter 23 ∞.)

Compound Presentation

A compound presentation is one in which there are two presenting parts, such as the occiput and fetal hand or the complete breech and fetal hand. Most compound presentations resolve themselves spontaneously, but others require additional manipulation at birth. Compound presentations occur in 1 in 377 to 1 in 1213 births (Lanni & Seeds, 2007).

Care of the Woman and Fetus at Risk for Macrosomia

Fetal **macrosomia** is defined as a newborn weight of more than 4000 g at birth (ACOG, 2000). The condition is more common with excessive maternal weight gain in pregnancy, maternal obesity, maternal diabetes, mothers with a previous infant who weighed more than 4000 g, and in cases of grand multiparity and prolonged gestation (Mahony, Foley, McAuliffe et al., 2007). Macrosomia is also more common in fetuses who have erythroblastosis fetalis. Some ethnic groups are prone to giving birth to larger babies (Mahony et al., 2007).

Risks of Macrosomia

Maternal implications of macrosomia include increased risk of CPD, dysfunctional labor, prolonged labor, soft tissue laceration during vaginal birth, and postpartum hemorrhage.

The most significant complication for the fetus-neonate with macrosomia is shoulder dystocia, an obstetric emergency in which, after the birth of the head, the anterior shoulder fails to deliver either spontaneously or with gentle traction (unresolved shoulder dystocia can lead to fetal death). Other risks include upper brachial plexus injury, fractured clavicle, meconium aspiration, asphyxia, hypoglycemia, polycythemia, and hyperbilirubinemia.

In addition, infants who are macrosomic at birth are more likely to become obese in childhood and adolescence. These children are also at risk to develop diabetes in later life (Landon, Catalano, & Gabbe, 2007).

Clinical Therapy

The occurrence of maternal and fetal problems associated with excessively large infants may be lessened somewhat by identifying macrosomia before the onset of labor. If a large fetus is suspected, the maternal pelvis should be evaluated carefully. Fetal size can be estimated by palpating the crown-to-rump length of the fetus in utero and by ultrasound. Clinical studies have demonstrated that palpation and ultrasound are equally effective assessments of fetal weight. Routine use of ultrasound to predict fetal weight is not recommended; however, ultrasound does have predictive value in ruling out macrosomia (Magliore & Copel, 2007). When the uterus appears excessively large, either hydramnios, an oversized fetus, or a multiple gestation must be considered as the possible cause. If so, evaluation of the etiology should include ultrasonography.

When fetal weight is estimated to be 4500 g or more, a cesarean birth is usually planned. The best method of birth for an estimated fetal weight of 4000 to 4500 g is debated. The discussion centers primarily on the incidence of shoulder dystocia during vaginal birth and the difficulty in accurately estimating the fetal weight. Unexpected shoulder dystocia during vaginal birth can be a grave problem. As an emergency measure the physician/CNM may ask the nurse to assist the woman into the McRoberts maneuver (sharp flexion of the thighs toward the hips and abdomen) or to apply suprapubic pressure in an attempt to aid in the birth of the fetal shoulders. Fundal pressure should never be used because it can further wedge the anterior shoulder under the symphysis pubis.

Nursing Care Management

The nurse assists in identifying women who are at risk for carrying a large fetus or those who exhibit signs of macrosomia. Because these women are prime candidates for dystocia and its complications, the nurse frequently assesses the FHR for indications of nonreassuring fetal status and evaluates the rates of cervical dilatation and fetal descent.

The fetal monitor is applied for continuous fetal evaluation. Early decelerations (caused by fetal head compres-

sion) could mean size disproportion at the bony inlet. Any sign of labor dysfunction or nonreassuring fetal status is reported to the physician/CNM immediately. Lack of fetal descent is another indicator that should alert the nurse to the possibility that the infant is too large for a vaginal birth.

The nurse provides support for the laboring woman and her partner and information about the implications of macrosomia and possible associated problems. During the birth, the nurse continues to provide support and encouragement to the woman or the couple.

The nurse inspects macrosomic newborns after birth for cephalohematoma, Erb's palsy, and fractured clavicles and informs the nursery staff of any problems so that the newborn is observed closely for cerebral, neurologic, and motor problems.

In a woman with a macrosomic fetus, the uterus has been stretched farther than it would have been with an average size fetus. The overstretching may lead to contractile problems during labor or after birth. After birth the overstretched uterus may not contract well (uterine atony) and will feel boggy (soft). In this case, uterine hemorrhage is likely. The fundus of the uterus is massaged to stimulate contraction, and IV or IM Pitocin may be needed. Maternal vital signs are closely monitored for deviation suggestive of shock.

Care of the Woman and Fetus in the Presence of Nonreassuring Fetal Status

When the oxygen supply is insufficient to meet the physiologic needs of the fetus, a nonreassuring fetal status may result. This status may be transient or chronic, and may be prompted by a variety of factors. The most common are cord compression and uteroplacental insufficiency, possibly caused by preexisting maternal or fetal disease or placental abnormalities. If the resulting hypoxia persists and metabolic acidosis occurs, the situation could cause permanent damage to, or be life threatening for, the fetus.

Early signs of nonreassuring fetal status are variations from the normal heart rate pattern and decreased fetal movement. Meconium-stained amniotic fluid and the presence of ominous FHR patterns, such as persistent late decelerations (regardless of the depth of deceleration), persistent severe variable decelerations (especially if the return to baseline is prolonged), and prolonged decelerations are signs of nonreassuring fetal status. Meconium-stained fluid can only be determined after the membranes have ruptured. Other signs of nonreassuring fetal status include tachycardia, bradycardia, and loss of variability. When these patterns are detected, **intrauterine resuscitation** (corrective measures used to optimize the oxygen exchange within the maternal-fetal circulation) should be started without delay. Treatment of maternal hypotension involves having the woman turn to a left lateral position (right lateral may also be tried), beginning an intravenous infusion or increasing the flow rate if an infusion is already in place, or, if cord prolapse is suspected, having the woman assume a knee-chest position. The nurse should maintain position changes that result in an increase in the fetal heart rate and perform a vaginal examination to attempt to detect a prolapsed cord. If a prolapsed cord is discovered, the examiner applies pressure to the presenting part to relieve the additional pressure on the cord. Uterine activity can be decreased by discontinuing intravenous Pitocin administration or administering a tocolytic agent (such as terbutaline) to decrease contraction frequency and intensity. Oxygen is also administered to the woman via facial mask.

Caregivers can obtain additional information about the condition of the fetus by performing fetal scalp stimulation or fetal acoustical stimulation (see Chapter 18 ∞). The management scheme for nonreassuring fetal status is illustrated in Figure 22–9 ■.

Maternal Implications

Indications of a nonreassuring fetal status greatly increase the psychologic stress of a laboring woman and her family members. Professional staff members may become so involved in assessing fetal status and initiating corrective measures that they fail to provide the woman and her partner with explanations and emotional support. It is imperative to offer both. In many instances, if birth is not imminent, the woman must undergo cesarean birth. This method of birth may be a source of fear and of frustration, too, if the couple prepared for a shared vaginal birth experience.

Clinical Therapy

Treatment centers on improving the blood flow to the fetus by correcting maternal hypotension, decreasing the intensity and frequency of contractions if present, providing IV fluids to the woman as needed, administering oxygen, and gathering further information about fetal status. Fetal

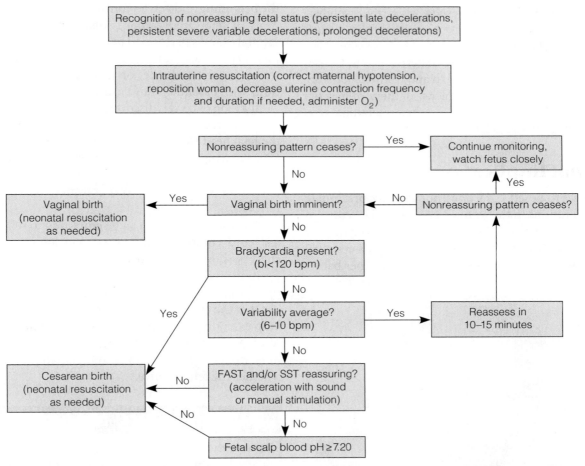

FIGURE 22–9 Intrapartal management of nonreassuring fetal status. Note: bl = baseline; FAST = fetal acoustic stimulation test; SST = scalp stimulation test.
Source: From Zuspan, F. P., & Quilligan, E. J. (1998). *Handbook of obstetrics, gynecology, and primary care.* Copyright 1998, Mosby reprinted with permission from Elsevier Science.

response to intrauterine resuscitation measures dictates subsequent actions.

Nursing Care Management

The nurse reviews the woman's prenatal history and notes the presence of any conditions (such as preeclampsia, diabetes, renal disease, IUGR) that may be associated with decreased uteroplacental-fetal blood flow. When the membranes rupture, the nurse assesses the FHR immediately and notes the characteristics of the amniotic fluid. As labor progresses, the nurse is especially alert to suspicious changes in the FHR. At all times, the nurse encourages and supports maternal positioning that maximizes uteroplacental-fetal blood flow.

Care of the Woman and Fetus with a Prolapsed Umbilical Cord

A **prolapsed umbilical cord** results when the umbilical cord precedes the fetal presenting part. When this occurs, pressure is placed on the umbilical cord as it is trapped between the presenting part and the maternal pelvis. Consequently the vessels carrying blood to and from the fetus are compressed (Figure 22–10 ■). Prolapse of the cord may occur with rupture of the membranes if the presenting part is not well engaged in the pelvis.

Maternal Implications

Although a prolapsed cord does not directly precipitate physical alterations in the woman, her immediate concern for the baby creates enormous stress. The woman may need to deal with some unusual interventions, a cesarean birth, and, in some circumstances, the death of her baby.

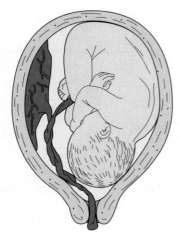

FIGURE 22–10 Prolapse of the umbilical cord.

Fetal-Neonatal Implications

Compression of the cord results in decreased blood flow and leads to nonreassuring fetal status. If labor is underway, the cord is compressed further with each contraction. If the pressure on the cord is not relieved, the fetus will die.

Clinical Therapy

Preventing the occurrence of prolapse of the cord is the preferred medical approach. A laboring woman with a confirmed rupture of membranes will be kept horizontal, usually in bed, until the fetal head is well engaged and the risk of a prolapse is significantly decreased. If a prolapse occurs, relieving the compression on the cord is critical to fetal outcome. The medical and nursing team must work together to facilitate birth.

Bed rest is indicated for all laboring women with a history of ruptured membranes, until engagement with no cord prolapse has been documented. Furthermore, with spontaneous rupture of membranes or amniotomy, the FHR should be auscultated for at least a full minute and at the beginning and end of contractions for several contractions. If fetal bradycardia is detected on auscultation, a vaginal exam is performed to rule out cord prolapse. In the presence of cord prolapse, electronic monitor tracings show severe, moderate, or prolonged variable decelerations with baseline bradycardia.

If a loop of cord is discovered, the examiner's gloved fingers must remain in the vagina to provide firm pressure on the fetal head (to relieve compression) until the physician/CNM arrives. This is a lifesaving measure. The mother is given oxygen via face mask, and the FHR is monitored to determine whether the cord compression is adequately relieved.

The force of gravity can be employed to relieve umbilical cord compression. The woman assumes the knee-chest position or the bed is adjusted to the Trendelenburg position, and the woman is transported to the birthing or operating room in this position. The nurse must remember that the cord may be occultly prolapsed with an actual loop extending into the vagina or lying alongside the presenting part. It may be pulsating strongly or so weakly that it is difficult to determine on palpation of the cord whether the fetus is alive.

Nursing Care Management

Because there are few outward signs of cord prolapse, each pregnant woman is advised to call her physician or certified nurse-midwife when the membranes rupture and to go to the office, clinic, or birthing facility. A sterile vaginal examination determines if there is danger of cord prolapse. If the presenting part is well engaged, the risk of cord prolapse is minimal, and the woman may ambulate as desired. If the presenting part is not well engaged, bed rest is recommended to prevent cord prolapse.

Because cord prolapse can be associated with fetal death, some physicians/CNMs insist that bed rest be maintained after rupture of membranes regardless of fetal engagement. This can lead to conflict if the laboring woman and her partner do not hold the same opinions. The nurse can ease this situation by assisting communication between the physician/CNM and the couple.

During labor, any alteration of the FHR or the presence of meconium in the amniotic fluid indicates the need to assess for cord prolapse. Vaginal birth is possible with prolapsed cord if the cervix is completely dilated and pelvic measurements are adequate. In order for a vaginal birth to be attempted, birth should be imminent. In most cases, a vaginal birth is performed only if it results in a shorter time period than the preparations would take for a cesarean birth.

If these conditions are not present, cesarean birth is the method of choice. The woman is transported to the operating room, and the examiner continues to relieve the pressure on the cord until the infant is born.

Care of the Woman and Fetus at Risk Because of Anaphylactoid Syndrome of Pregnancy

Anaphylactoid Syndrome of Pregnancy

In the presence of a small tear in the amnion or chorion high in the uterus, a small amount of amniotic fluid may leak into the chorionic plate and enter the maternal system as an **amniotic fluid embolism**, which is currently known as anaphylactoid syndrome of pregnancy. Anaphylactoid syndrome of pregnancy is a rare labor complication, but it has a 60% to 80% mortality rate (Demianczuk & Corbetti, 2005). The fluid can also enter at areas of placental separation or cervical tears. Under pressure from the contracting uterus, the fluid is driven into the maternal circulation and then the maternal lungs. The more debris in the amniotic fluid (such as meconium), the greater the maternal problems. This condition frequently occurs during or after the birth when the woman has had a difficult, rapid labor.

Maternal Implications

The woman with anaphylactoid syndrome of pregnancy experiences a sudden onset of respiratory distress, circulatory collapse, acute hemorrhage, and cor pulmonale as the embolism blocks the vessels of the lungs. She exhibits dyspnea and cyanosis leading to hemorrhagic shock and coma. Birth must be facilitated immediately to obtain a live fetus.

Clinical Therapy

Any woman exhibiting chest pain, dyspnea, cyanosis, frothy sputum, tachycardia, hypotension, and massive hemorrhage requires the cooperation of every member of the healthcare team if her life is to be saved. Medical interventions are supportive. Recovery is contingent on return of the mother's cardiovascular and respiratory stability. If necessary, a cesarean birth is performed.

Nursing Care Management

In the absence of the physician/CNM, the nurse administers oxygen under positive pressure until medical help arrives. An intravenous line is quickly established. If respiratory and cardiac arrest occurs, cardiopulmonary resuscitation (CPR) is initiated immediately. The anesthesiologist should be called immediately.

The nurse readies the equipment necessary for blood transfusion and for the insertion of the CVP line. As the blood volume is replaced, using fresh whole blood to provide clotting factors, the CVP is monitored frequently. In the presence of cor pulmonale, fluid overload could easily occur.

Care of the Woman with Cephalopelvic Disproportion (CPD)

The birth passage includes the maternal bony pelvis, beginning at the pelvic inlet and ending at the pelvic outlet, and the maternal soft tissues within these anatomic areas. A contracture (narrowed diameter) in any of the described areas can result in **cephalopelvic disproportion (CPD)** if the fetus is larger than the pelvic diameters. Abnormal fetal presentations and positions occur in CPD as the fetus moves to accommodate its passage through the maternal pelvis.

The gynecoid and anthropoid pelvic types are usually adequate for vertex birth, but the android and platypelloid types are predisposed to CPD. Certain combinations of types also can result in pelvic diameters inadequate for

CRITICAL THINKING

A fetal heart tracing demonstrates the following: baseline heart rate of 140 with variability of 6 to 10 bpm. When you compare the FHR with the uterine contractions, you note that there is a slowing of the FHR at the time of the contraction and that the FHR tracing looks like the contraction curve, but it is upside down. Based on this tracing, what would you do?

Answers can be found in Appendix F ∞.

MyNursingKit | Dangers of Early Umbilical Cord Clamping

MyNursingKit | Cephalopelvic Disproportion

vertex birth. (See Chapter 17 ∞ for a description of pelvic types and their implications for childbirth.)

Types of Contractures

The pelvic inlet is contracted if the shortest anterior-posterior diameter is less than 10 cm (3.9 in.) or the greatest transverse diameter is less than 12 cm (4.7 in.). The anterior-posterior diameter may be approximated by measuring the diagonal conjugate, which in the contracted inlet is less than 11.5 cm (4.5 in.). Clinical pelvimetry is used to determine the smallest anterior-posterior diameter through which the fetal head must pass. Clinical pelvimetry is a learned skill where an examiner performs a vaginal examination to determine the pelvic measurements. X-rays are no longer performed on a pregnant woman to determine the adequacy of her pelvis. Soft-tissue dystocia can occur as a result of fibroids, Bandl's ring, stool, or a full bladder. Anomalies of the reproductive tract can also affect a woman's ability to have a vaginal birth.

The treatment goal is to allow the natural forces of labor to push the biparietal diameter of the fetal head beyond the potential interspinous obstruction. Although forceps may be used, they cause difficulty because pulling on the head destroys flexion, and the space is further diminished. A bulging perineum and crowning indicate that the obstruction has been passed.

An interischial tuberous diameter of less than 8 cm (3.1 in.) constitutes an outlet contracture. Outlet and mid-pelvic contractures frequently occur simultaneously. Whether vaginal birth can occur depends on the woman's interischial tuberous diameters and the fetal posterosagittal diameter.

Maternal Implications

Labor is prolonged in the presence of CPD. Membrane rupture can result from the force of the unequally distributed contractions being exerted on the fetal membranes. In obstructed labor, in which the fetus cannot descend, uterine rupture can occur. With delayed descent, necrosis of maternal soft tissues can result from pressure exerted by the fetal head. Eventually, necrosis can cause fistulas from the vagina to other nearby structures. Difficult, forceps-assisted births can also result in damage to maternal soft tissue.

Fetal-Neonatal Implications

If the membranes rupture and the fetal head has not entered the inlet, there is a danger of cord prolapse. Excessive molding of the fetal head can result. Traumatic, forceps-assisted birth can damage the fetal skull and central nervous system. Facial bruising, facial nerve trauma, and damage to the eye sockets can also occur.

Clinical Therapy

Fetopelvic relationships can be assessed by comparing pelvic measurements obtained by a manual exam before labor. An estimated weight of the fetus can be obtained by ultrasound measurements.

When the pelvic diameters are borderline or questionable, a trial of labor (TOL) may be advised. In this process, the woman continues to labor and careful, frequent assessments of cervical dilatation and fetal descent are made. Internal uterine and fetal scalp electrode monitoring may be used to more accurately assess uterine and fetal status. As long as there is continued progress, the TOL continues. Oxytocin should only be used if CPD is not suspected. When CPD is suspected, oxytocin should be discontinued. If progress ceases, the decision for a cesarean birth is made.

Nursing Care Management

The adequacy of the maternal pelvis for a vaginal birth should be assessed both during and before labor. During the intrapartal assessment, the size of the fetus and its presentation, position, and lie must also be considered. (See Chapter 18 ∞ for intrapartal assessment techniques.)

The nurse should suspect CPD when labor is prolonged, cervical dilatation and effacement are slow, and engagement of the presenting part is delayed. The couple may need support in coping with the stresses of this complicated labor. The nurse keeps the couple informed of what is happening and explains the procedures being used.

Nursing actions during the TOL are similar to care during any labor except that cervical dilatation and fetal descent are assessed more frequently. Both contractions and the fetus should be monitored continuously. Any signs of nonreassuring fetal status are reported to the physician/CNM immediately.

The mother may be positioned in a variety of ways to increase the pelvic diameters. Sitting or squatting increases the outlet diameters and may be effective when there is failure of or slow fetal descent. Changing from one side to the other or maintaining a hands-and-knees position may assist the fetus in the occiput-posterior position to change to an occiput-anterior position. The mother may instinctively want to assume one of these positions. If not, the nurse may encourage a change of position.

Care of the Woman with a Complication of the Third or Fourth Stage of Labor

Common complications of the third and fourth stages of labor include retained placenta, lacerations, and placenta accreta.

Retained Placenta

Retention of the placenta beyond 30 minutes after birth is termed **retained placenta**. It occurs in 1 in 100 to 1 in 200 vaginal births (Francois & Foley, 2007). Bleeding as a result of a retained placenta can be excessive. If placenta expulsion does not occur, a manual removal of the placenta by the physician/CNM is attempted. In women who do not have an epidural in place, intravenous sedation may be required because of the discomfort caused by the procedure. Failure to retrieve the placenta via manual removal usually necessitates surgical removal by curettage. If the woman does not have an epidural in place, the procedure can be performed under general anesthesia. Retained placenta may be a symptom of an accreta, increta, or percreta (to be discussed shortly).

Lacerations

Lacerations of the cervix or vagina may be indicated when bright-red vaginal bleeding persists in the presence of a well-contracted uterus. The incidence of lacerations is higher when the childbearing woman is young or a nullipara, has an epidural, has forceps-assisted birth and an episiotomy, and has not done perineal massage or preparation during pregnancy. Vaginal and perineal lacerations are often categorized in terms of degree, as follows:

- First-degree laceration is a superficial tear limited to the fourchette, perineal skin, and vaginal mucous membrane.
- Second-degree laceration involves the perineal skin, vaginal mucous membrane, underlying fascia, and muscles of the perineal body; it may extend upward on one or both sides of the vagina.
- Third-degree laceration extends through the perineal skin, vaginal mucous membranes, and perineal body and involves the anal sphincter.
- Fourth-degree laceration is the same as third degree but extends through the rectal mucosa to the lumen of the rectum; it may be called a third-degree laceration with a rectal wall extension.

Placenta Accreta

The chorionic villi attach directly to the myometrium of the uterus in *placenta accreta*. Two other types of placental adherence are *placenta increta,* in which the myometrium is invaded, and *placenta percreta,* in which the myometrium is penetrated. The adherence itself may be total, partial, or focal, depending on the amount of placental involvement. The incidence of placenta accreta is 1 in 533 births (Francois & Foley, 2007). It is the most common type, accounting for 78% of adherent placentas. Major risk factors include placenta previa and a previous uterine incision. Other risk factors include increasing maternal age and parity, previous uterine surgery, and endometrial defects. Risk increases as the number of cesarean births increase.

The primary complication with placenta accreta is maternal hemorrhage and failure of the placenta to separate following birth of the infant. An abdominal hysterectomy is performed in two-thirds of women (Francois & Foley, 2007). The need for a hysterectomy depends on the amount and depth of involvement.

Care of the Family Experiencing Perinatal Loss

Perinatal loss is death of a fetus or infant from the time of conception through the end of the newborn period 28 days after birth. Spontaneous abortion (miscarriage) in the antepartal period is discussed in Chapter 15 ∞; this section discusses intrauterine fetal death (IUFD) after 20 weeks' gestation, often referred to as *stillbirth* or *fetal demise.*

Common Causes of Perinatal Loss

Antepartal fetal deaths, although infrequent, account for about half of all perinatal mortality in the United States (Druzin, Smith Jr., Gabbe, & Reed, 2007). The *perinatal mortality rate (PMR)* is defined by the National Center for Health Statistics as late fetal deaths (over 28 gestational weeks) plus the first 6 days of life (National Center for Health Statistics, 2006). It is estimated that 70% to 90% of stillbirths occur before the onset of labor, with more than 50% occurring between 20 and 28 weeks' gestation (Druzin et al., 2007). The cause may be unknown, or it may result from any of a number of physiologic maladaptations including asphyxia; congenital malformations; superimposed pregnancy complications including preeclampsia or eclampsia, abruptio placentae, placenta previa, diabetes, renal disease, cord accidents, fetal growth restriction, and alloimmunization. Perinatal loss associated with birth defects can occur as a result of congenital anomalies or may occur if the fetus is exposed to teratogens late in the pregnancy (Blackburn, 2007). Other fetal deaths may occur with no apparent cause. See Key Facts to Remember: Factors Associated with Perinatal Loss.

Perinatal loss in industrialized countries has declined in recent years as early diagnosis of congenital anomalies and advances in genetic testing techniques have increased the use of elective termination. Surprisingly, other reproductive advances have increased the incidence of fetal death. It appears fetal death occurs more frequently in monochorionic twins. Because most monochorionic twins are conceived naturally, they have a higher incidence of loss. Most twins conceived via assisted reproductive technology are dichorionic placentation (Sperling, Kiil, Larsen et al., 2006). Pregnancies conceived by in vitro fertilization had higher rates of pregnancy loss, pregnancy complications (placenta abruption, fetal loss after 24 weeks' gestation, gestational hypertension, placenta previa, and cesarean births) (Shevell, Malone, Vidaver et al., 2005). In addition, certain genetic testing procedures such as amniocentesis and chorionic villus sampling (CVS) can actually cause fetal loss.

In developing countries, infection plays a significant role in fetal mortality. Ascending bacterial organisms include *Escherichia coli*, group B streptococci, and *Ureaplasma urealyticum*. These infections can occur either before or after the membranes have ruptured, resulting in fetal demise. Viral causes of fetal demise include parvovirus and coxsackievirus. *Toxoplasma gondii, Listeria monocytogenes*, and the organisms that cause leptospirosis, Q fever, and Lyme disease have also been identified as causative factors for stillbirth. Untreated syphilis is associated with a high stillbirth rate as is malaria infection when contracted for the first time by the mother during the pregnancy (Gibbs & Roberts, 2007). These infections carry a much higher morbidity and mortality rate in developing countries.

KEY FACTS TO REMEMBER

Factors Associated with Perinatal Loss

Fetal Factors

Chromosomal disorders
Birth defects, not chromosomal in nature
Anencephaly, open neural tube defects, isolated
    hydrocephalus, congenital heart defects
Nonimmune hydrops fetalis
Infections
Complications of multiple gestations

Maternal Factors

Prolonged pregnancy
Diabetes
Chronic hypertension
Preeclampsia/eclampsia
Advanced maternal age
Hereditary thrombophilias
Antiphospholipid syndrome
Uterine rupture
RH disease
Ascending bacteria from the vagina

Placental and Other Factors

Placenta previa
Abruptio placentae
Cord accident
Premature rupture of membranes
Substance abuse
Unknown factors

Paternal causes of fetal death are also being examined. One recent study determined that paternal exposure to pesticides resulted in a higher rate of fetal deaths when compared with pregnancies conceived by men who were not exposed to pesticides occupationally (Ronda, Regidor, Garcia & Dominguez, 2005).

Certain maternal conditions can also be associated with higher rates of fetal death. Past maternal exposure to some bacterial and viral antigens can produce an autoimmune response that can result in fetal death (Silver, 2007). Women with acquired and immune thrombophilia have higher rates of miscarriage and fetal demise than those without hematologic alterations (Michels & Tiu, 2007).

Maternal Physiologic Implications

Prolonged retention of the dead fetus may lead to the development of disseminated intravascular coagulation (DIC), also called consumption coagulopathy, in the mother. After the release of thromboplastin from the degenerating fetal tissues into the maternal bloodstream, the extrinsic clotting system is activated, triggering the formation of multiple tiny blood clots. Fibrinogen and factors V and VII are subsequently depleted, and the woman begins to display symptoms of DIC. Fibrinogen levels begin a linear descent 3 to 4 weeks after the death of the fetus and continue to decrease in the absence of appropriate medical intervention.

Besides DIC, other adverse outcomes can also occur if the onset of labor and subsequent birth are delayed. Women with prolonged retention of a dead fetus are more prone to infection. A resulting infection can cause endometritis or sepsis. The longer the pregnancy continues, the higher the incidence of maternal infection.

Although immediate induction is routinely performed, there may be situations in which induction is delayed, such as maternal refusal or the presence of a multiple gestation. In these cases, fibrinogen levels are monitored weekly or biweekly to recognize and prevent progressive coagulopathy from occurring (Lindsey, 2006). In cases of fetal death in the presence of a multiple gestation, some perinatologists may opt to do a single set of coagulation labs, whereas others do not do any laboratory assessment. DIC rarely occurs in cases of multiple gestations where the remaining fetus(es) are allowed to grow and mature (Lindsey, 2006).

Clinical Therapy

Many women first report an absence of fetal activity, although some women may fail to recognize this change in fetal activity. Diagnosis of IUFD is confirmed by visualization of the fetal heart with absence of heart action on ultrasound. Some practitioners routinely have a second ultrasound performed or have a second practitioner verify the absence of cardiac activity before making the diagnosis. When a fetal demise occurs, maternal estriol levels fall. Without medical intervention, most women have spontaneous labor within 2 weeks of fetal death. The once common practice of waiting for the onset of labor has largely been abandoned in recent years because the risks of complications increase with delaying the birth. It is estimated that 60% of fetal deaths have no known case. In 25% of all fetal deaths, the cause remains unknown even after an autopsy (Lindsey, 2006). The specific cause is more difficult to identify if the time since the death is prolonged. Prompt birth increases the ability to identify the cause of death.

In modern practice, most women with a diagnosed fetal demise are given the option of waiting a few days or scheduling an induction procedure immediately. Most women will elect for an induction within a day or two of the final diagnosis. One study determined that women who waited more than 24 hours experienced more prolonged anxiety compared with women who underwent induction within 6 hours of diagnosis (Lindsey, 2006). The mode of induction is dependent upon the gestational age of the fetus, the readiness of the cervix, and the previous mode of birth. In women who have had a previous cesarean birth, a repeat cesarean may be performed because the use of Pitocin or prostaglandin agents can increase the risk of a uterine rupture. Women with an unfavorable cervix may be given vaginal prostaglandin agents, misoprostol, or laminaria tents. Women whose gestations are less than 16 gestational weeks may have a laminaria tent inserted into the cervix before a dilatation and extraction procedure. *Laminaria tents* are made from the stems of brown seaweed which are cut, shaped, dried, sterilized, and packaged in specific sizes. Laminaria tents work by drawing water out of the cervical tissue, allowing the cervix to soften and dilate. They are commonly used to dilate the cervix in preterm gestations when induction is warranted. They may be placed before surgical procedures or inductions of labor.

Women less than 28 weeks' gestation are typically given prostaglandin E_2 (PGE_2) 10 to 20 mg vaginal suppositories every 4 to 6 hours or oral or vaginal misoprostol 400 mcg every 4 to 6 hours until spontaneous labor occurs (Lindsey, 2006). Because PGE_2 suppositories can cause severe vomiting and diarrhea, women are commonly pretreated with antiemetic and antidiarrheal preparations to prevent or lessen these unpleasant side effects (Lindsey, 2006). Recent studies have shown that misoprostol is more effective than other regimens with fewer side effects and shorter times to childbirth (Prairie, Lauria, Kapp et al., 2007).

Women who are term and have not had a previous cesarean birth or other uterine scar may undergo an induction of labor. Women with an unfavorable cervix may be given cervical ripening agents, such as vaginal prostaglandin agents. Induction with Pitocin can be performed following the same protocol as any other term induction of labor.

Postbirth Evaluation

Identifying the causative factor of fetal loss assists many families in progressing through the grieving process. Information obtained from a postmortem examination or postmortem studies can provide vital information related to the cause of the fetal death, the possibility for reoccurrence, and closure for the couple. The information can also be used to help with recurrence and future preconceptional counseling, pregnancy management, prenatal diagnostic procedures, and neonatal management (Lindsey, 2006). The types of studies and tests performed depend on the parents' past history, medical history, and the couple's preferences for the depth of testing desired. Chromosome studies should be considered if the couple has a history of other second or third trimester losses or if either parent has a suspected balanced translocation or mosaic chromosomal pattern. Fetuses who are dysmorphic have growth retardation, are hydropic, or have anomalies or other signs of chromosomal abnormalities may be candidates for chromosomal studies (anomalies) (Lindsey, 2006).

If an intra-amniotic infection is the suspected cause, cultures of both the placenta and the fetus should be obtained. If specific infections are being considered, both IgM and IgG antibodies should be drawn to determine if an acute infectious process has occurred.

Certainly, all stillborn infants should have a careful visual inspection at the time of birth for obvious defects or abnormalities. The placenta and membranes should also be closely examined and the placenta should be sent to pathology for further testing. The umbilical cord should be inspected for true knots, a velamentous insertion, lack of Wharton's jelly, or a short cord to determine if a cord accident was the cause. If a specific cause is suspected, blood tests and x-rays can be performed to verify the suspicions (Lindsey, 2006). An autopsy is the best mechanism to determine the cause of death; however, in the event that the parents decline an autopsy, an MRI can also provide detailed information (Lindsey, 2006).

Most practitioners perform a CBC and antibody screen upon admission. Because diabetes is a causative factor, a random or postpartum glucose level can be obtained to rule out this cause. If diabetes is identified, a hemoglobin A1C should be performed. Additional maternal factors can also be evaluated. Additional tests that may be performed are listed in Table 22–1.

Phases of Grief

Grief is an individual's total response to a loss, including physical symptoms, thoughts, feelings, functional limitations, and spiritual reactions. It may be manifested by certain behaviors and rituals of **mourning**, such as weeping or visiting a gravesite, which help the person experience,

TABLE 22-1	Tests to Determine Cause of Fetal Loss	
Fetal Testing	**Maternal Testing**	
Fetal blood tests and X-rays	Diabetes testing	
Autopsy or MRI	CBC with platelet count	
Placental studies	Kleihauer-Betke test	
Chromosomal studies (if indicated)	Abnormal antibody testing (lupus anticoagulant, anticardiolipin antibodies)	
	TSH levels	
	Infectious disease testing (rubella, syphilis, malaria, toxoplasmosis, cytomegalovirus)	
	Hereditary thrombophilia testing	
	Toxicology testing	

accept, and adjust to the loss. The period of adjustment to loss is known as **bereavement**.

The behaviors that couples exhibit while mourning may be associated with the five stages of grieving described by Kubler-Ross (1969). Often the first stage is *denial* of the death of the fetus. Even when the initial healthcare provider suspects fetal demise, the couple is hoping that a second opinion may be different. Some couples may not be convinced of the death until they see and hold the stillborn infant after birth. The second stage is *anger,* resulting from feelings of loss, loneliness, and perhaps guilt. The anger may be projected at significant others and healthcare team members, or it may be absent when the death is sudden and unexpected. The mother may attempt to identify a specific event that caused the death and may blame herself. *Bargaining,* the third stage, may or may not be present, depending on the couple's preparation for the death of the fetus. If the death is unanticipated, the couple may not have time for bargaining. Bargaining is more commonly seen when the death is expected, such as in the case of a known lethal congenital anomaly. It is marked by the couple making mental trade-offs in exchange for the fetus being healthy. In the fourth stage, *depression* is evidenced by preoccupation, weeping, and withdrawal. Changing hormonal levels in the first 24 to 48 hours after the birth may compound the depression and associated grief. The final stage, *acceptance,* occurs when resolution occurs. This stage is highly individualized and may take months to years to complete.

Nursing Care Management

Nursing Assessment and Diagnosis

Cessation of fetal movement reported by the mother to the nurse is frequently the first indication of fetal death. It is followed by a gradual decrease in the signs and symptoms of pregnancy. Fetal heart tones are absent, and fetal movement is no longer palpable. Once fetal demise

is established, the nurse assesses the family members' ability to adapt to their loss. Open communication between the mother, her partner, and the healthcare team members contributes to a realistic understanding of the medical condition and its associated treatments. The nurse may discuss prior experiences the family has had with loss and what they feel were their perceived coping abilities at that time. Identifying the family's social supports and resources is also important.

Perinatal loss may also occur in the intrapartum period as a result of an intrapartum complication, such as an unresolved shoulder dystocia, prolapsed umbilical cord, abruptio placentae, or other complication. In such emergency situations, healthcare team members often focus on the physical needs of the mother and an attempt to save the fetus's life. Commonly, the family is not advised a perinatal death has occurred until the infant is delivered. Thus, the parents are faced with the sudden and completely unanticipated death of their infant. The most common reaction is protest or disbelief. Although the physician or CNM informs the family of the death, the nurse continues one-on-one care with the family, providing both physical and emotional support throughout this crucial period. The nurse assists the family in the grief process and explores their immediate wishes for viewing and holding their deceased child.

Nursing diagnoses that may apply include the following:

- *Anticipatory Grieving* related to imminent loss of a child
- *Powerlessness* related to lack of control in current situational crisis
- *Ineffective Denial* related to the unexpected death of the fetus
- *Compromised Family Coping* related to death of a child/unresolved feelings regarding perinatal loss
- *Interrupted Family Processes* related to fetal demise
- *Hopelessness* related to sudden, unexpected fetal loss
- *Risk for Spiritual Distress* related to intense suffering secondary to unexpected fetal loss

Nursing Plan and Implementation

Most facilities have an established protocol to follow in the event of perinatal death. It typically provides a holistic focus for family-centered nursing care. It is often helpful for the nurse to view the stillborn baby before talking to the parents so they are prepared for what to expect regarding the baby's appearance. The nurse can then point out normal things about the baby. It is important that the entire healthcare team is notified so multidisciplinary care can be initiated. When fetal death has been confirmed before admission, the entire staff on the unit is informed so they can avoid making inappropriate remarks. Many facilities have a symbol, such as a card with a leaf or a cluster of flowers, which is placed on the mother's door so that all staff members are aware of the loss.

HINTS FOR PRACTICE

No matter who you are or how much nursing experience you have, when an expectant family is in pain because of their loss, and you feel you do not know the right thing to say, "I'm so sorry, I don't know what to say" is a start.

Preparing the Family for the Birth

Upon arrival to the facility, the couple with a known or suspected fetal demise should immediately be placed in a private room. When possible, the woman should be in a room that is farthest away from other laboring women. Care should be taken not to leave the couple in the waiting room with other expectant parents or visitors waiting for news from other women in labor.

The couple should be allowed to remain together as much as they wish. The nurse provides privacy as needed and maintains a supportive environment. The couple should be given complete information about what to expect and what will happen. Questions should be encouraged and answered. The nurse stays with the couple so they do not feel alone and isolated; however, cues that the couple want to be alone should be assessed continuously. Some couples may want outside support, such as family members or friends, to be present during the labor. The nurse facilitates the couple's wishes.

When possible, the same nurse should provide care for the couple so a therapeutic relationship can be established. As the relationship develops, the nurse provides solace by listening to the couple without offering explanations. The nurse also provides ongoing opportunities for the couple to ask questions. It is not uncommon for the family to ask the same questions repeatedly. This is part of the initial grief process. The nurse should provide clear explanations and straightforward answers. The nurse also arranges for other members of the multidisciplinary team to interact with the family. If a grief counselor is available, an initial interaction with the couple should be arranged. If the family desires to see a spiritual advisor, the nurse offers to contact the hospital chaplain or another cleric for them. A social worker is commonly involved. The nurse typically coordinates members of the multidisciplinary team so a comprehensive plan of care can be initiated.

The nurse explains details of the plan of care and allows the family to ask questions and make decisions for their labor and birth preferences. The availability of anesthesia and analgesia should be reviewed. The woman typically can have pain medication whenever she desires. The nurse facilitates the participation of the woman and her partner in the labor and birth process.

It is important to remember that, in contrast to a typical birth experience, the birth of a stillborn infant marks both the beginning and the end. For this reason, it is imperative that the couple and family have all wishes and preferences respected. The family may be overwhelmed and may have difficulty making decisions in this period. The nurse needs to assist the couple to explore their feelings and help them to make decisions about who is present and what rituals will occur during and following the birth. Examples of birth preferences include:

- Use of music, dimmed lighting, or other environmental preferences
- Laboring or birthing in a specific position
- Having the infant placed on the mother's chest immediately after birth
- Allowing the father to cut the umbilical cord
- Including other family members or friends at the birth

Sometimes couples worry that others may view their preferences as "strange" or "wrong." The nurse can reassure the family that it is their experience and that there are no right or wrong feelings or wishes.

The couple may have waves of overwhelming grief, disbelief, or sadness. The nurse needs to encourage the couple to experience the grief that they feel. It is not uncommon for one partner to attempt to put on a "brave front," feeling that, by showing grief, he or she will make the other partner feel worse. It is also not uncommon for partners to have intense feelings that they feel unable to share. Encourage partners to express their emotions freely to the extent they are able. Help them understand that they may each experience different feelings.

Supporting the Family in Viewing the Stillborn Infant

Advocates of seeing the stillborn infant believe that viewing assists in dispelling denial and enables the couple to progress to the next step in the grieving process. If they choose to see their stillborn infant, prepare the couple for what they will see by saying, "She is going to feel cold," "He is going to be blue," or other appropriate statements. If the parents have shared with the nurse the name they had chosen for their baby, use that name in discussing the baby (e.g., "Jessie's face is bruised."). Another common practice is to wrap the infant in a blanket or apply a hat to cover birth defects. This allows the parents an opportunity to view the infant before seeing the birth defect. Most parents will eventually remove the covering to inspect the infant; however, applying a covering allows them time to adjust to the appearance at their own pace.

Some families hold their infant for a short time before returning him or her to the nurse, whereas others wish to spend a great deal of time with their infant. The nurse allows the infant to remain with the family for as long as the family desires. Some parents may elect to bathe or dress their stillborn; the nurse supports them in their choice. Some couples may want other family members, friends, or their other children to see the infant. The nurse acts as an advocate to ensure the family's wishes are respected.

Providing Discharge Care

Most facilities prepare a remembrance box or package for the family to take home. This typically consists of a photograph taken of the infant or the family, a card with the baby's footprints, a crib card, identification band, a lock of hair, and possibly a blanket or clothing worn by the infant. In the event that the couple declines the package, it is common for the hospital to retain these items for a specific period of time in case the parents change their minds.

After the birth, the couple can be given the option of an early discharge (as early as 6 to 8 hours after the birth). Facility protocol will dictate where mothers are transferred after a perinatal loss. Some hospitals have the women remain on the labor and birthing unit; others will give the mother the option of choosing a postpartum room or one on a medical unit. If the mother is transferred to a postpartum unit, care is given to put her in a room far away from other rooms and the newborn nursery. Again, it is imperative that all staff members, as well as student nurses, are notified of the mother's status.

Discharge focuses on the physical considerations and adaptation of the mother. The nurse provides the mother with postpartum directions for follow-up care, written materials, and a phone number for questions. The woman should also be given information on her milk coming in and interventions to follow to decrease the discomfort associated with engorgement.

Additional information should be given on the grief process (Figure 22–11 ■). The nurse can prepare the couple to return home by stressing that others may not know what to say, and that even loved ones may make inappropriate comments because they do not know how to respond to grief and loss. This can prepare the couple for the reactions of others. If there are siblings, each will usually progress through age-appropriate grieving. Provide the parents with information about normal mourning reactions, both psychologic and physiologic.

When caring for a family suffering from a perinatal loss, it is important to remember that the nurse experiences many of the same grief reactions as the parents of a stillborn infant. It is important to have colleagues and family members available for counseling and support.

Facilitating the Family's Grief Work

The parents of a stillborn infant suffer a devastating experience that precipitates an intense emotional trauma. During the pregnancy, the couple has already begun the attachment process, which now must be terminated through the grieving process. Facilitating the family's grief work is thus a critical nursing intervention—one that requires skill, sensitivity, and compassion.

Following discharge, some families may need closure of the intrapartum event in order to continue their grief

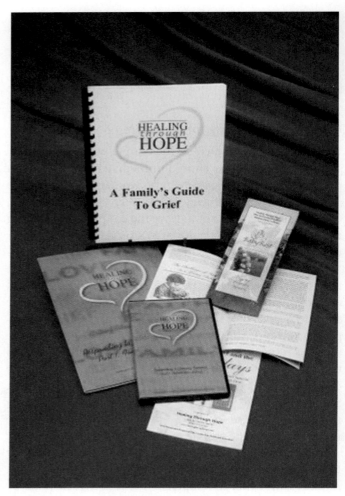

FIGURE 22–11 Bereavement literature.
Source: Healing through Hope.

work. A consultation can be scheduled with the practitioner that cared for them during the pregnancy and birth. Families may also wish to read the results of tests performed during the intrapartum period and the autopsy report. The couple should be provided with a copy of the medical record and encouraged to ask questions, express their feelings, and ask for clarification.

Families are routinely referred for counseling services after a perinatal loss has occurred. A counselor who specializes in perinatal issues can provide expertise and assist the couple in their grieving. Partners should be allowed to verbalize fears and concerns about future pregnancies. When appropriate, referrals to genetic counselors, religious support persons, and social service agencies also should be provided.

Besides referral information, the woman should receive scheduled follow-up phone calls to assess the family's functioning and their progress with grief work. During these follow-up phone calls, pertinent information can be given and additional resources can be identified.

As the grief process ensues, families should be encouraged to implement cultural, religious, or social customs that will assist them in grieving and mourning. The nurse should advise the family that certain upcoming milestones, such as holidays, future birthdays, baby showers, Mother's Day, Father's Day, and other social events, may trigger their grief. The family can better cope with these events if they are adequately prepared.

Referring the Family to Community Services

Although most facilities have an established protocol for families experiencing perinatal loss, more comprehensive programs are being established in communities to provide a step-by-step intervention program to assist these families. Community support groups that focus on perinatal loss can provide an important support network and resources. Specialized groups, such as those focused on early pregnancy loss, stillbirth, and perinatal loss associated with specific congenital anomalies, allow families the opportunity to interact with peers who have lost infants under similar circumstances. The nurse provides the group name, contact person (if possible), and phone number. Various books written by mothers who have lost children are available in bookstores and are valuable resources for grieving parents.

Internet technology has allowed large numbers of individuals to share resources and information, and participate in online support groups. Internet resources can be effective for all families and may be the only resources available for families in rural underserved areas.

Specialized community outreach programs are another community resource that can provide assistance to grieving families. One example is an early community intervention program that provides counseling to parents whose fetus has a known lethal congenital anomaly. In perinatal hospice programs, parents are given the opportunity to explore options, such as elective termination or waiting for the onset of spontaneous labor or a medically indicated induced labor. For families wishing to continue their pregnancies, the program typically assigns a multidisciplinary team who provides compassionate care, ongoing counseling, referral to support groups, and spiritual guidance (Ramer-Chrastek & Thygesen, 2005).

Care of the Couple Who Has Experienced Loss in a Previous Pregnancy

Couples who have had a previous perinatal loss typically enter a subsequent pregnancy with conflicting feelings and may experience ambivalence, fear, and anxiety. Many times, their past experience is relived when another pregnancy occurs. Some couples conceive soon after a loss whereas others wait years. Some couples enter a subsequent pregnancy with grief work largely completed whereas others are still experiencing unresolved grief.

The nurse caring for a couple who has had a previous loss needs to be kind, compassionate, and patient. Couples need specific information and clear explanations of all prenatal information. Referrals to a genetic counselor should be made when appropriate. Some couples may wish to have a consultation with a perinatologist. If unresolved grief issues are present or the family experiences extreme anxiety, counseling may be beneficial.

Interventions to decrease anxiety can help the couple tremendously. At the first visit, an early ultrasound can be performed to verify the presence of the fetal heart. In early pregnancy, women may be fearful when first trimester pregnancy symptoms begin to resolve. It may be helpful for these women to come in for weekly visits for a period of time simply to hear the fetal heart beat. This intervention may continue to be helpful until the woman begins to feel fetal movement. Throughout the pregnancy, the office or clinic nurse can play a key role by providing reassurance and answering questions that the woman may have.

Women with a previous loss typically receive additional antepartum testing throughout the pregnancy. Ultrasounds can be used to provide reassurance and assess fetal growth and development, placental functioning, and cord variations. Nonstress testing and biophysical profiles can be performed weekly after 32 weeks' gestation to ensure fetal well-being. Fetal kick counts should be initiated at 28 weeks and continue until the birth occurs. Women with a previous loss should give birth to their child at their expected date of birth or when the pregnancy is at term and should not go over their due date, because placental functioning can decline in postdate pregnancies.

Many women who have had a previous perinatal loss continue to have ongoing stress and anxiety, even after a subsequent birth of a healthy infant (Ramer-Chrastek & Thygesen, 2005). Postpartum and nursery nurses should assess for ongoing stress and anxiety and be prepared to provide additional support to these families.

Evaluation

Anticipated outcomes of nursing care include the following:

- Family members express their feelings about the death of their baby.
- Family members participate in decision making regarding preferences for the labor, birth, and the immediate postpartum period.
- Family members participate in the decision of whether to see their baby and other decisions about the baby.
- The family has resources available for continued support.
- Family members know the community resources available and have names and phone numbers to use if they choose.
- The family is moving into and through the grieving process.

Nursing care of a family experiencing perinatal loss is further described in the accompanying Nursing Care Plan.

Nursing Care Plan For a Family Experiencing Perinatal Loss

CLIENT SCENARIO

Irina Borodina, age 26, G1P0 at 27 weeks' gestation, arrives with her husband, Anton, at the labor and birthing unit stating she has been cramping over the last 3 hours and does not feel the baby move. Fetal heart tones are absent. Additional assessments, including an ultrasound, confirm a fetal demise. The physician informs Irina and Anton of the loss and they decide to undergo an immediate induction. The nurse explains what will occur during labor and the care that will be given to the body of their deceased child after birth.

During labor Irina is quiet, and she and her husband periodically weep. During the birth the room is darkened and quiet. Anton asks to see the baby, a male. The nurse explains that the baby is very small, wraps the tiny body in a blanket, and gives it to the father to hold. Irina turns away, crying, and asks the nurse why her baby died. She sobs that she did everything the doctors advised, and does not understand what went wrong. "It's not fair!" she says. "Why did God do this to me?" The nurse explains that tests can be performed to help determine why their baby died, but Irina withdraws and does not appear to be listening. She tells the nurse she is exhausted, and asks to be alone with her husband. The nurse removes the body from the room and informs the couple that they can ask for the baby back if they choose.

When the nurse checks on the couple a few minutes later, they seem calmer. However, when she asks them whether they would like to view the baby now, Irina bursts into tears again and shouts at the nurse, "Why can't you just leave us alone?" Her husband quietly suggests that they phone their priest and ask him to bless the baby, but she shakes her head despondently. "I prayed so hard all these months, and God took our baby away anyway! Why should I turn to Him now?"

ASSESSMENT

Subjective: Exhaustion, crying, states feelings of bewilderment.

Objective: Hyperventilation during admission, anorexia, pulse 120, respirations 20, restless. Refuses to view baby. Refuses visit from priest. States, "It's not fair!" Blames God for "taking our baby away."

Nursing Diagnosis	Spiritual Distress as evidenced by refusal to view or hold baby, statement of anger at God for taking baby away, and refusal to participate in customary religious practices*
Client Goal	The client will participate in seeing and holding the baby, while verbalizing thoughts and feelings associated with the loss.
AEB:	• Openly expresses feelings concerning the loss. • Verbalizes understanding of cause of the baby's death. • Requests to see and hold baby. • Accepts offer of visit from spiritual advisor.

NURSING INTERVENTIONS

RATIONALES

1. Provide factual information as soon as it is available about the cause of the fetal demise if known.

   Rationale: Promotes understanding of the physiologic etiology of the loss and acceptance of the loss as real.

2. Provide consistency in the nursing staff assignments for the client.

   Rationale: Promotes establishment of a therapeutic relationship. Continuity of care builds trust and familiarity between the nurse and the parents. This will allow the nurse to assess over time how the couple is coping with the loss. A supportive relationship helps to facilitate the grieving process.

3. Prepare the baby for viewing.

   Rationale: The nurse should dress the baby like the other babies in the nursery with a T-shirt, hat, and diaper and wrap the child in a clean soft blanket.

Nursing Care Plan   For a Family Experiencing Perinatal Loss *(Continued)*

NURSING INTERVENTIONS

4. Encourage the parents to see, touch, and name the baby.

5. Offer remembrances of the baby for the parents to keep.

6. Provide an opportunity for religious or spiritual counseling and practices.

RATIONALES

Rationale: Grief work begins when the parents begin to accept the loss as a reality. Spending time seeing and holding their baby may help the parents begin to accept the reality of the baby's birth and death. The parents should be informed of the baby's appearance before viewing. Naming the baby also helps parents accept the loss. The nurse uses the name to reflect support and acknowledgment of the loss that the parents are experiencing.

Rationale: Small tokens of remembrance such as a lock of hair, baby bracelet, footprints or handprints, or even a photo help parents accept the reality of their baby's death and promote the grieving process. Parents will appreciate the fact that someone acknowledges their baby. If parents prefer not to have a photo they should be told that the photo and other keepsake items are kept on file and they are welcome to have one if they decide otherwise.

Rationale: Support can be provided to the parents by offering to contact a spiritual advisor, or to arrange for a place and time to carry out a religious ritual. Allow privacy for the couple when clergy is present.

Evaluation of Client Goal

- The client communicates feelings of sadness, helplessness, and anger.
- The client verbalizes understanding of physiologic etiology of her loss.
- The client views, holds, and calls baby by name while saying good-bye.
- The client accepts visit from spiritual advisor and verbalizes spiritual comfort.

CRITICAL THINKING QUESTIONS

1. How can the nurse promote the grieving process for a couple who has experienced perinatal loss?

Answer: The nurse can respond to grieving parents by acknowledging the loss of their baby; by calling the baby by name; being empathetic; participating in prayer, a blessing, or other religious ritual at the request of the family; and providing the parents with some tokens of remembrance such as a lock of hair, baby bracelet, footprints or handprints, a baby blanket, and a photo. The nurse can also encourage family members to share their thoughts and feelings about the loss and be accepting of any type of emotional response. In some facilities the nurse can perform an emergency baptism upon the family's request if a spiritual advisor is not available.

2. What types of nursing behaviors might squelch the grieving process?

Answer: Failure of the nursing staff to acknowledge the pregnancy or loss may impede grief work. Encouraging the parents not to cry or talk about their loss, or prohibiting

contact between the baby and the parents, also impedes grief work. Isolating the mother on a nonmaternity floor *against* her wishes promotes a feeling of helplessness. Encouraging the use of tranquilizers or sedatives to numb the pain may prolong the denial and, therefore, the grieving process. These behaviors do not allow the parents to receive support or grieve for their loss.

3. What are some factors that might affect the grief reaction to a perinatal loss?

Answer: Factors affecting grief reactions may include differences between the father's and mother's reactions. Males typically internalize grief, whereas women are more expressive of and want to talk about their grief. Previous losses, either with another pregnancy or a recent loss or death of another family member, make the current loss more difficult. Cultural influences may also affect grief reactions to a perinatal loss, because mourning behaviors vary.

*For your reference, this care plan is an example of how one nursing diagnosis might be addressed.

- Psychologic disorders such as depression and acute anxiety may have a profound effect on labor, particularly when complications that might jeopardize the mother or fetus occur.
- A hypertonic labor pattern is characterized by painful contractions that are not effective in effacing and dilating the cervix. It usually leads to a prolonged latent phase.
- Hypotonic labor patterns begin normally and then progress to infrequent, less intense contractions.
- Precipitous labor is extremely rapid labor and birth that lasts less than 3 hours. It is associated with an increased risk to the mother and newborn.
- Postterm pregnancy is one that extends more than 294 days or 42 weeks past the first day of the last menstrual period.
- The occiput-posterior position of the fetus during labor prolongs the labor process, causes severe back discomfort in the laboring woman, and predisposes her to vaginal and perineal trauma and lacerations during birth.
- The types of fetal malpresentations include face, brow, breech, shoulder, and compound.
- A fetus or newborn weighing more than 4000 g is termed macrosomic. Problems with a fetus this size may occur during labor, birth, and the early neonatal period.
- Multiple-gestation pregnancies carry an increased risk of pregnancy-related complications.
- Nonreassuring fetal status is indicated by persistent late decelerations, persistent severe variable decelerations, and prolonged decelerations. If nonreassuring fetal status is recognized and treated appropriately, the fetus may not experience permanent damage.
- Prolapsed umbilical cord results when the umbilical cord precedes the fetal presenting part. This places pressure on the umbilical cord and diminishes blood flow to the fetus.

- Amniotic fluid embolism is an extremely rare event that occurs when a bolus of amniotic fluid enters the maternal circulation and then the maternal lungs. The maternal mortality rate is very high with this complication.
- Hydramnios (also known as polyhydramnios) occurs when there is more than 2000 mL of amniotic fluid contained within the amniotic membranes. Hydramnios is associated with fetal malformations that affect fetal swallowing and with maternal diabetes mellitus, Rh sensitization, and multiple-gestation pregnancies.
- Oligohydramnios is present when there is a severely reduced volume of amniotic fluid. Oligohydramnios is associated with IUGR, with postmaturity, and with fetal renal or urinary malfunctions. The fetus is more likely to experience variable decelerations because the amniotic fluid is insufficient to keep pressure off the umbilical cord.
- CPD occurs when there is a narrowed diameter in the maternal pelvis. The narrowed diameter is called a contracture and may occur in the pelvic inlet, the midpelvis, or the outlet. If pelvic measurements are borderline, a trial of labor may be attempted. Failure of cervical dilatation or fetal descent necessitates a cesarean birth.
- Third- and fourth-stage complications usually involve hemorrhage. The causes of hemorrhage include retained placenta, lacerations of the birth canal or cervix, placenta accrete, and retained placenta.
- Perinatal loss poses a major nursing challenge to provide support and care for the parents.

CHAPTER REFERENCES

Albers, L. L. (2007). The evidence for physiologic management of the active phase of the first stage of labor. *Journal of Midwifery & Women's Health, 52*(3), 207–215.

American College of Obstetricians & Gynecologists (ACOG). (2000). *Fetal macrosomia.* ACOG Practice Bulletin No. 22. Washington, DC: Author.

American College of Obstetricians & Gynecologists (ACOG). (2003). *Dystocia and augmentation.* ACOG Practice Bulletin No. 49. Washington, DC: Author.

American College of Obstetricians & Gynecologists (ACOG). (2004). *Management of postterm pregnancy.* ACOG Practice Bulletin No. 55. Washington, DC: Author.

American College of Obstetricians & Gynecologists (ACOG). (2006). *Mode of term singleton breech delivery.* ACOG Committee Opinion No. 340. Washington, DC: Author.

Battista, L. R., & Wing, D. H. (2007). Abnormal labor and induction of labor. In S. G. Gabbe, J. R. Niebyl, & J. L. Simpson (Eds.), *Obstetrics: Normal and problem pregnancies* (5th ed.). Philadelphia: Churchill Livingstone.

Blackburn, S. T. (2007). *Maternal, fetal, and neonatal physiology: A clinical perspective* (3rd ed.). Philadelphia: Saunders.

Coyle, M. E., Smith, C. A., & Peat, B. (2005). Cephalic version by moxibustion for breech presentation. *Cochrane Database of Systematic Reviews,* Issue 2. Art. No.: CD003928. DOI: 10.1002/14651858.CD003928.pub2.

Cunningham, F. G., Leveno, K.,J., Bloom, S., & Hauth, J. C. (2005). *Williams obstetrics* (22nd ed.). Stamford, CT: Appleton & Lange.

Demianczuk, C.E., & Corbetti, T. F. (2005). Successful pregnancy after amniotic fluid embolism: A case report. *Journal of Obstetrics & Gynecology Canada, 27*(7), 699–701.

Druzin, M. L., Smith, J. F., Gabbe, S. G., & Reed, K. L. (2007) Antepartum fetal evaluation. In S. G. Gabbe, J. R. Niebyl, & J. L. Simpson (Eds.), *Obstetrics: Normal and problem pregnancies* (5th ed.). Philadelphia: Churchill Livingstone.

Family Practice Notebook. (2007). Brow presentation. Retrieved November 9, 2007, from http://www.fpnotebook.com/OB102.htm

Fox, A. J., & Chapman, M. G. (2006). Longitudinal ultrasound assessment of fetal presentation: A review of 1010 consecutive cases. *The Australian & New Zealand Journal of Obstetrics & Gynaecology, 46* (4), 341–344.

Francois, K. E., & Foley, M. R. (2007). Antepartum and postpartum hemorrhage. In S. G. Gabbe, J. R. Niebyl, & J. L. Simpson (Eds.), *Obstetrics: Normal and problem pregnancies* (5th ed.). Philadelphia: Churchill Livingstone.

Gibbs, R. S., & Roberts, D. J. (2007). Case records of the Massachusetts General Hospital. Case 27-2007. A 30-year-old pregnant woman with intrauterine fetal death. *New England Journal of Medicine, 357*(9), 918–925.

Gilbert, W. M., Hicks, S. M., Boe, N. M., & Danielson, B. (2003). Vaginal versus cesarean delivery for breech presentation: A population-based study. *Obstetrics & Gynecology, 102,* 911–917.

Kubler-Ross, E. (1969). *On death and dying.* New York: MacMillian.

Landon, M. B., Catalano, P. M., & Gabbe, S. G. (2007). Diabetes mellitus complicating pregnancy. In S. G. Gabbe, J. R. Niebyl, & J. L. Simpson (Eds.), *Obstetrics: Normal and problem pregnancies* (5th ed.). Philadelphia: Churchill Livingstone.

Lanni, S. M., & Seeds, J. W. (2007). Malpresentations. In S. G. Gabbe, J. R. Niebyl, & J. L. Simpson (Eds.), *Obstetrics: Normal and problem pregnancies* (5th ed.). Philadelphia: Churchill Livingstone.

Le Ray, C., Serres, P., Schmitz, T., Cabrol, D., & Goffinet, F. (2007). Manual rotation in occiput posterior or transverse positions: Risk factors and consequences on the cesarean delivery rate. *Obstetrics & Gynecology, 110*(4), 873–879.

Lindsey, J. L. (2006). Evaluation of fetal death. *E-medicine.* Retrieved November 27, 2007, from http://www.emedicine.com/med/topic3235.htm

Magliore, L., & Copel, J. A. (2007). Ultrasound clinics. Role of U/S during labor and induction. *Contemporary OB/GYN, 52*(5), 81–82, 84, 86.

Mahony, R., Foley, M., McAuliffe, F., & O'Herlihy, C. (2007). Maternal weight characteristics influence recurrence of fetal macrosomia in women with normal glucose tolerance. *The Australian & New Zealand Journal of Obstetrics & Gynaecology, 47*(5), 399–401; PMID: 17877598.

Michels, T. C., & Tiu, A. Y. (2007). Second trimester pregnancy loss. *American Family Physician, 1;76*(9), 1341–1346.

National Center for Health Statistics. (2006). Chartbook on trends on the health of Americans. Retrieved November 14, 2007, from http://www.cdc.gov/nchs/hus.htm

National Institute of Mental Health (NIMH). (2008). Statistics. Retrieved August 20, 2008 from www.nimh.gov/health/statistics/index.shtml

Parker, J., & Napolitano, P.G. (2005). Brow presentation. E-medicine. Retrieved November 9, 2007, from http://www.emedicine.com/med/topic3274.htm

Prairie, B. A., Lauria, M. R., Kapp, N., Mackenzie, T., Baker, E. R., & George, K. E. (2007). Mifepristone versus laminaria: A randomized controlled trial of cervical ripening in midtrimester termination. *Contraception. 76*(5), 383–388.

Ramer-Chrastek, J., & Thygesen, N. V. (2005). A perinatal hospice for an unborn child with a life-limiting condition. *International Journal of Palliative Nursing, 11*(6), 274–276.

Ronda, E., Regidor, E., García, A. M., & Domínguez, V. (2005). Association between congenital anomalies and paternal exposure to agricultural pesticides depending on mother's employment status. *Journal of Occupational Environmental Medicine, 47*(8), 826–28.

Shevell, T., Malone, F. D., Vidaver, J., Porter, T. F., Luthy, D. A., Comstock, C. H., et al. (2005). Assisted reproductive technology and pregnancy outcome. *Obstetrics & Gynecology, 106*(5 Pt 1), 1039–1045.

Silver, R. M. (2007). Fetal death. *Obstetrics & Gynecology, 109*(1), 153–167.

Sperling, L., Kiil, C., Larsen, L. U., Ovist, Q., Schwartz, M., Jorgenson, C., et al. (2006). Naturally conceived twins with monochorionic placentation have the highest risk of fetal loss. *Ultrasound in Obstetrics & Gynecology, 5,* 644–652.

CHAPTER 23

Birth-Related Procedures

Labor and birth today are remarkably safe for both the mother and her baby. With all of our advanced technology, we in healthcare have the ability to make enormous strides toward our outcome goals. But the bigger challenge is to do all of that and still honor the truly life-changing, miraculous nature of the birth experience.

—Labor and Delivery RNC

LEARNING OUTCOMES

23-1. Explain the methods, purpose, criteria, and contraindications of external version in determining nursing care management.

23-2. Describe the use of amniotomy and the nursing care management of woman and fetus.

23-3. Explain the indications, contraindications, labor readiness, and methods in determining the nursing care management for women during labor induction.

23-4. Describe the indications for amnioinfusion and the nursing care of the woman during amnioinfusion.

23-5. Delineate the measures to prevent episiotomy, factors that predispose women to episiotomy, and types of episiotomy in determining the nursing care management.

23-6. Explain the indications, maternal and neonatal risks, and nursing care management during forceps-assisted birth.

23-7. Describe the nursing care management of the woman and newborn during vacuum-assisted birth.

23-8. Explain the indications for cesarean birth, impact on the family unit, preparation and teaching needs, and associated nursing care.

23-9. Examine the risks, guidelines, and nursing care of the woman undergoing vaginal birth following cesarean birth.

KEY TERMS

Most births occur without the need for operative obstetric intervention. In some instances, however, procedures are necessary to maintain the safety of the woman and the fetus. The most common of these procedures are amniotomy, induction of labor, episiotomy, cesarean birth, and vaginal birth following a previous cesarean birth.

Generally, women are aware of the possible need for an obstetric procedure during their labor and birth. However, some women expect to have a "natural" experience and feel disappointed, angry, or even guilty when an unanticipated procedure is needed. This conflict between expectation and the need for intervention presents a challenge to maternity nurses. The nurse provides information regarding any procedure to help the woman and her partner understand what is proposed, the anticipated benefits and possible risks, and any alternatives.

Care of the Woman During Version

Version, or turning the fetus, is a procedure used to change the fetal presentation by abdominal or intrauterine manipulation. The most common type of version is **external cephalic version (ECV)**, in which the fetus is changed from a breech to a cephalic presentation by external manipulation of the maternal abdomen (Figure 23–1 ■). A less common type of version, called **podalic version**, is used only with the second fetus during a vaginal twin birth and only if the twin does not descend readily or if the heart rate is nonreassuring. In a podalic version medication is used to relax the uterus. The obstetrician then places a hand inside the uterus, grabs the fetus's feet, and draws them down through the cervix. The use of podalic versions are declining as more women with a second twin in a non-vertex presentation are counseled to undergo a cesarean birth (Bjelic-Radisic, Pristauz, Haas et al., 2007). The success rates of ECV in singleton pregnancies ranges from 51% to 65% (Lanni & Seeds, 2007; Zeck, Walcher, & Lang, 2008).

Criteria for External Version

If breech or shoulder presentation (transverse lie) is detected in the later weeks of pregnancy, an external version may be attempted. Before the external version is begun, an ultrasound is used to locate the placenta and to confirm fetal presentation.

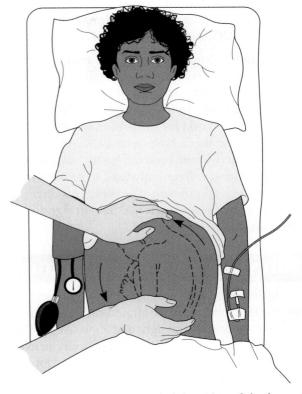

FIGURE 23–1 External (or cephalic) version of the fetus. A new technique involves applying pressure to the fetal head and buttocks so that the fetus completes a "backward flip" or "forward roll."

The following criteria should be met before performing external version:

• The pregnancy is 36 or more weeks' gestation. A version may result in complications that require immediate birth by cesarean (Lanni & Seeds, 2007).
• A nonstress test (NST), obtained immediately before performing the version, is reactive. A reactive NST indicates fetal well-being.
• The fetal breech is not engaged. Once the presenting part is engaged it is difficult, if not impossible, to do a version.

Contraindications for External Version

Contraindications include the following:

• Maternal problems, such as uterine anomalies, uncontrolled preeclampsia, or third-trimester bleeding

- Complications of pregnancy, such as rupture of membranes, oligohydramnios, hydramnios, or placenta previa or vasa previa
- Previous cesarean birth or other significant uterine surgery
- Multiple gestations
- Nonreassuring fetal heart rate (FHR) or other evidence of uteroplacental insufficiency
- Fetal abnormalities, such as intrauterine growth restriction (IUGR) or nuchal cord

Before the external version begins, an intravenous line may be established to administer medications in case of difficulty. The woman may receive terbutaline subcutaneously to relax the uterus. Some physicians may also order regional anesthesia for the procedure. Both tocolytics and regional anesthesia have been associated with higher success rates and lower cesarean births (Lanni & Seeds, 2007). Ultrasound is frequently used to provide information about the fetal position. The version is discontinued in the presence of severe maternal pain or significant fetal bradycardia or decelerations.

Nursing Care Management

On admission the nurse begins a thorough assessment by verifying that there are no contraindications to the version procedure. Maternal vital signs and a reactive NST are obtained. This initial assessment period provides an ideal time for educating the woman and her partner and for addressing their concerns. They can be encouraged to express their understanding and expectations of the procedure. At the same time, the possibility of failure of the ECV and slight risk of cesarean birth if the FHR becomes nonreassuring should also be discussed. Explaining what will occur in either of these circumstances will better prepare the woman and her partner if intervention becomes necessary. Although the physician is ultimately responsible for obtaining informed consent, it is also the nurse's role to ensure that the woman understands the procedure and has the opportunity to ask questions and voice her concerns or fears.

The nurse places an intravenous line before beginning the procedure to maintain intravenous (IV) access in case of a complication. Throughout the procedure, the nurse continues to monitor maternal blood pressure, pulse, and comfort level frequently (because the mother may experience pain during the procedure). Fetal well-being is ascertained before, intermittently during, and for (at least) 30 minutes following the procedure, using electronic fetal monitoring (EFM), ultrasound, or both. The nurse also assesses maternal-fetal response to the tocolytic. Aftercare instructions, which may include maternal monitoring for contractions and fetal movement (fetal kick counts), are provided as well.

Care of the Woman During Amniotomy

Amniotomy is the artificial rupture of the amniotic membranes (AROM). It is probably the most common invasive procedure in obstetrics. Because the amniotomy requires that an instrument, called an amnihook, be inserted through the cervix, at least 2 cm (0.8 in.) of cervical dilatation is required.

Amniotomy has been used as a means to shorten labor. A recent study that examined amniotomy and the length of labor did show a reduction in the first stage of labor as well as differences in maternal satisfaction or low Apgar scores (Smyth, Alldred, & Markham, 2007). Amniotomy can also be used at any time during the first stage to augment labor (accelerate the progress). Amniotomy is more effective in multiparous women (Battista & Wing, 2007). This is because the cervix is more pliable. Amniotomy manipulates both hormones and mechanical factors to stimulate labor. Upon rupturing the membranes, natural prostaglandins are released which stimulate uterine contractions. The escape of amniotic fluid allows the presenting part to descend and place direct pressure on the cervix, thus resulting in an acceleration of dilatation.

Amniotomy may also be done during labor to apply an internal fetal heart monitoring electrode to the scalp, to insert an intrauterine pressure catheter, or to obtain a fetal scalp blood sample for acid-base determination and fetal pH monitoring. In addition, amniotomy allows assessment of the color and composition of amniotic fluid. Amniotomy performed when the presenting part is not well applied to the cervix increases the risk of umbilical cord prolapse (see Chapter 22 ∞).

AROM Procedure

While performing a vaginal examination, the physician or certified nurse-midwife (CNM) introduces an amnihook into the vagina and makes a small tear in the amniotic membrane, which allows amniotic fluid to escape.

Nursing Care Management

The nurse explains the AROM procedure to the woman and then assesses fetal presentation, position, and station, because amniotomy is usually delayed until engagement has occurred. The woman is asked to assume a semi-reclining position and is draped to provide privacy. The FHR is assessed just before and immediately after the amniotomy, and the two FHR assessments are compared. If there are marked changes, the nurse should check for prolapse of the cord (see Chapter 22 ∞). The amniotic fluid is inspected for amount, color, odor, and the presence of meconium or blood. While wearing disposable gloves, the nurse cleanses and dries the perineal area and changes the underpads as needed. Because there is now an open pathway for organisms to ascend into the uterus the number of vaginal exams must be kept to a minimum to reduce the chance of introducing an infection. In addition, the woman's temperature is monitored a minimum of every 2 hours. The nurse needs to provide information regarding the expected effects of the amniotomy. It is important for the woman to know that amniotic fluid is constantly produced, because some women may worry that they will experience a "dry birth."

HINTS FOR PRACTICE

Before the AROM procedure, place several layers of disposable pads under the woman's buttocks and a folded towel between the woman's legs. The towel readily absorbs the fluid released during the procedure and prevents soiling of the bed linens. After the procedure, remove the towel as well as all layers of absorbent pads that have been soiled. Several clean absorbent pads should be placed under the woman's buttocks because amniotic fluid will continue to leak from the vagina. This increases the woman's comfort.

Care of the Woman During Cervical Ripening

Cervical ripening is softening and effacing of the cervix. It may be used for the pregnant woman who is at term or late preterm when there is a medical or obstetric indication for induction of labor. Pharmacologic methods of cervical ripening include prostaglandin agents and Cytotec.

Prostaglandin Agents

The most commonly used ripening agent is Prepidil gel, which contains 0.5 mg dinoprostone, a prostaglandin E_2 (PGE_2) agent. It is placed either intracervically or intravaginally. Prostaglandin agents placed intravaginally are superior to intracervical placement (Boulvain, Kelly, & Irion, 2008). A similar agent called Cervidil is packaged as a 2 cm (0.8 in.) square vaginal insert that resembles a thin piece of cardboard. It releases 10 mg of dinoprostone at a rate of 0.3 mg/hour over 12 hours. In a study by Facchinetti and colleagues (2007), women who received the Cervidil vaginal insert had more vaginal births within 24 hours of administration and shorter hospitalizations than those who re-

ceived the prostaglandin gel. There is often a reduction of time to childbirth in multiparous women who receive the gel preparation (Marconi, Bozzetti, Morabito et al., 2008).

Prostaglandin agents have been demonstrated to cause cervical ripening, to shorten labor, and to lower requirements for Pitocin during labor induction (Facchinetti et al., 2007; Marconi et al., 2008). Prostaglandin agents are typically used when labor induction is indicated, but not emergent, such as maternal gestational diabetes, postdates, or large-for-gestational-age fetuses who warrant birth occurring in the near future. For example, a woman who is over 41 weeks but has a very unfavorable cervix may be given prostaglandin gel to ripen her cervix before a Pitocin induction is scheduled.

Prostaglandin gel is administered in a hospital setting where women can be monitored for approximately 2 hours (depending on agency protocol) after the administration of the medication. The woman is then sent home and an induction is scheduled in the near future. Complications such as hyperstimulation and nonreassuring fetal status typically occur in the first hour after administration and peak at 4 hours. If the fetal heart rate remains unchanged during the initial 2 hour assessment and uterine activity has not become regular, the woman may be discharged once appropriate follow-up instructions and warning signs are provided. See Drug Guide: Dinoprostone (Prepidil) Vaginal Gel for additional information.

Women receiving the Cervidil vaginal insert are observed in the hospital setting and have continuous fetal monitoring while the insert is in place. The woman should remain incumbent for 2 hours after administration. The insert should be removed immediately if uterine hyperstimulation or non-reassuring fetal status occurs. A beta-adrenergic agent should also be administered if hyperstimulation occurs (Forrest Pharmaceuticals, 2007).

TEACHING TIP

Advise the woman that prostaglandin agents commonly cause uterine stimulation after insertion. Review the signs of labor that warrant further assessment after discharge home. The woman should be taught the difference between common reactions to the prostaglandin agents (such as cramping, uterine irritability, and gel leakage) versus the true signs of labor (strong regular contractions, rupture of membranes) before leaving the hospital.

Misoprostol (Cytotec)

Misoprostol (Cytotec) is a synthetic PGE_1 analogue that some healthcare agencies use to ripen the cervix and induce labor. It is available as a tablet and can be administered using several routes including the following: oral, vaginal, rectal, sublingually, or buccally. Although the last two routes are effective, they are rarely used. The rectal route is primarily used when attempting to control postpartum hemorrhaging

Drug Guide Dinoprostone (Prepidil) Vaginal Gel

Overview of Maternal-Fetal Action

Pregnancy Risk Category: C

Dinoprostone is a naturally occurring form of prostaglandin E_2. Dinoprostone can be used at term to ripen the cervix and can stimulate the smooth muscle of the uterus to enhance uterine contractions. Prepidil can be administered endocervically (Pfizer Pharmaceuticals, Inc., 2008).

Route, Dosage, Frequency
The gel contains 0.5 mg of dinoprostone. The gel is placed in the posterior fornix of the vagina, and the client is kept supine for 2 hours, after which time she may ambulate. Continuous electronic monitoring is typically used for 2 hours after administration. Women who show no signs of labor and have a reassuring fetal monitoring strip may be discharged after 2 hours of administration.

Contraindications

- Client with known sensitivity to prostaglandins
- Presence of nonreassuring fetal status
- Unexplained bleeding during pregnancy
- Strong suspicion of cephalopelvic disproportion
- Client already receiving Pitocin
- Client who is not anticipated to be able to give birth vaginally
- Previous cesarean birth, uterine scar, or uterine rupture (Battista & Wing, 2007).

Dinoprostone vaginal gel should be used with CAUTION in clients with ruptured membranes, a fetus in breech presentation, presence of glaucoma, or history of asthma (Pfizer Pharmaceuticals, Inc., 2008).

Maternal Side Effects
Uterine hyperstimulation with or without nonreassuring fetal status has occurred in a very small number (6.6%) of clients. Other reported maternal side effects include gastrointestinal disturbance (fewer than 1% of clients have experienced fever, nausea, vomiting, diarrhea, or abdominal pain) (Wilson, Shannon & Shields., 2009).

Effects on Fetus/Newborn
Nonreassuring fetal heart rate patterns

Nursing Considerations

- Assess for presence of contraindications.
- Monitor maternal vital signs, cervical dilatation, and effacement carefully.
- Monitor fetal status for presence of reassuring fetal heart rate pattern (baseline 110 to 160 bpm, presence of variability, presence of accelerations with fetal movement, absence of late or variable decelerations).
- Prepare to administer terbutaline if uterine hyperstimulation, sustained uterine contractions, nonreassuring fetal status, or any other adverse reactions occur.

(Tang, Gemzell-Danielsson, & Ho, 2007). Practitioners may opt to administer the medication using different routes. One study showed that oral administration reduced hyperstimulation and had a lower cesarean birth rate when compared with vaginal administration (Cheng, Ming, & Lee, 2008). However, previous studies stated the opposite, that the vaginal route had higher rates of vaginal births (Cunningham, Leveno, Bloom et al., 2005). Other studies report that the low dosages used in current practice are all associated with a lower incidence of hyperstimulation (Weeks, Alfirevic, Faúndes et al., 2007). Although conflicting research findings can be confusing, it is important to note that Cytotec is delivered via various routes and yields successful results.

During the 1990s, when Cytotec was widely used for cervical ripening and labor induction, several reports associated its use with higher rates of uterine hyperstimulation and subsequent rupture. It has also been associated with amniotic fluid embolism, which is also a rare complication (FDA, 2008). Since that time, the drug has been contraindicated for inducing labor in women who have had a previous cesarean birth or have a scar on their uterus (Cheng et al., 2008). Although quite rare, Cytotec has also been associated with uterine rupture in women who have no previous scar on their uterus (Matsuo, Scanlon, Atlas et al., 2008). Other risk factors for uterine rupture include a high dose regimen (100 mcg or higher), advanced gesta-

tional age, and five or more previous pregnancies (ACOG, 2003; FDA, 2008). Other risks of Cytotec include fetal tachycardia, nonreassuring fetal status, and meconium passage (FDA, 2008). After a careful review of the literature and current studies, ACOG (2003) issued the following recommended guidelines for Cytotec administration:

- Use only during the third trimester for cervical ripening or labor induction.
- One-fourth tablet or 25 mcg should be the initial dosage.
- Recurrent administration should not exceed dosing intervals of more than 3 to 6 hours.
- Pitocin should not be administered less than 4 hours after the last Cytotec dose.
- Continuous fetal and uterine monitoring should be performed in a hospital setting.

Absolute contraindications for the use of Cytotec include the following:

- Presence of uterine contractions three times in 10 minutes
- Significant maternal asthma (Shiraishi, Asano, Niimi et al., 2008)
- History of previous cesarean birth or other uterine scar
- Bleeding during the pregnancy
- Presence of placenta previa
- Nonreassuring fetal heart rate tracing

Nursing Care Management

Physicians, certified nurse-midwives (CNMs), and birthing room nurses who have had special education and training may administer agents for cervical ripening. The woman and her support person(s) are provided information about the procedure, and any questions are answered. Baseline maternal vital signs are assessed, and an electronic fetal monitor is applied. The EFM tracing should indicate minimal or absent uterine activity, a reassuring FHR pattern, and a reactive NST. If uterine contractions are not occurring regularly, the ripening agent is inserted into the vagina. Prepidil can be administered every 6 hours. If prescribed, Cytotec is administered every 3 to 6 hours until adequate cervical change occurs (Cheng et al., 2008). The nurse instructs the woman to lie supine with a right hip wedge for a specified time (usually at least 1 hour). The woman can then assume any comfortable position. As discussed previously, the nurse monitors the woman for uterine hyperstimulation and FHR abnormalities (changes in baseline rate, variability, presence of decelerations) for at least 2 hours following insertion. During administration of PGE_2, if nausea and vomiting are present or contractions occur more frequently than every 2 minutes (and/or last greater than 75 seconds), the gel is removed.

Care of the Woman During Labor Induction

ACOG defines **labor induction** as the stimulation of uterine contractions before the spontaneous onset of labor, with or without ruptured fetal membranes, for the purpose of accomplishing birth. Induction may be indicated in the presence of the following (Battista & Wing, 2007):

- Diabetes mellitus
- Renal disease
- Preeclampsia/eclampsia
- Chronic pulmonary disease
- Premature rupture of membranes (PROM)
- Chorioamnionitis
- Postterm gestation greater than 42 weeks
- Mild abruptio placentae without evidence of nonreassuring fetal status
- Intrauterine fetal demise (IUFD)
- Intrauterine fetal growth restriction (IUGR)
- Alloimmunization
- Oligohydramnios
- Nonreassuring fetal status
- Nonreassuring antepartum testing

Relative indications include chronic hypertension, systemic lupus erythematosus, gestational diabetes, hypercoagulation disorders, cholestasis of pregnancy, polyhydramnios,

fetal anomalies requiring specialized neonatal care, logistical factors (risk of rapid birth, distance from hospital, psychologic factors, advanced cervical dilatation), previous stillbirth, and postterm gestation greater than 41 weeks (Battista & Wing, 2007).

All contraindications to spontaneous labor and vaginal birth are contraindications to the induction of labor. Maternal contraindications include but are not limited to the following (Battista & Wing, 2007):

- Client refusal
- Placenta previa or vasa previa
- Transverse fetal lie
- Prior classic uterine incision (or any vertical incision in the upper portion of the uterus)
- Active genital herpes infection
- Umbilical cord prolapse
- Absolute cephalopelvic disproportion

Relative contraindications include cervical carcinoma; malpresentation, such as breech; and funic presentation. A **funic presentation** is when the umbilical cord is interposed between the cervix and the presenting part. It can be located by clinical evaluation or by ultrasound (Battista & Wing, 2007).

Labor Readiness

Before induction is attempted, appropriate assessment must indicate that both the woman and fetus are ready for the onset of labor. This includes evaluation of fetal maturity and cervical readiness.

Fetal Maturity

The gestational age of the fetus is best evaluated by accurate maternal menstrual dating and early ultrasounds. Amniotic fluid studies also provide valuable information in assessing fetal lung maturity (see Chapter 14 ∞).

Cervical Readiness

The findings on vaginal examination help determine whether cervical changes favorable for induction have occurred. Bishop (1964) developed a prelabor scoring system that is helpful in predicting the potential success of induction (Table 23–1). Components evaluated are cervical dilatation, effacement, consistency, and position, as well as the station of the fetal presenting part. A score of 0, 1, 2, or 3 is given to each assessed characteristic. The higher the total score for all the criteria, the more likely it is that labor will occur. The lower the total score, the higher the failure rate. A favorable cervix is the most important criterion for a successful induction (Cheng et al., 2008). The presence of a cervix that is anterior, soft, 50% effaced, and dilated at least 2 cm (0.8 in.), with the fetal head at −1 to +1 station or lower (Bishop score of 8 or 9), is favorable for successful induction

MyNursingKit | Induction of Labor

TABLE 23–1	Prelabor Status Evaluation Scoring System			
	Assigned Value			
Factor	0	1	2	3
Cervical dilatation	Closed	1 to 2 cm	3 to 4 cm	5 cm or more
Cervical effacement	0% to 30%	40% to 50%	60% to 70%	80% or more
Fetal station	–3	–2	–1, 0	+1, or lower
Cervical consistency	Firm	Moderate	Soft	
Cervical position	Posterior	Midposition	Anterior	

Source: Bishop, E. H. (1964). Pelvic scoring for elective inductions. *Obstetrics & Gynecology, 24,* 266.

(Mbele, Makin, & Pattinson, 2007). If the cervix is unfavorable, a method of cervical ripening may be tried.

Methods of Inducing Labor

When the cervix is favorable, the most frequently used methods of induction are amniotomy (discussed previously), stripping the amniotic membranes, intravenous Pitocin infusion, and complementary methods.

Stripping the Membranes

A nonpharmacologic method of induction frequently used by physicians/CNMs is *stripping* (or *sweeping*) *the amniotic membranes.* The practitioner inserts a gloved finger into the internal os and rotates it 360 degrees twice, separating the amniotic membranes that are lying against the lower uterine segment. This is thought to release prostaglandins that stimulate uterine contractions. The procedure is usually uncomfortable and can result in cramping, uterine contractions, and vaginal bleeding.

Pitocin Infusion

Administration of Pitocin is an effective method of initiating uterine contractions to induce labor and may also be used to enhance ineffective contractions (*labor augmentation*). A primary line of 1000 mL of electrolyte solution (e.g., lactated Ringer's solution) is started intravenously. Ten units of Pitocin are added to a secondary line of intravenous (IV) fluid so the resulting mixture will contain 10 milliunits/mL of Pitocin (1 milliunit/min, or 6 mL/h), and the prescribed dose can be calculated easily. After the primary infusion is started, the Pitocin solution is piggybacked into the primary tubing port closest to the catheter insertion. The infusion is then administered using an infusion pump to control the flow rate precisely. The rate of infusion is based on physician/CNM protocol and careful assessment

of the contraction pattern. The goal for induction is to achieve stable contractions every 2 to 3 minutes that last 40 to 60 seconds. The uterus should relax to full baseline resting tone between each contraction. Progress is determined by changes in the effacement and dilatation of the cervix and station of the presenting part.

Pitocin induction is not without some associated risks, including hyperstimulation of the uterus, resulting in uterine contractions that are too frequent or too intense, with an increased resting tone. Hypertonic contractions may lead to decreased placental perfusion and nonreassuring fetal status. Other risks include uterine rupture, water intoxication, fetal hypoxia, and in rare circumstances fetal death (Wilson et al., 2009).

Complementary Methods

In addition to the medical (allopathic) methods just discussed, a variety of more natural, noninvasive methods to initiate contractions may also be used. These methods include sexual intercourse; self or partner nipple or breast stimulation; the use of herbs, castor oil, or enemas; acupuncture; and mechanical dilatation of the cervix with balloon catheters (Tenore, 2003). The cautions and contraindications are the same as those for medical induction of labor.

Although not frequently presented in medical (allopathic) or nursing texts, the natural methods can be effective, although some of them may not have undergone as rigorous scientific research as pharmacologic agents. Many certified nurse-midwives and their clients desire a less medical approach to birth and want to use natural methods when possible. It is important for basic nursing students, nurses, and clients to be aware of all aspects of pregnancy care.

Sexual intercourse is a logical method of inducing cervical ripening and uterine contractions; female orgasm stimulates contractions, and male ejaculate is a rich source of prostaglandins. Penetration during intercourse can also stimulate the lower uterine segment and cause uterine contractions. In addition, breast and nipple stimulation, which are often part of lovemaking, cause the production of endogenous oxytocin, which in turn stimulates the uterus to contract (Tenore, 2003).

Herbal preparations and other homeopathic solutions have not been scientifically studied to the same extent as other natural methods. The caregiver needs a thorough personal knowledge or ongoing consultation with a homeopathic physician to safely recommend the use of these approaches during late pregnancy (Tenore, 2003).

Although castor oil has been used for many years it has not been frequently studied as a method of labor induction. The mechanism by which castor oil stimulates uterine contractions is not understood. Some practitioners consider it to be an old-fashioned, nonuseful substance, whereas others have noted that it is especially effective for primigravidas.

COMPLEMENTARY AND ALTERNATIVE THERAPIES

Evening primrose oil is a natural substance that is extracted from the plant's seeds. It has been widely used for centuries by midwives as a means of softening the cervix, vagina, and perineum to facilitate the onset of labor. Evening primrose oil contains a fatty acid called gamma linolenic acid, which is converted into a prostaglandin compound. Prostaglandins play a key role in ripening the cervix so labor can begin. Women can be advised to begin evening primrose oil supplementation during the 36th week of pregnancy. The recommended dose is 2500 mg per day taken either orally or vaginally until birth. Side effects are rare but can include headaches, nausea, or skin rashes. Women who experience side effects should be counseled to discontinue the supplement unless advised otherwise by their physician (Midwifery Today E-News, 2002).

CRITICAL THINKING

You are a birthing center nurse caring for Wendy Johnson, G2P1, during a Pitocin infusion to induce her labor. Wendy has been receiving the medication via infusion pump for 4 hours and currently is receiving 6 milliunits/min (36 mL/hr). You have just completed your assessments and found the following: BP 120/80, pulse 80, respirations 16; contractions every 3 minutes lasting 60 seconds and of strong intensity; the FHR baseline is 144 to 150 with average variability; and cervical dilatation is 6 cm (2.4 in.). Will you continue the same infusion rate, increase the rate, or decrease the rate?

Answers can be found in Appendix F ∞.

For additional information about nursing interventions during use of Pitocin, see Drug Guide: Oxytocin (Pitocin) and the Nursing Care Plan for Induction of Labor.

Nursing Care Management

Aspects to address during client teaching about induction of labor include the purpose, the procedure itself, nursing care that will be provided, assessments, comfort measures, and a review of breathing techniques that may be used during labor. Regardless of the induction method used, close observation and accurate, ongoing assessments are mandatory to provide safe, optimal care for both woman and fetus. A qualified clinician should be readily accessible to manage any complications that may occur.

As contractions are established, vaginal examinations are done to evaluate cervical dilatation, effacement, and station. The frequency of vaginal examinations primarily depends on the woman's parity, comfort level, and strength of her contractions. If evaluating the need for analgesia, a vaginal examination should be performed to avoid giving the medication too early and increasing the risk of prolonging labor. This examination also helps identify advanced dilatation and imminent birth.

Pitocin induction protocols recommend obtaining baseline data (maternal temperature, pulse, respirations, blood pressure), a 20- to 30-minute EFM recording demonstrating a reassuring FHR, a reactive NST, and the contraction status before the induction is started. The fetal monitor is used to provide continuous data.

Before each increase of the Pitocin infusion rate the nurse assesses the following:

- Maternal blood pressure, pulse, respirations, temperature, and pain level
- Contraction status including frequency, duration, intensity, and resting tone
- FHR baseline, variability, and reactivity, noting the presence of accelerations, any decelerations, or bradycardia

Care of the Woman During Amnioinfusion

Amnioinfusion (AI) is a technique by which warmed, sterile normal saline or Ringer's lactate solution is introduced into the uterus through an intrauterine pressure catheter (IUPC). Amnioinfusion can be used intrapartally to increase the volume of fluid in cases of oligohydramnios, in which cord compression causes FHR deceleration and nonreassuring fetal status. It provides an extra cushion of fluid that relieves pressure on the umbilical cord and promotes increased perfusion to the fetus. AI is also implemented to dilute moderate to heavy meconium released in utero; when used for meconium dilution, amnioinfusion has resulted in a significant decrease of meconium below the cords (aspiration of meconium below the vocal cords that results from inhalation of meconium when the infant takes its initial breath). At birth, if the infant inhales any meconium present in the amniotic fluid, serious breathing problems and pneumonia may result. Amnioinfusion may also be indicated for preterm labor with premature rupture of membranes.

Nursing Care Management

The nurse is often the first person to detect changes in fetal heart rate associated with cord compression or to observe meconium-stained amniotic fluid. When cord compression is suspected, the immediate intervention is to assist the laboring woman to another position. If this intervention is not successful in restoring the FHR, an amnioinfusion may be considered.

The nurse helps administer the AI, assesses the woman's vital signs and contraction status, and monitors the fetal heart rate by continuous EFM. It is important to provide

MyNursingKit | Amnioinfusion

Drug Guide Oxytocin (Pitocin)

Overview of Obstetric Action Oxytocin (Pitocin) exerts a selective stimulatory effect on the smooth muscle of the uterus and blood vessels. Oxytocin affects the myometrial cells of the uterus by increasing the excitability of the muscle cell, increasing the strength of the muscle contraction, and supporting propagation of the contraction (movement of the contraction from one myometrial cell to the next). Its effect on the uterine contraction depends on the dosage used and on the excitability of the myometrial cells. During the first half of gestation, there is little excitability of the myometrium, and the uterus is fairly resistant to the effects of oxytocin. However, from midgestation on, the uterus responds increasingly to exogenous intravenous oxytocin. Cautious use of diluted oxytocin administered intravenously at term results in a slow rise of uterine activity.

The circulatory half-life of oxytocin is 3 to 5 minutes. It takes approximately 40 minutes for a particular dose of oxytocin to reach a steady-state plasma concentration (Wilson et al., 2006).

The effects of oxytocin on the cardiovascular system can be pronounced. Blood pressure initially may decrease but after prolonged administration increase by 30% above the baseline. Cardiac output and stroke volume increase. With doses of 20 milliunits/min or above, oxytocin exerts an antidiuretic effect decreasing free water exchange in the kidney and markedly decreasing urine output.

Oxytocin is used to induce labor at term and to augment uterine contractions in the first and second stages of labor. Oxytocin may also be used immediately after birth to stimulate uterine contraction and thereby control uterine atony.

Route, Dosage, Frequency For induction of labor: Add 10 units of Pitocin (1 mL) to 1000 mL of intravenous solution. (The resulting concentration is 10 mU oxytocin per 1 mL of intravenous fluid.) Using an infusion pump, administer IV, starting at 0.5–1 milliunit/min and increase by 1–2 milliunits/min every 40–60 minutes. Alternatively, start at 1–2 milliunits/min and increase by 1 milliunit/min every 15 minutes until a good contraction pattern (every 2–3 minutes and lasting 40–60 seconds) is achieved.

Maternal Contraindications

- Severe preeclampsia-eclampsia
- Predisposition to uterine rupture (in nullipara over 35 years of age, multigravida 4 or more, overdistention of the uterus, previous major surgery of the cervix or uterus)
- Cephalopelvic disproportion
- Malpresentation or malposition of the fetus, cord prolapse
- Preterm infant
- Rigid, unripe cervix; total placenta previa
- Presence of nonreassuring fetal status

Maternal Side Effects Hyperstimulation of the uterus results in hypercontractility, which in turn may cause the following:

- Abruptio placentae
- Impaired uterine blood flow, leading to fetal hypoxia
- Rapid labor, leading to cervical lacerations
- Rapid labor and birth, leading to lacerations of cervix, vagina, or perineum, uterine atony; fetal trauma
- Uterine rupture
- Water intoxication (nausea, vomiting, hypotension, tachycardia, cardiac arrhythmia) if oxytocin is given in electrolyte-free solution or at a rate exceeding 20 milliunits/min; hypotension with rapid IV bolus administration postpartum

Effect on Fetus-Newborn

- Fetal effects are primarily associated with the presence of hypercontractility of the maternal uterus. Hypercontractility decreases the oxygen supply to the fetus, which is reflected by irregularities or decrease in fetal heart rate (FHR).
- Hyperbilirubinemia (Wilson et al., 2010) when administered for augmentation of labor
- Trauma from rapid birth

Nursing Considerations

- Explain induction or augmentation procedure to client.
- Apply fetal monitor, and obtain 15- to 20-minute tracing and nonstress test (NST) to assess FHR before starting IV oxytocin.
- For induction or augmentation of labor, start with primary IV, and piggyback secondary IV with oxytocin and infusion pump.
- Ensure continuous monitoring of the fetus and uterine contractions.
- The maximum rate is 40 milliunits/min (Blackburn, 2007). Not all protocols recommend a maximum dose. When indicated, the maximum dose is generally between 16 and 40 milliunits/min. Decrease oxytocin by similar increments once labor has progressed to 5–6 cm dilatation. Protocols may vary from one agency to another.
  0.5 milliunit/min = 3 mL/hr
  1.0 milliunit/min = 6 mL/hr
  1.5 milliunit/min = 9 mL/hr
  2 milliunit/min = 12 mL/hr
  4 milliunit/min = 24 mL/hr
  6 milliunit/min = 36 mL/hr
  8 milliunit/min = 48 mL/hr
  10 milliunit/min = 60 mL/hr
  12 milliunit/min = 72 mL/hr
  15 milliunit/min = 90 mL/hr
  18 milliunit/min = 108 mL/hr
  20 milliunit/min = 120 mL/hr
- Assess FHR, maternal blood pressure, pulse, frequency and duration of uterine contractions, and uterine resting tone before each increase in the oxytocin infusion rate.
- Record all assessments and IV rate on monitor strip and on client's chart.

Drug Guide   Oxytocin (Pitocin) *(Continued)*

- Record oxytocin infusion rate in milliunits/min and mL/hr (e.g., 0.5 milliunits/min [3 mL/hr]).
- Record on monitor strip all client activities (such as change of position, vomiting), procedures done (amniotomy, sterile vaginal examination), and administration of analgesic agents to allow for interpretation and evaluation of tracing.
- Assess cervical dilatation as needed.
- Apply nursing comfort measures.
- Discontinue IV oxytocin infusion and infuse primary solution when (1) nonreassuring fetal status is noted (bradycardia, late or variable decelerations; (2) uterine contractions are more frequent than every 2 minutes; (3) duration of contractions exceeds more than 60 seconds; or (4) insufficient relaxation of the uterus between contractions or a steady increase in resting tone are noted (Blackburn, 2007). In addition to discontinuing IV oxytocin infusion, turn client to side, and if nonreassuring fetal status is present, administer oxygen by tight face mask at 7–10 L/min; notify physician.
- Maintain intake and output record.

For augmentation of labor:

Prepare and administer IV Pitocin as for labor induction. Increase rate until labor contractions are of good quality. The flow rate is gradually increased at no less than every 30 minutes to a maximum of 10 milliunits/min (Blackburn, 2007). In some settings or in a situation when limited fluids may be administered, a more concentrated solution may be used. When 10 units Pitocin are added to 500 mL IV solution, the resulting concentration is 1 milliunit/min = 3 mL/hr. If 10 units Pitocin are added to 250 mL IV solution, the concentration is 1 milliunit/min = 1.5 mL/hr.

For administration after expulsion of placenta:

- One dose of 10 units of Pitocin (1 mL) is given intramuscularly or added to IV fluids for continuous infusion.
- Assess FHR, maternal blood pressure, pulse, frequency and duration of uterine contractions, and uterine resting tone before each increase in oxytocin infusion rate.
- Record all assessments and IV rate on monitor strip and on client's chart. Record oxytocin infusion rate in milliunits/min and mL/hr (e.g., 0.5 milliunits/min [3 mL/hr]).
- Record on monitor strip all client activities (such as change of position, vomiting), procedures done (amniotomy, sterile vaginal examination), and administration of analgesic agents to allow for interpretation and evaluation of tracing.
- Assess cervical dilatation as needed.
- Apply nursing comfort measures.
- Maintain intake and output record. Assess intake and output every hour.

---

ongoing information to the laboring woman and her partner and to answer questions as they arise. Comfort measures and positioning are vital because the woman is now on bed rest. Frequent changing of disposable underpads and perineal care are also needed because of the constant leakage of fluid from the vagina. The nurse ensures that fluids that are infused into the uterus are being adequately expelled. Fluid expulsion is evaluated by counting sanitary pads and visual observation during perineal care.

Care of the Woman During an Episiotomy

An **episiotomy** is a surgical incision of the perineal body to enlarge the outlet. The second most common procedure in maternal-child care, the episiotomy has long been thought to minimize the risk of lacerations of the perineum and the overstretching of perineal tissues. However, episiotomy may actually increase the risk of fourth-degree perineal lacerations (Dudding, Vaizey, &, Kamm, 2008). Though very common, the routine use of episiotomy has been seriously questioned for several years. Research suggests that (1) rather than protecting the perineum from lacerations, the presence of an episiotomy makes it more likely that the woman will have anal sphincter tears and (2) perineal lacerations heal more quickly than deep perineal tears (Wheeler & Richter, 2007). In clinical practice, research has shown that the incidence of major perineal trauma (extension to or through the anal sphincter) is more likely to happen if a midline episiotomy is done (Roberts, Ely, & Ward, 2007). Women with previous episiotomies that resulted in a third- or fourth-degree extension were more likely to have a repeat occurrence when episiotomy was used initially compared with those women who had a spontaneous

(Continued on page 546)

Nursing Care Plan For Induction of Labor

CLIENT SCENARIO

Lakshmi Pandey is being admitted to labor and childbirth this morning for an induction. She is accompanied by her husband, Nitya. Lakshmi is a primigravida at 40 weeks' gestation. She has been experiencing Braxton Hicks contractions over the last week, but a contraction pattern has not been established. Lakshmi's membranes are intact and vital signs are within normal limits. Her cervix is soft and pliable, 20% effaced, and 1 cm (0.4 in.) dilated. Fetal station is –1. The nurse places Lakshmi on the external fetal monitor to obtain a baseline fetal heart rate pattern and evaluate uterine activity.

ASSESSMENT

Subjective: Braxton Hicks contractions, restless, backache, apprehensive. Pain level reported as 5 out of 10.

Objective: Cervix is 1 cm (0.4 in.) dilated, 20% effaced, –1 station, amniotic membranes are intact. BP 120/84, temperature 37.1°C (98.8°F), pulse 94, respirations 14, FHR 144 with average variability.

Nursing Diagnosis	Risk for Injury related to hyperstimulation of uterus caused by induction of labor*
Client Goal	Progression of labor without difficulty or complications
AEB:	• Contraction frequency every 2 to 3 minutes, duration 40 to 60 seconds, and moderate intensity
	• Progression of cervical dilation, effacement, and fetal descent
	• Resting tone returns to baseline between contractions
	• Vital signs remain within normal limits

NURSING INTERVENTIONS

1. Obtain a baseline for maternal blood pressure, pulse, respirations, temperature, and pain level.

2. Place client on external fetal monitor for 20 minutes to obtain a baseline for FHR and variability.

3. Perform nonstress test.

4. Insert IV line and begin primary infusion with 1000 mL of electrolyte solution.

5. Piggyback Pitocin solution into primary IV tubing, via pump, in the port closest to the IV insertion site.

6. Begin Pitocin infusion per agency protocol.

7. Monitor infusion pump and connections.

RATIONALES

Rationale: Pitocin induction can affect the cardiovascular system. Blood pressure may initially be decreased. If the induction is prolonged the blood pressure may increase by 30%. Respirations can become elevated because of pain sensation, anxiety, or physiological causes. Temperature is obtained to monitor for infection. The pain level is assessed continuously to determine if pain medication is warranted or changes in vital signs are caused by maternal discomfort.

Rationale: Assesses for fetal well-being. Normal FHR ranges from 110 to 160 bpm. Variability measuring three to five fluctuations in 1 minute is documented as average. Continuous EFM is performed during a Pitocin induction.

Rationale: A nonstress test is performed to assess the fetal heart rate in response to fetal movement. Accelerations of fetal heart rate with fetal movement may indicate the fetus has adequate oxygenation and an intact central nervous system. A reactive nonstress test indicates there were at least two accelerations of 15 bpm above baseline, lasting 15 seconds in a 20-minute period.

Rationale: An electrolyte solution such as lactated Ringer's is used for the primary solution. A primary IV allows continuous intravenous access and fluid infusion in the event the Pitocin drip needs to be discontinued.

Rationale: Pitocin is mixed in 1000 mL of an electrolyte solution (usually 5% dextrose in lactated Ringer's solution) and piggybacked to main IV line. A pump is used to ensure dosage accuracy.

Rationale: The rate to be used is determined by physician/CNM orders or agency protocol.

Rationale: This ensures adequate dosing. Early identification of problems with the infusion site, the piggyback connection, or flow rate will minimize effects on uterine contractions and FHR. If a problem is found, correct and restart infusion at the beginning dose.

Nursing Care Plan For Induction of Labor (Continued)

NURSING INTERVENTIONS

RATIONALES

8. Monitor and evaluate maternal blood pressure and pulse before each increase in the Pitocin infusion rate.

Rationale: Prolonged inductions may increase the blood pressure by 30%. The Pitocin infusion rate should not be advanced if maternal hypertension or hypotension is present or if there are any radical changes in pulse rate.

9. Evaluate urine output.

Rationale: There is an antidiuretic effect with dosages of Pitocin above 20 milliunits/min. This level decreases free water exchange in the kidneys, therefore markedly decreasing urine output.

10. Evaluate and document fetal heart rate before each increase in Pitocin infusion rate.

Rationale: During Pitocin infusion, fetal heart rate should range between 110 and 160 bpm. Hypercontractility of the maternal uterus may cause nonreassuring fetal status. Fetal bradycardia may occur along with a decrease in variability, leading to fetal hypoxia. Fetal tachycardia may also occur. If persistent fetal bradycardia or fetal tachycardia occurs, the Pitocin is discontinued.

11. Evaluate and document contraction pattern before each increase of the Pitocin infusion rate.

Rationale: Contractions every 2 to 3 minutes, lasting 40 to 60 seconds with moderate intensity, are considered adequate. Cervical dilatation progresses an average of 1.2 cm/hr to 1.5 cm/hr (0.5 in./hr to 0.6 in./hr) during the active phase of labor.

12. Increase Pitocin infusion dosage until adequate contractions are achieved or the maximum dose per agency protocol is reached.

Rationale: Pitocin may be increased every 20 to 40 minutes until an adequate contraction pattern is achieved.

13. Evaluate contraction frequency, duration, and intensity before increasing the infusion rate. Discontinue Pitocin infusion and infuse primary solution if signs of hyperstimulation of the uterus are detected.

Rationale: Signs of hyperstimulation include contraction frequency less than 2 minutes, duration exceeding 60 seconds, and increased resting tone. Hyperstimulation of the uterus puts the client at risk for abruptio placentae and uterine rupture.

14. Initiate treatment measures to reverse the effects of Pitocin infusion if fetal tachycardia or bradycardia occurs.

Rationale: When the FHR falls outside the normal range (110 to 160 bpm), treatment measures should be initiated. To reverse the effects of Pitocin, immediately discontinue Pitocin, infuse primary solution, administer oxygen by tight face mask at 7 to 10 L/min, place client in side-lying position, and notify physician/CNM.

Evaluation of Client Goal
- Contractions increased in frequency, duration, and intensity.
- Increase in cervical dilatation, effacement, and intensity was achieved.
- Uterus remains soft between contractions.

CRITICAL THINKING QUESTIONS

1. Lakshmi has been receiving Pitocin infusion for the past 4 hours and is currently receiving 6 milliunits/min. Your assessment of Lakshmi's contractions includes frequency every 3 minutes, lasting 60 seconds with moderate intensity. FHR ranges from 140 to 155 bpm with average variability. Cervix is now 6 cm (2.4 in.) dilated, 100% effaced, anterior, and the station is 0. Will you continue to monitor at the same infusion rate, increase the rate, or decrease the rate?

Answer: The contraction pattern has reached the desired frequency, duration, and strength. Now that the cervix is 6 cm (2.4 in.), the infusion rate can be maintained. Continue to monitor contraction pattern and cervical dilation. Adjust infusion rate to maintain adequate contraction pattern with FHR and variability remaining within normal limits.

2. While monitoring a client with a Pitocin infusion, you assess that the client's contractions are now every 2 minutes and fetal heart rate has dropped to 100 bpm with a decrease in variability. Several late decelerations are also assessed. What is your initial nursing action?

Answer: Discontinue Pitocin infusion and infuse primary solution. Also turn client to side-lying position, administer oxygen by tight face mask at 7 to 10 L/min, and notify physician/CNM.

*For your reference, this care plan is an example how one nursing diagnosis might be addressed.

laceration without the use of episiotomy (Edwards, Grotegut, Harmanli et al., 2006). Additional complications associated with episiotomy are blood loss, infection, pain, and perineal discomfort that may continue for days or weeks past birth, including painful intercourse (Ejegård, Ryding, & Sjögren, 2008).

Factors That Predispose Women to Episiotomy

Overall factors that place a woman at increased risk for episiotomy are primigravid status, large or macrosomic fetus, occiput-posterior position, use of forceps or vacuum extractor, and shoulder dystocia. Other factors that may be mitigated by nurses and physicians/CNMs include the following:

- Use of lithotomy and other recumbent positions (causes excessive and uneven stretching of the perineum)
- Encouraging or requiring sustained breath holding during second-stage pushing (causes excessive and rapid perineal stretching, can adversely affect blood flow in mother and fetus, and requires woman to be re-

sponsive to caregiver directions rather than to her own urges to push spontaneously)
- Arbitrary time limit placed by the physician/CNM on the length of the second stage

Preventative Measures

Following are some general tips to help reduce the incidence of routine episiotomies:

- Perineal massage during pregnancy for nulliparous women
- Natural pushing during labor, and avoiding the lithotomy position or pulling back on legs (which tightens the perineum)
- Side-lying position for pushing, which helps slow birth and diminish tears
- Warm or hot compresses on the perineum and firm counterpressure
- Encouraging a gradual expulsion of the infant at the time of birth by encouraging the mother to "push, take a breath, push, take a breath" thereby easing the infant out slowly
- Avoiding immediate pushing after epidural placement

EVIDENCE-BASED PRACTICE

Antenatal Perineal Massage for Reducing Perineal Trauma

Clinical Question
What is the effectiveness of antenatal perineal massage on the incidence of perineal trauma at birth, and its associated complications?

The Evidence
Perineal trauma following birth can be associated with both short- and long-term complications. This type of trauma can result from surgical episiotomy as well as spontaneous tears. Rates of trauma are particularly high in primiparous women. Pain from perineal trauma can last up to 3 months, and this pain may impair a return to normal sexual function. Perineal massage during the antenatal period has been proposed as one method of enabling the perineum to expand more easily during birth. A systematic review published in the Cochrane Database of Systematic Reviews provided data comparing perineal trauma in 2400 women who conducted antenatal perineal massage to women who did not. This type of rigorous, unbiased review of multiple randomized controlled trials represents the strongest evidence for practice.

What Is Effective?
Digital perineal massage performed by the woman herself or by her partner during the last 4 to 5 weeks of pregnancy reduced the number of needed episiotomies by about 15%. Perineal trauma—defined as an incidence of trauma requiring suturing—was also reduced when antenatal perineal massage

had been used. The benefit was greatest for women who were experiencing their first vaginal birth. When perineal trauma did occur, there was no difference in the extent of tearing in the group with perineal massage, so the advantage appears to be primarily in avoiding episiotomy. No differences were found in the incidence of instrument-assisted birth, resumption of sexual activity, or incontinence of urine or feces.

What Is Inconclusive?
The number of women in these studies who were multiparous was small, and so it cannot be definitively determined if perineal massage is as effective when it is not the first vaginal birth. No testing of massage devices was included in these studies. There was no specific type of perineal massage dictated, and so a particular method cannot be recommended.

Best Practice
You can suggest to primiparous women that perineal massage done by themselves or their partners will decrease the need for an episiotomy and may reduce the likelihood of perineal trauma with its associated ongoing perineal pain. Perineal massage should be performed for at least the final 4 to 5 weeks of pregnancy to assure optimal therapeutic effect.

Reference
Beckman, M., & Garrett, A. (2006). Antenatal perineal massage for reducing perineal trauma. *Cochrane Database of Systematic Reviews.* Issue 1.

Some practitioners routinely perform episiotomy as a standard of care. Therefore, nurses should provide information about episiotomy and encourage women to talk to their practitioner about the incidence of its use within the practice. Women who are opposed to an episiotomy should be encouraged to discuss their objection to the procedure with their healthcare provider at a prenatal visit before the onset of labor.

Episiotomy Procedure

The two types of episiotomy in current practice are midline and mediolateral (Figure 23–2 ■). Just before birth, when approximately 3 to 4 cm (1.2 to 1.6 in.) of the fetal head is visible during a contraction, the episiotomy is performed using sharp scissors with rounded points (Kilpatrick & Garrison, 2007). The midline incision begins at the bottom center of the perineal body and extends straight down the midline to the fibers of the rectal sphincter. The mediolateral incision begins in the midline of the posterior fourchette and extends at a 45-degree angle downward to the right or left.

The episiotomy is usually performed with regional or local anesthesia but may be done without anesthesia in emergency situations. It is generally proposed that as crowning occurs, the distention of the tissues causes numbing. Repair of the episiotomy (episiorrhaphy) and any lacerations is completed either during the period between birth of the newborn and before expulsion of the placenta or after expulsion of the placenta. Adequate anesthesia must be given for the repair.

Nursing Care Management

The woman needs to be supported during the episiotomy and the repair because she may feel some pressure, or pulling or tugging sensations. In the absence of adequate anesthesia she may feel pain. Placing a hand on the woman's shoulder and talking with her can provide comfort and distraction from the repair process. If the woman is having more discomfort than she can comfortably handle, the nurse needs to act as an advocate in communicating the woman's needs to the physician/CNM. At all times the woman needs to be the one who decides whether the amount of discomfort she is experiencing is tolerable. She should never be told, "This doesn't hurt." She is the person experiencing the discomfort, and her evaluation needs to be respected.

The type of episiotomy is recorded on the birth record. This information should also be included in a report to subsequent caregivers so that adequate assessments can be made and relief measures can be instituted.

Comfort measures may begin immediately after birth with the application of an ice pack to the perineum. For

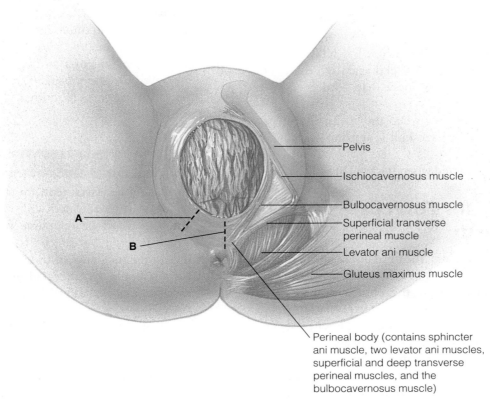

Pelvis

Ischiocavernosus muscle

Bulbocavernosus muscle

Superficial transverse perineal muscle

Levator ani muscle

Gluteus maximus muscle

Perineal body (contains sphincter ani muscle, two levator ani muscles, superficial and deep transverse perineal muscles, and the bulbocavernosus muscle)

FIGURE 23–2 The two most common types of episiotomies are midline and mediolateral. *A,* Right mediolateral. *B,* Midline.

optimal effect the ice pack should be applied for 20 to 30 minutes and removed for at least 20 minutes before being reapplied. The nurse assesses the perineal tissues frequently to prevent injury from the ice pack. The episiotomy site should be inspected every 15 minutes during the first hour after the birth for redness, swelling, tenderness, bruising, and hematomas. As part of postpartal care the mother will need instruction in perineal hygiene, self-care, and comfort measures.

It is important for nurses to recognize that perineal pain continues for a period of time, and may be significant. This pain should not be discounted: Women who experience prolonged perineal pain tend to have problems with breastfeeding and depression and are reluctant to reestablish sexual activity.

Nursing advocacy is needed to promote selective rather than routine episiotomy. It is imperative that each nurse stay current regarding new information and research in order to maintain current practice standards.

Care of the Woman During Forceps-Assisted Birth

Forceps are surgical instruments designed to assist in the birth of a fetus by providing either traction or the means to rotate the fetal head to an occiput-anterior position. In medical literature and practice, **forceps-assisted birth** is also known as instrumental delivery or operative vaginal delivery. Three categories of forceps application exist:

1. Outlet forceps are applied when the fetal skull has reached the perineum, the fetal scalp is visible, and the sagittal suture is not more than 45 degrees from the midline.
2. Low forceps are applied when the leading edge (presenting part) of the fetal skull is at a station of +2 or more.
3. Midforceps are applied when the fetal head is engaged.

Indications for Forceps-Assisted Birth

Forceps may be indicated in the presence of any condition that threatens the mother or fetus and that can be relieved by birth. Conditions that put the woman at risk include heart disease, pulmonary edema, infection, and exhaustion. Fetal conditions include premature placental separation and nonreassuring fetal status. Forceps may be used to shorten the second stage of labor and assist the woman's pushing effort. They may also be used when regional anesthesia has affected the woman's motor innervation and she cannot push effectively.

Before forceps are used, the following conditions must be met (Nielsen, Galan, Kilpatrick & Garrison, 2007):

- The cervix must be completely dilated and the exact position and station of the fetal head known.
- Membranes must be ruptured to allow a firm grasp on the fetal head, which must be engaged and in vertex or face presentation.
- The type of pelvis should be known, because certain pelvic types do not permit rotation.
- The maternal bladder should be empty and adequate anesthesia given.
- No degree of cephalopelvic disproportion can be present.
- The operator must have the knowledge to perform the procedure.
- Maternal anesthesia is available.
- Adequate staff is available with the ability to perform a cesarean birth if indicated.
- Maternal consent has been obtained.

Neonatal and Maternal Risks

Some newborns may develop a small area of ecchymosis and/or edema along the sides of the face as a result of forceps application. Facial lacerations and brachial plexus can also occur (Doumouchtsis & Arulkumaran, 2008). Caput succedaneum or cephalohematoma (with subsequent hyperbilirubinemia) may occur, as may transient facial paralysis. Although rare, cerebral hemorrhages, fractures, brain damage, and fetal death have also been reported (Doumouchtsis & Arulkumaran, 2008).

Maternal risks include possible lacerations of the birth canal; extensions of a midline episiotomy into the anus; increased bleeding, bruising, and perineal edema; and anal incontinence (Pretlove, Thompson, Toozs-Hobson et al., 2008).

Nursing Care Management

By using ongoing assessment, the nurse may note the variables that are associated with an increased rate of instrument-assisted or operative birth. Nursing care measures can then be directed toward variables that may reduce the incidence of these factors. For example, labor dystocia may be corrected by changing maternal position, ambulation, use of breast/nipple stimulation or an electric breast pump, and frequent bladder emptying. FHR abnormalities may be improved by position changes, increased fluid intake, and/or adequate oxygen exchange.

If a forceps-assisted birth is required, the nurse explains the procedure briefly to the woman. With adequate regional anesthesia the woman should feel

MyNursingKit Forceps Delivery

pressure during the procedure. The nurse ensures that adequate anesthesia is provided by alerting the physician if discomfort or pain occurs. The nurse encourages the woman to use breathing techniques that help prevent her from pushing during application of the forceps (Figure 23–3 ■).The nurse monitors contractions and advises the physician when one is present because traction is only applied with a contraction. With each contraction the physician provides traction on the forceps as the woman pushes. The nurse reinforces to the woman that she needs to push while traction is being applied, explaining that the combined efforts help with expulsion of the fetus. It is not uncommon to observe mild fetal

bradycardia as traction is being applied to the forceps. This bradycardia results from head compression and is transient.

Immediately following birth, the newborn is assessed for facial edema, bruising, caput succedaneum, cephalohematoma, and any signs of cerebral edema. In the fourth stage the nurse assesses the woman for perineal swelling, bruising, hematoma, excessive bleeding, and hemorrhage. In the postpartum period it is important to assess for signs of infection if lacerations occurred during the procedure. The nurse provides an opportunity for questions and reiterates explanations provided.

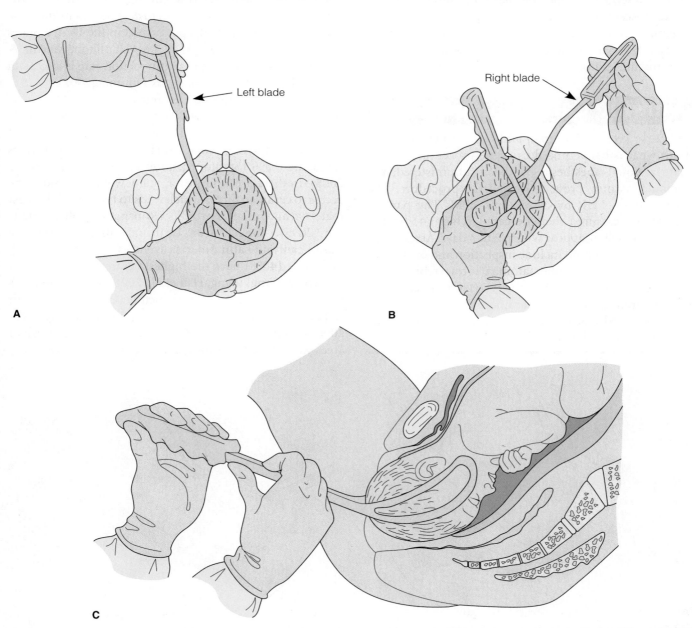

FIGURE 23–3 Application of forceps in occiput-anterior (OA) position. *A,* The left blade is inserted along the left side wall of the pelvis over the parietal bone. *B,* The right blade is inserted along the right side wall of the pelvis over the parietal bone. *C,* With correct placement of the blades, the handles lock easily. During uterine contractions, traction is applied to the forceps in a downward and outward direction to follow the birth canal.

Care of the Woman During Vacuum-Assisted Birth

Vacuum-assisted birth is an obstetric procedure used to facilitate the birth of a fetus by applying suction to the fetal head. The vacuum extractor is composed of a soft suction cup attached to a suction bottle (pump) by tubing. The suction cup, which comes in various sizes, is placed against the fetal occiput, and the pump is used to create negative pressure (suction) inside the cup. Traction is applied in coordination with uterine contractions, descent occurs, and the fetal head is born (Figure 23–4 ■). General recommendations include that there should be progressive descent with the first two pulls and that the procedure should be limited to prevent cephalohematomas, brain injury, and fetal death (Doumouchtsis & Arulkumaran, 2008).

Nursing Care Management

The nurse keeps the woman and her partner informed about what is happening during the procedure. If adequate regional anesthesia has been administered, the woman feels only pressure during the procedure. The nurse assesses FHR by continuous EFM. The parents need to be reassured that the caput (chignon) on the baby's head will disappear within 2 to 3 days. Assessment of the newborn should include inspection and continued observation for cephalohematomas, intracerebral hemorrhage, and retinal hemorrhages (Doumouchtsis & Arulkumaran, 2008). Because infants born via vacuum are at increased risk for jaundice, careful assessment of the infant's skin color is also needed.

Care of the Family During Cesarean Birth

Cesarean birth, the birth of the infant through an abdominal and uterine incision, is one of the oldest surgical procedures known. Until the twentieth century cesarean procedures were primarily used in an attempt to save the fetus of a dying woman. As the maternal and perinatal morbidity and mortality rates associated with cesarean birth steadily decreased throughout the twentieth century, the proportion of cesarean births increased. Beginning in the early 1970s the cesarean birth rate rose steadily for almost two decades. In 1989, however, in an effort to control healthcare costs, the number of cesarean births began to decline. But in 2006, the number of cesarean births performed in the United States reached an all-time high of 31.1% (Hamilton, Martin, & Ventura, 2007). Canada's cesarean section rate is also at an all-time high at 23.7% (Chaillet & Dumont, 2007).

Cesarean birth rates differ dramatically in other parts of the world. The worldwide rate is estimated to be 12% (Thomas, 2006). Worldwide, cesarean birth is the least common in the Sub-Sahara African countries with rates averaging 0.3% (Stanton, Dubourg, De Brouwere et al., 2005). In these areas, however, many women do not have access to cesarean births which leads to the world's highest maternal and infant morbidity (Ronsmans, Holtz, & Stanton, 2006). The cesarean birth rate in East Asia, the Caribbean, and Latin America averages 26%. Brazil (36%) and Chile (40%) have the highest cesarean birth rates in the world (Tang, Wang, Hsu et al., 2006). Other countries with cesarean rates over 30% include China, Iran, South Korea, Taiwan, and the Dominican Republic (Tang et al., 2006; Thomas, 2006). Worldwide, women living in urban areas were three times more likely to have a cesarean than

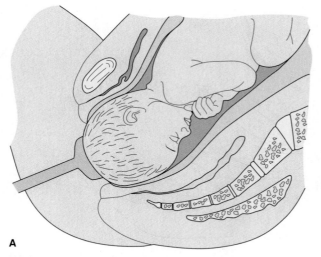
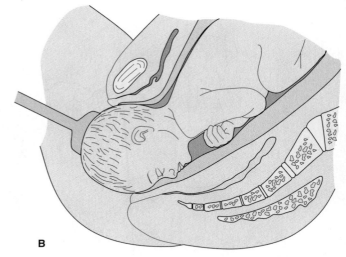

A **B**

FIGURE 23–4 Vacuum extractor traction. *A,* The cup is placed on the fetal occiput creating suction. Traction is applied in a downward and outward direction. Traction continues in a downward direction as the fetal head begins to emerge from the vagina. *B.* Traction is maintained to lift the fetal head out of the vagina.

women living in rural areas (Thomas, 2006). Countries with low cesarean birth rates include Austria (14.5%), the Netherlands (13.6%), and Norway (15.7%) (Häger, Øian, Nilsen et al., 2006; Kwee, Elferink-Stinkens, Reuwer, & Bruinse, 2007). Overall, the incidence of cesarean birth has continued to increase worldwide.

The increasing rate in the United States is linked to a rise in repeat cesarean births fueled by concerns regarding the risk of uterine rupture with a vaginal birth after a previous cesarean birth. There is also an increase in requests from women for cesarean births so that they can avoid the pain of labor and vaginal birth. The trend increased further when some medical literature stated that vaginal births could result in pelvic floor damage during the birth process (Samarasekera, Bekhit, Wright et al., 2008). There is also an emerging trend to "schedule" birth into busy routines to meet specific needs of the parents, such as coordinating work projects, arranging for babysitting of older children, or arranging for relatives who live in other geographic locations to travel to be present for the birth itself.

Over the last few years, there has been a rise in the number of nulliparous women requesting cesarean births (Wiklund, Edman, Ryding et al., 2008). This trend has led to further increases in the cesarean birth rate. Although cesarean birth on request is associated with a reduction in maternal hemorrhage risk, it is also associated with increases in neonatal respiratory problems, longer hospitalizations, and an increase in complications in subsequent pregnancies, including placenta implantation problems and uterine rupture (ACOG, 2007). Maternal request for a cesarean birth without medical indications should not be recommended for women desiring several children, for women less than 39 gestational weeks, or when pregnancy dating is unknown or may be inaccurate. It should also not be motivated by the lack of anesthesia availability in an institution (National Institute of Health, 2006). In some developing countries, such as Nigeria, cesarean by request is viewed as a guarantee that a woman will deliver a live infant (Chigbu & Iloabachie, 2007).

Many other factors have contributed to the rise in the cesarean birth rate and need to be considered in any discussion about decreasing the rate. These factors include an increased use of epidural anesthesia, maternal age over 35, failed inductions, decline in vaginal breech deliveries, decreases in operative vaginal deliveries, increased repeat cesarean rates, reduced vaginal birth after cesarean birth rates, increased physician scheduling of cesarean births for personal convenience, policy statements from professional organizations encouraging cesarean birth, political pressure from malpractice insurance carriers who attempt to dictate practice standards, and fear of litigation (ACOG, 2007; Landon, 2007).

Indications

Commonly accepted indications for cesarean birth include complete placenta previa, cephalopelvic disproportion, placental abruption, active genital herpes, umbilical cord prolapse, failure to progress in labor, nonreassuring fetal status, previous classical incision on the uterus (either previous cesarean birth or myomectomy), more than one previous cesarean birth, benign and malignant tumors that obstruct the birth canal, and cervical cerclage. Certain maternal medical conditions including cardiac disorders; severe maternal respiratory disease; central nervous system disorders that increase intracranial pressure; mechanical vaginal obstruction, such as an ovarian mass or lower uterine segment fibroids; and severe mental illness that results in an altered state of consciousness are all contraindications to a vaginal birth and warrant a cesarean birth (Landon, 2007). Other indications that are now commonly associated with cesarean birth, although in some circumstances they may be able to be delivered vaginally, include breech presentation, previous cesarean birth, major congenital anomalies, and severe Rh alloimmunization.

Maternal Mortality and Morbidity

Cesarean births have a higher maternal mortality rate than vaginal births. Women giving birth via cesarean are 3.6 times more likely to die in the postpartum period compared with women who give birth vaginally (Deneux-Tharaux, Carmona, Bouvier-Colle et al., 2006). Whereas approximately 2.1 per 100,000 women die during a vaginal birth, mortality is 5.9 per 100,000 for women who undergo an elective cesarean birth. Women who undergo an emergency cesarean birth face a significantly higher incidence of death, 18.2 per 100,000 (Hannah, 2004). Perinatal morbidity is often associated with infection, hypertensive disorders, reaction to anesthesia, blood clots, and bleeding problems (Moodley, 2008).

Countries vary widely regarding the percentage of women who die from birth-related complications. The worldwide maternal morbidity rate is 402 per 100,000 births, with 50% occurring in the Sub-Saharan Africa countries and 45% occurring in Asia (Hill, Thomas, AbouZahr et al., 2007). In the United States, 12.1 women per 100,000 giving birth to a live infant die in childbirth (Hoyert, 2007). In Albania, 6.9 women per 100,000 live births die annually as a result of childbirth, which is significantly lower than the reported 22.9 deaths in 2000 (World Health Organization, 2007).

In addition to the complications associated with cesarean birth, there are also risks that increase maternal mortality and morbidity in subsequent pregnancies. Women who have previously given birth via cesarean have a 1% risk of uterine rupture in subsequent pregnancies (Shipp, Zelop, & Lieberman, 2008). Women who have had a previous cesarean birth have an increased risk of bleeding problems in future pregnancies. The risk of placenta previa in subsequent pregnancies is 15 per 1000, while the risk of abruptio placentae is 13 per 1000 (Odibo, Cahill, Stamilio et al., 2007). There is also an increase in fetal demise and in neonatal respiratory distress and the need for oxygen administration in fetuses whose mothers have previously given birth via cesarean (Gray, Quigley, Hockley, et al., 2007).

Skin Incisions

The skin incision for a cesarean birth is either transverse (Pfannenstiel) or vertical and is not indicative of the type of incision made into the uterus. The transverse incision is made across the lowest and narrowest part of the abdomen. Because the incision is made just below the pubic hairline, it is almost invisible after healing. The limitation of this type of skin incision is that it does not allow for extension of the incision if needed. This incision is used when time is not of the essence (e.g., with failure to progress and stable fetal and maternal status), because it usually requires more time to make and repair.

The vertical incision is made between the navel and the symphysis pubis. This type of incision is quicker and is therefore preferred in cases of nonreassuring fetal status when rapid birth is indicated, with preterm or macrosomic infants, or when the woman is significantly obese (Landon, 2007). Time factors, client preference, previous vertical skin incision, or physician preference determines the type of skin incision.

Uterine Incisions

The type of uterine incision depends on the need for the cesarean. The choice of incision affects the woman's opportunity for a subsequent vaginal birth and her risks of a ruptured uterine scar with a subsequent pregnancy.

The two major locations of uterine incisions are in the lower uterine segment and in the upper segment of the uterine corpus. The lower uterine segment incision most commonly used is a transverse incision (Figure 23–5 ■). The lower uterine segment incision is preferred for the following reasons (Cunningham et al., 2005):

1. The lower segment is the thinnest portion of the uterus and involves less blood loss.
2. It requires only moderate dissection of the bladder from underlying myometrium.
3. It is easier to repair, although repair takes longer.
4. The site is less likely to rupture during subsequent pregnancies.

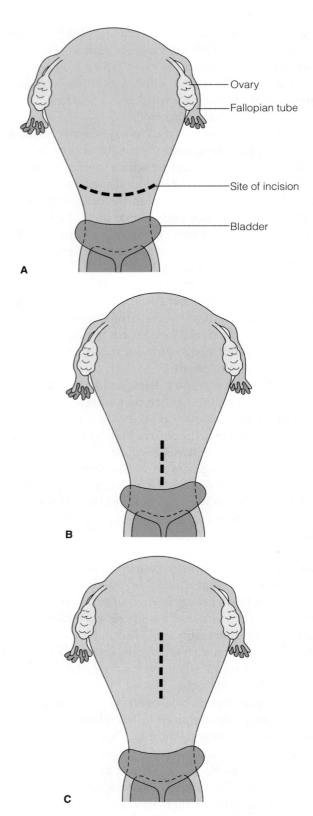

FIGURE 23–5 Uterine incisions for a cesarean birth. *A,* This transverse incision in the lower uterine segment is called a Kerr incision. *B,* The Sellheim incision is a vertical incision in the lower uterine segment. *C,* This view illustrates the classic uterine incision that is done in the body (corpus) of the uterus. The classic incision was commonly done in the past and is associated with increased risk of uterine rupture in subsequent pregnancies and labor.

5. There is a decreased chance of adherence of bowel or omentum to the incision line.

Disadvantages are as follows:

1. It takes longer to make a transverse incision.
2. It is limited in size because of the presence of major vessels on either side of the uterus.
3. It has a greater tendency to extend laterally into the uterine vessels.
4. The incision may stretch and become a thin window, but it usually does not create problems clinically until subsequent labor ensues.

The lower uterine segment vertical incision is preferred for multiple gestation, abnormal presentation, placenta previa, nonreassuring fetal status, and preterm and macrosomic fetuses. Disadvantages of this incision are as follows:

1. The incision may extend downward into the cervix.
2. More extensive dissection of the bladder is needed to keep the incision in the lower uterine segment; hemostasis and closure are more difficult.
3. The vertical incision carries a higher risk of rupture with subsequent labor. Consequently, once a vertical incision is performed, future births need to be via cesarean.

One other incision, the classic incision, was the method of choice for many years but is used infrequently now. This vertical incision was made into the upper uterine segment. More blood loss resulted and it was more difficult to repair. Most important, it carried an increased risk of uterine rupture with subsequent pregnancy, labor, and birth because the upper uterine segment is the most contractile portion of the uterus.

Analgesia and Anesthesia

There is no perfect anesthesia for cesarean birth. Each has its advantages, disadvantages, possible risks, and side effects. Goals for analgesia and anesthesia administration include safety, comfort, and emotional satisfaction for the client (see Chapter 20 ∞).

CULTURAL PERSPECTIVES

Women from other countries who have had a previous cesarean birth typically have a vertical skin incision; however, the skin incision does not provide data on the type of uterine incision that was performed. Careful explanation is provided and an operative report is obtained when possible. Operative reports in other languages need to be translated by personnel familiar with medical terminology. In the event an operative report cannot be obtained, which is common, a thorough explanation regarding the need for a repeat cesarean is provided.

Nursing Care Management

Preparation for Cesarean Birth

Because one of every four births is a cesarean, preparation for this possibility should be an integral part of all prenatal education. Pregnant women and their partners should be encouraged to discuss the possibility of a cesarean birth with their physician/CNM and at the same time discuss their specific needs and desires under those circumstances. Their preferences may include the following:

- Participating in the choice of anesthetic
- Father (or significant other) being present during the procedures and/or birth
- Father (or significant other) being present in the recovery or postpartum room
- Video recording and/or taking pictures of the birth
- Delayed instillation of eye drops to promote eye contact between parent and infant in the first hours after birth
- Physical contact or holding the infant while in the operating and/or recovery room (by the father if the mother cannot hold the newborn)
- Breastfeeding in the recovery area within the first hour of birth

Information that couples need about cesarean birth includes the following:

- What preparatory procedures to expect
- Description or viewing of the birthing room
- Types of anesthesia for birth and analgesia available postpartum
- Sensations that may be experienced
- Roles of significant others
- Interaction with newborn
- Immediate recovery phase
- Postpartum phase

Preparing the woman and her family for birth involves more than the procedures of establishing an intravenous line, instilling a urinary indwelling catheter, and performing an abdominal prep. As discussed previously, good communication skills are essential in preparing the woman and her support person. The use of therapeutic touch and direct eye contact (if culturally acceptable and possible) assist the woman in maintaining a sense of control and lessen anxiety.

If the cesarean birth is scheduled and not an emergency, the nurse has ample time for preoperative teaching. The context in which this information is relayed should be birth oriented rather than surgery oriented. This provides an opportunity for the woman to express her concerns, ask questions, and develop a relationship with the nurse.

In preparation for surgery, the woman is given nothing by mouth. To reduce the likelihood of serious pulmonary damage if gastric contents are aspirated, antacids may be administered within 30 minutes of surgery. If epidural anesthesia is used, the nurse may assist with the procedure, monitor the woman's blood pressure and response, and continue EFM. An abdominal and perineal prep is done, and an indwelling catheter is inserted to prevent bladder distention. An intravenous line is started with a large bore needle to permit blood administration if it becomes necessary. Preoperative medication may be ordered. The pediatrician should be notified and preparation made to receive the new baby. The nurse ensures that the infant warmer is working and that resuscitation equipment is available.

The nurse assists in positioning the woman on the operating table. Fetal heart rate is assessed before surgery and during preparation because fetal hypoxia can result from the supine position. The operating room table is adjusted so it slants slightly to one side or a hip wedge (folded blanket or towels) is placed under the right hip to tip the uterus slightly and reduce compression of blood vessels. The uterus should be displaced 15 degrees from the midline. This helps relieve the pressure of the heavy uterus on the vena cava and lessens the incidence of vena cava compression and maternal supine hypotension. The suction should be in working order and the urine collection bag should be positioned under the operating table to obtain proper drainage. Auscultation or EFM of the fetal heart rate is continued until immediately before the procedure. A last-minute check is done to ensure that the fetal scalp electrode has been removed if the fetus was internally monitored.

The nurse continues to provide reassurance and describe the various procedures being performed along with a rationale to ease anxiety and give the woman a sense of control.

TEACHING TIP

Women undergoing elective cesarean birth can be taught many aspects of postoperative teaching before their birth experience. Important components of client education that can be emphasized before birth include dealing with postoperative discomfort, splinting the incision to decrease pain, frequent deep breathing and coughing, and the importance of early ambulation. Women who receive this information before the birth are more apt to remember it when it is reviewed in the early postpartum period.

Preparation for Repeat Cesarean Birth

When a couple is anticipating a repeat cesarean birth, they have a general understanding of what will occur, which can help them make informed choices about their birth experience. Couples who have had previous negative experiences need an opportunity to describe what they felt. They can be encouraged to identify what they would like

to be different and to list options that would make the experience more positive. Those who have already had positive experiences need reassurance that their needs and desires will be met in a similar manner. In addition, an opportunity should be provided to discuss any fears or anxieties. The positive aspects of a repeat cesarean birth should be emphasized. For women who previously labored and then had an unexpected cesarean birth, the experience may be perceived as negative. Positive aspects that should be emphasized include participation in selecting the birth date, lack of fatigue related to labor, ability to prepare and make arrangements for other children, and ability for other family members or friends to be present at the hospital during or immediately after birth if desired by the couple.

Preparation for Emergency Cesarean Birth

When the need for a cesarean birth emerges suddenly, the period preceding surgery must be used to its greatest advantage. It is imperative that caregivers use their most effective communication skills in supporting the couple. The nurse describes what the couple may anticipate during the next few hours. Asking the couple "What questions or concerns do you have about the decision?" gives them an opportunity for clarification. The nurse can prepare the woman in stages, giving her information and the rationale for interventions before beginning any procedure. It is essential to tell the woman (1) what is going to happen, (2) why it is being done, and (3) what sensations she may experience. This allows the woman to be informed and to consent to the procedure, which gives her a sense of control and reduces her feelings of helplessness.

Supporting the Father or Partner

Every effort should be made to include the father or partner in the birth experience. When attending the cesarean birth, the partner wears protective coverings similar to those worn by others in the operating suite. A stool can be placed beside the woman's head so that the partner can sit nearby to provide physical touch, visual contact, and verbal reassurance.

To promote the participation of the father who chooses not to be in the operating suite, the nurse can do the following:

1. Allow the father to be nearby, where he can hear the newborn's first cry.
2. Encourage the father to carry or accompany the infant to the nursery for the initial assessment.
3. Involve the father in postpartum care in the recovery room.

In some emergency circumstances, a support person may not be permitted in the operating room. Some facilities have policies that prohibit a support person from being in the operating room if the woman requires general anesthesia or if an emergency birth is being performed. In these situations, the support person should receive a thorough explanation of what is happening and why, be advised when the staff will return to provide information, know the expected length of time for the procedure, and be reassured that the mother is receiving the care she and the baby need. Because this exclusion is stressful for family members, staff should try to provide information as soon as possible after providing emergency care to the mother.

Immediate Postnatal Recovery Period

After birth the nurse assesses the Apgar score and completes the same initial assessment and identification procedures used for vaginal births. Infant identification bands must be placed on the infant and the mother (as well as the third person, if present) before removing the infant from the operating room. Every effort should be made to assist the parents in bonding with their infant. If the mother is awake, one of her arms can be freed to enable her to touch and stroke the infant. The newborn may be placed on the mother's chest or held in an *en face* position. If physical contact is not possible, the nurse can provide a running narrative so the mother knows what is happening with her baby. The nurse assists the anesthesiologist or nurse anesthetist with raising the mother's head so she can see her infant immediately after birth. The parents can be encouraged to talk to the baby, and the father can hold the baby until she or he is taken to the nursery.

The nurse caring for the postpartum woman assesses the mother's vital signs every 5 minutes until they are stable, then every 15 minutes for an hour, then every 30 minutes until she is discharged to the postpartum unit. The nurse should remain with the woman until she is stable.

The nurse evaluates the dressing and perineal pad every 15 minutes for at least an hour. The fundus should be gently palpated to determine whether it is remaining firm; it may be palpated by placing a hand to support the incision. Intravenous Pitocin is usually administered to promote the contractility of the uterine musculature. If the woman has been under general anesthesia, she should be positioned on her side to facilitate drainage of secretions, turned, and assisted with coughing and deep breathing every 2 hours for at least 24 hours. If she has received a spinal or epidural anesthetic, the level of anesthesia is checked every 15 minutes until full sensation has returned. It is important for the nurse to monitor intake and output and to observe the urine for a bloody tinge, which could mean surgical trauma to the bladder. The physician prescribes medication to relieve the mother's pain and nausea, and it is administered as needed.

HINTS FOR PRACTICE

Bonding can be promoted by allowing the mother to hold or nurse the infant during this time period. If the infant has been moved to a separate area, such as the nursery, encourage maternal participation by allowing the support person to visit the infant and report back to the mother. The support person can take digital pictures or bring back the blanket that was used to wrap up the baby immediately after the birth. Frequent updates from the nurse such as "Your baby's doing just fine" provide reassurance to the mother if separation is needed.

Care of the Woman Undergoing Vaginal Birth After Cesarean (VBAC)

In the late 1990s there was an increasing trend to have a trial of labor and attempt **vaginal birth after cesarean (VBAC)** in cases of nonrecurring indications for a cesarean (such as umbilical cord prolapse, breech, placenta previa, or nonreassuring fetal status). This trend was influenced by consumer demand and studies that supported VBAC as a viable alternative to repeat cesarean. It resulted in a reduction in the cesarean section rate to 20.7% in 1996.

Recent media reports identifying risks of VBAC (discussed shortly) have reintroduced the debate regarding its safety. At the same time, trends in counseling women to have an elective repeat cesarean birth are driving cesarean births to an all-time high in the United States because of the reduction in VBACs.

The ACOG (2004) guidelines update states that the following aspects need to be considered for VBAC:

- A woman with one previous cesarean birth and a low transverse uterine incision may be counseled and encouraged to attempt VBAC.
- A clinically adequate pelvis is a requirement for VBAC.
- A woman with two previous cesareans who has also had a previous vaginal birth may attempt VBAC.
- It must be possible to perform a cesarean within 30 minutes.
- A physician, adequate staff, anesthesia, and facilities must be readily available throughout active labor to perform a cesarean birth if needed.
- A classic or T uterine incision is a contraindication to VBAC.

The most common risks associated with failed VBAC births are hemorrhage, uterine scar separation or uterine rupture, hysterectomy, surgical injuries, infant death, and

MyNursingKit | VBAC Bibliography

neurologic complications (see Chapter 21 ∞). It should be noted that these complications occur as a result of a uterine rupture. The incidence of uterine rupture is 0.9% of all trials of labors when the mother has had a previous cesarean birth (Shipp, Zelop, & Lieberman, 2008). Women who go into spontaneous labor have a much lower incidence of uterine rupture (1 per 100) compared with women who undergo Pitocin induction (1.4 per 100) (Grossetti, Vardon, Creveuil et al., 2007). Prostaglandin agents should not be used in women attempting a VBAC because of the increased risk of uterine rupture. The incidence of uterine rupture in women who receive a prostaglandin agent is as high as 2.2 per 100 (Grossetti et al., 2007). Conservative policies, such as awaiting spontaneous labor, avoiding prostaglandin agents, and avoiding elective inductions, can assist in reducing the incidence of uterine rupture. The incidence of uterine rupture in women before labor is 3 per 1000 (Grossetti et al., 2007).

Women who have a successful VBAC have lower incidences of infection, less blood loss, fewer blood transfusions, and shorter hospital stays. Healthcare costs are considerably lower for women who have a VBAC than for those who have a repeat cesarean birth (Odibo & Macones, 2003). After a woman had one successful VBAC, the risks of neonatal and maternal complications was low in subsequent attempts. An increasing number of VBACs are associated with greater VBAC success (Mercer, Gilbert, Landon et al., 2008).

Research shows a close correlation between maternal weight and success for VBACs (Juhasz, Gyamfi, Gyamfi et al., 2005). Obese women with a body mass index greater than 29 were 50% less likely to have a successful VBAC (Juhasz et al., 2005).

Nursing Care Management

The nursing care of a woman undergoing VBAC varies according to institutional protocols. Generally, a saline lock is inserted for IV access if needed or an intravenous infusion of fluids is started, continuous EFM is used, and clear fluids may be taken. A woman at higher risk may require additional precautionary measures, such as internal monitoring after the membranes have ruptured. Care must be taken to ensure that the woman and her partner feel safe but not unduly restricted by the VBAC status.

Supportive and comfort measures are very important. The woman may be excited about this opportunity to experience labor and vaginal birth, or she may be hesitant and frightened about the possibility of complications. The presence of the nurse is important in providing information and encouragement for the laboring woman and her partner.

CHAPTER HIGHLIGHTS

- An external (or cephalic) version may be done after 36 weeks' gestation to change a breech presentation to a cephalic presentation. Benefits of the version are that a lower risk vaginal birth may be anticipated. The version is accomplished with the use of tocolytics to relax the uterus.
- Amniotomy (AROM) is performed to hasten labor. The risks are prolapse of the umbilical cord and infection.
- Prostaglandin E_2 may be used to soften and efface the cervix (called cervical ripening).
- Labor is induced for many reasons. The medical (allopathic) methods include amniotomy, stripping the membranes, and intravenous Pitocin infusion. Nursing responsibilities are heightened during an induced labor.
- An amnioinfusion is a technique in which warmed solution is introduced into the uterine cavity during the intrapartum period. An amnioinfusion is used in cases of oligohydramnios, nonreassuring fetal heart rate patterns related to cord compression, nonreassuring fetal status, and when the fetus has passed thick meconium in utero.

- An episiotomy is an incision made to enlarge the outlet just before birth of the fetus. Although prevalent in the United States, its routine use is questioned.
- Forceps-assisted birth can be accomplished using outlet, low, or midforceps. Outlet forceps are the most common and are associated with few maternal-fetal complications.
- A vacuum extractor is a soft, pliable cup attached to suction that can be applied to the fetal head and used in much the same way as forceps.
- After declining for several years, the cesarean birth rate reached an all-time high of 26.1% in 2002. The nurse has a vital role in providing information, support, and encouragement to the couple participating in a cesarean birth.
- Preparation for cesarean birth requires establishing an intravenous line, instilling a urinary indwelling catheter, and performing an abdominal/perineal prep as well as providing preoperative client teaching.
- Vaginal birth after cesarean (VBAC) is the subject of more controversy now than in the past.

CHAPTER REFERENCES

American College of Obstetricians and Gynecologists (ACOG). (2003). *New U.S. Food and Drug Administration labeling on Cytotec (misoprostol) use and pregnancy* (ACOG Committee Opinion No. 283). Washington, DC: Author.

American College of Obstetricians and Gynecologists (ACOG). (2004). *Vaginal birth after previous cesarean delivery* (Practice Bulletin No. 54). Washington, DC: Author.

American College of Obstetricians and Gynecologists (ACOG). (2007). *Cesarean delivery upon maternal request* (ACOG Committee Opinion No. 394). Washington, DC: Author.

Battista, L. R., & Wing, D. A. (2007). Abnormal labor and induction of labor. In S. G. Gabbe, J. R. Niebyl, & J. L. Simpson (Eds.), *Obstetrics: Normal and problem pregnancies* (5th ed., pp. 322–343). Philadelphia, PA: Churchill Livingstone/Elsevier.

Bishop, E. H. (1964). Pelvic scoring for elective inductions. *Obstetrics and Gynecology, 24,* 266.

Bjelic-Radisic, V., Pristauz, G., Haas, J., Giuliani, A., Tamussino, K., Bader, A., Lang, U., & Schlembach, D. (2007). Neonatal outcome of second twins depending on presentation and mode of delivery. *Twin Research & Human Genetics, 10*(3), 521–527.

Boulvain, M., Kelly, A., & Irion, O. (2008). Intracervical prostaglandins for induction of labour. *Cochrane Database Systematic Review, 23*(1), CD006971.

Chaillet, N., & Dumont, A. (2007). Evidenced-based strategies for reducing cesarean section rates: A meta-analysis. *Birth, 34*(1), 53–64.

Cheng, S. Y., Ming, H., & Lee, J. C. (2008). Titrated oral compared with vaginal misoprostol for labor induction: A randomized controlled trial. *Obstetrics & Gynecology, 111*(1), 119–125.

Chigbu, C. O., & Iloabachie, G. C. (2007). The burden of caesarean section refusal in a developing country setting. *British Journal Obstetrics and Gynecology, 114*(10), 1261–1265.

Cunningham, F. G., Leveno, K. J., Bloom, S. L., Hauth, J. C., Gilstrap, L. C., & Wenstrom, K. D. (2005). *Williams obstetrics* (22nd ed.). Norwalk, CT: Appleton & Lange.

Deneux-Tharaux, C., Carmona, E., Bouvier-Colle, M. H., & Bréart, G. (2006). Postpartum maternal mortality and cesarean delivery. *Obstetrics & Gynecology, 108*(3), 541–548.

Doumouchtsis, S. K., & Arulkumaran, S. (2008). Head trauma after instrumental births. *Clinics in Perinatology, 35*(1), 69–83.

Dudding, T., Vaizey, C., & Kamm, M. (2008). Obstetrics anal sphincter injury: Incidence, risk factors, and management. *Annuals Surgery, 247*(2), 224–237.

Edwards, H., Grotegut, C., Harmanli, O. H., Rapkin, D., & Dandolu, V. (2006). Is severe perineal damage increased in women with prior anal sphincter injury? *Journal of Maternal Fetal Neonatal Medicine, 19*(11), 723–727.

Ejegård, H., Ryding, E. L., & Sjögren, B. (2008). Sexuality after delievery with episiotomy: A long-term follow-up. *Gynecologic and Obstetric Investigation, 66*(1), 1–7.

Facchinetti, F., Venturini, P., Fazzio, M., & Volpe, A. (2007). Elective cervical ripening in women beyond the 290th day of pregnancy: A randomized trial comparing 2 dinoprostone preparations. *Journal of Reproductive Medicine, 52*(10), 945–949.

Food & Drug Administration (FDA). (2008). Cytotec. Retrieved February 18, 2008, from http://www.fda.gov/cder/foi/label/2002/19268slr037.pdf

Forrest Pharmaceuticals, Inc. (2007). *Cervidil dinoprostone 10 mg vaginal insert.* St. Louis: Forrest Pharmaceutical Laboratories.

Grossetti, E., Vardon, D., Creveuil, C., Herlicoviez, M., & Dreyfus, M. (2007). Rupture of the scarred uterus. *Acta Obstet Gynecol Scand, 86*(5), 572–578.

Gray, R., Quigley, M. A., Hockley, C., Kurinczuk, J. J., Goldacre, M., & Brocklehurst, P. (2007). Caesarean delivery and risk of stillbirth in subsequent pregnancy: A retrospective cohort study in an English population. *British Journal of Obstetrics & Gynecology, 114*(3), 264–270.

Häger, R., Øian, P., Nilsen, S. T., Holm, H. A., & Berg, A. B. (2006). The breakthrough series on Cesarean section. *Tidsskr Nor Laegeforen, 126*(2), 173–175.

Hamilton, B. E., Martin, J. A., & Ventura, S. J. (2007). Births: Preliminary data for 2006. *National Vital Statistics Reports, 56*(7), 1–50.

Hannah, M. E. (2004). Planned elective cesarean: A reasonable choice for some women. *Canadian Medical Association Journal, 170*(5), 813–814.

Hill, K., Thomas, K., AbouZahr, C., Walker, N., Say, L., Inoue, M., & Suzuki, E. (2007). Estimates of maternal mortality worldwide between 1990 and 2005: An assessment of available data. *Lancet, 13;370*(9595), 1311–1319.

Hoyert, D. L. (2007). Maternal mortality and related concepts. National Center for Health Statistics. *Vital Health Statistics, 3*(33), 1–15.

Juhasz, G., Gyamfi, C., Gyamfi, P., & Stone, C. L. (2005). Effect of body mass index and excessive weight gain on success of vaginal birth after cesarean. *Obstetrics & Gynceology, 106*(4), 741–746.

Kilpatrick, S., & Garrison, E. (2007). Normal labor and delivery. In S. G. Gabbe, J. R. Niebyl, & J. L. Simpson (Eds.), *Obstetrics: Normal and problem pregnancies* (5th ed., pp. 303–321). Philadelphia, PA: Churchill Livingstone/Elsevier.

Kwee, A., Elferink-Stinkens, P. M., Reuwer, P. J., & Bruinse, H. W. (2007). Trends in obstetric interventions in the Dutch obstetrical care system in the period 1993–2002. *European Journal of Obstetrics, Gynecology & Reproductive Biology, 132*(1), 70–75.

Landon, M. B. (2007). Cesarean delivery. In S. G. Gabbe, J. R. Niebyl, & J. L. Simpson (Eds.), *Obstetrics: Normal and problem pregnancies* (5th ed., pp. 486–520). Philadelphia, PA: Churchill Livingstone/Elsevier.

Lanni, S. M., & Seeds, J. W. (2007). Malpresentations. In S. G. Gabbe, J. R. Niebyl, & J. L. Simpson (Eds.), *Obstetrics: Normal and problem pregnancies* (5th ed., pp. 428–455). Philadelphia, PA: Churchill Livingstone/Elsevier.

Marconi, A. M., Bozzetti, P., Morabito, A., & Pardi, G. (2008). Comparing two dinoprostone agents for cervical ripening and induction of labor: A randomized trial. *European Journal Obstetric Gynecology Reproductive Biology, 138*(20): 135–140.

Matsuo, K., Scanlon, J. T., Atlas, R. O., & Kopelman, J. N. (2008). Staircase sign: A newly described uterine contraction pattern seen in rupture of unscarred gravid uterus. *Journal of Obstetrics & Gynaecology, 34*(1), 100–104.

Mbele, A. M., Makin, J. D., & Pattinson, R. C. (2007). Can the outcome of induction of labour with oral misoprostol be predicted? *South Africa Medical Journal, 97*(4), 289–292.

Mercer, B. M., Gilbert, S., Landon, M. B., Spong, C. Y., Leveno, K. J., Rouse, D. J., et al. (2008). Labor outcomes with increasing number of prior vaginal births after cesarean delivery. *Obstetrics & Gynecology, 111*(2), 285–291.

Midwifery Today E_News. (2002). *Herbs. Midwifery Today Forums, 1,* 44. Retrieved July 20, 2004 from http://www.midwiferytoday.com/enews

Moodley, J. (2008). Maternal deaths due to hypertensive disorders in pregnancy. *Best Practices in Research & Clinical Obstetrics & Gynaecology* (2008 Feb 15); E-pub ahead of print.

National Institute of Health. (2006). NIH State-of-the-Science Conference Statement on cesarean delivery on maternal request. *NIH Consensus State Science Statements. 23*(1), 1–29.

Nielson, P. E., Galan, H. L., Kilpatrick, S., & Garrison, E. (2007). Operative vaginal delivery.

In S. G. Gabbe, J. R. Niebyl, & J. L. Simpson (Eds.), *Obstetrics: Normal and problem pregnancies* (5th ed., pp. 344–363). Philadelphia, PA: Churchill Livingstone/Elsevier.

Odibo, A. O., Cahill, A. G., Stamilio, D. M., Stevens, E. J., Peipert, J. F., & Macones, G. A. (2007). Predicting placental abruption and previa in women with a previous cesarean delivery. *American Journal of Perinatology, 24*(5), 299–305.

Odibo, A. O., & Macones, G. A. (2003). Current concepts regarding vaginal birth after cesarean delivery. *Current Opinion in Obstetrics and Gynecology, 15*(6), 479–482.

Pfizer Pharmaceuticals, Inc. (2008). Dinoprostone (Prepidil) Vaginal Gel insert. New York, NY: Pfizer Pharmaceutical Laboratories.

Pretlove, S. J., Thompson, P. J., Toozs-Hobson, P. M., Radley, S., & Khan, K. S. (2008). Does the mode of delivery predispose women to anal incontinence in the first year postpartum? A comparative systematic review. *British Journal of Obstetrics & Gynecology, 115*(4), 421–434.

Roberts, L. L., Ely, J. W., & Ward, M. M. (2007). Factors contributing to maternal birth-related trauma. *American Journal of Medical Quality, 22*(5), 334–343.

Ronsmans, C., Holtz, S., & Stanton, C. (2006). Socioeconomic differentials in caesarean rates in developing countries: A retrospective analysis. *The Lancet, 368*(9546), 1472–1473.

Samarasekera, D. N., Bekhit, M. T., Wright, Y., Lowndes, R. H., Stanley, K. P., Preston, J. P., Preston, P., & Speakman, C. T. (2008, February 29). Long-term anal continence and quality of life following postpartum anal sphincter injury. *Colorectal Disease.* Retrieved

July 16, 2008 from http://www.ncbi.nlm.nih.gov/pubmed/8266886. epub ahead of print.

Shiraishi, Y., Asano, K., Niimi, K., Fukunaga, K., Wakaki, M., Kagyo, J., et al. (2008). Cyclooxygenase-2/prostaglandin D2/CRTH2 pathway mediates double-stranded RNA-induced enhancement of allergic airway inflammation. *Journal of Immunology, 180*(1), 541–549.

Shipp, T. D., Zelop, C., & Lieberman, E. (2008). Assessment of the rate of uterine rupture at the first prenatal visit: A preliminary evaluation. *Journal of Maternal Fetal & Neonatal Medicine, 21*(2), 129–133.

Smyth, R. M. D., Alldred, S. K., & Markham, C. (2007). Amniotomy for shortening spontaneous labor. *Cochrane Database of Systematic Reviews 2007*, Issue 4., Art. No.: CD006167. DOI: 10.1002/14651858.CD006167.pub2

Stanton, C. K., Dubourg, D., De Brouwere, D., Pujades, M., & Ronsmans, C. (2005). Reliability of data on caesarean sections in developing countries. *Bulletin of the World Health Organization, 83*, 449–459.

Tang, C. H., Wang, H. I., Hsu, C. S., Su, H. W., Chen, M. J., & Lin, H. C. (2006). Risk-adjusted cesarean section rates for the assessment of physician performance in Taiwan: A population-based study. *Bio-Medical Central Public Health, 6*, 246.

Tang, O. S., Gemzell-Danielsson, K., & Ho, P. C. (2007). Misoprostol: Pharmacokinetic profiles, effects on the uterus and side-effects. *International Journal of Gynaecology & Obstetrics, 99*, Suppl 2:S160-7. Epub 2007 Oct 26.

Tenore, J. L. (2003). Methods for cervical ripening and induction of labor. *American Family Physician, 67*, 2123–2128.

Thomas, J. (2006). Rates of cesarean delivery in developing countries suggest unequal access. *International Family Planning Perspectives, 32*(2). Retrieved February 26, 2008, from http://www.guttmacher.org/pubs/journals/3210506.html

Weeks, A., Alfirevic, Z., Faúndes, A., Hofmeyr, G. J., Safar, P., & Wing, D. (2007). Misoprostol for induction of labor with a live fetus. *International Journal of Gynaecology & Obstetrics, 99* Suppl 2: S194-7. Epub 2007 Oct 25.

Wheeler, T. L., & Richter, H. E. (2007). Delivery method, anal sphincter tears and fecal incontinence: New information on a persistent problem. *Current Opinions in Obstetrics & Gynecology, 19*(5), 474–479.

Wilkund, I., Ryding, E. G., & Andolf, E. (2008). Expectation and experience of childbirth in primiparae with caesarean section. *British Journal of Obstetrics and Gynaecology, 115*(3), 324–331.

Wilson, B. A., Shannon, M. T., & Shields, K. M. (Eds.). (2009). *Nursing drug guide: 2009.* Upper Saddle River, NJ: Prentice Hall.

World Health Organization [WHO]. (2007). *Making pregnancy safer towards the European strategy for making pregnancy safer: Improving maternal and perinatal health.* Country profile: Albania. Copenhagen, Denmark: WHO.

Zeck W., Walcher, W., & Lang, U. (2008). External cephalic version in singleton pregnancies at term: A retrospective analysis. *Gynecology & Obstetric Investigation, 66*(1), 18–21.

PART FIVE

The Newborn

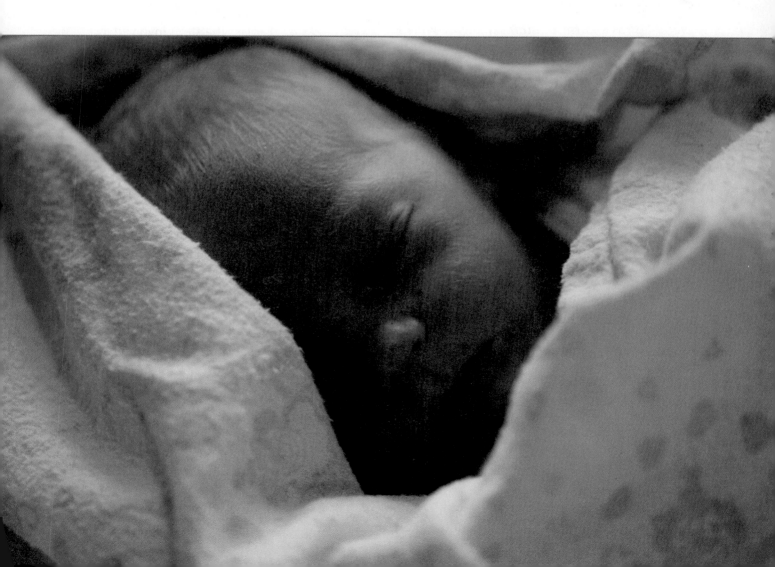

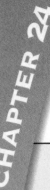

CHAPTER 24

The Physiologic Responses of the Newborn to Birth

I had been a nurse for nine years when my youngest sister asked me to be her labor coach. I thought I remembered my maternity nursing rotation, but it is so different when it is family. My sister was great, however, and my niece was active and beautiful. I was struck by the reality that the transition babies must make to the world is simply staggering. You know, I love the work I do as a nurse, but this experience vividly reminded me that nursing is about life and death, joy and suffering, and everything in between.

—Hospice Nurse

LEARNING OUTCOMES

24-1. Explain the respiratory and cardiovascular changes that occur during the newborn's transition to extrauterine life and during stabilization in determining the nursing care of the newborn.

24-2. Compare the factors that modify the newborn's blood values to the corresponding results.

24-3. Relate the process of thermogenesis in the newborn and the major mechanisms of heat loss to the challenge of maintaining newborn thermal stability.

24-4. Explain the steps involved in conjugation and excretion of bilirubin in the newborn.

24-5. Identify the reasons a newborn may develop jaundice and nursing interventions to decrease the probability of jaundice.

24-6. Delineate the functional abilities of the newborn's gastrointestinal tract and liver.

24-7. Relate the development of the newborn's kidneys to the newborn's ability to maintain fluid and electrolyte balance.

24-8. Describe the characteristics of newborn urinary function.

24-9. Describe the immunologic response available to the newborn.

24-10. Explain the physiologic and behavioral characteristics of newborn neurologic function, patterns of behavior during the periods of reactivity, and possible nursing interventions.

24-11. Describe the normal sensory-perceptual abilities and behavioral states seen in the newborn period and the associated nursing care.

The newborn period is the time from birth through the 28th day of life. During this period, the newborn adjusts from intrauterine to extrauterine life. The nurse needs to be knowledgeable about a newborn's normal physiologic and behavioral adaptations and to be able to recognize alterations from normal.

The first few hours of life, in which the newborn stabilizes respiratory and circulatory functions, are called **neonatal transition**. All other newborn body systems change their level of functioning and become established over a longer period of time during the neonatal period.

Respiratory Adaptations

To begin life as a separate being, the baby must immediately establish respiratory gas exchange in conjunction with marked circulatory changes. These radical and rapid changes are crucial to the maintenance of extrauterine life.

Intrauterine Factors Supporting Respiratory Function

Even before the significant respiratory events occur at birth, certain intrauterine factors also enhance the newborn's ability to breathe. Adequate fetal lung development allows the newborn to expand his or her lungs and exchange oxygen and carbon dioxide gases. Even before birth the fetus practices breathing movements, which allow him or her to breathe immediately after birth.

Fetal Lung Development

The respiratory system is in an ongoing state of development during fetal life, and lung development continues into early childhood. During the first 20 weeks' gestation, development is limited to the differentiation of pulmonary, vascular, and lymphatic structures. At 20 to 24 weeks, alveolar ducts begin to appear, followed by primitive alveoli at 24 to 28 weeks. During this time, the alveolar epithelial cells begin to differentiate into type I cells (structures necessary for gas exchange) and type II cells (structures that provide for the synthesis and storage of surfactant). **Surfactant** is composed of surface-active phospholipids (lecithin and sphingomyelin), which are critical for alveolar stability.

At 28 to 32 weeks' gestation, the number of type II cells increases further, and surfactant is produced by a choline pathway within them. Surfactant production by this pathway peaks at about 35 weeks' gestation and remains high until term, paralleling late fetal lung development. At this time, the lungs are structurally developed enough to permit maintenance of lung expansion and adequate exchange of gases.

Clinically, the peak production of lecithin—one component of surfactant—corresponds closely to the marked decrease in the incidence of respiratory distress syndrome for babies born after 35 weeks' gestation. Production of sphingomyelin (the other component of surfactant) remains constant during gestation. The newborn born before the lecithin/sphingomyelin (L/S) ratio is 2:1 will have varying degrees of respiratory distress. (See discussion of L/S ratio in Chapter 29 ∞.)

Fetal Breathing Movements

The newborn's ability to breathe air immediately after his or her birth appears to result from weeks of intrauterine practice. In this respect, breathing can be seen as a continuation of an intrauterine process; the lungs convert from a fluid-filled organ to a gas-filled organ capable of gas exchange.

Fetal breathing movements (FBMs) occur as early as 11 weeks' gestation (see Biophysical Profile in Chapter 14 ∞ for discussion). These breathing movements are essential for developing the chest wall muscles and the diaphragm and, to a lesser extent, for regulating lung fluid volume and resultant lung growth.

Initiation of Breathing

To maintain life, the lungs must function immediately after birth. Two radical changes must take place for the lungs to function:

1. Pulmonary ventilation must be established through lung expansion following birth.
2. A marked increase in the pulmonary circulation must occur.

The first breath of life—the gasp in response to mechanical and reabsorptive, chemical, thermal, and sensory changes associated with birth—initiates the serial opening of the alveoli. So begins the transition from a fluid-filled environment to an air-breathing, independent, extrauterine life. Figure 24–1 ■ summarizes the initiation of respiration.

Mechanical and Reabsorptive Processes

During the latter half of gestation, the fetal lungs continuously produce fluid. This fluid expands the lungs almost completely, filling the air spaces. Some of the lung fluid moves up into the trachea and into the amniotic fluid and is then swallowed by the fetus.

In preparation for birth, lung fluid production normally decreases and fetal breathing movement decreases 24 to 36 hours before the onset of true labor (Knuppel, 2007). However, approximately 80 to 100 mL of lung fluid remains in the respiratory passages of a normal full-term fetus at the time of birth. This lung fluid must be removed from the lungs to permit adequate movement of air (Polin, Fox, & Abman, 2004).

As the fetus experiences labor there is a fetal gasp and active exhalation that initiates the removal of fluid from the lungs (Rosenberg, 2007). During birth the fetal chest is compressed, increasing intrathoracic pressure, and squeezing a small amount of the fluid out of the lungs. After the birth of the newborn's trunk, the chest wall recoils. This chest recoil creates a negative intrathoracic pressure, which is thought to produce a small, passive inspiration of air that replaces the fluid in the large airways that is squeezed out. The significance of the "thoracic squeeze" is controversial and it is now thought that the process of labor is primarily responsible for the initial movement of lung fluid out of the lungs (Rosenberg, 2007).

After this first inspiration, the newborn exhales, with crying, against a partially closed glottis, creating positive intrathoracic pressure. The high positive intrathoracic pressure distributes the inspired air throughout the alveoli and begins to establish *functional residual capacity* (FRC), the air left in the lungs at the end of a normal expiration. The higher intrathoracic pressure also increases absorption of fluid via the capillaries and lymphatic system. The negative intrathoracic pressure created when the diaphragm moves down with inspiration causes lung fluid to flow from the alveoli across the alveolar membranes into the pulmonary interstitial tissue.

At birth the alveolar epithelium is temporarily more permeable. This, combined with decreased cellular resistance at the onset of breathing, may facilitate passive liquid absorption. With each succeeding breath, the lungs con-

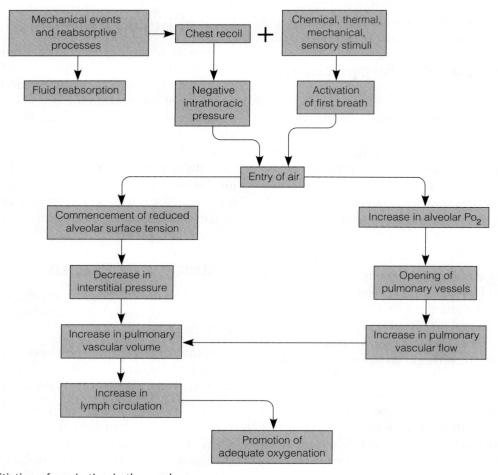

FIGURE 24–1 Initiation of respiration in the newborn.

tinue to expand, stretching the alveolar walls and increasing the alveolar volume. Protein molecules are too large to pass through capillary walls. The presence of more protein molecules in the pulmonary capillaries than in the interstitial tissue creates oncotic pressure. This pressure draws the interstitial fluid into the capillaries and lymphatic tissue to balance the concentration of protein. Lung expansion helps the remaining lung fluid move into the interstitial tissue. As pulmonary vascular resistance decreases, pulmonary blood flow increases, and more interstitial fluid is absorbed into the bloodstream. In the healthy term newborn, lung fluid moves rapidly into the interstitial tissue but may take several hours to move into the lymph and blood vessels. Most of the lung fluid is reabsorbed within 2 hours after birth, and it is completely absorbed within 12 to 24 hours after birth (Rosenberg, 2007).

Although the initial chest recoil assists in clearing the airways of accumulated fluid and permits further inspiration, most clinicians believe mucus and fluid should be suctioned from the newborn's mouth, nose, and throat. They use a bulb or mucous trap attached to suction as soon as the newborn's head and shoulders are born and again as the newborn adapts to extrauterine life and stabilizes (see Clinical Skill: Performing Nasal Pharyngeal Suctioning on page 456).

Newborns may have problems clearing the fluid in the lungs and beginning respiration for a variety of reasons:

- The lymphatic system may be underdeveloped, thus decreasing the rate at which the fluid is absorbed from the lungs.
- Complications that occur before or during labor and birth can interfere with adequate lung expansion and cause failure to decrease pulmonary vascular resistance, resulting in decreased pulmonary blood flow. These complications include inadequate compression of the chest wall in very small newborns (small for gestational age [SGA] or very low birth weight [VLBW]) because of immature muscular development; the absence of chest wall compression in a newborn born by cesarean birth, although this compression can be externally applied by skilled physicians as they deliver the newborn from the uterus; respiratory depression because of maternal analgesia or anesthesia agents; or aspiration of amniotic fluid, meconium, or blood.

Chemical Stimuli

An important chemical stimulator that contributes to the onset of breathing is transitory asphyxia of the fetus and newborn. The first breath is an inspiratory gasp, the result of central nervous system reaction to sudden pressure, temperature change, and other external stimuli (Knuppel, 2007). This first breath is triggered by the slight elevation in PCO_2 and decrease in pH and PO_2, which are the natural result of a normal vaginal labor and birth. These changes, which are present in all newborns to some degree, stimulate the aortic and carotid chemoreceptors, initiating impulses that trigger the medulla's respiratory center. Although this brief period of asphyxia is a significant stimulator, prolonged asphyxia is abnormal and depresses respiration. Another chemical factor may result from clamping the umbilical cord that may cause a drop in levels of a prostaglandin that inhibits respirations (Bloom, 2006). As a result newborns can vigorously cry and be active before the cord is clamped or the placenta separates.

Thermal Stimuli

A significant decrease in environmental temperature after birth, 37°C to 21°C–23.9°C (98.6°F to 70°F–75°F), results in sudden chilling of the moist newborn (Cheffer, 2004). The cold stimulates skin nerve endings, and the newborn responds with rhythmic respirations. Normal temperature changes that occur at birth are apparently within acceptable physiologic limits. Excessive cooling may result in profound depression and evidence of cold stress (see Chapter 29 ∞ for discussion of cold stress).

Sensory Stimuli

During intrauterine life, the fetus is in a dark, sound-dampened, fluid-filled environment and is nearly weightless. After birth the newborn experiences light, sounds, and the effects of gravity for the first time. As the fetus moves from a familiar, comfortable, quiet environment to one of sensory abundance, a number of physical and sensory influences help respiration begin. They include the numerous tactile, auditory, and visual stimuli of birth. Joint movement results in enhanced proprioceptor stimulation to the respiratory center to sustain respirations. Thoroughly drying the newborn and placing the baby in skin-to-skin contact with the mother's chest and abdomen provide ample stimulation in a far more comforting way and also decrease heat loss.

HINTS FOR PRACTICE

Gentle physical contact by thoroughly drying the newborn and placing the baby in skin-to-skin contact with the mother's chest and abdomen is emphasized when using external stimulation means for the first breaths. These methods provide ample stimulation in a comforting way and also decrease heat loss.

Factors Opposing the First Breath

Three major factors may oppose the initiation of respiratory activity: (1) the contracting force between alveoli—called *alveolar surface tension*; (2) viscosity of lung fluid within the respiratory tract, which is influenced by surfactant levels; and (3) the ease with which the lung is able to fill with air—called *lung compliance*.

Alveolar surface tension is the contracting force between the moist surfaces of the alveoli. This tension, which is necessary for healthy respiratory function, would nevertheless cause the small airways and alveoli to collapse between each inspiration were it not for the presence of surfactant. By reducing the attracting force between alveoli, surfactant prevents the alveoli from completely collapsing with each expiration and thus promotes lung expansion. Similarly, surfactant promotes lung compliance, the ability of the lung to fill with air easily. When surfactant decreases, compliance also decreases, and the pressure needed to expand the alveoli with air increases.

Resistive forces of the fluid-filled lung, combined with the small radii of the airways, necessitate pressures of 30 to 40 cm (11.8 to 15.7 in.) of water to open the lung initially (Thureen, Deacon, Hernandez, & Hall, 2005).

The first breath usually establishes FRC that is 30% to 40% of the fully expanded lung volume. This FRC allows alveolar sacs to remain partially expanded on expiration, decreasing the need for continuous high pressures for each of the following breaths. Subsequent breaths require only 6 to 8 cm H_2O pressure to open alveoli during inspiration. Therefore, the first breath of life is usually the most difficult.

Cardiopulmonary Physiology

The onset of respiration stimulates changes in the cardiovascular system that are necessary for successful transition to extrauterine life, hence the term **cardiopulmonary adaptation**. As air enters the lungs, P_{O_2} rises in the alveoli, which stimulates the relaxation of the pulmonary arteries and triggers a decrease in pulmonary vascular resistance. As pulmonary vascular resistance decreases, the vascular flow in the lung increases rapidly and achieves 100% normal flow at 24 hours of life. This delivery of greater blood volume to the lungs contributes to the conversion from fetal circulation to newborn circulation.

After pulmonary circulation is established, blood is distributed throughout the lungs, although the alveoli may or may not be fully open. For adequate oxygenation to occur, the heart must deliver sufficient blood to functional, open alveoli. Shunting of blood is common in the early newborn period. Bidirectional blood flow, or right-to-left shunting through the ductus arteriosus, may divert a significant amount of blood away from the lungs, depending on the pressure changes of respiration, crying, and the cardiac cycle. This shunting in the newborn period is also responsible for the unstable transitional period in cardiopulmonary function.

Oxygen Transport

The transportation of oxygen to the peripheral tissues depends on the type of hemoglobin in the red blood cells. In the fetus and newborn, a variety of hemoglobins exist, the most significant being fetal hemoglobin (HbF) and adult hemoglobin (HbA). Approximately 70% to 90% of the hemoglobin in the fetus and newborn is of the fetal variety. The greatest difference between HbF and HbA relates to the transport of oxygen.

Because HbF has a greater affinity for oxygen than does HbA, the oxygen saturation in the newborn's blood is greater than in the adult's, but the amount of oxygen available to the tissues is less. This situation is beneficial prenatally, because the fetus must maintain adequate oxygen uptake in the presence of very low oxygen tension (umbilical venous P_{O_2} cannot exceed the uterine venous P_{O_2}). Because of this high concentration of oxygen in the blood, hypoxia in the newborn is particularly difficult to recognize. Clinical manifestations of cyanosis do not appear until low blood levels of oxygen are present. In addition, alkalosis (increased pH) and hypothermia can result in less oxygen being available to the body tissues, whereas acidosis, hypercarbia, and hyperthermia can result in less oxygen being bound to hemoglobin and more oxygen being released to the body tissues.

Maintaining Respiratory Function

The lung's ability to maintain oxygenation and ventilation (the exchange of oxygen and carbon dioxide) is influenced by such factors as lung compliance and airway resistance. Lung compliance is influenced by the elastic recoil of the lung tissue and anatomic differences in the newborn. The newborn has a relatively large heart and mediastinal structures that reduce available lung space. Also, the newborn chest is equipped with weak intercostal muscles and a rigid rib cage with horizontal ribs and a high diaphragm, which restricts the space available for lung expansion. The large abdomen further encroaches on the high diaphragm to decrease lung space. Another factor that limits ventilation is airway resistance, which depends on the radii, length, and number of airways. Airway resistance is increased in the newborn when compared with adults.

Characteristics of Newborn Respiration

The normal newborn respiratory rate is 30 to 60 breaths per minute. Initial respirations may be largely diaphragmatic, shallow, and irregular in depth and rhythm. The abdomen's movements are synchronous with the chest movements. When the breathing pattern is characterized by pauses lasting 5 to 15 seconds, **periodic breathing** is occurring. Periodic breathing is rarely associated with differences in skin color or heart rate changes, and it has no prognostic significance. Tactile or other sensory stimulation increases the inspired oxygen and converts periodic breathing patterns to normal breathing patterns during neonatal transition. With deep sleep, the pattern is reasonably regular. Periodic breathing occurs with rapid-eye-movement (REM) sleep, and grossly irregular breathing is evident with motor activity, sucking, and crying. Cessation of breathing lasting more than 20 seconds is defined as *apnea* and is abnormal in term newborns. Apnea may or may not be associated with changes in skin color or heart rate (drop below 100 beats per minute). Apnea always needs to be further evaluated.

Newborns tend to be obligatory nose breathers because the nasal route is the primary route of air entry. This is because of the high position of the epiglottis and the position of the soft palate (Blackburn, 2007). Although many term newborns can breathe orally, with nasal occlusion, nasal obstructions can cause respiratory distress. Therefore, it is important to keep the nose and throat clear. Immediately after birth, and for about the next 2 hours, respiratory rates of 60 to 70 breaths per minute are normal. Some cyanosis and acrocyanosis are normal for several hours; thereafter the infant's color improves steadily. If respirations drop below 30 or exceed 60 per minute when the infant is at rest, or if retractions, cyanosis, or nasal flaring and expiratory grunting occur, the clinician should be notified. Any increased use of the intercostal muscles (retractions) may indicate respiratory distress. (See Chapter 29 and Table 29–1 ∞ for signs of respiratory distress.)

Cardiovascular Adaptations

As described earlier, the onset of respiration triggers increased blood flow to the lungs after birth. This greater blood volume contributes to the conversion from fetal circulation to neonatal circulation.

Fetal-Newborn Transitional Physiology

During fetal life, blood with the higher oxygen content is diverted to the heart and brain. Blood in the descending aorta is less oxygenated and supplies the kidney and intestinal tract before it is returned to the placenta. Limited amounts of blood, pumped from the right ventricle toward the lungs, enter the pulmonary vessels. In the fetus, increased pulmonary resistance forces most of this blood through the ductus arteriosus into the descending aorta (Table 24–1).

Marked changes occur in the cardiovascular system at birth. Expansion of the lungs with the first breath decreases pulmonary vascular resistance and increases pulmonary blood flow. Pressure in the left atrium increases as blood returns from the pulmonary veins. Pressure in the right atrium drops, and systematic vascular resistance increases as umbil-

TABLE 24–1	Fetal and Neonatal Circulation	
System	Fetal	Neonatal
Pulmonary blood vessels	Constricted, with very little blood flow; lungs not expanded	Vasodilation and increased blood flow; lungs expanded; increased oxygen stimulates vasodilation.
Systemic blood vessels	Dilated, with low resistance; blood mostly in placenta	Arterial pressure rises because of loss of placenta; increased systemic blood volume and resistance.
Ductus arteriosus	Large, with no tone; blood flow from pulmonary artery to aorta	Reversal of blood flow; now from aorta to pulmonary artery because of increased left atrial pressure. Ductus is sensitive to increased oxygen and body chemicals and begins to constrict.
Foramen ovale	Patent, with increased blood flow from right atrium to left atrium	Increased pressure in left atrium attempts to reverse blood flow and shuts one-way valve.

ical venous blood flow is halted when the cord is clamped. These physiologic mechanisms mark the transition from fetal to neonatal circulation and show the interplay of cardiovascular and respiratory systems (Figure 24–2 ■).

Five major areas of change occur in cardiopulmonary adaptation (Figure 24–3 ■):

1. *Increased aortic pressure and decreased venous pressure.* Clamping of the umbilical cord eliminates the placental vascular bed and reduces the intravascular space. Consequently, aortic (systemic) blood pressure increases. At the same time, blood return via the inferior vena cava decreases, resulting in a decreased right atrial pressure and a small decrease in pressure within the venous circulation.

2. *Increased systemic pressure and decreased pulmonary artery pressure.* With the loss of the low-resistance placenta, systemic resistance pressure increases, resulting in greater systemic pressure. At the same time, lung expansion increases pulmonary blood flow, and the increased blood PO_2 associated with initiation of respirations dilates pulmonary blood vessels. The combination of vasodilation and increased pulmonary blood flow decreases pulmonary artery resistance. As the pulmonary vascular beds open, the systemic vascular pressure increases, enhancing perfusion of the other body systems.

3. *Closure of the foramen ovale.* Closure of the foramen ovale is a function of changing atrial pressures. In utero, pressure is greater in the right atrium, and the foramen ovale is open after birth. Decreased pulmonary resistance and increased pulmonary blood flow increase the pulmonary venous return into the left

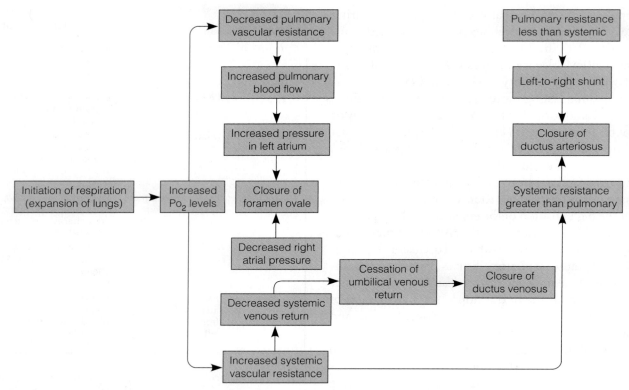

Figure 24–2 Transitional circulation: conversion from fetal to neonatal circulation.

atrium, thereby increasing left atrial pressure slightly. The decreased pulmonary vascular resistance and the decreased umbilical venous return to the right atrium also decrease right atrial pressure. The pressure gradients across the atria are now reversed, with the left atrial pressure now greater, and the foramen ovale is functionally closed 1 to 2 hours after birth. However, a slight right-to-left shunting may occur in the early newborn period. Any increase in pulmonary resistance or right atrial pressure, such as occurs with crying, acidosis, or cold stress, may cause the foramen ovale to reopen, resulting in a temporary right-to-left shunt. Anatomical closure occurs within 30 months (Blackburn, 2007).

4. *Closure of the ductus arteriosus.* Initial elevation of the systemic vascular pressure above the pulmonary vascular pressure increases pulmonary blood flow by reversing the flow through the ductus arteriosus. Blood now flows from the aorta into the pulmonary artery. Furthermore, although the presence of oxygen causes the pulmonary arterioles to dilate, an increase in blood PO_2 triggers the opposite response in the ductus arteriosus—it constricts.

In utero, the placenta provides prostaglandin E_2 (PGE_2), which causes ductus vasodilation. With the loss of the placenta and increased pulmonary blood flow, PGE_2 levels drop, leaving the active constriction by PO_2 unopposed. If the lungs fail to expand or if PO_2 levels drop, the ductus remains patent. Functional closure starts by 10 to 15 hours after birth, and fibrosis of

the ductus occurs within 4 weeks after birth (Blackburn, 2007).

5. *Closure of the ductus venosus.* Although the mechanism initiating closure of the ductus venosus is not known, it appears to be related to mechanical pressure changes after severing of the cord, redistribution of blood, and cardiac output. Closure of the bypass forces perfusion of the liver. Fibrosis of the ductus venosus occurs within 2 months. Figure 24–3 depicts the changes in blood flow and oxygenation as the fetal cardiopulmonary circulation adapts to extrauterine life.

Characteristics of Cardiac Function

Evaluation of the newborn's heart rate, blood pressure, heart sounds, and cardiac workload provides data for evaluating cardiac function.

Heart Rate

Shortly after the first cry and the start of changes in cardiopulmonary circulation, the newborn heart rate can accelerate to 180 beats per minute. The average resting heart rate in the first week of life is 120 to 160 beats per minute in a healthy, full-term newborn but may vary significantly during deep sleep or active awake states. In the full-term newborn, the heart rate may drop to 80 to 100 beats per minute during deep sleep (Creehan, 2008).

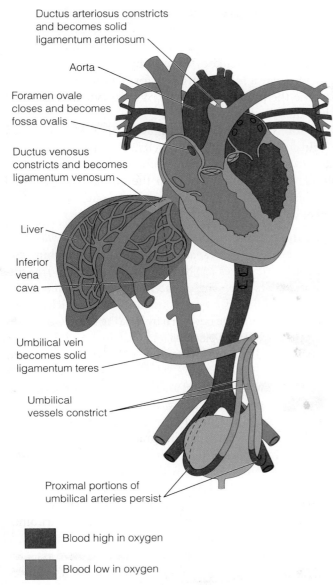

Ductus arteriosus constricts
and becomes solid
ligamentum arteriosum

Aorta

Foramen ovale
closes and becomes
fossa ovalis

Ductus venosus
constricts and becomes
ligamentum venosum

Liver

Inferior
vena
cava

Umbilical vein
becomes solid
ligamentum teres

Umbilical
vessels constrict

Proximal portions of
umbilical arteries persist

Blood high in oxygen

Blood low in oxygen

FIGURE 24–3 Major changes that occur in the newborn's circulatory system.
Source: Hole, J. W. (1993). *Human anatomy and physiology* (6th ed.). Dubuque, IA: W. C. Brown. All rights reserved. Reprinted by permission.

Apical pulse rates should be obtained by auscultation for a full minute, preferably when the newborn is asleep. The heart rate should be evaluated for abnormal rhythms or beats. Peripheral pulses of all extremities should also be evaluated to detect any inequalities or unusual characteristics (Creehan, 2008). Peripheral pedal pulses may be difficult to palpate in the newborn. They can be assessed when blood pressure is measured if blood pressure readings are taken on all four extremities.

Blood Pressure

The blood pressure tends to be highest immediately after birth and then descends to its lowest level at about 3 hours of age. By days 4 to 6, the blood pressure rises and plateaus at a

level approximately the same as the initial level. Blood pressure is sensitive to the changes in blood volume that occur in the transition to newborn circulation (Figure 24–4 ■). Peripheral perfusion pressure is a particularly sensitive indicator of the newborn's ability to compensate for alterations in blood volume before changes in blood pressure. Capillary refill should be less than 2 to 3 seconds when the skin is blanched.

Blood pressure values during the first 12 hours of life vary with the birth weight and gestational age. The average mean blood pressure is 50 to 55 mm Hg in the full-term, resting newborn over 3 kg during the first 12 hours of life (Thureen et al., 2005). In the preterm newborn, the average blood pressure varies according to weight. Crying may cause an elevation of 20 mm Hg in both the systolic and diastolic blood pressure; thus accuracy is more likely in the quiet newborn. The measurement of blood pressure is best accomplished by using the Doppler technique or a 1- to 2-in. cuff and a stethoscope over the brachial artery. The routine assessment of blood pressure in screening of well, term newborns is no longer recommended (American Academy of Pediatrics (AAP) and the American Academy of Obstetricians and Gynecologists (ACOG), 2007. Four point extremity blood pressure assessment is warranted in the presence of any cardiovascular symptoms (tachycardia, persistent murmur, abnormal pulses, poor perfusion, or abnormal precordial activity) (Creehan, 2008). Blood pressure in the lower extremities is usually higher than that in the upper extremities.

Heart Murmurs

Murmurs are produced by turbulent blood flow. Murmurs may be heard when blood flows across an abnormal valve or across a stenosed valve, when there is an atrial or ventricular septal defect, or when there is increased flow across a normal valve.

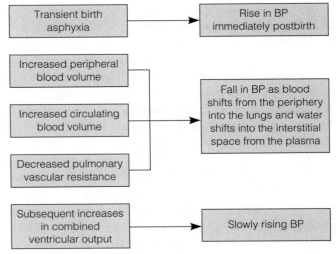

| Transient birth asphyxia | → | Rise in BP immediately postbirth |

| Increased peripheral blood volume |
| Increased circulating blood volume | → | Fall in BP as blood shifts from the periphery into the lungs and water shifts into the interstitial space from the plasma |
| Decreased pulmonary vascular resistance |

| Subsequent increases in combined ventricular output | → | Slowly rising BP |

FIGURE 24–4 Response of blood pressure (BP) to neonatal changes in blood volume.

In newborns, 90% of all murmurs are transient *and not associated with anomalies.* They usually involve incomplete closure of the ductus arteriosus or foramen ovale. Soft murmurs may be heard as the pulmonary branch arteries increase their blood flow from 7% to 50% of the combined ventricular output during transition, causing a physiologic peripheral pulmonary stenosis. Clicks may normally be heard at the lower left sternal border as the great vessels dilate to accommodate systolic blood flow in the first few hours of life. Because of the current practice of early discharge, murmurs associated with ventricular septal defect and patent ductus arteriosus are not often picked up until the first well-baby checkup at 4 to 6 weeks of age. Murmurs are sometimes absent even in seriously malformed hearts.

Cardiac Workload

Before birth the right ventricle does approximately two-thirds of the cardiac work, resulting in increased size and thickness of the right ventricle at birth. In the first 2 hours after birth, when the ductus arteriosus remains mostly patent, about one-third of the left ventricular output is returned to the pulmonary circulation. As a result, the left ventricle has a significantly greater increase in volume load than the right ventricle after birth and it needs to progressively increase in size and thickness. This may explain why right-sided heart defects are better tolerated than left-sided ones and why left-sided heart defects rapidly become symptomatic after birth.

Hematopoietic System

In the first days of life, hematocrit may rise 1 to 2 g/dL above fetal levels as a result of placental transfusion, low oral fluid intake, and diminished extracellular fluid volume. By 1 week postnatally, peripheral hemoglobin is comparable to fetal blood counts. The hemoglobin level declines progressively over the first 2 months of life (Polin, Fox, & Abman, 2004). This initial decline in hemoglobin creates a phenomenon known as **physiologic anemia of infancy**. A factor that influences the degree of physiologic anemia is the nutritional status of the newborn. Supplies of vitamin E, folic acid, and iron may be inadequate given the amount of growth in the later part of the first year of life. Hemoglobin values fall, mainly from a decrease in red cell mass rather than from the dilutional effect of increasing plasma volume. The fact that red cell survival is lower in newborns than in adults, and that red cell production is less, also contributes to this anemia. Neonatal RBCs have a life span of 80 to 100 days, approximately two-thirds the life span of adult RBCs. The normal RBC count in a term newborn is in the range of 5.1 to 5.3 million per milliliter during the first 24 to 48 hours of life (Bagwell, 2007).

Leukocytosis is a normal finding, because the stress of birth stimulates increased production of neutrophils during the first few days of life. Neutrophils then decrease to 35% of the total leukocyte count by 2 weeks of age. Lymphocytes play a role in antibody formation and eventually become the predominant type of leukocyte and the total white blood cell count falls.

Blood volume is approximately 85 mL/kg of body weight for a term infant (Bagwell, 2007). For example, an 3.6 kg (8 lb) newborn has a blood volume of 306 mL. Blood volume varies based on the amount of placental transfusion received during the delivery of the placenta, as well as other factors, including the following:

1. *Delayed cord clamping and the normal shift of plasma to the extravascular spaces.* Newborn hemoglobin and hematocrit values are higher when a placental transfusion occurs after birth. Placental vessels contain about 75 to 125 mL of blood at term, most of which can be transfused into the newborn by holding the newborn below the level of the placenta and delaying clamping of the cord. Blood volume increases by 61% with delayed cord clamping (Bagwell, 2007). The increase is reflected by a rise in hemoglobin level and an increase in the hematocrit. For greatest accuracy, the initial hemoglobin and hematocrit levels should be measured in the cord blood, although this is not a routine practice. In term newborns a delay in clamping the umbilical cord appears to offer protection from anemia without harmful effects (Mercer, Erickson-Owens, Graves, & Haley, 2007). In preterm or SGA newborns delay in cord clamping may have risks. It can speed and worsen symptoms of hyperbilirubinemia and cause hypervolemia.

2. *Gestational age.* There appears to be a positive association between gestational age, RBC numbers, and hemoglobin concentration.

3. *Prenatal and/or perinatal hemorrhage.* Significant prenatal or perinatal bleeding decreases the hematocrit level and causes hypovolemia.

4. *The site of the blood sample.* Hemoglobin and hematocrit levels are significantly higher in capillary blood than in venous blood. Sluggish peripheral blood flow creates RBC stasis, thereby increasing RBC concentration in the capillaries. Consequently, blood samples taken from venous blood sites are more accurate than those from capillary sites.

CULTURAL PERSPECTIVES

In aboriginal cultures cords and placentas were sometimes left to dry attached to the newborn.

TABLE 24–2	Normal Term Newborn Cord Blood Values
Laboratory Data	Normal Range
Hemoglobin	14 to 20 g/dL
Hematocrit	43% to 63%
WBC	10,000 to 30,000/mm³
Neutrophils	40% to 80%
Platelets	150,000 to 350,000/mm³
RBC	5,100,000 to 5,300,000/mL
Reticulocytes	3% to 7%
Blood volume	82.3 mL/kg (third day after early cord clamping)
	92.6 mL/kg (third day after delayed cord clamping)
Sodium	129 to 144 mEq/L
Potassium	3.4 to 9.9 mEq/L
Chloride	103 to 111 mEq/L
Calcium	8.2 to 11.1 mg/dL
Glucose	45 to 96 mg/dL

Source: Fanaroff, A. A., & Martin, R. J. (Eds.). (2006). *Neonatal-perinatal medicine* (7th ed., pp. 1801, 1810). St. Louis: Mosby.

The concentration of serum electrolytes in the blood indicates the fluid and electrolyte status of the newborn. See Table 24–2 for normal term newborn electrolyte and blood values.

Temperature Regulation

Temperature regulation is the maintenance of thermal balance by the loss of heat to the environment at a rate equal to the production of heat. Newborns are *homeothermic;* they attempt to stabilize their internal (core) body temperatures within a narrow range in spite of significant temperature variations in their environment.

Thermoregulation in the newborn is closely related to the rate of metabolism and oxygen consumption. Within a specific environmental temperature range, called the **neutral thermal environment (NTE)** zone, the rates of oxygen consumption and metabolism are minimal, and internal body temperature is maintained because of thermal balance (Thureen et al., 2005) (see Table Neutral Thermal Environmental Temperature on WEB). For an unclothed, full-term newborn, the NTE is an ambient environmental temperature range of 32°C to 34°C (89.6°F to 93.2°F) within 50% relative humidity. The limits for an adult are 26°C to 28°C (78.8°F to 82.4°F) (Polin, Fox, & Abman, 2004). Thus the normal newborn requires higher environmental temperatures to maintain a thermoneutral environment.

Several newborn characteristics affect the establishment of thermal stability:

- The newborn has less subcutaneous fat than an adult and a thin epidermis.

- Blood vessels in the newborn are closer to the skin than those of an adult. Therefore, the circulating blood is influenced by changes in environmental temperature and in turn influences the hypothalamic temperature-regulating center.
- The flexed posture of the term newborn decreases the surface area exposed to the environment, thereby reducing heat loss.

Size and age may also affect the establishment of a NTE. For example, the preterm or small-for-gestational-age (SGA) newborn has less adipose tissue and is hypoflexed, and therefore requires higher environmental temperatures to achieve a neutral thermal environment. Larger, well-insulated newborns may be able to cope with lower environmental temperatures. If the environmental temperature falls below the lower limits of the NTE, the newborn responds with increased oxygen consumption and metabolism, which results in greater heat production. Prolonged exposure to the cold may result in depleted glycogen stores and acidosis. Oxygen consumption also increases if the environmental temperature is above the NTE.

Heat Loss

A newborn is at a distinct disadvantage in maintaining a normal temperature. With a large body surface in relation to mass and a limited amount of insulating subcutaneous fat, the full-term newborn loses about four times the heat of an adult. The newborn's poor thermal stability is primarily because of excessive heat loss rather than impaired heat production. Because of the risk of hypothermia and possible cold stress, minimizing heat loss in the newborn after birth is essential (see Provision of Initial Newborn Care in Chapters 19 and 26 ∞ for nursing measures).

Two major routes of heat loss are from the internal core of the body to the body surface and from the external surface to the environment. Usually the core temperature is higher than the skin temperature, resulting in continuous transfer or conduction of heat to the surface. The greater the difference in temperature between core and skin, the more rapidly heat transfers. The transfer is accomplished through an increase in oxygen consumption, depletion of glycogen stores, and metabolization of brown fat.

Heat loss from the body surface to the environment takes place in four ways—by convection, radiation, evaporation, and conduction (Figure 24–5 ■).

- **Convection** is the loss of heat from the warm body surface to the cooler air currents. Air-conditioned rooms, air currents with a temperature below the infant's skin temperature, oxygen by mask, and removal from an incubator for procedures increase convective heat loss in the newborn.

MyNursingKit | Neonatal Thermoregulation

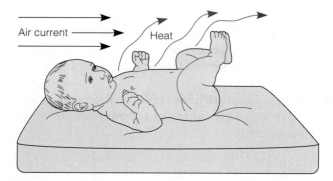

A. Convection

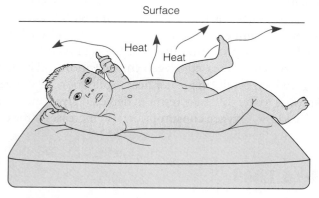

B. Radiation

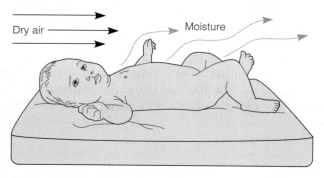

C. Evaporation

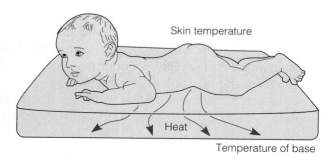

D. Conduction

FIGURE 24–5 Methods of heat loss. *A,* Convection. *B,* Radiation. *C,* Evaporation. *D,* Conduction.

- **Radiation** losses occur when heat transfers from the heated body surface to cooler surfaces and objects not in direct contact with the body. The walls of a room or of an incubator are potential causes of heat loss by radiation, even if the ambient temperature of the incubator is within the thermal neutral range for that infant. Placing cold objects (such as ice for blood gases) onto the incubator or near the infant in the radiant warmer will increase radiant losses.
- **Evaporation** is the loss of heat incurred when water is converted to a vapor. The newborn is particularly prone to lose heat by evaporation immediately after birth (when the baby is wet with amniotic fluid), and during baths; thus drying the newborn is critical.
- **Conduction** is the loss of heat to a cooler surface by direct skin contact. Chilled hands, cool scales, cold examination tables, and cold stethoscopes can cause loss of heat by conduction. Even if objects are warmed to the incubator temperature, the temperature difference between the infant's core temperature and the ambient temperature may be significant. This difference results in heat transfer.

Once the infant has been dried after birth, the highest losses of heat generally result from radiation and convection, because of the newborn's large body surface compared with weight, and from thermal conduction, because of the marked difference between core temperature and skin temperature. The newborn can respond to the cooler environmental temperature with adequate peripheral vasoconstriction, but this mechanism is not entirely effective because of the minimal amount of fat insulation present, the large body surface, and ongoing thermal conduction. Because of these factors, minimizing the baby's heat loss and preventing hypothermia are imperative. (See Chapter 29 ∞ for nursing measures to prevent hypothermia.)

Heat Production (Thermogenesis)

When exposed to a cool environment, the newborn requires additional heat. The newborn has several physiologic mechanisms that increase heat production, or *thermogenesis.* These mechanisms include increased basal metabolic rate, muscular activity, and chemical thermogenesis (also called *nonshivering thermogenesis [NST]*) (Rosenberg, 2007).

Nonshivering thermogenesis is an important mechanism of heat production unique to the newborn. It occurs when skin receptors perceive a drop in the environmental temperature and, in response, transmit sensations to stimulate the sympathetic nervous system. NST uses the newborn's stores of **brown adipose tissue (BAT)** (also called brown fat) to provide heat. Brown fat receives its name from the dark color caused by its enriched blood supply, dense cellular content, and abundant nerve endings. These

EVIDENCE-BASED PRACTICE

Thermoregulation and Heat Loss Prevention in Neonates

Clinical Question

What is the best way to support thermoregulation in the newborn immediately after birth?

The Evidence

Neonates have several risk factors for hypothermia after birth—a large surface-to-mass ratio, minimal subcutaneous tissue, and wet skin. The challenge of thermoregulation is increased if the infant is low birth weight, preterm, or sick. Cold stress can lead to harmful side effects or even death. Several systematic reviews of research on newborn thermoregulation have been published by professional groups interested in neonatal health—the Association of Women's Health, Obstetric and Neonatal Nurses, the American College of Nurse Midwives, and the American College of Pediatricians. These reviews have focused on healthy newborns as well as neonates at risk. Multiple systematic reviews of multi-site randomized trials provide the strongest level of evidence for nursing practice.

What Is Effective?

Skin-to-skin contact of the newborn with its mother after birth is recommended as the mainstay of thermoregulation for most healthy newborns. When placed skin-to-skin, the baby gets heat directly from its mother via conduction. Skin-to-skin care is associated with both short- and long-term benefits, and has been shown to be an effective method of thermoregulation for babies as small as 1200 grams. For smaller babies, or babies who are too ill to be placed on their mother's skin, resuscitation and other treatments may allow evaporative heat loss. Prewarming the delivery suite to 80 degrees Fahrenheit and placing the infant in a plastic bag up to the neck during physiological stabilization prevents heat loss in high-risk babies. Other barrier methods, such as stockinet caps, were not shown to be effective in reducing heat loss. Heated mattresses have also been shown to be effective in preventing hypothermia.

What Is Inconclusive?

While plastic barriers have been shown to avoid hypothermia in high-risk neonates, no studies have demonstrated that these interventions reduce the long-term risk of death, brain injury, mean duration of oxygen therapy, or hospitalization. Some barrier methods (such as occlusive dressings) resulted in hyperthermia. Continuous monitoring of the neonate's body temperature should accompany any of the heat loss barrier methods.

Best Practice

Family-centered birth care provides the best environment for the neonate, including support of thermoregulation. You can avoid hypothermia in healthy newborns by drying the baby with a towel, placing the bare newborn in direct contact with the mother's bare skin, and placing a blanket over them both. Babies that are too small or too sick for skin-to-skin contact should be dried, placed on a heated mattress, and wrapped in plastic wrap up to the neck. A small cut can be made in the plastic for access to the umbilicus. In the case of plastic barriers, continuous monitoring of the baby's temperature is necessary to avoid over-heating.

References

Knobel, R., & Holditch-Davis, D. 2007. Thermoregulation and heat loss prevention after birth and during neonatal intensive-care unit stabilization of extremely low-birthweight infants. *JOGNN: The Journal of Gynecological, Obstetric, and Neonatal Nursing.* 36(3):280–287.

Lyon, A. 2007. Temperature control in the neonate. *Paediatrics and Child Health.* 18(4):155–160.

McCall, E., Alderdice, F., Halliday, H., Jenkins, J., & Vohra, S. 2008. Interventions to prevent hypothermia at birth in preterm and/or low birthweight infants. *Cochrane Database of Systematic Reviews.* Issue 1.

Mercer, J., Erickson-Owens, D., Graves, B., & Haley, M. 2007. Evidence-based practices for the fetal to newborn transition. *Journal of Midwifery and Womens Health.* 52(3):262–272.

characteristics of brown fat cells promote rapid metabolism, heat generation, and heat transfer to the peripheral circulation. The large numbers of brown fat cells increase the speed with which triglycerides are metabolized to produce heat.

Thus, NST from BAT is the primary source of heat in the hypothermic newborn. It first appears in the fetus at about 26 to 30 weeks' gestation and continues to increase until 2 to 5 weeks after the birth of a term infant, unless the fat is depleted by cold stress. Brown fat is deposited in the midscapular area, around the neck, and in the axillas, with deeper placement around the trachea, esophagus, abdominal aorta, kidneys, and adrenal glands (Figure 24–6 ■). BAT constitutes 2% to 6% of the newborn's total body weight.

Shivering, a form of muscular activity common in the cold adult, is rarely seen in the newborn, although it has been observed at ambient temperatures of 15°C (59°F) or less (Polin et al., 2004). If the newborn shivers, it means the newborn's metabolic rate has already doubled. The extra muscular activity does little to produce needed heat.

Thermographic studies of newborns exposed to cold show an increase in the skin heat produced over the newborn's brown fat deposits between 1 and 14 days of age (Polin et al., 2004). However, if the brown fat supply has been depleted, the metabolic response to cold is limited or lacking. An increase in basal metabolism as a result of hypothermia results in an increase in oxygen consumption. A decrease in the environmental temperature of 2°C, from 33°C to 31°C, is a drop sufficient to double the oxygen consumption of a term newborn. Keeping the normal newborn warm promotes normal oxygen requirements, whereas chilling can cause the newborn to show signs of respiratory distress.

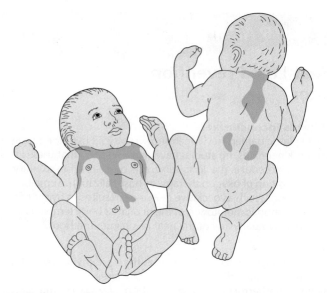

FIGURE 24–6 The distribution of brown adipose tissue (brown fat) in the newborn.
Source: Adapted from Davis, V. (1980, November–December). Structure and function of brown adipose tissue in the neonate. *Journal of Obstetric, Gynecologic, and Neonatal Nursing, 9,* 364.

When exposed to cold, the normal term newborn is usually able to cope with the increase in oxygen requirements, but the preterm newborn may be unable to increase ventilation to the necessary level of oxygen consumption. (See Chapter 29 ∞ for a discussion of cold stress.) Because oxidation of fatty acids depends on the availability of oxygen, glucose, and adenosine triphosphate (ATP), the newborn's ability to generate heat can be altered by pathologic events such as hypoxia, acidosis, and hypoglycemia or by medication that blocks the release of norepinephrine. Meperidine (Demerol) given to a laboring woman or as a newborn analgesic could slow or prevent metabolism of newborn brown fat and can lead to a greater fall in the newborn's body temperature during the neonatal period. The potential effect of meperidine on brown fat can be lessened if the mother and the newborn are well hydrated and in a neutral thermal environment. Newborn hypothermia prolongs as well as potentiates the effects of many analgesic and anesthetic drugs in the newborn.

Response to Heat

Sweating is the term newborn's usual initial response to hyperthermia. The newborn sweat glands have limited function until after the fourth week of extrauterine life; heat is lost through peripheral vasodilation and evaporation of insensible water loss. The term infant will be flaccid and assume a position of extension to facilitate heat loss (Blackburn, 2007). Oxygen consumption and metabolic rate also increase in response to hyperthermia. Severe hyperthermia can lead to death or to gross brain damage if the baby survives.

Hepatic Adaptations

In the newborn, the liver is frequently palpable 2 to 3 cm below the right costal margin. It is relatively large and occupies about 40% of the abdominal cavity. The newborn liver plays a significant role in iron storage, carbohydrate metabolism, conjugation of bilirubin, and coagulation.

Iron Storage and RBC Production

As RBCs are destroyed after birth, the iron is stored in the liver until needed for new RBC production. Newborn iron stores are determined by total body hemoglobin content and length of gestation. The term newborn has about 270 mg of iron at birth, and about 140 to 170 mg of this amount is in the hemoglobin. If the mother's iron intake has been adequate, enough iron will be stored to last until the infant is about 5 months of age. After about 6 months of age, foods containing iron or iron supplements must be given to prevent anemia.

Carbohydrate Metabolism

At term, the newborn's cord blood glucose level is 15 mg/dL lower than maternal blood glucose level (Rosenberg, 2007). Newborn carbohydrate reserves are relatively low. One-third of this reserve is in the form of liver glycogen. Newborn glycogen stores are twice those of the adult. The newborn enters an energy crunch at the time of birth, with the removal of the maternal glucose supply and the increased energy expenditure associated with the birth process and extrauterine life. Fuel sources are consumed at a faster rate because of the work of breathing, loss of heat when exposed to cold, activity, and activation of muscle tone. Glucose is the main source of energy in the first 4 to 6 hours after birth. During the first 2 hours of life, the serum blood glucose level declines, then rises, and finally reaches a steady state by 3 hours after birth (Rosenberg, 2007).

The nurse may assess the glucose level on admission if risk factors are present or per agency protocol. As stores of liver and muscle glycogen and blood glucose decrease, the newborn compensates by changing from a predominantly carbohydrate metabolism to fat metabolism. Energy can be derived from fat and protein, as well as from carbohydrates. The amount and availability of each of these "fuel substrates" depend on the ability of immature metabolic pathways (which lack specific enzymes or hormones) to function in the first few days of life.

Conjugation of Bilirubin

Conjugation of bilirubin is the conversion of yellow lipid-soluble pigment into water-soluble pigment. Unconjugated (indirect) bilirubin is a breakdown product derived from hemoglobin released primarily from destroyed RBCs. Unconjugated bilirubin is not in excretable form and is a potential toxin. **Total serum bilirubin** is the sum of conjugated (direct) and unconjugated (indirect) bilirubin.

Fetal unconjugated bilirubin crosses the placenta to be excreted, so the fetus does not need to conjugate bilirubin. Total bilirubin at birth is usually less than 3 mg/dL unless an abnormal hemolytic process has been present in utero. After birth the newborn's liver must begin to conjugate bilirubin. This produces a normal rise in serum bilirubin levels in the first few days of life.

The bilirubin formed after RBCs are destroyed is transported in the blood bound to albumin. The bilirubin is transferred into the hepatocytes and bound to intracellular proteins. These proteins determine the amount of bilirubin held in a liver cell for processing and consequently determine the amount of bilirubin uptake into the liver. The activity of uridine-diphosphoglucuronosyl transferase (UDPGT) enzyme results in the attachment of unconjugated bilirubin to glucuronic acid (product of liver glycogen), producing conjugated (direct) bilirubin. Direct bilirubin is excreted into the tiny bile ducts, then into the common duct and duodenum. The conjugated (direct) bilirubin then progresses down the intestines, where bacteria transform it into urobilinogen (urine bilirubin) and stercobilinogen. Stercobilinogen is not reabsorbed but is excreted as a yellow-brown pigment in the stools.

Even after the bilirubin has been conjugated and bound, it can be changed back to unconjugated bilirubin via the enterohepatic circulation. In the intestines β-glucuronidase enzyme acts to split off (deconjugate) the bilirubin from glucuronic acid if it has not first been acted on by gut bacteria to produce urobilinogen; the free bilirubin is reabsorbed through the intestinal wall and brought back to the liver via portal vein circulation. This recycling of the bilirubin and decreased ability to clear bilirubin from the system are prevalent in babies with very high β-D-glucuronidase activity levels, those who are exclusively breastfed, and those with delayed bacterial colonization of the gut (such as with the use of antibiotics). This further increases the newborn's susceptibility to jaundice (Figure 24–7 ■).

The newborn liver has relatively less glucuronyl transferase activity in the first few weeks of life than an adult liver. This reduction in hepatic activity, along with a relatively large bilirubin load, decreases the liver's ability to conjugate bilirubin and increases susceptibility to jaundice.

Physiologic Jaundice

Physiologic jaundice is caused by accelerated destruction of fetal RBCs, impaired conjugation of bilirubin, and increased bilirubin reabsorption from the intestinal tract. This condition does not have a pathologic basis but is a normal biologic response of the newborn.

Maisels (2005) describes six factors—several of which can also be related to pathologic events—whose interaction may give rise to physiologic jaundice.

1. *Increased amounts of bilirubin delivered to the liver.* The increased blood volume because of delayed cord clamping combined with faster RBC destruction in the newborn leads to an increased bilirubin level in the blood. A proportionately larger amount of nonerythrocyte bilirubin forms in the newborn. Therefore, newborns have two to three times greater production or breakdown of bilirubin than do adults. The use of forceps or vacuum extraction, which sometimes causes facial bruising or cephalohematoma (entrapped hemorrhage), can increase the amount of bilirubin to be handled by the liver.
2. *Defective hepatic uptake of bilirubin from the plasma.* If the newborn does not ingest adequate calories, the formation of hepatic binding proteins diminishes, resulting in higher bilirubin levels.
3. *Defective conjugation of the bilirubin.* Decreased uridine-diphosphoglucuronosyl activity as in hypothyroidism or inadequate caloric intake causes the intracellular binding proteins to remain saturated and results in greater unconjugated bilirubin levels in the blood. The fatty acids in breast milk are thought to compete with bilirubin for albumin-binding sites and therefore impede bilirubin processing.
4. *Defect in bilirubin excretion.* A congenital infection may cause impaired excretion of conjugated bilirubin. Delay in introduction of bacterial flora and decreased intestinal motility can also delay excretion and increase enterohepatic circulation of bilirubin.
5. *Inadequate hepatic circulation.* Decreased oxygen supplies to the liver associated with neonatal hypoxia or congenital heart disease lead to a rise in the bilirubin level.
6. *Increased reabsorption of bilirubin from the intestine.* Reduced bowel motility, intestinal obstruction, or delayed passage of meconium increases the circulation of bilirubin in the enterohepatic pathway, thereby resulting in higher bilirubin values.

About 50% of full-term and 80% of preterm newborns exhibit physiologic jaundice on about the second or third

MyNursingKit | Neonatal Jaundice

MyNursingKit | Jaundice in the Newborn

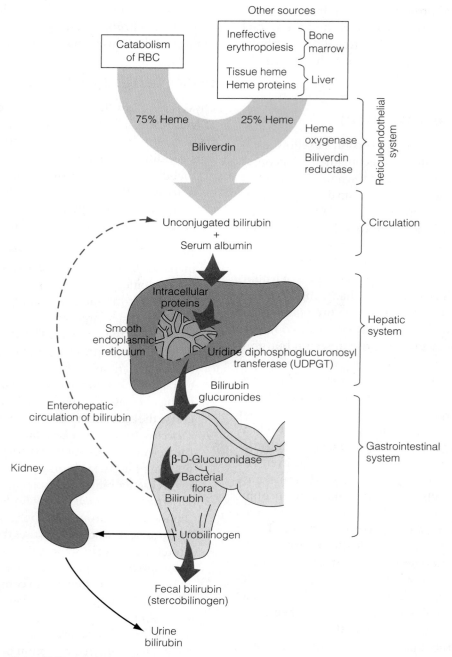

FIGURE 24–7 Conjugation of bilirubin in newborns.
Source: Adapted from Avery, G. B., Fletcher, M. A., & MacDonald, M. G. (1999). *Neonatology: Pathophysiology and management of the newborn* (5th ed., p. 767, Fig. 38–5). Philadelphia: Lippincott Williams & Wilkins.

day after birth. The characteristic yellow color results from increased levels of unconjugated (indirect) bilirubin, which are a normal product of RBC breakdown and reflect the body's temporary inability to eliminate bilirubin. Serum levels of bilirubin are about 4 to 6 mg/dL before the yellow coloration of the skin and sclera appear. *The signs of physiologic jaundice appear after the first 24 hours postnatally.* This time frame differentiates physiologic jaundice from pathologic jaun-

dice (see Chapter 29 ∞), which is clinically seen at birth or within the first 24 hours of postnatal life. Major risk factors for developing severe hyperbilirubinemia in late preterm and term infants are total serum (TSB) or transcutaneous (TcB) level in the high-risk zone on the bilirubin nomogram (Figure 24–8 ■).

There is no consistent definition of neonatal hyperbilirubinemia; what is considered to be in that range varies with population characteristics and

EVIDENCE IN ACTION

Universal screening for hyperbilirubinemia and not visual inspection alone is necessary to identify elevated bilirubin levels in newborns.
(AWHONN, Clinical Position Statement, 2005)

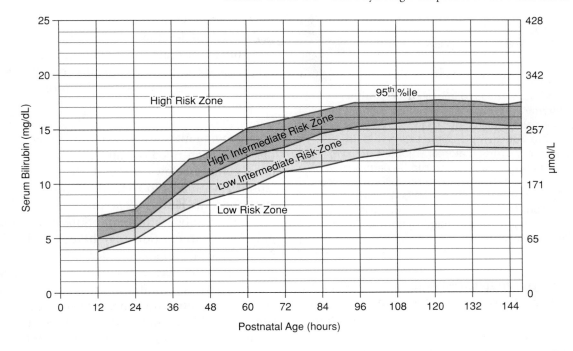

FIGURE 24–8 Postnatal hour-specific bilirubin nomogram. Note: Nomogram for designation of risk in 2840 well newborns at 36 or more weeks' gestational age with birth weight of 2000 g or more or 35 or more weeks' gestational age and birth weight of 2500 g or more based on the hour-specific serum bilirubin values. The serum level was obtained before discharge, and the zone in which the value fell predicted the likelihood of a subsequent bilirubin level exceeding the 95th percentile (high-risk zone) as shown in Appendix 3, Table 4. Used with permission from Bhutani et al. See Appendix 1 for additional information about this nomogram, which should not be used to represent the natural history of neonatal hyperbilirubinemia.
Source: American Academy of Pediatrics Subcommittee on Hyperbilirubinemia. (2004). Management of hyperbilirubinemia in the newborn infant 35 or more weeks of gestation. *Pediatrics, 114*(1), 297–316 (Fig. 2. p. 301).

postbirth age (Blackburn, 2007). Peak bilirubin levels are reached between days 3 and 5 in the full-term infant and between days 5 and 7 in the preterm infant. These values are established for European and American Caucasian newborns. Chinese, Japanese, Korean, and Native American newborns have considerably higher bilirubin levels that are not as apparent and that persist for longer periods with no apparent ill effects (Maisels, 2005).

The nursery or postpartum room environment, including lighting, may hinder the early detection of the degree and type of jaundice. Pink walls and artificial lights mask the beginning of jaundice in newborns. Daylight assists the observer in early recognition by eliminating distortions caused by artificial light.

If jaundice is suspected, the nurse can quickly assess the newborn's coloring by pressing the skin, generally on the forehead or nose, with a finger. As blanching occurs, the nurse can observe the icterus (yellow coloring).

Several newborn care procedures will decrease the probability of high bilirubin levels.

- Maintain the newborn's skin temperature at 36.5°C (97.8°F) or above, because cold stress results in acidosis. Acidosis in turn decreases available serum albumin-binding sites, weakens albumin-binding powers, and causes elevated unconjugated bilirubin levels.

- Monitor stool for amount and characteristics. Bilirubin is eliminated in the feces; inadequate stooling may result in reabsorption and recycling of bilirubin. Early breastfeeding should be encouraged because the laxative effect of colostrum increases excretion of meconium and transitional stool.

- Encourage early feedings to promote intestinal elimination and bacterial colonization and provide caloric intake necessary for formation of hepatic binding proteins.

If jaundice becomes apparent, nursing care is directed toward keeping the newborn well hydrated and promoting intestinal elimination. (For specific nursing management and therapies, see the Nursing Care Plan for a Newborn with Hyperbilirubinemia in Chapter 29 ∞.)

Physiologic jaundice may be very upsetting to parents; they require emotional support and thorough explanation of the condition. If the baby is placed under phototherapy (see Chapter 29 ∞), a few additional days of hospitalization may be required, which may also be disturbing to parents. They can be encouraged to provide for the emotional needs of their newborn by continuing to feed, hold, and caress the infant. If the mother is discharged, the parents are encouraged to return for feedings and feel free to telephone or visit when possible. In many instances, the mother, especially if she is breastfeeding, may elect to remain hospitalized with her newborn; the nurse should support this decision. If insurance limitations make this unrealistic, it may be possible to find an empty room for the discharged mother and her family to use while visiting the newborn. As an alternative to continued hospitalization, the newborn may be treated with home phototherapy. (See Phototherapy in Chapter 29 ∞ for more information.)

Breastfeeding Jaundice and Breast Milk Jaundice

Breastfeeding is implicated in prolonged jaundice in some newborns. *Breastfeeding jaundice* occurs in the first days of life in breastfed newborns. It appears to be associated with poor feeding practices and not with any abnormality in milk composition (Shrago, 2006). Prevention of early breastfeeding jaundice includes encouraging frequent (every 2 to 3 hours) breastfeeding, avoiding supplementation, and accessing maternal lactation counseling.

In *breast milk jaundice*, the bilirubin level begins to rise after the first week of life, when physiologic jaundice is waning after the mother's milk has come in. The level peaks at 5 to 10 mg/dL at 2 to 3 weeks of age and declines over the first several months of life (Maisels, 2005).

In contrast to breastfeeding jaundice, breast milk jaundice is related to milk composition. Some women's breast milk contains several times the normal concentration of certain free fatty acids. These free fatty acids may compete with bilirubin for binding sites on albumin and inhibit the conjugation of bilirubin or increase lipase activity, which disrupts the RBC membrane. Increased lipase activity enhances absorption of bile across the gastrointestinal tract membrane, thereby increasing the enterohepatic circulation of bilirubin. In the past it was thought that the breast milk of women whose newborns have breast milk jaundice contained an enzyme that inhibited glucuronyl transferase, but this hypothesis has not been proven (Thureen et al., 2005).

Newborns with breastfeeding jaundice appear well, and at present development of kernicterus (toxic levels of bilirubin in the brain) has not been documented. Temporary cessation of breastfeeding may be advised if bilirubin reaches presumed toxic levels of approximately 20 mg/dL or if the interruption is necessary to establish the cause of the hyperbilirubinemia. Most physicians believe that breastfeeding may be resumed once other causes of jaundice have been ruled out and as long as serum bilirubin levels remain below 20 mg/dL. In cases of breast milk jaundice, within 24 to 36 hours after breastfeeding is discontinued, the newborn's serum bilirubin levels begin to fall dramatically. With resumption of breastfeeding, the bilirubin concentration may have a slight rise of 2 to 3 mg/dL, with a subsequent decline. Breastfeeding mothers need encouragement and support in their desire to breastfeed their infants, assistance and instruction regarding pumping and expressing milk during the interrupted nursing period, and reassurance that nothing is wrong with their milk or mothering abilities. (See Key Facts to Remember: Factors in Physiologic, Breast Milk, and Breastfeeding Jaundice.)

TEACHING TIP

Breastfeeding mothers need encouragement and support in their desire to breastfeed their infants, assistance and instruction about pumping and expressing milk during the interrupted breastfeeding period, and reassurance that nothing is wrong with their milk or mothering abilities.

KEY FACTS TO REMEMBER

Factors in Physiologic, Breast Milk, Breastfeeding Jaundice

Physiologic Jaundice

Physiologic jaundice occurs after the first 24 hours of life.
During the first week of life, bilirubin should not exceed 13 mg/dL. Some pediatricians allow levels up to 15 mg/dL.
Bilirubin levels peak at 3 to 5 days in term infants.

Breast Milk Jaundice

Bilirubin levels begin to rise after the first week of life when mature breast milk comes in.
Peak of 5 to 10 mg/dL is reached at 2 to 3 weeks of age.
It may be necessary to interrupt breastfeeding for a short period when bilirubin reaches 20 mg/dL.

Breastfeeding Jaundice

Bilirubin levels rise after the first 24 hours of age.
Peaks on third or fourth day of life and declines through first month to normal levels.
Incidence can be decreased by increasing the number of breastfeeding episodes to 8 to 12 in 24 hours.

MyNursingKit | Breastfeeding and Jaundice

Coagulation

The liver plays an important part in blood coagulation during fetal life and continues this function following birth. Coagulation factors II, VII, IX, and X (synthesized in the liver) are activated under the influence of vitamin K and therefore are considered vitamin K dependent. The absence of normal flora needed to synthesize vitamin K in the newborn gut results in low levels of vitamin K and creates a transient blood coagulation alteration between the second and fifth day of life. From a low point at about 2 to 3 days after birth, these coagulation factors rise slowly, but they do not approach adult levels until 9 months of age or later ranges (Luchtman-Jones, L., Schwartz, A., & Wilson, D., 2006). Other coagulation factors with low umbilical cord blood levels are XI, XII, and XIII. Fibrinogen and factors V and VII are near adult.

Although newborn bleeding problems are rare, an injection of vitamin K (AquaMEPHYTON) is given prophylactically on the day of birth to combat potential clinical bleeding problems. (Chapter 26 ∞ discusses administration of vitamin K to newborns and Chapter 29 ∞ discusses hemorrhagic disease of the newborn in greater depth.)

Platelet counts at birth are in the same range as for older children, but newborns may manifest mild transient difficulty in platelet aggregation functioning. This platelet problem is accentuated by phototherapy. Prenatal maternal therapy with phenytoin sodium (Dilantin) or phenobarbital also causes abnormal clotting studies and newborn bleeding in the first 24 hours after birth. Infants born to mothers receiving warfarin (Coumadin) compounds may bleed, because these agents cross the placenta and accentuate existing vitamin K-dependent factor deficiencies. Transient neonatal thrombocytopenia may occur in infants born to mothers with severe hypertension or HELLP syndrome (hemolysis, elevated liver enzymes, and low platelet count) and in infants born to mothers who have idiopathic isoimmune thrombocytopenic purpura.

Gastrointestinal Adaptations

By 36 to 38 weeks' gestation, the gastrointestinal system is adequately mature, with enzymatic activity and the ability to transport nutrients.

Digestion and Absorption

The full-term newborn has sufficient intestinal and pancreatic enzymes to digest most simple carbohydrates, proteins, and fats. The carbohydrates requiring digestion in the newborn are usually disaccharides (lactose, maltose, sucrose), which are split into monosaccharides (galactose, fructose, and glucose) by the enzymes of the intestinal mucosa. Lactose is the primary carbohydrate in the breastfeeding newborn and is generally easily digested and well absorbed. The only enzyme lacking is pancreatic amylase, which remains relatively deficient during the first few months of life. Newborns have trouble digesting starches (changing more complex carbohydrates into maltose) so they should not eat until after the first few months of life.

Although proteins require more digestion than carbohydrates, they are well digested and absorbed from the newborn intestine. The newborn digests and absorbs fats less efficiently because of the minimal activity of the pancreatic enzyme lipase. The newborn excretes about 10% to 20% of the dietary fat intake, compared with 10% for the adult. The newborn absorbs the fat in breast milk more completely than the fat in cows' milk, because breast milk consists of more medium-chain triglycerides and contains lipase. (See Chapter 27 ∞ for further discussion of newborn nutrition.)

By birth, the newborn has experienced swallowing, gastric emptying, and intestinal propulsion. In utero, fetal swallowing is accompanied by gastric emptying and peristalsis of the fetal intestinal tract. By the end of gestation, peristalsis becomes much more active in preparation for extrauterine life. Fetal peristalsis is also stimulated by anoxia, causing the expulsion of meconium into the amniotic fluid in more mature fetuses.

Air enters the stomach immediately after birth. The small intestine is filled with air within 2 to 12 hours and the large bowel within 24 hours. The salivary glands are immature at birth, and the newborn produces little saliva until about age 3 months. The newborn's stomach has a capacity of about 50 to 60 mL. It empties intermittently, starting within a few minutes of the beginning of a feeding and ending 2 to 4 hours after feeding. Bowel sounds are present within the first 30 to 60 minutes of birth and the newborn can successfully feed during this time. The newborn's gastric pH becomes less acidic about a week after birth and remains less acidic than that of adults for the next 2 to 3 months. *lower esophageal sphincter*

The cardiac sphincter is immature, as is neural control of the stomach, so some regurgitation may be noted in the newborn period. Regurgitation of the first few feedings during the first day or two of life can usually be lessened by avoiding overfeeding and by burping the newborn well during and after the feeding.

When no other signs and symptoms are evident, vomiting is limited and ceases within the first few days of life. Continuous vomiting or regurgitation should be observed closely. If the newborn has swallowed bloody or purulent amniotic fluid, lavage of the stomach may be indicated in the term newborn to relieve the problem. Bilious vomiting is abnormal and must be evaluated thoroughly because it might represent a condition that warrants prompt surgical intervention.

Adequate digestion and absorption are essential for newborn growth and development. If optimal nutritional support is available, postnatal growth should parallel intrauterine growth; that is, after 30 weeks' gestation, the fetus gains 30 g per day and adds 1.2 cm (0.5 in.) to body length daily. To gain weight at the intrauterine rate, the term newborn requires 120 cal/kg/day. After birth, caloric intake is often insufficient for weight gain until the newborn is 5 to 10 days old. During this time, there may be a weight loss of 5% to 10% in term newborns. A shift of intracellular water to extracellular space and insensible water loss account for the 5% to 10% weight loss; thus failure to lose weight when caloric intake is inadequate may indicate fluid retention.

Elimination

Term newborns usually pass meconium within 8 to 24 hours of life and almost always within 48 hours. **Meconium** is formed in utero from the amniotic fluid and its constituents, intestinal secretions, and shed mucosal cells. It is recognized by its thick, tarry black or dark green appearance. Transitional (thin brown to green) stools consisting of part meconium and part fecal material are passed for the next day or two, and then the stools become entirely fecal. Generally the stools of a breastfed newborn are pale yellow (but may be pasty green); they are more liquid and more frequent than those of formula-fed newborns, whose stools are paler (Figure 24–9 ■). Frequency of bowel movement varies but ranges from one every 2 to 3 days to as many as 10 daily. Totally breastfed infants often progress to stools that occur every 5 to 7 days. Mothers should be counseled that the newborn is not constipated as long as the bowel movement remains soft. (See Key Facts to Remember: Physiologic Adaptations to Extrauterine Life.)

Urinary Tract Adaptations

Kidney Development and Function

Certain physiologic features of the newborn's kidneys influence the newborn's ability to handle body fluids and excrete urine.

1. The term newborn's kidneys have a full complement of functioning nephrons by 34 to 36 weeks' gestation.
2. The glomerular filtration rate of the newborn's kidney is low compared with the adult rate. Because of this physiologic decrease in kidney glomerular filtration, the newborn's kidney is unable to dispose of water rapidly when necessary.
3. The juxtamedullary portion of the nephron has limited capacity to reabsorb HCO_3^+ and H^+ and concentrate urine (reabsorb water back into the blood). The limitation of tubular reabsorption can lead to inappropriate loss of substances present in the glomerular filtrate, such as amino acids, bicarbonate, glucose, and sodium.

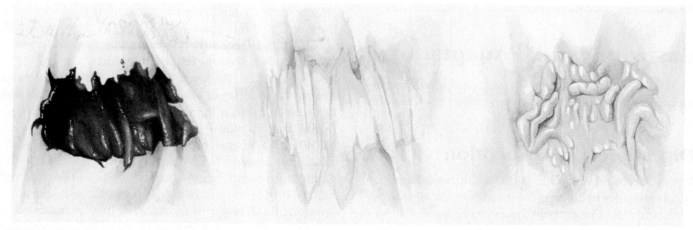

FIGURE 24–9 Newborn stool samples. *A,* Meconium stool. *B,* Breast milk stool. *C,* Cow's milk stool.

Full-term newborns are less able than adults to concentrate urine because the tubules are short and narrow. Also the reduced ability to concentrate urine is caused by the limited tubular reabsorption of water and limited excretion of solutes (principally sodium, potassium, chloride, bicarbonate, urea, and phosphate) in the growing newborn. The ability to concentrate urine fully is attained by 3 months of age. Feeding practices may affect the osmolarity of the urine but have limited effect on concentration of the urine.

Because the newborn has difficulty concentrating urine, the effect of excessive insensible water loss or restricted fluid intake is unpredictable. The newborn kidney is also limited in its dilutional capabilities. Concentrating and dilutional limitations of renal function are important considerations in monitoring fluid therapy to prevent dehydration or overhydration.

Characteristics of Newborn Urinary Function

Many newborns void immediately after birth, and the voiding frequently goes unnoticed. Among normal newborns, 93% void by 24 hours after birth and 100% void by 48 hours after birth (Thureen et al., 2005). A newborn who has not voided by 48 hours should be assessed for adequacy of fluid intake, bladder distention, restlessness, and symptoms of pain. The appropriate clinical personnel should be notified if indicated.

The initial bladder volume is 6 to 44 mL of urine. Unless edema is present, normal urinary output is often limited, and the voidings are scanty until fluid intake increases. (The fluid of edema is eliminated by the kidneys, so infants with edema have a much higher urinary output.) The first 2 days postnatally, the newborn voids two to six times daily, with a urine output of 15 mL/kg/day. The newborn subsequently voids 5 to 25 times every 24 hours, with a volume of 25 mL/kg/day.

Following the first voiding, the newborn's urine frequently appears cloudy (because of mucus content) and has a high specific gravity, which decreases as fluid intake increases. Occasionally pink stains ("brick dust spots") appear on the diaper. These are caused by urates and are innocuous. Blood may occasionally be observed on the diapers of female newborns. This *pseudomenstruation* is related to the withdrawal of maternal hormones. Males may have bloody spotting from a circumcision if performed. In the absence of apparent causes for bleeding, the clinician should be notified. During early infancy, normal urine is straw colored and almost odorless, although odor occurs when certain drugs are given, metabolic disorders exist, or infection is present. Table 24–3 contains urinalysis values for the normal newborn.

TABLE 24–3	Newborn Urinalysis Values

Protein less than 5 to 10 mg/dL
WBC less than 2 to 3/hpf
RBC 0
Casts 0
Bacteria 0
Color pale yellow

Immunologic Adaptations

The newborn's immune system is not fully activated until sometime after birth. Limitations in the newborn's inflammatory response result in failure to recognize, localize, and destroy invasive bacteria. Thus the signs and symptoms of infection are often subtle and nonspecific in the newborn. The newborn also has a poor hypothalamic response to pyrogens; therefore fever is not a reliable indicator of infection. In the neonatal period, hypothermia is a more reliable sign of infection.

Of the three major types of immunoglobulins that are primarily involved in immunity—IgG, IgA, and IgM—only IgG crosses the placenta. The pregnant woman forms antibodies in response to illness or immunization. This process is called **active acquired immunity**. When IgG antibodies are transferred to the fetus in utero, **passive acquired immunity** results, because the fetus does not produce the antibodies itself. IgG antibodies are very active against bacterial toxins.

Because the maternal IgG is transferred primarily during the third trimester, preterm newborns (especially those born before 34 weeks' gestation) may be more susceptible to infection. In general, newborns have immunity to tetanus, diphtheria, smallpox, measles, mumps, poliomyelitis, and a variety of other bacterial and viral diseases. The period of resistance varies: Immunity against common viral infections such as measles may last 4 to 8 months, whereas immunity to certain bacteria may disappear within 4 to 8 weeks.

The normal newborn can produce a protective immune response to vaccines, such as hepatitis B immunoglobulin vaccine, given as early as a few hours after birth. It is customary to begin the majority of routine immunizations at 2 months of age so that the infant can develop active acquired immunity. For discussion of newborn immunization see Chapter 26 ∞.

IgM antibodies are produced in response to blood group antigens, gram-negative enteric organisms, and some viruses in the expectant mother. Because IgM does not normally cross the placenta, most or all of it is produced by the fetus beginning at 10 to 15 weeks' gestation. Elevated levels of IgM at birth may indicate placental leaks or, more commonly, antigenic stimulation in utero.

Consequently elevations suggest that the newborn was exposed to an intrauterine infection such as syphilis or TORCH syndrome (toxoplasmosis, rubella, cytomegalovirus, herpesvirus hominis type 2 infection). (For further discussion, see Chapter 16 ∞.) The lack of available maternal IgM in the newborn also accounts for the susceptibility to gram-negative enteric organisms such as *Escherichia coli*.

The functions of IgA immunoglobulins are not fully understood. IgA appears to provide protection mainly on secreting surfaces such as the respiratory tract, gastrointestinal tract, and eyes. Serum IgA does not cross the placenta and is not normally produced by the fetus in utero. Unlike the other immunoglobulins, IgA is not affected by gastric action. Colostrum, the forerunner of breast milk, is very high in the secretory form of IgA. Consequently it may be of significance in providing some passive immunity to the infant of a breastfeeding mother. Newborns begin to produce secretory IgA in their intestinal mucosa about 4 weeks after birth.

Neurologic and Sensory-Perceptual Functioning

The newborn's brain is about one-quarter the size of an adult's, and myelination of nerve fibers is incomplete. Unlike the cardiovascular and respiratory systems, which undergo tremendous changes at birth, the nervous system is minimally influenced by the actual birth process.

Because many biochemical and histologic changes have yet to occur in the newborn's brain, the postnatal period is considered a time of risk with regard to the development of the brain and nervous system. For neurologic development—including development of intellect—to proceed, the brain and other nervous system structures must mature in an orderly, unhampered fashion. (For discussion of cranial nerves, see Chapter 25 ∞.)

Intrauterine Factors Influencing Newborn Behavior

Newborns respond to and interact with the environment in a predictable pattern of behavior that is somewhat shaped by their intrauterine experience. This intrauterine experience is affected by intrinsic factors such as maternal nutrition and external factors such as the mother's physical environment. Depending on the newborn's intrauterine experience and individual temperament, neonatal behavioral responses to different stresses vary. Some newborns react quietly to stimulation, others become overreactive and tense, and some may exhibit a combination of the two.

Factors such as exposure to intense auditory stimuli in utero can eventually be manifested in the behavior of the newborn. For example, the fetal heart rate (FHR) initially increases when the pregnant woman is exposed to auditory stimuli, but repetition of the stimuli leads to decreased FHR. Thus the newborn who was exposed to intense noise during fetal life is significantly less reactive to loud sounds postnatally.

Characteristics of Newborn Neurologic Function

Normal newborns are usually in a position of partially flexed extremities with the legs near the abdomen. When awake, the newborn may exhibit purposeless, uncoordinated bilateral movements of the extremities. The organization and quality of the newborn's motor activity are influenced by a number of factors, including the following (Brazelton, 1984):

- Sleep-alert states
- Presence of environmental stimuli, such as heat, light, cold, and noise
- Conditions causing a chemical imbalance, such as hypoglycemia
- Hydration status
- State of health
- Recovery from the stress of labor and birth

Eye movements are observable during the first few days of life. An alert newborn is able to fixate on faces and geometric objects or patterns such as black-and-white stripes. A bright light shining in the newborn's eyes elicits the blinking reflex.

The cry of the newborn should be lusty and vigorous. High-pitched cries, weak cries, and no cries are causes for concern.

The newborn's body growth progresses in a cephalocaudal (head-to-toe), proximal-distal fashion. The newborn is somewhat hypertonic; that is, there is resistance to extending the elbow and knee joints. Muscle tone should be symmetrical. Diminished muscle tone and flaccidity may indicate neurologic dysfunction.

Specific symmetrical deep tendon reflexes can be elicited in the newborn. The knee jerk reflex is brisk; a normal ankle clonus may involve three to four beats. Plantar flexion is present. Other reflexes, including the Moro, grasping, Babinski, rooting, and sucking reflexes, are characteristic of neurologic integrity (Table 24–4 provides a summary of stimulus for, and response for, the common newborn reflexes). (For discussion of reflexes see Chapter 25 ∞.)

Performance of complex behavioral patterns reflects the newborn's neurologic maturation and integration. Newborns who can bring a hand to their mouth may be demonstrating motor coordination as well as a self-quieting technique, thus increasing the complexity of the behavioral response. Newborns also possess complex, organized defen-

TABLE 24–4	Common Reflexes of the Newborn	
Reflex Name	Evoking Stimulus	Response
Blinking reflex	Light flash	Eyelids close.
Pupillary reflex	Light flash	Pupil constricts.
Rooting reflex	Light touch of finger on cheek close to mouth	Head rotates toward stimulation; mouth opens and attempts to suck finger. Disappears by about 4 months of age.
Sucking reflex	Finger (or nipple) inserted into mouth	Rhythmic sucking occurs.
Moro reflex	Infant lying on back: slightly raised head suddenly released; infant held horizontally, lowered quickly about 6 in., and stopped abruptly	Arms are extended, head is thrown back, fingers are spread wide; arms are then brought back to center convulsively with hands clenched; spine and lower extremities are extended. Disappears by about 6 months of age.
Startle reflex	Loud noise	Similar to Moro reflex flexion in arms; fists are clenched.
Grasping reflex	Finger placed in palm of hand	Infant's fingers close around and grasp object.
Tonic neck reflex	Head turned to one side while infant lies on back	Arm and leg are extended on the side the infant faces. Opposite arm and leg are flexed.
Abdominal reflex	Tactile stimulation or tickling	Abdominal muscles contract.
Withdrawal reflex	Slight pinprick to the sole of the infant's foot	Leg flexes.
Walking reflex	Infant supported in an upright position with feet lightly touching a flat surface	Rhythmic stepping movement. Disappears at about 4 to 8 weeks of age.
Babinski reflex	Gentle stroking on the sole of each foot	Fanning and extension of the toes (adults respond to this stimulation with flexion of toes).
Plantar, or toe-grasping, reflex	Pressure applied with the finger against the balls of the infant's feet	A plantar flexion of all toes. Disappears by the end of the first year of life.

Source: Adapted from Mott, S. R., James, S. R., & Sperhac, A. M. (1990). *Nursing care of children and families: A holistic approach* (2nd ed.). Menlo Park, CA: Addison-Wesley Nursing.

sive motor patterns, as exhibited by the ability to remove an obstruction, such as a cloth across the face.

Periods of Reactivity

The baby usually shows a predictable pattern of behavior during the first several hours after birth, characterized by two **periods of reactivity** separated by a sleep phase.

First Period of Reactivity

The first period of reactivity lasts approximately 30 minutes after birth. During this period the newborn is awake and active and may appear hungry and have a strong sucking reflex. This is a natural opportunity to initiate breastfeeding if the mother has chosen it. Bursts of random, diffuse movements alternating with relative immobility may occur. Respirations are rapid, as high as 80 breaths per minute, and there may be retraction of the chest, transient flaring of the nares, and grunting. The heart rate is rapid, and the rhythm may be irregular. Bowel sounds are usually absent.

Period of Inactivity to Sleep Phase

After approximately half an hour the newborn's activity gradually diminishes, and the heart rate and respirations decrease as the newborn enters the sleep phase. The sleep phase may last from a few minutes to 2 to 4 hours. During this period, the newborn will be difficult to awaken and will show no interest in sucking. Bowel sounds become audible, and cardiac and respiratory rates return to baseline values.

Second Period of Reactivity

During the second period of reactivity, the newborn is again awake and alert. This period lasts 4 to 6 hours in the normal newborn. Physiologic responses are variable during this stage. The heart and respiratory rates increase; however, the nurse must be alert for apneic periods, which may cause a drop in the heart rate. The newborn is stimulated to continue breathing during such times. The newborn may develop rapid color changes and become mildly cyanotic or mottled during these fluctuations. Production of respiratory and gastric mucus increases, and the newborn responds by gagging, choking, and regurgitating.

Continued close observation and intervention may be required to maintain a clear airway during this period of reactivity. The gastrointestinal tract becomes more active. The newborn often passes the first meconium stool and may also have an initial voiding. The newborn will indicate readiness for feeding by such behaviors as sucking, rooting, and swallowing. If feeding was not initiated in the first period of reactivity, it is done at this time. (See Chapter 27 ∞ for further discussion of this first feeding.)

MyNursingKit | Sleep Patterns and States

Behavioral States of the Newborn

The behavior of the newborn can be divided into two categories, the sleep state and the alert state (Brazelton, 1999). These postnatal behavioral states are similar to those that have been identified during pregnancy. Subcategories are identified under each major category.

Sleep States

The sleep states are as follows:

1. *Deep or quiet sleep.* Deep sleep is characterized by closed eyes with no eye movements; regular, even breathing; and jerky motions or startles at regular intervals. Behavioral responses to external stimuli are likely to be delayed. Startles are rapidly suppressed, and changes in state are not likely to occur. Heart rate may range from 100 to 120 beats per minute.
2. *Active rapid eye movement (REM).* The baby has irregular respirations; eyes closed, with REM; irregular sucking motions; minimal activity; and irregular but smooth movement of the extremities. Environmental and internal stimuli may initiate a startle reaction and a change of state.

Newborn sleep cycles have been recognized and defined according to duration. The length of the sleep cycle depends on the age of the newborn. At term, REM active sleep and quiet sleep occur in intervals of 50 to 60 minutes (Gardner & Goldson, 2006). About 45% to 50% of the newborn's total sleep is active sleep, 35% to 45% is quiet sleep, and 10% is transitional between these two periods. Growth hormone secretion depends on regular sleep patterns. Any disturbance of the sleep-wake cycle can result in irregular spikes of growth hormone. REM sleep stimulates the highest peaks of growth hormone and the growth of the neural system. Over a period of time, the newborn's sleep-wake patterns become diurnal; that is, the newborn sleeps at night and stays awake during the day. (See Newborn Behavioral Assessment in Chapter 25 ∞ for a short discussion of Brazelton's assessment of newborn states.)

Alert States

In the first 30 to 60 minutes after birth, many newborns display a quiet alert state, characteristic of the first period of reactivity (Figure 24–10 ■). Nurses should use these alert states to encourage bonding and breastfeeding. These periods of alertness tend to be short the first 2 days after birth to allow the baby to recover from the birth process. Subsequent alert states are of choice or of necessity (Brazelton, 1999). Increasing choice of wakefulness by the newborn indicates a maturing capacity to achieve and maintain consciousness. Heat, cold, and hunger are but a few of the stimuli that can cause wakefulness by necessity. Once the disturbing stimuli are removed, the baby tends to fall back asleep.

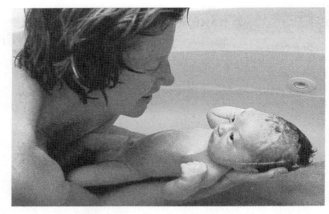

FIGURE 24–10 Mother and newborn gaze at each other. This quiet, alert state is the optimum state for interaction between baby and parents.

The following are subcategories of the alert state (Brazelton, 1999).

1. *Drowsy or semidozing.* The behaviors common to the drowsy state are open or closed eyes; fluttering eyelids; semidozing appearance; and slow, regular movements of the extremities. Mild startles may be noted from time to time. Although the reaction to a sensory stimulus is delayed, a change of state often results.
2. *Wide awake.* In the wide-awake state, the newborn is alert and follows and fixates on attractive objects, faces, or auditory stimuli. Motor activity is minimal, and the response to external stimuli is delayed.
3. *Active awake.* In the active-awake state the newborn's eyes are open and motor activity is quite intense, with thrusting movements of the extremities. Environmental stimuli increase startles or motor activity, but individual reactions are difficult to distinguish because of the generally high activity level.
4. *Crying.* Intense crying is accompanied by jerky motor movements. Crying serves several purposes for the newborn. It may be a distraction from disturbing stimuli such as hunger and pain. Fussiness often allows the newborn to discharge energy and reorganize behavior. Most important, crying elicits an appropriate response of help from the parents.

Behavioral and Sensory Capacities of the Newborn

The newborn has several behavioral capacities that assist in adaptation to extrauterine life. For example, **self-quieting ability** is the ability of newborns to use their own resources to quiet and comfort themselves. Their repertoire includes hand-to-mouth movements, sucking on a fist or tongue, and attending to external stimuli. Neurologically impaired newborns are unable to use self-quieting activities and require more frequent comforting from caregivers when stimulated. For example, drug-positive newborns often exhibit abnormal sleep and feeding patterns and irritability.

Habituation is the newborn's ability to process and respond to complex stimulation. For example, when a bright light is flashed into the newborn's eyes, the initial response is blinking, constriction of the pupil, and perhaps a slight startle reaction. However, with repeated stimulation, the newborn's response repertoire gradually diminishes and disappears. The capacity to ignore repetitious disturbing stimuli is a newborn defense mechanism readily apparent in the noisy, well-lit nursery.

Sensory abilities include visual, auditory, olfactory, taste, and tactile capacities.

Visual Capacity

Orientation is the newborn's ability to be alert to, to follow, and to fixate on appealing and attractive complex visual stimuli. The newborn prefers the human face and eyes and bright shiny objects. As the face or object comes into the line of vision, the newborn responds with bright, wide eyes, still limbs, and fixed staring. This intense visual involvement may last several minutes, during which time the newborn is able to follow the stimulus from side to side. Figure 24–11 ■ illustrates this response. The newborn uses this sensory capacity to become familiar with family, friends, and surroundings.

Auditory Capacity

The newborn responds to auditory stimulation with a definite, organized behavior repertoire. The stimulus used to assess auditory response should be selected to match the state of the newborn. A rattle is appropriate for light sleep, a voice for an awake state, and a clap for deep sleep. As the

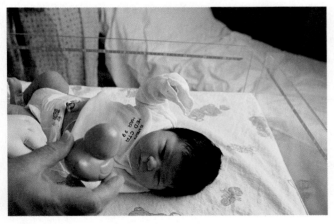

FIGURE 24–11 Head turning to follow movement.

newborn hears the sound, the cardiac rate rises, and a minimal startle reflex may be seen. If the sound is appealing, the newborn will become alert and search for the site of the auditory stimulus. Lack of auditory development is associated with an increased risk of SIDS. The AAP currently recommends that newborns receive hearing screening before discharge from the hospital; universal hearing screening before 1 month of age is a goal of *Healthy People 2010* (Creehan, 2008).

Olfactory Capacity

Newborns can select their mother by smell and are apparently able to select people by smell (Klaus, Kennell, & De Pompei, 2006). Newborns are able to distinguish their mothers' breast pads from those of other mothers at just 1 week postnatally.

Taste and Sucking

The newborn responds differently to varying tastes. Sugar, for example, increases sucking. Newborns fed with a rubber nipple versus the breast also show sucking pattern variations. When breastfeeding, the newborn sucks in bursts, with frequent regular pauses. The bottle-fed newborn tends to suck at a regular rate, with infrequent pauses.

When awake and hungry, the newborn displays rapid searching motions in response to the rooting reflex. Once feeding begins, the newborn establishes a sucking pattern according to the method of feeding. Finger sucking is seen in utero as well as after birth. The newborn frequently uses nonnutritive sucking as a self-quieting activity, which assists in the development of self-regulation. For bottle-fed infants, there is no reason to discourage nonnutritive sucking with a pacifier. Pacifiers should be offered to breastfed infants only after breastfeeding is well established. If the pacifier is offered too soon, a phenomenon called "nipple confusion" may occur in which the breastfed infant has difficulty learning to suck from the breast and will nurse less (see Supplementary Bottle Feeding in Chapter 27 ∞).

Tactile Capacity

The newborn is very sensitive to being touched, cuddled, and held. Often a mother's first response to an upset or crying newborn is touching or holding. Swaddling, placing a hand on the abdomen, or holding the arms to prevent a startle reflex are other methods of soothing the newborn. The quieted newborn is then able to attend to and interact with the environment.

- Newborn respiration could be initiated by internal chemical and mechanical stimulation, but also in association with thermal and sensory stimulation and the presence of sympathetic nervous system hormones.
- The production of surfactant is crucial to keeping the lungs expanded during expiration by reducing alveolar surface tension.
- The newborn is an obligatory nose breather. Respirations change from being primarily shallow, irregular, and diaphragmatic to synchronous abdominal and chest breathing. Normal respiratory rate is 30 to 60 beats per minute.
- Periodic breathing is normal, and newborn sleep states affect breathing patterns.
- The status of the cardiopulmonary system may be measured by evaluating the heart rate, blood pressure, and presence or absence of murmurs. The normal heart rate is 120 to 160 beats per minute.
- Oxygen transport in the newborn is significantly affected by the presence of greater amounts of HbF (fetal hemoglobin) than HbA (adult hemoglobin); HbF holds oxygen easier but releases it to the body tissues only at low PO_2 levels.
- Blood values in the newborn are modified by several factors, such as the site of the blood sample, gestational age, prenatal and/or perinatal hemorrhage, and the timing of the clamping of the umbilical cord.
- The newborn is considered to have established thermoregulation when oxygen consumption and metabolic activity are minimal.
- Evaporation is the primary heat loss mechanism in newborns who are wet from amniotic fluid or a bath. In addition, excessive heat loss occurs from radiation and convection, because of the newborn's larger surface area compared with weight, and from thermal conduction, because of the marked difference between core temperature and skin temperature.
- The primary source of heat in the cold-stressed newborn is brown adipose tissue.
- The early onset form of breastfeeding jaundice is thought to be primarily caused by the process of feeding whereas late onset form jaundice is less common and believed to be primarily caused by the characteristics of breast milk.
- Blood glucose levels should reach a steady state by 3 hours of age.
- The newborn's liver plays a crucial role in iron storage, carbohydrate metabolism, conjugation of bilirubin, and coagulation.
- The normal newborn possesses the ability to digest and absorb nutrients necessary for newborn growth and development.
- The newborn's stools change from meconium (thick, tarry, dark green) to transitional stools (thin, brown-to-green) and then to the distinct forms for either breastfed newborns (yellow-gold, soft, or mushy) or formula-fed newborns (pale yellow, formed, and pasty). Most newborns pass their first stool within 48 hours of birth.
- The newborn's kidneys are characterized by a decreased rate of glomerular flow, limited tubular reabsorption, limited excretion of solutes, and limited ability to concentrate urine. Most newborns void within 48 hours of birth.
- The immune system in the newborn is not fully activated until some time after birth, but the newborn possesses some immunologic abilities.
- Neurologic and sensory-perceptual functioning in the newborn is evident from the newborn's interaction with the environment, presence of synchronized motor activity, and well-developed sensory capacities.
- The first period of reactivity lasts for 30 minutes after birth. The newborn is alert and hungry at this time, making this a natural opportunity to promote attachment.
- The second period of reactivity requires close monitoring and may require intervention by the nurse if apnea, decreased heart rate, gagging, choking, and regurgitation occur. Nurses assist parents in resolving symptoms which compromise newborn well-being.
- The behavioral states in the newborn can be divided into sleep states and alert states.
- Sensory development proceeds in a specific order: tactile/vestibular, olfactory/gustatory, and auditory/visual.

CHAPTER REFERENCES

American Academy of Pediatrics (AAP) & American College of Obstetricians and Gynecologists (ACOG). (2007). *Guidelines for perinatal care* (6th ed.). Elk Grove Village, IL: Author.

Association of Women's Health, Obstetric and Neonatal Nurses (AWHONN). (2005). Clinical position statement: Universal screening for hyperbilirubinemia [Position Statement]. Washington, DC: Author.

Bagwell, G. A. (2007). Hematologic system. In C. Kenner & J. W. Lott, *Comprehensive neonatal care: An interdisciplinary approach* (4th ed., pp. 221–253). St. Louis: Saunders.

Blackburn, S. T. (2007). *Maternal, fetal, & neonatal physiology: A clinical perspective* (3rd ed.). St. Louis: Saunders.

Bloom, R. (2006). Delivery room resuscitation of the newborn: Part I Overview and initial management. In A. A. Fanaroff, R. J. Martin, & M. C. Walsh (Eds.), *Fanaroff and Martin's neonatal-perinatal medicine* (8th ed., pp. 483–491). St. Louis, MO: Mosby.

Brazelton, T. B. (1984). *Neonatal behavioral assessment scale* (2nd ed.). London: Heineman.

Brazelton, T. B. (1999). Behavioral competence. In G. B. Avery, M. A. Fletcher, & M. G. MacDonald (Eds.), *Neonatology: Pathophysiology and management of the newborn* (5th ed., pp. 321–332). Philadelphia: Lippincott.

Cheffer, N. D. (2004). Adaptation to extrauterine life and immediate nursing care. In S. Mattson & J. E. Smith (Eds.), *Core curriculum for maternal-newborn nursing* (3rd ed., pp. 421–436). St. Louis: Saunders.

Creehan, P. A. (2008). Newborn physical assessment. In K. R. Simpson & P. A. Creehan, *Perinatal nursing* (3rd ed., pp. 546–574). Philadelphia: Lippincott Williams & Wilkins.

Gardner, S. L., & Goldson, E. (2006). The neonate and the environment: Impact on development. In G. B. Merenstein & S. L. Gardner (Eds.), *Handbook of neonatal intensive care* (6th ed., pp. 273–349). St. Louis: Mosby.

Hannon, P. R., Willis, S. K., & Scrimshaw, S. C. (2001). Persistence of maternal concerns surrounding neonatal jaundice. An exploratory study. *Archives of Pediatrics & Adolescent Medicine*, 155, 1357–1363.

Klaus, M. H., Kennell, J. H., & De Pompei, P. M. (2006). Care of the mother, father, and infant. In A. A. Fanaroff, R. J. Martin, & M. C. Walsh (Eds.), *Fanaroff and Martin's neonatal-perinatal medicine* (8th ed., pp. 645–659). St. Louis, MO: Mosby.

Knuppel, R. A. (2007). Maternal-placental-fetal unit: Fetal & early neonatal physiology. In A. H. DeCherney, L. Nathan, T. M. Goodwin, & N. Laufer (Eds.), *Current obstetric & gynecologic diagnosis & treatment* (10th ed., pp. 159–186). New York: Lang Medical Books/McGraw-Hill.

Luchtman-Jones, L., Schwartz, A., & Wilson, D. (2006). Hematologic problems in the fetus and neonate. In R. Martin, A. Fanaroff, & M. Walsh (Eds.), *Fanaroff and Martin's neonatal-perinatal medicine* (8th ed., pp. 1287–1343). St. Louis, MO: Mosby.

Maisels, M. J. (2005). Jaundice. In M. G. MacDonald, M. D. Mullett, & M. Seshia (Eds.), *Avery's neonatology: Pathophysiology & management of the newborn.* (6th ed., pp. 768–846). Philadelphia: Lippincott Williams & Wilkins.

Mercer, J. S., Erickson-Owens, D. A., Graves, B., & Haley, M. (2007). Evidence-based practices for the fetal to newborn transition. *Journal of Midwifery and Women's Health, 52*(3), 262–272.

Polin, R. A., Fox, W. W., & Abman, S. H. (2004). *Fetal and neonatal physiology* (3rd ed.). Philadelphia: Saunders.

Rosenberg, A. A. (2007). The neonate. In S. G. Gabbe, J. R. Niebyl, & J. L. Simpson (Eds.). *Obstetrics: Normal and problem pregnancies.* (5th ed., pp. 523–565). Philadelphia, PA: Churchill Livingstone/Elsevier.

Shrago, L. C., Reisnider, E., & Insel, E. (2006). The neonatal bowel output study: Indicators of adequate breast milk intake neonates. *Pediatric Nursing, 32*(3), 195–201.

Thureen, P. J., Deacon, J., Hernandez, J., & Hall, D. M. (2005). *Assessment and care of the well newborn* (2nd ed.). Philadelphia: Saunders.

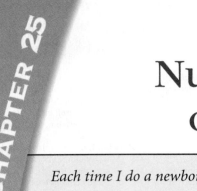
Nursing Assessment of the Newborn

Each time I do a newborn's first bath I am struck anew by the magic of human life. It is one of my favorite parts of the day.

—Newborn Nursery Nurse

LEARNING OUTCOMES

25-1. Describe the physical and neuromuscular maturity characteristics assessed to determine the gestational age of the newborn.

25-2. Explain the components and methods of a systematic physical assessment of the newborn.

25-3. Describe the normal physical characteristics and normal variations of the newborn considered in a newborn assessment.

25-4. Compare abnormal findings in a newborn physical assessment to possible causes and nursing responses.

25-5. Explain the components and methods for assessing neurologic/ neuromuscular status and reflexes.

25-6. Describe the normal neurologic/ neuromuscular characteristics and reflexes of the newborn considered in a newborn neurologic assessment.

25-7. Compare abnormal findings in a newborn neurologic assessment to possible causes and nursing responses.

25-8. Explain the components and methods of a behavioral assessment of the newborn.

25-9. Describe the normal behavioral characteristics and normal variations of the newborn considered in a newborn behavioral assessment.

25-10. Compare abnormal findings in a newborn behavioral assessment to possible causes and nursing responses.

25-11. Use the assessment procedure and results of the newborn physical, neurologic, and behavioral assessments to teach and involve parents in the care of the newborn.

KEY TERMS

U nlike the adult, the newborn communicates needs primarily by behavior. Because nurses are the most consistent professional observers of the newborn, they can translate this behavior into information about the newborn's condition and respond with appropriate nursing interventions. This chapter focuses on the assessment of the newborn and the interpretation of these findings.

Assessment of the newborn is a continuous process designed to evaluate development and adjustments to extrauterine life. In the birth setting, the Apgar scoring procedure (see Chapter 19 ∞ for discussion) and careful observation form the basis of assessment and are correlated with information such as the following:

- Maternal prenatal care history
- Birthing history
- Maternal analgesia and anesthesia
- Complications of labor or birth
- Treatment instituted immediately after birth, in conjunction with determination of clinical gestational age
- Consideration of the classification of newborns by weight and gestational age and by neonatal mortality risk
- Physical examination of the newborn

The nurse incorporates data from these sources with the assessment findings during the first 1 to 4 hours after birth to formulate a plan for nursing intervention.

The various newborn assessments and the data obtained from them are valuable only to the degree to which they are shared with the parents. The parents must be included in the assessment process from the moment of their child's birth. The *Apgar score* and its meaning should be explained immediately to the family. As soon as possible, the parents should take part in the physical and behavioral assessments as well.

The nurse encourages the parents to identify the unique behavioral characteristics of their newborn and to learn nurturing activities. Attachment is promoted when parents have an opportunity to explore their newborn in private and identify individual physical and behavioral characteristics.

The nurse's supportive responses to parents' questions and observations are essential throughout the assessment process. The newborn physical examination is the beginning of newborn health surveillance and health education for the newborn's family that continues into the community setting.

Timing of Newborn Assessments

During the first 24 hours of life, the newborn makes the critical transition from intrauterine to extrauterine life. The risk of mortality and morbidity is statistically high during this period. Assessment of the newborn is essential to ensure that the transition proceeds successfully.

There are three major time frames for assessments of newborns while they are in the birth facility.

- The first assessment is done in the birthing area immediately after birth to determine the need for resuscitation or other interventions. The stable newborn can stay with the family after birth to initiate early attachment. The newborn with complications is usually taken to the nursery for further evaluation and intervention.
- A second assessment is done by the nursery nurse as part of routine admission procedures. During this assessment, the nurse carries out a brief physical examination to estimate gestational age and evaluate the newborn's adaptation to extrauterine life. No later than 2 hours after birth, the admitting nursery nurse should evaluate the newborn's status and any problems that place the newborn at risk (American Academy of Pediatrics [AAP] & American College of Obstetricians and Gynecologists [ACOG], 2007).
- Before discharge, a certified nurse-midwife, physician, or nurse practitioner will carry out a behavioral assessment and a complete physical examination to detect any emerging or potential problems. A general assessment is also done at this time. See Key Facts to Remember: Timing and Types of Newborn Assessments.

KEY FACTS TO REMEMBER
Timing and Types of Newborn Assessments

Assess immediately after birth: need for resuscitation or if newborn is stable and can be placed with parents to initiate early attachment and bonding.

Assessments within 1 to 4 hours after birth:
- Progress of newborn's adaptation to extrauterine life
- Determination of gestational age
- Ongoing assessment for high-risk problems

Assessment procedures within first 24 hours or before discharge:
- Complete physical examination (Depending on agency protocol, the nurse may complete some components independently or with the certified nurse-midwife, physician, or nurse practitioner completing the exam before discharge.)
- Nutritional status and ability to formula-feed or breastfeed satisfactorily
- Behavioral state organization abilities

This chapter presents the procedures for estimating gestational age and performing the complete physical examination and behavioral assessment. Chapter 19 ∞ discusses the immediate postbirth assessment. Chapter 26 ∞ describes the brief assessment performed during the first 4 hours of life.

Estimation of Gestational Age

The nurse must establish the newborn's gestational age in the first 4 hours after birth so that careful attention can be given to age-related problems. Traditionally, a newborn's gestational age was determined from the date of the pregnant woman's last menstrual period. However, this method was accurate only 75% to 85% of the time. Because of the problems that develop with the preterm newborn or the newborn whose weight is inappropriate for gestational age, a more accurate system was developed to postnatally evaluate the newborn. Once learned, the procedure can be done in a few minutes. *It is essential that the nurse wear gloves when assessing the newborn in these early hours after birth and before the first bath until amniotic fluid, as well as vaginal and bloody secretions, on the skin are removed.*

Clinical **gestational age assessment tools** have two components: (1) external physical characteristics and (2) neurologic or neuromuscular development. Physical characteristics generally include sole creases, amount of breast tissue, the amount of lanugo, cartilaginous development of the ear, and testicular descent and scrotal rugae or labial development. These objective clinical criteria are not influenced by labor and birth and do not change significantly within the first 12 hours after birth.

Neurologic examination facilitates assessment of functional or physiologic maturation in addition to physical development. However, the newborn's nervous system is unstable during the first 24 hours of life. Therefore, neurologic evaluation findings based on reflexes or assessments dependent on the higher brain centers may not be reliable. If the neurologic findings drastically deviate from the gestational age derived by evaluation of external characteristics, a second assessment is done in 24 hours.

The neurologic assessment components (excluding reflexes) can aid in assessing the gestational age of newborns of less than 34 weeks' gestation. Between 26 and 34 weeks, neurologic changes are significant, whereas significant physical changes are less evident. One significant neuromuscular change is that muscle tone progresses from extensor tone to flexor tone in the extremities as the neurological system matures in a *caudocephalad* (tail-to-head) progression.

Ballard, Khoury, Wedig et al. (1991) developed the *estimation of gestational age by maturity rating*, a simplified version of the well-researched **Dubowitz tool**. The Ballard tool omits some of the neuromuscular tone assessments, such as head lag, ventral suspension (which is difficult to assess in very ill newborns or those on respirators), and leg recoil. In the Ballard tool, each physical and neuromuscular finding is given a value, and the total score is matched to a gestational age (Figure 25–1 ■). The maximum score on the Ballard tool is 50, which corresponds to a gestational age of 44 weeks.

For example, on completion of a gestational assessment of a 1-hour-old newborn, the nurse gives a score of 3 to all the physical characteristics, for a total of 18, and gives a score of 3 to all neuromuscular assessments, for a total of 18. The physical characteristics score of 18 is added to the neurologic score of 18 for a total score of 36, which correlates with 38+ weeks' gestation. Because all newborns vary slightly in the development of physical characteristics and maturation of neurologic function, scores usually vary instead of all being 3, as in this example.

Postnatal gestational age assessment tools can overestimate preterm gestational age and underestimate postterm gestational age. The tools have been shown to lose accuracy when newborns of less than 28 weeks' or more than 43 weeks' gestation are assessed. Ballard et al. (1991) in the **New Ballard Score (NBS)** added criteria for more accurate assessment of the gestational age of newborns between 20 and 28 weeks' gestation and less than 1500 g. They suggest that the assessments should be made within 12 hours of birth to optimize accuracy, especially in infants of less than 26 weeks' gestational age. Also the Ballard assessment may be overstimulating to infants of less than 27 weeks' gestation. Some maternal conditions, such as preeclampsia, diabetes,

NEWBORN MATURITY RATING & CLASSIFICATION

ESTIMATION OF GESTATIONAL AGE BY MATURITY RATING
Symbols: X - 1st Exam O - 2nd Exam

NEUROMUSCULAR MATURITY

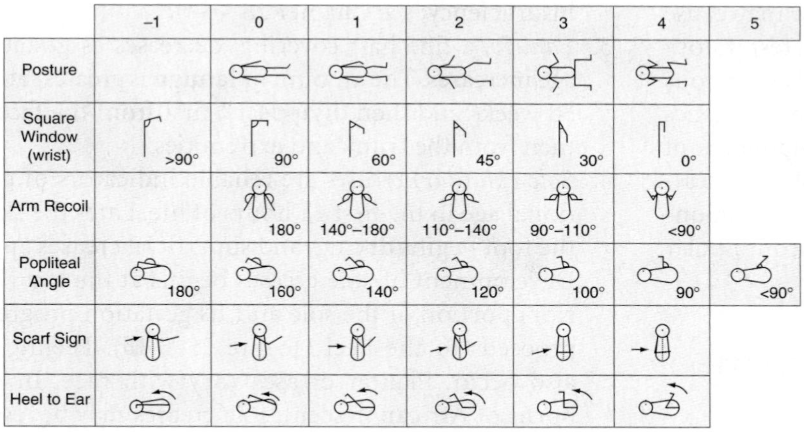

	−1	0	1	2	3	4	5
Posture							
Square Window (wrist)	>90°	90°	60°	45°	30°	0°	
Arm Recoil		180°	140°–180°	110°–140°	90°–110°	<90°	
Popliteal Angle	180°	160°	140°	120°	100°	90°	<90°
Scarf Sign							
Heel to Ear							

Gestation by Dates _____ wks

_____

Birth Date _____ Hour _____ a.m. / p.m.

APGAR _____ 1 min _____ 5 min

MATURITY RATING

score	weeks
−10	20
−5	22
0	24
5	26
10	28
15	30
20	32
25	34
30	36
35	38
40	40
45	42
50	44

PHYSICAL MATURITY

	−1	0	1	2	3	4	5
Skin	sticky friable transparent	gelatinous red, translucent	smooth pink, visible veins	superficial peeling &/or rash, few veins	cracking pale areas rare veins	parchment deep cracking no vessels	leathery cracked wrinkled
Lanugo	none	sparse	abundant	thinning	bald areas	mostly bald	
Plantar Surface	heel-toe 40–50 mm:−1 <40 mm:−2	>50 mm no crease	faint red marks	anterior transverse crease only	creases ant. 2/3	creases over entire sole	
Breast	imperceptible	barely perceptible	flat areola no bud	stippled areola 1–2 mm bud	raised areola 3–4 mm bud	full areola 5–10 mm bud	
Eye/Ear	lids fused loosely:−1 tightly:−2	lids open pinna flat stays folded	sl. curved pinna; soft; slow recoil	well curved pinna; soft but ready recoil	formed & firm instant recoil	thick cartilage ear stiff	
Genitals male	scrotum flat, smooth	scrotum empty faint rugae	testes in upper canal rare rugae	testes descending few rugae	testes down good rugae	testes pendulous deep rugae	
Genitals female	clitoris prominent labia flat	prominent clitoris small labia minora	prominent clitoris enlarging minora	majora & minora equally prominent	majora large minora small	majora cover clitoris & minora	

SCORING SECTION

	1st Exam = X	2nd Exam = 0
Estimating Gest Age by Maturity Rating	_____Weeks	_____Weeks
Time of Exam	Date _____ Hour___ a.m. p.m.	Date _____ Hour___ a.m. p.m.
Age at Exam	_____ Hours	_____ Hours
Signature of Examiner	_____ M.D.	_____ M.D.

FIGURE 25–1 Newborn maturity rating and classification. If a 1-hour-old newborn is given a score of 3 for each of the physical characteristics and neuromuscular assessments, the newborn's total score would be 36. A total score of 36 correlates with 38 or more weeks' gestation.
Source: Ballard, J. L., Khoury, J. C., Wedig, K., Wang, L., Eilers-Walsmann, B. L., & Lipp, R. (1991). New Ballard score, expanded to include extremely premature infants. *Journal of Pediatrics, 119*(3), 417.

and maternal analgesia and anesthesia, may affect certain gestational assessment components and warrant further evaluation. Maternal diabetes, although it appears to accelerate fetal physical growth, seems to retard maturation. Maternal hypertension states, which retard fetal physical growth, seem to speed maturation.

Newborns of women with preeclampsia have a poor correlation with the criteria involving active muscle tone and edema. Maternal analgesia and anesthesia may cause respiratory depression in the baby. Babies with respiratory distress syndrome (RDS) tend to be flaccid and edematous and to assume a "froglike" posture. These characteristics affect the scoring of the neuromuscular components of the assessment tool used. The NBS gestational age assessment tool will be used throughout the chapter to demonstrate the assessment of the physical and neuromuscular criteria associated with gestational age.

Assessment of Physical Maturity Characteristics

The nurse first evaluates observable characteristics without disturbing the baby. Selected physical characteristics common to the Dubowitz and Ballard gestational assessment tools are presented here in the order in which they might be most effectively evaluated:

1. *Resting posture,* although a neuromuscular component, should be assessed as the baby lies undisturbed on a flat surface (Figure 25–2 ■).

2. *Skin* in the preterm newborn appears thin and transparent, with veins prominent over the abdomen early in gestation. As the newborn approaches term, the skin appears opaque because of increased subcutaneous tissue. Disappearance of the protective vernix caseosa promotes skin desquamation; this is commonly seen in postmature infants (infants of more than 42 weeks' gestational age) and those showing signs of placental insufficiency; see Chapter 28 ∞).

3. *Lanugo,* a fine hair covering, decreases as gestational age increases. The amount of **lanugo** is greatest at 28 to 30 weeks and then disappears, first from the face and then from the trunk and extremities.

4. *Sole (plantar) creases* are reliable indicators of gestational age in the first 12 hours of life. Later the skin of the foot begins drying, and superficial creases appear. Development of sole creases begins at the top (anterior) portion of the sole and, as gestation progresses, proceeds to the heel (Figure 25–3 ■). Peeling may also occur. Plantar creases vary with race. In newborns of African descent, sole creases may be less developed at term.

5. The nurse inspects the *areola* and gently palpates the *breast bud tissue* by applying the forefinger and middle finger to the breast area and measuring the tissue between them in centimeters or millimeters (Figure 25–4 ■). At term gestation, the tissue measures between 0.5 and 1 cm (5 and 10 mm). During the assessment, the nipple should not be grasped firmly because skin and subcutaneous tissue will prevent accurate estimation of size. The nurse

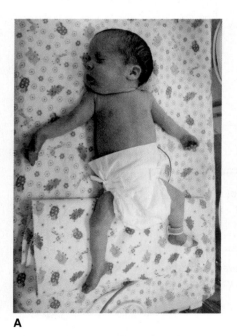
A

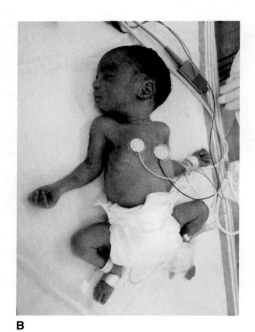
B

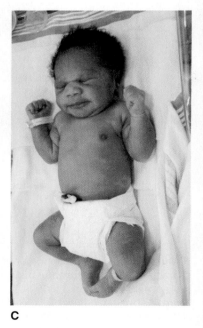
C

Figure 25–2 Resting posture. *A,* Newborn exhibits beginning of flexion of the thigh (score 1 or 2). The gestational age is approximately 31 weeks. Note the extension of the upper extremities. *B,* Newborn exhibits stronger flexion of the arms, hips, and thighs (score 3). The gestational age is approximately 35 weeks. *C,* The full-term newborn exhibits hypertonic flexion of all extremities (score 4).

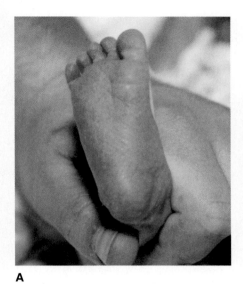
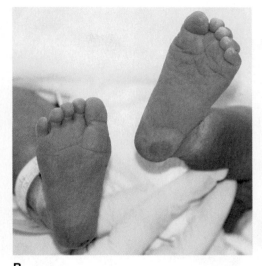
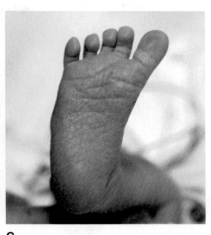

A   **B**   **C**

FIGURE 25–3 Sole creases. *A,* Newborn has a few sole creases on the anterior portion of the foot. Note the slick heel (score 2). The gestational age is approximately 35 weeks. *B,* Newborn has a deeper network of sole creases on the anterior two-thirds of the sole. Note the slick heel (score 3). The gestational age is approximately 37 weeks. *C,* The term newborn has deep sole creases down to and including the heel as the skin loses fluid and dries after birth (score 4). Sole (plantar) creases can be seen even in preterm newborns.

must do this procedure gently to avoid causing trauma to the breast tissue.

As gestation progresses, the breast tissue mass and areola enlarge. However, a large breast tissue mass can occur as a result of specific conditions other than advanced gestational age or the effects of maternal hormones on the baby. In the large-for-gestational-age infant, a diabetic mother's accelerated develop-

ment of breast tissue is a reflection of subcutaneous fat deposits. Small-for-gestational-age (SGA) term or postterm newborns may have used subcutaneous fat (which would have been deposited as breast tissue) to survive in utero; as a result, their lack of breast tissue may indicate a gestational age of 34 to 35 weeks, even though other factors indicate a term or postterm newborn.

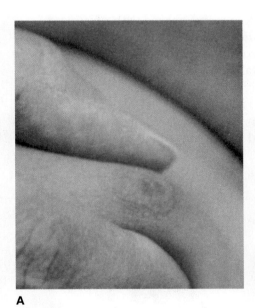
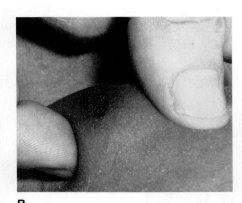
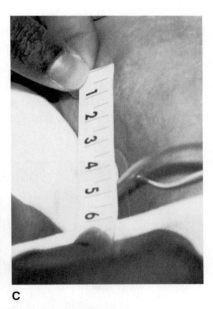

A   **B**   **C**

FIGURE 25–4 Breast tissue. *A,* Newborn has steppled areola, a visible raised area of 0.75 cm (0.3 in.) diameter (score 3). The gestational age is 38 weeks. *B,* Newborn has 10 mm breast tissue area (score 4). The gestational age is 40 to 44 weeks. *C,* Gently compress the tissue between the middle and index fingers and measure the tissue in centimeters or millimeters. Absence of or decreased breast tissue often indicates premature or small-for-gestational-age newborn.
Source: B from Dubowitz, L., & Dubowitz, V. (1977). *The gestational age of the newborn.* Menlo Park, CA: Addison-Wesley. Reprinted by permission of V. Dubowitz, MD, Hammersmith Hospital, London, England.

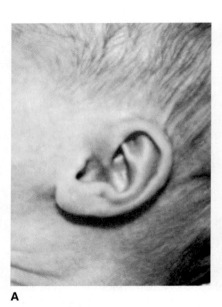 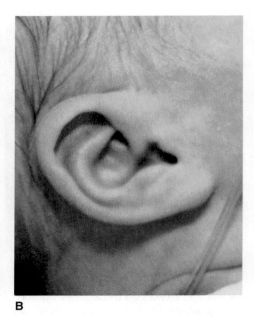 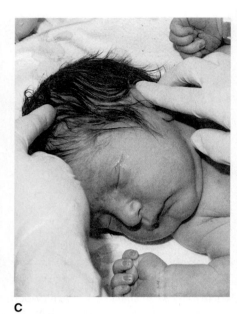

A   **B**   **C**

FIGURE 25–5 Ear form and cartilage. *A,* The ear of the infant at approximately 36 weeks' gestation shows incurving of the upper two-thirds of the pinna (score 2). *B,* Infant at term shows well-defined incurving of the entire pinna (score 3). *C,* If the auricle stays in the position in which it is pressed or returns slowly to its original position, it usually means the gestational age is less than 38 weeks.

6. *Ear form and cartilage distribution* develop with gestational age. The cartilage gives the ear its shape and substance (Figure 25–5 ■). In a newborn of less than 34 weeks' gestation, the ear is relatively shapeless and flat; it has little cartilage, so the ear folds over on itself and remains folded. By approximately 36 weeks' gestation, some cartilage and incurving of the upper pinna are present, and the pinna springs back slowly when folded. (The nurse tests this response by holding the top and bottom of the pinna together with the forefinger and thumb and then releasing them or by folding the pinna of the ear forward against the side of the head, releasing it, and observing the response.) By term, the newborn's pinna is firm, stands away from the head, and springs back quickly from the folding.

7. *Male genitals* are evaluated for size of the scrotal sac, presence of rugae (wrinkles and ridges in the scrotum), and descent of the testes (Figure 25–6 ■). Before 36 weeks, the scrotum has few rugae, and the testes are palpable in the inguinal canal. By 36 to 38 weeks, the testes are in the upper scrotum, and rugae have developed over the anterior portion of the scrotum. By term, the testes are generally in the lower scrotum, which is pendulous and covered with rugae.

8. The appearance of the *female genitals* depends in part on subcutaneous fat deposition and therefore relates to fetal nutritional status (Figure 25–7 ■). The clitoris varies in size, and occasionally is so swollen that it is difficult to identify the sex of the newborn. This swelling may be caused by adrenogenital syndrome, which causes the adrenals

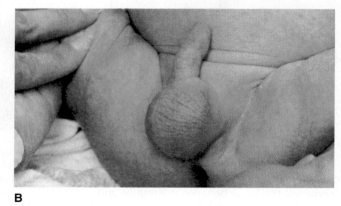

A   **B**

FIGURE 25–6 Male genitals. *A,* Preterm newborn's testes are not within the scrotum. The scrotal surface has few rugae (score 2). *B,* Term newborn's testes are generally fully descended. The entire surface of the scrotum is covered by rugae (score 3).

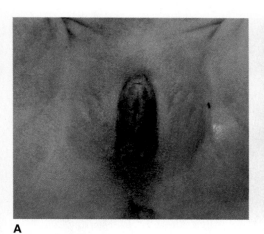
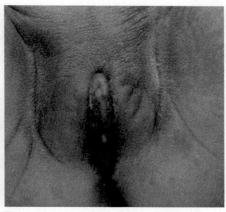
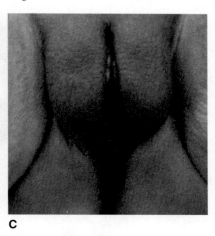

A   **B**   **C**

FIGURE 25–7 Female genitals. *A,* Newborn has a prominent clitoris. The labia majora are widely separated, and the labia minora, viewed laterally, would protrude beyond the labia majora (score 1). The gestational age is 30 to 36 weeks. *B,* The clitoris is still visible. The labia minora and labia majora are equally prominent (score 2). The gestational age is 36 to 40 weeks. *C,* The term newborn has developed large labia majora that cover both clitoris and labia minora (score 3).

to secrete excessive amounts of androgen and other hormones. At 30 to 32 weeks' gestation, the clitoris is prominent, and the labia majora are small and widely separated. As gestational age increases, the labia majora increase in size. At 36 to 40 weeks, they nearly cover the clitoris. At 40 weeks and beyond, the labia majora cover the labia minora and clitoris.

Other physical characteristics assessed by some gestational age scoring tools include the following:

1. *Vernix* covers the preterm newborn. The postterm newborn has no vernix. After noting vernix distribution, the birthing area nurse (wearing gloves) dries the newborn to prevent evaporative heat loss, thus disturbing the vernix and potentially altering this gestational age criterion.
2. *Hair* of the preterm newborn has the consistency of matted wool or fur and lies in bunches rather than in the silky, single strands of the term newborn's hair.
3. *Skull firmness* increases as the fetus matures. In a term newborn the bones are hard, and the sutures are not easily displaced. The nurse should not attempt to displace the sutures forcibly.
4. *Nails* appear and cover the nail bed at about 20 weeks' gestation. Nails extending beyond the fingertips may indicate a postterm newborn.

Assessment of Neuromuscular Maturity Characteristics

The central nervous system of the fetus matures at a fairly constant rate. Tests have been designed to evaluate neurologic status as manifested by development of neuromuscular tone. As noted earlier, neuromuscular tone in the fetus develops in a caudocephalic direction, from the lower to the upper extremities.

The neuromuscular evaluation requires more manipulation and disturbances than the physical evaluation of the newborn. The neuromuscular evaluation (see Figure 25–1) is best performed when the infant has stabilized.

1. The *square window sign* is elicited by gently flexing the newborn's hand toward the ventral forearm until resistance is felt. The angle formed at the wrist is measured (Figure 25–8 ■).
2. *Recoil* is a test of flexion development. Because flexion first develops in the lower extremities, recoil is first tested in the legs. The nurse places the newborn on its back on a flat surface. With a hand on the newborn's knees, the nurse places the baby's legs in flexion, then extends them parallel to each other and flat on the surface. The response to this maneuver is recoil of the newborn's legs. According to gestational age, they may not move or they may return slowly or quickly to the flexed position. Preterm infants have less muscle tone than term infants, so preterm infants have less recoil.

   Arm recoil is tested by flexion at the elbow and extension of the arms at the newborn's side. While the baby is in the supine position, the nurse completely flexes both elbows, holds them in this position for 5 seconds, extends the arms at the baby's side, and releases them. On release, the elbows of a full-term newborn form an angle of less than 90 degrees and rapidly recoil back to a flexed position. The elbows of a preterm newborn have slower recoil time and form an angle greater than 90 degrees. Arm recoil is also slower in healthy but fatigued newborns after birth; therefore arm recoil is best elicited after the first hour of birth, when the baby has had time to recover from the stress of the birth. The deep sleep state also

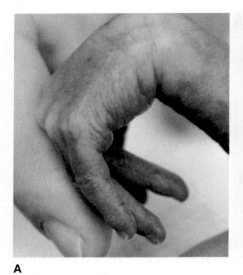
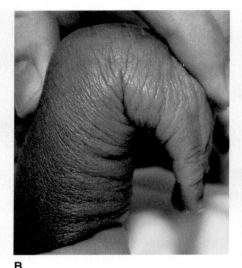
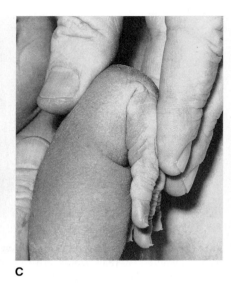

A   B   C

FIGURE 25–8 Square window sign. *A,* This angle is 90 degrees and suggests an immature newborn of 28 to 32 weeks' gestation (Score 0). *B,* A 30- to 40-degree angle is commonly found from 38 to 40 weeks' gestation (score 2 to 3). *C,* A 0-degree angle can occur from 40 to 42 weeks' gestation (score 4).
Source: C is from Dubowitz, L, & Dubowitz, V. (1977). The gestational age of the newborn. Menlo Park, CA: Addison-Wesley. Reprinted by permission of V. Dubowitz, MD, Hammersmith Hospital, London, England.

decreases the arm recoil response. Assessment of arm recoil should be bilateral to rule out brachial palsy.

3. The *popliteal angle* (degree of knee flexion) is determined with the newborn flat on its back. The thigh is flexed on the abdomen and chest, and the nurse places the index finger of the other hand behind the newborn's ankle to extend the lower leg until resistance is met. The angle formed is then measured. Results vary from no resistance in the very immature newborn to an 80-degree angle in the term newborn.

4. The *scarf sign* is elicited by placing the newborn supine and drawing an arm across the chest toward the new-

born's opposite shoulder until resistance is met. The location of the elbow is then noted in relation to the midline of the chest (Figure 25–9 ■). A preterm infant's elbow will cross the midline of the chest, whereas a full-term infant's elbow will not cross midline.

5. The *heel-to-ear extension* is performed by placing the newborn in a supine position and then gently drawing the foot toward the ear on the same side until resistance is felt. The nurse should allow the knee to bend during the test. It is important to hold the buttocks down to keep from rolling the baby. Both the proximity of foot to ear and the degree of knee extension are assessed. A preterm,

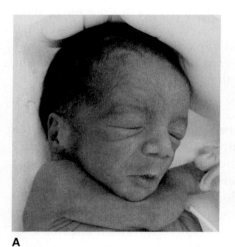
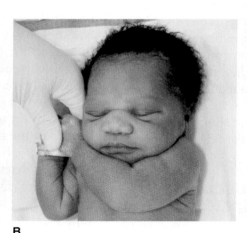
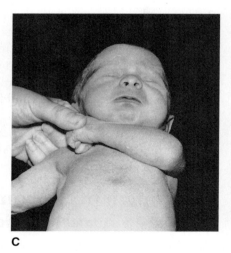

A   B   C

FIGURE 25–9 Scarf sign. *A,* No resistance is noted until after 30 weeks' gestation. The elbow moves readily past the midline (score 1). *B,* The elbow is at midline at 36 to 40 weeks' gestation (score 2). *C,* Beyond 40 weeks' gestation the elbow will not reach the midline (score 4).
Source: C is from Dubowitz, L, & Dubowitz, V. (1977). The gestational age of the newborn. Menlo Park, CA: Addison-Wesley. Reprinted by permission of V. Dubowitz, MD, Hammersmith Hospital, London, England.

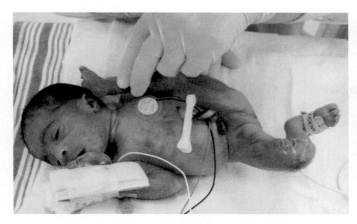

FIGURE 25–10 Heel to ear. No resistance. Leg fully extended (score 0).

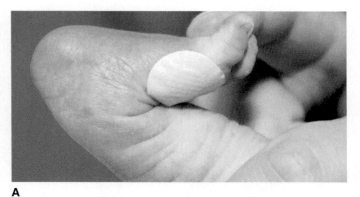

A

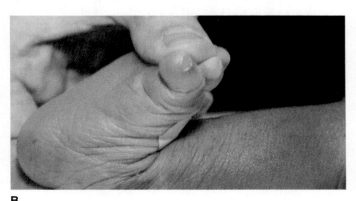

B

FIGURE 25–11 Ankle dorsiflexion. *A,* A 45-degree angle indicates 32 to 36 weeks' gestation. A 20-degree angle indicates 36 to 40 weeks' gestation (score 2 to 3). *B,* A 15- to 0-degree angle is common at 40 weeks' or more gestational age (score 4).

immature newborn's leg will remain straight and the foot will go to the ear or beyond (Figure 25–10 ■). With advancing gestational age, the newborn demonstrates increasing resistance to this maneuver. Maneuvers involving the lower extremities of newborns who had frank breech presentation should be delayed to allow for resolution of leg positioning.

6. *Ankle dorsiflexion* is determined by flexing the ankle on the shin. The nurse uses a thumb to push on the sole of the newborn's foot while the fingers support the back of the leg. Then the angle formed by the foot and the interior leg is measured (Figure 25–11 ■). This sign can be influenced by intrauterine position and congenital deformities.

7. *Head lag* (neck flexor) is measured by pulling the newborn to a sitting position and noting the degree of head lag. Total lag is common in newborns up to 34 weeks' gestation, whereas postterm newborns (42+ weeks) hold their heads in front of their body lines. Full-term newborns can support their heads momentarily.

8. *Ventral suspension* (horizontal position) is evaluated by holding the newborn prone on the nurse's hand. The position of the head and back and the degree of flexion in the arms and legs are noted. Some flexion of arms and legs indicates 36 to 38 weeks' gestation; fully flexed extremities, with head and back even, are characteristic of a term newborn.

9. *Major reflexes* such as sucking, rooting, grasping, Moro, tonic neck, Babinski, and others are evaluated during the newborn exam. These reflexes are discussed later in the chapter.

A supplementary method for estimating gestational age (done by the physician or nurse practitioner) is to view the vascular network of the cornea with an ophthalmoscope. The nurse may need to delay administration of prophylactic eye ointment in preterm infants until after

this vascular eye exam is done. The amount of vascularity present over the surface of the lens assists in identifying infants of 27 through 34 weeks' gestational age (Rosenberg, 2007).

When the gestational age determination and birth weight are considered together, the newborn can be identified as one whose growth is *below the 10th percentile, or small for gestational age (SGA); appropriate for gestational age (AGA); or above the 90th percentile, which is large for gestational age (LGA)* (Figure 25–12 ■). This determination enables the nurse to anticipate possible physiologic problems. This information is used in conjunction with a complete physical examination, to establish a plan of care appropriate for the individual newborn. For example, an SGA or LGA newborn often requires frequent glucose monitoring and early feedings started soon after birth as they are at risk for hypoglycemia. (See Chapter 28 ∞ for more complete discussion of these categories and the potential problems associated with them.)

The nurse also plots the gestational age against the newborn's length, head circumference, and weight on the appropriate growth chart to determine if these measurements fall within the average range—the 10th to 90th percentile

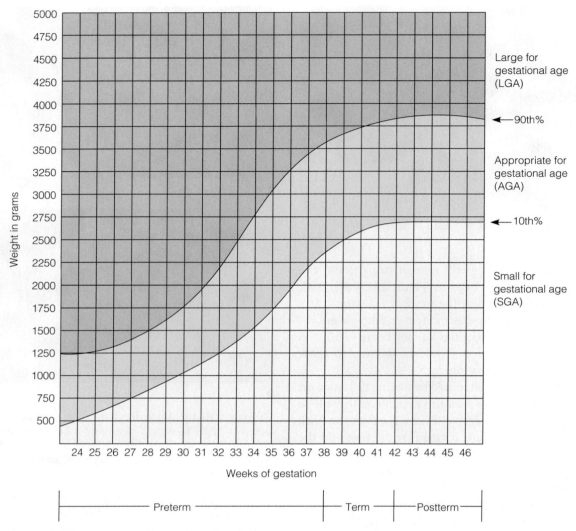

FIGURE 25–12 Classification of newborns by birth weight and gestational age. The nurse places the newborn's birth weight and gestational age on the graph and classifies the newborn as large for gestational age (LGA), appropriate for gestational age (AGA), or small for gestational age (SGA).
Source: Battaglia, F. C., & Lubchenco, L. O. (1967). A practical classification of newborn infants by weight and gestational age. *Journal of Pediatrics, 71*, 161.

for the corresponding gestational age (Figure 25–13 ■). These correlations further document the level of maturity and appropriate category for the newborn. The comparison of the infant's weight-length ratio further facilitates identification of SGA infants as having symmetrical or asymmetrical growth restriction. (See Chapter 28 ∞ for further discussion.) Measuring weight and height often aggravates newborns and may alter their vital signs. For better accuracy, take the newborn's vital signs before weighing and measuring the infant.

Physical Assessment

After the initial determination of gestational age and related potential problems, the nurse carries out a more extensive physical assessment in a warm, well-lit area that is free of drafts. Completing the physical assessment in the presence of the parents provides an opportunity to acquaint them with their unique newborn. The examination is performed in a systematic, head-to-toe manner, and all findings are recorded. When assessing the physical and neurologic status of the newborn, the nurse should first consider general appearance and then proceed to specific areas.

The Assessment Guide: Newborn Physical Assessment on pages 616–627 outlines how to systematically assess the newborn. Normal findings, alterations, and related causes are presented and correlated with suggested nursing responses. The findings are typical for a full-term newborn.

General Appearance

The newborn's head is disproportionately large for its body. The neck looks short because the chin rests on the chest. Newborns have a prominent abdomen, sloping shoulders,

CLASSIFICATION OF NEWBORNS—
BASED ON MATURITY AND INTRAUTERINE GROWTH

Symbols: X-1st Exam O-2nd Exam

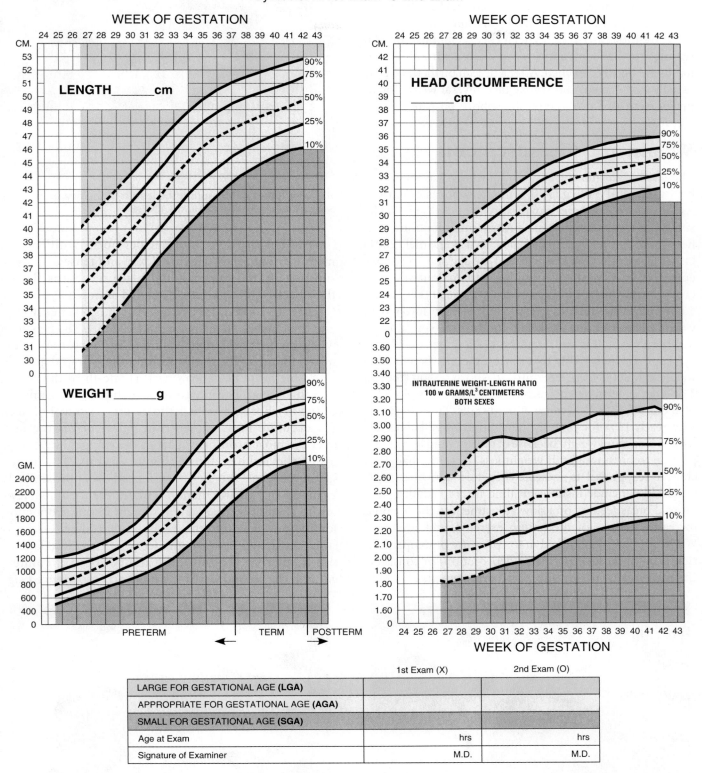

	1st Exam (X)	2nd Exam (O)
LARGE FOR GESTATIONAL AGE **(LGA)**		
APPROPRIATE FOR GESTATIONAL AGE **(AGA)**		
SMALL FOR GESTATIONAL AGE **(SGA)**		
Age at Exam	hrs	hrs
Signature of Examiner	M.D.	M.D.

FIGURE 25–13 Classification of newborns based on maturity and intrauterine growth.
Source: Adapted from Lubchenco, L. O., Hansman, C., & Boyd, E. (1966). Intrauterine growth in length and head circumference as estimated from live births at gestational ages from 26 to 42 weeks. *Pediatrics, 37,* 403–408; Battaglia, F. C., & Lubchenco, L. O. (1967). A practical classification of newborn infants by weight and gestational age. *Journal of Pediatrics, 71,* 159.

narrow hips, and rounded chests. The center of the baby's body is the umbilicus rather than the symphysis pubis as in the adult. The body appears long and the extremities short.

Newborns tend to stay in a flexed position similar to the one maintained in utero and will offer resistance when the extremities are straightened. This flexed position contributes to the short appearance of the extremities. The hands are tightly clenched. After a breech birth, the feet are usually dorsiflexed, and it may take several weeks for the newborn to assume the typical newborn posture.

Weight and Measurements

The normal full-term Caucasian newborn has an average birth weight of 3405 g (7 lb, 8 oz). Newborns of African, Asian, or Mexican American descent are usually somewhat smaller at term whereas Native American infants are often heavier at term (Mandleco, 2004; Wu & Daniel, 2001). Other factors that influence weight are age and size of parents, health of mother (smoking and malnutrition decrease birth weight), and the interval between pregnancies (short intervals, such as every year, result in lower birth weight). After the first week, and for the first 6 months, the newborn's weight increases about 198 g (7 oz) weekly.

Approximately 70% to 75% of the newborn's body weight is water. During the initial newborn period (the first 3 or 4 days), term newborns have a physiologic weight loss of about 5% to 10% because of fluid shifts. This weight loss may reach 15% for preterm newborns. Large babies also tend to lose more weight because of greater fluid loss in proportion to birth weight. If weight loss is greater than 10%, clinical reappraisal is indicated. Factors contributing to weight loss include insufficient fluid intake resulting from delayed breastfeeding or a slow adjustment to the formula, increased volume of meconium excreted, and urination. Weight loss may be marked in the presence of temperature elevation (because of associated dehydration) or consistent chilling (because of nonshivering thermogenesis).

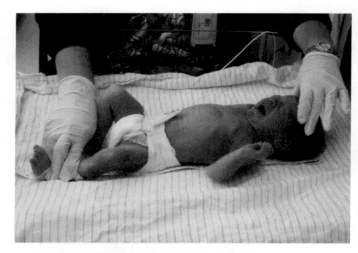

FIGURE 25–14 Measuring the length of the newborn.
Source: Courtesy of Vanessa Howell, RNC, BSN.

The length of the normal newborn is difficult to measure because the legs are flexed and tensed. To measure length, the nurse should place newborns flat on their backs with their legs extended as much as possible (Figure 25–14 ■). The average length is 50 cm (20 in.), and the range is 46 to 56 cm (18 to 22 in.). The newborn will grow approximately 2.5 cm (1 in.) a month for the next 6 months. This is the period of most rapid growth.

At birth the newborn's head is one-third the size of an adult's head. The circumference (biparietal diameter) of the newborn's head is 32 to 37 cm (12.5 to 14.5 in.). For accurate measurement, the nurse places the tape over the most prominent part of the occiput and brings it just above the eyebrows (Figure 25–15A ■). The circumference of the newborn's head is approximately 2 cm (0.8 in.) greater than the circumference of the newborn's chest at birth, and will remain in this proportion for the next few months. (Factors that alter this measurement are discussed in the section titled Head later in this chapter.) It is best to take another head circumference on the second day if the newborn experienced sig-

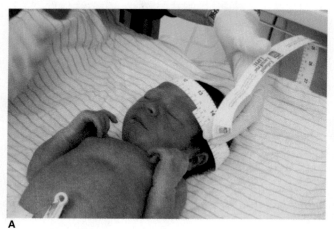

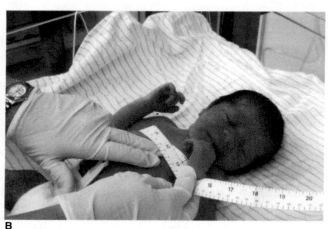

A **B**
FIGURE 25–15 *A,* Measuring the head circumference of the newborn. *B,* Measuring the chest circumference of the newborn.
Source: Courtesy of Vanessa Howell, RNC, BSN.

KEY FACTS TO REMEMBER

Newborn Measurements

Weight

Average: 3405 g (7 lb, 8 oz)

Range: 2500 to 4000 g (5 lb, 8 oz to 8 lb, 13 oz)

Weight is influenced by racial origin and maternal age and size.

Physiologic weight loss 5% to 10% for term newborns, up to 15% for preterm newborns

Growth: 198 g (7 oz) per week for first 6 months

Length

Average: 50 cm (20 in.)

Range: 46 to 56 cm (18 to 22 in.)

Growth: 2.5 cm (1 in.) per month for first 6 months

Head Circumference

32 to 37 cm (12.5 to 14.5 in.)

Approximately 2 cm larger than chest circumference

Chest Circumference

Average: 32 cm (12.5 in.)

Range: 30 to 35 cm (12 to 14 in.)

---

nificant head molding or developed a caput from the birth process.

The average circumference of the chest is 32 cm (12.5 in.) and ranges from 30 to 35 cm (12 to 14 in.). Chest measurements are taken with the tape measure placed at the lower edge of the scapulas and brought around anteriorly, directly over the nipple line (Figure 25–15B). The abdominal circumference, or girth, may also be measured at this time, by placing the tape around the newborn's abdomen at the level of the umbilicus, with the bottom edge of the tape at the top edge of the umbilicus. (See Key Facts to Remember: Newborn Measurements.)

Temperature

Initial assessment of the newborn's temperature is critical. In utero, the temperature of the fetus is about the same as, or slightly higher than, the expectant mother's. When babies enter the outside world, their temperature can suddenly drop as a result of exposure to cold drafts and the skin's heat loss mechanisms.

If no heat conservation measures are started, the normal term newborn's deep body temperature falls 0.1°C (0.2°F) per minute; skin temperature drops 0.3°C (0.5°F) per minute. Skin temperature markedly decreases within 10 minutes after exposure to room air. The temperature should stabilize within 8 to 12 hours. Temperature is monitored when the newborn is admitted to the nursery and at least every 30 minutes until the newborn's status has remained stable for 2 hours. Thereafter, the nurse should as-

sess temperature at least once every 8 hours, or according to institutional policy (AAP & ACOG, 2007). In infants who have been exposed to group B hemolytic streptococcus, more frequent temperature monitoring may be required. (See Chapter 24 ∞ for a discussion of the physiology of temperature regulation.)

Temperature can be assessed by the axillary skin method, a continuous skin probe, the rectal route, or a tympanic thermometer. Axillary temperature reflects body (core) temperature and the body's compensatory response to the thermal environment. Axillary temperatures are the preferred method and are considered to be a close estimation of the rectal temperature. In preterm and term newborns, there is less than 0.1°C (0.2°F) difference between temperatures between the two sites and the axillary method is preferred. With the axillary method, the thermometer must remain in place at least 3 minutes unless an electronic thermometer is used (Figure 25–16 ■). Axillary temperature ranges from 36.5°C to 37.0°C (97.7°F to 98.6°F). The nurse should keep in mind that axillary temperatures can be misleading, because the friction caused by apposition of the inner arm skin and upper chest wall and the nearness of brown fat to the probe may elevate the temperature.

Skin temperature is measured most accurately by means of continuous skin probe, especially for small newborns or newborns maintained in incubators or under radiant warmers. Normal skin temperature is 36°C to 36.5°C (96.8°F to 97.7°F). Continuous assessment of skin temperature allows time for initiation of interventions before a more serious fall in core temperature occurs (Figure 25–17 ■).

Rectal temperature is assumed to be the closest approximation to core temperature, but the accuracy of this method depends on the depth to which the thermometer is inserted. Normal rectal temperature is 36.6°C to 37.2°C (97.8°F to 99°F). The rectal route is *not* recommended as a routine method, because it may irritate the rectal mucosa and increase chances of perforation (Blackburn, 2007).

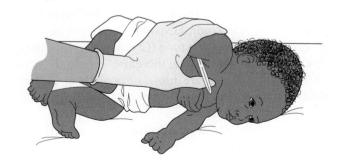

FIGURE 25–16 Axillary temperature measurement. The thermometer should remain in place for 3 minutes. The nurse presses the newborn's arm tightly but gently against the thermometer and the newborn's side, as illustrated.

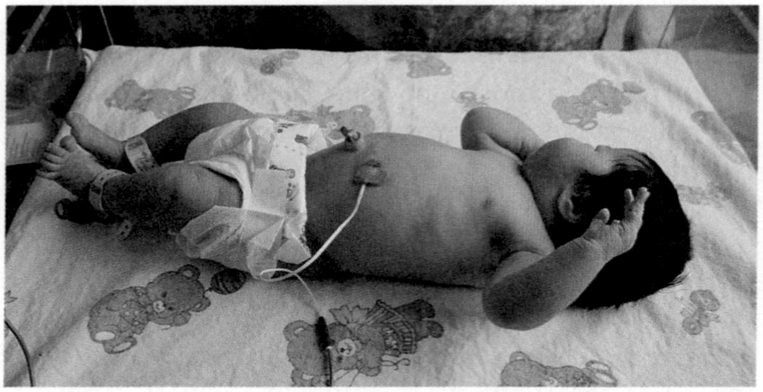

FIGURE 25–17 Temperature monitoring for the newborn. A skin thermal sensor is placed on the newborn's abdomen, upper thigh, or arm and secured with porous tape or a foil-covered foam pad.

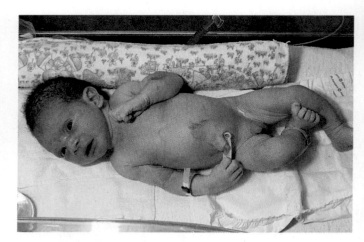

FIGURE 25–18 Acrocyanosis.

Temperature instability, a deviation of more than 1°C (2°F) from one reading to the next, or a subnormal temperature may indicate an infection. In contrast to an elevated temperature in older children, an increased temperature in a newborn may indicate a reaction to too many coverings, too hot a room, or dehydration. Dehydration, which tends to increase body temperature, occurs in newborns whose feedings have been delayed for any reason. Newborns may respond to overheating (a temperature greater than 37.5°C [99.5°F]) by increased restlessness and eventually by perspiration after 35 to 40 minutes of exposure (Blackburn, 2007). The perspiration appears initially on the head and face and then on the chest.

Skin Characteristics

Although the newborn's skin color varies with genetic background, all healthy newborns have a pink tinge to their skin. The ruddy hue results from increased red blood cell concentrations in the blood vessels and limited subcutaneous fat deposits.

Skin pigmentation is slight in the newborn period, so color changes may be seen even in darker skinned babies. Caucasian newborns have a pinkish red skin tone a few hours after birth, and African-American newborns have a reddish-brown skin color. Hispanic and Asian newborns have an olive or yellow skin tone (Creehan, 2008). Skin pigmentation deepens over time; therefore, variations in skin color indicating illness are more difficult to evaluate in African-American and Asian newborns (Creehan, 2008). A newborn who is cyanotic at rest and pink only with crying may have *choanal atresia* (congenital blockage of the passageway between the nose and pharynx). If crying increases the cyanosis, heart or lung problems should be suspected. Very pale newborns may be anemic or have hypovolemia (low BP) and should be evaluated for these problems.

Acrocyanosis (bluish discoloration of the hands and feet) may be present in the first 2 to 6 hours after birth (Figure 25–18 ■). This condition is caused by poor peripheral circulation, which results in vasomotor instability and capillary stasis, especially when the baby is exposed to cold. Blue hands and nails are a poor indicator of decreased oxygenation in a newborn. If the central circulation is adequate, the blood supply should return quickly (2 to 3 seconds) to the extremity after the skin is blanched with a finger. The nurse should assess the face and mucous membranes for pinkness that reflects adequate oxygenation.

Mottling (lacy pattern of dilated blood vessels under the skin) occurs as a result of general circulation fluctuations. It may last several hours to several weeks or may come and go periodically. Mottling may be related to chilling or prolonged apnea, sepsis, or hypothyroidism.

Harlequin sign (clown) color change is occasionally noted: A deep red color develops over one side of the newborn's body while the other side remains pale, so that the skin resembles a clown's suit. This color change results from a vasomotor disturbance in which blood vessels on one side dilate while the vessels on the other side constrict. It usually lasts from 1 to 20 minutes. Affected newborns may have single or multiple episodes, but they are transient and clinically insignificant. The nurse should document each occurrence.

Jaundice is first detectable on the face (where skin overlies cartilage) and the mucous membranes of the mouth and has a head-to-toe progression (Creehan, 2008). Jaundice advances from head to toe and regresses in the opposite direction. It is evaluated by blanching the tip of the nose, the forehead, the sternum, or the gum line. This procedure must be carried out in appropriate lighting. If jaundice is present, the area will appear yellowish immediately after blanching. Another area to assess for jaundice is the sclera. Evaluation and determination of the cause of jaundice must be initiated immediately to prevent possibly serious sequelae. The jaundice may be related to breastfeeding (some cases but extremely rare), hematomas, immature liver function, or bruises from forceps, or may be caused by blood incompatibility, oxytocin

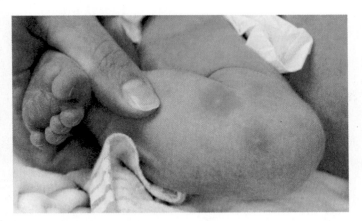

FIGURE 25–19 Erythema toxicum on leg.

(Pitocin) augmentation or induction, or a severe hemolysis process. Any jaundice noted before a newborn is 24 hours of age should be reported to the physician or neonatal nurse practitioner. (For discussion of various types of jaundice see Chapter 24 ∞ and for detailed discussion of causes and treatment for jaundice, see Chapter 29 ∞.)

Erythema toxicum is an eruption of lesions in the area surrounding a hair follicle that are firm, vary in size from 1 to 3 mm, and consist of a white or pale yellow papule or pustule with an erythematous base. It is often called "newborn rash" or "flea bite" dermatitis. The rash may appear suddenly, usually over the trunk and diaper area, and is frequently widespread (Figure 25–19 ■). The lesions do not appear on the palms of the hands or the soles of the feet. The peak incidence is at 24 to 48 hours of life. The condition rarely presents at birth or after 5 days of life. The cause is unknown, and no treatment is necessary. Some clinicians believe it may be caused by irritation from clothing. The lesions disappear in a few hours or days. If a maculopapular rash appears, a smear of the aspirated papule will show numerous eosinophils on staining; no bacteria will be cultured.

Milia, which are exposed sebaceous glands, appear as raised white spots on the face, especially across the nose (Figure 25–20 ■). No treatment is necessary, because they

will clear spontaneously within the first month. Infants of African heritage have a similar condition called transient neonatal pustular melanosis (Thureen, Deacon, Hernandez, & Hall, 2005).

Skin turgor is assessed to determine hydration status, the need to initiate early feedings, and the presence of any infectious processes. The usual place to assess skin turgor is over the abdomen, forearm, or thigh. Skin should be elastic and should return rapidly to its original shape.

Vernix caseosa, a whitish, cheeselike substance, covers the fetus while in utero and lubricates the skin of the newborn. The skin of the term or postterm newborn has less vernix and is frequently dry; peeling is common, especially on the hands and feet.

Forceps marks may be present after a difficult forceps birth. The newborn may have reddened areas over the cheeks and jaws. It is important to reassure the parents that these marks will disappear, usually within 1 or 2 days. Transient facial paralysis resulting from the forceps pressure is a rare complication. Vacuum extractor suction marks on the vertex of the scalp are often seen when vacuum extractors are used to assist with the birth. These marks are benign and do not indicate underlying brain lesions.

Birthmarks

Telangiectatic nevi (stork bites) appear as pale pink or red spots and are frequently found on the eyelids, nose, lower occipital bone, and nape of the neck (Figure 25–21 ■). These lesions are common in newborns with light complexions and are more noticeable during periods of crying. These areas have no clinical significance and usually fade by the second birthday.

Mongolian spots are macular areas of bluish black or gray-blue pigmentation on the dorsal area and the buttocks (Figure 25–22 ■). They are common in newborns of Asian, Hispanic, and African descent and other dark-skin races. They gradually fade during the first or second year

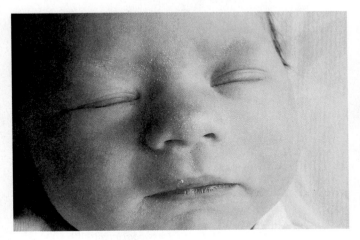

FIGURE 25–20 Facial milia.

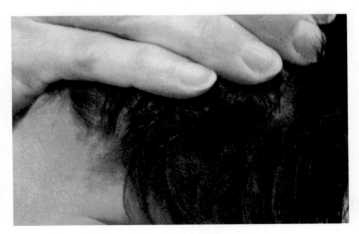

FIGURE 25–21 Stork bites on nape of neck.

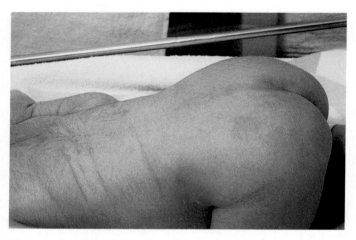

FIGURE 25–22 Mongolian spots.

of life. They may be mistaken for bruises and should be documented in the newborn's chart.

Nevus flammeus (port-wine stain) is a capillary angioma directly below the epidermis. It is a nonelevated, sharply demarcated, red-to-purple area of dense capillaries (Figure 25–23 ■). In infants of African descent, it may appear as a purple-black stain. The size and shape vary, but it commonly appears on the face. It does not grow in size, does not fade with time, and does not blanch as a rule. The birthmark may be concealed by using an opaque cosmetic cream. If convulsions and other neurologic problems accompany the nevus flammeus, the clinical picture is suggestive of *Sturge-Weber syndrome*, with involvement of the fifth cranial nerve (the ophthalmic branch of the trigeminal nerve).

Nevus vasculosus (strawberry mark) is a capillary hemangioma. It consists of newly formed and enlarged capillaries in the dermal and subdermal layers. It is a raised, clearly delineated, dark red, rough-surfaced birthmark commonly found in the head region. Such marks usually grow (often rapidly) starting during the second or third week of life and may not reach their fullest size for 1 to 3 months (Thureen, Deacon, Hernandez et al., 2005).

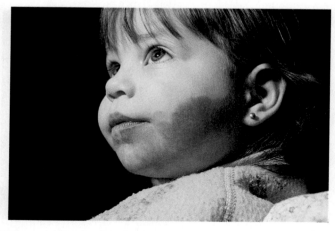

FIGURE 25–23 Port-wine stain.

They begin to shrink and start to resolve spontaneously several weeks to months after they reach peak growth. A pale purple or gray spot on the surface of the hemangioma signals the start of resolution. The best cosmetic effect is achieved when the lesions are allowed to resolve spontaneously.

Birthmarks are frequently a cause of concern for parents. The mother may be especially anxious, fearing that she is to blame ("Is my baby 'marked' because of something I did?"). Guilt feelings are common in the presence of misconceptions about the cause. Birthmarks should be identified and explained to the parents. By providing appropriate information about the cause and course of birthmarks, the nurse frequently relieves the fears and anxieties of the family. The nurse should note any bruises, abrasions, or birthmarks seen on admission to the nursery.

Head

General Appearance

The newborn's head is large (approximately one-fourth of the body size), with soft, pliable skull bones. For most term infants, the occipital-frontal circumference (OFC) is 32 to 37 cm (12.6 to 14.6 in.). The head may appear asymmetrical in the newborn of a vertex birth. This asymmetry, called **molding**, is caused by the overriding of the cranial bones during labor and birth (Figure 25–24 ■). The degree of

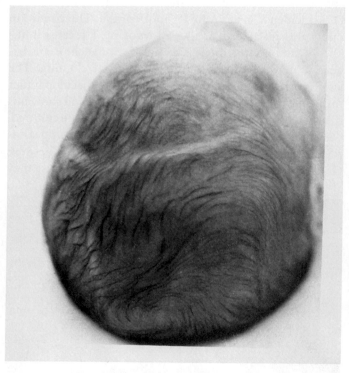

FIGURE 25–24 Overlapped cranial bones produce a visible ridge in a small, premature newborn. Easily visible overlapping does not occur often in term infants.
Source: Korones, S. B. (1986). *High-risk newborn infants* (4th ed.). St. Louis: Mosby.

molding varies with the amount and length of pressure exerted on the head. Within a few days after birth, the overriding usually diminishes and the suture lines become palpable. Because head measurements are affected by molding, a second measurement is indicated a few days after birth. The heads of breech-born newborns and those born by elective cesarean are characteristically round and well-shaped because no pressure was exerted on them during birth. Any extreme differences in head size may indicate microcephaly (abnormally small head) or hydrocephalus (an abnormal buildup of fluid in the brain). Variations in the shape, size, or appearance of the head measurements may be caused by *craniosynostosis* (premature closure of the cranial sutures), which will need to be corrected through surgery to allow brain growth, and *plagiocephaly* (asymmetry caused by pressure on the fetal head during gestation) (Thureen, Deacon, Hernandez et al., 2005).

Two *fontanelles* ("soft spots") may be palpated on the newborn's head. Fontanelles, which are openings at the juncture of the cranial bones, can be measured with the fingers. Accurate measurement necessitates that the examiner's finger be measured in centimeters. The assessment should be carried out with the newborn in a sitting position and not crying. The *diamond-shaped anterior fontanelle* is approximately 3 to 4 cm long by 2 to 3 cm wide. It is located at the juncture of the frontal and parietal bones. The *posterior fontanelle, smaller and triangular,* is formed by the parietal bones and the occipital bone and is 0.5 by 1 cm. Because of molding, the fontanelles are smaller immediately after birth than several days later. The anterior fontanelle closes within 18 months, whereas the posterior fontanelle closes within 8 to 12 weeks.

The fontanelles are a useful indicator of the newborn's condition. The anterior fontanelle may swell when the newborn cries or passes a stool or may pulsate with the heartbeat, which is normal. A bulging fontanelle usually signifies increased intracranial pressure, and a depressed fontanelle indicates dehydration (Creehan, 2008).

The sutures between the cranial bones should be palpated for the amount of overlapping. In newborns whose growth has been restricted the sutures may be wider than normal, and the fontanelles may also be larger because of impaired growth of the cranial bones. In addition to inspecting the newborn's head for degree of molding and size, the nurse should evaluate it for soft tissue edema and bruising.

Cephalohematoma

Cephalohematoma is a collection of blood resulting from ruptured blood vessels between the surface of a cranial bone (usually parietal) and the periosteal membrane (Figure 25–25 ■). The scalp in these areas feels loose and slightly edematous. These areas emerge as defined hematomas between the first and second day. Although

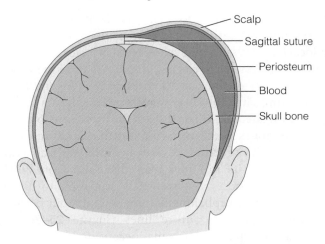

Scalp
Sagittal suture
Periosteum
Blood
Skull bone

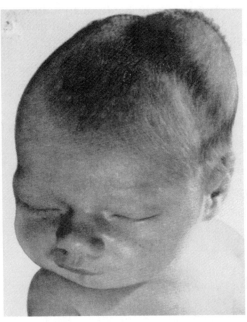

FIGURE 25–25 Cephalohematoma is a collection of blood between the surface of a cranial bone and the periosteal membrane. This is a cephalohematoma over the left parietal bone.
Source: Potter, E. L., & Craig, J. M. (1975). *Pathology of the fetus and infant* (3rd ed.). Chicago: Year Book Medical Publishers. Reproduced with permission.

external pressure may cause the mass to fluctuate, it does not increase in size when the newborn cries. Cephalohematomas may be unilateral or bilateral and do not cross suture lines. They are relatively common in vertex births and may disappear within 2 weeks to 3 months. They may be associated with physiologic jaundice, because extra red blood cells are being destroyed within the cephalohematoma. A large cephalohematoma can lead to anemia and hypotension.

Caput Succedaneum

Caput succedaneum is a localized, easily identifiable, soft area of the scalp, generally resulting from a long and difficult labor or vacuum extraction. The sustained pressure of the presenting part against the cervix results in compression of local blood vessels, and venous return is slowed. Slowed venous return in turn causes an increase in tissue fluids, an edematous swelling, and occasional bleeding under the periosteum. The caput may vary from a small area to a severely elongated head. The fluid in the caput is reabsorbed within 12 hours to a few days after birth. Caputs resulting from vacuum extractors are sharply outlined, circular areas up to 2 cm (0.8 in.) thick. They disappear more slowly than naturally occurring edema. It is possible to distinguish between a cephalohematoma and a caput because the caput overrides suture lines (Figure 25–26 ■), whereas the cephalohematoma, because of its location, never crosses a suture line. Also, caput succedaneum is present at birth, whereas cephalohematoma generally is not. See Table 25–1.

TABLE 25–1	Comparison of Cephalohematoma and Caput Succedaneum

Cephalohematoma

Collection of blood between cranial (usually parietal) bone and periosteal membrane

Does not cross suture lines

Does not increase in size with crying

Appears on first and second day

Disappears after 2 to 3 weeks or may take months

Caput Succedaneum

Collection of fluid, edematous swelling of the scalp

Crosses suture lines

Present at birth or shortly thereafter

Reabsorbed within 12 hours or a few days after birth

Hair

The term newborn's hair is smooth with texture variations depending on ethnic background (Creehan, 2008). Scalp hair is usually high over the eyebrows. Assessment of the newborn's hair characteristics such as color, quantity, texture, hairlines, direction of growth, and hair whorles can identify genetic, metabolic, and neurologic disorders. For example, coarse, brittle, and dry hair may indicate hypothyroidism.

Face

The newborn's face is well designed to help the newborn suckle. Sucking (fat) pads are located in the cheeks, and a labial tubercle (sucking callus) is frequently found in the center of the upper lip. The chin is recessed, and the nose is flattened. The lips are sensitive to touch, and the sucking reflex is easily initiated.

Symmetry of the eyes, nose, and ears is evaluated. See the Newborn Physical Assessment Guide on pages 616–627 for deviations in symmetry and variations in size, shape, and spacing of facial features. Facial movement symmetry should be assessed to determine the presence of facial palsy.

Facial paralysis appears when the newborn cries; the affected side is immobile, and the palpebral (eyelid) fissure widens (Figure 25–27 ■). Paralysis may result from forceps-assisted birth or pressure on the facial nerve from the maternal pelvis during birth. Facial paralysis usually disappears within a few days to 3 weeks, although in some cases it may be permanent.

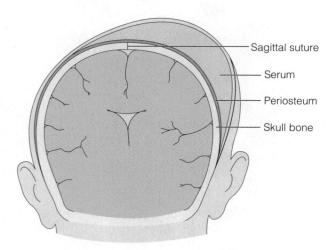

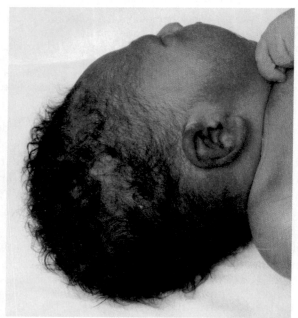

FIGURE 25–26 Caput succedaneum is a collection of fluid (serum) under the scalp.

Eyes

The eyes of the newborn of northern European descent are a blue-gray or slate blue-gray color. Dark-skin newborns tend to have dark eyes at birth. Scleral color tends to be bluish white because of its relative thinness. A blue

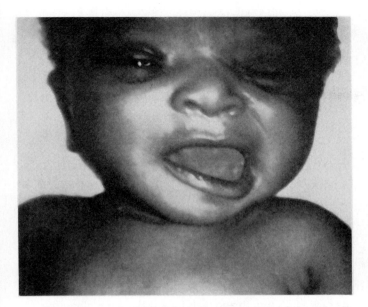

FIGURE 25–27 Facial paralysis. Paralysis of the right side of the face from injury to right facial nerve.
Source: Courtesy of Dr. Ralph Platow. From Potter, E. L., & Craig, J. M. (1975). *Pathology of the fetus and infant* (3rd ed.). Chicago: Year Book Medical Publishers. Reproduced with permission.

sclera is associated with osteogenesis imperfecta. The infant's eye color is usually established at approximately 3 months, although it may change any time up to 1 year.

The eyes should be checked for size, equality of pupil size, reaction of pupils to light, blink reflex to light, and edema and inflammation of the eyelids. The eyelids are usually edematous during the first few days of life because of the pressure associated with birth.

Erythromycin is frequently used prophylactically instead of silver nitrate and usually does not cause chemical irritation of the eye. The instillation of silver nitrate drops in the newborn's eyes may cause edema, and **chemical conjunctivitis** may appear a few hours after instillation, but it disappears in 1 to 2 days. Tetracycline is still used in some institutions (AAP & ACOG, 2007). If infectious conjunctivitis exists, the newborn has the same purulent (greenish yellow) discharge exudate as in chemical conjunctivitis, but it is caused by gonococcus, *Chlamydia,* staphylococci, or a variety of gram-negative bacteria. It requires treatment with ophthalmic antibiotics. Onset is usually after the second day. Edema of the orbits or eyelids may persist for several days, until the newborn's kidneys can eliminate the fluid.

Small **subconjunctival hemorrhages** appear in about 10% of newborns and are commonly found on the sclera. These hemorrhages are caused by the changes in vascular tension or ocular pressure during birth. They will remain for a few weeks and are of no pathologic significance. Parents need reassurance that the newborn is not bleeding from within the eye and that vision will not be impaired.

The newborn may demonstrate transient strabismus caused by poor neuromuscular control of eye muscles

(Figure 25–28 ■). It gradually regresses in 3 to 4 months. The "doll's eye" phenomenon is also present for about 10 days after birth. As the newborn's head position is changed to the left and then to the right, the eyes move to the opposite direction. "Doll's eye" results from underdeveloped integration of head-eye coordination.

The nurse should observe the newborn's pupils for opacities or whiteness and for the absence of a normal red retinal reflex. Red retinal reflex is a red-orange flash of color observed when an ophthalmoscope light reflects off the retina. In a newborn with dark skin color, the retina may appear paler or more grayish. Absence of red reflex occurs with cataracts. Congenital cataracts should be suspected in newborns of mothers with a history of rubella, cytomegalic inclusion disease, or syphilis. Brushfield spots (black or white spots on the periphery of the iris) can be associated with Down syndrome (Creehan, 2008).

The cry of the newborn is commonly tearless because the lacrimal structures are immature at birth and are not usually fully functional until the second month of life. However, some babies produce tears during the newborn period.

Poor oculomotor coordination and absence of accommodation limit visual abilities, but newborns have peripheral vision, can fixate on objects near (20.3 to 25.4 cm [8 to 10 in.]) and in front of their face for short periods, can accommodate to large objects (7.6 cm [3 in.] tall by 7.6 cm [3 in.] wide), and can seek out high-contrast geometric shapes. Newborns can perceive faces, shapes, and colors and begin to show visual preferences early. Newborns generally blink in response to bright lights, to a tap on the bridge of the nose (glabellar reflex), or to a light touch on the eyelids. Pupillary light reflex is also present. Examination of the eye is best accomplished by rocking the newborn from an upright position to the horizontal a few

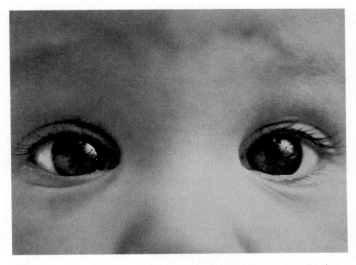

FIGURE 25–28 Transient strabismus may be present in the newborn because of poor neuromuscular control.
Source: Photo courtesy of Mead Johnson Laboratories, Evansville, IN.

times or by other methods, such as diminishing overhead lights, which elicit an opened-eye response.

Nose

The newborn's nose is small and narrow. Infants are characteristically nose breathers for the first few months of life and generally remove obstructions by sneezing. Nasal patency is ensured if the newborn breathes easily with the mouth closed. If respiratory difficulty occurs, the nurse checks for choanal atresia (congenital blockage of the passageway between nose and pharynx). Historically, choanal atresia can be checked by attempting to gently pass a soft #5 French catheter into both nostrils. Because of possible trauma, a cold, flat metal object may also be held under the nose to observe for fogging (Thureen et al., 2005).

The newborn has the ability to smell after the nasal passages are cleared of amniotic fluid and mucus. Newborns demonstrate this ability by the search for milk. Newborns turn their heads toward a milk source, whether bottle or breast. Newborns react to strong odors, such as alcohol, by turning their heads away or blinking.

Mouth

The lips of the newborn should be pink, and a touch on the lips should produce sucking motions. Saliva is normally scant. The taste buds develop before birth, and the newborn can easily discriminate between sweet and bitter flavors.

The easiest way to examine the mouth completely is to stimulate infants to cry by gently depressing their tongue, thereby causing them to open the mouth fully. It is extremely important to examine the entire mouth to check for a cleft palate, which can be present even in the absence of a cleft lip. The examiner moves a gloved index finger along the hard and soft palate to feel for any openings (Figure 25–29 ■). Glove powder should always be removed before examining the newborn's mouth.

Occasionally, an examination of the gums will reveal *precocious teeth* over the area where the lower central incisor will erupt. If they appear loose, they should be removed to prevent aspiration. Gray-white lesions (inclusion cysts) on the gums may be confused with teeth. On the hard palate and gum margins, **Epstein's pearls**, small glistening white specks (keratin-containing cysts) that feel hard to the touch, are often present. They usually disappear in a few weeks and are of no significance. **Thrush** may appear as white patches that look like milk curds adhering to the mucous membranes and bleeding may occur when patches are removed. Thrush is caused by *Candida albicans,* often acquired from an infected vaginal tract during birth, antibiotic use, or poor handwashing when the mother handles her newborn. Thrush is treated with a preparation of nystatin (Mycostatin).

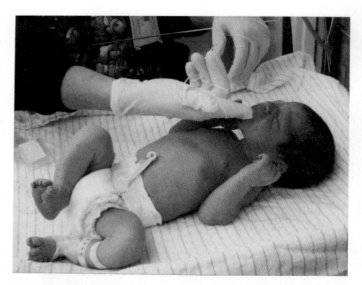

FIGURE 25–29 The nurse inserts a gloved index finger into the newborn's mouth and feels for any openings along the hard and soft palates.
Note: Gloves or a finger cot are always worn to examine the palate.
Source: Courtesy of Vanessa Howell, RNC, BSN.

A newborn who is tongue-tied has a ridge of frenulum tissue attached to the underside of the tongue at varying lengths from its base, causing a heart shape at the tip of the tongue. "Clipping the tongue," or cutting the ridge of tissue, is not recommended. This ridge does not affect speech or eating, but cutting creates an entry for infection.

Transient nerve paralysis resulting from birth trauma may be manifested by asymmetrical mouth movements when the newborn cries or by difficulty with sucking and feeding.

Ears

The ears of the newborn are soft and pliable and should recoil readily when folded and released. In the normal newborn, the top of the ear (pinna) should be parallel to the outer and inner canthus of the eye. The ears should be inspected for shape, size, firmness of cartilage, and position. *Low-set ears* are characteristic of many syndromes and may indicate chromosomal abnormalities (especially trisomies 13 and 18), mental retardation, and internal organ abnormalities, especially bilateral renal agenesis as a result of embryologic developmental deviations (Figure 25–30 ■). *Preauricular skin tags* may be present just in front of the ear. Visualization of the tympanic membrane is not usually done soon after birth because blood and vernix block the ear canal.

Following the first cry, the newborn's hearing becomes acute as mucus from the middle ear is absorbed, the eustachian tube becomes aerated, and the tympanic membrane becomes visible. The newborn's hearing initially can be evaluated by noting the baby's response to loud or moderately loud noises that are not accompa-

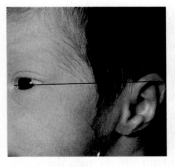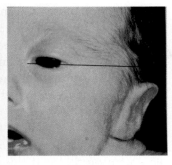

FIGURE 25–30 The position of the external ear may be assessed by drawing a line across the inner and outer canthus of the eye to the insertion of the ear. *A,* Normal position. *B,* True low-set position.
Source: Photo courtesy of Mead Johnson Laboratories, Evansville, IN.

nied by vibrations. The sleeping newborn should stir or awaken in response to nearby sounds. (This is not a very accurate test, but it may alert the examiner to a possible problem.) The newborn can discriminate the individual characteristics of the human voice and is especially sensitive to sound levels within the normal conversational range. The newborn in a noisy nursery may habituate to the sounds and not stir unless the sound is sudden or much louder than usual.

The AAP has endorsed universal newborn hearing screening (UNHS) before discharge from the birthing unit as the standard of care (Creehan, 2008). If the birth occurs in the home or an alternative birthing center, referral for screening should be made within 1 month of birth. The current goal is to screen all infants by 1 month of age, confirm hearing loss with audiologic examination by 3 months of age, and treat with comprehensive early intervention services before 6 months of age (AAP & ACOG, 2007). Families need to be educated about appropriate interpretation of screening test results and the appropriate steps for follow-up.

Neck

A short neck, creased with skin folds, is characteristic of the normal newborn. Because muscle tone is not well developed, the neck cannot support the full weight of the head, which rotates freely. The head lags considerably when the newborn is pulled from a supine to a sitting position, but the prone newborn is able to raise the head slightly. The neck is palpated for masses and the presence of lymph nodes and is inspected for webbing. Adequacy of range of motion and neck muscle function is determined by fully extending the head in all directions. Injury to the sternocleidomastoid muscle (congenital torticollis) must be considered in the presence of neck rigidity.

The nurse evaluates the clavicles for evidence of fractures, which occasionally occur during difficult births or

in newborns with broad shoulders. The normal clavicle is straight. If fractured, a lump and a grating sensation (crepitus) during movements may be palpated along the course of the side of the break. The nurse also elicits the Moro reflex (page 614) to evaluate bilateral equal movement of the arms. If the clavicle is fractured, the response will be demonstrated only on the unaffected side.

Chest

The thorax is cylindric and symmetric at birth, and the ribs are flexible. The general appearance of the chest should be assessed. A protrusion at the lower end of the sternum, called the xiphoid cartilage, is frequently seen. It is under the skin and will become less apparent after several weeks as adipose tissue accumulates.

Engorged breasts occur frequently in both male and female newborns. This condition, which occurs by the third day, is a result of maternal hormonal influences and may last up to 2 weeks (Figure 25–31 ■). A whitish secretion from the nipples may also be noted. The newborn's breast should not be massaged or squeezed, because this may cause a breast abscess. Extra nipples, or supernumerary nipples, are occasionally noted below and medial to the true nipples. These harmless pink or brown (in dark-skin newborns) spots vary in size and do not contain glandular tissue. Accessory nipples can be differentiated from a pigmented nevi (mole) by placing the fingertips alongside the accessory nipple and pulling the adjacent tissue laterally. The accessory nipple will appear dimpled. At puberty the accessory nipple may darken.

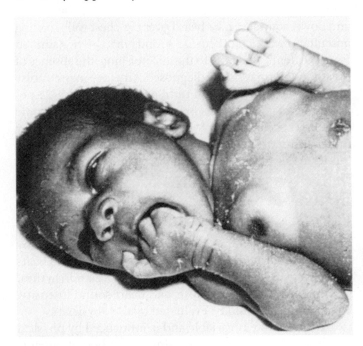

FIGURE 25–31 Breast hypertrophy.
Source: Korones, S. B. (1986). *High-risk newborn infants* (4th ed.). St. Louis: Mosby.

Cry

The newborn's cry should be strong, lusty, and of medium pitch. A high-pitched, shrill cry is abnormal and may indicate neurologic disorders or hypoglycemia. Periods of crying usually vary in length after consoling measures are used. Babies' cries are an important method of communication and alert caregivers to changes in their condition and needs.

HINTS FOR PRACTICE

Vital sign assessments are most accurate if the newborn is at rest, so measure pulse and respirations first if the baby is quiet. To soothe a crying baby, try placing your moistened gloved finger in the baby's mouth, and then complete your assessment while the baby suckles.

Respiration

MyNursingKit | Neonatal Airway Assessment

Normal breathing for a term newborn is 30 to 60 respirations per minute and is predominantly diaphragmatic, with associated rising and falling of the abdomen during inspiration and expiration. The nurse should note any signs of respiratory distress, nasal flaring, intercostal or xiphoid retraction, expiratory grunt or sigh, seesaw respirations, or tachypnea (greater than 60 breaths per minute). Hyperextension (chest appears high) or hypoextension (chest appears low) of the anteroposterior diameter of the chest should also be noted. Both the anterior and posterior chest are auscultated. Some breath sounds are heard best when the newborn is crying, but localizing and identifying breath sounds are difficult in the newborn. Upper airway noises and bowel sounds can be heard over the chest wall, making auscultation difficult. Because sounds may be transmitted from the unaffected lung to the affected lung, the absence of breath sounds may not be diagnosed. Air entry may be noisy in the first couple of hours until lung fluid resolves, especially after cesarean births. Brief periods of apnea (episodic breathing) occur, but no color or heart rate changes occur in healthy, term newborns. Sepsis should be suspected in full-term newborns experiencing apneic episodes.

Heart

Heart rates can be as rapid as 180 beats per minute in newborns and fluctuate a great deal, especially if the baby moves or is startled. The normal range is 120 to 160 beats per minute. The heart is examined for rate and rhythm, position of the apical impulse, and heart sound intensity. Dysrhythmias should be evaluated by the physician.

The pulse rate is variable and is influenced by physical activity, crying, state of wakefulness, and body temperature. Auscultation is performed over the entire heart region (precordium), below the left axilla, and below the

scapula. Apical pulse rates are obtained by auscultation for a full minute, preferably when the newborn is asleep.

The placement of the heart in the chest should be determined when the newborn is in a quiet state. The heart is relatively large at birth and is located high in the chest, with its apex somewhere between the fourth and fifth intercostal space.

A shift of heart tones in the mediastinal area to either side may indicate pneumothorax, dextrocardia (heart placement on the right side of the chest), or a diaphragmatic hernia. The experienced nurse can detect these and many other problems early with a stethoscope. The nurse should auscultate heart sounds using both the bell and diaphragm of the stethoscope. Normally, the heart beat has a "toc tic" sound. A slur or slushing sound (usually after the first sound) may indicate a *murmur*. Although 90% of all murmurs are transient and are considered normal, they should be monitored closely by a physician. Many murmurs are secondary to closing of patent ductus arteriosus or patent foramen ovale, which should close 1 to 2 days after birth.

In newborns, a low-pitched, musical murmur just to the right of the apex of the heart is fairly common. Occasionally, significant murmurs are heard, such as the murmur of a patent ductus arteriosus, aortic or pulmonary stenosis, or small ventricular septal defect. (See Chapter 28 ∞ for a discussion of congenital heart defects.)

Peripheral pulses (brachial, femoral, pedal) are also evaluated to detect any lags or unusual characteristics. Brachial pulses are palpated bilaterally for equality and compared with the femoral pulses. Femoral pulses are palpated by applying gentle pressure with the middle finger over the femoral canal (Figure 25–32 ■). Decreased or absent femoral pulses may indicate coarctation of the aorta or hypovolemia and require additional evaluation. A wide difference in blood pressure between the upper and lower extremities also indicates coarctation of aorta.

The measurement of blood pressure is best accomplished by using a noninvasive blood pressure device (Figure 25–33 ■). If a blood pressure cuff is used, the newborn's extremities must be immobilized during the assessment, and the cuff should cover two-thirds of the upper arm or upper leg. Movement, crying, and inappropriate cuff size can give inaccurate measurements of the blood pressure.

HINTS FOR PRACTICE

If possible, obtain blood pressure measurement during quiet sleep or sleep state. Place the cuff on the infant's arm or leg and give the infant time to quiet. Obtain an average of two to three measurements when making clinical decisions. Follow mean blood pressure to monitor changes, as it is less likely to be erroneous. Noninvasive blood pressure may overestimate blood pressure in very low-birth-weight infants.

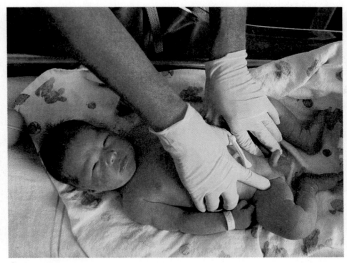

A

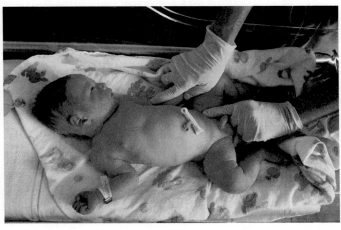

B

FIGURE 25–32 *A,* Bilaterally palpate the femoral arteries for rate and intensity of the pulses. Press fingertip gently at the groin as shown. *B,* Compare the femoral pulses to the brachial pulses by palpating the pulses simultaneously for comparison of rate and intensity.

Blood pressure may not be measured routinely on healthy newborns, but it is essential for newborns who are having distress, are premature, or are suspected of having a cardiac anomaly (Thureen et al., 2005). Infants who have birth asphyxia and are on ventilators have significantly lower systolic and diastolic blood pressures than healthy infants. If a cardiac anomaly is suspected, blood pressure is measured in all four extremities. (See Key Facts to Remember: Newborn Vital Signs.) At birth, systolic values usually range from 70 to 50 mm Hg and diastolic values from 45 to 30 mm Hg. By the tenth day of life, blood pressure rises to 90/50 mm Hg.

Abdomen

The nurse can learn a great deal about the newborn's abdomen without disturbing the infant. The abdomen

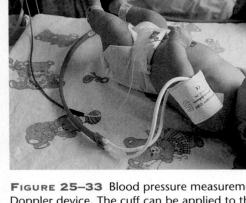

FIGURE 25–33 Blood pressure measurement using a Doppler device. The cuff can be applied to the upper arm or thigh.

should be cylindrical, protrude slightly, and move with respiration. A certain amount of laxness of the abdominal muscles is normal. A scaphoid (hollow-shaped) appearance suggests the absence of abdominal contents, often seen in diaphragmatic hernias. No cyanosis should be present, and few if any blood vessels should be apparent to the eye. There should be no gross distention or bulging. The more distended the abdomen, the tighter the skin becomes, with engorged vessels appearing. Distention is the first sign of many gastrointestinal abnormalities.

Before palpation of the abdomen, the nurse should auscultate for the presence or absence of bowel sounds in

---

KEY FACTS TO REMEMBER
Newborn Vital Signs

Pulse

120 to 160 bpm
During sleep as low as 80 to 100 bpm; if crying, up to 180 bpm
Apical pulse counted for 1 full minute

Respirations

30 to 60 respirations/minute
Predominantly diaphragmatic but synchronous with abdominal movements
Respirations are counted for 1 full minute

Blood Pressure

70–50/45–30 mm Hg at birth
90/50 mm Hg at day 10

Temperature

Normal range: 36.5°C to 37.5°C (97.7°F to 99.4°F)
Axillary: 36.4°C to 37.2°C (97.5°F to 99°F)
Skin: 36°C to 36.5°C (96.8°F to 97.7°F)
Rectal: 36.6°C to 37.2°C (97.8°F to 99°F)

all four quadrants. Bowel sounds may be present by 1 hour after birth. Palpation can cause a transient decrease in bowel sounds intensity.

Abdominal palpation should be done systematically. The nurse palpates each of the four abdominal quadrants and moves in a clockwise direction until all four quadrants have been palpated for softness, tenderness, and the presence of masses. The nurse should place one hand under the back for support during palpation.

Umbilical Cord

Initially the umbilical cord is white and gelatinous in appearance, with the two umbilical arteries and one umbilical vein readily apparent. Because a single umbilical artery is frequently associated with congenital anomalies, the nurse should count the vessels during the newborn assessment. The cord begins drying within 1 or 2 hours of birth and is shriveled and blackened by the second or third day. Within 7 to 10 days it sloughs off, although a granulating area may remain for a few days longer.

Cord bleeding is abnormal and may result because the cord was inadvertently pulled or the cord clamp was loosened. Foul-smelling drainage is also abnormal and is generally caused by infection, which requires immediate treatment to prevent septicemia. If the newborn has a patent urachus (abnormal connection between the umbilicus and bladder), moistness or draining urine may be apparent at the base of the cord. Another umbilical cord anomaly that can occur is umbilical cord hernia and associated patent omphalomesenteric duct (Figure 25–34 ■). Umbilical hernias are more common in infants of African American descent than in Caucasian infants (Thureen et al., 2005).

Serous or serosanguineous drainage that continues after the cord falls off may indicate a granuloma. It appears as a small red button deep in the umbilicus. Treatment involves cauterization by a healthcare provider with a topical silver nitrate stick (Thureen et al., 2005).

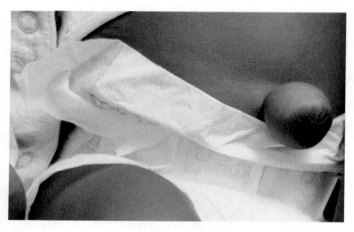

FIGURE 25–34 Umbilical hernia.

Genitals

Female Infants

The nurse examines the labia majora, labia minora, and clitoris and notes the size of each as appropriate for gestational age. A vaginal tag or hymenal tag is often evident and will usually disappear in a few weeks. During the first week of life, the female newborn may have a vaginal discharge composed of thick, whitish mucus. This discharge, which can become tinged with blood, is called **pseudomenstruation** and is caused by the withdrawal of maternal hormones. *Smegma*, a white, cheeselike substance, is often present between the labia. Removing it may traumatize tender tissue.

Male Infants

The nurse inspects the penis to determine whether the urinary orifice is correctly positioned. *Hypospadias* occurs when the urinary meatus is located on the ventral surface of the penis or *epispadius* (meatus is on the dorsal surface of the glans). Hypospadius occurs most commonly among people of Western European descent. *Phimosis* is a condition in which the opening of the foreskin (prepuce) is small and the foreskin cannot be pulled back over the glans at all. This condition may interfere with urination, so the adequacy of the urinary stream should be evaluated.

The scrotum is inspected for size and symmetry. Scrotal color variations are especially prominent in African American, Indian, and Hispanic newborns (Creehan, 2008). The scrotum should be palpated to verify the presence of both testes and to rule out *cryptorchidism* (failure of testes to descend). The testes are palpated separately between the thumb and forefinger, with the thumb and forefinger of the other hand placed together over the inguinal canal. Scrotal edema and discoloration are common in breech births. *Hydrocele* (a collection of fluid surrounding the testes in the scrotum) is common in newborns and should be identified. It usually resolves without intervention. The presence of a discolored or dusky scrotum and solid testis should raise the suspicion of testicular torsion which should be reported immediately.

Anus

The anal area is inspected to verify that it is patent and has no fissure. Imperforate anus and rectal atresia may be ruled out by observation. Digital examination, if necessary, is done by a physician or nurse practitioner. The nurse also notes the passage of the first meconium stool. Atresia of the gastrointestinal tract or meconium ileus with resultant obstruction must be considered if the newborn does not pass meconium in the first 24 hours of life.

HINTS FOR PRACTICE

Always examine more closely any infant who is reluctant to move an extremity. Fractures are often asymptomatic in the newborn: paralytic injuries are characterized by immobility of an extremity.

Extremities

Extremities are examined for gross deformities, extra digits or webbing, clubfoot, and range of motion. Normal newborn extremities appear short, are generally flexible, and move symmetrically.

Arms and Hands

Nails extend beyond the fingertips in term newborns. The nurse should count fingers and toes. *Polydactyly* is the presence of extra digits on either the hands or the feet. *Syndactyly* refers to fusion (webbing) of fingers or toes. The hands are inspected for normal palmar creases. A single palmar crease, called *simian line* (see Figure 7–18B ∞), is frequently present in children with Down syndrome.

Brachial palsy, paralysis of portions of the arm, results from trauma to the brachial plexus during a difficult birth. It occurs commonly when strong traction is exerted on the head of the newborn in an attempt to deliver a shoulder lodged behind the symphysis pubis in the presence of shoulder dystocia. Brachial palsy may also occur during a breech birth if an arm becomes trapped over the head and traction is exerted.

The portion of the arm affected is determined by the nerves damaged. **Erb-Duchenne paralysis (Erb's palsy)** involves damage to the upper arm (fifth and sixth cervical nerves) and is the most common type. Injury to the eighth cervical and first thoracic nerve roots and the *lower portion* of the plexus produces the relatively rare lower arm injury. The *whole-arm type* results from damage to the entire plexus.

With Erb-Duchenne paralysis the newborn's arm lies limply at the side. The elbow is held in extension, with the forearm pronated. The newborn is unable to elevate the arm, and the Moro reflex cannot be elicited on the affected side (Figure 25–35 ■). Lower arm injury causes paralysis of the hand and wrist; complete paralysis of the limb occurs with the whole-arm type.

The nurse carefully instructs the parents in the correct method of performing passive range of motion exercises (to prevent muscle contractures and restore function) and

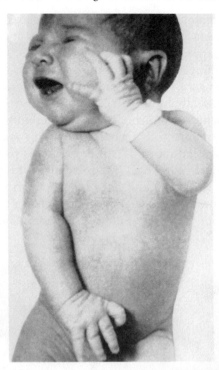

FIGURE 25–35 Right Erb's palsy resulting from injury to the fifth and sixth cervical roots of the brachial plexus.
Source: Potter, E. L., & Craig, J. M. (1975). *Pathology of the fetus and infant* (3rd ed.). Chicago: Year Book Medical Publishers. Reproduced with permission.

arranges supervised practice sessions for the parents and referral to physical therapy follow-up within 2 weeks of discharge. In more severe cases, splinting of the arm is indicated until the edema decreases. The arm is held in a position of abduction and external rotation with the elbow flexed 90 degrees, often called the "Statue of Liberty" position. The "Statue of Liberty" splint is commonly used, although similar results are obtained by attaching a strip of muslin to the head of the crib and tying the other end around the wrist, thereby holding the arm up.

Prognosis is related to the degree of nerve damage resulting from trauma and hemorrhage within the nerve sheath. Complete recovery occurs within a few months with minimal trauma. Moderate trauma may result in partial paralysis. Recovery is unlikely with severe trauma, and muscle wasting may develop.

Legs and Feet

The legs of the newborn should be of equal length, with symmetrical skin folds. However, they may assume a "fetal posture" secondary to position in utero, and it may take several days for the legs to relax into a normal position. To evaluate for hip dislocation or hip instability, the Ortolani and Barlow maneuvers are performed. The nurse (or more commonly, the physician or nurse practitioner) performs the **Ortolani's maneuver** to rule out the possibility of developmental dysplastic hip, also called congenital hip dysplasia (hip dislocatability). With the newborn relaxed and quiet on a firm surface, with hips and knees flexed at a 90-degree angle, the experienced nurse grasps the infant's thigh with the middle finger over the greater trochanter and lifts the thigh to bring the femoral head from its posterior position toward the acetabulum. With gentle abduction of the thigh, the femoral head is returned to the acetabulum. Simultaneously, the examiner feels a sense of reduction or a "clunk" as the femoral head returns. This reduction is palpable and may be heard. With **Barlow's maneuver**, the healthcare provider grasps and adducts the infant's thigh and applies gentle downward pressure. Dislocation is felt as the femoral head slips out of the acetabulum. The femoral head is then returned to the acetabulum using the Ortolani's maneuver, confirming the diagnosis of an unstable or dislocatable hip (Figure 25–36 ■).

The feet are then examined for evidence of a talipes deformity (clubfoot). Intrauterine position frequently causes the feet to appear to turn inward (Figure 25–37 ■); this is termed a "*positional*" *clubfoot.* If the feet can easily be returned to the midline by manipulation, no treatment is indicated and the nurse teaches range of motion exercises to the family. Further evaluation is indicated when the foot will not turn to a midline position or align readily. This is considered the most severe type of "true clubfoot," or talipes equinovarus.

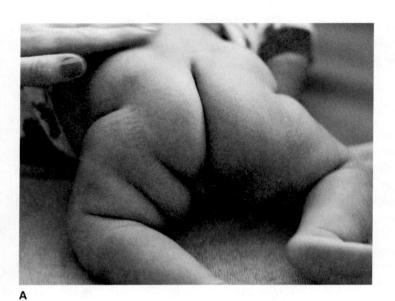

A

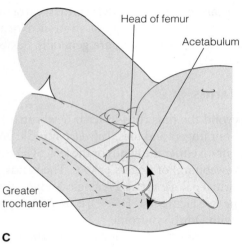

Head of femur

Acetabulum

Greater trochanter

C

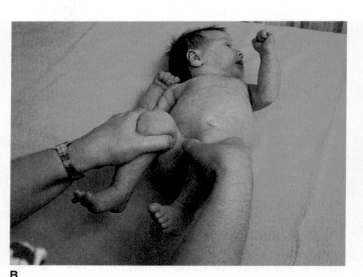

B

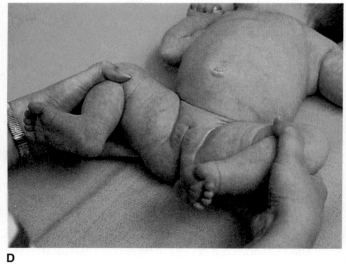

D

Figure 25–36 *A,* The asymmetry of gluteal and thigh fat folds seen in infant with left developmental dysplasia of the hip. *B,* Barlow's (dislocation) maneuver. Baby's thigh is grasped and adducted (placed together) with gentle downward pressure. *C,* Dislocation is palpable as femoral head slips out of acetabulum. *D,* The Ortolani's maneuver puts downward pressure on the hip and then inward rotation. If the hip is dislocated, this maneuver will force the femoral head back into the acetabular rim with a noticeable "clunk."

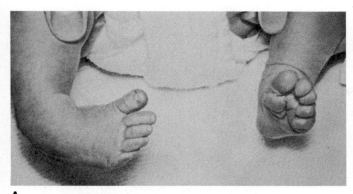

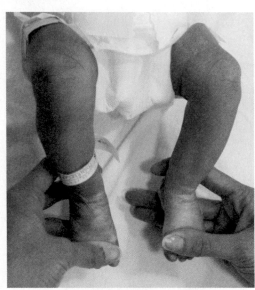

FIGURE 25–37 *A,* Unilateral talipes equinovarus (clubfoot). *B,* To determine the presence of clubfoot, the nurse moves the foot to the midline. Resistance indicates true clubfoot. *Source: A.* Used with permission from Mead Johnson Nutritionals, Evansville, IN.

Back

With the newborn prone, the nurse examines the back. The spine should appear straight and flat, because the lumbar and sacral curves do not develop until the newborn begins to sit. The base of the spine is examined for a dermal sinus. A nevus pilosus ("hairy nerve") is occasionally found at the base of the spine in newborns. It is significant because it is frequently associated with spina bifida. A pilonidal dimple should be examined to ascertain that there is no connection to the spinal canal.

Assessment of Neurologic Status

The nurse should begin the neurologic examination with a period of observation, noting the general physical characteristics and behaviors of the newborn. Important behaviors to assess are the *state of alertness, resting posture, cry,* and *quality of muscle tone and motor activity.*

The usual position of the newborn is with partially flexed extremities, with the legs abducted to the abdomen. When awake, the newborn may exhibit purposeless, uncoordinated bilateral movements of the extremities. If these movements are absent, minimal, or obviously asymmetrical, neurologic dysfunction should be suspected. Eye movements are observable during the first few days of life. An alert newborn is able to fixate on faces and brightly colored objects. Shining a bright light in the newborn's eyes elicits the blinking response.

The nurse evaluates muscle tone by moving various parts of the body while the head of the newborn is in a neutral position. The newborn is somewhat hypertonic; that is, there should be resistance to extending the elbow and knee joints. Muscle tone should be symmetrical. Diminished muscle tone and flaccidity require further evaluation.

Tremors or jitteriness (tremor-like movements) in the full-term newborn must be evaluated to differentiate the tremors from convulsions. Tremors may also be related to hypoglycemia, hypocalcemia, or substance withdrawal. Environmental stimuli may initiate tremors. Jitteriness may be distinguished from tonic-clonic seizure activity because it usually can be stopped by the infant's sucking on the extremity or by the nurse holding or flexing the involved extremity. A fine jumping of the muscle is likely to be a central nervous system disorder and requires further evaluation. Newborn seizures may consist of no more than chewing or swallowing movements, deviations of the eyes, rigidity, or flaccidity because of CNS immaturity. In contrast to tremors, seizures are not usually initiated by stimuli, and cannot be stopped by holding.

Specific deep tendon reflexes can be elicited in the newborn but have limited value unless they are obviously asymmetric. The knee jerk is typically brisk; a normal ankle clonus may involve three or four beats. Plantar flexion is present.

The immature CNS of the newborn is characterized by a variety of reflexes. Because the newborn's movements are uncoordinated, methods of communication are limited, and control of bodily functions is restricted, the reflexes serve a variety of purposes. Some are protective (blink, gag, sneeze), some aid in feeding (rooting, sucking) and may not be very active if the infant has eaten recently, and some stimulate human interaction (grasping). See Newborn Physical Assessment Guide in this chapter for a summary of stimulus for, alternations for, and possible causes of common newborn reflexes.

The most common reflexes found in the normal newborn are the following:

- The **tonic neck reflex** (fencer position) is elicited when the newborn is supine and the head is turned to one side. In response, the extremities on the same side straighten, whereas on the opposite side they flex (Figure 25–38 ■).

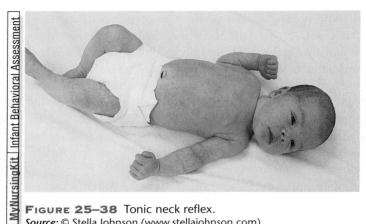

FIGURE 25–38 Tonic neck reflex.
Source: © Stella Johnson (www.stellajohnson.com).

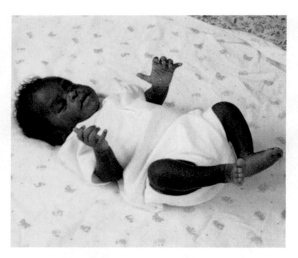

FIGURE 25–40 Moro reflex.

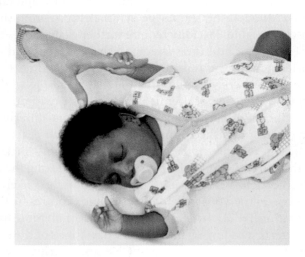

FIGURE 25–39 Palmar grasp.

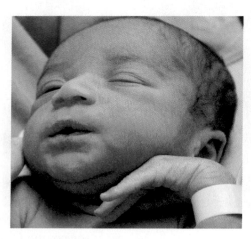

FIGURE 25–41 Rooting reflex.

This reflex may not be seen during the early newborn period, but once it appears it persists until about the third month.

- The palmar **grasping reflex** is elicited by stimulating the newborn's palm with a finger or object; the newborn grasps and holds the object or finger firmly enough to be lifted momentarily from the crib (Figure 25–39 ■).
- The **Moro reflex** is elicited when the newborn is startled by a loud noise or lifted slightly above the crib and then suddenly lowered. In response, the newborn straightens arms and hands outward while the knees flex. Slowly the arms return to the chest, as in an embrace. The fingers spread, forming a C, and the newborn may cry (Figure 25–40 ■). This reflex may persist until about 6 months of age.
- The **rooting reflex** is elicited when the side of the newborn's mouth or cheek is touched. In response, the newborn turns toward that side and opens the lips to suck (if not fed recently) (Figure 25–41 ■).
- The **sucking reflex** is elicited when an object is placed in the newborn's mouth or anything touches the lips. Newborns suck even while sleeping; this is called nonnutritive sucking, and it can have a quieting effect on the baby.

- The **Babinski reflex (response)**, or fanning and hyperextension of all toes and dorsiflexion of the big toe, occurs when the lateral aspect of the sole is stroked from the heel upward across the ball of the foot (Mandleco, 2004). In children older than 24 months, an abnormal response is extension or fanning of the toes; this Babinski response indicates upper motor neuron abnormalities (Figure 25–42 ■).
- **Trunk incurvation (Galant reflex)** is seen when the newborn is prone. Stroking the spine causes the pelvis to turn to the stimulated side.

In addition to these reflexes, newborns can *blink, yawn, cough, sneeze,* and *draw back from pain* (protective reflexes). They can even move a little on their own. When placed on their stomachs, they push up and try to crawl (prone crawl). When held upright with one foot touching a flat surface, the newborn puts one foot in front of the other and "walks" (*stepping reflex*) (Figure 25–43 ■). This reflex is more pronounced at birth and is lost in 4 to 8 weeks.

The nurse uses the following steps to assess CNS integration:

1. Insert a gloved finger into the newborn's mouth to elicit a sucking reflex.
2. As soon as the newborn is sucking vigorously, assess hearing and vision responses by noting changes in sucking in the presence of a light, a rattle, and a voice.
3. The newborn should respond to such stimuli with a brief cessation of sucking, followed by continuous sucking with repetitious stimulation.

This CNS integration exam demonstrates auditory and visual integrity as well as the capability of complex behavioral interactions.

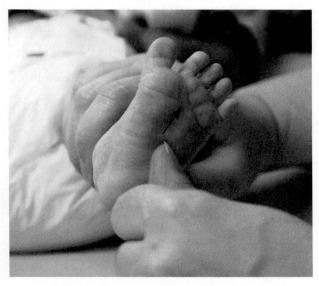

FIGURE 25–42 The Babinski reflex (response).

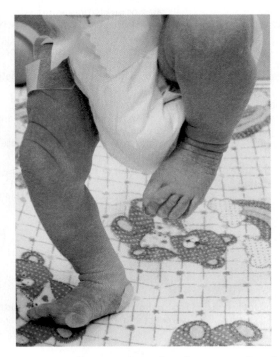

FIGURE 25–43 The stepping reflex disappears after about 4 to 8 weeks of age.

TABLE 25–2	Potential Birth Injuries
Classification	Examples*
Soft-tissue injuries	Lacerations, abrasions, bruising, fat necrosis
Skull injuries	Cephalohematoma*, fractures
Scalp laceration	Fetal scalp electrode
Scalp abscess	Fetal scalp electrode
Intracranial hemorrhage	Subdural, subarachnoid
Eye injuries	Subconjunctival* and retinal hemorrhages
Fractures	Clavicle,* facial bones, humerus, femur
Dislocations	Hips
Torticollis	Sternocleidomastoid muscle
Nerve injuries	Facial nerve*, brachial plexus*, phrenic nerve, recurrent laryngeal nerve (vocal cord paralysis), Horner syndrome
Spinal cord injuries	Spina bifida
Visceral rupture	Liver, spleen
*Most common birth injuries seen in newborns.	

As healthcare providers carry out the newborn physical and neurologic assessment, they are always on the alert to recognize possible alterations and possible injuries related to the birth process that require further investigation and intervention. (See Table 25–2 for potential birth injuries.)

Newborn Physical Assessment Guide

Following is a guide for systematically assessing the newborn (pages 616–627). Normal findings, alterations, and related causes are presented and correlated with suggested nursing responses. The findings are typical for a full-term newborn.

Newborn Behavioral Assessment

Two conflicting forces influence parents' perceptions of their newborn. One is their preconception, based on hopes and fears, of what their newborn will be like. The other is their initial reaction to the baby's temperament, behaviors, and physical appearance. Nurses can assist parents in identifying their baby's specific behaviors.

CRITICAL THINKING

Maria Reyes, a 19-year-old G2 (now P2) mother, delivered a 40-week-old female newborn 24 hours ago. The newborn exam was normal. Mrs. Reyes asks about the newborn's exam. She says she has noticed that the baby cries more than her first child did and seems to require holding for longer periods of time after feeding before "quieting down." She is concerned that there is something she is doing wrong and wants to know when her newborn will start to act like her first baby. What should you discuss with her about newborn behavior?

Answers can be found in Appendix F ∞.

ASSESSMENT GUIDE NEWBORN PHYSICAL ASSESSMENT

Physical Assessment/ Normal Findings	Alterations and Possible Causes*	Nursing Responses to Data†
Vital Signs		
Blood pressure (BP) At birth: 70–50/ 45–30 mm Hg	Low BP (hypovolemia, shock)	Monitor BP in all cases of distress, prematurity, or suspected anomaly.
Day 10: 90/50 mm Hg (may be unable to measure diastolic pressure with standard sphygmomanometer)		Low BP: Refer to physician immediately so measures to improve circulation are begun.
Pulse: 120 to160 bpm (if asleep, as low as 100 bpm; if crying, up to 180 bpm)	Weak pulse (decreased cardiac output) Bradycardia (severe asphyxia) Tachycardia (over 160 bpm at rest) (infection, CNS problems, arrhythmia, stress, hypovolemia)	Assess skin perfusion by blanching (capillary refill test-normal 2-3 sec.). Correlate finding with BP assessments; refer to physician. Carry out neurologic and thermoregulation assessments. Check blood pressure and Hct.
Respirations: 30 to 60 breaths/minute Synchronization of chest and abdominal movements	Tachypnea (pneumonia, respiratory distress syndrome [RDS])	Identify sleep-wake state; correlate with respiratory pattern.
Diaphragmatic and abdominal breathing	Rapid, shallow breathing (hypermagnesemia caused by large doses given to mothers with preeclampsia) Respirations below 30 breaths/minute (maternal anesthesia or analgesia)	Evaluate for all signs of respiratory distress; report findings to physician.
Transient tachypnea	Expiratory grunting, subcostal and substernal retractions; flaring of nares (respiratory distress); apnea (cold stress, respiratory disorder)	Evaluate for cold stress. Report findings to physician/neonatal nurse practitioner.
Crying: Strong and lusty Moderate tone and pitch	High pitched, shrill (neurologic disorder, hypoglycemia)	Discuss newborn's use of cry for communication.
Cries vary in length from 3 to 7 minutes after consoling measures are used	Weak or absent (CNS disorder, laryngeal problem)	Assess and record abnormal cries. Reduce environmental noises.
Temperature: Axilla 36.4°C to 37.2°C (97.5°F to 99°F)	Elevated temperature (room too warm, too much clothing or covers, dehydration, sepsis, brain damage) Subnormal temperature (brainstem involvement, cold, sepsis)	Notify physician of elevation or drop. Counsel parents on possible causes of elevated or low temperatures, appropriate home-care measures, when to call physician.
Heavier newborns tend to have higher body temperatures	Swings of more than 2°F from one reading to next or subnormal temperature (infection)	Teach parents how to take rectal and/or axillary temperature; assess parents' information regarding use of thermometer; provide teaching as needed.
Weight: 2500 to 4000 g (5 lb. 8 oz to 8 lb. 13 oz)	Less than 2748 g (less than 6 lb) = SGA or preterm infant Greater than 4050 g (greater than 9 lb) = LGA or infants of diabetic mothers	Plot weight and gestational age on growth chart to identify high-risk infants. Ascertain body build of parents. Counsel parents regarding appropriate caloric intake.
Within first 3 to 4 days, normal weight loss of 5% to 10% Large babies tend to lose more because of greater fluid loss in proportion to birth weight except infants of diabetic mother	Loss greater than 15% (low fluid intake, loss of meconium and urine, feeding difficulties, diabetes insipidus)	Notify physician of net losses or gains. Calculate fluid intake and losses from all sources (insensible water loss, radiant warmers, and phototherapy lights).
Length: 46 to 56 cm (18 to 22 in.)	Less than 45 cm (congenital dwarf)	Assess for other signs of dwarfism.
Grows 10 cm (3 in.) during first 3 months	Short/long bones proximally (achondroplasia) Short/long bones distally (Ellis-van Creveld syndrome)	Determine other signs of skeletal system adequacy. Plot progress at subsequent well-baby visits.
	*Possible causes of alterations are identified in parentheses.	†This column provides guidelines for further assessment and initial nursing interventions.

ASSESSMENT GUIDE NEWBORN PHYSICAL ASSESSMENT *(Continued)*

Physical Assessment/ Normal Findings	Alterations and Possible Causes*	Nursing Responses to Data†
Posture		
Body usually flexed, hands may be tightly clenched, neck appears short as chin rests on chest	Only extension noted, inability to move from midline (trauma, hypoxia, immaturity)	Record spontaneity of motor activity and symmetry of movements.
In breech births feet are usually dorsiflexed	Constant motion (maternal caffeine intake or drug withdrawal)	If parents express concern about newborn's movement patterns, reassure and evaluate further if appropriate.
Skin		
Color: Color consistent with genetic background	Pallor of face, conjunctiva (anemia, hypothermia, anoxia)	Discuss with parents common skin color variations to allay fears.
Newborns of European descent: pink-tinged or ruddy color over face, trunk, extremities	Beefy red (hypoglycemia, immature vasomotor reflexes, polycythemia)	Document extent and time of occurrence of color change.
Newborns of African or Native American descent: pale pink with yellow or red tinge		
Newborns of Asian descent: pink or rosy red to yellow tinge		
Common variations: acrocyanosis, circumoral cyanosis, Mongolian spots, or harlequin color change	Meconium staining (nonreassuring fetal status)	Obtain Hb and hematocrit values, obtain bilirubin levels.
	Jaundice (hemolytic reaction from blood incompatibility within first 24 hours, sepsis)	Assess for respiratory difficulty. Differentiate between physiologic and pathologic jaundice.
Mottled when undressed	Cyanosis (choanal atresia, CNS damage or trauma, respiratory or cardiac problem, cold stress)	Assess degree of (central or peripheral) cyanosis and possible causes; refer to physician.
Minor bruising: over buttocks in breech presentation and over eyes and forehead in facial presentations		Discuss with parents cause and course of minor bruising related to labor and birth.
Texture: Smooth, soft, flexible, may have dry, peeling hands and feet	Generalized cracked or peeling skin (SGA or postterm; blood incompatibility; metabolic, kidney dysfunction)	Report to physician. Instruct parents to shampoo the scalp and anterior fontanelle areas daily with soap; rinse well; avoid use of oil.
	Seborrheic-dermatitis (cradle cap) Absence of vernix (postmature) Yellow vernix (bilirubin staining)	
Turgor: Elastic, returns to normal shape after pinching	Maintains tent shape (dehydration)	Assess for other signs and symptoms of dehydration.
Pigmentation: Clear; milia across bridge of nose, forehead, or chin will disappear within a few weeks		Advise parents not to pinch or prick these pimplelike areas.
Café-au-lait spots (one or two)	Six or more (neurologic disorder such as von Recklinghausen's disease, cutaneous neurofibromatosis)	If there are six or more café-au-lait spots, refer for genetic and neurologic consult.
Mongolian spots common over dorsal area and buttocks in dark-skin infants		Assure parents of normalcy of this pigmentation; it will fade in first year or two.
Erythema toxicum	Impetigo (group A ß-hemolytic streptococcus or *Staphylococcus aureus* infection)	If impetigo occurs, instruct parents about handwashing and linen precautions during home care.
Telangiectatic nevi	Hemangiomas: Nevus flammeus (port-wine stain) Nevus vascularis (strawberry hemangioma) Cavernous hemangiomas	Collaborate with physician. Counsel parents about birthmark's progression to allay misconceptions. Record size and shape of hemangiomas. Refer for follow-up at well-baby clinic.
	*Possible causes of alterations are identified in parentheses.	†This column provides guidelines for further assessment and initial nursing interventions.

(Continued on next page)

ASSESSMENT GUIDE NEWBORN PHYSICAL ASSESSMENT (Continued)

Physical Assessment/ Normal Findings	Alterations and Possible Causes*	Nursing Responses to Data†
Skin (Continued)		
Rashes	Rashes (infection)	Assess location and type of rash (macular, papular, vesicular). Obtain history of onset, prenatal history, and related signs and symptoms.
Petechiae of head or neck (breech presentation, cord around neck)	Generalized petechiae (clotting abnormalities)	Determine cause; advise parents if further health care is needed.
Head		
General appearance, size, movement Round, symmetric, and moves easily from left to right and up and down; soft and pliable	Asymmetric, flattened occiput on either side of the head (plagiocephaly) Head held at angle (torticollis) Unable to move head side to side (neurologic trauma)	Instruct parents to change infant's positions frequently when awake. When awake, needs to spend "tummy time." Infants should be placed supine for sleep per "Back to sleep" guidelines. Determine adequacy of all neurologic signs.
Circumference 32 to 37 cm (12.5 to 14.5 in.); 2 cm greater than chest circumference Head one-fourth of body size	Extreme differences in size may be microencephaly (Cornelia de Lange syndrome, cytomegalic inclusion disease [CID], rubella, toxoplasmosis, chromosome abnormalities), hydrocephalus (meningomyelocele, achondroplasia), anencephaly (neural tube defect) Head is 3 cm or more larger than chest circumference (preterm, hydrocephalus)	Measure circumference from occiput to frontal area using metal or paper tape. Measure chest circumference using metal or paper tape and compare to head circumference. Record measurements on growth chart. Reevaluate at well-baby visits.
Common variations: Molding	Cephalohematoma (trauma during birth, may persist up to 3 months)	Evaluate neurologic response. Observe for hyperbilirubinemia. Check Hct.
Breech and cesarean newborns' heads are round and well shaped	Caput succedaneum (long labor and birth; disappears in 1 week)	Reassure parents regarding common manifestations caused by birth process and when they should disappear.
Fontanelles: Palpation of juncture of cranial bones	Overlapping of anterior fontanelle (malnourished or preterm newborn)	Discuss normal closure times with parents and care of "soft spots" to allay misconceptions.
Anterior fontanelle: 3 to 4 cm long by 2 to 3 cm wide, diamond shaped	Premature closure of sutures (craniosynotiosis)	Refer to physician.
Posterior fontanelle: 1 to 2 cm at birth, triangle shaped Slight pulsation	Late closure (hydrocephalus)	Observe for signs and symptoms of hydrocephalus. Refer to physician.
	Moderate to severe pulsation (vascular problems)	
Moderate bulging noted with crying, stooling, or pulsations with heartbeat	Bulging (increased intracranial pressure, meningitis) Sunken (dehydration)	Evaluate hydration status. Evaluate neurologic status. Report to physician.
Hair		
Texture: Smooth with fine texture variations (Note: Variations depend on ethnic background.)	Coarse, brittle, dry hair (hypothyroidism) White forelock (Waardenburg syndrome)	Instruct parents regarding routine care of hair and scalp.
Distribution: Scalp hair high over eyebrows (Spanish Mexican hairline begins mid-forehead and extends down back of neck.)	Low forehead and posterior hairlines may indicate chromosomal disorders	Assess for other signs of chromosomal aberrations. Refer to physician.
Face		
Symmetric movement of all facial features, normal hairline, eyebrows and eyelashes present		Assess and record symmetry of all parts, shape, regularity of features, sameness or differences in features.
	*Possible causes of alterations are identified in parentheses.	†This column provides guidelines for further assessment and initial nursing interventions.

ASSESSMENT GUIDE   NEWBORN PHYSICAL ASSESSMENT *(Continued)*

Physical Assessment/ Normal Findings	Alterations and Possible Causes*	Nursing Responses to Data†
Spacing of features: Eyes at same level, nostrils equal size, cheeks full, and sucking pads present	Eyes wide apart—ocular hypertelorism (Apert syndrome, Cri du chat, Turner syndrome)	Observe for other signs and symptoms indicative of disease states or chromosomal aberrations.
Lips equal on both sides of midline	Abnormal face (Down syndrome, cretinism, gargoylism)	
Chin recedes when compared with other bones of face	Abnormally small jaw—micrognathia (Pierre Robin syndrome, Treacher Collins syndrome)	Maintain airway; do not position supine. Initiate surgical consultation and referral.
Movement: Makes facial grimaces	Inability to suck, grimace, and close eyelids (cranial nerve injury)	Initiate neurologic assessment and consultation.
Symmetric when resting and crying	Asymmetry (paralysis of facial cranial nerve)	Assess and record symmetry of all parts, shape, regularity of features, and sameness or differences in features.

Eyes

Physical Assessment/ Normal Findings	Alterations and Possible Causes*	Nursing Responses to Data†
General placement and appearance: Bright and clear; even placement; slight nystagmus (involuntary cyclical eye movements)	Gross nystagmus (damage to third, fourth, and sixth cranial nerves)	
Concomitant strabismus	Constant and fixed strabismus	Reassure parents that strabismus is considered normal up to 6 months.
Move in all directions Blue or slate blue-gray	Lack of pigmentation (albinism) Brushfield spots may indicate Down syndrome (a light or white speckling of the outer two-thirds of the iris)	Discuss with parents any necessary eye precautions. Assess for other signs of Down syndrome.
Brown color at birth in dark-skin infants		Discuss with parents that permanent eye color is usually established by 3 months of age.
Eyelids: Position: above pupils but within iris, no drooping	Elevation of (hydrocephalus) or retraction of upper lid (hyperthyroidism). "Sunset sign" lid elevation and downward gaze (hydrocephalus), ptosis (congenital or paralysis of oculomotor muscle)	Assess for signs of hydrocephalus and hyperthyroidism. Evaluate interference with vision in subsequent well-baby visits.
Eyes on parallel plane	Upward slant in non-Asians (Down syndrome)	Assess for other signs of Down syndrome.
Epicanthal folds in Asians and 20% of newborns of northern European descent	Epicanthal folds (Down syndrome, Cri du chat syndrome)	
Movement: Blink reflex in response to light stimulus. Eyes open wide in dimly lighted room	Blink absent (CNS injury)	Evaluate neurologic status. Refer to physician.
Inspection: Edematous for first few days of life, resulting from birth; no lumps or redness	Purulent drainage (infection); infectious conjunctivitis (gonococcus, chlamydia, staphylococcus, or gram-negative organisms) Marginal blepharitis (lid edges red, crusted, scaly)	Initiate good handwashing. Refer to physician. Evaluate infant for seborrheic dermatitis; scales can be removed easily.
Cornea: Clear	Ulceration (herpes infection); large cornea or corneas of unequal size (congenital glaucoma)	Refer to ophthalmologist.
Corneal reflex present	Clouding, opacity of lens (cataract)	Assess for other manifestations of congenital herpes; institute nursing care measures.
Sclera: May appear bluish in newborn, then white; slightly brownish color frequent in newborns of African descent	True blue sclera (osteogenesis imperfecta)	Refer to physician.

*Possible causes of alterations are identified in parentheses.

†This column provides guidelines for further assessment and initial nursing interventions.

(Continued on next page)

ASSESSMENT GUIDE NEWBORN PHYSICAL ASSESSMENT (Continued)

Physical Assessment/ Normal Findings	Alterations and Possible Causes*	Nursing Responses to Data†
Eyes (Continued)		
Pupils: Pupils equal in size, round, and react to light by accommodation	Anisocoria—unequal pupils (CNS damage) Dilation or constriction (intracranial) damage, retinoblastoma; glaucoma Pupils nonreactive to light or accommodation (brain injury)	Refer for neurologic examination.
Slight nystagmus in newborn who has not learned to focus Pupil light reflex demonstrated at birth or by 3 weeks of age	Nystagmus (labyrinthine disturbance, CNS disorder)	
Conjunctiva: Chemical conjunctivitis Subconjunctival hemorrhage	Pale color (anemia)	Obtain hematocrit and hemoglobin.
Palpebral conjunctiva (red but not hyperemic)	Inflammation or edema (infection, blocked tear duct)	Reassure parents that chemical conjunctivitis will subside in 1 to 2 days and subconjunctival hemorrhage disappears in a few weeks.
Vision: 20/200 Tracks moving object to midline Fixed focus on objects at a distance of about 10 to 20 in.; may be difficult to evaluate in newborn Prefers faces, geometric designs, and black and white to colors	Cataracts (congenital infection)	Record any questions about visual acuity, and initiate follow-up evaluation at first well-baby checkup.
Lashes and lacrimal glands: Presence of lashes (lashes may be absent in preterm newborns)	No lashes on inner two-thirds of lid (Treacher Collins syndrome); bushy lashes (Hurler syndrome); long lashes (Cornelia de Lange syndrome)	
Cry commonly tearless	Excessive tearing (plugged lacrimal duct, natal narcotic withdrawal), glaucoma	Demonstrate to parents how to milk blocked tear duct. Refer to ophthalmologist if tearing is excessive before third month of life.
Nose		
Appearance of external nasal aspects: May appear flattened as a result of birth process	Continued flat or broad bridge of nose (Down syndrome)	Arrange consultation with specialist. May be normal racial variation—Asian or African ancestry
Small and narrow in midline, even placement in relationship to eyes and mouth	Low bridge of nose, beaklike nose (Apert syndrome, Treacher Collins syndrome) Upturned (Cornelia de Lange syndrome)	Initiate evaluation of chromosomal abnormalities.
Patent nares bilaterally (nose breathers)	Blockage of nares (mucus and/or secretions), choanal atresia	Inspect for obstruction of nares.
Sneezing common to clear nasal passages	Flaring nares (respiratory distress)	Maintain oral airway until surgical correction is made.
Responds to odors, may smell breast milk	No response to stimulating odors	Inspect for obstruction of nares.
Mouth		
Function of facial, hypoglossal, glossopharyngeal, and vagus nerves: Symmetry of movement and strength	Mouth draws to one side (transient seventh cranial nerve paralysis caused by pressure in utero or trauma during birth, congenital paralysis) Fishlike shape (Treacher Collins syndrome)	Initiate neurologic consultation. Administer artificial tears if eye on affected side of face is unable to close.
Presence of gag, swallowing, coordinated with sucking reflexes Adequate salivation	Suppressed or absent reflexes	Evaluate other neurologic functions of these nerves.
	*Possible causes of alterations are identified in parentheses.	†This column provides guidelines for further assessment and initial nursing interventions.

ASSESSMENT GUIDE NEWBORN PHYSICAL ASSESSMENT (Continued)

Physical Assessment/ Normal Findings	Alterations and Possible Causes*	Nursing Responses to Data†
Palate (soft and hard): Hard palate dome-shaped. Uvula midline with symmetrical movement of soft palate	High-steepled palate (Treacher Collins syndrome), bifid uvula (congenital anomaly)	Assess for other congenital anomalies.
Palate intact, sucks well when stimulated	Clefts in either hard or soft palate (polygenic disorder)	Initiate a surgical consultation referral.
Epithelial (Epstein's) pearls appear on mucosa		Assure parents that these are normal and will disappear at 2 or 3 months of age.
Esophagus patent, some drooling common in newborn	Excessive drooling or bubbling (esophageal atresia)	Test for patency of esophagus.
Tongue: Free moving in all directions, midline	Lack of movement or asymmetric movement (neurologic damage) Tongue-tied Fasciculations (fine tremors) Spinal muscular atrophy	Further assess neurologic functions. Test reflex elevation of tongue when depressed with tongue blade.
Pink color, smooth to rough texture, noncoated	Deviations from midline (cranial nerve damage)	Check for signs of weakness or deviation.
	White cheesy coating (thrush)	Differentiate between thrush and milk curds by wiping patches: if white patches don't come off easily, it is thrush.
	Tongue has deep ridges	Reassure parents that tongue pattern may change from day to day.
Tongue proportional to mouth	Large tongue with short frenulum (cretinism, Down syndrome, other syndromes)	Evaluate in well-baby clinic to assess development delays. Initiate referrals.
Ears		
External ear: Without lesions, cysts, or nodules	Nodules, cysts, or sinus tracts in front of ear Adherent earlobes Low set ears (genetic anomaly or syndrome) Preauricular skin tags	Evaluate characteristics of lesions. Counsel parents to clean external ear with washcloth only; discourage use of cotton-tip applicators. Refer to physician for ligation.
Hearing: Eustachian tubes are cleared with first cry		
Absence of all risk factors for hearing loss	Presence of one or more risk factors	Assess history of risk factors for hearing loss.
Attends to sounds; sudden or loud noise elicits Moro reflex	No response to sound stimuli (deafness)	Test for Moro reflex.
Neck		
Appearance: Short, straight, creased with skin folds	Abnormally short neck (Turner syndrome) Arching or inability to flex neck (meningitis, congenital anomaly)	Report findings to physician.
Posterior neck lacks loose extra folds of skin	Webbing of neck (Turner syndrome, Down syndrome, trisomy 18)	Assess for other signs of the syndromes.
Clavicles: Straight and intact	Knot or lump on clavicle (fracture during difficult birth)	Obtain detailed labor and birth history; apply figure-8 bandage. Consider oral analgesics.
Moro reflex elicitable	Unilateral Moro reflex response on unaffected side (fracture of clavicle, brachial palsy, Erb-Duchenne paralysis)	Collaborate with physician.
Symmetric shoulders	Hypoplasia	
	*Possible causes of alterations are identified in parentheses.	†This column provides guidelines for further assessment and initial nursing interventions.

(Continued on next page)

Physical Assessment/ Normal Findings	Alterations and Possible Causes*	Nursing Responses to Data†
Chest		
Appearance and size: Circumference: 32.5 cm (12.8 in.), 1 to 2 cm (0.4 to 0.8 in.) less than head Wider than it is long		Measure at level of nipples after exhalation.
Normal shape without depressed or prominent sternum	Funnel chest (congenital or associated with Marfan syndrome)	Determine adequacy of other respiratory and circulatory signs.
Lower end of sternum (xiphoid cartilage) may be protruding; is less apparent after several weeks	Continued protrusion of xiphoid cartilage (Marfan syndrome, "pigeon chest")	Assess for other signs and symptoms of various syndromes.
Sternum 8 cm (3.1 in.) long	Barrel chest	
Expansion and retraction: Bilateral expansion	Unequal chest expansion (pneumonia, pneumothorax, respiratory distress)	Assess respiratory effort regularity, flaring of nares, difficulty on both inspiration and expiration.
No intercostal, subcostal, or supracostal retractions	Retractions (respiratory distress) See-saw respirations (respiratory distress)	
Auscultation: Breath sounds are louder in infants	Decreased breath sounds (decreased respiratory activity, atelectasis, pneumothorax)	Obtain transillumination. Record finding and consult physician.
Chest and axillae clear on crying	Increased breath sounds (resolving pneumonia or in cesarean births)	Perform assessment and report to physician any positive findings.
Bronchial breath sounds (heard where trachea and bronchi closest to chest wall, above sternum and between scapulae):		

Bronchial sounds bilaterally
   Air entry clear
   Rales may indicate normal newborn atelectasis
   Cough reflex absent at birth, appears in 2 or more days
	Adventitious or abnormal sounds (respiratory disease or distress)	Evaluate color for pallor or cyanosis. Report to physician.

Breasts: Flat with symmetric nipples	Lack of breast tissue (preterm or SGA)	
Breast tissue diameter 5 cm (2 in.) or more at term	Discharge	Evaluate for infection.
Distance between nipples 8 cm (3.1 in.)	Breast abscesses	
Breast engorgement occurs on third day of life; liquid discharge may be expressed in term newborns	Enlargement	Reassure parents of normality of breast engorgement.
Nipples	Supernumerary nipples Dark-colored nipples	No intervention is necessary.
Heart		
Auscultation: Location: lies horizontally, with left border extending to left of midclavicle		
Regular rhythm and rate	Arrhythmia (anoxia), tachycardia, bradycardia	Refer all arrhythmia and gallop rhythms. Initiate cardiac evaluation.
Determination of point of maximal impulse (PM1)	Malpositioning (enlargement, abnormal placement, pneumothorax, dextrocardia, diaphragmatic hernia)	
Usually lateral to midclavicular line at third or fourth intercostal space		
Functional murmurs	Location of murmurs (possible congenital cardiac anomaly)	Evaluate murmur: location, timing, and duration; observe for accompanying cardiac pathology symptoms; ascertain family history.
No thrills		
Horizontal groove at diaphragm shows flaring of rib cage to mild degree	Inadequacy of respiratory movement Marked rib flaring (vitamin D deficiency)	Initiate cardiopulmonary evaluation; assess pulses and blood pressures in all four extremities for equality and quality.
	*Possible causes of alterations are identified in parentheses.	†This column provides guidelines for further assessment and initial nursing interventions.

Physical Assessment/ Normal Findings	Alterations and Possible Causes*	Nursing Responses to Data†
Abdomen		
Appearance: Cylindrical with some protrusion, appears large in relation to pelvis, some laxness of abdominal muscles	Distention, shiny abdomen with engorged vessels (gastrointestinal abnormalities, infection, congenital megacolon)	Examine abdomen thoroughly for mass or organomegaly. Measure abdominal girth.
No cyanosis, few vessels seen Diastasis recti—common in infants of African descent	Scaphoid abdominal appearance (diaphragmatic hernia)	Report deviations of abdominal size.
	Increased or decreased peristalsis (duodenal stenosis, small bowel obstruction)	Assess other signs and symptoms of obstruction.
	Localized flank bulging (enlarged kidneys, ascites, or absent abdominal muscles)	Refer to physician.
Umbilicus: No protrusion of umbilicus (protrusion of umbilicus common in infants of African descent)	Umbilical hernia Patent urachus (congenital malformation)	Measure umbilical hernia by palpating the opening and record; it should close by 1 year of age; if not, refer to physician.
Bluish white color	Omphalocele (covered defect) Gastroschisis (uncovered defect)	Cover omphalocele and gastroschisis with sterile, moist dressing or plastic sterile bag.
Cutis navel (umbilical cord projects), granulation tissue present in navel	Redness or exudate around cord (infection) Yellow discoloration (hemolytic disease, meconium staining)	Instruct parents on cord care and hygiene.
Two arteries and one vein apparent	Single umbilical artery (congenital anomalies)	Refer anomalies to physician.
Begins drying 1 to 2 hours after birth		
No bleeding	Discharge or oozing of blood from the cord	
Auscultation and percussion all four gradients: Soft bowel sounds heard shortly after birth every 10 to 30 seconds	Bowel sounds in chest (diaphragmatic hernia) Absence of bowel sounds Hyperperistalsis (intestinal obstruction)	Collaborate with physician. Assess for other signs of dehydration and/or infection.
Femoral pulses: Palpable, equal bilateral	Absent or diminished femoral pulses (coarctation of aorta)	Monitor blood pressure in upper and lower extremities.
Inguinal area: No bulges along inguinal area	Inguinal hernia	Initiate referral.
No inguinal lymph nodes felt		Continue follow-up in well-baby clinic.
Bladder: Percusses 1 to 4 cm (0.4 to 1.6 in.) above symphysis	Failure to void within 24 to 48 hours after birth	Check whether baby voided at birth.
Emptied about 3 hours after birth; if not, at time of birth	Exposure of bladder mucosa (exstrophy of bladder)	Obtain urine specimen if infection is suspected.
Urine—inoffensive, mild odor	Foul odor (infection)	Consult with clinician.
Genitals		
Gender clearly delineated	Ambiguous genitals	Refer for genetic consultation.
Male		
Penis: Slender in appearance, about 2.5 cm (1 in.) long, 1 cm (0.4 in.) wide at birth	Micropenis (congenital anomaly) Meatal atresia	Observe and record first voiding.
Normal urinary orifice, urethral meatus at tip of penis	Hypospadias, epispadias	Collaborate with physician in presence of abnormality. Delay circumcision.
	*Possible causes of alterations are identified in parentheses.	†This column provides guidelines for further assessment and initial nursing interventions.

(Continued on next page)

ASSESSMENT GUIDE NEWBORN PHYSICAL ASSESSMENT *(Continued)*

Physical Assessment/ Normal Findings	Alterations and Possible Causes*	Nursing Responses to Data†
Noninflamed urethral opening	Urethritis (infection)	Palpate for enlarged inguinal lymph nodes and record painful urination.
Foreskin adheres to glans	Ulceration of meatal opening (infection, inflammation)	Evaluate whether ulcer is because of diaper rash; counsel regarding care.
Uncircumcised foreskin tight for 2 to 3 months	Phimosis—if still tight after 3 months	Instruct parents on how to care for uncircumcised penis.
Circumcised		Teach parents how to care for circumcision.
Erectile tissue present		
Scrotum: Skin loose and hanging or tight and small; extensive rugae and normal size	Large scrotum containing fluid (hydrocele) Red, shiny scrotal skin (orchitis)	Shine a light through scrotum (transilluminate) to verify diagnosis.
Normal skin color Scrotal discoloration common in breech	Minimal rugae, small scrotum	Assess for prematurity.
Testes: Descended by birth; not consistently found in scrotum	Undescended testes (cryptorchidism)	If testes cannot be felt in scrotum, gently palpate femoral, inguinal, perineal, and abdominal areas for presence.
Testes size 1.5 to 2 cm (0.6 to 0.8 in.) at birth	Enlarged testes (tumor) Small testes (Klinefelter syndrome or adrenal hyperplasia)	Refer and collaborate with physician for further diagnostic studies.

Female

Mons: Normal skin color, area pigmented in dark-skin infants		
Labia majora cover labia minora in term and postterm newborns; symmetric size appropriate for gestational age	Hematoma, lesions (trauma) Labia minora prominent	Evaluate for recent trauma. Assess for prematurity.
Clitoris: Normally large in newborn Edema and bruising in breech birth ·	Hypertrophy (hermaphroditism)	Refer for genetic workup.
Vagina: Urinary meatus and vaginal orifice visible (0.5 cm [0.2 in.] circumference)	Inflammation; erythema and discharge (urethritis) Congenital absence of vagina	Collect urine specimen for laboratory examination. Refer to physician.
Vaginal tag or hymenal tag disappears in a few weeks		
Discharge; smegma under labia	Foul-smelling discharge (infection)	Collect data and further evaluate reason for discharge.
Bloody or mucoid discharge	Excessive vaginal bleeding (blood coagulation defect)	

Buttocks and Anus

Buttocks symmetric	Pilonidal dimple	Examine for possible sinus. Instruct parents about cleansing this area.
Anus patent and passage of meconium within 24 to 48 hours after birth	Imperforate anus, rectal atresia (congenital gastrointestinal defect)	Evaluate extent of problems. Initiate surgical consultation.
No fissures, tears, or skin tags	Fissures	Perform digital examination to ascertain patency if patency uncertain.

Extremities and Trunk

Short and generally flexed, extremities move symmetrically through range of motion but lack full extension	Unilateral or absence of movement (spinal cord involvement) Fetal position continued or limp (anoxia)	Review birth record to assess possible cause.
All joints move spontaneously; good muscle tone of flexor type, birth to 2 months	Spasticity when infant begins using extensors (cerebral palsy)	Collaborate with physician.

*Possible causes of alterations are identified in parentheses.

†This column provides guidelines for further assessment and initial nursing interventions.

ASSESSMENT GUIDE NEWBORN PHYSICAL ASSESSMENT (Continued)

Physical Assessment/ Normal Findings	Alterations and Possible Causes*	Nursing Responses to Data†
Arms: Equal in length	Brachial palsy (difficult birth)	Report to clinician.
Bilateral movement	Erb-Duchenne paralysis	
Flexed when quiet	Muscle weakness, fractured clavicle Absence of limb or change of size (phocomelia, amelia)	
Hands: Normal number of fingers	Polydactyly (Ellis-van Creveld syndrome) Syndactyly—one limb (developmental anomaly) Syndactyly—both limbs (genetic component)	Report to clinician.
Normal palmar crease	Simian line on palm (Down syndrome)	Refer for genetic workup.
Normal size hands	Short fingers and broad hand (Hurler syndrome)	Evaluate for history of distress in utero.
Nails present and extend beyond fingertips in term newborn	Cyanosis and clubbing (cardiac anomalies) Nails long or yellow stained (postterm)	Carry out cardiac and respiratory assessments. Check pulse oximetry.
Spine: C-shaped spine	Spina bifida occulta (nevus pilosus)	Evaluate extent of neurologic damage; initiate care of spinal opening.
Flat and straight when prone	Dermal sinus	
Slight lumbar lordosis	Myelomeningocele	
Easily flexed and intact when palpated		
At least half of back devoid of lanugo		
Full-term infant in ventral suspension should hold head at 45-degree angle, back straight	Head lag, limp, floppy trunk (neurologic problems)	Elicit reflex to assess degree of involvement.
Hips: No sign of instability	Sensation of abnormal movement, jerk, or snap of hip dislocation	Physician or nurse practitioner examines all newborn infants for dislocated hip before discharge from birthing center.
Hips abduct to more than 60 degrees	Limited abduction (developmental dysplasia of hip)	If this is suspected, refer to orthopedist for further evaluation. Reassess at well-baby visits.
Inguinal and buttock skin creases: Symmetric inguinal and buttock creases	Asymmetry (dislocated hips)	Refer to orthopedist for evaluation. Counsel parents regarding symptoms of concern, and discuss therapy.
Legs: Legs equal in length	Shortened leg (dislocated hips)	Refer to orthopedist for evaluation.
Legs shorter than arms at birth	Lack of leg movement (fractures, spinal defects)	Counsel parents regarding symptoms of concern, and discuss therapy.
Feet: Foot is in straight line	Talipes equinovarus (true clubfoot)	Discuss differences between positional and true clubfoot with parents.
Positional clubfoot—based on position in utero		Teach parents passive manipulation of foot.
		Refer to orthopedist if not corrected by 3 months of age.
Fat pads and creases on soles of feet	Incomplete sole creases in first 24 hours of life (premature)	
Talipes planus (flat feet) normal under 3 years of age		Reassure parents that flat feet are normal in infants.
	*Possible causes of alterations are identified in parentheses.	†This column provides guidelines for further assessment and initial nursing interventions.

(Continued on next page)

ASSESSMENT GUIDE   NEWBORN PHYSICAL ASSESSMENT *(Continued)*

Physical Assessment/ Normal Findings	Alterations and Possible Causes*	Nursing Responses to Data†
Neuromuscular		
Motor function: Symmetric movement and strength in all extremities	Limp, flaccid, or hypertonic (CNS disorders, infection, dehydration, fracture)	Appraise newborn's posture and motor functions by observing activities and motor characteristics.
May be jerky or have brief twitching	Tremors (hypoglycemia, hypocalcemia, infection, neurologic damage)	Evaluate for electrolyte imbalance, hypoglycemia, and neurologic functioning.
Head lag not over 45 degrees	Delayed or abnormal development (preterm, neurologic involvement)	
Neck control adequate to maintain head erect briefly	Asymmetry of tone or strength (neurologic damage)	Refer for genetic evaluation.
Reflexes		
Blink: Stimulated by flash of light; response is closure of eyelids	Lack of blink response (damage to cranial nerve, CNS injury)	Assess neurologic status.
Pupillary reflex: Stimulated by flash of light; response is constriction of pupil	Lack of reflex (damage to cranial nerve, CNS injury)	
Moro: Response to sudden movement or loud noise should be one of symmetric extension and abduction of arms with fingers extended; then return to normal relaxed flexion	Asymmetry of body response (fractured clavicle, injury to brachial plexus)	Discuss normality of this reflex in response to loud noises and/or sudden movements.
Infant lying on back: slightly raised head suddenly released; infant held horizontally, lowered quickly about 6 in., and stopped abruptly Fingers form a C Present at birth; disappears by 6 months of age	Consistent absence (brain damage)	Absence of reflex requires neurologic evaluation.
Rooting and sucking: Turns in direction of stimulus to cheek or mouth; opens mouth and begins to suck rhythmically when finger or nipple is inserted into mouth; difficult to elicit after feeding; disappears by 4 to 7 months of age	Poor sucking or easily fatigable (preterm, breastfed infants of drug-addicted mothers, possible cardiac problem) Absence of response (preterm, neurologic involvement, depressed newborns)	Evaluate strength and coordination of sucking. Observe newborn during feeding, and counsel parents about mutuality of feeding experience and newborn's responses.
Sucking is adequate for nutritional intake and meeting oral stimulation needs		
Palmar grasp: Fingers grasp adult finger when palm is stimulated and held momentarily; lessens at 3 to 4 months of age	Asymmetry of response (neurologic problems)	Evaluate other reflexes and general neurologic functioning.
Plantar grasp: Toes curl downward when sole of foot is stimulated; lessens by 8 months	Absent (defects of lower spinal column)	Assess for other lower extremity neurologic problems.
Stepping: When held upright and one foot touching a flat surface, will step alternately; disappears at 4 to 8 weeks of age	Asymmetry of stepping (neurologic abnormality)	Evaluate muscle tone and function on each side of body. Refer to specialist.
Babinski: Fanning and extension of all toes when one side of sole is stroked from heel upward across ball of foot; disappears at about 12 months	Absence of response (low spinal cord defects)	Refer for further neurologic evaluation.
Tonic neck: Fencer position—when head is turned to one side, extremities on same side extend and on opposite side flex; this reflex may not be evident during early neonatal period; disappears at 3 to 4 months of age	Absent after 1 month of age or persistent asymmetry (cerebral lesion)	Assess neurologic functioning.
Response often more dominant in leg than in arm		

*Possible causes of alterations are identified in parentheses.

†This column provides guidelines for further assessment and initial nursing interventions.

ASSESSMENT GUIDE NEWBORN PHYSICAL ASSESSMENT (Continued)

Physical Assessment/ Normal Findings	Alterations and Possible Causes*	Nursing Responses to Data†
Prone crawl: While on abdomen, newborn pushes up and tries to crawl	Absence or variance of response (preterm, weak, or depressed newborns)	Evaluate motor functioning. Refer to specialist.
Trunk incurvation (Galant): In prone position, stroking of spine causes pelvis to turn to stimulated side	Failure to rotate to stimulated side (neurologic damage)	
	*Possible causes of alterations are identified in parentheses.	†This column provides guidelines for further assessment and initial nursing interventions.

The **Brazelton Neonatal Behavioral Assessment Scale** provides valuable guidelines for assessing the newborn's state changes, temperament, and individual behavior patterns. It provides a way for the nurse, in conjunction with the parents (primary caregivers), to identify and understand the individual newborn's states and capabilities. Families learn which responses, interventions, or activities best meet the special needs of their newborn, and this understanding fosters positive attachment experiences.

The assessment tool identifies the newborn's repertoire of behavioral responses to the environment and also documents the newborn's neurologic adequacy and capabilities. The examination usually takes 20 to 30 minutes and involves about 30 tests. Some items are scored according to the newborn's response to specific stimuli. Others, such as consolability and alertness, are scored as a result of continuous behavioral observations throughout the assessment. (For a complete discussion of all test items and maneuvers, see Brazelton & Nugent, 1995.)

Because the first few days after birth are a period of behavioral disorganization, the complete assessment should be done on the third day after birth. The nurse should make every effort to elicit the best response. This may be accomplished by repeating tests at different times or by testing during situations that facilitate the best possible response, such as when the parents are holding, cuddling, rocking, and/or singing to their baby.

Assessment of the newborn should be carried out initially in a quiet, dimly lighted room, if possible. The nurse should first determine the newborn's state of consciousness, because scoring and introduction of the test items are correlated with the sleep or waking state. The newborn's state depends on physiologic variables, such as the amount of time from the last feeding, positioning, environmental temperature, and health status; presence of such external stimuli as noises and bright lights; and the wake-sleep cycle of the infant. An important characteristic of the newborn period is the pattern of states, as well as the transitions from one state to another. The pattern of states is a predictor of the newborn's receptivity and ability to respond to stimuli in a cognitive manner. Babies learn best in a quiet, alert state and in an environment that is supportive and protective and that provides appropriate stimuli.

The nurse should observe the newborn's sleep-wake patterns (as discussed in Chapter 24 ∞), including the rapidity with which the newborn moves from one state to another, the ability to be consoled, and the ability to diminish the impact of disturbing stimuli. The following questions may provide the nurse with a framework for assessment:

- Does the newborn's response style and ability to adapt to stimuli indicate a need for parental interventions that will alert the newborn to the environment so that he or she can grow socially and cognitively?
- Are parental interventions necessary to lessen the outside stimuli, as in the case of the baby who responds to sensory input with intensity?
- Can the baby control the amount of sensory input that he or she must deal with?

The behaviors, and the sleep-wake states in which they are assessed, are categorized as follows:

- *Habituation.* The nurse assesses the newborn's ability to diminish or shut down innate responses to specific repeated stimuli, such as a rattle, bell, light, or pinprick to heel.
- *Orientation to inanimate and animate visual and auditory assessment stimuli.* The nurse observes how often and where the newborn attends to auditory and visual stimuli. Orientation to the environment is determined by an ability to respond to clues given by others and by a natural ability to fix on and follow a visual object horizontally and vertically. This capacity and parental appreciation of it are important for positive communication between infant and parents; the parents' visual (*en face*) and auditory (soft, continuous voice) presence stimulates their newborn to orient to them. Inability or lack of response may indicate visual or auditory problems. It is important for parents to know

that their newborn can turn to voices soon after birth or by 3 days of age and can become alert at different times with a varying degree of intensity in response to sounds.

- *Motor activity.* Several components are evaluated. Motor tone of the newborn is assessed in the most characteristic state of responsiveness. This summary assessment includes overall use of tone as the newborn responds to being handled—whether during spontaneous activity, prone placement, or horizontal holding—and overall assessment of body tone as the newborn reacts to all stimuli.

- *Variations.* Frequency of alert states, state changes, color changes (throughout all states as examination progresses), activity, and peaks of excitement are assessed.

- *Self-quieting activity.* This assessment is based on how often, how quickly, and how effectively newborns can use their resources to quiet and console themselves when upset or distressed. Considered in this assessment are such self-consolatory activities as putting hand to mouth, sucking on a fist or the tongue, and attuning to an object or sound (Figure 25–44 ■). The newborn's need for outside consolation must also be considered (e.g., seeing a face; being rocked, held, or dressed; using a pacifier; being swaddled).

- *Cuddliness or social behaviors.* This area encompasses the newborn's need for, and response to, being held. Also considered is how often the newborn smiles.

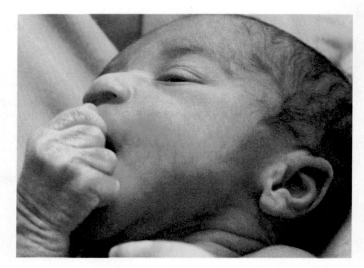

FIGURE 25–44 The newborn can bring hand to mouth as a self-soothing activity.

These behaviors influence the couple's self-esteem and feelings of acceptance or rejection. Cuddling also appears to be an indicator of personality. Cuddlers appear to enjoy, accept, and seek physical contact; are easier to placate; sleep more; and form earlier and more intense attachments. Noncuddlers are active, restless, have accelerated motor development, and are intolerant of physical restraint. Smiling, even as a grimace reflex, greatly influences parent-newborn feedback. Parents identify this response as positive.

CHAPTER HIGHLIGHTS

- A perinatal history, determination of gestational age, physical examination, and behavior assessment form the basis for a complete newborn assessment.

- The common physical characteristics included in the gestational age assessment are skin, lanugo, sole (plantar) creases, breast tissue and size, ear form and cartilage, and genitalia.

- The neuromuscular components of gestational age scoring tools are usually posture, square window sign, popliteal angle, arm recoil, heel-to-ear extension, and scarf sign.

- By assessing the physical and neuromuscular components specified in a gestational age tool, the nurse can determine the gestational age of the newborn.

- After determining the gestational age of the baby, the nurse can assess how the newborn will make the transition to extrauterine life and anticipate potential physiologic problems.

- The nurse identifies the newborn as small for gestational age (SGA), appropriate for gestational age (AGA), or large for gestational age (LGA), and prioritizes individual needs.

- Normal ranges for vital signs assessed in the newborn are as follows: heart rate, 120 to 160 beats per minute; respirations, 30 to 60 respirations per minute; axillary tempera-

ture, 36.4°C to 37.2°C (97.5°F to 99°F); skin temperature, 36°C to 36.5°C (96.8°F to 97.7°F); rectal temperature, 36.6°C to 37.2°C (97.8°F to 99°F); and blood pressure at birth, 70–50/45–30 mm Hg (at birth).

- Normal newborn measurements are as follows: weight range, 2500 to 4000 g (5 lb, 8 oz to 8 lb, 13 oz), with weight dependent on maternal size and age; length range, 46 to 56 cm (18 to 22 in.); and head circumference range, 32 to 37 cm (12.5 to 14.5 in.)—approximately 2 cm (0.8 in.) larger than the chest circumference.

- Commonly elicited newborn reflexes are tonic neck, Moro, grasp, rooting, sucking, and blink.

- Newborn behavioral abilities include habituation, orientation to visual and auditory stimuli, motor activity, cuddliness, and self-quieting activity.

- An important role of the nurse during the physical and behavioral assessments of the newborn is to teach parents about their newborn and involve them in their baby's care. This involvement facilitates the parents' identification of their newborn's uniqueness and allays their concerns.

CHAPTER REFERENCES

American Academy of Pediatrics (AAP), Committee on Fetus and Newborn, & American College of Obstetricians and Gynecologists (ACOG), Committee on Obstetrics. (2007). *Guidelines for perinatal care* (6th ed.). Evanston, IL: Author.

Ballard, J. L., Khoury, J. C., Wedig, K., Wang, L., Eilers-Walsmann, B. L., & Lipp, R. (1991). New Ballard score, expanded to include extremely premature infants. *Journal of Pediatrics, 119*(3), 417–423.

Blackburn, S. T. (2007). *Maternal, fetal, neonatal physiology: A clinical perspective* (3rd ed.). St. Louis: Saunders.

Brazelton, T. B., & Nugent, J. K. (1995). *The neonatal behavioral assessment scale* (3rd ed.). London: MacKeith.

Creehan, P. A. (2008). Newborn physical assessment. In K. R. Simpson & P. A. Creehan, *Perinatal nursing* (3rd ed., pp. 546–574). Philadelphia: Lippincott Williams & Wilkins.

Mandleco, B. L. (2004). *Growth and development handbook: Newborn through adolescence.* Clifton Park, NY: Thomson/Delmar Learning.

Rosenberg, A. A. (2007). The neonate. In S. G. Gabbe, J. R. Niebyl, & J. L. Simpson (Eds.). *Obstetrics: Normal and problem pregnancies.* (5th ed., pp. 523–565). Philadelphia, PA: Churchill Livingstone/Elsevier.

Thureen, P. J., Deacon, J., Hernandez, J. A., & Hall, D. M. (2005). *Assessment and care of the well newborn* (2nd ed.). St. Louis: Elsevier.

Wu, T.-Y., & Daniel, L. (2001). Growth of immigrant Chinese infants in the first year of life. *American Journal of Maternal Child Nursing, 26*(4), 202–207.

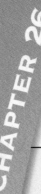
Normal Newborn: Needs and Care

I've been a postpartum nurse for about 6 years. A large part of my job involves teaching or enhancing parenting skills. I get enormous satisfaction out of watching a hesitant dad change his newborn for the first time or helping a mother breastfeed this baby, when she wasn't able to with her last one. I only wish I had more time to spend with each family.

—Mother-Baby Nurse

LEARNING OUTCOMES

26-1. Explain essential information from the prenatal period and the newborn's birth experience from the labor/birth and transition record to predict the newborn's ability to transition to the extrauterine environment.

26-2. Explain how the physiologic and behavioral responses of the newborn during the first 4 hours after birth (admission and transitional period) determines the nursing care management of the newborn.

26-3. Explain how the physiologic and behavioral responses of the newborn after the transition period to discharge determines the nursing care management of the newborn.

26-4. Describe the nurse's role in the care of the parents and newborn before, during, and after circumcision.

26-5. Examine the nurse's role in enhancing parent-newborn attachment.

26-6. Discuss how cultural practices of parents influence the nursing care management of the newborn.

26-7. Describe common concerns of families regarding their newborns.

26-8. Describe topics and related content to be included in discharge planning and parent teaching on daily newborn and infant care.

26-9. Discuss opportunities to individualize parent teaching and enhance each parent's abilities and confidence while providing infant care in the birthing unit.

At the moment of birth, numerous physiologic adaptations begin to take place in the newborn's body. Because of these dramatic changes, newborns require close observation to determine how smoothly they are making the transition to extrauterine life. Newborns also require specific care that enhances their chances of making the transition successfully.

The two broad goals of nursing care during this period are: (1) to promote the physical well-being of the newborn, and (2) to support the establishment of a well-functioning family unit. The nurse meets the first goal by providing comprehensive care to the newborn in the mother-baby unit. The nurse meets the second goal by teaching family members how to care for their new baby and by supporting their efforts so that they feel confident and competent. Thus the nurse must be knowledgeable about family adjustments that need to be made as well as the healthcare needs of the newborn. It is important that the family return home with the positive feeling that they have the support, information, and skills to care for their newborn. Equally important is the need for each member of the family to begin a unique relationship with the newborn. The cultural and social expectations of individual families and communities affect the way in which normal newborn care is carried out.

The previous two chapters presented an informational database of the physiologic and behavioral changes occurring in the newborn and the pertinent nursing assessments that are needed. This chapter discusses the nursing care management while the newborn is in the birthing unit. The Clinical Pathway: Newborn Care feature starts on page 632.

Nursing Care During Admission and the First Four Hours of Life

Immediately after birth, the baby is formally admitted to the healthcare facility.

Nursing Assessment and Diagnosis

Before the birth of an infant, the nurse reviews the mother's prenatal record for information concerning possible risk factors for the infant. These include infectious diseases screening results, drug or alcohol use by the mother, gestational diabetes, and any other data determined to be of use in anticipating the needs of the newborn. In addition, the nurse reviews the birth record for prolonged rupture of membranes, instrument or vacuum childbirth, use of narcotic analgesia, presence of meconium, and any other data that may impact the infant's ability to successfully transition to the extrauterine environment.

During the first 4 hours after birth, the nurse carries out a preliminary physical examination, including an assessment of the newborn's physiologic adaptations. In many birthing units, the nurse performs and documents the initial head-to-toe physical assessment during the first hour of transition. The nurse is responsible for notifying the physician or nurse practitioner of any deviation from normal. A complete physical examination is also performed later by the physician or nurse practitioner, within 24 hours after birth and within 24 hours before discharge. This can be accomplished with one physical examination (American Academy of Pediatrics [AAP] & American College of Obstetricians and Gynecologists [ACOG], 2007) (see Chapter 25 ∞).

Nursing diagnoses are based on an analysis of the assessment findings. Physiologic alterations of the newborn form the basis of many nursing diagnoses, as does the family members' incorporation of them in caring for their new baby. Nursing diagnoses that may apply to newborns include the following:

- *Ineffective Airway Clearance* related to presence of mucus and retained lung fluid
- *Risk for Imbalanced Body Temperature* related to evaporative, radiant, conductive, and convective heat losses
- *Acute Pain* related to heel sticks for glucose or hematocrit tests or vitamin K injection

As discussed in Chapter 25 ∞, the newborn's physiologic adaptation to extrauterine life occurs rapidly and all body systems are affected. (See Key Facts to Remember: Signs of Newborn Transition.) Therefore, many of these nursing diagnoses and associated interventions must be identified and implemented in a very short period.

Nursing Plan and Implementation

The nurse initiates newborn admission procedures and evaluates the newborn's need to remain under observation. This evaluation may take place in a special transition area or at the mother's bedside. It includes the following:

- Maternal and birth history
- Airway clearance
- Vital signs
- Body temperature
- Neurologic status
- Ability to feed
- Evidence of complications

Clinical Pathway   NEWBORN CARE

FIRST 4 HOURS	4 TO 8 HOURS PAST BIRTH	8 TO 24 HOURS PAST BIRTH
REFERRAL		
Review labor/birth record Review transitional nursing record Check ID bands and security alarms if present Consult prn: orthopedics, genetics, infectious disease	Check ID bands and security alarms Transfer to mother-baby care at 4 to 6 hours of age if stable As parents desire, obtain circumcision permit after their discussion with physician Lactation consult prn	Check ID bands and security alarm q shift **Expected Outcomes** Mother/baby ID bands correlate at time of discharge, security alarms in place at all times; consults completed prn
ASSESSMENTS		
Continue assessments begun first hour after birth Vital sign: TPR, BP prn, q1h × 4 (skin temp 36°C to 36.5°C [96.8°F to 97.7°F], resp may be irregular but within 30 to 60 per min) **Newborn Assessments** • Respiratory status with resp. distress scale × 1 then prn. If resp. distress, assess q5–15 min • Cord: bluish white color, clamp in place and free from skin • Color: skin, mucous membranes, extremities, trunk pink with slight acrocyanosis of hands and feet • Wt (5 lb. 8 oz to 8 lb. 13 oz) 2500 to 4000 g, length (18 to 22 in.) 46 to 56 cm, HC (12.5 to 14.5 in.) 32 to 37 cm, CC (32.5 cm, 1 to 2 cm less than head) • Extremity movement—may be jerky or brief twitches • Gestational age classification—term AGA • Anomalies (cong. anomalies can interfere with normal extrauterine adaptation)	Assess newborn's progress through periods of reactivity Vital signs: TPR q8h and prn, or per agency protocol, BP prn **Newborn Assessments** • Skin color q4h prn (circulatory system stabilizing, acrocyanosis decreased) • Eyes for drainage, redness, hemorrhage • Auscultate lungs q4h (noisy, wet breath sounds clear and equal) • Increased mucus production (normal in second period of reactivity) • Check apical pulse q4h • Check umbilical cord base for redness, drainage, foul odor, drying, clamp in place • Extremity movements q4h • Check for expected reflexes (suck, rooting, Moro, grasp, blink, yawn, sneeze, tonic neck, Babinski) • Note common normal variations • Assess suck and swallow during feeding • Note behavioral characteristics • Check temp before and after admission bath	VS q8h; normal ranges: T, 36.4°C to 37.2°C (97.5°F to 99°F) P, 120 to 160; R, 30 to 60; BP, 90–60/50–40 mm Hg **Continue Newborn Assessments** • Skin color q4h • Signs of drying or infection in cord area • Check that clamp is in place until removed before discharge • Check circ. for bleeding after procedure, then q30min × 2, then q4h and prn Observe for jaundice. Obtain total serum bili (TsB) if infant visibly jaundiced before 24 hours of age. Obtain transcutaneous bili on all infants not previously tested before discharge. **Expected Outcomes** Vital signs medically acceptable, color pink, assessments WNL, circ. site without s/s infection, cord site without s/s of infection and clamp removed; newborn behavior WNL
TEACHING/PSYCHOSOCIAL		
Admission activities performed at mother's bedside if possible, orient to nursery prn, handwashing, assess teaching needs Teach parents use of bulb syringe, signs of choking, positioning, and when to call for assistance Teach reasons for use of radiant warmer, infant hat, and warmed blankets when out of warmer Discuss/teach infant security, identification	Reinforce teaching about choking, bulb syringe use, positioning, temperature maintenance with clothing and blankets Teach infant positioning to facilitate breathing and digestion Teach new parents holding and feeding skills Teach parents soothing and calming techniques Teach parents about introducing newborn to sibling	Final discharge teaching: diapering, normal void and stool patterns, bathing, nail and cord care, circumcision/uncircumcised penis/genital care and normal characteristics, rashes, jaundice, sleep-wake cycles, soothing activities, taking temperatures, thermometer reading Explain s/s of illness and when to call healthcare provider Infant safety: car seats, immunizations, metabolic screening **Expected Outcomes** Mother/family verbalize comprehension of teaching; demonstrate care capabilities

Clinical Pathway   NEWBORN CARE (Continued)

FIRST 4 HOURS	4 TO 8 HOURS PAST BIRTH	8 TO 24 HOURS PAST BIRTH
NURSING CARE MANAGEMENT AND REPORTS		
Place under radiant warmer Place hat on newborn (decreases convection heat loss) Suction nares/mouth with bulb syringe prn Keep bulb syringe with infant Attach security sensor Obtain lab tests: blood glucose; as needed Obtain blood type, Rh, Coombs on cord blood, HSV culture if parental hx Notify physician's office of infant's birth and any change in status Maintain Standard Precautions	Wean from radiant warmer (T 37°C [98°F] axillary) Chemstrips prn; BP prn Oxygen saturation prn Bathe infant if temp greater than 36.5°C (97.7°F) Position on side Suction nares prn (esp. during second period of reactivity) Obtain peripheral Hct per protocol Cord care per protocol Fold diaper below cord (for plastic diapers, turn plastic layer away from skin)	Check for hearing test results Weigh before discharge Cord assessment q shift DC cord clamp before discharge Perform newborn metabolic screening blood tests before discharge Circumcision if indicated; circumcision care: change diaper prn, noting ability to void; follow policy for circumcision damp or Plastibell care **Expected Outcomes** Newborn maintains temp, lab test WNL, cord dry without s/s of infection and clamp removed, screening tests accomplished, circ. site without s/s of infection or bleeding
ACTIVITY AND COMFORT		
Place under radiant warmer or wrap in prewarmed blankets until stable or maintain skin-to-skin contact with mother Soothe baby as needed with voice, touch, cuddling, nesting in warmer	Leave in warmer until stable, then swaddle Position on back after each feeding	Place in open crib Swaddle to allow movement of extremities in blanket, including hands to face **Expected Outcomes** Infant maintains temp WNL in open crib, infant attempts self-calming behaviors
NUTRITION		
Assist newborn to breastfeed as soon as mother/baby condition allows Supplement breast only when medically indicated or per agency policy Initiate formula-feeding within first hour Gavage feed if necessary to prevent hypoglycemia	Breastfeed on demand, at least q3–4h Teach positions, observe/assist with feeding, breast/nipple care, establishing milk supply, breaking suction, feeding cues, latching-on techniques, nutritive suck, burping Formula-feed on demand, at least q3–4h Determine readiness to feed and feeding tolerance	Continue breastfeeding or formula-feeding pattern Assess feeding tolerance q4h Discuss normal feeding requirements, signs of hunger and satiation, handling feeding problems, and when to seek help **Expected Outcomes** Mother verbalizes knowledge of feeding information; breastfeeds on demand without supplement; bottle—tolerates formula-feeding, nipples without problems
ELIMINATION		
Note first void and stool if not noted at birth	Note all voids, amount and color of stools q4h	Evaluate all voids and stool color q8h **Expected Outcomes** Voids qs; stools qs without difficulty; stool character WNL diaper area without s/s of skin breakdown or rashes
MEDICATION		
Prophylactic ophthalmic ointment both after baby makes eye contact with parents and within 1 hr after birth Administer AquaMEPHYTON IM, dosage according to infant weight per MD/NP order and within 1 hr of birth	Hepatitis B injection as ordered by physician after consent signed by parents	Hepatitis B vaccine within 2 hrs of birth or before discharge **Expected Outcomes** Baby has received ophthalmic ointment and vitamin K injection; baby has received first Hep B vaccine if ordered and parental permission received

(Continued on next page)

Clinical Pathway   NEWBORN CARE *(Continued)*

FIRST 4 HOURS	4 TO 8 HOURS PAST BIRTH	8 TO 24 HOURS PAST BIRTH
DISCHARGE PLANNING/HOME CARE		
Hepatitis B consent signed Hearing screen consent signed Plan discharge call with parent or guardian in 24 hr to 2 days Assess parents' discharge plans, needs, and support systems	Review/reinforce teaching with mother and significant other Review home preparedness Present birth certificate instructions	Initial newborn screening tests (hearing, blood tests, metabolic screen [i.e., PKU]) before discharge Bath and feeding classes, videos, or written information given Give written copy of discharge instructions Newborn photographs Set up appointment for follow-up PKU test Have car seat available before discharge All discharge referrals made, follow-up appt scheduled **Expected Outcomes** Infant discharged home with family; mother verbalizes follow-up appt time/date
FAMILY INVOLVEMENT		
Facilitate early investigation of baby's physical characteristics (maintain temp during unwrapping), hold infant *en face* Dim lights to help infant keep eyes open	Assess parents' knowledge of newborn behaviors, such as alertness, suck and rooting, attention to human voice, response to calming techniques	Assess mother-baby bonding/interaction Incorporate father and siblings in care Enhance parent-infant interaction by sharing characteristics and behavioral assessment Support positive parenting behaviors Identify community referral needs and refer to community agencies **Expected Outcome** Demonstrates caring and family incorporation of infant
DATE		

AGA, average for gestational age; Appt, appointment; CC, chest circumference; cong., congenital; esp., especially; HC, head circumference; Hct, hematocrit; Hx, history; ID, identification; PKU, phenylketonuria; qs, quantity sufficient; s/s, signs and symptoms; temp, temperature; TPR, temperature, pulse, respirations; VS, vital signs; WNL, within normal limits.

If the evaluation is normal, the baby is successfully making the transition to extrauterine life and may need less frequent observations. In some settings, this may also be a time for moving the mother and baby to another care unit.

Initiation of Admission Procedures

After birth the baby is formally admitted to the healthcare facility. The admission procedures include a review of prenatal and birth information for possible risk factors, a gestational age assessment, and an assessment to ensure that the newborn's adaptation to extrauterine life is proceeding normally. This evaluation of the newborn's status and risk factors must be done no later than 2 hours after birth (AAP & ACOG, 2007).

If the initial assessment indicates that the newborn is not at risk physiologically, the nurse performs many of the routine admission procedures in the presence of the parents in the birthing area. Some care measures indicated by the assessment findings may be performed by the nurse or by the family members under the guidance of the nurse in an effort to educate and support the family. Other interventions may be delayed until the newborn has been transferred to an observational nursery.

The nurse responsible for the newborn first checks and confirms the newborn's identification with the mother's identification and then obtains and records all significant information. The essential data to be recorded on the newborn's chart are as follows:

1. *Condition of the newborn.* Pertinent information includes the newborn's Apgar scores at 1 and 5 minutes, resuscitative measures required in the birthing area, physical examination, vital signs, voidings, and passing of

KEY FACTS TO REMEMBER

Signs of Newborn Transition

Normal findings for the newborn during the first few days of life include the following:

Pulse: 120 to 160 beats/minute

    During sleep as low as 100 beats/minute

    If crying, up to 180 beats/minute

    Apical pulse is counted for 1 full minute because rate may fluctuate

Respirations: 30 to 60 respirations/minute

    Predominantly diaphragmatic but synchronous with abdominal movements

    Brief periods of apnea (less than 15 seconds) with no color or heart rate changes

Temperature:

    Axillary: 36.4°C to 37.2°C (97.5°F to 99°F)

    Skin: 36°C to 36.5°C (96.8°F to 97.7°F)

Blood pressure: 90–60/50–40 mm Hg at birth; 100/50 mm Hg at day 10

Blood glucose: greater than or equal to 40 mg%

Hematocrit: less than 65% to 70% central venous sample

---

meconium. Complications to be noted are excessive mucus, delayed spontaneous respirations or responsiveness, abnormal number of cord vessels, and obvious physical abnormalities.

2. *Labor and birth record.* A copy of the labor and birth record should be placed in the newborn's chart or be accessible on the computer. The record contains the significant data about the birth, for example, duration, course, and status of mother and fetus throughout labor and birth and any analgesia or anesthesia administered to the mother. Particular care is taken to note any variation or difficulties, such as prolonged rupture of membranes, abnormal fetal position, presence or absence of meconium-stained amniotic fluid, signs of nonreassuring fetal heart rate during labor, nuchal cord (cord around the newborn's neck at birth), precipitous birth, use of forceps or vacuum extraction assisted device, maternal analgesics and anesthesia received within 1 hour before birth, and administration of antibiotics during labor.

3. *Antepartal history.* Any maternal problems that may have compromised the fetus in utero, such as preeclampsia, spotting, illness, recent infections (evidence of chorioamnionitis), blood type, rubella status, serology results, hepatitis B screen results, colonization with group B streptococci or intrapartum maternal antibiotic therapy; maternal medications (including tocolytics and corticosteroids), a history of maternal substance abuse are of immediate concern in newborn assessment. The chart should also include information about maternal age, estimated date of birth (EDB), previous pregnancies, and presence of any congenital anomalies. A human immunodeficiency virus (HIV) test result, if obtained, is also relevant (AAP & ACOG, 2007).

4. *Parent-newborn interaction information.* The nurse notes parents' interactions with their newborn and their desires regarding care, such as rooming-in, circumcision, and the type of feeding. Information about other children in the home, available support systems, interactional patterns within each family unit, situations that compromise lactation (breast surgery, previous lactation failure), and any high risk circumstances (adolescent mother, domestic violence, history of child abuse) assists the nurse in providing comprehensive care (AAP & ACOG, 2007).

As part of the admission procedure, the nurse weighs the newborn in both grams and pounds. In the United States, parents understand weight best when it is stated in pounds and ounces (Figure 26–1 ■). The nurse cleans and covers the scales each time a newborn is weighed to prevent cross infection and heat loss from conduction.

The nurse then measures the newborn, recording the measurements in both centimeters and inches. The three routine measurements are length, circumference of the head, and circumference of the chest. In some facilities, abdominal girth may also be measured. The nurse rapidly assesses the baby's color, muscle tone, alertness, and general state. Remember that the first period of reactivity may have concluded, and the baby may be in the sleep-inactive phase, which makes the infant hard to arouse. The nurse does basic assessments for estimating gestational age and completes the physical assessment (see Chapter 25 ∞).

In addition to obtaining vital signs, the nurse may perform a hematocrit and blood glucose evaluation on at-risk newborns or as clinically indicated (such as for small-for-gestational-age [SGA] or large-for-gestational-age [LGA] infants, or if the newborn is jittery). These procedures

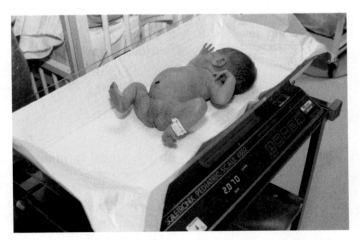

FIGURE 26–1 Weighing of newborn: The scale is cleaned and balanced before each weighing, with the protective pad in place.

may be done on admission or within the first 2 hours after birth (AAP & ACOG, 2007.) (See the Clinical Skill in Chapter 29 ∞, pages 768–769.)

Maintenance of a Clear Airway and Stable Vital Signs

Free flow oxygen should be readily available. The nurse positions the newborn on his or her back (or side, if infant has copious secretions). If necessary, the nurse should use a bulb syringe or DeLee wall suction (see the Clinical Skill in Chapter 19 ∞) to remove mucus from the stomach to help prevent possible aspiration. When possible, this procedure should be delayed for 10 to 15 minutes after birth, reducing the potential for severe vasovagal reflex apnea.

In the absence of any newborn distress, the nurse continues with the admission by taking the newborn's vital signs. The initial temperature is taken by the axillary method. A wider range of normal exists for axillary temperature, specifically 36.4°C to 37.2°C (97.5°F to 99°F).

Once the initial temperature is taken, the nurse monitors the core temperature either by obtaining axillary temperatures at intervals or by placing a skin sensor on the newborn for continuous reading. The usual skin sensor placement site is the newborn's abdomen, but placement on the upper thigh or arm can give a reading closely correlated with the mean body temperature. The vital signs for a healthy term newborn should be monitored at least every 30 minutes until the newborn's condition has remained stable for 2 hours (AAP & ACOG, 2007). The newborn's respirations may be irregular yet still be normal. Brief periods of apnea, lasting only 5 to 10 seconds with no color or heart rate changes, are considered normal. The normal pulse range is 120 to 160 beats per minute (bpm), and the normal respiratory range is 30 to 60 respirations per minute.

Maintenance of a Neutral Thermal Environment

A neutral thermal environment is essential to minimize the newborn's need for increased oxygen consumption and use of calories to maintain body heat in the optimal range of 36.4°C to 37.2°C (97.5°F to 99°F). If the newborn becomes hypothermic, the body's response can lead to metabolic acidosis, hypoxia, and shock.

A neutral thermal environment is best achieved by performing the newborn assessment and interventions with the newborn unclothed and under a radiant warmer. The radiant warmer's thermostat is controlled by the thermal skin sensor taped to the newborn's abdomen, upper thigh, or arm (Figure 26–2 ■). The sensor indicates when the newborn's temperature exceeds or falls below the acceptable temperature range. The nurse should be aware that leaning over the newborn may block the radiant heat waves from reaching the newborn.

It is common practice in some institutions to cover the newborn's head with a cap made of insulated fabrics, wool, or polyolefin; lined with Gamgee; or insulated with a plastic liner to prevent further evaporative heat loss, in addition to placing the baby under a radiant warmer (Blackburn, 2007). (See Temperature Regulation in Chapter 24 ∞ and Clinical Skill: Thermoregulation of the Newborn.)

When the newborn's temperature is normal and vital signs are stable (about 2 to 4 hours after birth), the baby may be given a sponge bath. However, this admission bath may be postponed for some hours if the newborn's condition dictates or the parents wish to give the first bath. In light of early discharge practices (12 to 48 hours), healthy term infants can be safely bathed immediately after the admission assessment is completed. The baby is bathed while still under the radiant warmer; the bathing may be done in the parents' room and by the parents (Medves & O'Brien, 2004). Bathing the newborn offers an excellent opportunity for teaching and welcoming parents' involvement in the care of their baby.

The nurse rechecks the baby's temperature after the bath and, if it is stable, dresses the newborn in a shirt, diaper, and cap; wraps the baby; and places the newborn in an open crib at room temperature. If the baby's axillary temperature is below 36.5°C (97.7°F), the nurse returns the baby to the radiant warmer. The rewarming process should be gradual to prevent hyperthermia. Once the newborn is rewarmed, the nurse implements measures to prevent further neonatal heat loss, such as keeping the newborn dry, swaddled in one or two blankets with hat on, and away from cool surfaces or instruments. The nurse also protects the newborn from drafts, open windows or doors, and air conditioners. Blankets and clothing are stored in a warm place. (See Chapter 25 ∞ and Key Facts to Remember: Maintenance of Stable Newborn Temperature.) Newborns are often "double-wrapped" in two or more blankets for temperature maintenance.

Prevention of Vitamin K Deficiency Bleeding

A prophylactic injection of vitamin K_1 (AquaMEPHYTON) is recommended to prevent hemorrhage, which can

Clinical Skill Thermoregulation of the Newborn

NURSING ACTION	RATIONALE

Preparation

1. Prewarm the incubator or radiant warmer. Make sure warm towels and/or lightweight blankets are available.

2. Maintain the temperature of the birthing room at 22°C (71°F), with a relative humidity of 60% to 65%.

The change from a warm, moist intrauterine environment to a cool, dry, drafty environment stresses the newborn's immature thermoregulation system.

Equipment and Supplies

- Prewarmed towels or blankets
- Infant stocking cap
- Servocontrol probe
- Infant T-shirt and diaper
- Open crib

Procedure

1. Don gloves.

Gloves are worn whenever there is the possibility of contact with body fluids—in this case, a newborn wet with amniotic fluid, vernix, and maternal blood.

2. Place the newborn under the radiant warmer. Wipe the newborn free of blood, fluid, and excess vernix, especially from the head, using prewarmed towels.

The radiant warmer creates a heat-gaining environment. Drying is important to prevent the loss of body heat through evaporation.

3. If the newborn is stable, wrap him or her in a prewarmed blanket, apply a stocking cap, and carry the newborn to the mother. The mother and her support person can hold and enjoy the newborn together. Alternatively, carry the newborn wrapped to the mother, loosen the blanket, and place the infant skin-to-skin on the mother's chest under a warmed blanket.

Use of a prewarmed blanket reduces convection heat loss and facilitates maternal-newborn contact without compromising the newborn's thermoregulation. Skin-to-skin contact with the mother or father helps maintain the newborn's temperature.

4. After the newborn has spent time with the parents, return him or her to the radiant warmer and apply a diaper. Leave the newborn uncovered (except for the cap and diaper) under the radiant warmer.

Radiant heat warms the outer skin surface, so the skin needs to be exposed.

5. Tape a servocontrol probe on the newborn's anterior abdominal wall, with the metal side next to the skin. Do not place it over the ribs. Secure the probe with porous tape or a foil-covered aluminum heat deflector patch. Figure 26–2 shows a newborn with a skin probe. Note that in this picture the newborn is no longer wearing a stocking cap.

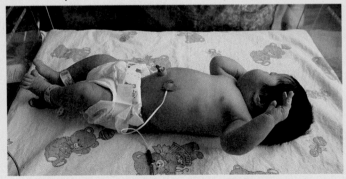

FIGURE 26–2 Temperature monitoring for the newborn. A skin thermal sensor is placed on the newborn's abdomen, upper thigh, or arm and secured with porous tape or a foil-covered foam pad.
Source: Photographer, Elena Dorfman.

(Continued on next page)

Clinical Skill Thermoregulation of the Newborn *(Continued)*

NURSING ACTION	RATIONALE
6. Turn the heater to servocontrol mode so that the abdominal skin is maintained at 36.4°C to 37.2°C (97.5°F to 99°F).	
7. Monitor the newborn's axillary and skin probe temperatures per agency protocol.	*The temperature indicator on the radiant warmer continually displays the newborn's probe temperature. The axillary temperature is checked to ensure that the machine is accurately recording the newborn's temperature.*
8. When the newborn's temperature reaches 37.2°C (99°F), add a T-shirt, double-wrap the infant (two blankets), and place the newborn in an open crib.	
9. Recheck the newborn's temperature in 1 hour and regularly thereafter according to agency policy.	*It is important to monitor the newborn's ability to maintain his or her own thermoregulation.*
10. If the newborn's temperature drops below 36.1°C (97°F), rewarm the infant gradually. Place the infant (unclothed except for a diaper) under the radiant warmer with a servocontrol probe on the anterior abdominal wall.	*Rapid heating can lead to hyperthermia, which is associated with apnea, increased insensible water loss, and increased metabolic rate.*
11. Recheck the newborn's temperature in 30 minutes, then hourly.	
12. When the temperature reaches 37.2°C (99°F), dress the newborn, remove him or her from the radiant warmer, double-wrap, and place in an open crib. Check the temperature hourly until stable, then regularly according to agency policy.	

Note: An infant who repeatedly requires rewarming should be observed for other signs and symptoms of illness and a physician should be notified, because the situation may warrant screening for infection.

◆ KEY FACTS TO REMEMBER

Maintenance of Stable Newborn Temperature

Take action to help the newborn maintain a stable temperature:

- Keep the newborn's clothing and bedding dry.
- Double-wrap the newborn and put a stocking cap on him or her.
- Use the radiant warmer during procedures.
- Reduce the newborn's exposure to drafts.
- Warm objects that will be in contact with the newborn (e.g., stethoscope).
- Encourage the mother to snuggle with the newborn under blankets or to breastfeed the newborn with hat and light cover on.

---

occur because of low prothrombin levels in the first few days of life (see Drug Guide: Vitamin K_1 Phytonadione [AquaMEPHYTON] on page 639). The potential for hemorrhage is considered to result from the absence of gut bacterial flora, which influences the production of vitamin K_1 in the newborn (see Chapter 29 ∞ for further discussion). Newborns should receive a single parenteral dose of 0.5 to 1 mg of natural vitamin K_1 oxide (phytonadione) within 1 hour of birth or this dose may be delayed until af-

ter the first breastfeeding in the childbirth/birthing area (AAP & ACOG, 2007; Wilson, Shannon, & Shields, 2009). Current recommendations underscore the need for treatment in infants who are exclusively breastfed (Blackburn, 2007).

The vitamin K_1 injection is given intramuscularly in the middle third of the vastus lateralis muscle, located in the lateral aspect of the thigh (Figure 26–3 ■). Before injecting, the nurse must thoroughly clean the newborn's skin site for the injection with a small alcohol swab. The nurse uses a 25 gauge, 5/8-in. needle for the injection. An alternate site is the rectus femoris muscle in the anterior aspect of the thigh. However, this site is near the sciatic nerve and femoral artery; therefore, injections here should be done with caution (Figure 26–4 ■).

Prevention of Eye Infection

The nurse is also responsible for giving the legally required prophylactic eye treatment for *Neisseria gonorrhoeae*, which may have infected the newborn of an infected mother during the birth process. A variety of topical agents appear to be equally effective. Ophthalmic ointments that are used include 0.5% erythromycin (Ilotycin Ophthalmic) (see Drug Guide: Erythromycin Ophthalmic Ointment [Ilotycin Ophthalmic]), 1% tetracycline, or per

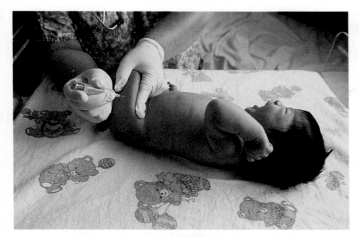

FIGURE 26–3 Procedure for vitamin K injection. Cleanse area thoroughly with alcohol swab and allow skin to dry. Bunch the tissue of the upper outer thigh (vastus lateralis muscle) and quickly insert a 25 gauge, 5/8-in. needle at a 90-degree angle to the thigh. Aspirate, then slowly inject the solution to distribute the medication evenly and minimize the baby's discomfort. Remove the needle and gently massage the site with an alcohol swab.
Source: Photgrapher, Elena Dorfman.

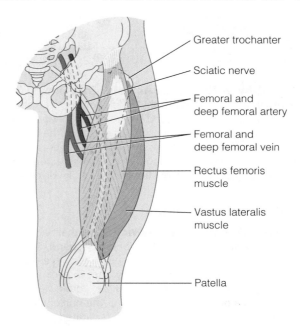

FIGURE 26–4 Injection sites. The middle third of the vastus lateralis muscle is the preferred site for intramuscular injection in the newborn. The middle third of the rectus femoris is an alternate site, but its proximity to major vessels and the sciatic nerve requires caution in using this site for injection.

agency protocol (AAP & ACOG, 2007). All are also effective against chlamydia, which has a higher incidence rate than gonorrhea.

Successful eye prophylaxis requires that the medication be instilled into the lower conjunctival sac of each eye (Figure 26–5 ■). The nurse massages the eyelid gently to distribute the ointment. Instillation may be delayed up to 1 hour after birth to allow eye contact during parent-newborn bonding.

Eye prophylaxis medications can cause chemical conjunctivitis, which gives the newborn some discomfort and may interfere with the ability to focus on the parents' faces. The resulting edema, inflammation, and discharge may cause concern if the parents have not been informed that the side effects will clear in 24 to 48 hours and that this prophylactic eye treatment is necessary for the newborn's well-being.

Drug Guide Vitamin K₁ Phytonadione (AquaMEPHYTON)

Overview of Neonatal Action Phytonadione is used in prophylaxis and treatment of vitamin K deficiency bleeding (VKDB), formerly known as hemorrhagic disease of the newborn. It promotes liver formation of the clotting factors II, VII, IX, and X. At birth, the newborn does not have the bacteria in the colon that are necessary for synthesizing fat-soluble vitamin K₁. Therefore, the newborn may have decreased levels of prothrombin during the first 5 to 8 days of life, reflected by a prolongation of prothrombin time.

Pregnancy Risk Category: C

Route, Dosage, Frequency Intramuscular injection is given in the vastus lateralis thigh muscle. A one-time-only prophylactic dose of 0.5 to 1 mg is given intramuscularly within 1 hour of birth or may be delayed until after the first breastfeeding in the delivery/birthing area (AAP & ACOG, 2007, Wilson, Shannon, & Shields, 2009).

If the mother received anticoagulants during pregnancy, an additional dose may be ordered by the physician and is given 6 to 8 hours after the first injection. IM concentration: 1 mg/0.5 mL (neonatal strength); can use 10 mg/mL concentration to minimize volume injected.

Neonatal Side Effects Pain and edema may occur at the injection site. Allergic reactions, such as rash and urticaria, may also occur.

Nursing Considerations

- Protect drug from light
- Give vitamin K₁ before circumcision procedure
- Observe for signs of local inflammation
- Observe for bleeding (usually occurs on second or third day). Bleeding may be seen as generalized ecchymoses or bleeding from umbilical cord, circumcision site, nose, or gastrointestinal tract. Results of serial prothrombin time (PT) and international normalized ratio (INR) should be assessed.
- Observe for jaundice and kernicterus, especially in preterm infants.

Drug Guide Erythromycin Ophthalmic Ointment (Ilotycin Ophthalmic)

Overview of Neonatal Action Erythromycin (Ilotycin Ophthalmic) is used as prophylactic treatment of ophthalmia neonatorum, which is caused by the bacteria *Neisseria gonorrhoeae*. Preventive treatment of gonorrhea in the newborn is required by law. Erythromycin is also effective against ophthalmic chlamydial infections. It is either bacteriostatic or bactericidal, depending on the organisms involved and the concentration of drug.

Pregnancy Risk Category: B

Route, Dosage, Frequency Ophthalmic ointment (0.5%) is instilled as a narrow ribbon or strand, 1 cm long, along the lower conjunctival surface of each eye, starting at the inner canthus. It is instilled only once in each eye (AAP & ACOG, 2007). The ointment may be administered in the birthing area or, alternatively, later in the nursery so that eye contact between infant and parent is facilitated and the bonding process immediately after birth is not interrupted. After administration, gently close the eye and manipulate to ensure the spread of ointment (Wilson, Shannon, & Shields, 2009).

Neonatal Side Effects Sensitivity reaction; may interfere with ability to focus and may cause edema and inflammation. Side effects usually disappear in 24 to 48 hours.

Nursing Considerations

- Wash hands immediately before instillation to prevent introduction of bacteria.
- Do not irrigate the eyes after instillation. Use new tube or single-use container for ophthalmic ointment administration shortly after birth. May wipe away excess after 1 minute with sterile cotton (AAP & ACOG, 2007).
- Observe for hypersensitivity.
- Teach parents about need for eye prophylaxis. Educate them regarding side effects and signs that need to be reported to the healthcare provider.

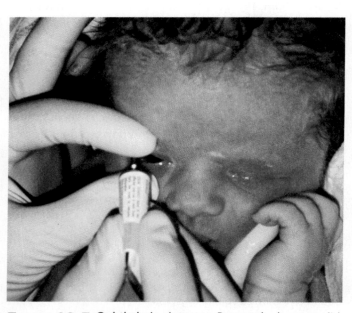

FIGURE 26–5 Ophthalmic ointment. Retract the lower eyelid outward to instill a 1/4-in. (1 cm) long strand of ointment from a single-dose tube along the lower conjunctival surface. *Make sure that the tip of the tube does not touch the eye.*

Early Assessment of Neonatal Distress

During the first 24 hours of life, the nurse is constantly alert for signs of distress. If the newborn is with the parents during this period, the nurse must take extra care to teach them how to maintain their newborn's temperature, recognize the hallmarks of newborn distress, and respond immediately to signs of respiratory problems. The parents learn to observe the newborn for changes in color or activity, grunting or "sighing" sounds with breathing, rapid breathing with chest retractions, or facial grimacing. Their interventions include nasal and oral suctioning with a bulb syringe, positioning, and vigorous fingertip stroking of the newborn's spine to stimulate respiratory activity if necessary. The nurse must be available immediately if the newborn develops distress. (See Key Facts to Remember: Signs of Newborn Distress.)

A common cause of neonatal distress is early onset group B streptococcal (GBS) disease. Infected mothers transmit GBS infection to their infants during labor and birth; thus it is recommended that at-risk mothers re-

KEY FACTS TO REMEMBER
Signs of Newborn Distress

Increased respiratory rate (more than 60/minute) or difficult respirations
Sternal retractions
Nasal flaring
Grunting
Excessive mucus
Facial grimacing
Cyanosis (central: skin, lips, tongue)
Abdominal distention or mass
Vomiting of bile-stained material
Absence of meconium elimination within 24 hours of birth
Absence of urine elimination within 24 hours of birth
Jaundice of the skin within 24 hours of birth or because of a hemolytic process
Temperature instability (hypothermia or hyperthermia)
Jitteriness or glucose less than 40 mg%

Source: Adapted from Tappero, E. P., & Honeyfield, M. E. (1996). *Physical assessment of the newborn* (2nd ed.). Petaluma, CA: NICU Inc.

ceive intrapartum antimicrobial prophylaxis (IAP) for GBS disease. All infants of mothers identified as at risk should be assessed and observed for signs and symptoms of sepsis (see Chapter 16 ∞ for discussion of maternal care).

Initiation of First Feeding

The timing of the first feeding varies depending on whether the newborn is to be breastfed or formula-fed and whether there were any complications during pregnancy or birth, such as maternal diabetes or intrauterine growth restriction (IUGR). Mothers who choose to breastfeed their newborns should be encouraged to put their baby to the breast during the first period of reactivity. This practice should be encouraged because successful, long-term breastfeeding during infancy appears to be related to beginning breastfeedings in the first few hours of life. Sleep-wake states affect feeding behavior and need to be considered when evaluating the newborn's sucking ability (Karl, 2004).

Formula-fed newborns usually begin the first feedings by 5 hours of age, during the second period of reactivity when they awaken and appear hungry. Signs indicating newborn readiness for the first feeding are licking of the lips, placing a hand in or near the mouth, active bowel sounds, absence of abdominal distention, and a lusty cry that quiets with rooting and sucking behaviors when a stimulus is placed near the lips. Observing the earlier, more subtle cues that the baby is ready to nurse provides an opportunity for the nurse to teach the parents to recognize these cues and respond before the baby is frustrated and crying.

Facilitation of Parent-Newborn Attachment

To facilitate **parent-newborn attachment**, eye-to-eye contact between the parents and their newborn is extremely important during the early hours after birth, when the newborn is in the first period of reactivity. The newborn is alert during this time, the eyes are wide open, and the baby often makes direct eye contact with human faces within optimal range for visual acuity (7 to 8 in.). It is theorized that this eye contact is an important foundation in establishing attachment in human relationships (Klaus & Klaus, 1985). Consequently, administration of the prophylactic eye medication is often delayed, but no more than 1 hour, to provide an opportunity for a period of eye contact between parents and their newborn, thus facilitating the attachment process (AAP & ACOG, 2007). Parents who cannot be with their newborns in this first period because of maternal or infant distress may need reassurance that the bonding process can proceed normally as soon as both mother and baby are stable.

Another situation that can facilitate attachment is the interactive bath. While bathing their newborn for the first time, parents attend closely to their baby's behavior. In this way, the newborn becomes an active participant and parents are drawn into an interaction with their newborn. The nurse can interpret the infant's behavior, model ways to respond to the behavior, and support parental strategies for doing so (Karl, 2004).

Evaluation

When evaluating the nursing care provided during the period immediately after birth, the nurse may anticipate the following outcomes:

- The newborn baby's adaptation to extrauterine life is successful as demonstrated by all vital signs within acceptable parameters.
- The baby's physiologic and psychologic integrity is supported.
- Positive interactions between parent and infant will be supported

Nursing Care of the Newborn Following Transition

Once a healthy newborn has demonstrated successful adaptation to extrauterine life, he or she needs appropriate observations for the first 6 to 12 hours after birth and the remainder of the stay in the birthing facility.

Nursing Diagnosis

Examples of nursing diagnoses that may apply during daily care of the newborn include the following:

- *Risk for Ineffective Breathing Pattern* related to periodic breathing
- *Imbalanced Nutrition: Less than Body Requirements* related to limited nutritional and fluid intake and increased caloric expenditure
- *Impaired Urinary Elimination* related to meatal edema secondary to circumcision
- *Risk for Infection* related to umbilical cord healing, circumcision site, immature immune system, or potential birth trauma (forceps or vacuum extraction birth)
- *Health-Seeking Behaviors* related to lack of information about basic baby care, male circumcision, and breastfeeding and/or formula-feeding
- *Interrupted Family Processes* related to integration of newborn into family or demands of newborn care and feeding
- *Risk for Injury* related to reabsorption of bilirubin and decreased defecation

CRITICAL THINKING

Aisha Khan gave birth to a healthy girl 2 hours ago. Now she calls you to her room. She sounds frightened and says her baby can't breathe. You find Aisha cradling her newborn in her arms. The baby is mildly cyanotic, is waving her arms, and has mucus coming from her nose and mouth. What would you do?

Answers can be found in Appendix F ∞.

Nursing Plan and Implementation

Maintenance of Cardiopulmonary Function

The nurse assesses vital signs every 6 to 8 hours or more, depending on the newborn's status. The newborn should be placed on the back (supine) for sleeping. A bulb syringe is kept within easy reach should the baby need oral-nasal suctioning. If the newborn has respiratory difficulty, the nurse clears the airway. Vigorous fingertip stroking of the baby's spine will frequently stimulate respiratory activity. A cardiorespiratory monitor can be used on newborns that are not being observed at all times and are at risk for decreased respiratory or cardiac function. Indicators of risk are pallor, cyanosis, ruddy color, apnea, and other signs of instability. Changes in skin color may indicate the need for closer assessment of temperature, cardiopulmonary status, hematocrit, glucose, and bilirubin levels.

Maintenance of a Neutral Thermal Environment

The nurse makes every effort to maintain the newborn's temperature within the normal range. The nurse must make certain the newborn is dried completely after the bath, dressed, and exposed to the air as little as possible. A head covering should be used for the small newborn that has less subcutaneous fat to act as insulation in maintaining body heat. Ambient temperature of the room where the newborn is kept should be monitored to prevent excessive cooling. Parents may be advised to dress the newborn in one more layer of clothing than is necessary for an adult to maintain thermal comfort. The use of layering allows for flexibility as the infant is moved from one area to another.

A newborn whose temperature falls below optimal level uses calories to maintain body heat rather than for growth. Chilling also decreases the affinity of serum albumin for bilirubin, thereby increasing the likelihood of newborn jaundice. In addition, it increases oxygen use and may cause respiratory distress.

An overheated newborn will increase activity and respiratory rate in an attempt to cool the body. Both measures deplete caloric reserves, and the increased respiratory rate leads to increased insensible fluid loss (Blackburn, 2007).

Promotion of Adequate Hydration and Nutrition

Newborn nutrition is addressed in depth in Chapter 27 ∞. The nurse records caloric and fluid intake and enhances adequate hydration by maintaining a neutral thermal environment and offering early and frequent feedings. Early feedings promote gastric emptying and increase peristalsis, thereby decreasing the potential for hyperbilirubinemia by decreasing the amount of time fecal material is in contact with enzyme β-glucuronidase in the small intestine. This enzyme frees the bilirubin from the feces, allowing it to be reabsorbed into the vascular system. The nurse records voiding and stooling patterns. The first voiding should occur within 24 hours and the first passage of stool within 48 hours. When they do not occur, the nurse continues the normal observation routine while assessing for abdominal distention, bowel sounds, hydration, fluid intake, and temperature stability.

The newborn is weighed at the same time each day for accurate comparisons and must be kept warm during the weighing. A weight loss of up to 10% for term newborns is considered within normal limits during the first week of life. This weight loss is the result of limited intake, loss of excess extracellular fluid, and passage of meconium. Parents should be told about the expected weight loss, the reason for it, and the expectations for regaining the birth weight. Birth weight is usually regained by 2 weeks if feedings are adequate.

Excessive handling can cause an increase in the newborn's metabolic rate and caloric use and cause fatigue. The nurse should be alert to the newborn's subtle cues of fatigue, including a decrease in muscle tension and activity in the extremities and neck, as well as loss of eye contact, which may be manifested by fluttering or closure of the eyelids. The nurse quickly ceases stimulation when signs of fatigue appear. The nurse should demonstrate to parents the need to be aware of newborn cues and to wait for periods of alertness for contact and stimulation. The nurse is also responsible for assessing the woman's comfort and latching-on techniques if breastfeeding, or the bottle-feeding techniques.

Promotion of Skin Integrity

Newborn skin care, including bathing, is important for the health and appearance of the individual newborn and for infection control within the nursery. Ongoing skin care involves cleansing the buttock and perianal areas with fresh water and cotton or a mild soap and water with diaper changes. If commercial baby wipes are used, those without alcohol should be selected. Perfumed and latex-free wipes are also available.

The umbilical cord is assessed for signs of bleeding or infection. Removal of the cord clamp within 24 to 48 hours of birth reduces the chance of tension injury to

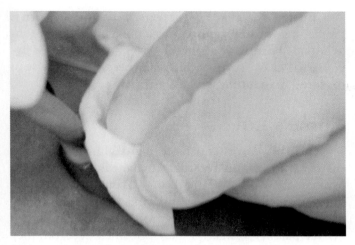

FIGURE 26–6 The umbilical cord base is carefully cleansed.

the area. Keeping the umbilical stump clean and dry can reduce the chance for infection (Figure 26–6 ■). Many types of routine cord care are practiced, including the use of triple dye, an antimicrobial agent such as bacitracin, or application of 70% alcohol to the cord stump. These practices are largely based on tradition rather than current research findings. The skin absorption and toxicity of triple-dye agents in newborns have not been carefully studied. Studies have shown that alcohol used alone is not effective in preventing umbilical cord colonization and infection (omphalitis) (AAP & ACOG, 2007). Folding the diaper down to avoid covering the cord stump can prevent contamination of the area and promote drying. The nurse is responsible for cord care per agency policy. It is also the nurse's responsibility to instruct parents in caring for the cord and observing for signs and symptoms of infection after discharge, such as foul smell, redness and drainage, localized heat and tenderness, or bleeding.

Promotion of Safety

Safety of the newborn is paramount. It is essential that the nurse and other caregivers verify the identity of the newborn by comparing the numbers and names on the identification bracelets of mother and newborn before giving a baby to a parent (AAP & ACOG, 2007; Askin, 2008). An additional form of identification band has a built-in sensor unit that sounds an alarm if the baby is transported beyond set birthing-unit boundaries. Individual birthing units should practice safety measures to prevent infant abduction and provide information to parents regarding their role in this area and in general newborn safety measures. Parental measures to prevent abduction and provide for safety include the following:

SECURITY

- Parents should check that identification bands are in place as they care for their infant and, if missing, they should ask that they be replaced immediately.

- They should only allow people with proper birthing unit picture identification to bring and/or remove the baby from the room. If parents don't know the staff person, they should call the nurse for assistance.
- Parents should report the presence of any suspicious people on the birthing unit.

SAFETY

- Parents should never leave their baby alone in their room. If they walk in the halls or take a shower, parents should have a family member watch the baby or return the baby to the nursery.
- If a parent feels weak, faint, or unsteady on his or her feet, he or she should not lift the baby. Instead, the parent should call for assistance.
- Parents should always keep an eye and hand on the baby when he or she is out of the crib.
- Newborns need protection from infection even though they do possess some immunity. Parents should ask visitors to leave if they have any of the following: cold, diarrhea, discharge from sores, or contagious disease.

Prevention of Complications

Newborns are at continued risk for the complications of hemorrhage, late-onset cardiac symptoms, and infection. Pallor may be an early sign of hemorrhage and must be reported to the physician. The newborn is placed on a cardio-respiratory monitor to permit continuous assessment. Several newborn conditions put newborns at risk for hemorrhage. Cyanosis that is not relieved by oxygen administration requires emergency intervention, may indicate a congenital cardiac condition or shock, and requires ongoing assessment.

Infection in the nursery is best prevented by requiring that all personnel who have direct contact with newborns scrub for 2 to 3 minutes from the fingertips to and including the elbows at the beginning of each shift. The hands must also be washed with soap and rubbed vigorously for 15 seconds before and after contact with every newborn and after touching any soiled surface such as the floor or one's hair or face. Parents are instructed to practice good handwashing and/or use of an antiseptic hand cleaner before touching the baby. They are also instructed that anyone holding the baby should practice good handwashing, even after the family returns home. In some clinical settings family members are asked to wear gowns (preferably disposable) over their street clothes during their contact with infants. These are good opportunities for the nurse to reinforce the efficacy of handwashing in preventing the spread of infection.

Jaundice in newborns is caused by the accumulation of the pigment *bilirubin* in the skin. Jaundice occurs in most newborn infants. Most jaundice is benign, but because of the potential toxicity of bilirubin, newborn infants must be monitored to identify those who might develop severe hyperbilirubinemia and, in rare cases, acute bilirubin encephalopathy or kernicterus (see Chapter 29 ∞ for more detailed discussion) (AAP & ACOG, 2007). Current recommendations include obtaining a total serum bilirubin level in any infant that is visibly jaundiced in the first 24 hours of life, and obtaining either a serum or transcutaneous bilirubin level before discharge. Nomograms for evaluating risk factors based on bilirubin levels and age of infant are available (see Chapter 24 ∞ for discussion).

Circumcision

Circumcision is a surgical procedure in which the prepuce, an epithelial layer covering the penis, is separated from the glans penis and excised. This procedure permits exposure of the glans for easier cleaning.

Circumcision was originally a religious rite practiced by Jews and Muslims. The practice gained widespread cultural acceptance in the United States but is much less common in Europe. Many parents choose circumcision because they want their male child to have a physical appearance similar to that of his father or the majority of other children or they may feel that it is expected by society. Another commonly cited reason for circumcising newborn males is to prevent the need for anesthesia, hospitalization, pain, and trauma if the procedure is needed later in life (AAP & ACOG, 2007). During the prenatal period, the nurse ensures that parents have clear and current information regarding the risks and benefits of circumcision.

Families make the decision about circumcision for their newborn male child. In most cases the choice is based on cultural, social, and family tradition. To ensure informed consent, parents should be advised during the prenatal period about possible long-term medical effects of circumcision and noncircumcision.

Current Recommendations

As in the past, recommendations regarding circumcision have varied. The 1999 AAP policy statement was reaffirmed in 2005 and does not recommend *routine* circumcision but acknowledges that medical indications for circumcision still exist (AAP & ACOG, 2007). The policy recommends that analgesia (dorsal penile nerve block [DPNB], or subcutaneous ring block) be used during circumcision to decrease procedural pain (AAP & ACOG, 2007). The DPNB and subcutaneous ring block are the most effective options (AAP & CPS, 2006). If a circumcision is to be performed, it should be done using the least painful method. Recent studies show that using oral sucrose for painful procedures can be effective in reducing pain for newborns and it should be used with other non-pharmacologic measures to enhance its effectiveness (AAP & CPS, 2006).

Circumcision *should not be performed* if the newborn is premature or compromised, has a known bleeding problem, or is born with a genitourinary defect such as hypospadias or epispadias, which may necessitate the use of the foreskin in future surgical repairs.

Nurse's Role

The nurse plays an essential role in providing parents with current information regarding the medical, social, and psychologic aspects of newborn circumcision. A well-informed nurse can allay parents' anxiety by sharing information and allowing them to express their concerns. In order for parents to make a truly informed decision, they must be knowledgeable about the potential risks and outcomes of circumcision. Hemorrhage, infection, difficulty in voiding, separation of the edges of the circumcision, discomfort, and restlessness are early potential problems. Later there is a risk that the glans and urethral meatus may become irritated and inflamed from contact with the ammonia from urine. Ulcerations and progressive stenosis may develop. Adhesions, entrapment of the penis, and damage to the urethra are all potential complications that could require surgical correction (AAP & ACOG, 2007).

The parents of an uncircumcised male infant require information from the nurse about good hygienic practices. They are told that the foreskin and glans are two similar layers of cells that separate from each other. The separation process begins prenatally and is normally completed between 3 to 5 years of age. In the process of separation, sterile sloughed cells build up between the layers. This buildup looks similar to the smegma secreted after puberty, and it is harmless. Occasionally during the daily bath, the parent can gently test for retraction. If retraction has occurred, daily gentle washing of the glans with soap and water is sufficient to maintain adequate cleanliness. The parents should teach the child to incorporate this practice into his daily self-care activities. Most uncircumcised males have no difficulty doing so.

If circumcision is desired, the procedure is performed when the newborn is well stabilized and has received his initial physical examination by a healthcare provider. The parents may also choose to have the circumcision done after discharge. However, they need to be advised that if the baby is older than 1 month, the current practice is to hospitalize him for the procedure.

Before a circumcision, the nurse ensures that the physician has explained the procedure, determined whether the parents have any further questions about the procedure, and verified that the circumcision permit is signed. As with any surgical procedure, the infant's identification band should be checked to verify his identity before the procedure begins. The nurse gathers the equipment and prepares the newborn by removing the diaper and placing him on a padded circumcision board or some other type of restraint, but restraining only the legs. These restraint measures along with the application of warm blankets to the upper body increase infant comfort during the procedure (Thureen et al., 2005). In Jewish circumcision ceremonies, the infant is held by the father or godfather and given wine before the procedure.

A variety of devices (Gumco clamp, Plastibel, Mogen clamp) are used for circumcision (Figures 26–7 ■ and 26–8 ■), and all produce minimal bleeding. Therefore the nurse should make special note of infants with a family history of bleeding disorders or with mothers who took anticoagulants, including aspirin, prenatally. During the procedure, the nurse assesses the newborn's response. One important consideration is pain experienced by the newborn. A DPNB or ring block using 1% lidocaine without epinephrine or similar anesthetic significantly minimizes the pain and shifts in behavioral patterns such as crying, irritability, and erratic sleep cycles associated with circumcision. Other studies are investigating the use of topical anesthetic applied 60 to 90 minutes before prepuce removal, acetaminophen, and cryoanalgesia. Studies indicate that a combination of methods is most effective in reducing pain during circumcision (AAP & CPS, 2006). Also see Evidence-Based Practice: Feeding to Control Procedural Pain in Newborns.

During the procedure, the nurse provides comfort measures such as swaddling, lightly stroking the baby's head, providing a pacifier for nonnutritive sucking, and talking to him. Following the circumcision, the infant should be held and comforted by a family member or the nurse. The nurse must be alert to any behavioral cues that these measures are overstimulating the newborn instead of comforting him. Such cues include turning away of the head, increased generalized body movement, skin color changes, hyperalertness, and hiccoughing.

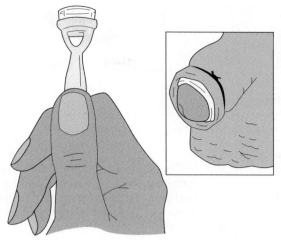

FIGURE 26–8 Circumcision using the Plastibell. The bell is fitted over the glans. A suture is tied around the bell's rim and the excess prepuce is cut away. The plastic rim remains in place for 3 to 4 days until healing occurs. The bell may be allowed to fall off; it is removed if still in place after 8 days.

Ideally, the circumcision should be assessed every 30 minutes for at least 2 hours following the procedure. It is important to observe for the first voiding after a circumcision to evaluate for urinary obstruction related to penile injury and/or edema. Petroleum ointment and gauze may be applied to the site immediately following the procedure to help prevent bleeding and can be used to protect the healing tissue afterward.

The nurse must also teach family members how to assess for unusual bleeding, how to respond if it is present, and how to care for the newly circumcised penis. Parents of babies circumcised with a method other than Plastibell should receive the following information:

- Clean with warm water with each diaper change.
- Apply petroleum ointment for the next few diaper changes to help prevent further bleeding (Figure 26–9 ■).
- If bleeding does occur, apply light pressure with a sterile gauze pad to stop the bleeding within a short time. If this is not effective, contact the physician immediately, or take the baby to the caregiver's office.
- The glans normally has granulation tissue (a yellowish film) on it during healing. Continued application of a petroleum ointment (or ointment suggested by the healthcare provider) can help protect the granulation tissue that forms as the glans heals.
- Report to the care provider any signs or symptoms of infection, such as increasing swelling, pus drainage, and cessation of urination.
- When diapering, ensure that the diaper is not loose enough to cause rubbing with movement, or tight enough to cause pain.

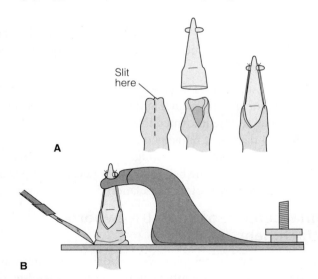

FIGURE 26–7 Circumcision using a circumcision clamp. *A,* The prepuce is drawn over the cone and *B,* the clamp is applied. Pressure is maintained for 3 to 4 minutes, and then excess prepuce is cut away.

EVIDENCE-BASED PRACTICE

Feeding to Control Procedural Pain in Newborns

Clinical Question
What nonpharmacological methods can help reduce the pain associated with common neonatal procedures?

The Evidence
Pain assessment and management are important issues in neonatal care. Most newborns will experience a venipuncture or heel lance for blood sampling during their hospital stay. Although clinicians agree that newborn infants are capable of responding to painful stimuli, most do not administer medication to control the short-term pain associated with these common procedures. Two systematic reviews of 26 research studies investigated the use of feeding—specifically the oral administration of breast milk or a sucrose solution—to control the pain associated with common procedures. Multiple systematic reviews with this quantity of randomized trials represent the strongest level of evidence for nursing practice.

What Is Effective?
Newborns who were feeding during heel lance or venipuncture demonstrated fewer physiological and behavioral signs of pain. Actual feeding at the breast was associated with a reduction in heart rate change, percentage time crying, duration of crying, and improvement in validated neonatal pain measures. The latter two outcomes were also improved with the administration of sucrose, either by slow administration with an oral syringe or by dipping a pacifier in a sucrose solution. Some of the physiological indicators of pain (specifically heart rate and blood pressure) were improved equally by the mother holding and feeding the baby and an assistant holding the baby with a pacifier in its mouth. All groups that were fed during the procedure—whether it was breast milk

from the mother, expressed breast milk, or sucrose—had better pain control than babies who were swaddled, positioned, or given a pacifier without being held.

What Is Inconclusive?
It does not appear that any of these measures completely eliminated the pain of routine procedures. Additionally, these studies were focused on healthy newborns undergoing minimally invasive, singular painful procedures. The effectiveness of either breast milk or sucrose for repeated painful procedures was not studied. With regard to preterm or sick newborns, there is insufficient evidence to support the safety of breast milk or sucrose as a routine, repeated comfort measure. For preterm and sick full-term newborns who are subjected to repeated painful procedures during hospitalization, the ideal analgesic has not yet been identified.

Best Practice
Newborns undergoing single painful procedures such as venipuncture or heel lance should be breastfed by the mother during the procedure if at all possible. If not, you can feed the baby expressed breast milk or a sucrose solution with a syringe, a bottle, or by dipping a pacifier in the solution. Holding the baby while doing so achieves the best pain control.

References
Leef, K. (2006). Evidence-based review of oral sucrose administration to decrease the pain response in newborn infants. *Neonatal Network, 25*(4), 275–284.

Shah, P., Aliwalas, L., & Shah, V. (2007). Breastfeeding or breast milk for procedural pain in neonates. *Cochrane Database of Systematic Reviews*, Issue 4.

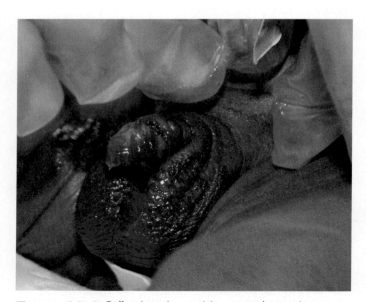

FIGURE 26–9 Following circumcision, petroleum ointment may be applied to the site for the next few diaper changes.

- If the infant's care provider recommends oral analgesics, follow instructions for proper measuring and administration.

If the Plastibell is used, parents should receive information about normal appearance and how to observe for infection. The parents are informed that the Plastibell should fall off within 8 days. If it remains on after 8 days, they should consult with their physician. Though no ointments or creams should be used while the bell remains, application of petroleum ointment may protect granulation tissue afterward.

Enhancement of Parent-Newborn Attachment

The nurse encourages parent-newborn attachment by involving all family members with the new member of the family. (For specific interventions see Chapters 19 and 31 ∞ and Client Teaching: Enhancing Attachment.) Infant massage is a common childcare practice in

Infant Naming in Kenya

In Kenya, the naming of the child is an important event. Names are commonly selected to mirror important or current events. For example, an infant who is born while traveling may be given a name that means "wanderer" or "traveler." Other names may be chosen after a relative who is among the "living-dead" (deceased). It is believed that this results in a partial reincarnation of that relative, especially if the child has characteristics in common with that individual. It is also believed there is a connection between newborns and the spirit world. In some parts of the country, the name is chosen when the child is crying. Different names of the living-dead are called, and if the child quits crying when a particular name is called, that is the given name. In some areas, the name is given on the third day and is marked by a celebration with feasting and rejoicing. On the fourth day, the father of the child commonly hangs an iron necklace on the child's neck. It is at this time that the infant is considered a full human being and the connection with the spirit world is lost.

many parts of the world, especially Africa and Asia, and has recently gained attention in the United States. Parents can be taught to use infant massage as a method to facilitate the bonding process and to reduce the stress and pain associated with teething, constipation, inoculations, and colic. Infant massage not only induces relaxation for the infant but also provides a calming and "feel-good" interaction for the parents that foster the development of warm, positive relationships. See Cultural Perspectives: Infant Naming in Kenya.

The nurse can discuss waking activities such as talking with the baby while making eye contact, holding the baby in an upright position (sitting or standing), gently bending the baby back and forth while grasping under the knees and supporting the head and back with the other hand, or gently rubbing the baby's hands and feet. Quieting activities may include swaddling or bundling the baby to increase a sense of security; using slow, calming movements; and talking softly, singing, or humming to the baby (Figure 26–10 ■). (See the Teaching Card: Teaching Techniques for Waking and Quieting Newborns in the center of this text.) The nurse must also be aware of cultural variations in newborn care such as naming the newborn, giving compliments about the baby, and using good luck charms (see Cultural Perspectives: Examples of Cultural Beliefs and Practices Regarding Baby Care). The nurse plays a vital role in fostering parent-infant attachment. It is important to be sensitive to the cultural beliefs and values of the family.

Client Teaching ENHANCING ATTACHMENT

Content	Teaching Method
• Present information on periods of reactivity and expected newborn responses.	Focus on open discussion.
• Describe normal physical characteristics of the newborn.	Present slides showing newborn characteristics.
• Explain the bonding process, its gradual development, and the reciprocal interactive nature of the process.	
• Discuss the infant's capabilities for interaction, such as nonverbal communication abilities. The nonverbal communications include movement, gaze, touch, facial expressions, and vocalizations—including crying. Emphasize that eye contact is considered one of the cardinal factors in developing infant-parent attachment and will be integrated with touching and vocal behaviors.	Show a video on the interactive capabilities of newborns.
• Explain that touching, including stroking, patting, massaging, and kissing, will progress to interactive touch between the parents and their infant; discuss their need to assimilate these behaviors into their daily routine with the baby.	Provide handouts, and use a doll to demonstrate behaviors.
• Describe and demonstrate comforting techniques, including the use of sound, swaddling, rocking, massage, and stroking.	Demonstrate the techniques and ask for a return demonstration.
• Describe the progression of the infant's behaviors as the infant matures, and the importance of the parents' consistent response to their infant's cues and needs.	Allow time for questions and discussion.
• Provide information about available pamphlets, videos, and support groups in the community.	

A Letter From Your Baby

Dear Parents:

I come to you a small, immature being with my own style and personality. I am yours for only a short time; enjoy me.

1. Please take time to find out who I am, how I differ from you, and how much I can bring you joy.

2. Please feed me when I am hungry. I never knew hunger in the womb, and clocks and time mean little to me.

3. Please hold, cuddle, kiss, touch, stroke, and croon to me. I was always held closely in the womb and was never alone before.

4. Please don't be disappointed when I am not the perfect baby that you expected, nor disappointed with yourselves that you are not the perfect parents.

5. Please don't expect too much from me as your newborn baby, or too much from yourself as a parent. Give us both six weeks as a birthday present—six weeks for me to grow, develop, mature, and become more stable and predictable, and six weeks for you to rest and relax and allow your body to get back to normal.

6. Please forgive me if I cry a lot. Bear with me and in a short time, as I mature, I will spend less and less time crying and more time socializing.

7. Please watch me carefully and I can tell you the things that soothe, console and please me. I am not a tyrant who was sent to make your life miserable, but the only way I can tell you that I am not happy is with my cry.

8. Please remember that I am resilient and can withstand the many natural mistakes you will make with me. As long as you make them with love, you cannot ruin me.

9. Please take care of yourself and eat a balanced diet, rest, and exercise so that when we are together, you have the health and strength to take care of me.

10. Please take care of your relationship with others. Relationships that are good for you, support both you and me.

Although I may have turned your life upside down, please realize that things will be back to normal before long.

Thank you,

Your Loving Child

FIGURE 26–10 A letter from your baby.

Evaluation

When evaluating the nursing care provided during the newborn period, the nurse may anticipate the following outcomes:

- The baby's physiologic and psychologic integrity is supported by maintaining stable vital signs and interactions based on normal newborn behaviors.
- The newborn feeding pattern will be satisfactorily established.
- The parents express understanding of the bonding process and display attachment behaviors.

Nursing Management in Preparation for Discharge

Although the adjustment to parenting is a normal process, going home presents a critical transition for the family. The parents become the primary caregivers for the newborn and must provide a nurturing environment in which the emotional and physical needs of the newborn can be met. Nursing interventions focus on promoting health and preventing possible problems.

Nursing Assessment and Diagnosis

When preparing for discharge, assess whether parents have realistic expectations of the newborn's behavior and the depth of their knowledge in caring for their newborn.

Nursing diagnoses that may apply to the newborn's family include the following:

- *Readiness for Enhanced Parenting* related to appropriate behavioral expectations for the newborn.
- *Readiness for Enhanced Family Processes* related to integration of newborn into family unit or demands of newborn care and feeding.

Planning and Implementation

Parent Teaching

To meet the parent's need for information, the nurse who is responsible for the care of the mother and newborn should assume the primary responsibility for parent education. Nearly every contact with the parents presents an opportunity for sharing information that can facilitate their sense of competence in newborn care. The nurse also needs to recognize and respect the many good ways of providing safe care. Unless their care methods are harmful to the newborn, the parents' methods of giving care should be reinforced rather than contradicted.

CULTURAL PERSPECTIVES

Examples of Cultural Beliefs and Practices Regarding Baby Care*

Umbilical Cord

People of Latin American, Filipino, Haitian cultural background may use an abdominal binder or bellyband to protect against dirt, injury, and umbilical hernia. They may also apply oils to the stump of the cord or tape metal to the umbilicus to ward off evil spirits (D'Avanza & Geissler, 2008).

People of northern European ancestry may expect a sterile cutting of the cord at birth. They may allow the stump to air-dry and discard the cord once it falls off.

Some Latin American parents cauterize the stump with a candle flame, hot coal, or burning stick (WHO, 1999).

In Ecuador, the cord stump is left long in girls to prevent a small uterus and problems with childbirth (WHO, 1999).

Parent-Infant Contact

People of Asian ancestry may pick up the baby as soon as it cries, or they may carry the baby at all times.

Several native North American nations people, notably the Navajos, may use cradle boards, so the infant can be with family even during work and feel secure (Andrews, 2008).

The Muslim father traditionally calls praise to Allah in the newborn's right ear and cleans the infant after birth (Hedayat, 2001).

Feeding

Some women of Asian heritage may breastfeed their babies for the first 1 to 2 years of life. Many Cambodian refugees practice breastfeeding on demand without restriction, or, if formula-feeding, provide a "comfort bottle" in between feedings (Lipson & Dibble, 2008).

People of Iranian heritage may breastfeed female babies longer than male babies. Many Muslim women will not breastfeed in public.

Some people of African ancestry may wean their babies after they begin to walk.

Some Asians, Haitian, Hispanics, Eastern Europeans, and Native Americans may delay breastfeeding because they believe colostrum is "bad" (D'Avanzo & Geissler, 2008).

Haitian mothers may believe that "strong emotions" spoil breast milk (Lipson & Dibble, 2008).

Circumcision

People of Muslim and Jewish ancestry practice circumcision as a religious ritual (Ott, Al-Khadhuri, & Al-Junaibi, 2003; Lipson & Dibble, 2008).

Many natives of Africa and Australia practice circumcision as a puberty rite.

Native Americans and people of Asian and Latin American cultures rarely perform circumcision (Lipson & Dibble, 2008).

As of 2006, global estimates about 30% of males are circumcised (WHO, 2008).

Health and Illness

Some people from Latin American cultural backgrounds may believe that touching the face or head of an infant when admiring it will ward off the "evil eye." They may also neglect to cut the baby's nails to avoid nearsightedness and instead put mittens on the baby's hands to prevent scratching. They also may believe that fat babies are healthy.

Some people of Asian heritage may not allow anyone to touch the baby's head without asking permission.

Some Orthodox Jews believe that saying the baby's name before the formal naming ceremony will harm the baby.

Some Asians and Haitians delay naming their infants until after confinement month (D'Avanzo & Geissler, 2008).

Some people of Vietnamese ancestry believe that cutting a baby's hair or nails will cause illness.

*Note: The information is meant only to provide examples of the behaviors that may be found within certain cultures. Not all members of a culture practice the behaviors described.

Caring for newborns in the hospital setting means that the nurse will have contact with clients from a wide variety of racial, religious, and cultural backgrounds. Though it may not be possible to be conversant with all cultures, the nurse can demonstrate cultural competence with both colleagues and patients when she or he:

- Shows respect for the inherent dignity of every human being, whatever the person's age, gender, or religion.
- Accepts the rights of individuals to choose their care provider, participate in care, and refuse care.
- Acknowledges personal biases and prevents them from interfering with the delivery of quality care to persons of other cultures.
- Recognizes cultural issues and interacts with clients from other cultures in culturally sensitive ways.

- Incorporates cultural preferences, health beliefs and behaviors, and traditional practices into the management plan.
- Develops client-appropriate educational materials that address the language and cultural beliefs of the client.
- Accesses culturally appropriate resources to deliver care to clients from other cultures.
- Assists clients to access quality care within a dominant culture.

(Green-Hernandez, Quinne, Falkenstern et.al., 2004)

The nurse must be sensitive to the cultural beliefs and values of the family (see Cultural Perspectives: Examples of Cultural Beliefs and Practices Regarding Baby Care).

The information that follows is provided to increase the nurse's knowledge of newborn care and can also be used to meet parents' needs for information. Parents may be familiar with handling and caring for infants, or this may be their first time to interact with a newborn. If they are new parents, the sensitive nurse gently teaches them by example and provides instructions geared to their needs and previous knowledge about the various aspects of newborn care.

The length of stay in the birthing unit for mother and baby after birth is often 48 hours or less. The challenge for the nurse is to use every opportunity to teach, guide, and support individual parents, fostering their capabilities and confidence in caring for their newborn. Including mother-baby care and home care instruction on the night shift assists with education needs for early discharge parents.

The nurse observes how parents interact with their newborn during feeding and caregiving activities. Even during a short stay, there are opportunities for the nurse to provide information and observe whether the parents are comfortable with changing the diapers of, wrapping, handling, and feeding their newborn (Figure 26–11 ■). Do both parents get involved in the newborn's care? Is the mother depending on someone else to help her at home? Does the mother give reasons (e.g., "I'm too tired," "My stitches hurt," or "I'll learn later") for not wanting to be involved in her baby's care? As the family provides care, the nurse can enhance parental confidence by giving them positive feedback. If the parents encounter problems, the nurse can express confidence in their abilities to master the new skill or information, suggest alternatives, and serve as a role model. All these factors need to be considered when evaluating the educational needs of the parents.

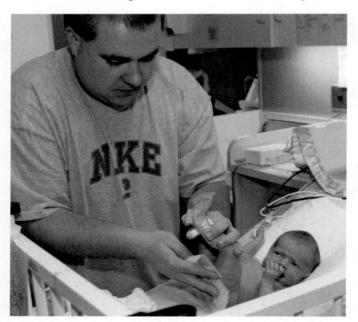

FIGURE 26–11 A father demonstrates competence and confidence in diapering his newborn daughter.

Several methods may be used to teach families about newborn care. Daily newborn care videos and classes are nonthreatening ways to convey general information. Individual instruction is helpful to answer specific questions or to clarify an item that may have been confusing in class. Currently many birthing centers have 24-hour educational video channels or videos to be viewed in the mother's room on a variety of postpartum and newborn care issues.

> **TEACHING TIP**
>
> For clients who are hearing impaired, videotapes with information in both spoken and signed formats are most helpful. Birthing centers should have handouts available for families who do not speak English and either birthing center interpreters (not family members) or language interpreter phones.

One-to-one teaching while the nurse is in the mother's room is the most effective educational method. Both first-time and experienced postpartum parents rate individual teaching as the most effective method of instruction. Individual instruction is helpful both to answer specific questions and to clarify something that the parents may have found confusing in the educational video. With shorter stays, most teaching unfortunately tends to focus on infant feeding and immediate physical care needs of the mothers, with limited anticipatory guidance provided in other areas. To address this deficit, Table 26–1 includes a broad range of information important to share with new parents. These topics are discussed in detail here. Also see the Teaching Card: Teaching Infant Discharge Care inserted in the center of this text and Key Facts to Remember: When Parents Should Call Their Healthcare Provider.

General Instructions for Newborn Care

One of the first concerns of anyone who has not had the experience of picking up a baby is how to do it correctly. The newborn is easily picked up by sliding one hand under the neck and shoulders and the other hand under the buttocks or between the newborn's legs and then gently lifting upward. This technique provides security and support for the head (which the newborn is unable to support until 3 or 4 months of age).

The nurse can be an excellent role model for families in the area of safety. Safety topics include the proper positioning of the newborn on the back to sleep and correct use of the bulb syringe (discussed shortly). The baby should never be left alone anywhere but in the crib. The mother is reminded that while she and her newborn are together in the birthing unit, she should never leave her baby alone for security reasons and because newborns spit up frequently the first day or two after birth. Other newborn safety measures are discussed in detail in Chapter 32 ∞.

Demonstrating a bath (see Chapter 32 ∞), cord care, and temperature assessment is the best way for the nurse

TABLE 26-1 | What to Tell Parents About Infant Care

Immediate Safety Measures for the Newborn

Watch for excessive mucus: use bulb syringe to remove mucus.

Have baby sleep on his or her back in crib or in someone's arms.

Voiding and Stool Characteristics and Patterns

Urine is straw to amber color without foul smell. Small amounts of uric acid crystals are normal in first days of life (may be mistaken by parents as blood in diaper because of reddish "brick dust" appearance).

At least 6 to 10 wet diapers a day after the first few days of life.

Normal progression of stool changes: (1) meconium (thick, tarry, dark green); (2) transitional stools (thin, brown to green); (3a) breastfed infant: yellow gold, soft or mushy stools; (3b) formula-fed infant: pale yellow, formed and pasty stools.

Only one to two stools a day for formula-fed baby.

Six to 10 small, loose yellow stools per day or only one stool every few days after breastfeeding is well established (after about 1 month).

Cord Care

Wash hands with clean water before and after care. Keep the cord dry and exposed to air or loosely covered with clean clothes. (If cultural custom demands binding of the abdomen, a sanitary method such as the use of a clean piece of gauze can be recommended.)

Clean cord and skin around base with a cotton swab or cotton ball. Clean two to three times a day or with each diaper change. Touching the cord, applying unclean substances to it, and applying bandages should be avoided. Do not give tub baths until cord falls off in 7 to 14 days.

Fold diapers below umbilical cord to air-dry the cord (contact with wet or soiled diapers slows the drying process and increases the possibility of infection).

Check cord each day for any odor, oozing of greenish yellow material, or reddened areas around the cord. Expect tenderness around the cord and darkening and shriveling of cord. Report to healthcare provider any signs of infection.

Normal changes in cord: Cord should look dark and dry up before falling off. A small drop of blood may present when cord falls off.

Never pull the cord or attempt to loosen it.

Care Required for Circumcision and Uncircumcised Infants

Circumcision Care:

Squeeze water over circumcision site once a day.

Rinse area off with warm water and pat dry.

Apply a small amount of petroleum jelly (unless a Plastibell is in place) with each diaper change.

Fasten diaper over penis snugly enough so that it does not move and rub the tender glans.

Because the glans is sensitive, avoid placing baby on his stomach for the first day after the procedure.

Check for any foul-smelling drainage or bleeding at least once a day.

Let Plastibell fall off by itself (about 8 days after circumcision).

Plastibell should not be pulled off.

Light, sticky, yellow drainage (part of healing process) may form over head of penis.

Uncircumcised Care:

Clean uncircumcised penis with water during diaper changes and with bath.

Do not force foreskin back over the penis; foreskin will retract normally over time (may take 3 to 5 years).

Techniques for Waking and Quieting Newborns

Techniques for Waking Baby:

Loosen clothing, change diaper.

Hand-express milk onto baby's lips.

Talk with baby while making eye contact.

Hold baby in upright position (sitting or standing).

Have baby do sit-ups (gently and rhythmically bend baby back and forth while grasping the baby under his or her knees and supporting baby's head and back with your other hand).

Play patty-cake with baby.

Stimulate rooting reflex (brush one cheek with hand or nipple).

Increase skin contact (gently rub hands and feet).

Techniques for Quieting Baby:

Check for soiled diaper.

Hold swaddled baby upright against mid-chest, supporting bottom and back of head. Baby can hear heartbeat, feel warmth, and hear your softly spoken words or calming sounds.

Use slow, calming movements with baby.

Softly talk, sing, or hum to baby.

Signs of Illness and Use of Thermometer

See Key Facts to Remember: When Parents Should Call Their Healthcare Provider to provide information on these topics to parents. Parents should be told to call their healthcare provider if redness, foul odor, bright red bleeding, or greenish yellow drainage occurs at the cord site or if the area remains unhealed 2 to 3 days after the cord stump has sloughed off. No single method of umbilical cord care (topical antimicrobials [triple-dye, iodophor ointment, or hexachlorophene powder] or alcohol) has been proven to be superior in preventing colonization and disease (AAP & ACOG, 2007). The use of sterile water or air drying results in umbilical cords separating more quickly than those treated with alcohol (Askin, 2008). See Table 26–1.

The nurse demonstrates and reviews the taking of axillary or tympanic temperatures and discourages the use of mercury thermometers. It is important that families understand the differences and know how to select a thermometer. The newborn's temperature needs to be taken only when signs of illness are present. Parents are advised to call their physician or pediatric nurse practitioner immediately if they observe any signs of illness.

Nasal and Oral Suctioning

Most newborns are obligatory nose breathers for the first months of life. They generally maintain air passage patency by coughing or sneezing. During the first few days of life, however, the newborn has increased mucus, and gentle suctioning with a bulb syringe may be indicated. The nurse can demonstrate the use of the bulb syringe in the mouth and nose and have the parents do a return demonstration. The parents should repeat this demonstration of suctioning and cleansing the bulb before discharge so they feel confident in performing the procedure. Care should be taken to apply only gentle suction to prevent nasal bleeding.

To suction the newborn, the bulb syringe is compressed before the tip is placed in the nostril. The nurse or parent must take care not to occlude the passageway. The

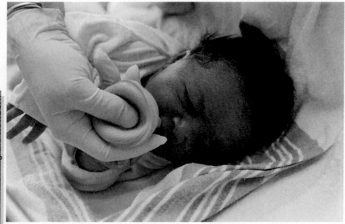

FIGURE 26–12 Nasal and oral suctioning. The bulb is compressed, the tip is placed in either the mouth or the nose, and the bulb is released.
Source: © Stella Johnson (www.stellajohnson.com).

MyNursingKit | Swaddling the Newborn

bulb is permitted to reexpand slowly by releasing the compression on the bulb (Figure 26–12 ■). The bulb syringe is removed from the nostril, and drainage is then compressed out of the bulb and onto a tissue. The bulb syringe may also be used in the mouth if the newborn is spitting up and unable to handle the excess secretions. The bulb is compressed, the tip of the bulb syringe is placed about 1 inch to one side of the newborn's mouth, and compression is released. This draws up the excess secretions. The procedure is repeated on the other side of the mouth. The roof of the mouth and the back of the throat are avoided because suction in these areas might stimulate the gag reflex. The bulb syringe should be washed in warm, soapy water and rinsed in warm water daily and as needed after use. Rinsing with a half-strength white vinegar solution followed by clear water may help to extend the useful life of the bulb syringe by inhibiting bacterial growth. A bulb syringe should always be kept near the newborn. New parents and nurses who are inexperienced with babies may fear that the baby will choke and are relieved to know how to take action if such an event occurs. They should be advised to turn the newborn's head to the side or hold the newborn with his or her head down as soon as there is any indication of gagging or vomiting and to use the bulb syringe as needed.

Some infants may have transient edema of the nasal mucosa following suctioning of the airway after birth. The nurse can demonstrate the use of normal saline to loosen secretions, and instruct parents in the gentle and moderate use of the bulb syringe to avoid further irritation of the mucous membranes. If parents will be using humidifiers at home, they should be instructed to follow the manufacturer's cleaning instructions carefully so that molds, spores, and bacteria from a dirty humidifier do not enter the baby's environment.

Swaddling the Newborn

Swaddling (wrapping) helps the newborn maintain body temperature, provides a feeling of closeness and security, and may be effective in quieting a crying baby by having the newborn's hands near their mouth to allow for sucking (Roach, 2004). A blanket is placed on the crib (or secure surface) in the shape of a diamond. The top corner of the blanket is folded down slightly, and the newborn's body is placed with the head at the upper edge of the blanket. The right corner of the blanket is wrapped around the newborn and tucked under the left side (not too tightly—the newborn needs a little room to move and to allow for hands to get to the mouth). The bottom corner is then pulled up to the chest, and the left corner wrapped around the baby's right side (Figure 26–13 ■). The nurse can show this wrapping technique to a new mother so she will feel more skilled in handling her baby.

HINTS FOR PRACTICE

Remember that left-handed people tend to hold the baby over their right shoulder, and right-handed people do the opposite. This keeps the dominant hand free. However, most health personnel wear their nametags on the left side. To avoid scratching the baby's face, wear your nametag on the same side as your dominant hand.

Sleep and Activity

The National Institute of Child Health and Human Development and the American Academy of Pediatrics recommend that healthy term infants be placed on their back to sleep. Parents are taught the importance of following "Back to Sleep Guidelines" to reduce the incidence of sudden infant death syndrome (SIDS) (American Academy of Pediatrics [AAP] Task Force on Sudden Infant Death Syndrome, 2005). Though infants may need to be placed on their sides initially because of copious or thick secretions, placing them on their backs in the newborn period serves to educate parents regarding infant positioning. Studies indicate that parents position their babies in the same positions they observe in the hospital setting, so nurses must demonstrate this behavior to reduce the risk of SIDS. If exceptions are warranted, these should be explained to families so they do not misinterpret what they observe. The placement of babies in a prone position during wakeful play sessions "Tummy time" should be encouraged as well (AAP & ACOG, 2007).

Perhaps nothing is more individual to each baby than the sleep-activity cycle. It is important for the nurse to recognize the individual variations of each newborn and to assist parents as they develop sensitivity to their infant's communication signals and rhythms of activity and sleep. See Chapter 25 ∞ for a more detailed discussion of sleep-wake activity.

Car Safety Considerations

Half of the children killed or injured in automobile accidents could have been protected by the use of federally approved car seats. Newborns must go home from the birthing unit in a car seat adapted to fit them (Figure 26–14 ■). Babies should never be placed in the front seat of a car equipped with a passenger-side airbag. The car seat should be positioned to face the rear of the car until the baby is 1 year old or weighs 9.09 kg (20 lb) (AAP, 2008). Nurses need to ensure that all parents are knowledgeable about the benefits of child safety seat use and proper installation. Nurses can encourage parents to have their infant safety seats checked by local groups trained specifically for that purpose. The Seat Check Initiative provides locations and information about child safety seats.

Newborn Screening and Immunization Programs

Before the newborn and mother are discharged from the birthing unit, the nurse informs the parents about the **newborn screening tests** and tells them when to return to the birthing center or clinic if further tests are needed.

MyNursingKit | National SIDS/Infant Death Resource Center

MyNursingKit | Car Seat Safety

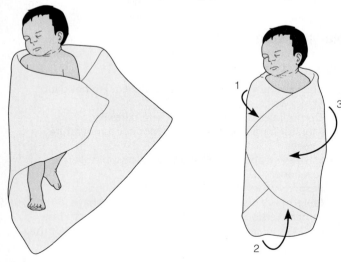

FIGURE 26–13 Steps in wrapping a baby.

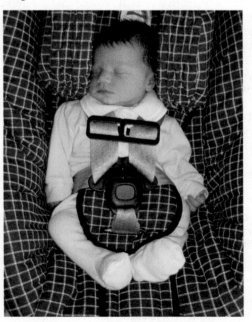

FIGURE 26–14 Infant car restraint for use from birth to about 12 months of age.

Some of the disorders that can be identified from a few drops of blood obtained by a heel stick are cystic fibrosis, galactosemia, congenital adrenal hyperplasia, congenital hypothyroidism, maple syrup urine disease, phenylketonuria (PKU), sickle cell trait, biotinidase deficiency, and hemoglobinopathies.

The Expanded Newborn Screening Program allows parents to have their babies screened for more than 20 disorders. Early newborn discharge puts infants at risk for delayed or even missed diagnosis of PKU and congenital hypothyroidism because of decreased sensitivity of screening before 24 hours of age. Newborns should be retested by 2 weeks of age if the first test was done before 24 hours of age. New technology is quickly increasing the number of metabolic and other disorders that can be detected in the newborn period. Although controversy exists over the need for such comprehensive testing, it is recommended that states test for a core panel of 29 treatable congenital conditions and an additional 25 conditions that may be detected by screening (AAP, Newborn Screening Authoring Committee, 2008). Some states are now screening for more than 50 congenital conditions. Phenylketonuria and congenital hypothyroidism are the only tests that are performed in all 50 states and the District of Columbia (ACOG Committee on Genetics, 2003). PKU and select metabolic disorders are discussed further in Chapter 28 ∞.

Hearing loss is found in 1 to 3 per 1000 infants in the normal newborn population (Thureen, Deacon, Hernandez et al., 2005). The recommended initial newborn hearing screening should be accomplished before discharge from the birthing unit with appropriate follow-up if the newborn fails to pass the initial screen in all hospitals providing obstetric services (AAP & ACOG, 2007, Creehan, 2008). (For further discussion see Chapter 25 ∞.)

Immunization programs against the hepatitis B virus during the newborn period and infancy are in place in many states, at least 20 countries, and high-incidence areas such as American Samoa. Universal vaccination of infants is recommended. Infants should receive the first dose of hepatitis B (Hep B) vaccine at birth to 2 months of age. The second dose should be administered at least 1 month after the first dose. The third dose should be administered at least 4 months after the first dose and at least 2 months after the second dose, but not before 6 months of age (AAP & ACOG, 2007). See Drug Guide: Hepatitis B Vaccine (Engerix-B, Recombivax HB). Parents need to be advised whether their birthing center provides newborn hepatitis vaccination so that an adequate follow-up program can be set in motion.

Early discharge has affected both the timing of newborn metabolic screening tests and the acquisition of subsequent immunization. For example, the accuracy of the

---

Drug Guide Hepatitis B Vaccine (Engerix-B, Recombivax HB)

Overview of Neonatal Action Recombinant hepatitis B vaccine is used as a prophylactic treatment against all subtypes of hepatitis B virus. It provides passive immunization for newborns of HBsAg-negative and HBsAg-positive mothers. Hepatitis B can be transmitted across the placenta, but most newborns are infected during birth.

The vaccine is produced from baker's yeast and plasmid containing the HBsAg gene.

Hepatitis B (thimerosal free) vaccine contains more than 95% HBsAg protein and is an inactivated (noninfective) product. Universal immunization is recommended.

Infants of HBsAg-positive mothers should concurrently receive 0.5 mL of hepatitis B immunoglobulin (HBIG) prophylaxis at separate injection sites (AAP & ACOG, 2007, Wilson, Shannon, & Shields, 2009).

Pregnancy Risk Category: C

Route, Dosage, Frequency The first dose of 0.5 mL (10 mcg) is given intramuscularly into the anterolateral thigh within 12 hours of birth for infants born to HBsAg-positive mothers. The second dose of vaccine is given at least 1 month after the first dose and followed by a final dose at least 4 months after the first dose and at least 3 months after the second dose, but not before 6 months of age.

Infants born to HBsAg-negative mothers receive their first dose of vaccine at birth, the second dose at 1 to 2 months, and the third dose at 6 to 18 months (AAP & ACOG, 2007).

Infants whose mother's HBsAg status is unknown should receive the same doses of vaccine as infants born to HBsAg-positive mothers.

Neonatal Side Effects The only common side effect is soreness at the injection site. Occasionally, there is erythema, swelling, warmth, and induration at the injection site, irritability, or a low-grade fever (37.7°C [99.8°F]).

Nursing Considerations Delay administration during active infection, as the vaccine will not prevent infection during its incubation period.

- The vaccine should be used as supplied. Do not dilute. Shake well.
- Do not inject intravenously or interdermally.
- Monitor for adverse reactions. Monitor temperature closely.
- Have epinephrine available to treat possible allergic reactions.
- Responsiveness to the vaccine is age dependent. Preterm infants weighing less than 1000 g have lower seroconversion rates. Consider delaying the first dose until the infant is term postconceptual age (PCA) or use a four-dose schedule.

test for PKU is directly related to the newborn's age. The likelihood of detecting PKU increases as the infant grows older; the infant must be at least 24 hours old for a valid test. A second test is required in most states, usually between 1 week and 1 month of age, to minimize the chance of a positive child going undetected.

The nurse should teach the family all necessary caregiving methods before discharge. A checklist may be helpful to determine whether the teaching has been completed and to verify the parents' knowledge on leaving the birthing unit (Figure 26–15 ■). The nurse needs to review all areas for understanding or answer outstanding questions with the mother and father, without rushing, and take time to resolve all queries. Any concerns of the parents or nurse are noted.

Community-Based Nursing Care

The nurse discusses with parents ways to meet their newborn's needs, ensure safety, and appreciate the newborn's unique characteristics and behaviors. By assisting parents in establishing links with their community-based healthcare provider, the nurse can get the new family off to a good start. Parents also need to know the signs of illness, how to reach the pediatrician or after-hours clinic, and the importance of follow-up after discharge. (See Key Facts to Remember: When Parents Should Call Their Healthcare Provider and the Teaching Card: Teaching Signs of Possible Illness During the Newborn Period inserted in the center of this text.) Parents should also check with their clinician for advice about over-the-counter medications to be kept in the medicine cabinet.

The family should have the care provider's phone number, address, and any specific instructions. Having the birthing unit or nursery phone number is also reassuring to a newborn's family. They are encouraged to call with questions. Follow-up calls lend added support by providing another opportunity for parents to have their questions answered.

Some institutions have initiated postpartum and/or newborn follow-up home visits especially for infants discharged before 48 hours after birth. The follow-up infant examination should be within 48 hours of discharge (AAP & ACOG, 2007) when the family is unable to visit their primary care physician within that time period. The home visit focuses on normal newborn care, assessment for hyperbilirubinemia (jaundice), extreme weight loss, feeding

---

◆

KEY FACTS TO REMEMBER
When Parents Should Call Their Healthcare Provider

Temperature above 38°C (100.4°F) axillary or below 36.6°C (97.8°F) axillary

Continual rise in temperature

More than one episode of forceful vomiting or frequent vomiting over a 6-hour period

Refusal of two feedings in a row

Lethargy (listlessness), difficulty in awakening baby

Cyanosis (bluish discoloration of skin) with or without a feeding

Absence of breathing longer than 20 seconds

Inconsolable infant (quieting techniques are not effective) or continuous high-pitched cry

Discharge or bleeding from umbilical cord, circumcision, or any opening (except vaginal mucus or pseudomenstruation)

Two consecutive green, watery stools or black stools or increased frequency of stools

No wet diapers for 18 to 24 hours or fewer than six to eight wet diapers per day after 4 days of age

Development of eye drainage

---

problems, and knowledge related to newborn care and feeding within the family unit.

Routine well-baby visits should be scheduled with the clinic, pediatric nurse practitioner, or physician. Regardless of the type of follow-up services available in the community, the nurse contributes to the newborn's health by stressing the importance of routine care and by helping families who have no follow-up plans to connect to local resources for care (for detail discussion of home care, see Chapter 32).

Evaluation

When evaluating the nursing care provided in preparation for discharge, the nurse may anticipate the following outcomes:

- The parents demonstrate safe techniques in caring for their newborn.
- Parents verbalize developmentally appropriate behavioral expectations of their newborn and knowledge of community-based newborn follow-up care.

		FOR NURSES ONLY

NURSERY TEACHING CHECKLIST

Please read the *Mother/Baby* information booklet given to you after birth. After reading it, please go through the following list and check whether you understand each topic or need to know more.

		I know this already	Doesn't apply to me	I need to know more	Taught/ reviewed/ demonstrated
Baby Care	What to do if baby is choking or gagging				
	Safety				
	How to do skin care/cord care				
	How to take care of the circumcision or genital area				
	How to know if my baby is sick and what to do				
	What is jaundice and how to detect it				
	Use of thermometer				
	Use of bulb syringe				
	How and when to burp baby				
	Newborn behavior: crying/comforting				
	How to position baby after feeding				
	What does demand scheduling mean				
Breastfeeding	I attended breastfeeding class/watched breastfeeding video	YES ☐	NO ☐		
	How to position baby for feeding				
	How to get baby to latch on to my nipple properly				
	When and how long to breastfeed				
	Removal of baby from my nipple				
	What is the supply and demand concept				
	What is the let-down reflex				
	When does breast milk come in				
	Supplementing				
	Proper diet for breastfeeding mothers				
	Prevention and comfort measures for sore nipples				
	Prevention and comfort measures for engorgement				
	When and how to use a breast pump				
	How to express milk by hand				
	How to go back to work and continue to breastfeed				
Bottle-Feeding	How to feed my baby a bottle				
	Reasons for NOT propping bottles				
	How to clean nipple/bottle				
	How to mix formula				
	What formula should my baby drink				
Safety	**Use of infant car seat**				
	Back to Sleep				
	Shaken Baby Syndrome				

Other information:

_____

_____

_____

_____

_____

I have received and understand the instructions given on the above topics.

_____   _____
MOTHER'S SIGNATURE   DATE

Videos viewed/ Literature given:

_____

Language Spoken by Mother:

☐ English ☐ Spanish ☐ Other _____

Interpreter Used? ☐ Yes ☐ No ☐ Family Interprets

Nurse's Signature(s):

_____

_____

_____

FIGURE 26–15 An infant teaching checklist is completed by the time of discharge.
Source: Adapted from Presbyterian/St. Luke's Medical Center, Denver, CO.

- The overall goal of newborn nursing care is to provide comprehensive care while promoting the establishment of a well-functioning family unit.
- In the period immediately after birth, during which adaptation to extrauterine life occurs, the newborn requires close monitoring to identify any deviations from normal.
- Nursing goals during the first 4 hours after birth (admission and transitional period) are to maintain a clear airway, maintain a neutral thermal environment, prevent hemorrhage and infection, initiate oral feedings, and facilitate attachment.
- The newborn is routinely given prophylactic vitamin K to prevent possible hemorrhagic disease of the newborn.
- Prophylactic eye treatment for *Neisseria gonorrhoeae* is legally required for all newborns.
- Nursing goals for ongoing newborn care include maintenance of cardiopulmonary function, maintenance of neutral thermal environment, promotion of adequate hydration and nutrition, prevention of complications, promotion of safety, and enhancement of attachment and family knowledge of child care.
- Essential daily care includes assessing vital signs, weight, overall color, intake, output, umbilical cord and circumcision, newborn nutrition, parent education, and attachment.
- Following a circumcision, the newborn must be observed closely for signs of bleeding, inability to void, and signs of infection and pain.
- Signs of illness in newborns include temperature above 38°C (100.4°F) axillary or below 36.6°C (97.8°F) axillary, more than one episode of forceful vomiting, refusal of two feedings in a row, lethargy, cyanosis with or without a feeding, and absence of breathing for longer than 20 seconds.
- Newborn screening for congenital hypothyroidism and phenylketonuria may be done on all newborns in the first 1 to 3 days.

EXPLORE PEARSON **mynursingkit**™

MyNursingKit is your one stop for online chapter review materials and resources. Prepare for success with additional NCLEX®-style practice questions, interactive assignments and activities, web links, animations and videos, and more!

Register your access code from the front of your book at
www.mynursingkit.com

CHAPTER REFERENCES

American Academy of Pediatrics (AAP). (2008). Car safety seats: A guide for families 2008. Retrieved April 20, 2008, from www.aap.org/family/carseatguide

American Academy of Pediatrics (AAP) & Canadian Paediatric Society (CPS). (2006). Prevention and management of pain in the neonate: An update. *Pediatrics, 118*(5), 2231–2241.

American Academy of Pediatrics (AAP), Committee on Fetus and Newborn & American College of Obstetricians and Gynecolgists (ACOG) Committee on Obstetrics. (2007). *Guidelines for perinatal care* (6th ed.). Evanston, IL: Author.

American Academy of Pediatrics (AAP), Newborn Screening Authoring Committee. (2008). Newborn screening expands: Recommendations for pediatricians and medical homes—implications for the system. *Pediatrics, 121*(1), 192–217.

American Academy of Pediatrics (AAP). Task Force on Sudden Infant Death Syndrome. (2005). The changing concept of sudden infant death syndrome: Diagnostic coding shifts, controversies regarding the sleeping environment, and new variables to consider in reducing risk. *Pediatrics, 116*(5), 1245–1255.

American College of Obstetricians and Gynecologists (ACOG), Committee on Genetics. (2003). Newborn screening (ACOG Committee Opinion No. 287). *Obstetric Gynecology, 102*, 887–889.

Andrews, M. M. (2008). Transcultural perspectives in the nursing care of children and adolescents.

In M. M. Andrews & J. S. Boyle (Eds.), *Transcultural concepts in nursing care* (5th ed., pp. 116–145). Philadelphia: Lippincott.

Askin, D. (2008). Newborn adaptations to extrauterine life. In K. R. Simpson & P. A. Creehan, *Perinatal nursing* (3rd ed., pp. 527–545). Philadelphia: Lippincott Williams & Wilkins.

Association of Women's Health, Obstetric and Neonatal Nurses (AWHONN). (2001). *Evidence-based clinical practice guideline: Neonatal skin care.* Washington, DC: Author.

Blackburn, S. T. (2007). *Maternal, fetal, & neonatal physiology: A clinical perspective* (3rd ed.). St. Louis: Saunders.

Creehan, P. A. (2008). Newborn physical assessment. In K. R. Simpson & P. A. Creehan, *Perinatal nursing.* (3rd ed., pp. 546–574). Philadelphia: Lippincott Williams & Wilkins.

D'Avanzo, C. E., & Geissler, E. M. (2008). *Pocket guide to cultural assessment* (4th ed.). St. Louis, MO: Mosby.

Green-Hernandez, G., Quinne, A., Falkenstern, S., Denman-Vitale, S., & Judge-Ellis, T. (2004). Making nursing care culturally competent. *Holistic Nursing Practice,* July/August, 215–218.

Hedayat, K. M. (2001). Issues in Islamic biomedical ethics: A primer for the pediatrician. *Pediatrics, 108*(4), 965–971.

Karl, D. J. (2004). Using principles of newborn behavioral state organization to facilitate breastfeeding. *MCN American Journal of Maternal Child Nursing, 29*(5), 292–298.

Klaus, M., & Klaus, P. (1985). *The amazing newborn.* Menlo Park, CA: Addison-Wesley.

Lipson, J. G., & Dibble, S. L. (2008). Culture & Clinical Care. (7th ed.). San Francisco, CA: The Regents, University of California.

Medves, J. M., & O'Brien, B. (2004). The effect of bather and location of first bath on maintaining thermal stability in newborns. *Journal of Obstetric, Gynecologic, and Neonatal Nursing, 33*(2), 175–182.

Ott, B., Al-Khadhuri, J., & Al-Junaibi, S. (2003). Preventing ethical dilemmas: Understanding Islamic health care practices. *Pediatrics, 29*(3), 227–230.

Roach, J. A. (2004). Newborn stimulation: Preventing over-stimulation is key for optimal growth & well-being. *AWHONN Lifelines, 7*(6), 531–535.

Thureen, P. J., Deacon, J., Hernandez, J. A., & Hall, D. M. (2005). *Assessment and care of the well newborn.* (2nd ed.). St. Louis: Elsevier Saunders.

Wilson, B. A., Shannon, M. T., & Shields, K. M. (2009). *Prentice Hall nurse's drug guide 2009.* Upper Saddle River, NJ: Pearson Education, Inc.

World Health Organization. (1999). Care of the umbilical cord: A review of the evidence [On-line]. Retrieved June 21, 2008 from www.who.int/rht/documents/MSM98-4

World Health Orgnization (2008). Male circumcision information package. [On-line]. Retrieved June 20, 2008 from www.who.int/hiv/pub/malecircumcision/infopack/en/index.html

CHAPTER 27

Newborn Nutrition

As a lactation educator my goal is to ensure that breastfeeding is well established before the couplet (mom and baby) is discharged. I try to set the groundwork for trust and rapport, so that after they go home the family is not afraid to call me if questions arise. Sometimes I see the mom and baby weeks or even months later, and they will thank me for getting them off to a good start.

—Hospital Lactation Nurse

LEARNING OUTCOMES

27-1. Compare the nutritional value and composition of breast milk and formula preparations in relation to the nutritional needs of the newborn.

27-2. Explain the advantages and disadvantages of breastfeeding and formula-feeding in determining the nursing care of both mother and newborn.

27-3. Examine practices used in the nursing care of both breastfeeding and formula-feeding mothers that promote successful feeding of infants in the hospital-based and community-based setting.

27-4. Formulate a teaching plan related to infant feeding based on the evaluation of the mother's knowledge-deficits, method of feeding, concerns, and cultural values.

27-5. Explain the nutritional needs of the unborn and normal growth patterns in the nutritional assessment of the infant and educate parents on these.

27-6. Explain the influence of cultural values on infant care, especially feeding practices, in nursing care of the mother/family with a newborn.

KEY TERMS

$\mathbf{E}$arly nutrition has a significant impact on the present and future health and well-being of the infant because this is a period of rapid growth and brain development. Good nutrition fosters physical growth and helps maintain a healthy immune system. In addition, infant feeding itself is an important component of newborn socialization that promotes cognitive and emotional development.

Whether choosing to breastfeed or use infant formula, parents find feeding their newborn an exciting, satisfying, but often worrisome task. Meeting this essential need of their new child helps parents strengthen their attachment to their baby and fosters their self-images as nurturers and providers. It is important that the nurse is well informed about infant nutrition and feeding methods, because the parents look to the nurse for this guidance. Parents need accurate and consistent information from the nursing staff. They need to learn the skills to feed their infant successfully. Through each interaction with the parents, there is an opportunity for the nurse to support the parents and promote the family's sense of confidence.

In this chapter an emphasis is placed on feeding the full-term healthy infant of normal birth weight during the neonatal period. We will look at the nutritional needs of the newborn in the context of both breast milk and formula composition, discuss feeding methods, explore community-based nursing care, and finally look at a nutritional assessment of the newborn.

Nutritional Needs and Milk Composition

The newborn's diet must supply all the nutrients required by the body in the proper quantities to meet the newborn's rapid rate of physical and neurologic growth and development. A newborn's diet should provide adequate hydration and sufficient calories and include protein, carbohydrates, fat, vitamins, and minerals. Exclusive breast milk and/or iron-fortified 20-calorie/ounce formula are sufficient as sole sources of nutrition to meet the dietary needs of the newborn from birth up to 6 months of age. Complementary solid foods are introduced in the second half of the first year, and the infant continues to receive breast milk and/or formula until at least 12 months of age (American Academy of Pediatrics Section on Breastfeeding, 2005).

This next section will discuss the nutritional requirements of the newborn and how these are met by breast milk and cow's milk-based formula. There are three categories of commercial infant formulas: (1) standard cow's milk-based formulas, (2) soy protein-based formulas, and (3) specialized or therapeutic formulas. Further information on the latter two may be found in the following section on specialty formulas.

Dietary Reference Intakes

Before discussing the nutritional needs of the infant, the nurse should note that the new title *dietary reference intake (DRI)* is an updated generic term that replaces the well-known nutritional reference term *recommended dietary allowances (RDAs)*. The term *RDA* previously served as a benchmark for nutritional adequacy in the United States, but it reflected primarily disease prevention from nutrient deficiency. The term *DRI* encompasses four aspects of nutrient-based reference values: (1) estimated average requirement (EAR), (2) recommended dietary allowance (RDA), (3) adequate intake (AI), and (4) tolerable upper intake level (UL). The DRIs represent a framework that links nutrition and health across the lifespan (Gregory, 2005).

Growth

It is normal for both breastfed and formula-fed infants to lose weight in the first 3 to 4 days of life. Formula-feeding infants generally lose up to 3.5% of their birth weight; breastfeeding infants should not exceed a weight loss greater than 7% of their birth weight (Association of Women's Health, Obstetric and Neonatal Nurses (AWHONN), 2007; International Lactation Consultant Association, 2005). Infants lose weight with the passage of meconium and because their fluid intake is normally low in the first few days while transitioning to enteral feedings. This loss is normal and does not result in dehydration, as infants draw on their extracellular water reserves. Infants should begin gaining weight by day of life 5 or sooner and should be at or above birth weight by 10 to 14 days of age. Weight gain during the first 4 weeks should be about 10 g/kg/day or 5 to 7 oz/week (Riordan, 2005).

Breastfed and formula-fed babies have different growth rates. This is understandable because the compositions of breast milk and formula are different. Most physicians (as well as formula companies) consider breastfeeding as the "gold standard" from which to compare nutritional outcomes (AAP, 2005; Lawrence & Lawrence, 2005).

Formula-fed infants tend to regain their birth weight earlier than breastfed infants because the formula-fed infant has a greater fluid intake early on. The breastfeeding infant's fluid intake depends on the mother's milk supply and breastfeeding efficiency. It is noteworthy that breastfeeding infants born to multiparous mothers often do not lose much weight as infants born to primiparous mothers, because the multiparous mother's milk typically "comes in" quicker (Lawrence & Lawrence, 2005). If a healthy full-term infant with normal birth weight has a weight loss exceeding 7%, then a feeding evaluation is indicated. If an infant has a weight loss of 10% or greater then an evaluation, intervention, and follow-up is indicated to

---

◇

KEY FACTS TO REMEMBER

Newborn Caloric and Fluid Needs

Following are newborn caloric and fluid needs:
- Caloric intake: 45.5 to 52.5 kcal/lb/day or 100 to 115 kcal/kg/day
- Fluid requirements: 64 to 73 mL/lb/day or 140 to 160 mL/kg/day
- First 6 months weight gain:
  Formula-fed—1 oz/day;
  Breastfed—0.5 oz/day

---

make certain that the infant receives sufficient fluid and calories. In this case, a follow-up weight check is recommended to ascertain if the feeding problem is resolved.

Growth rates for breastfed and formula-fed infants are somewhat different once feedings are established. Exclusively breastfed infants have the same or slightly higher weight gain than their formula-fed and mixed-fed peers in the first 3 to 4 months. Thereafter, formula-fed and mixed-fed infants have a greater weight gain pattern compared with breastfed infants. This characteristic weight gain pattern results in a leaner body build in the breastfed group by the latter half of the first year of life (Riordan, 2005). Measurements of length and head circumference are the same for both groups. An infant typically grows 2.5 cm (1 in.) per month in the first 6 months, and then 1.3 cm (0.5 in.) for the next 6 months. Length is a greater indicator of growth than is weight. Infants generally double their birth weight by 5 months, triple their birth weight by 1 year of age, and quadruple their birth weight by 2 years (Riordan, 2005). Growth charts for tracking an infant's weight, length, and head circumference can be downloaded from The Centers for Disease Control and Prevention website (http://www.cdc.gov/growthcharts).

Fluid

Requirements

Fluid requirements during the neonatal period are high (140 to 160 mL/kg/day) because of the newborn's decreased ability to concentrate urine and increased overall metabolic rate. Although the infant's total body water content is high (75% to 80%) compared with an adult (60%), the infant has an increased surface area to mass ratio and decreased renal absorptive capacity that makes the infant more susceptible to dehydration from insufficient fluid intake or increased fluid loss caused by diarrhea, vomiting, or another source of fluid loss. Parents and caretakers should be aware of the signs of dehydration. Dry or chapped lips, dry oral cavity, decreased urine output, concentrated urine, general weakness, lethargy, poor skin turgor, sunken eyes, and sunken fontanelle are some of the

signs of dehydration. The infant's fluid intake will need to be increased above the baseline fluid needs when the infant has a fever or is in a warm environment for an extended period of time. For infants under 6 months of age, increased fluid requirements should be met with additional breast milk or formula, rather than water.

Milk Composition

Breast milk and formula contain almost 90% water, which meets the infant's water needs. Feeding supplemental water is not recommended routinely for infants under 6 months of age who are still on an exclusively milk diet (breast milk or formula), because the increased water can cause hyponatremia and may result in seizures if water consumption is excessive. In some cases in which the infant has become more severely dehydrated or will not tolerate increased breast milk or formula, a physician may recommend use of a water/electrolyte solution for initial rehydration.

Energy

Requirements

The basal metabolic rate (BMR) refers to the energy needed for thermoregulation, cardiorespiratory function, cellular activity, and growth. The healthy full-term infant's BMR is about twice that of an adult, based on body weight (Rolfes, Pinna, & Whitney, 2006). A newborn requires 100 to 115 kcal/kg/day at 1 month and 85 to 95 kcal/kg/day from 6 to 12 months of age. When infants do not receive sufficient calories, they risk losing weight, may experience tissue breakdown, and are at risk for delayed growth and development (Gregory, 2005).

Milk Composition

Healthy full-term newborns derive about half of their required calories from fat (breast milk 52%, formula 49%). The remaining calories are derived from carbohydrates (breast milk 42%, formula 43%) and to a lesser extent from protein (breast milk 6%, formula 8%) (Mead-Johnson, 2004; Ross, 2007). Often, calories derived from protein are not counted in the total daily caloric intake as there is a metabolic cost to breaking down protein that at least partially negates the caloric benefits.

Fats

Requirements

As noted, infants receive approximately 50% of their calories from fat. Fats also help the body absorb the fat-soluble vitamins A, D, E, and K. Fats are a precursor of prostaglandins and other hormones. Essential fatty acids and their derivitives docosahexaenoic acid (DHA) and arachidonic acid (ARA) are associated with improved visual acuity and cognitive ability (Riordan, 2005).

Milk Composition

Triglycerides make up 98% to 99% of milk fat. Triglycerides break down to free fatty acids and glycerol. The lipid fraction of breast milk provides essential fatty acids, including linoleic acid and linolenic acid, as well as their longer chain derivatives docosahexaenoic acid (DHA) and arachidonic acid (ARA). In 2001 the Food and Drug Administration (FDA) approved the addition of DHA and ARA to infant formula. Fat content is the most variable component in breast milk, ranging from 30 to 50 grams/liter. It is influenced by maternal parity, duration of pregnancy, the stage of lactation, diurnal regulation, and changes in fat content even during a single feeding. Multiparous mothers produce milk with a lower content of fatty acids. Mothers of preterm infants have a greater concentration of long-chain polyunsaturated fatty acids (LCPUFAs) in their milk compared with mothers of term infants. Phospholipids and cholesterol levels are higher in colostrum compared with mature milk, although overall fat content is higher in mature breast milk compared with colostrum. Fat content is generally higher in the evening and lower in the early morning. Within a single feeding session an infant initially receives the low-fat foremilk before receiving the higher calorie, high-fat hindmilk. Finally, the fat content of breast milk is also affected by maternal diet and maternal fat stores. Mothers on low-fat diets have increased production of medium chain fatty acids (C6-C10), and mothers with high levels of body fat produce breast milk with a higher fat content (Lawrence & Lawrence, 2005).

The fats in the milk-based formulas are modified to parallel the fat profile of breast milk by removing the butterfat from cow's milk and adding vegetable oils. There are quite a few differences in the fat sources and amounts used among the major formula brands. The different blends of fats all provide a fatty acid profile in the end that is similar to breast milk in terms of amount of saturated, monounsaturated, and polyunsaturated fats present. In 2002, the formula companies in the United States added long-chain polyunsaturated fatty acids (LCPUFAs), namely docosahexaenoic acid (DHA) for brain development and arachidonic acid (ARA) for visual acuity (Cloherty, Eichenwald & Stark, 2008).

Carbohydrates

Requirements

Carbohydrates (sugars) serve as the other main source of energy for the infant, providing about 40% of the calories in the infant's diet. By weight, both breast milk and formula contain more carbohydrate than fat, but the caloric value of carbohydrate is 4 calories/gram whereas fat provides 9 calories/gram.

Milk Composition

In breast milk, the primary carbohydrate is lactose. In addition to providing energy, lactose also functions to enhance the absorption of calcium, magnesium, and zinc (Lawrence & Lawrence, 2005). Breast milk also contains trace amounts of other carbohydrates such as glucosamines and nitrogen-containing oligosaccharides. Glucosamines are one of the building blocks for connective tissues and help strengthen and hold together ligaments and tendons. Oligosaccharides promote the growth of *Lactobacillus bifidus,* which promotes an intestinal acidic environment creating a hostile environment for bacteria to thrive (Riordan, 2005).

In comparing carbohydrates among the milk-based formulas, both Enfamil® and Similac® provide all of their carbohydrate calories from lactose. Carnation Good Start® uses a blend of 70% lactose and 30% maltodextrin (a table sugar-like carbohydrate) (Sears, 2008).

Protein

Requirements

Proteins are the building blocks for muscle and organ structure. They are key to just about every metabolic process in the body including energy metabolism, cell-signaling, growth, and immune function. Some dietary proteins are absorbed intact, although the majority are broken down into component amino acids and utilized by the infant to build new proteins to support rapid growth and repair of body cells. The protein requirement for an infant is about 0.8 to 0.9 grams per deciliter (Riordan, 2005).

Milk Composition

Milk proteins are often grouped into whey proteins and casein. Casein is the major phosphoprotein found in milk. It is not easily denatured and is relatively insoluble in water. It is the predominant protein that forms the curds seen when milk interacts with acid or the enzyme rennin in the stomach. Whey proteins are the remaining proteins suspended in the liquid portion of milk after curds are formed. Cow's milk contains a high amount of casein (a low ratio of whey to casein—approximately 20:80) compared with human milk (60:40 whey:casein). Because of its tendency to form curds, milk with high amounts of casein is less easily digested. Cow's milk-based formulas are usually modified to get closer to the whey:casein ratio of human milk. For example, the whey:casein ratio in Enfamil® is 60:40. Although Similac® has a ratio of 48:52, the company claims this produces an amino acid profile in the blood that is closer to that found in the breastfeeding infant. Carnation Good Start®

contains hydrolyzed whey protein, which the company states decreases the incidence of constipation, but which makes comparison difficult (Sears, 2008). It should also be noted that the whey and casein components in breast milk are not static and change over time to meet the needs of the growing infant. In early lactation, the whey:casein ratio is 90:10. As lactation progresses, the whey:casein ratio in mature breast milk is 60:40. Finally, during late lactation, the whey:casein ratio is 50:50 (Riordan, 2005).

Whey protein in breast milk is composed of five major components: (1) alpha-lactalbumin, (2) serum albumin, (3) lactoferrin, (4) immunoglobulins, and (5) lysozyme. The latter three components are involved in immunologic activities. Breast milk contains many other kinds of proteins as well. These include enzymes, growth modulator, and hormones (Blackburn, 2007). The major whey components in cow's milk-based formula are beta-lactoglobulin and alpha-lactalbumin. The former can trigger allergic reactions in some infants (Vonlanthen, 1998).

Vitamins, Minerals, and Trace Elements

Vitamins

REQUIREMENTS Vitamins can be grouped into fat-soluble and water-soluble vitamins. The fat-soluble vitamins are vitamins A, D, E, and K and are found in both cow's milk-based formula and breast milk. Vitamin K is also synthesized in the infant's intestinal tract by bacteria that are colonized there. After absorption via the lymphatic system, vitamins enter the blood and are transported to the various tissues where they are needed. Excess fat-soluble vitamins are stored in adipose tissue and the liver (Rolfes, Pinna, & Whitney, 2006). Excessive amounts of fat-soluble vitamins may result in toxicity, and there is general agreement that no routine fat-soluble vitamin supplementation is needed with the exception of vitamin D. To prevent rickets the AAP recommends that deeply pigmented breastfed infants or those with inadequate exposure to sunlight receive 200 international units of oral vitamin D drops daily during the first 2 months of life (AAP & ACOG, 2007). The infants should continue to take the vitamin supplement until feeding at least 500 mL per day (about 16.6 oz/day) of vitamin D-fortified formula or milk. Most healthy, full-term formula-feeding infants of average birth weight will receive sufficient vitamin D intake before they are 2 months old, and therefore may not require vitamin D supplementation.

MILK COMPOSITION Breast milk is naturally low in vitamin D (25 international units/L or less), and may be of concern particularly among breastfeeding infants who have limited sunlight exposure. Factors that place an infant at high risk for vitamin D deficiency include: having increased skin pigmentation, living in a geographic location where there is little sunlight, having one's skin consistently covered with clothing or sunscreen, not spending much time outdoors, living in an area that consistently has heavy pollution that blocks sunlight, and having a mother who is vitamin D deficient. Some breastfeeding advocates argue that an infant requires only a few minutes of sunlight exposure per day to stimulate vitamin D production in the skin to protect the infant from vitamin-D deficiency (Mohrbacher & Stock, 2003). The AAP contends that it is difficult to know what is adequate sunlight exposure for an individual, and they also recommend against direct, sunlight exposure of infants (AAP & ACOG, 2007).

The vitamin B complex and vitamin C are water-soluble vitamins that pass readily from serum to breast milk. However, mothers who follow a strict vegetarian diet or macrobiotic diet may have insufficient vitamin B_{12} in their milk. In that case the exclusively breastfed infant should receive vitamin B_{12} supplementation. Formula is fortified with adequate amounts of the water-soluble vitamins to meet the DRI. Unlike fat-soluble vitamins, any excess water-soluble vitamins ingested are simply excreted and the threat of toxicity is low (Lawrence & Lawrence, 2005).

Minerals

REQUIREMENTS Minerals have diverse regulatory functions throughout the body. For example, calcium is important in the clotting mechanisms; phosphorus is a component in ATP, DNA, RNA, and phospholipids; calcium and phosphorus are necessary for bone formation; sodium is involved in fluid balance; calcium, sodium, and potassium are needed for nerve and muscle function; chlorine is involved in acid-base balance; cobalt works with vitamin B_{12} to form blood cells; copper and iron aid in extracting energy from the citric acid cycle and are also involved in blood production; iodine is needed for thyroid hormone synthesis; and magnesium, manganese, and zinc are needed to help with many enzymatic processes.

Iron is an important mineral required by the body to make hemoglobin and is needed for neurologic function. Neurotransmitters require adequate iron levels to function properly and therefore infants with chronic anemia are at risk for cognitive and developmental delays. Infants deficient in iron may look pale, appear sleepy or tire easily while feeding, and be tachycardic or tachypneic at rest. The infant's iron status is affected by the amount of iron accumulated in utero, the infant's diet after birth, and the general health of the infant. The amount of iron transferred to the fetus during the third trimester of pregnancy is influenced by maternal iron status (O'Brien, Zavaleta, Abrams, & Caulfield, 2003).

MILK COMPOSITION Both breast milk and infant formulas contain several major and trace minerals to satisfy the needs of the growing infant. The mineral content of breast milk does not appear to be influenced by maternal diet. The vitamins and minerals among the three formulas being compared are essentially the same, although all generally contain higher levels of minerals than breast milk to compensate for their lower bioavailability.

Much has been written about the iron content of breast milk and formula and its bioavailability to the infant. The American Academy of Pediatrics does not advocate the use of low-iron fortified formulas because of the increased risk for anemia associated with their use (AAP & ACOG, 2007). Low-iron formula is fortified with only 2 mg of iron per liter compared with "iron-fortified" formula which is fortified with 12 mg of iron per liter. It should be noted that the iron concentration in breast milk is 0.5 to 1.0 mg per liter, which is considerably lower than in iron-fortified formulas. However, the iron in breast milk is much more completely absorbed—the infant receiving breast milk absorbs 50% to 80% of the iron in breast milk compared with less than 12% of the iron in formula. Researchers continue to study iron nutrition to determine the best level of iron fortification in infant formula. Healthy term infants with normal birth weights receiving breast milk or an iron-fortified infant formula during the first 5 to 6 months of life are unlikely to develop iron-deficiency anemia because these infants have sufficient iron stores to sustain them until they start solid feedings in the second half of the first year of life (Riordan, 2005).

Nurses have a responsibility to educate parents who have a misconception that infants fed iron-fortified formula are likely to have constipation. The iron added to formula is in an ionic form and does not cause constipation (Katz, Levin, Cotton, Patrick-Miller, Tesoro, & Rose, 2007). The casein in formula (which is different than the casein in breast milk) creates large, rubbery curds that are slow to metabolize and have been associated with constipation in formula-fed infants. In addition, there is evidence that palm olein oil (an additive to some formulas) also may contribute to constipation. Palm olein oil is added to some formulas to provide palmitic acid in an attempt to match the natural palmitic acid profile in breast milk. However, the chemical arrangements are different. Palmitic acid derived from olein oil is poorly absorbed. The unabsorbed palmitic acid in formula reacts with calcium to create insoluble soaps during digestion and increases the hardness of the stool (Ross Products Division, 2006).

Trace Elements

New additives to formulas not yet mentioned include nucleotides (building blocks for DNA and RNA that appear to enhance the immune system, among other things), carnitine (derived from the amino acid lysine and functioning in part to transport fatty acids to the mitochondria for oxida-

tion), and taurine (a conditionally essential non-protein sulfur amino acid with a number of functions including a role in growth, and in CNS and auditory function development). There are many other breast milk components not yet duplicated in formula (and many will never be because of the cost). Also, not all components in breast milk have been identified. In general, though, formula companies are always striving to improve their products to develop the best "humanized" milk possible. There is no question that formulas today are far superior to formulas from the past.

Specialty Formula

If an infant has medical problems related to inability to metabolize components of breast milk or standard formula, or if the parents are vegans, the family should consult with the baby's healthcare provider to discuss the issue of supplements or switching their infant to another infant formula.

Soy protein-based formulas (e.g., Enfamil Prosobee LIPIL®, Isomil®, Isomil Advance®, Isomil DF®, and Good Start Supreme Soy®) do not contain any bovine protein or lactose. Soy protein-based formulas use a soy protein harvested from soybeans and supplemented with methionine (an essential amino acid), carnitine, and taurine. Because soy protein-based formulas do not contain lactose, the formula is usually sweetened with corn syrup or sucrose. The latter may cause dental decay after teeth have erupted. Phytates present in soy formulas decrease the absorption of iron, calcium, and zinc, so greater concentrations of minerals and vitamins are added to soy formulas.

Soy protein-based formula is not intended as a first-choice formula except for infants with primary lactase deficiency or galactosemia and for term infants of formula-feeding vegan parents. The AAP states that the "isolated soy protein-based formulas are safe and effective alternatives to provide appropriate nutrition for normal growth and development" for term infants whose nutritional needs are not being met from breast milk or cow's milk-based formulas. According to the AAP, there is no proof that soy protein-based formula will prevent or lessen the symptoms of colic or prevent atropic disease, and infants who have a sensitivity to cow's milk protein may have a sensitivity to soy protein as well. Therefore, the AAP does not recommend routinely switching an infant from cow's milk-based formula to soy-based formula (Greer, Sicherer, Burks, & Committee on Nutrition and Section on Allergy and Immunology, 2008).

Infants with an allergic response to standard formulas may require a hypoallergenic "hydrolysate" formula. Hydrolyzed formulas (i.e., Nutramigen®, Alimentum®, and Pregestimil®) are sometimes referred to as "predigested" formulas because the dietary proteins have been broken down in a process that mimics digestion (hydrolysis). The simple protein compounds are usually too small to be recognized by the infant's immune system as an antigen, thereby decreasing the infant's allergic response. These formulas are also used in infants who have difficulties with normal digestion or absorption.

The other group of hypoallergenic formulas is the elemental amino acid-based formulas, such as Neocate® and Elecare®. The proteins in these formulas have been completely broken down to their amino acid constituents. These formulas are the most hypoallergenic formulas available and virtually eliminate the possibility of allergic reaction. They are intended for severely allergenic infants with multiple dietary protein intolerances or infants with severe absorption disorders.

Other specialized formulas are intended for infants with particular medical conditions and should be fed to infants only under a physician's supervision. There are specific specialized formulas intended for infants born prematurely to promote rapid growth. There are other specialized formulas for infants with heart disease, kidney disease, malabsorption syndromes, metabolic diseases, and allergies. These formulas vary in caloric content, nutrient composition and ingredients, digestibility, taste/odor, and cost.

The sole or primary carbohydrate in breast milk and humanized milk-based formulas is lactose. However, some of the specialty formulas use other carbohydrates such as corn syrup solids, sucrose, tapioca starch, and dextrose. This raises concerns about the long-term use of lactose-free formulas when an infant's sole source of food is formula. All too often, fussy breastfeeding or cow's milk-based formula-fed infants are switched to a lactose-free formula because of concerns about lactose intolerance. It is important to distinguish true lactose intolerance from cow's milk protein allergy or some other source of feeding intolerance.

Lactose intolerance is defined as a "deficiency of the intestinal enzyme lactase that splits lactose into two smaller sugars, glucose and galactose, and allows lactose to be absorbed from the intestine" (Marks, 2008). This condition causes diarrhea, flatulence, abdominal pain, and sometimes abdominal bloating, abdominal distention, and nausea. There are three causes of lactose intolerance: (1) congenital lactase deficiency, (2) secondary lactose intolerance, and (3) developmental or acquired lactose intolerance (Marks, 2008).

Congenital lactase deficiency is common in premature infants because of an inability to produce the enzyme lactase until they have matured. It is exceedingly rare in term infants and is due to a mutation of lactose producing gene. Symptoms of congenital deficiency begins shortly after birth (Marks, 2008). Secondary lactose intolerance occurs as a result of damage to the mucosal lining of the small intestine, where the lactase enzyme is produced. Any condition that causes gastroenteritis, especially if prolonged, can create this condition. Following a severe bout of diarrhea,

transient lactose intolerance may persist for a brief time until the brush border of the intestinal mucosa heals.

The most common cause of lactose intolerance is developmental or acquired. Many parents will assume that their infant has lactose intolerance because they or the child's older sibling has lactose intolerance. However, this is an age-related condition that develops after 2 to 5 years of age and, therefore, is not a common condition affecting newborns. Its prevalence and onset varies by ethnicity. Nearly 100% of Asians, 80% to 100% of Native Americans, up to 80% of African Americans and Latinos, and up to 20% of American Caucasians acquire lactose intolerance during their lifetime (Marks, 2008).

Infants with symptoms similar to those of lactose intolerance are more likely to be reacting to cow's milk protein (mostly because of the beta-lactoglobulin component in cow's milk) or to some other antigen. This can occur even with exclusively breastfed infants who are allergic to bovine protein, as some of the cow's milk protein antigens consumed by the mother can pass into her breast milk. Elimination of the antigen from the mother's diet may resolve the problem.

Choice of Feeding: Breast versus Formula

The Evolution of Formula

Finding an acceptable breast milk substitute following maternal death, infant abandonment, low milk supply, and other situations has been a challenge for centuries. There is physical evidence of societies using alternative feedings dating back to 2000 B.C. Spouted feeding cups and other feeding receptacles have been found in the graves of infants throughout Europe. Records from written works show that from 1500 to 1700, "wet nurses" (lactating women whose purpose of employment was to nurse another woman's infant, sometimes abandoning her own infant to gain employment) were hired at foundling homes (orphanages) and by wealthy European women, because it was customary for noblewomen to delegate all physical work, including infant care (Lawrence & Lawrence, 2005).

By the nineteenth century wet nursing was falling out of favor, and "dry nursing" was attempted. Dry nursing is the practice of feeding an infant milk obtained from another mammal (goats, cows, mares, donkeys, etc.) (Schuman, 2003). Cow's milk was most commonly used because of its availability, not because it was closer in composition to human milk. This practice was used in foundling homes and was associated with very high infant mortality (Lawrence & Lawrence, 2005).

Recognizing the need for an improved alternative breast milk substitute, a few physicians continued attempts to develop a "humanized" animal milk substitute. Around the 1860s, the first commercially available baby food and infant formula was developed in Europe; it became available in the United States by the 1870s. The first formula was comprised of only malt, cow's milk, and wheat flour and required reconstitution with water (Schuman, 2003). Between 1860 and 1920 additional scientific discoveries contributed to overall infant survival among non-breastfeeding infants. These included discovery of the germ theory and subsequent development of pasteurization of milk, the invention of the bottle and rubber nipple to replace feeding devices that required skill to use and were difficult to clean, and the invention of the "ice box" to refrigerate the baby milk (Baumslag & Michels, 1995).

Two of the biggest commercial advances in milk science were the invention of sweetened condensed milk in the 1830s and evaporated milk in 1883. The invention of sweetened condensed milk and evaporated milk meant that for the first time in history, a family did not have to have access to a cow in order to feed their infant milk (if not breastfeeding). The evaporated milk formula gained acceptance because it was affordable, widely available, and appeared to support growth equal to that of breastfed infants. It is estimated that by 1960 about 80% of formula-fed infants were being fed with evaporated milk formula and given supplements of vitamins and iron. However, poor infant outcomes were still being observed.

Artificial baby milk that was originally intended as a lifesaving product for extreme situations was now being aggressively marketed as a food for all infants. In the 1960s proprietary commercial formulas began to gain acceptance because parents were impressed with the advances in science and wanted to raise their children scientifically "by the book." By this time more and more women were working outside the home than ever before. In addition to a changing social climate in America, advances in agriculture created a surplus of cow's milk and offered a new marketing opportunity for global commercialization of formula (Baumslag & Michels, 1995).

One of their marketing tactics was to provide free formula to hospitals, enabling hospitals to phase out their formula preparation rooms. Mothers viewed commercial formula as an acceptable breast milk substitute that appeared to have medical endorsement, was easy to use, and was affordable. It also freed her up to do other things such as work outside the home. By 1972, formula use peaked and breastfeeding rates in the United States plummeted (only 25% of women were breastfeeding at hospital discharge) (Schuman, 2003). Again, the public was led to believe that commercial formula was as good as, if not better than, breast milk.

Research efforts beginning in the 1970s showed that breast milk was unquestionably superior to evaporated milk and proprietary infant formulas as evidenced by a sig-

nificant rise in infant morbidity and mortality, especially in developing countries (Baumslag & Michels, 1995). The revelation of the research findings from the 1970s up to the present has led to a resurgence in breastfeeding. By 2003, 66% of mothers in the United States were breastfeeding at hospital discharge. However, only 33% of infants were still receiving some breast milk at 6 months of age (Ross, 2007).

Over the last 50 years or so, considerable time, effort, and money have been allocated to the development of commercial infant formulas in an attempt to better imitate the content and performance of human milk. In 1954, the Executive Board of the American Academy of Pediatrics established a Committee on Nutrition to set the standards for nutritional requirements and feeding practices for infants, children, and adolescents. This committee makes recommendations for nutritional requirements in infant formulas to the Federal Food and Drug Administration. In 1971 the FDA created the first regulation for commercial formula, which established minimum requirements for fat, protein, linoleic acid, and vitamins and minerals (Schuman, 2003). In 1980 Congress passed the Infant Formula Act, which was later amended in 1986. The safety and nutritional quality of formula are now significantly regulated.

Although breastfeeding is increasing in popularity, formula-feeding continues to be a viable and nurturing choice, particularly in developed countries, and meets the goal of successful growth of the baby. The closeness and warmth that can occur during breastfeeding is also an integral part of formula-feeding. An advantage of formula-feeding is that parents can share equally in this nurturing, caring experience with their baby.

Advantages of Breast Milk

In their breastfeeding policy statement, the American Academy of Pediatrics recommends exclusive breastfeeding as the preferred feeding for all infants, with a few exceptions, for the first 6 months and continued breastfeeding during the introduction of solids until the infant is 12 months old or older, as desired. There is overwhelming scientific evidence that shows that breastfeeding provides newborns and infants with specific nutritional, immunologic, and psychosocial advantages over formula-feeding (AAP & ACOG, 2007).

Nutritional Advantages

Human milk provides optimum nutrition for the human infant because it is species specific. The macronutrients such as protein, fat, and carbohydrates (lactose) are synthesized by the mother in the alveoli of the breasts by specialized secretory cells. Micronutrient elements such as vitamins and minerals are derived from the circulating maternal plasma. There are more than

MyNursingKit | Breastfeeding

200 distinct components in breast milk, with more remaining to be identified (Lawrence & Lawrence, 2005).

Lactose is the primary carbohydrate in mammalian milk and plays a crucial role in the nourishment of our offspring. Human milk has a very high lactose content compared with the milk of other mammal species. After lactose is hydrolyzed into galactose and glucose, the galactose is used in the formation of cerebral galactolipids and contributes to brain and central nervous system development. Glucose is used by many tissues, but especially by the brain, which consumes 20% of the body's energy requirements and derives this almost exclusively from glucose. In addition to providing a cellular energy source, lactose enhances the absorption of calcium, magnesium, and zinc (Lawrence & Lawrence, 2005).

Approximately 98% of the human milk fat is in the form of triglycerides, and a very small but clinically significant amount is from cholesterol. Some researchers believe that the cholesterol in breast milk may play a role in myelination and neurologic development. Cholesterol levels in breast milk may also stimulate the production of enzymes that lead to more efficient metabolism of cholesterol, thereby reducing its harmful long-term effects on the cardiovascular system.

Fatty acids are another key component to brain development. Prenatally, fatty acids transfer across the placenta. Postnatally, they are obtained from the diet. Omega-3 and omega-6 fatty acids are two classes of essential fatty acids found in breast milk, although the level can vary with maternal diet. Fish is a rich source of these kinds of fatty acids.

Docosahexaenoic acid (DHA) and arachidonic acid (ARA) are long-chain polyunsaturated fatty acids (LCPUFAs) derived from linoleic acid and α-linolenic acid. They are major components of the cell membranes of the retina, brain, and other neural tissues. Along with oleic acid, these LCPUFAs are needed for myelination of the spinal cord and other nerves, and they have an impact on visual acuity and cognitive and behavioral functions. Since 2002 some infant formulas have been supplemented with DHA and ARA. However, breast milk still contains 167 other fatty acids of uncertain function and which are absent from formula (Cloherty et al., 2008). It seems reasonable that many of these will turn out to be important as well.

Another advantage of breast milk is that its composition varies according to gestational age and stage of lactation. For example, the milk of a mother who delivers a preterm infant has a greater concentration of DHA and ARA than does the milk of a mother who gives birth to a full-term infant. Babies born prematurely miss receiving the continuous placental transfer of DHA and ARA while developing during the third trimester. By receiving breast milk, these preterm infants receive the increased concentrations of DHA and ARA intended for the premature in-

fant (Lawrence & Lawrence, 2005). See Evidence-Based Practice: Breastfeeding for Low-Birth-Weight and Premature Newborns.

Breast milk provides newborns with minerals in more appropriate doses than do formulas (Blackburn, 2007). As mentioned earlier in this chapter, the iron found in breast milk, even though much lower in concentration than that of prepared formulas, is much more readily and fully absorbed and appears sufficient to meet the infant's iron needs for the first 6 months. Additional iron that is not absorbed may increase the growth of pathogenic bacteria as well as cause cellular oxidative injury. In addition, formula does not contain lactoferrin, an iron-binding protein that scavenges iron in the gut and enhances its absorption (Lawrence & Lawrence, 2005).

There is research supporting additional health advantages for the breastfed infant. Breastfed infants have a reduced risk of developing type 1 or type 2 diabetes melitus, lymphoma, leukemia, Hodgkin's disease, obesity, hypercholesterolemia, and asthma. Finally, the mother who breastfeeds has health advantages as well. After childbirth there is decreased postpartum bleeding and more rapid uterine involution. The breastfeeding mother has a decreased risk of developing breast cancer and ovarian cancer, and may have a decreased risk of developing postmenopausal osteoporosis (AWHONN, 2007).

Immunologic Advantages

The immunologic advantages of breast milk include varying degrees of protection from respiratory tract and gastrointestinal tract infections, necrotizing enterocolitis, urinary tract infections, otitis media, bacterial meningitis, bacteremia, and allergies (AWHONN, 2007). Transplacental passage of maternal immunoglobulin gradually diminishes over the first 6 months of life until the infant can begin to produce his or her own immunoglobulins. Breast milk-derived immunologic protection helps supplement this protection.

Secretory IgA, an immunoglobulin present in colostrum and breast milk, has antiviral, antibacterial, and antigenic-inhibiting properties, specifically across mucosal surfaces such as the intestinal tract. Secretory IgA plays a role in decreasing the permeability of the small intestine to help prevent large protein molecules from triggering an allergic response. Other constituents of colostrum and breast milk that act to inhibit the growth of bacteria or viruses are *Lactobacillus bifidus,* lysozymes, lactoperoxidase, lactoferrin, transferrin, and various immunoglobulins.

Some mothers wonder if there are special considerations for breastfed infants regarding immunizations, in particular the oral poliovirus vaccination because it is a live virus vaccine. These mothers worry that their antibod-

EVIDENCE-BASED PRACTICE

Breastfeeding for Low-Birth-Weight and Premature Newborns

Clinical Question

Does breastfeeding low-birth-weight and premature newborns while they are in the NICU demonstrate improved outcomes for the baby?

The Evidence

The benefits of breastfeeding for newborns up to 6 months of age are well documented. However, when these babies require treatment in the Neonatal Intensive Care Unit (NICU), breastfeeding presents challenges for mothers, newborns, and nurses. Research shows that it is possible to successfully establish breastfeeding in more than 90% of preterm and low-birth-weight babies. Several authors in both the United States and internationally used various experimental designs to determine if the efforts made to provide breastfeeding to babies in the NICU resulted in improved outcomes over babies who were not afforded this type of nutrition. Several randomized trials have focused on the outcomes of breastfed high-risk newborns, and one longitudinal study followed a group of 50 breastfed low-birth-weight premature infants to determine if there were long-term benefits of breast milk feeding. The replication of these experiments across settings represents strong evidence for nursing practice.

What Is Effective?

These studies revealed that more than half of the babies who receive breast milk in the NICU will continue breastfeeding after discharge. Premature and low-birth-weight newborns who were fed breast milk in the NICU and continued breastfeeding after discharge had higher scores on a measure of mental development and an index of physical development at 6 months of age. The infants with the higher scores were not necessarily exclusively fed breast milk, but were consistently receiving human milk in some amount from birth to 6 months corrected age. Family support, timely breastfeeding information, and a supportive and encouraging neonatal intensive care unit environment are needed for women to succeed in breastfeeding their hospitalized newborns. The NICU is an ideal environment to instruct and support mothers about human milk feeding because of low nurse/patient-family ratios that allow the nurse to have extended contact with the family. The NICU provides opportunities for teaching and instruction about the health benefits of human milk. Getting started with breastfeeding soon after birth is a critical point.

What Is Inconclusive?

The amount of breast milk needed to achieve these outcomes is unclear; these studies did not measure the quantity of milk but rather whether any breast milk was given at all. Alternatives for the nearly 10% of NICU babies for whom breast milk is not an option were not explored.

Best Practice

You can help mothers of premature and low-birth-weight babies in the NICU to breastfeed to achieve optimal outcomes for the baby. To promote breastfeeding in vulnerable infants, help the mother make an informed decision, establish and maintain her milk supply, feed the baby breast milk that has been pumped, and prepare both the mother and baby for a transition to breastfeeding after discharge.

References

Akerstrom, S., Asplund, I., & Norman, M. (2007). Successful breastfeeding after discharge of preterm and sick newborn infants. *Acta Paediatrica, 96*(10), 1450–1454.

Lessen, R., & Crivelli-Kovach, A. (2007). Prediction of initiation and duration of breastfeeding for neonates admitted to the neonatal intensive care unit. *Journal of Perinatal and Neonatal Nurses, 21*(3), 256–266.

Zukowsky, K. (2007). Breast-fed low-birth-weight premature neonates: Developmental assessment and nutritional intake in the first 6 months of life. *Journal of Perinatal and Neonatal Nurses, 21*(3), 242–249.

---

ies will inactivate the live poliovirus. The Centers for Disease Control and Prevention recommend that all babies be on the same schedule; there is no indication for withholding breastfeeding in relationship to OPV administration, and no extra doses of the vaccine are indicated. Furthermore, breastfed babies actually have better antibody responses to parenteral and oral vaccines than formula-fed infants (Lawrence & Lawrence, 2005).

Psychosocial Benefits of Breastfeeding

The psychosocial advantages of breastfeeding are primarily those associated with maternal-infant attachment. For some mothers the attachment process begins when the decision to become pregnant is made. The hormonal changes associated with pregnancy strengthen that bond. Events that occur during pregnancy, such as hearing the fetal heart beat, feeling the fetus move within her, and watching her abdomen grow bigger, further promote the bonding. At birth there may be intense bonding. For other mothers bonding develops over the next few days (Lawrence & Lawrence, 2005). Some hospital practices inadvertently interfere with the attachment process. Rooming-in and breastfeeding have been shown to increase maternal-infant attachment.

When a mother chooses to breastfeed, she often has more frequent direct skin-to-skin contact with her infant than if she were bottle feeding (bottle-feeding parents should be encouraged to have frequent skin-to-skin contact too, however.) Infants with skin-to-skin contact have greater physiologic stability, cry less, sleep longer, and tend to breastfeed better. The newborn's sense of touch is highly developed at birth and is a primary means of communication. The tactile stimulation associated with breastfeeding can communicate warmth, closeness, and comfort. The increased closeness provides both new-born and mother with the opportunity to learn each other's behavioral cues and needs. Mothers may feel more affectionate toward their newborns, have improved let-down response while pumping, and breastfeed more frequently and for longer periods of time (Klaus, 1998; Mohrbacher & Stock, 2003).

The mother who breastfeeds has a different hormonal state compared with the mother who does not breastfeed. Prolactin levels double each time the infant suckles at the breast, regardless of the age of the infant or duration of lactation. If a mother does not stimulate her breasts by breastfeeding or pumping, her prolactin levels return to prepregancy levels by 14 days postpartum (Lawrence & Lawrence, 2005). Prolactin increases feelings of relaxation and euphoria. Oxytocin levels also increase with breastfeeding. Oxytocin produces feelings of relaxation and sleepiness, heightens responsiveness and receptivity toward the infant, and increases the frequency of nurturing behaviors (Lawrence & Lawrence, 2005).

Another psychological advantage to the breastfeeding mother is satisfaction derived from the knowledge that she is providing her infant with the optimal nutritional start in life. For many mothers breastfeeding takes effort, understanding, and an emotional commitment to endure the demands of this lifestyle choice. The mother's sense of accomplishment in being able to satisfy her baby's needs for nourishment and comfort can be a tremendous source of personal satisfaction.

There are significant cost savings for the family that chooses breastfeeding. The cost of standard formula is approximately $1,200 annually per infant. There are also healthcare cost savings for families resulting from the decreased incidence of illness in the infant. Because breast-fed babies access healthcare resources less often, the family saves money on medical visits and prescription medications and loses less time from work.

Potential societal benefits to breastfeeding include decreased spending on public assistance programs (e.g., WIC), and environmental benefits in terms of use of natural resources and solid waste disposal. Breastfeeding is not dependent on modern technology and can provide the infant with a fresh, clean, naturally warm source of nutrition independent of transportation, supply, electricity, refrigeration, clean water, bottles, nipples, etc.

EVIDENCE IN ACTION

Infant to mother skin-to-skin care immediately following birth supports breastfeeding and bonding.

(Metanalysis) (Moore, Anderson, & Bergman, 2007)

There are also substantial medical cost savings to society, estimated to be approximately $400 in excess medical costs per never-breastfed infant (AWHONN, 2007). With current breastfeeding initiation rates of approximately 66%, this amounts to an additional $544 million per year in potential healthcare costs that could be saved by breastfeeding.

Potential Disadvantages and Contraindications to Breastfeeding

Disadvantages

The following is a list of sometimes cited potential disadvantages to breastfeeding:

1. *Pain with breastfeeding.* Breastfeeding is a natural process but requires a certain knowledge base that formerly was passed on from generation to generation. With the decline in the extended family structure, this source of knowledge and assistance is often missing for the new mother. Nipple tenderness is the most common source of discomfort and is usually related to improper positioning and/or not obtaining a proper attachment of the infant on the breast. Pain can also be related to engorgement or infection. Breastfeeding with proper technique should not hurt and these mothers should be encouraged to seek assistance from a knowledgeable person skilled in lactation.
2. *Leaking milk.* Some women will leak milk when their breasts are full and it is nearly time to breastfeed again or whenever they experience "let-down," which can be triggered by hearing, seeing, or even thinking of their babies. If this causes concern to the mother, she can be instructed on how to apply gentle pressure directly over her nipple for a minute or so to stop the leaking momentarily. The use of nursing pads (with instructions to change wet pads frequently), wearing printed tops that camouflage small leaks, and reassurance that the problem lessens with time may help alleviate this problem.
3. *Embarrassment.* Some mothers feel uncomfortable about breastfeeding because they are modest, or they may feel embarrassed because our society views breasts as sexual objects. In addition, an unfriendly social environment may make it difficult to breastfeed in public. This is not an easy issue to overcome. Some mothers will feel some reassurance after learning how to breastfeed discreetly while in public.
4. *Stress.* Finding time and feeling tied down to the demands of breastfeeding can be stressful, especially for

the mother attending school or working outside of the home. This is a common reason mothers cite for weaning their infant prematurely. Mothers can be offered the option to decrease the frequency of pumping rather than quitting altogether. Of course this will decrease the mother's milk supply, but there are numerous studies showing that babies who receive some breast milk are still healthier than babies who do not receive any breast milk at all.

5. *Unequal feeding responsibilities/fathers left out.* Some parents want feedings to be a shared responsibilty. The parents should be informed that it is advisable for the father to wait to bottle-feed the baby with expressed breast milk until after breastfeeding is established. In the meantime, encourage the father to be supportive of the breastfeedng mother, to have a lot of skin-to-skin contact with his infant, and to share the responsibilities of all other aspects of infant care (bathing, dressing, diapering, burping, rocking, etc.).

6. *Diet restriction.* Some mothers think that they have to give up eating certain foods when they breastfeed. This is, for the most part, a myth. Generally, mothers can still eat all the foods they are accustomed to eating. There are rare instances in which some infants are intolerant to something in the mother's milk. The most common problem comes from dairy products. In this case switching to cow's milk-based formula will not help as the infant will react to the cow's milk proteins in the formula. Often these infants will have cross-reaction to other types of proteins and will not tolerate soy-based formulas either. These babies may need to be on an expensive specialty formula such as a "predigested" hydrolysate formula if the mother quits breastfeeding. Again, this is not a common problem, but when it comes up, it is advisable to refer the mother to a lactation consultant for its management.

7. *Limited hormonal birth control options.* Some mothers think that they cannot use a hormonal method of birth control while breastfeeding. Mothers should be informed that using birth control pills containing progesterone and estrogen can cause a decrease in milk volume and may affect the quality of breast milk. It is preferred that the mother who wants to use a hormonal birth control method consider using the progestin-only mini pill (i.e., Nicronor®, Nor-QD®, Aygestin®, or Norlutate®); receive Depo-Provera®, a progestin-only injection administered every 90 days; or have a progestin-only implant. Although progestin-only hormonal birth control is compatible with lactation, they should not be started at the time of discharge. It is recommended that the mother wait 6 weeks before taking the hormonal medication to en-

sure a good milk supply (AAP & ACOG, 2007). Mothers can be reassured that barrier methods of birth control and natural family planning do not interfere with lactation at all and are good options to consider as well.

8. *Vaginal dryness associated with breastfeeding.* Some mothers experience vaginal dryness related to a low level of estrogen while lactating. Mothers can be given reassurance that this is only a temporary side effect while breastfeeding. A water-based lubricant such as K-Y® jelly or Astroglide® can be used during intercourse until the mother weans and estrogen levels increase again.

9. *Medications and breastfeeding.* Some mothers are concerned about the safety of breastfeeding while they are taking medications. Mothers can be reassured that most prescription and over-the-counter medications are safe for the breastfeeding infant. However, the mother needs to inform her healthcare provider and her infant's healthcare provider that she needs to take a medication for a period of time. The healthcare provider has a responsibility to research the medication, look at alternatives if indicated, and inform the mother whether the medication is compatible with breastfeeding. If the medication is not compatible with breastfeeding but is needed for only a short time, the mother can use a breast pump to maintain lactation and discard the milk.

Potential Contraindications

There are some instances when breastfeeding is or may be contraindicated:

- Mother who is HIV-positive or has AIDS is counseled against breastfeeding except in countries where the risk of neonatal death from diarrhea and other disease (excluding AIDS) is high (AWHONN, 2007).
- Mother uses illicit drugs (i.e., cocaine, heroin).
- Mother is an alcoholic.
- Maternal smoking can result in breast milk concentrations of nicotine of 1.5 to 3 times the maternal plasma concentration. Although there is no documented infant health risk related to breastfeeding and smoking, smoking cessation is urged for maternal health reasons (Thureen, Deacon, Hernandez, & Hall, 2005).
- Specific medications (e.g., radioactive isotopes, antimetabolites, chemotherapy drugs, and a few others) may cause concerns. A mother with a diagnosis of breast cancer should not breastfeed so that she can begin treatment immediately.
- Mother has active, untreated tuberculosis.
- Infant has galactosemia.

- Mother has active herpes on her breast—the infant may still feed on the unaffected side only until the lesion has healed.
- Mother has varicella.
- Mother is HTLV1–positive (human T-cell leukemia virus type 1).
- Mother has other illness, on a case-by-case basis.

In addition concern is expressed about whether women with breast implants should breastfeed or are able to breastfeed. Some research on breast augmentation using the periareolar approach suggests increased incidence of lactation insufficiency (inadequate expressed milk volume and/or infant growth). Factors that may influence the ability of a mother with breast augmentation to breastfeed include: the surgical approach used, alterations in nipple sensation, amount of breast tissue present, and lack of or little breast changes during pregnancy with little or no postpartum engorgement (Hill, Wihelm, Aldag, & Chatterton, 2004).

Another concern is related to the possible toxicity of the silicone in some breast implants. The silicone concentrations in formula and cow's milk is higher than that found in the milk of mothers with implants; therefore silicone breast implants are not a contraindication to breastfeeding (Thureen, Deacon, Hernandez et al., 2005).

Medications

It has long been recognized that medications taken by the breastfeeding mother may penetrate breast milk to some degree. Over the past 20 years, numerous studies have been published providing a better understanding of the kinetics of drug entry into breast milk, as well as factors influencing its bioavailability to the nursing infant. Understanding medications in breast milk and the implications to the infant is important, because use of medication has been identified as a barrier to breastfeeding and a major reason women cite for discontinuing it (Hale, 2006).

It should be noted that (1) most drugs pass into breast milk, (2) almost all medications appear in only small amounts in human milk (usually less than 1% of the maternal dosage), and (3) very few drugs are contraindicated for breastfeeding women (AAP Committee on Drugs, 2001; Briggs, Freeman, & Yaffe, 2005; Hale, 2006; Lawrence & Lawrence, 2005). The properties of a drug influence its passage into breast milk, as does the amount of the drug taken, the frequency and route of administration, and the timing of the dose in relationship to infant feeding. The drug's effects are influenced by the infant's age, the feeding frequency, the volume of milk taken, and the degree of absorption through the gastrointestinal tract.

Five adjustments should be made when administering drugs to a nursing mother to decrease the effects on the infant (Blackburn, 2007).

1. Avoid long-acting forms of drugs. The infant may have difficulty metabolizing and excreting them, and accumulation may be a problem.
2. Consider absorption rates and peak blood levels in scheduling the administration of the drugs. Less of the drug crosses into the milk if the infant is fed before the mother is given the oral medication.
3. Use preparations that can be given at longer intervals (once versus three to four times per day).
4. When alternatives are available, select the drug that shows the least tendency to pass into breast milk.
5. Use single-symptom drugs versus multisymptom drugs (e.g., a decongestant for allergy rather than a multisymptom drug, especially because liquid forms may contain alcohol).

The mother should be advised to inform her healthcare provider that she is breastfeeding when a drug is prescribed for her. In counseling the breastfeeding mother, the healthcare provider should weigh the benefits of the medication against the possible risk to the infant and its possible effects on the breastfeeding process. The potential risk to the infant must also be weighed against the effect of interrupting breastfeeding. Table 27–1 compares several factors for parents to consider when choosing between breastfeeding and formula-feeding.

Potential Problems in Breastfeeding

Because mothers are discharged from the birthing unit before breastfeeding is well established, they are frequently alone when they encounter changes in the breastfeeding process. Many women stop nursing if the situations they encounter seem to pose problems. Nurses can offer anticipatory guidance regarding common breastfeeding phenomena and provide resources for the woman's use after discharge. See Chapter 31 ∞ for a detailed discussion of self-care measures the nurse can suggest to a woman with a breastfeeding problem after discharge from the birthing unit.

The Feeding Process

Breast Milk Production

Breast Anatomy

The female breast is divided into 15 to 20 lobes, separated from one another by fat and connective tissue, and interspersed with blood vessels, lymphatic vessels, and nerves. These lobes are subdivided into lobules composed of small units called alveoli where milk is synthesized by the alveolar secretory epithelium. The lobules have a system of lactiferous ductules that join larger ducts and eventually open onto the nipple surface. Mothers are often surprised to see milk coming out multiple nipple pores

TABLE 27–1	Comparison of Breastfeeding and Formula-Feeding
Breastfeeding	**Formula (Iron-Enriched)-Feeding**

Infant Nutrition

Breastfeeding	Formula (Iron-Enriched)-Feeding
Species specific. An ideal balance of nutrients, efficiently absorbed. High bioavailability of iron leaves lower iron for bacterial growth, cell injury.	Derived from bovine milk and/or plant sources. Lower bioavailability of nutrients requires higher concentrations in milk. Additives may cause intolerance.
Higher levels of essential fatty acids, lactose, cystine, and cholesterol, necessary for brain and nerve growth.	Still missing numerous ingredients. Formulas do not contain cholesterol. Soy and hydrolysate formulas do not contain lactose. DHA & ARA now added.
Composition varies according to gestational age and stage of lactation, meeting changing nutritional needs.	Nutritional value not varied. Nutritional adequacy depends on proper preparation/dilution.
Long-term decreased incidence of diabetes, cancer, obesity, asthma.	
Contains unsaturated fats.	Contains saturated fats.
Infants determine the volume of milk consumed.	Parents or healthcare provider determine the volume consumed. Over-feeding may occur if caregiver is determined that baby empty bottle.
Frequency of feeding is determined by infant cues. May feed more frequently as milk digestion faster.	Frequency of feeding is determined by infant's cues. May feed less frequently as milk digestion is slower.

Immunologic Properties

Breastfeeding	Formula (Iron-Enriched)-Feeding
Contains immunoglobulins, enzymes, and leukocytes that protect against pathogens. Nutrients promote growth of *Lactobacillus,* protective bacteria. Lower rates of urinary tract infections, otitis media, and other infectious diseases.	No anti-infective properties. Formula is linked to an increased incidence of gastrointestinal and respiratory tract infections.
Anti-infective properties present in the milk permit longer storage duration.	Potential for bacterial contamination exists during preparation and storage.
Breast milk is hypoallergenic, with minimal risk of protein allergy/intolerance.	Cow's milk protein allergy relatively common.

Maternal Health

Breastfeeding	Formula (Iron-Enriched)-Feeding
Faster return to prepregnancy weight.	Provides infant nutrition when breast milk not available because of maternal illness, medication/drug use, or lactation failure (breast surgery, endocrine disease).
Breastfeeding associated with lower risk of breast, ovarian cancer.	

Psychosocial Aspects

Breastfeeding	Formula (Iron-Enriched)-Feeding
Skin-to-skin contact enhances bonding.	Both parents can participate in positive parent-infant interaction during feeding.
Hormones of lactation promote maternal feelings and sense of well-being.	Father can assume feeding responsibilities.
The value system of modern society can create barriers to successful breastfeeding.	
Some mothers may feel ashamed or embarrassed.	
Breastfeeding after returning to work may be difficult.	

Cost

Breastfeeding	Formula (Iron-Enriched)-Feeding
Healthy diet for mother.	Formula cost per year: $1200 for standard formula, $2500/year for hypoallergenic formulas.
Savings for infant medical costs: approximately $400 average in first year of life.	Ancillary costs: bottles or bottle liners, nipples, cleaning costs.
Ancillary costs: nursing pads, nursing bras.	Refrigeration is needed if preparing more than one bottle at a time.
A breast pump may be needed.	
Refrigeration is necessary for storing expressed milk.	

Convenience

Breastfeeding	Formula (Iron-Enriched)-Feeding
Milk is always the perfect temperature. No preparation time is needed.	Formula must be purchased commercially. Preparation is time consuming. Less convenient for traveling or for night feedings.
The mother must be available to feed or will need to provide expressed milk to be given in her absence.	Mother need not be present—anyone can feed the infant.
If she misses a feeding, the mother must express milk to maintain lactation.	
The mother may experience slight discomfort in the early days of lactation.	

when they express their milk. See Figure 27–1 ■ to view the anatomy of the breast.

Lactogenesis

During pregnancy, increased levels of estrogen stimulate breast duct proliferation and development, and elevated progesterone levels promote the development of lobules and alveoli in preparation for lactation. Prolactin levels rise from approximately 10 ng/mL pre-pregnancy to 200 ng/mL at term. However, lactation is suppressed during pregnancy by elevated progesterone levels secreted by the placenta. Once the placenta is expelled at birth, progesterone levels fall and

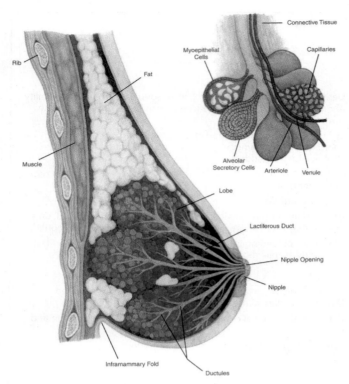

FIGURE 27–1 Anatomy of the breast.
Source: From Riordan, J. (2005). *Breastfeeding and human lactation* (3rd ed.). Boston: Jones & Bartlett. Copyright 2005 Jones and Bartlett Publishers, Sudbury, MA, www.jbpub.com. Reprinted with permission.

the inhibition is removed, triggering milk production. This occurs whether the mother has breast stimulation or not. However, if by the third or fourth day breast stimulation is not occurring, prolactin levels begin to drop. By 2 weeks postpartum, prolactin levels will be back to prepregnancy levels and milk production will cease.

Physiologic Control of Breastfeeding

Initially, lactation is under endocrine control. The hormone **prolactin** is released from the anterior pituitary in response to breast stimulation from suckling or the use of a breast pump. Prolactin stimulates the milk secreting cells in the alveoli to produce milk, then rapidly drops back to baseline. If more than approximately 3 hours occurs between stimulation, prolactin levels begin to drop below baseline. To reverse the overall decline in prolactin level, the mother can be encouraged to stimulate her breasts more frequently (e.g., every 1.5 to 2 hours). Mothers should be strongly encouraged to stimulate their breasts frequently if their infants are not effective feeders or if they are separated from their infants. Prolactin receptors are established during the first 2 weeks postpartum in response to frequency of breast stimulation (Human Milk Banking Association of North America, 2005). Inadequate development of prolactin receptors during this time is likely to negatively impact the mother's long-term milk volume.

The milk that flows from the breast at the start of a feeding or pumping session is called **foremilk**. The foremilk is watery milk high in protein and low in fat (1% to 2%). This milk has trickled down from the alveoli between feedings to fill the lactiferous ducts. It is low-fat milk because the fat globules made in the alveoli stick to each other and to the walls of the alveoli and do not trickle down. In addition to prolactin release, stretching of the nipple and compression of the areola signal the hypothalamus to trigger the posterior pituitary gland to release oxytocin. **Oxytocin** acts on the myoepithelial cells surrounding the alveoli in the breast tissue to contract, ejecting milk, including the fat globules present, into the ducts. This process is called the milk-ejection reflex, better known in lay terms as the **"let-down" reflex (response)**. The average initial let-down response occurs about 2 minutes after an infant begins to suckle, and there will be 4 to 10 let-down responses during a feeding session. The milk that flows during "let-down" is called hindmilk. As noted, **hindmilk** is rich in fat (can exceed 10%) and therefore high in calories. In a sample of expressed breast milk, the average total fat concentration is about 4% and the total caloric content is about 20 calories/ounce.

By 6 months of breastfeeding prolactin levels are only 5 to 10 ng/mL (Neville, 1999) yet milk production continues. A whey protein called feedback inhibitor of lactation (FIL) has been identified as influencing milk production through a negative feedback loop. FIL is present in breast milk and functions to decrease milk production. The more milk that remains in the breast for a longer period of time, the more milk production is decreased. On the other hand, the more often the breasts are emptied, the lower the level of FIL and the faster milk is produced. This mechanism of regulating milk at the local level is called autocrine control. This process is key to understanding how a mother maintains or loses her milk supply (Blackburn, 2007).

There are a number of factors that can delay or impair lactogenesis. Maternal factors include cesarean birth, postpartum hemorrhage, type 1 diabetes, untreated hypothyroidism, obesity, polycystic ovary syndrome, retained placenta fragments, vitamin B_6 deficiency, history of previous breast surgery, insufficient glandular breast tissue, and significant stress (Mohrbacher & Stock, 2003; Riordan, 2005). Other factors that can interfere with breastfeeding include smoking and use of alcohol, as well as some prescription and over-the-counter medications (e.g., antihistamines, combined birth control pills).

Stages of Human Milk

During the establishment of lactation there are three stages of human milk: colostrum, transitional milk, and mature milk.

Colostrum is the initial milk that begins to be secreted during midpregnancy and is immediately available to the baby at birth. It provides the infant with all the nutrition required until the mother's milk becomes more abundant in a few days. No routine supplementation of other fluids is necessary unless there is a medical indication. Colostrum is a thick, creamy yellowish fluid with concentrated amounts of protein, fat-soluble vitamins, and minerals, and it has lower amounts of fat and lactose compared with mature milk. It also contains antioxidants and high levels of lactoferrin and secretory IgA. It promotes the establishment of *Lactobacillus bifidus* flora in the digestive tract, which helps to protect the infant from disease and illness. Colostrum also has a laxative effect on the infant, which helps the baby pass meconium stools, which in turn helps decrease hyperbilirubinemia.

Between day 2 and day 5, maternal milk production normally becomes noticeably more abundant. The milk "coming in" is called transitional milk. **Transitional milk** has qualities intermediate to colostrum and mature milk. It is still light yellow in color but is more copious than colostrum and contains more fat, lactose, water-soluble vitamins, and calories. By day 5, most mothers are producing about 500 mL/day.

Mature milk is white or slightly blue-tinged in color. It is present by 2 weeks postpartum and continues thereafter until lactation ceases. Mature milk contains about 13% solids (carbohydrates, proteins, and fats) and 87% water. Although mature human milk appears similar to skim cow's milk and may cause mothers to question whether their milk is "rich enough," mothers should be reassured that this is the normal appearance of mature human milk and that it provides the infant with all the necessary nutrients. Although gradual changes in composition do occur continuously over periods of weeks to accommodate the needs of the growing newborn, in general the composition of mature milk is fairly consistent with the exception of the fat content as noted previously. Milk production continues to increase slowly over the first month. By 6 months postpartum a mother produces about 800 mL/day (Blackburn, 2007).

Timing of Newborn Feedings

The timing of newborn feedings is ideally determined by physiologic and behavioral cues rather than a set schedule.

Initial Feeding

The nurse should assess for active bowel sounds, absence of abdominal distention, and a lusty cry that quiets and is replaced with rooting and sucking behaviors when a stimulus is placed near the lips. These signs indicate that the newborn is hungry and physically ready to tolerate the initial feeding.

If there are no complications at the birth and the mother is not overly sedated, the infant may be placed on the mother's chest after birth. Throughout the first 2 hours after birth, but especially during the first hour of life, the infant is usually alert and ready to breastfeed. Because colostrum is not irritating if aspirated (which may occur because of the newborn's initial uncoordinated sucking and swallowing abilities) and is readily absorbed by the respiratory system, breastfeeding can usually begin immediately after birth. The mother benefits psychologically from early breastfeeding through enhancement of maternal-infant bonding and physiologically by the release of oxytocin, which helps contract the uterus, expelling the placenta and decreasing the risk of postpartum hemorrhage. Early feedings benefit the newborn because they help prevent hypoglycemia, promote the passage of meconium, provide the immunologic protection of colostrum, and begin to stimulate further maternal milk production, helping prevent later feeding difficulties.

If the mother plans to bottle-feed, she and her newborn can still enjoy skin-to-skin contact initially. Bottle-feedings are not typically initiated in the birthing room. Bottle-fed newborns are offered formula as soon as they show an interest/feeding cues or per hospital policy. For both breastfed and bottle-fed infants, early feeding enhances maternal-infant attachment and stimulates peristalsis, helping to eliminate the by-products of bilirubin conjugation (which decreases the risk of jaundice).

Assessment of the newborn's physiologic status is a primary and ongoing concern to the nurse throughout the first feeding. Extreme fatigue coupled with rapid respiration, circumoral cyanosis, and diaphoresis of the head and face may indicate cardiovascular complications and should be assessed further.

The first feeding also provides an opportunity for the nurse to assess the effectiveness of the newborn's suck, swallow, and gag reflexes. The nurse should also remain alert to the possibility of medical problems during this time, including respiratory disorders, congenital cardiovascular problems, or more rare disorders such as tracheoesophageal fistula and esophageal atresia (Chapter 28 ∞). Findings associated with esophageal anomalies include maternal polyhydramnios and increased oral mucus in the infant. In cases of esophageal atresia, the feeding is taken well initially, but as the esophageal pouch fills, the feeding is quickly regurgitated unchanged by stomach contents. If a fistula is present, the infant gags, chokes, regurgitates mucus, and may become cyanotic as fluid passes through the fistula into the lungs.

It is not unusual for the newborn to regurgitate some mucus and water following a feeding, even if it was taken without difficulty, because of initial uncoordinated suck and swallow abilities. It is important to observe the newborn closely and position the baby on the side after the feeding to aid drainage and facilitate gastric emptying. Once the infant is tolerating feeding, the child's normal position after feeding is on his or her back.

Establishing a Feeding Pattern

An "on-demand" feeding program facilitates each baby's own rhythm and helps a new mother establish lactation. The newborn rapidly digests breast milk and may want to nurse 8 to 10 times in a 24-hour period. After the initial period of alertness and eagerness to suckle, the infant progresses to light sleep, then deep sleep, followed by increased wakefulness and interest in breastfeeding. As wakefulness and interest in nursing increase, the infant will often cluster 5 to 10 feeding episodes over 2 to 3 hours, followed by a 4- to 5-hour deep sleep. After this cluster of minifeeds and deep sleep, the infant will feed frequently but at more regular intervals. Crying is considered a late feeding cue. Often newborn arousal from sleep is the first sign of hunger. Early feeding cues include rooting, smacking, or attempting to suck on anything near his mouth (especially his hand). Although people often accept crying as normal and healthy behavior for newborns, it may actually delay the transition to extrauterine life. Crying involves a Valsalva maneuver that increases pulmonary vascular pressure, which may cause unoxygenated blood to be shunted into systemic circulation through the foramen ovale and ductus arteriosus. If no one has responded to the newborn by this time, then the infant may begin to fuss and eventually work up to a full cry. A newborn that is left to cry and not given the opportunity to feed at this point may subsequently become very disorganized and have a difficult time latching-on to the breast or coordinating his suck correctly.

Certain hospital practices/policies may contribute to delays in feeding by prolonging the feeding intervals and even decreasing the number of feedings in a 24-hour period. Couplet care or rooming-in practices promote cue-based feedings. Therefore, it may be advantageous for the baby to be in the room with the mother; she will respond to the baby's needs more quickly than the nursery staff may be able to, resulting in less infant crying.

Couplet care permits the mother to learn about and respond to her infant's early feeding cues. Early cues that indicate a newborn is interested in feeding include hand-to-mouth or hand-passing-mouth motion, whimpering, sucking, and rooting (Mulford, 1992). Satiety behaviors can include withdrawal of head from nipple, falling asleep, relaxation of hands, and relief of body tension. When couplet care is not available, a supportive nursing staff and flexible nursery policies allow the mother to feed her infant on cue. It is very frustrating to a new mother to attempt to feed a newborn who is sound asleep because he or she is either not hungry or exhausted from crying.

Feeding intervals are counted from the start of one feeding to the start of the next feeding. Breastfeeding babies typically feed every 1.5 to 3 hours (8 to 12 times in a

24-hour period), but often in an irregular pattern known as "cluster feeding," in which the infant feeds as frequently as every hour for a few feedings followed by a longer sleep period. The normal newborn sleeps a total of 16 to 18 hours per day, but generally with no more than one sleep stretch of up to 5 hours in length. It is more important to focus on the number of feedings in 24 hours than the exact feeding interval time. Formula-fed infants generally eat every 3 to 4 hours and typically 6 to 8 times per day. It is important that families are taught about the normal feeding/sleeping pattern of a newborn, as many parents are distressed by their infant's early erratic feeding pattern. Parents need to be informed that their infant will have a more predictable sleep and feeding pattern when he is 2 to 4 months of age.

Maternal medications received during labor may affect newborn feeding behavior by delaying these early cluster feedings. Delays in normal feeding patterns depend on the specific drug and its half-life. Newborns whose mothers received epidural analgesia have been noted to be irritable and demonstrate reduced motor organization, poor self-quieting skills, and decreased visual skills and alertness. Because breastfeeding infants generally have only one long sleep stretch in a 24-hour period, parents can help their infant to take the long sleep stretch at night if they attempt to awaken their infant during the day when the infant is in a light state of sleep and has already slept longer than 3 hours. Parents can attempt to encourage cluster feedings during the day, and, after awhile, the infant may sleep a 5-hour sleep stretch at night. In the meantime, the mother can be encouraged to take "cat naps" during the day while her infant is sleeping. At night the mother can keep stimulation down (lights low, noise low, and diaper change only when necessary).

Both breastfeeding and formula-feeding infants have the same fluid requirements, but because they have different diets, their rates of digestion are different. Digestion of formula produces large, rubbery curds that take about 4 hours to digest compared with the softer, smaller curds produced by breast milk. For this reason formula-fed newborns generally sleep longer at a stretch and awaken to feed every 3 to 4 hours. It is not uncommon that formula-fed newborns may take one or two 5-hour sleep stretches in a 24-hour period. As a result they will often take a larger volume at each feed. Babies may begin skipping the night feeding about 8 to 12 weeks after birth. The need for a night feeding is individual and depends on the infant's size and development.

Satiety behaviors are the same for formula-fed babies as for breastfed babies. These behaviors include longer pauses toward the end of the feeding and noticeable total body relaxation (the baby lies limp with hands down at his side and unclenched). The infant may also release his mother's nipple or the bottle nipple, and may fall asleep. If a baby is satiated and content following feedings, is meeting daily output expectations, and is gaining weight as expected, then feedings are going well.

Both breastfed and formula-fed infants experience growth spurts at certain times and require increased feeding. The breastfeeding mother may meet these increased demands by nursing more frequently to increase her milk supply. It takes about 72 hours for the milk supply to increase adequately to meet the new demand. A slight increase in feedings meets the formula-fed infant's needs.

Some mothers may find fixed feeding schedules attractive. These mothers should be informed that although strict feeding schedules may work for some babies, they often do not work for all babies because they do not take into account differences among breastfeeding women and differences among infants. There are documented cases of infants diagnosed with failure to thrive, poor weight gain, dehydration, breast milk supply failure, and involuntary early weaning associated with this feeding method (Aney, 1998). The American Academy of Pediatrics released a Media Alert in April 1998 reaffirming its position that "the best feeding schedules are ones babies design themselves. Scheduled feedings designed by parents may put babies at risk for poor weight gain and dehydration" (AAP, 1998).

Nourishing her newborn is a major concern of the new mother. Her feelings of success or failure may influence her self-concept as she assumes her maternal role. With proper instruction, support, and encouragement from professionals, feeding becomes a source of pleasure and satisfaction to both the parents and infant.

Client Education: Feeding Technique

Breastfeeding Positions and Latching-On

Breastfeeding is not instinctive, it is learned. It is a natural process, but it takes "know-how." Ideally, each breastfeeding mother should have a breastfeeding evaluation to determine any knowledge deficits, acknowledge any concerns, provide instructions, and assist with breastfeeding.

POSITIONING   There are many breastfeeding positions, but only the four classic breastfeeding positions will be discussed here. In addition, there are minor variations of hand placement and body position even among the four classic positions. The four positions discussed here include (1) modified cradle position, (2) cradle position, (3) football (or clutch) hold position, and (4) side-lying position (Figures 27–2 through 27–5 ■). After a mother has fed using one position, encourage her to try a different position when she offers her second breast. Alternating positions facilitates drainage of the breasts and changes the pressure points on the breast. This will provide some relief to the mother with sore nipples.

HINTS FOR PRACTICE

The cradle position is challenging, especially when attempted during early lactation by inexperienced mothers, because the mother is attempting to support her baby's head near the crook of her arm. This makes it difficult to control the head position and may allow the baby's head to bend forward (chin toward chest) making attachment difficult. It is better to have the infant's head lag slightly backward (chin tilted slightly upward) so that the infant leads into the breast chin first. Some mothers find it easier to start in the modifed cradle position and then switch into the cradle position.

LATCHING-ON   It is important to have the mother and baby positioned properly in order to achieve an optimal attachment. If, for example, the infant is lying flat on his back (supine position) to feed in the modified cradle position, cradle position, or side-lying position, the infant can obtain only a shallow latch (not attached far back onto

MyNursingKit | Video: Nursing in Action: Breastfeeding

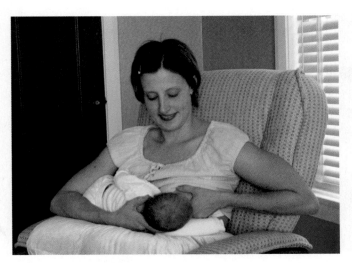

FIGURE 27–2 Modified cradle position.
Source: Courtesy of Brigette Hall, MSN, IBCLC.

- Have the mother sit comfortably in upright position using good body alignment. Use pillows for support (may use Boppy, body pillow, or standard bed pillows). Lap pillow should help bring the baby up to breast level so the mother does not lean over baby.
- Place the baby on the mother's lap and turn the baby's entire body toward the mother (the baby is in side-lying position). Position the baby's body so that the baby's nose lines up to the nipple. Maintain the baby's body in a horizontal alignment.
- To feed at left breast, the mother supports the baby's head with her right hand at nape of the baby's neck (allow head to slightly lag back); the mother's right thumb by the baby's left ear, and right forefinger near the baby's right ear.
- With the mother's free left hand, she can offer her left breast.

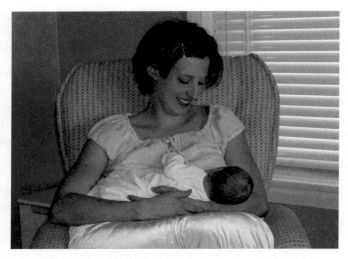

- Have the mother sit comfortably in upright position using good body alignment. Use pillows for support (may use Boppy, body pillow, or standard bed pillows). Lap pillow should help bring the baby up to breast level so the mother does not lean over the baby.
- Place the baby on the mother's lap and turn the baby's entire body toward the mother (the baby is in side-lying position). Position the baby's body so that the baby's nose lines up to the nipple. Maintain the baby's body in a horizontal alignment.
- If feeding from the left breast, have the mother cradle the baby's head near the crook of her left arm while supporting her baby's body with her left forearm.
- With the mother's free right hand, she can offer her left breast.

FIGURE 27–3 Cradle position.
Source: Courtesy of Brigette Hall, MSN, IBCLC.

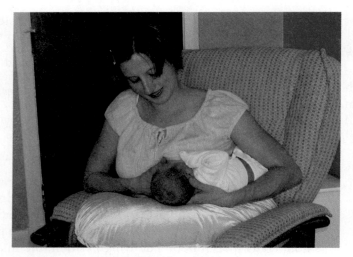

- Have the mother sit comfortably and use pillows to raise the baby's body to breast level. If using a Boppy and the Boppy is in "normal" position on the mother's lap, turn it counterclockwise slightly (if feeding at left breast) to provide extended support for the baby's body resting along the mother's left side and near the back of the mother's chair.
- If feeding at left breast, place the baby on the left side of the mother's body, heading the baby into position feet first. The baby's bottom should rest on the pillow near the mother's left elbow.
- Turn the baby slightly on her side so that she faces the breast.
- The mother's left arm clutches the baby's body close to the mother's body. The baby's body should feel securely tucked in under the mother's left arm.
- Have the mother support the baby's head with her left hand. With the mother's free right hand, she can offer her breast. (Good position for the mother with c-section.)

FIGURE 27–4 Football hold position.
Source: Courtesy of Brigette Hall, MSN, IBCLC.

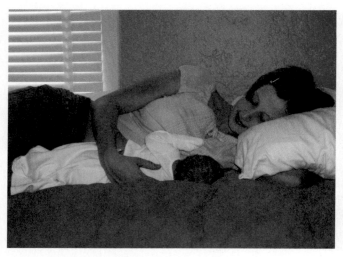

- Have the mother rest comfortably lying on her side (left side for this demonstration). Use pillows to support the mother's head and back, and provide support for the mother's hips by placing a pillow between her bent knees.
- Place the baby in side-lying position next to the mother's body. The baby's body should face the mother's body. The baby's nose should line up to the mother's nipple. Place a roll behind the baby's back, if desired.
- With the mother's free right hand, she can offer her left breast. After the baby is securely attached, mom can rest her right hand anywhere that is comfortable for her.

FIGURE 27–5 Side-lying position.
Source: Courtesy of Brigette Hall, MSN, IBCLC.

the areola). The infant's shoulder becomes an obstacle putting distance between the infant's mouth and his mother's breast. Anything that contributes to a shallow latch is going to cause sore nipples and other complications. Nipple trauma, although relatively common, is not normal. See Chapter 32 ∞ for a discussion of breastfeeding with inverted or flat nipples.

The infant needs to attach his lips onto the breast or, rather more accurately, far back onto the areola, not on the nipple. If the infant attaches just to the nipple, the mother will have sore nipples and pain may inhibit the let-down re-

flex. To obtain a deep latch, the mother needs to be taught how to elicit the infant's rooting reflex, stimulating the infant to open his mouth as widely as possible (like a big yawn). Once the infant does this, the mother should quickly but gently draw her baby in toward her. During the first few days of life, the newborn typically only opens his mouth widely for a second or so, and then he begins to close his mouth again. If the mother misses her chance to get her baby latched-on, she needs to simply start over again.

Figures 27–6 through 27–11 ■ demonstrate various positions and techniques used in latching-on.

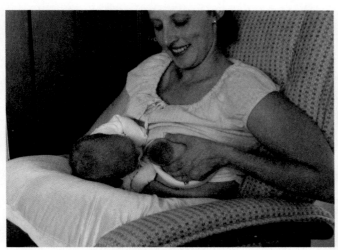

FIGURE 27–6 C-hold hand position.
Source: Courtesy of Brigette Hall, MSN, IBCLC.

To be ready to draw the baby's mouth onto the mother's breast, as soon as the baby opens her mouth widely enough, the mother needs to have her hand supporting her breast in the ready position. She can use various hand holds, but she needs to keep her fingers well behind the areola. One such hand position is called the "C-hold." In this hold, the thumb is placed on top of the breast near 12:00 position and the other four fingers are placed on the underside of the breast near the 6:00 position (depends on mother's hand size and length of fingers). The key point is to keep the fingers at least 1½ inches back from the base of the nipple as the fingers support the breast. Mothers are not often aware of where they place their fingers especially on the underside of the breast. If the fingers are too far forward (too close to the nipple), then the infant cannot grasp a large amount of areola in her mouth and this results in a "shallow" latch. A shallow latch is associated with nipple pain and ineffective drainage of the breast.

An alternate hand hold not shown is a "U-hold" hand position. The thumb and forefinger are near the 3 and 9 position on the breast again with fingers at least 1½ inches back from the base of the nipple; the body of the hand rests on the lower portion of the breast. Using this hand hold, the mother's arm position is down at her side rather than sticking outward as it is when supporting the breast using the C-hold position.

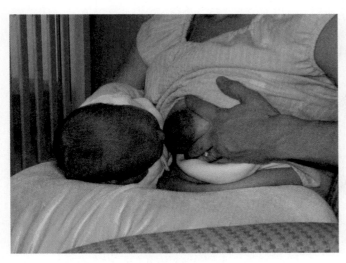

FIGURE 27–7 Scissor hold hand position.
Source: Courtesy of Brigette Hall, MSN, IBCLC.

The scissor hold is often discouraged because mothers (especially mothers with small hands) have a difficult time keeping their fingers off the areola or at least 1½ inches back from the base of the areola. Here, the mother is able to support her breast well without letting her fingers encroach onto the areola.

The mother should be instructed to gently support the breast and not press too deeply, which can obstruct the flow of milk through the ducts.

Before eliciting the rooting reflex, it is important to have the baby in good alignment. When the infant opens his mouth to latch on, the goal is to achieve a deep, asymmetric latch attachment. The goal is *not* to center the nipple in the baby's mouth. The rationale for this is to optimize oral-motor function. The jaw is a hinge joint. The upper jaw is immobile; the lower jaw compresses the breast. The breast is efficiently drained if more areola is drawn into the baby's mouth from the inferior aspect of the breast and a smaller amount drawn in from the superior aspect of the areola. Aligning the infant to the mother with baby's nose facing mother's nipple permits the jaw to be in a lower position. The next step is to let the infant drop his head back (head in "sniff position"), so that the infant leads into the breast with the chin.

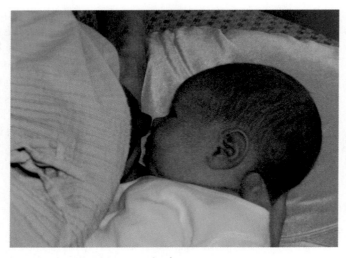

FIGURE 27–8 Nose to nipple.
Source: Courtesy of Brigette Hall, MSN, IBCLC.

To trigger the rooting reflex, teach the mother to use her nipple to stroke downward in a vertical motion across the middle of baby's lower lip. Initially, the infant may respond by licking or smacking. This is a normal response to the stimulus. Encourage the mother to keep stimulating the infant's lower lip until the infant finally opens his mouth widely. If the infant is not responding at all, then the infant is probably too sleepy and may need help waking up. After trying wake up techniques, the infant may be ready to try breastfeeding again.

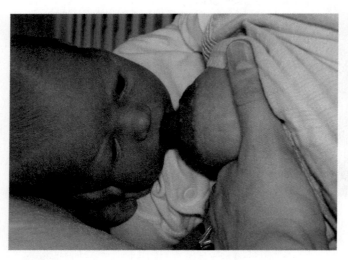

FIGURE 27–9 Initial attempt to elicit the rooting reflex.
Source: Courtesy of Brigette Hall, MSN, IBCLC.

Teach the mother to be patient and wait for the infant's mouth to gape open as widely as possible. Here the infant needs to open the mouth even wider before the mother draws her baby toward the breast. The mother should be encouraged to continue stroking the infant's lip until the infant opens the mouth wider.

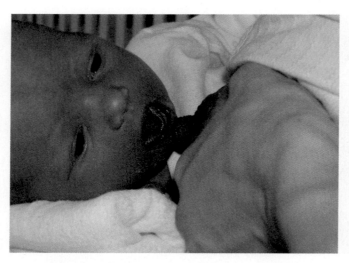

FIGURE 27–10 Continued attempt to elicit rooting reflex.
Source: Courtesy of Brigette Hall, MSN, IBCLC.

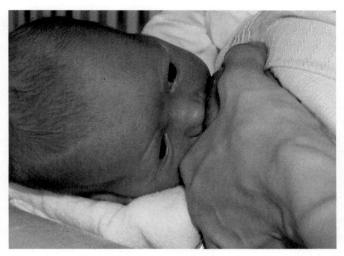

FIGURE 27–11 Baby is latched-on.
Source: Courtesy of Brigette Hall, MSN, IBCLC.

Once the baby has latched onto the breast, the mother should check that the baby is latched-on properly. The infant's chin should be embedded into the mother's breast. The infant's nose should be very close but not actually touching the breast. The nose should be centered. If the mother feels a little pinch on her areola, she can slowly release the hand supporting her breast so she can have a free hand to attempt to move her baby's jaw gently downward. To do this maneuver, the mother needs to place the thumb or forefinger of her free hand (the hand that just released the breast) on the baby's lower jaw (there is a horizontal groove to use as leverage—the groove on the baby's chin is parallel with the baby's lips). With gentle downward pressure the mother should feel relief of any persistent tenderness. This procedure opens the jaw wider and it also helps to roll out the infant's lower lip that may have been inadvertently drawn into the baby's mouth. As the baby begins to suckle, there should be no dimpling of the infant's cheeks and no smacking or clicking noises.

HINTS FOR PRACTICE

As you assist new mothers with breastfeeding, it is important to create a relaxed environment and approach to breastfeeding. Encourage the mother to get into a comfortable position, well supported with pillows. Remind her to bring the baby to her breast rather than leaning forward to the baby.

HINTS FOR PRACTICE

With a sleepy baby, unwrap the baby, encourage lots of skin-to-skin contact between mom and baby, and have mom rest with her baby near her breast so that the baby can feel and smell the breast. Encourage mom to watch for feeding cues, such as hand-to-mouth activity, fluttering eyelids, vocalization (but not necessarily crying), and mouthing activities.

Breastfeeding Assessment

During the birthing unit stay, the nurse must carefully monitor the progress of the breastfeeding pair. A systematic assessment of several breastfeeding episodes provides the opportunity to teach the new mother about lactation and the breastfeeding process, provide anticipatory guidance, and evaluate the need for follow-up care after discharge. Criteria for evaluating a breastfeeding session include maternal and infant cues, latch-on, position, let-down, nipple condition, infant response, and maternal response. The literature provides various tools to guide the assessment and documentation of the breastfeeding efforts. The LATCH Scoring Table is one example (Figure 27–12 ■). See Key Facts to Remember: Successful Breastfeeding Evaluation.

KEY FACTS TO REMEMBER

Successful Breastfeeding Evaluation

Babies are probably getting enough milk if:
- They are nursing at least eight times in 24 hours.
- In a quiet room, their mothers can hear them swallow while nursing.
- Their mothers' breasts appear to soften after breastfeeding.
- The number of wet diapers increases daily until the fourth or fifth day after birth, and there are at least six to eight wet diapers every 24 hours after day 5.
- Their stools are beginning to lighten in color by the third day after birth, or have changed to yellow no later than day 5.
- Offering a supplemental bottle is not a reliable indicator because most babies will take a few ounces even if they are getting enough breast milk.

Bottle-Feeding Breast Milk (Expression, Pumps, Storage)

There are a number of different reasons for bottle-feeding breast milk. The nurse should evaluate the indications in order to recommend the best technique for the mother and her particular need. Some mothers prefer to hand express their milk rather than use a breast pump, and many find that in the immediate post-partum period hand expression of milk may be a more effective method of removing drops of colostrum than using an electric breast pump. Nurses should teach all mothers the skill of hand expressing breast milk as it is possible the mother will find herself in a situation without a breast pump but needing to relieve herself from engorgement.

To hand express breast milk, have the mother follow steps 1 through 4 of the pumping instructions provided in

	0	*1*	*2*
L Latch	Too sleepy or reluctant No latch achieved	Repeated attempts Hold nipple in mouth Stimulate to suck	Grasps breast Tongue down Lips flanged Rhythmic sucking
A Audible swallowing	None	A few with stimulation	Spontaneous and intermittent > 24 hours old Spontaneous and frequent < 24 hours old
T Type of nipple	Inverted	Flat	Everted (after stimulation)
C Comfort (breast/ nipple)	Engorged Cracked, bleeding, large blisters or bruises Severe discomfort	Filling Reddened/small blisters or bruises Mild/moderate discomfort	Soft Nontender
H Hold (positioning)	Full assist (staff holds infant at breast)	Minimal assist (e.g., elevate head of bed, place pillows for support) Teach one side; mother does other Staff holds and then mother takes over	No assist from staff Mother able to position and hold infant

FIGURE 27–12 LATCH Scoring System. A breastfeeding charting and documentation tool, LATCH was created to provide a systematic method for breastfeeding assessment and charting. It can be used to assist the new mother in establishing breastfeeding and define areas of needed intervention.
Source: Used with permission from AWHONN. (1994). Jensen, D., Wallace, S., & Kelsay, P. A breastfeeding charting system and documentation tool. *Journal of Obstetric, Gynecologic, and Neonatal Nursing, 23*(1), 27–32. (Table 1 Latch Scoring Table, p. 29.) Washington, DC: Author. © 1994 by the Association of Women's Health, Obstetric and Neonatal Nurses. All rights reserved.

Table 27–2. Next the mother should use the Marmet technique of hand expression described next. It is important that the mother take care to place her hands exactly as directed. The steps are as follows:

1. The mother will position her thumb at the 12:00 position on the top edge of the areola (about 1 to 1½ inches back from the tip of her nipple) and her forefinger and middle finger pads at the 6:00 position on the bottom edge of the areola (about 1 to 1½ inches from the tip of her nipple). If positioned correctly, a line between the thumb and fingers will cross the nipple (see Figure 27–13 ■).
2. Next the mother will stretch her areola back toward her chest wall without lifting her fingers off her breast.
3. Now she should roll her thumb and fingers simultaneously forward. This action compresses the ducts beneath the areola and stimulates the breast to empty both manually and by triggering the let-down reflex.
4. The mother should repeat the sequence multiple times to completely drain her breasts. She should try to maintain a steady rhythm, cycling 45 to 60 times/minute. It is also more effective if the mother repositions her fingers to other positons on the same breast (3:00 and 9:00, 1:00 and 7:00, etc.) when the milk flow slows.

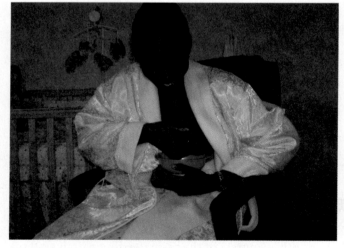

FIGURE 27–13 Hand expression.
Source: Courtesy of Brigette Hall, MSN, IBCLC.

The mother should take care not to traumatize her breasts or nipples. Hand expression should not be painful. Most mothers will need assistance in learning this technique initially. Reassure the mother that this skill is learned; with practice, she can become an expert at hand expression.

Although hand expression can be efficient, many mothers will choose to use a mechanical breast pump to express their milk. Not all breast pumps are of the same quality, even within the same category (see Table 27–3 and

---

TABLE 27–2   Pumping Instructions

1. Once a day rinse your breasts with water during your bath or shower. Avoid using soap on your nipples.
2. Wash your hands well with soap and water before preparing to pump.
3. Take a few minutes to massage your breasts and relax (e.g., do some deep breathing, think about your baby, look at a picture of your baby). Being relaxed is very important for letting down your milk. (Stress causes the release of adrenalin, which blocks receptors for let-down.)
4. You should sit up straight or lean slightly forward (perhaps even place a pillow behind your back so that your posture is tilted slightly forward), as gravity aids in the flow of your milk.
5. For single-sided pumping, pump each breast for 10-15 minutes. Some mothers find that they empty their breasts more efficiently if they switch back and forth from one side to the other as the milk flow diminishes until they have stimulated each breast for 15 minutes.
6. Pump your milk into glass or plastic bottle containers. Mothers of healthy infants may also use bottle bags/liners intended for breast milk storage to collect and store their milk. *[Because of the loss of antibodies that can occur with bottle bags/liners, mothers of preemies and fragile infants should probably avoid using these.]* Do not fill containers more than 3/4 full, because milk expands during freezing.
7. Feed freshly expressed breast milk when breastfeeding is not an option/choice. If the expressed breast milk is not needed immediately, store the expressed breast milk in the refrigerator if it is likely to be used within 5-8 days. (The sooner it is used the greater the quality of the milk.) Otherwise, freeze the expressed breast milk. Avoid placing breast milk in the freezer door or on the bottom of a self-defrosting freezer because the temperature fluctuates more in those areas.
8. Store expressed breast milk in volumes your infant is likely to feed at a single feeding or in a volume your infant will consume in a day.
9. Frozen breast milk can be thawed safely using one of two methods. To quickly thaw breast milk, remove the frozen bottle of breast milk from the freezer, place the bottle in a bowl in the sink, and run warm water over it. To thaw out more slowly, take the frozen bottle of breast milk, place it in the refrigerator and let it thaw out over several hours. The time it takes to do this depends on the volume in the bottle. Note that breast milk that has been sitting will normally separate. To re-mix it, simply swirl the bottle until the milk is evenly mixed. If the amount in the bottle is more than you will use in one feeding, pour the amount you want into a clean bottle, and put the rest back in the refrigerator. Take the bottle for feeding, place it in a bowl in the sink, and run warm water over it before feeding. The bottle should remain upright and not float in the bowl. The water level in the bowl should remain below the lid of the bottle/milk container. *Note: never use a microwave oven to thaw or warm breast milk.*
10. Thawed breast milk is good in the refrigerator for 24 hours.

TABLE 27–3   Types of Breast Pumps and Indications for Use

Indication	Manual Breast Pump (Figure 27–14)	Small Battery/Electric Breast Pump	Individual Double Electric Breast Pump	Hospital-Grade Multiuser Double Electric Breast Pump (Figure 27–15)
A missed feeding	■	◊		
An evening out	■	◊		
Working part-time	■	◊		
Convenience—occasional use	■	◊		
Working full-time			*	*
Premature/hospitalized infant				*
Low milk supply				*
Sore nipples/engorgement			*	*
Latch-on problems/infection			■	*
Drawing out flattish nipples	■	◊	*	*

■ Good ◊ Better *Best

Source: Adapted from the *Medela Breastfeeding Information Guide Tips and Products* (2002). Table: Which Breastpump Is Best for You? Pg. 3. Medela, Inc.

Figures 27–14 and 27–15 ■). Pumps generally cycle from low to high suction at a frequency similar to that of a breastfeeding infant (about 45 to 60 cycles per minute). However, differences in the quality of the pump motor or the presence or absence of controls over suction pressure mean that some pumps will generate inadequate pressure or cycle too slowly to be effective, whereas others may exert too high a suction that can cause injury. Flange size, proper fit, and comfort are other variables to consider. The nurse should refer the mother to a lactation consultant or other person knowledgable regarding different breast pumps. See breast pumping instruction on the Companion WEB. There are different guidelines for storage of expressed breast milk (EBM) depending on whether the infant is a healthy full-term infant or a premature or sick infant in the hospital. The guidelines in

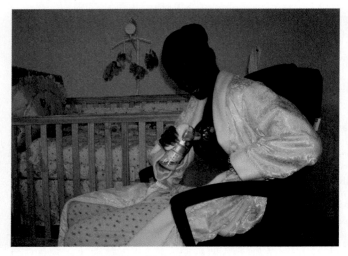

FIGURE 27–14 Manual breast pump.
Source: Courtesy of Brigette Hall, MSN, IBCLC.

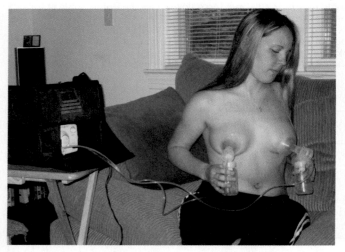

FIGURE 27–15 New mom using double electric breast pump at home.

TABLE 27–4	Storage Guidelines for Breast Milk and Formula	
Milk	Environment	Time Until Discard
Breast milk or Formula, opened/reconstituted	Being fed	Finish feed within 1 hour
Breast milk or Formula, opened/reconstituted	Environment/ 79 degrees	1 hour
Breast milk or Formula, opened/reconstituted	Room temperature	4 hours
Breast milk or Formula, opened/reconstituted	Cooler pack/ 59 degrees	24 hours
Thawed breast milk	Refrigerator	24 hours
Formula, opened/ reconstituted	Refrigerator	24 to 48 hours (see label)
Fresh breast milk	Refrigerator	8 days
Formula powder, opened can	Room temperature	1 month
Fresh breast milk	Freezer	3 month
Formula/powder in sealed container	Avoid excessive heat	Printed expiration date
Thawed breast milk	Freezer	Do not re-freeze
Formula	Freezer	Do not freeze

Source: Adapted from Human Milk Banking Association of North America (HMBANA). (2005). *Best practice for expressing, storing and handling human milk in hospitals, homes and child care settings.* Raleigh, NC: Author; Mead-Johnson Nutritionals. (2004). *Pediatric products handbook.* New York: Bristol-Myers Squibb Company. http://www.meadjohnson.com and Ross Products Division. (2004). *Pediatric nutritionals product guide.* Columbus, OH: Abbott Laboratories. http://www.ROSS.com.

Table 27–4 are intended as a resource for the mother of a healthy, full-term infant.

Supplementary Formula-Feeding

Supplementary formula-feedings for the breastfeeding infant after birth are not recommended routinely. Routine supplementation has been strongly implicated in early breastfeeding termination (AWHONN, 2007). Routine supplements are not only unnecessary, they can also contribute to maternal and infant health problems, including delayed early maternal milk production, maternal engorgement after her milk production has increased, infant milk-protein intolerance, and difficulties with learning to breastfeed.

"Nipple confusion" or "nipple preference" can occur in some babies causing them to develop an incorrect sucking technique, or to simply refuse to breastfeed again. This potential problem occurs because the techniques for breastfeeding and bottle-feeding are different. In breastfeeding, the infant has to open his mouth very wide in order to latch-

on. To transfer milk he has to extend his tongue forward, cupping the nipple and drawing it from back to front in a milking motion. With bottle-feeding, the infant keeps the tongue retracted and uses the tip of the tongue to block the flow of milk, which otherwise drips rapidly. Some babies can switch back and forth between breast and bottle without obvious difficulty, but for other infants, it is a problem. To reduce this possibility, experts in the field of lactation recommend introducing the bottle when the infant is able to latch on and breastfeeding is well established (usually after one month of age) with only the assistance of the mother (AWHONN, 2007). Evidence suggests that pacifier use may have a protective effect against SIDS. At one month of age, parents should consider offering a pacifier at nap and bedtime (Janke, 2008). To decrease risk of infection, pacifiers should be cleaned often and replaced regularly.

At times there are valid medical indications for supplementation of the breastfeeding infant. These include delayed lactogenesis; unavailability of the mother because of severe illness or separation; primary lactation failure; hypoglycemia; significant dehydration; weight loss of 8% to 10% with exclusive breastfeeding; delayed passage of stool (presence of meconium on day 5); hyperbilirubinemia related to poor intake, prematurity, or low birth weight; and refusal of or ineffective breastfeeding.

For those times when supplementation is indicated, the first choice is to use the mother's own milk (fresh, previously expressed, or frozen/thawed). If maternal breast milk is not available, pasteurized donor milk is the next choice, and then formula. Supplementation can be administered using a bottle or one of the following alternative feeding methods: cup feeding, spoon feeding, eyedropper or syringe feeding, or a nursing supplementer. The method chosen is based on the particular situation and parental preference.

Parents are often concerned because they have no visual assurance of the amount of breast milk consumed. The mother should be taught to observe the infant for effective breastfeeding. The infant should have a rhythmic suckling pattern (the slight pause between jaw compressions on the breast permits the mouth to fill with milk before swallowing). To note if the jaw compressions are strong enough, the mother should observe or feel if there is movement at the bilateral temporomandibular joints located in front of the infant's ears. The infant should maintain a rhythmic feeding pattern with only brief pauses (lasting only seconds, not minutes) between spurts of active feeding, with the feeding session typically lasting for 10 to 20 minutes on the first breast. The infant may feed only a few minutes on the second breast or not at all. The mother should visually observe for swallowing and later, as her milk is abundant, she will hear the infant's swallows. Discourage the mother from watching the clock to determine when the infant needs to switch breast sides but rather encourage her to watch the newborn's feeding pattern to note when active feeding ceases. When the infant is satiated, he will either pull away from the breast or fall asleep. The infant will be extremely relaxed at the end of the feeding and will sleep until the next feeding is due (at least an hour). As the infant matures, the feeding intervals will lengthen. Another indicator of breastfeeding efficiency is softening of the mother's breasts, although this is not a reliable indicator in the first few days postpartum while breast milk volume is low. Within a week however, this is a good indicator of milk transfer.

The infant who feeds well will have a characteristic output. See Figure 27–16 ■ for breastfeeding intake and output expectations. The infant should also have the characteristic weight loss followed by weight gain pattern discussed earlier in this chapter.

Finally, the most reliable measurement of effective breastfeeding is measuring the breast milk that actually transfers. This is done by obtaining pre- and post-breastfeeding weight checks using an accurate infant scale. The difference in pre-feed and post-feed weights is the amount of milk transferred to the infant and may be useful with assessing weight gain in late preterm infants.

Formula-Feeding Technique

With more attention placed on promoting and assisting breastfeeding mothers, the teaching needs of the mother who is formula-feeding may inadvertently get overlooked. Nurses may assume that families can simply follow the formula preparation instructions on the side of the formula containers. However, research shows that these parents also need teaching, counseling, and support. In a systematic review of five studies from developed countries looking at how parents prepare formula, all the studies revealed "errors in reconstition with a tendency to over-concentrate feeds, although under-concentrating also occurred" (Renfrew, Ansell, & Macleod, 2003). Parents need to learn about the feeding pattern for a formula-feeding infant, the intake and output expectations, the recommended type of formula for their infant, how to prepare and store formula, what equipment they will need, feeding technique, and safety precautions.

Commercial formulas are available in three forms: powder, concentrate, and ready-to-feed. There are situations in which one formula may be better to use than another, but in general, convenience and cost usually influence the parents' decision.

- *Powdered formula* is the least expensive type of formula. This formula can be made up one bottle at a time, or multiple bottles can be prepared, but they must be used within 24 to 48 hours. Standard powdered formula is made by adding one level scoop of powdered formula to 60 mL of water (the powder is added to the water). Powdered formulas are not sterile. Powdered formula is made from pasteurized liquid that is then freeze-spray dried into a powder; contamination with microorganisms can occur in the final stages of production. Preparation of any infant formula, but especially powdered formulas, requires careful handling to avoid contamination with microorganisms.
- *Formula concentrate* is more expensive than powder but is not as expensive as ready-to-feed formula. Formula concentrate is commercially sterile. This formula must be diluted with an equal part of water. By adding boiled water that has been cooled, sterility can be maintained.
- *Ready-to-feed* formula is the easiest to use because it is does not require any mixing; however, this convenience comes at a cost—it is the most expensive formula. It is indicated for use when adequate water is not available, when the infant is immunocompromised and requires commercially sterile (pasteurized) formula, when an inexperienced babysitter will be feeding the infant, and for convenience.

Whatever the type of formula chosen, the nurse should underscore the importance of proper preparation and prompt refrigeration. Parents will need to be briefed on safety precautions during formula preparation. A primary concern is proper mixing to reconstitute formula. Parents need clear instructions to avoid unintentional harm to their

Breastfeeding Intake and Output Expectations

- Baby should breastfeed 8 to 12 times/day and appear satisfied after feeding.
- Colostrum is all that the newborn needs in the first few days of life in most cases.
- It is normal for the infant to lose up to 7% (or between 5% and 10%) of birth weight in the first few days of life.
- Baby should gain 10 grams/kg/day after the milk is abundant (about day 4 of life).
- Baby should be back to birth weight by 2 weeks of age.
- Baby's stool should change in color, consistency, and frequency during the first few days of life. The color of stools changes from tarry black to dark greenish-black, to greenish-brown, to brownish-yellow, to light greenish-yellow, to bright yellow or yellowish-orange. The consistency of stools changes from tarry-sticky to thinner consistencies to curdy or seedy and "explosive." Volume of stool increases as volume of intake increases.

Day 1 and Day 2

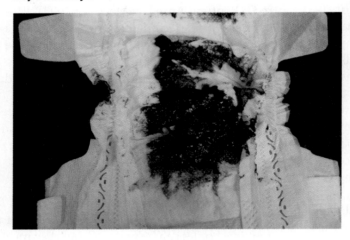

Minimum Output:

On day 1, the infant should produce at least one wet diaper and one meconium stool by 24 hours of age.

On day two, the infant should produce at least two wet diapers and 2 meconium stools. The stools may be thinning but remain dark (tarry black to greenish-brown).

Day 3 and Day 4

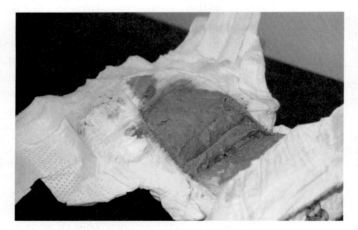

On day 3, the infant should produce at least three wet diapers and three transitional stools.

On day 4, the infant should produce at least four wet diapers and three to four transitional stools. The transitional stools are greenish-brown to greenish-yellow. Some infants will have transitioned to bright yellow milk stools by now.

Day 5

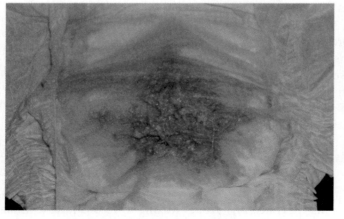

On day 5, the infant should produce at least five wet diapers and three to four yellow, milk stools.

Hereafter, breastfeeding babies will always produce at least six well-saturated wet diapers per day. They typically produce at least three to four stools per day (not uncommon to have up to 10 stools per day) for the first month of life. After a month of age, breastfeeding infants may drastically reduce the number of stools per day, even skipping several days.

Because stools are an indicator of caloric intake, low stool output (especially in the first couple of weeks of life) warrants a weight check and evaluation.

FIGURE 27–16 Breastfeeding intake and output expectations.
Source: Courtesy of Brigette Hall MSN, IBCLC.

infant. Parents should be instructed to follow the directions on the formula can label precisely as written. They should know that adding too much water during preparation dilutes the nutrients and caloric density. This contributes to undernourishment, insufficient weight gain, and possibly water intoxication, which can cause hyponatremia and seizures. Not adding enough water concentrates nutrients and calories and can tax an infant's immature kidneys and digestive system as well as cause dehydration (Morin, 2005). See Table 27–4 for storage guidelines for breast milk and formula.

Some recommended sanitary precautions and additional safety precautions are listed here:

- Check the expiration date on the formula container.
- Ensure good handwashing before preparing formula; never dip into the can without clean hands.
- Clean bottles, nipples, rings, disks, and bottle caps
  a. Washing in a dishwasher when available (small items and heat-sensitive items on top rack secured in a basket), or
  b. Boiling briefly (1 to 2 minutes) in a pot of water, or
  c. Cleaning using a microwave sterilization kit, or
  d. Cleaning using very warm soapy water and a nipple and bottle brush.
- Wash the top of the formula container before piercing the lid.
- Shake the liquid formulas well before pouring off the desired amount.
- Shake prepared milk that has been sitting in the refrigerator before feeding.
- Allow tap water to run for 1 minute before obtaining water to use for mixing—this helps clear any lead standing in the pipes. Also, always use cold tap water as warm water tends to contain higher levels of lead as well. Water should be warmed (or cooled after boiling) before being added to the formula.
- Use only the scoop supplied in the can of formula when formula preparation instructions call for a "scoop" of powdered formula.
  a. A scoop should not be "packed" and should be leveled off (i.e., with the back of a knife).
- Do not add anything else to the bottle, except under direction of the baby's healthcare provider.
- Warm-up milk in a bottle should be warmed by placing the bottle in a bowl of warm tap water. Do not fill the bowl with water higher than the rim of the bottle. (Babies can take cold formula but most young infants will prefer it warm.)
- Do not freeze formula.
- Allow freshly prepared (unused) formula to sit out at room temperature for no longer than two hours; use an insulated pack to transport formula. Milk left over in the bottle after a feeding should be discarded.

- In warm weather, transport reconstituted or formula concentrate from an open can in an insulated pack with frozen gel packs.
- Travel with water and formula separated—carry premeasured water bottles and bottles with premeasured amounts of powdered formula, or carry premeasured commercially prepared formula packets, or have the can of formula available.
- Inspect and replace bottle nipples as soon as they show wear—worn nipples can break apart and can become a choking hazard.
- Holding the infant during feeding (even when the infant can hold the bottle for himself) promotes bonding and prevents supine feedings.
- Do not allow the infant to bottle-feed in a supine position because this increases the risk of otitis media and dental caries in the older infant.
- Never prop a bottle—this is a choking hazard.
- Allow infants to take what they want AND to stop when they want. Overfeeding can lead to obesity.

Parents also need guidance about what kind of water to use to reconstitute formula (see Table 27–5 to review types of water sources) and should discuss with their infant's healthcare provider whether to boil the water before use. If boiling is used, parents need to be instructed to heat the water until it reaches a rolling boil, continue to let the water boil for 1 to 2 minutes, and, most importantly, to allow

TABLE 27–5	Water Sources
Type	Description
Distilled water	Minerals and most other impurities have been removed. It will not contain any flouride. An acceptable water source for reconstituting formula.
Filtered tap water	Some minerals and impurities removed during filtration, including flouride. This is an acceptable water source for reconstituting formula.
Natural mineral water	Comes from protected ground water and by law cannot be treated. Naturally contains high levels of minerals and sodium and so is not suitable for infants or for reconstituting formula.
Spring water	Comes from a single non-polluted ground water source, but unlike natural mineral water, it can be further treated. Because there is no regulation requiring the mineral content to be printed on the bottle label, it is best to avoid this water source for reconstituting formula.
Tap water	Water from the municipal water supply, and regulated by drinking water regulations. It is treated and considered safe for use in reconstituting formula.
Well water	Needs to be tested before use. Higher risk of nitrate poisoning. Untested water is not recommended for use in reconstituting formula.

the water to cool before using it to reconstitute the formula. Parents should also be instructed not to let the water boil down to a low level in the pan because this can cause minerals in the water to become concentrated.

Use of distilled bottle water and filtered tap water raises concerns with regard to flouride. The American Academy of Pediatrics recommends that no fluoride supplements should be given to an infant before 6 months of age, but does recommend supplementary flouride for infants and children ages 6 months to 3 years of age if the water source contains less than 0.3 ppm (AAP & ACOG, 2007). Parents should be encouraged to read the labels on bottled water to see if flouride has been added and to determine if the water source is suitable for their infant depending on his or her age (Table 27–5).

Parents often have questions about the kind of bottles and nipples to purchase. Plastic, glass, or disposable bottle bags may all be used based on preference. Mothers who bottle-feed expressed breast milk may want to avoid the use of bottle liners/bottle bags, especially if they have a fragile infant. Research shows that up to 60% of secretory immunoglobulin A (SIgA) found in breast milk binds to the polyethylene material used in these and is therefore lost to the infant (Lawrence & Lawrence, 2005). There are no human antibodies in formula so this is not a concern for bottle-feeding formula.

There are many different bottle nipples on the market. Parents will want to consider a slow-flow nipple for all newborns and for older breastfeeding babies learning to bottle-feed—over time the infant will graduate to medium-flow and high-flow nipples. Nipples come in different shapes. Generally, nipple shape plays a greater importance for breastfeeding babies receiving expressed breast milk or supplemental formula in a bottle. Breastfed babies transition best going from breast to bottle and back to breast again when using a bottle nipple that has a relatively wide base (to help maintain a wide open latch) and a medium to long nipple length. Another variable to consider is nipple construction. Nipples are generally made from either rubber or silicone. Families with a sensitivity to latex are advised to use silicone nipples. Silicone nipples also have less of an odor, which may be an issue for some infants who are breastfed.

Many newly designed bottles are marketed to lessen air intake while an infant feeds. There is not a particular bottle design that is best for all babies. Different families find different bottles and nipple assembly products better than others. A key point to emphasize to the families is feeding technique. Parents should try to avoid situations in which an infant is crying for a prolonged time. Crying results in increased ingestion of air even before the infant has started feeding. Infants who are very hungry also gulp more air. For these situations, instruct the parents to burp their infant frequently to prevent the infant from having a large emesis (see Figure 27–17 ■).The parent may even want to

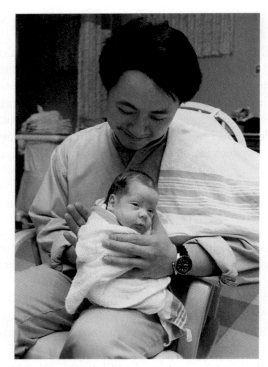

FIGURE 27–17 Burping time.
Source: © Stella Johnson (www.stellajohnson.com).

attempt to pat the baby's back briefly before starting the feeding to calm the infant and possibly burp as well. Another tip to avoid excessive ingestion of air is to have the parent hold his or her infant cradled in the arms while bottle-feeding and have the parent tilt the baby's bottle at a 45-degree angle (at least) in order for fluid to cover the nipple. This prevents the infant from sucking in air and swallowing it. See Figure 27–18 ■ to view this technique.

To know if an infant is bottle feeding well, the nurse needs to observe a bottle-feeding session. Parents should be informed that if the infant is sucking effectively, the parents should observe bubbles rising in the fluid (except if they are using plastic-lined bottles which contract as they empty). If the parent unintentionally placed the bot-

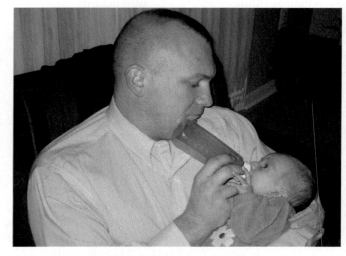

FIGURE 27–18 Dad feeding his baby a bottle.

tle nipple under the infant's tongue, preventing him from sucking, the infant may make sucking efforts but will not receive any fluid and no bubbles will be visualized. Infants who persistently leak milk from the side of the mouth may be getting fluid too quickly. The nurse could suggest using a slower flowing nipple. If symptoms persist, the infant should have an oral evaluation. The infant could have a short lingual frenulum (tongue-tie) and not be able to properly cup his tongue under the nipple and channel fluid to the back of his throat, or he may have an oral-motor dysfunction and need speech therapy or occupational therapy evaluation.

HINTS FOR PRACTICE

Parents should be instructed not to put honey or corn syrup on their infant's pacifier to encourage an infant to accept it. Honey and possibly corn syrup may be contaminated with *Clostridium botulinum*, a bacteria that causes infantile botulism. This is not a risk for the older child. Botulism is rare, but when it occurs it causes serious illness.

Community-Based Nursing Care

Promotion of Successful Infant Feeding

To promote a supportive hospital environment for breast-feeding, some hospitals have applied for Certificates of Intent to become "Baby Friendly." The World Health Organization (WHO) and the United Nations Children's Fund (UNICEF) have collaborated to create a global program, the Baby-Friendly Hospital Initiative, to recognize hospitals and birthing centers that offer optimal lactation services (WHO/UNICEF, 1994). Only hospitals that have been certified as complying with the 10 steps outlined in Table 27–6 have been awarded the designation as "Baby Friendly." Baby-Friendly status is not easy to achieve. One obstacle, among many, is having to agree not to accept free or low-cost formula. Currently there are approximately 63 hospitals in the United States with Baby-Friendly designation as of February 2008 according to an update on the Baby-Friendly Hospital Initiative USA website (BFHI USA, 2008).

Childbirth and the beginning of motherhood are critical times in a woman's life, so physical, psychologic, and social supports are of paramount importance. The nurse needs to explore the family's social support base. The father or other partner is the most important support person for her, although the baby can also provide some support in the form of positive feedback. However, extensive family support systems may not be available. Mother, mother-in-law, sisters, and other females who could mentor and care for the new mother may live at a distance or work full-time.

TABLE 27–6 Baby-Friendly Requirements

Baby-Friendly 10 Steps to Successful Breastfeeding

- Have a written breastfeeding policy that is routinely communicated to all healthcare staff.
- Train all healthcare staff in skills necessary to implement this policy.
- Inform all pregnant women about the benefits and management of breastfeeding.
- Help mothers initiate breastfeeding within one half-hour of birth.
- Show mothers how to breastfeed and maintain lactation, even if they should be separated from their infants.
- Give newborn infants no food or drink other than breast milk, unless medically indicated.
- Practice rooming in—that is, allow mothers and infants to remain together 24 hours a day.
- Encourage breastfeeding on demand.
- Give no artificial teats or pacifiers (also called dummies or soothers) to breastfeeding infants.
- Foster the establishment of breastfeeding support groups and refer mothers to them on discharge from the hospital or clinic.

Source: World Health Organization/United Nations Children's Emergency Fund (WHO/UNICEF). (1994). *U.S. committee for UNICEF interim program in the United States to promote the Baby-Friendly ten steps to successful breastfeeding.* Washington, DC: Government Printing Office.

Many families will have adequate income, a good knowledge base, and good coping skills to handle problems. Some families will have support from a large extended family group, friends, church, or other organization. However, that is not the case for everyone; as evidenced by the frequent discontinuing of breastfeeding in the early postpartum weeks, there is a need for assistance and follow-up in this area. When inadequate support is identified, it may be beneficial to request a referral for the family to have an outpatient case manager involved to make sure the mother knows how to access the community resources and is making a good adjustment. Nurses, dietitians, childbirth educators, certified nurse-midwives, lactation consultants, mother-to-mother support groups, and physicians must collaborate to provide consistent, timely information and support and to attend to the new mother's special needs.

Breastfeeding mothers who work outside the home and are supported in their decision tend to breastfeed their infants for longer periods than mothers who work but do not receive support. A baby-friendly workplace needs to be seen as another item in a benefit package offered by a company. Families and nurses who believe in breastfeeding need to be part of the solution to breastfeeding and workplace issues by educating employers in their communities (Rojjanasrirat, 2004).

With a national nursing shortage and the trend toward earlier discharge from the birthing center, there is limited time for inpatient education. Teaching moments, when they occur, may not be optimal because of the distraction of visitors and the mother's being sleep deprived, uncomfortable, or feeling the effects of an analgesic. It is important that parents receive verbal and written instructions and community resource information to which they can later refer. See also Chapter 32 ∞ for a complete discussion of self-care measures the nurse can suggest to a woman with a breastfeeding problem after discharge from the birthing center.

When parents leave the birthing center, the center staff need to have the name and phone number for both mother and baby's healthcare provider and know the indications that suggest they should contact them. The breastfeeding mother needs a list of lactation resources available in the community. If no resource handout is available, the mother should be given the phone number to **La Leche League International** or the International Lactation Consultant Association, which can provide assistance with finding the closest lactation support. Many hospitals around the country have a lactation program and may provide lactation services for a fee to anyone seeking services. Some cities have outpatient lactation centers that provide comprehensive lactation services including consultation services, breastfeeding classes, and an infant scale for assessing baby's weight, as well as telephone-based lactation advice. Some cities have lactation consultants in private practice who have an outpatient office or may do home visits. The Women Infant Children (WIC) Supplemental Nutrition Program may have a lactation consultant on staff or may have a contract with a lactation consultant in private practice in the community. Another potential resource is a home health agency. Some home health agencies provide outpatient lactation services in the patient's home. Some military facilities provide lactation services to their service members and dependents. The local library is also an excellent resource, and there are many books available commercially. Finally, the Internet can be a tremendous resource, although the quality of information cannot always be ensured. It is very helpful to have a handout listing some good sites that have been reviewed for accuracy.

Both breastfeeding and formula-feeding mothers who may be eligible for WIC should be encouraged to enroll themselves and their infants in the WIC nutrition program. WIC provides a specific number of cans of powdered formula to eligible mothers free of charge. The number of cans the mother receives is based on an agreement in the current government contract that WIC has with one of the two major formula companies (Mead-Johnson, the maker of Enfamil®; or Ross, the maker of Similac®) and whether a mother is partially breastfeeding (in this case she usually receives 4 cans per month) or entirely formula-feeding (usually receives 9 to 10 cans per month, depending on the formula ordered and how many ounces of formula the can provides). The breastfeeding mother can also receive additional food vouchers for herself. The amount of formula the mother receives *does not* increase as the infant grows. The parents need to understand that 10 cans will not be sufficient over time and that they will need to purchase the difference when the infant's needs exceed the amount supplied. Mothers with an extremely low income who lack family support may need the numbers for emergency food assistance programs in the area. These might include local food banks, local churches (including The Salvation Army), and United Way programs. Low-income mothers also need to be reminded to enroll their infant in The Food Stamp Program so they can receive additional food vouchers each month.

Cultural Considerations in Infant Feeding

All groups of people are influenced by their cultural background. Every culture shares a set of values, beliefs, behaviors, and a language unique for that group. These are learned characteristics shared among their members. A person's culture influences every aspect of his or her life. By learning about other cultures, the nurse will gain an understanding of the "context," or unstated assumptions that influence behavior, thus avoiding misunderstanding and improving the nurse's ability to communicate with the person. Of course, it is also true that not all individuals within a particular cultural group subscribe to each of the values, beliefs, and behaviors characteristic of that group. People need to be seen as individuals within the context of their culture (Callister, 2008).

Within the United States, many people agree that breastfeeding is the optimum infant feeding method. However, breast exposure is often viewed in a sexual context, leading to disapproval of the mother who attempts to breastfeed in public. Although this norm may be changing, it is important for the nurse to recognize that not only do "others" often hold these views, but the mother herself may feel this way. It is therefore important to determine the attitudes of the mother—based on her feelings, it may be very important or not important at all to spend time discussing methods of breastfeeding discreetly.

With regard to the feeding of colostrum, although many recognize that it has properties uniquely suited to the newborn, there are people who consider colostrum "unclean" and do not offer it to their newborns. This belief is found among some groups of Hispanics, Navajo Indians, Filipinos, and Vietnamese (Galanti, 2004; D'Avanzo & Geissler, 2008). In a situation like this, in which a cultural custom is harmful or denies the infant benefits, it is the nurse's responsibility to try to educate the family about the value of colostrum. A possible approach to this situation is as follows. First, reinforce the parents' desire to protect their baby from infection. Next, validate the assumption that since colostrum looks similar to pus from a wound, it makes sense that one might think it is also unclean. Next, point out that the reason pus looks the way it does is because of the white cells that the body sends to fight infection. Last, explain that as in the case of a wound, colostrum *is* one of the body's ways of helping fight infection—only in this case it is sending the white cells to the baby even before there is an infection. This last point again reinforces the initial validation of the parents' concern for infection but now uses that concern as motivation to feed the colostrum, rather than avoid it.

In these cultures and in some countries (Guinea, Pakistan, Bagladesh), breastfeeding begins only after milk flow is established (Riordan, 2005). In many Asian cultures, the newborn is given boiled water until the mother's milk flows. The newborn is fed on demand, and cries are responded to immediately. If the crying continues, evil spirits may be blamed and a priest's blessing may be sought. Although many of the Hmong women of Laos combine breastfeeding with some formula-feeding, they usually find expressing their milk or pumping their breasts unacceptable. Thus other methods of providing relief should be suggested if breast engorgement develops. Most Muslim mothers breastfeed because the Qur'an (Koran) encourages it until the child is 2 years old (Ott, Al-Khadhuri, & Al-Junaibi, 2003). Japanese women are returning to breastfeeding as the method of feeding for the baby's first year.

Language is one of the most culturally sensitive behaviors and the source of much confusion. African Americans may refer to their infant as "greedy," which may be interpreted as a concern that the infant is taking too much. However, rather than an expression of concern, this term is often used as an expression of approval of the infant's vigorous feeding. African American culture tends to emphasize plentiful feeding, and solid foods are introduced early—possibly even added to the infant's formula. If the nurse misinterprets the expression, he or she may think that the mother is limiting the baby's feeding and may attempt to convince the mother that she should be encouraging higher intake, which could lead to overfeeding. African American mothers view frequent feeding as an expression of hardiness and a positive behavioral characteristic for their children for the future. For traditional Mexicans, a fat baby is considered healthy and infants are fed on demand. "Spoiling" is encouraged.

These are but a few of the multitude of cultural influences related to feeding (see Cultural Perspectives: Breastfeeding in Other Cultures). When faced with an infant care practice different from the ones to which they are accustomed, nurses need to evaluate the effect of the practice. Different practices are not necessarily inferior. The nurse should intervene only if the practice is actually harmful to the mother or baby.

CULTURAL PERSPECTIVES

Breastfeeding in Other Cultures

Some people of Asian heritage may breastfeed their babies for the first 1 to 2 years of life. Many Cambodian refugees practice breastfeeding on demand without restriction, or, if formula-feeding, provide a "comfort bottle" in between feedings (Lipson & Dibble, 2008).

People of Iranian heritage may breastfeed female babies longer than male babies. Many Muslim women will not breastfeed in public (Hedayat, 2001; Ott, Al-Khadhuri, & Al-Junaibi, 2003).

Some people of African ancestry may wean their babies after they begin to walk.

Some Asians, Haitian, Hispanics, Eastern Europeans, and Native Americans may delay breastfeeding because they believe colostrum is "bad" (Riordan, 2005; D'Avanzo & Geissler, 2008).

Haitain mothers may believe that "strong emotions" spoil breast milk; and that thick breastmilk causes skin rashes and thin milk results in diarrhea (Callister, 2008; Lipson & Dibble, 2008).

In Malaysia, the ingestion of breast milk represents a great deal more than simple nutrition for newborn infants. It is believed that the mother's milk enters the baby's blood. This is thought to cultivate a long life. Breast milk is thought to bind the mother and baby together, creating a sense of respect and closeness. Although milk develops the infant's spirit and body, it also develops faith and character. It is thought that the consumption of breast milk formulates a maternal-infant bond that lasts throughout life. This bond cannot be broken by any means. Breastfeeding mothers drink "jamu" (a drink consisting of egg yolk, palm sugar, tamarind, and herbs) to ensure an adequate milk supply.

Complementary and Alternative Therapies

Herbs for Breastfeeding

Herbs (galactogogues) thought to increase milk supply include alfalfa, dandelion, fennel seeds, horsetail, red raspberry, fenugreek, goat's rue, milk thistle, basil, blessed thistle, marshmallow, caraway, and anise to name a few (Academy of Breastfeeding Medicine [ABM], 2004). The mother may drink caraway tea to reduce colic in the breastfeeding infant. Caraway tea also may be given directly to infants to treat colic (Skidmore-Roth, 2006). Most of the herbal galactogogues are taken as a tea, although capsules are also available. Fenugreek is probably the most commonly used herbal galactagogue because it seems to have the fewest adverse side effects. Women who drink it as a tea generally drink 2 to 3 cups per day. The tea is made by adding 1/4 teaspoon of fenugreek seeds steeped in 8 ounces of water for 10 minutes. Women who take the capsules generally take one to four capsules (580 to 610 mg capsules) three to four times per day (ABM, 2004). Mothers usually notice an increase in their milk production in 2 to 3 days. Goat's rue, fennel seed, or milk thistle (not blessed thistle) tea is made with 1 teaspoon of dried leaves steeped in 8 ounces of water for 10 minutes; women usually have 2 to 3 cups of tea per day (Wagner, Graham, & Hope, 2006). There are anti-galactogogue herbs (i.e., sage, parsley, and peppermint) that may or may not be used in combination with cabbage leaves and ice to decrease severe engorgement, to diminish an oversupply, and to "dry up" when weaning an infant from the breast. The following anti-galactogogue herbs may decrease milk supply, so they should be avoided until a woman is no longer breastfeeding: black walnut, sage, parsley, and yarrow (Skidmore-Roth, 2006). Black cohosh, blessed thistle, cascara sagrada, horseradish, garlic, cinnamon bark, kava kava, and senna are also contraindicated during lactation.

Nutritional Assessment

A nutritional assessment is an integral part of a thorough health appraisal and is commonly performed by the infant's primary care provider, a nurse, a lactation consultant, a registered dietician, or a speech therapist. The nutritional assessment will include all or some of the following parameters to measure wellness:

- Nutritional intake (i.e., breast milk, type of formula, other foods)
- Anthropometric measurements (i.e., measurements of weight, length, and head circumference)
- Biochemical status (i.e., the newborn metabolic screening, iron level, etc.)
- Physical examination (i.e., vital signs, total body examination, developmental milestones)
- Sociodemographic data (i.e., parity, maternal age, impact of cultural practices on feeding)

Parents will be asked to present a feeding diary for the provider to review, or the parents will need to recall the infant's feeding pattern over the last 24 to 48 hours. The parents will also be asked to describe the infant's urine and stool output, including quantity and quality. The healthcare professional is interested in the infant's behavior pattern, especially during and immediately after feeding. If the newborn is not gaining sufficient weight, the infant's feeding history must be examined more closely. If the infant is breastfeeding, a relevant maternal history is needed to determine if the mother is having breastfeeding difficulties and to help determine the root cause of the problem. If the infant is formula-feeding, the healthcare professional will first want to investigate the family's formula-feeding practices (including formula preparation technique). While gathering this data, the healthcare professional should be sensitive to the family's cultural practices. However, if a cultural practice has harmful ef-

fects, then the provider needs to tactfully educate the family to that fact.

The provider should plot the infant's measurements for length, head circumference, and weight on a growth chart denoting the infant's individual percentile measurement compared with the general population. Because there are variations among infants at the same age, it is important to monitor the infant's individual growth pattern over time. Ideally, the provider wants to see an infant track along the same growth curve. A drop of 20 percentile or more on the growth curve is cause for concern.

As the healthcare provider begins the infant's physical exam, the provider first obtains a subjective impression of the infant's overall appearance. The provider performs a head-to-toe physical examination carefully noting any deviations from normal. The physical exam helps identify any nutritional disorders. If the infant's primary healthcare provider has any concerns about the infant's nutritional status, the provider may order relevant laboratory studies (i.e., hemoglobin, hematocrit, transferrin, albumin, creatinine, nitrogen, and others), may evaluate the infant for malabsorption disorders, and may see a need to refer the infant to a pediatric gastroenterologist for further evaluation.

With all the infant data available, it is now possible to determine an infant's nutritional status and potential risks.

The following example shows the effectiveness of these assessments and interventions:

Scenario: *Baby girl Torres was born at 37 weeks' gestation to an 18-year-old, G1P0 via cesarean section. Baby Torres is now 76 hours postpartum and she and her mother are expected to go home today. While weighing the infant for a discharge weight, the mother mentions that she does not think her daughter is getting much breast milk when she feeds because her infant keeps falling asleep at the breast during the feeding. Baby Torres weighed 3542 grams at birth and her present weight is 3173 grams. (The difference is 369 grams. 369/3542 = 0.104 × 100 = 10.4% weight loss.) A quick assessment of the mother's breasts reveals soft breasts and normal-shaped nipples, with nipples intact. After contacting the infant's healthcare provider to report the significant weight loss, the nurse is now ready to formulate a plan of care.*

The nurse makes the following nursing diagnoses:
Ineffective Breastfeeding related to:

- Mother's lack of knowledge about breastfeeding
- Mother's not responding to infant's feeding cues
- Mother's inability to facilitate effective breastfeeding as evidenced by a weight loss of 10.4% in baby

Risk for Ineffective Breastfeeding related to:

- *Insufficient knowledge* regarding newborn's reflexes and breastfeeding techniques

- Lack of support by father of baby or other support persons
- Lack of maternal self-confidence
- Maternal fatigue
- Maternal ambivalence
- Poor infant sucking reflex
- Difficulty waking the sleepy baby

Risk for Imbalanced Nutrition: Less than Body Requirements related to:

- Mother's increased caloric and nutrient needs status post cesarean section
- Infant's inability to correctly latch-on and transfer milk

Expected Outcomes of Care
The expected outcomes for the infant include:

- Infant will arouse to feed at least every 3 hours and will stay awake until the end of each feeding.
- The infant will correctly latch on to the breasts and effectively breastfeed 8 to 12 times/day.
- The infant will maintain weight and will gain at least 10 g/kg/day.
- The infant will have four wet diapers, three to four bowel movements on day 4; five wet diapers, three to four bowel movements on day 5; and six to eight wet diapers, three to four bowel movements every day thereafter during the first month of life.
- Infant's stools will transition from black to yellow by day 5 and will change in consistency from thick and sticky to loose and explosive with small curds or seedy appearance.
- Infant will not have any uric acid crystals in her diaper after day 4.
- Infant will be satiated after feeding, as evidenced by relaxed muscle tone and sleepiness.

The expected outcomes for the mother include:

- Mother will verbalize/demonstrate an understanding of breastfeeding technique including positioning and latch-on, signs of adequate feeding, self-care.
- Mother will breastfeed pain-free.
- Mother will express satisfaction with the breastfeeding experience.
- Mother will consume a nutritionally balanced diet with appropriate caloric and fluid intake to support breastfeeding.

Plan of Care and Interventions

1. Review mother's history
   - Maternal demographics (e.g., mother's date of birth, parity, marital status)
   - Pregnancy history (e.g., complications during pregnancy, gestation at childbirth)
   - Complications of childbirth (e.g., cesarean section, excessive blood loss)
   - Current medical issues (e.g., hypothyroidism?, diabetes?)
   - History of breast surgery or radiation (e.g., breast reduction, radiation to treat previous breast cancer)
   - Use of medications, herbs, alcohol, cigarettes
   - Psychosocial history (maternal support system, hx of depression?, etc.)
   - History of previous breastfeeding experience
2. Maternal assessment
   - Assessment of breasts and nipples
   - Obtain a description of lochia drainage
3. Infant assessment
   - Obtain infant's weight and compare with previous weight measurements [*If this were an older infant, then it would be appropriate to obtain head circumference, length, and weight measurements and track the infant's trend on the growth chart; however, because this infant is only 3 days old, daily tracking of the other growth parameters is not applicable for this situation.*]
   - Infant exam with emphasis on oral anatomy and oral-motor function, infant reflexes, overall behavior, skin color (jaundice)
   - Assess infant for signs of dehydration
4. Infant feeding history
   - Diet
   - Feeding frequency and duration
   - History of supplementation
   - Review elimination pattern
     - Number of wet diapers, quality of urine
     - Number of bowel movements, quality of stool
5. Pre- and post-breastfeeding weight check
   - Calculate milk transfer during breastfeeding [*Post-feed weight minus pre-feed weight = net breast milk transfer. Note: The nurse must use a digital electronic scale accurate within 2 grams. The infant does not have to be naked but the clothing and diaper the infant is wearing cannot be changed during this test measurement.*]
6. Observation of breastfeeding technique
   - Positioning and latch-on technique, infant responses, suckling pattern, satiated after feeding
7. Review feeding requirement/caloric requirement based on infant's birth weight (3.542 kg)
   - Fluid requirement: 140 to 160 mL/kg/day
     - Should be up to full volume by day 6; should then receive 496 mL to 567 mL/day. [To calculate mL to oz: take 496 mL divided by 30 mL/oz = 16.5.] The infant should receive 16.5 to 18.9 oz/day.
     - The infant should feed 8 to 12 times/day. If the infant feeds 10 times/day, then the infant should feed 496/10 = 49.6 mL/feeding.
     - On day 3, the infant will not be expected to feed ~50 mL/feeding (minimum full volume); the

infant may only feed 30 mL/feeding but will be increasing volume daily as tolerated until up to full volume in the next couple of days.

- Caloric requirement 100 to 115 kcal/kg/day
  - Should be up to full caloric requirement by day 6; should receive 354 kcal/day to 407 kcal/day. Breast milk has 20 kcal/oz; standard infant formula has 20 kcal/oz. To determine how many ounces the infant will require per day, take 354 kcal/day divided by 20 = 17.7 oz/day. [Note: The infant should be gradually increasing her volume of milk each day and will soon be up to full volume.]

8. Assess teaching needs
   - Review benefits of breastfeeding
   - Review the process of breastfeeding (principle of supply and demand)
   - Review breastfeeding technique (reading infant cues, positioning, and latch-on)
   - Review infant intake and output expectations
   - Review infant weight gain expectations
   - Provide breast pump instructions and review collection and storage
   - Provide information on maternal nutrition and fluid requirements

9. Provide written instructions
   - *Provide frequent skin-to-skin contact.*

- *Watch infant for early feeding cues. If infant is too dehydrated and weak to exhibit these feeding behaviors, then help the infant to wake up at least every 3 hours.*
- *Start pumping each time the infant feeds (8 to 12 times/day),* if mother's breasts are still very soft and light (delay in milk coming in). All expressed breast milk should be fed to the infant. If mother is not able to express enough milk, then the infant should be supplemented with iron-fortified cow's milk-based formula unless specified otherwise.
- *Practice proper breastfeeding technique. Encourage the mother to breastfeed as often as possible and observe for signs of effective breastfeeding.*
- *Maintain a feeding diary to monitor infant's intake and output; call lactation consultant if infant is not meeting expectations.*
- *Rest as much as possible and be concerned only about self-care needs (prevention of engorgement, etc.), and caring for the infant right now.*
- *Eat healthy foods and drink plenty of fluids to thirst.*
- *Follow-up weight check on infant in 1 to 2 days and assess nutritional status.*

Follow-up lactation consultation visit follows in 2 days to determine milk transfer efficiency and evaluate maternal milk production.

CHAPTER HIGHLIGHTS

- The American Academy of Pediatrics (AAP) recommends exclusive breastfeeding for the first 6 months and continued breastfeeding until the infant is 1 year old or older.
- During the first few days after birth, the minimum output expectations for an exclusively breastfeeding infant will be: one wet/one stool on day 1; two wets/two stools on day 2; three wets/three to four stools on day 3; four wets/three to four stools on day 4; five wets/three to four stools on day 5. Thereafter, an exclusively breastfeeding infant has six to eight wet diapers and three to four yellow milk stools each day generally during the first month of life.
- Infants' stools start as black and sticky at birth and transition to yellow, curdy and seedy by day 5, or sooner.
- Formula-feeding infants lose about 3.5% of their birth weight. Breastfeeding infants lose up to 7% of their birth weight. A weight loss of more than 7% is excessive and requires an evaluation and follow-up. Infants should be back to their birth weight by 10 to 14 days of age.
- Growth rate over the life span is greatest during infancy. The healthy full-term infant gains approximately 10 g/kg/day for the first month of life. Exclusively breastfed infants have the same or slightly greater weight gain in the first 3 to 4 months of life than mixed-fed and formula-fed infants. Thereafter, formula-fed and mixed-fed infants are heavier than breastfed infants.

- Increases in body length and head circumference between breastfed and formula-fed infants is the same. An infant gains 1 inch per month in the first 6 months, and then 0.5 inches for the following 6 months. Length is a better indicator of growth than is weight.
- Generally, infants double their birth weight by 5 months, triple their birth weight by 1 year of age, and quadruple their birth weight by 2 years.
- The dietary reference intake (DRI) for calories for the newborn is 100 to 115 kcal/kg/day.
- The dietary reference intake (DRI) for fluid intake for the newborn is 140 to 160 mL/kg/day.
- Breast milk has immunologic and nutritional properties that make it the optimal food for the first year of life.
- Mature breast milk and standard commercially prepared formulas provide 20 kcal/oz.
- The breastfed infant's iron stores in full-term infants are usually depleted by the time the infant is 6 months old. The breastfeeding infant over 6 months of age who is eating supplementary foods rich in iron and infants consuming iron-enriched formula need no other vitamin or mineral supplements.
- There are three types of commercial infant formulas: cow's milk-based formula, soy milk-based formulas, and specialized formulas including hydrolysated formulas.

- Neither cow's milk nor soy milk should be given to infants before 1 year of age. The use of skim milk, or low-fat cow's milk, is not recommended for children under 2 years old.
- Signs indicating a newborn's readiness to feed include hand-to-mouth movements, rooting, smacking, fussing, and crying (a late feeding cue).
- By learning about cultural variations, the nurse will gain an understanding of the "context" or unstated assumptions that influence behavior, thus avoiding misunderstanding and improving the nurse's ability to communicate with clients.
- Infants should not receive water supplements until they start solid foods.
- Although most maternal medications are transmitted through breast milk, few are actually contraindicated. The bioavailability of transmitted drugs to the infant depends on a variety of factors, including route of administration, protein binding, degree of ionization, molecular weight, timing of the dose with respect to feeding time, and absorption across the infant's intestinal tract. Mothers should consult with a healthcare provider knowledgable about medications and lactation.
- Breastfeeding mothers should be taught to use proper positioning and latch-on technique. The mother should be advised to alternate feeding positions periodically to promote efficient drainage of all the ducts in the breast.
- The formula-feeding mother may need help learning about the types of formulas, and how to prepare and store formula. Like the breastfeeding mother, she will benefit from understanding feeding cues and proper technique for feeding her infant.
- Nutritional assessment of the infant includes the infant's dietary history, anthropometric measurements, physical examination, and laboratory tests if indicated.

CHAPTER REFERENCES

Academy of Breastfeeding Medicine (ABM). (2004). Protocol #9: Use of galactogogues initiating or augmenting maternal milk supply. *ABM News and Views, 10*(3), 20–22. Retrieved April 22, 2008, from http://www.bfmed.org/

American Academy of Pediatrics (AAP), Committee on Drugs. (2001). Transfer of drugs and other chemicals into human milk. *Pediatrics, 108*(3), 776–789. Retrieved April 20, 2008, from http://www.aap.org/healthtopics/breastfeeding.cfm

American Academy of Pediatrics (AAP), Committee on Fetus and Newborn & American College of Obstetricians and Gynecologists (ACOG), Committee on Obstetrics. (2007). *Guidelines for perinatal care* (6th ed.). Evanston, IL: Author.

American Academy of Pediatrics (AAP), Media Alert. (1998, April 20). *AAP addresses scheduled feedings vs. demand feedings.* Retrieved April 20, 2008, from http://www.ezzo.info/Aney/aapmediaalert.pdf

American Academy of Pediatrics (AAP), Section on Breastfeeding. (2005). Policy statement: Breastfeeding and the use of human milk. *Pediatrics, 115*(2), 496–506. Retrieved April 20, 2008, from http://www.aappolicy.aappublications.org

Aney, M. (1998). Commentary: 'Babywise' advice linked to dehydration, failure to thrive. *AAP News, 14*(4), 21. Retrieved April 22, 2008, from http://aapnews.aappublications.org/contentvol14/issue4/#COMMENTARY

Association of Women's Health, Obstetric and Neonatal Nurses (AWHONN). (2007). *Breastfeeding support: Prenatal care through the first year. Evidence-based clinical practice guideline* (2nd ed., pp. 1–89). Washington, DC: AWHONN.

Baby-Friendly Hospital Initiative USA (BFHI USA). (2008). *Implementing the UNICEF/WHO baby-friendly hospital initiative in the U.S.* Retrieved April 22, 2008, from http://www.babyfriendlyusa.org/eng/03.html

Baumslag, N., & Michels, D. L. (1995). *Milk, money, and madness: The culture and politics of breastfeeding.* Westport, CT: Bergin & Garvey.

Blackburn, S. T. (2007). *Maternal, fetal, & neonatal physiology: A clinical perspective* (3rd ed.). St. Louis, MO: Saunders.

Briggs, G. G., Freeman, R. K., & Yaffe, S. J. (2005). *Drugs in pregnancy and lactation: A reference guide to fetal and neonatal risk* (7th ed.). Baltimore: Lippincott Williams & Wilkins.

Callister, L. C. (2008). Integrating cultural beliefs and practices when caring for childbearing women and families. In K. R. Simpson & P. A. Creehan, *Perinatal nursing.* (3rd ed., pp. 29–57). Philadelphia: Lippincott Williams & Wilkins.

Cloherty, J. P., Eichenwald, E. C., & Stark, A. R. (2008). *Manual of neonatal care* (6th ed.). Philadelphia: Lippincott Williams & Wilkins.

D'Avanzo, C. E., & Geissler, E. M. (2008). *Pocket guide to cultural assessment* (4th ed.). St. Louis, MO: Mosby.

Galanti, G. A. (2004). *Caring for patients from different cultures* (3rd ed.). Philadelphia, PA: University of Pennsylvania Press.

Greer, F. R., Sicherer, S. H., Burks, W., & Committee on Nutrition and Section on Allergy and Immunology. (2008). Effects of early nutritional interventions on the development of atropic disease in infants and children: The role of maternal dietary restriction, breastfeeding, timing of introduction of complementary foods, and hydrolyzed formulas. *Pediatrics, 121*(1), 183–191.

Gregory, K. (2005). Update on nutrition for preterm and full-term infants. *Journal of Obstetric, Gynecologic, & Neonatal Nursing, 34*(1), 98–108.

Hale, T. W. (2006). *Medications and mothers' milk.* (12th ed.). Amarillo, TX: Pharmasoft Publishing.

Hedayat, K. M. (2001). Issues in Islamic biomedical ethics: A primer for the pediatrician. *Pediatrics, 108*(4), 965–991.

Hill, P. D., Wilhelm, P. A., Aldag, J. C., & Chatterton, R. T. (2004). Breast augmentation & lactation outcome: A case report. *American Journal of Maternal Child Nursing, 29*(4), 238–242.

Human Milk Banking Association of North America (HMBANA). (2005). *Best practice for expressing, storing and handling human milk in hospitals, homes and child care settings.* Raleigh, NC: Author.

International Lactation Consultant Association (ILCA) (2005). *Clinical guidelines for the* establishment of exclusive breastfeeding (2nd ed.). Raleigh, NC: Author. Retrieved April 20, 2008, from http://www.ilca.org/

Janke, J. (2008). Newborn nutrition. In K. R. Simpson & P. A. Creehan, *Perinatal nursing.* (3rd ed., pp. 582–611). Philadelphia: Lippincott Williams & Wilkins.

Katz, N., Levin, M. B., Cotton, J. M., Patrick-Miller, T. J., Tesoro, L. J., & Rose, H. M. (2007). *The pediatric group brochure on formula feeding: Formula feeding information.* Retrieved April 22, 2008, from http://www.pedgroup.com/frmlabrc.htm

Klaus, M. (1998). Mother and infant: Early emotional ties. *Pediatrics, 102*(5), 1244–1246.

Lawrence, R. A., & Lawrence, R. M. (2005). *Breastfeeding: A guide for the medical profession* (6th ed.). Philadelphia, PA: Mosby.

Lipson, J. G., & Dibble, S. L. (2008). Culture & Clinical Care. (7th ed.). San Francisco, CA: The Regents, University of California.

Marks, J. W. (2008). Lactose intolerance (lactase deficiency). (D. Lee, Ed.). *MedicineNet.com,* Retrieved June 22, 2008, from http://www.medicinenet.com/lactose_intolerance/article.htm

Mead-Johnson Nutritionals. (2004). *Pediatric products handbook.* New York: Bristol-Myers Squibb Company. Retrieved April 27, 2006, from http://www.meadjohnson.com

Mohrbacher, N., & Stock, J. (2003). *La Leche League International: The breastfeeding answer book* (3rd ed.). Schaumburg, IL: La Leche League International.

Moore, E. R., Anderson, G. C., & Bergman, N. (2007). Early skin-to-skin contact for mothers and their healthy newborn infants. [Cochrane Review]. In *Cochrane Database of Systemic Reviews,* 2007. Retrieved April 10, 2008, from The Cochrane Library, Wiley Interscience.

Morin, K. (2005). Information parents need about preparing formula. *The American Journal of Maternal/Child Nursing, 30*(5), 334.

Mulford, C. (1992). The mother-baby assessment (MBA): An "Apgar score" for breastfeeding. *Journal of Human Lactation, 8*(2), 79–82.

Neville, M. (1999). Physiology of lactation. In C. L. Wagner & D. M. Purohit (Eds.), *Clinics in perinatology: Clinical aspects of human milk and lactation* (pp. 251–279). Philadelphia: W.B. Saunders.

O'Brien, K. O., Zavaleta, N., Abrams, S. A., & Caulfield, L. E. (2003). Maternal iron status influences iron transfer to the fetus during the third trimester of pregnancy. *American Journal of Clinical Nutrition, 77*(4), 924–930.

Ott, B. B., Al-Khadhuri, J., & Al-Junaibi, S. (2003). Preventing ethical dilemmas: Understanding Islamic health care practices. *Pediatric Nursing, 29*(3), 227–230.

Renfrew, M. J., Ansell, P. L., & Macleod, K. L. (2003). Formula feed preparation: Helping reduce risks; a systematic review. *Archives of Diseases of Children, 88,* 855–858.

Riordan, J. (2005). *Breastfeeding and human lactation* (3rd ed.). Boston: Jones & Bartlett.

Rolfes, S. R., Pinna, K., & Whitney, E. (2006). *Understanding normal and clinical nutrition* (7th ed.). Belmont, CA: Thomson Wadsworth, a part of The Thomson Corporation.

Rojjanasrirat, W. (2004). Working women's breastfeeding experience. *MCN. American Journal of Maternal Child Nursing, 29*(4), 222–228.

Ross Products Division (2006, September). *Ross Infant Formula Applications: Prepared for Intermountain Healthcare Nutrition Departments Primary Children's Medical Center Salt Lake City, Utah.* Columbus, OH: Abbott.

Ross Products Division. (2007). *Pediatric nutritionals product guide.* Columbus, OH: Abbott

Schuman, J. (2003, February 1). A concise history of infant formula (twists and turns included). *Contemporary Pediatrics.* Retrieved October 4, 2005, from http://www.contemporarypediatrics.com/contpeds/article/articleDetail.jsp?id=111702

Sears, W. (2008). *A word about bottle-feeding.* Retrieved April 20, 2008, from http://www.askdrsears.com/html/0/T000100.asp#T031010

Skidmore-Roth, L. (2006). *Mosby's handbook of herbs and natural supplements.* (3rd ed.). St. Louis: Mosby.

Thureen, P. J., Deacon, J., Hernandez, J. A., & Hall, D. M. (2005). *Assessment and care of the well newborn* (2nd ed.). St. Louis: Elsevier-Saunders.

Vonlanthen, M. (1998). Lactose intolerance, diarrhea, and allergy. *Breastfeeding Abstracts, 18*(2), 11–12.

Wagner, C. L., Graham, E. M., & Hope, W. W. (2006). Counseling the breastfeeding mother. *e-Medicine.com., Inc.* Retrieved April 22, 2008, from http://www.emedicine.com/ped/topic2774.htm

World Health Organization/United Nations Children's Emergency Fund (WHO/UNICEF). (1994). *U.S. committee for UNICEF interim program in the United States to promote the Baby Friendly ten steps to successful breastfeeding.* Washington, DC: Government Printing Office.

CHAPTER 28

The Newborn at Risk: Conditions Present at Birth

When a newborn is admitted into my unit, and into my care, there is an initial flurry of activity where my entire universe, everything that I am, constricts down to focus on this one little being. Gradually, as the situation stabilizes, I become aware again of the other team members working in concert around me. And I am reassured that this new life is getting the very best care available.

—Neonatal Nurse Practitioner

LEARNING OUTCOMES

28-1. Explain the factors present at birth that indicate an at-risk newborn.

28-2. Compare the underlying etiologies of the physiologic complications of small-for-gestational-age (SGA) newborns and preterm appropriate-for-gestational-age (Pr AGA) newborns and the nursing care management for each.

28-3. Explain the impact that the common complications and clinical therapy of maternal diabetes mellitus has on the nursing care management of an infant of a diabetic mother.

28-4. Differentiate the characteristics, potential complications, and nursing care management of the postterm newborn and the newborn with postmaturity syndrome.

28-5. Compare the physiologic characteristics of the preterm newborn to the predisposition of each body system to various complications

28-6. Describe the nursing care management of the preterm newborn based on the physical and behavioral characteristics and gestational age of the preterm newborn.

28-7. Describe the steps and rationale for performing gavage feeding for the preterm newborn.

28-8. Compare selected congenital anomalies with the associated nursing assessment, goals, and interventions in the newborn period.

28-9. Explain the risks, abnormalities, complications, clinical therapy, and clinical manifestations of withdrawal for the infant of a substance-abusing mother in determining hospital and community-based nursing care management.

28-10. Explain the effects of maternal HIV/AIDS on the infant in the neonatal period and the issues for caregivers of infants at risk for HIV/AIDS in determining hospital-based and community-based nursing care management.

28-11. Compare the types of cardiac defects of the early newborn period with the clinical findings and medical/surgical management of each.

28-12. Explain the cause of and clinical therapy used to determine the nursing care management of newborns with an inborn error of metabolism.

The field of neonatology has expanded greatly. Many levels of nursery care have evolved in response to increasing knowledge about at-risk newborns: special care, intensive care, and convalescent or transitional care. Along with the newborn's parents, the nurse is an important caregiver in all these settings. As a member of the multidisciplinary healthcare team, the nurse is a technically competent professional who contributes the high-touch human care necessary in the high-tech perinatal environment.

In addition to the availability of a high level of newborn care, various other factors influence the outcome of at-risk infants, including the following:

- Birth weight
- Gestational age
- Type and length of newborn illness
- Environmental factors
- Maternal factors
- Maternal-infant separation

Identification of At-Risk Newborns

An at-risk newborn is one susceptible to illness (morbidity) or even death (mortality) because of dysmaturity, immaturity, physical disorders, or complications during or after birth. In most cases, the infant is the product of a pregnancy involving one or more predictable risk factors, including the following:

- Low socioeconomic level of the mother
- Limited access to health care or no prenatal care
- Exposure to environmental dangers, such as toxic chemicals and illicit drugs
- Preexisting maternal conditions such as heart disease, diabetes, hypertension, hyperthyroidism, and renal disease
- Maternal factors such as age and parity
- Medical conditions related to pregnancy and their associated complications
- Pregnancy complications such as abruptio placentae, oligohydramnios, preterm labor, premature rupture of membranes, preeclampsia

> ### EVIDENCE IN ACTION
> According to the American Academy of Pediatrics, Apgar scores that are low at 1 and 5 minutes are not definite indications of an acute intrapartum hypoxic event.
> (Policy statement) (Martin & Hankins, 2006)

Various risk factors and their specific effects on the pregnancy outcome are listed in Table 10–1 ∞. Because these factors and the perinatal risks associated with them are known, the birth of at-risk newborns can often be anticipated. The pregnancy can be closely monitored, treatment can be started as necessary, and arrangements can be made for birth to occur at a facility with appropriate resources to care for both mother and baby.

Whether or not prenatal assessment indicates that the fetus is at risk, the course of labor and birth and the infant's ability to withstand the stress of labor cannot be predicted. Thus, the nurse's use of electronic fetal heart monitoring or fetal heart auscultation by Doppler plays a significant role in detecting stress or distress in the fetus. Immediately after birth the Apgar score is a helpful tool for identifying the at-risk newborn, but it is not the only indicator of possible long-term outcome.

The newborn classification and neonatal mortality risk chart is another useful tool for identifying newborns at risk. Before this classification tool was developed, birth weight of less than 2500 g was the sole criterion for determining immaturity. Clinicians then recognized that a newborn could weigh more than 2500 g and still be immature. Conversely, an infant weighing less than 2500 g might be functionally at term or beyond. Thus birth weight and gestational age together are now the criteria used to assess neonatal maturity, morbidity, and mortality risk.

According to the newborn classification and neonatal mortality risk chart, gestation (postmenstrual age) is divided as follows:

- Preterm: less than 37 (completed) weeks
- Term: 37 to 41 6/7 (completed) weeks
- Postterm: greater than 42 weeks

Late preterm is an emerging classification that refers to subgroups of infants between 34 and 37 weeks' gestation; however, it is not yet used consistently for a single age range (Cloherty, Eichenwald, & Stark, 2008).

As shown in Figure 28–1 ■, large-for-gestational-age (LGA) newborns are those who plot above the 90th percentile curve on intrauterine growth curves. Appropriate-for-gestational-age (AGA) newborns are those that plot

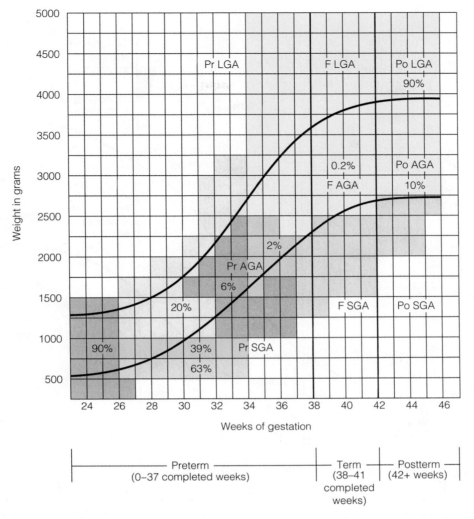

FIGURE 28–1 Newborn classification and neonatal mortality risk chart. Infants are classified according to weight as small for gestational age (SGA), appropriate for gestational age (AGA), or large for gestational age (LGA) and by weeks of newborn as preterm (Pr), term (F), or postterm (Po). Corresponding neonatal mortality risks are indicated by the percentage in the various colored regions.

Source: Koops, B. L., Morgan, L. P., & Battaglia, F. C. (1982). Neonatal mortality risk in relationship to birth weight and gestational age. *Journal of Pediatrics, 101(6),* 969.

between the 10th percentile and 90th percentile growth curves. Small-for-gestational-age (SGA) newborns are those that plot below the 10th percentile growth curve. A newborn is assigned to a category depending on birth weight, length, occipital-frontal head circumference, and gestational age. For example, a newborn classified as Pr SGA is preterm and small for gestational age. The full-term newborn whose weight is appropriate for gestational age is classified F AGA. It is important to note that intrauterine growth charts are influenced by altitude and the ethnicity of the newborn population used to create the chart. Also, the assigned newborn classification may vary according to the intrauterine growth curve chart used; therefore, the chart used should correlate with the characteristics of the client population.

Neonatal mortality risk is the infant's chance of death within the newborn period—that is, within the first 28 days

of life. As indicated in Figure 28–1 ■, the neonatal mortality risk decreases as both gestational age and birth weight increase. Infants who are preterm and small for gestational age have the highest neonatal mortality risk. The previously high mortality rates for LGA newborns have decreased at most perinatal centers because of both improved management of diabetes in pregnancy and increased recognition of potential complications of LGA newborns.

Neonatal morbidity can be anticipated based on birth weight and gestational age. In Figure 28–2 ■, the infant's birth weight is located on the vertical axis, and the gestational age in weeks is found along the horizontal axis. The area where the two meet on the graph identifies common problems. This tool assists in determining the needs of particular infants for special observation and care. For example, an infant of 2000 g at 40 weeks' gestation should be carefully assessed for evidence of

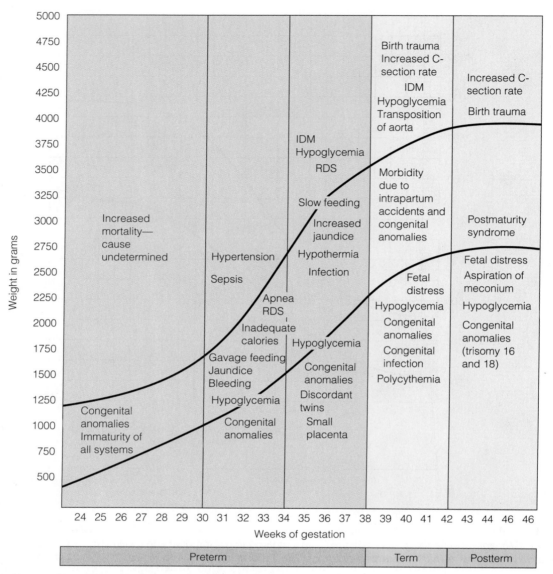

FIGURE 28–2 Neonatal morbidity by birth weight and gestational age.
Source: Lubchenco, L. O. (1976). *The high-risk infant* (p. 122). Philadelphia: Saunders.

neonatal distress, hypoglycemia, congenital anomalies, congenital infection, and polycythemia.

Identifying the nursing care needs of the at-risk newborn depends on minute-to-minute observations of the changes in the newborn's physiologic status. The organization of nursing care must be directed toward the following:

- Decreasing physiologically stressful situations
- Constantly observing for subtle signs of change in clinical condition
- Interpreting laboratory data and coordinating interventions
- Conserving the infant's energy for healing and growth
- Providing for developmental stimulation and maintenance of sleep cycles
- Assisting the family in developing attachment behaviors
- Involving the family in planning and providing care

Care of the Small-for-Gestational-Age/Intrauterine Growth Restriction Newborn

Currently infants are considered **small for gestational age (SGA)** when they are less than the 10th percentile for birth weight; very small for gestational age is when they are two standard deviations below the population norm or less than the third percentile (Baschat, Galan, Ross, & Gabbe, 2007) (Figure 28–3 ■). When possible, the birth weight charts used to assign the SGA classification to a newborn should be based on the local population into which the newborn is born (Baschat et al., 2007). A SGA newborn may be preterm, term, or postterm. An undergrown newborn may also be said to have **intrauterine growth restriction (IUGR)**, which describes pregnancy

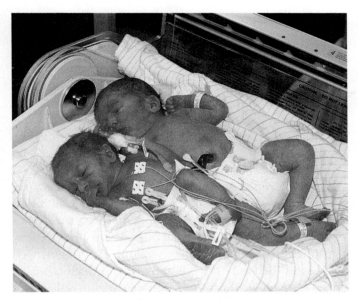

FIGURE 28-3 Thirty-five-week gestational age twins. Twin B (on left) is SGA and weighs 1260 g and twin A (on right) is AGA and weighs 2605 g.
Source: Courtesy of Carol Harrigan, RNC, MSN, NNP.

circumstances of advanced gestation and limited fetal growth. This classification of abnormal growth is also enhanced by looking at growth potential by adjusting birth-weight reference limits for first trimester maternal height, birth order, and sex. The terms *SGA* and *IUGR* are not necessarily interchangeable.

SGA infants are commonly seen with mothers who smoke or have high blood pressure, causing these infants to have an increased incidence of perinatal asphyxia and perinatal mortality when compared with AGA infants (Baschat et al., 2007). The incidence of polycythemia and hypoglycemia is also higher in this group of infants.

Factors Contributing to IUGR

IUGR may be caused by maternal, placental, or fetal factors and may not be apparent antenatally. Intrauterine growth is linear in the normal pregnancy from approximately 28 to 38 weeks' gestation. After 38 weeks, growth is variable, depending on the growth potential of the fetus and placental function (Baschat et al., 2007). The most common causes of growth restriction are as follows:

- *Maternal factors.* Primiparity, grand multiparity, multiple-gestation pregnancy (twins and higher-order multiples), lack of prenatal care, age extremes (< 16 years or > 40 years), and low socioeconomic status (which can result in inadequate health care, inadequate education, and inadequate living conditions) affect IUGR (Baschat et al., 2007). Before the third trimester, the nutritional supply to the fetus far exceeds its needs. Only in the third trimester are ma-

ternal malnutrition and drug abuse limiting factors in fetal growth.
- *Maternal disease.* Maternal heart disease, substance abuse (drugs, tobacco, alcohol), sickle cell anemia, phenylketonuria (PKU), lupus erythematosis, and asymptomatic pyelonephritis are associated with SGA. Complications associated with preeclampsia, chronic hypertensive vascular disease, and advanced diabetes mellitus can diminish blood flow to the uterus, thereby decreasing oxygen delivery to the fetus.
- *Environmental factors.* High altitude, exposure to X-rays, excessive exercise, work-related exposure to toxins, hyperthermia, and maternal use of drugs that have teratogenic effects, such as nicotine, alcohol, antimetabolites, anticonvulsants, narcotics, and cocaine, affect fetal growth (Baschat et al., 2007).
- *Placental factors.* Placental conditions such as small placenta, infarcted areas, abnormal cord insertions, placenta previa, and thrombosis may affect circulation to the fetus, which becomes more deficient with increasing gestational age.
- *Fetal factors.* Congenital infections such as TORCH infections (*t*oxoplasmosis, *o*ther, *r*ubella, *c*ytomegalovirus *h*erpes simplex virus), syphilis, congenital malformations, discordant twins (see Chapter 4 ∞), sex of the fetus (females tend to be smaller), chromosomal syndromes (trisomies 13, 18, 21), two vessel umbilical cord, and inborn errors of metabolism can predispose a fetus to fetal growth disturbances.

Identifying fetuses with IUGR is the first step in detecting common disorders associated with affected newborns. The perinatal history of maternal conditions, early dating of pregnancy by first-trimester ultrasound measurements, antepartal testing (nonstress test, contraction stress test, biophysical profile (see Chapter 14 ∞), Doppler velocimetry of placenta, gestational age assessment, and the physical and neurologic assessment of the newborn are also important (Cloherty et al., 2008).

HINTS FOR PRACTICE

In assessing a growth-restricted infant resulting from unexplained maternal etiology (e.g., hypertension, placental insufficiency), an in utero viral infection may be the cause.

Patterns of IUGR

Intrauterine growth occurs by an increase in both cell number and cell size. If insult occurs early during the critical period of organ development in the fetus, fewer new cells are formed, organs are small, and organ weight is subnormal. In contrast, growth failure that begins later in pregnancy does not affect the total number of cells, only their size. The organs are normal, but their size is diminished. There are two clinical pictures of IUGR newborns:

- *Symmetric (proportional) IUGR* is caused by long-term maternal conditions (such as chronic hypertension, severe malnutrition, chronic intrauterine viral infection, substance abuse [drugs, alcohol, tobacco], anemia) or fetal genetic abnormalities (Baschat et al., 2007). Symmetric IUGR can be noted by ultrasound in the first half of the second trimester. In symmetric IUGR there is chronic, prolonged restriction of growth in the size of organs, weight, length, and, especially, head circumference.

- *Asymmetric (disproportional) IUGR* is associated with an acute compromise of uteroplacental blood flow. Some associated causes are placental infarcts, preeclampsia, and poor weight gain in pregnancy. The growth restriction is usually not evident before the third trimester because, although weight is decreased, length and head circumference (used as a growth indicator) remain appropriate for that gestational age. After 36 weeks' gestation, the abdominal circumference of a normal fetus becomes larger than the head circumference. In asymmetric IUGR, the head circumference remains larger than the abdominal circumference. Thus measuring only the biparietal diameter on ultrasound will not reveal asymmetric IUGR. An early indicator of asymmetric SGA is a decrease in the growth rate of the abdominal circumference, reflecting subnormal liver growth, a reduction in glycogen stores, and a scarcity of subcutaneous fat (Baschat et al., 2007). Birth weight is below the 10th percentile, whereas head circumference and/or length may be between the 10th and 90th percentiles. Asymmetric SGA newborns are particularly at risk for asphyxia, pulmonary hemorrhage, hypocalcemia, and hypoglycemia in the newborn period.

Despite growth restriction, physiologic maturity develops according to gestational age. The SGA newborn's chances for survival are better than those of the preterm AGA newborn because of organ maturity, although this newborn still faces many potential difficulties.

Common Complications of the SGA Newborn

The complications occurring most frequently in the SGA newborn include the following:

- *Asphyxia.* The SGA newborn suffers chronic hypoxia in utero, which leaves little reserve to withstand the demands of normal labor and birth. Thus, intrauterine asphyxia, and its potential systemic problems, can occur. Cesarean birth may be necessary.

- *Aspiration syndrome.* In utero hypoxia can cause the fetus to gasp during birth, resulting in aspiration of amniotic fluid into the lower airways. It can also lead to relaxation of the anal sphincter and passage of meconium. This may result in aspiration of the meconium in utero or with the first breaths after birth.

- *Hypothermia.* Diminished subcutaneous fat (used for survival in utero), depletion of brown fat in utero, and a large surface area decrease the IUGR newborn's ability to conserve heat. The flexed position assumed by the term SGA newborn diminishes the effect of surface area.

- *Hypoglycemia.* An increase in metabolic rate in response to heat loss and poor hepatic glycogen stores causes hypoglycemia. In addition, the newborn is compromised by inadequate supplies of enzymes to activate gluconeogenesis (conversion of nonglucogen sources such as fatty acids and proteins to glucose).

- *Polycythemia.* The number of red blood cells is increased in the SGA newborn. This finding is considered a physiologic response to in utero chronic hypoxic stress. Polycythemia may contribute to hypoglycemia.

Newborns who have significant IUGR tend to have a poor prognosis, especially when born before 37 weeks' gestation. Factors contributing to poor outcome include the following:

- *Congenital malformations.* Congenital malformations occur in 5% of SGA infants (Cloherty et al., 2008). The more severe the IUGR, the greater the chance for malformation as a result of impaired mitotic activity and cellular hypoplasia.

- *Intrauterine infections.* When fetuses are exposed to intrauterine infections such as rubella and cytomegalovirus, they are profoundly affected by direct invasion of the brain and other vital organs by the offending virus, resulting in IUGR.

- *Continued growth difficulties.* SGA newborns tend to be shorter than newborns of the same gestational age. Asymmetric IUGR infants can be expected to catch up in weight and approach their inherited growth potential when given an optimal environment. Symmetric IUGR infants reportedly have varied growth potential but tend not to catch up to their peers (Baschat et al., 2007).

- *Cognitive difficulties.* Often SGA newborns can exhibit subsequent learning disabilities. The disabilities are characterized by hyperactivity, short attention span, and poor fine motor coordination (writing and drawing). Some hearing loss and speech defects also occur (Kahn, Hobbins, & Galan, 2008).

Clinical Therapy

The goal of medical therapy for SGA infants is early recognition and implementation of the medical management of potential problems.

Nursing Care Management

Nursing Assessment and Diagnosis

The nurse is responsible for assessing gestational age and identifying signs of potential complications associated with SGA infants. All body parts of the symmetric IUGR infant are in proportion, but they are below normal size for the baby's gestational age. Therefore the head does not appear overly large or the length excessive in relation to the other body parts. These newborns are generally vigorous.

The asymmetric IUGR infant appears long, thin, and emaciated, with loss of subcutaneous fat tissue and muscle mass. The baby may have loose skin folds; dry, desquamating skin; and a thin and often meconium-stained cord. The head appears relatively large (although it approaches normal size) because the chest size and abdominal girth are decreased. The baby may have a vigorous cry and appear alert and wide-eyed.

Nursing diagnoses that may apply to the SGA newborn include the following:

- *Impaired Gas Exchange* related to aspiration of meconium
- *Hypothermia* related to decreased subcutaneous fat
- *Risk for Injury to Tissues* related to decreased glycogen stores and impaired gluconeogenesis
- *Risk for Altered Tissue Perfusion* related to increased blood viscosity
- *Altered Nutrition: Less than Body Requirements* related to SGA's increased metabolic rate
- *Risk for Altered Parenting* related to prolonged separation of newborn from parents secondary to illness

Nursing Plan and Implementation

Hospital-Based Nursing Care

Hypoglycemia, the most common metabolic complication of IUGR, produces such sequelae as CNS abnormalities and mental retardation. Conditions such as asphyxia, hyperviscosity, and cold stress may also affect the baby's outcome. Meticulous attention to physiologic parameters is essential for immediate nursing management and reduction of long-term disorders. (See Nursing Care Plan for a Small-for-Gestational-Age Newborn on pages 702–703.)

Community-Based Nursing Care

The long-term needs of the SGA newborn include careful follow-up evaluation of patterns of growth and possible disabilities that may later interfere with learning or motor functioning. Long-term follow-up care is essential for infants with congenital malformations, congenital infections, and obvious sequelae from physiologic problems.

Parents of the IUGR newborn need support, because a positive atmosphere can enhance the baby's growth potential and the child's ultimate outcome.

Evaluation

Expected outcomes of nursing care include the following:

- The SGA newborn is free from respiratory compromise.
- The SGA newborn maintains a stable temperature.
- The SGA infant is free from hypoglycemic episodes and maintains glucose homeostasis.
- The SGA newborn gains weight and takes breast or formula feedings without developing physiologic distress or fatigue.
- The parents verbalize their concerns about their baby's health problems and understand the rationale behind management of their newborn.

Care of the Large-for-Gestational-Age (LGA) Newborn

A newborn whose birth weight is at or above the 90th percentile on the intrauterine growth curve (at any week of gestation) is considered **large for gestational age (LGA)**. Some AGA newborns have been incorrectly categorized as LGA because of miscalculation of the date of conception caused by postconceptual bleeding. Careful gestational age assessment is essential to identify the potential needs and problems of these infants.

The most well-known condition associated with excessive fetal growth is maternal diabetes (White's classes A to C; see Table 15–4 ∞); however, only a small fraction of large newborns are born to diabetic mothers. The cause of the majority of cases of LGA newborns is unclear, but certain factors or situations have been found to correlate with their birth (Cloherty et al., 2008):

- Genetic predisposition is correlated proportionately to the mother's prepregnancy weight and to weight gain during pregnancy. Large parents tend to have large infants.
- Multiparous women have two to three times the number of LGA infants as primigravidas.
- Male infants are typically larger than female infants.
- Infants with erythroblastosis fetalis, Beckwith-Wiedemann syndrome (a genetic condition associated with omphalocele and neonatal hypoglycemia and hyperinsulinemia), or transposition of the great vessels are usually large.

The increase in the LGA infant's body size is characteristically proportional, although head circumference and

(Continued on page 704)

Nursing Care Plan | For a Small-for-Gestational-Age Newborn

CLIENT SCENARIO

Ellen, a term baby, was born 8 hours ago weighing 2500 g at 40 weeks' gestation. Two hours after birth Ellen's temperature was 37.1°C (98.8°F) under the radiant warmer. She was swaddled and placed in an open crib. One hour later Ellen returns to the radiant warmer with a falling temperature reading of 36.1°C (97°F). Acrocyanosis has also been detected. Glucose levels are 35 mg/dL. The nurse monitors the newborn for signs of hypothermia and hypoglycemia.

ASSESSMENT

Subjective: Alert and active.

Objective: 40 weeks' gestation, birth weight 2500 g, length 48.3 cm (19 in.), head circumference 30 cm (11.8 in.), chest circumference 28 cm (11 in.), temperature 36.1°C (97°F) axillary, pulse 140, respirations 45, vigorous cry, alert, wide-eyed, dry skin, thin meconium-stained umbilical cord, glucose level 35 mg/dL, and tremors.

Nursing Diagnosis #1	Hypothermia related to decrease in subcutaneous fat tissue and increased body surface exposure to environment.*
Client Goal	The newborn will maintain stable body temperature within normal range of 36.5°C to 37.4°C (97.7°F to 99.4°F) in an open crib.
AEB:	• Temperature is within normal limits in open crib. • No signs of acrocyanosis, mottling, or lethargy are present.

NURSING INTERVENTIONS

1. Monitor axillary temperature every 4 hours and PRN.

2. Monitor pulse and respirations every 4 hours and PRN.

3. Assess skin color and temperature every 15 to 30 minutes in presence of color change.

4. Place newborn under radiant warmer if temperature falls below 36.5°C (97.7°F).

5. Place newborn in incubator if temperature is unstable.

6. Initiate frequent feeding as tolerated.

RATIONALES

Rationale: The ability of the SGA newborn to conserve heat is compromised by the following: diminished subcutaneous fat, a depletion of brown fat in utero, and a large body surface area.

Rationale: Oxygen requirements increase because of the metabolic consequences of hypothermia. Therefore pulse and respirations will be elevated. Quick identification of alterations in pulse and respirations will allow for immediate treatment.

Rationale: Pallor, acrocyanosis, and mottling of skin may be indicative of hypothermia. If skin temperature is not increasing then more drastic measures can be implemented.

Rationale: Place a skin probe on the abdomen and adjust to maintain a neutral thermal environment. This will allow the newborn to warm up slowly. Check axillary temperature to make sure that the machine is accurately recording the newborn's temperature. Rapid temperature elevation may cause hypotension and apnea.

Rationale: To help stabilize newborn's temperature and maintain a neutral thermal environment by initiating efforts to reduce heat loss through evaporation, radiation, convection, and conduction. Adjust incubator for newborn size and gestation to maintain a neutral thermal environment.

Rationale: Small frequent feedings of high-calorie formula are used with SGA infants because of their limited gastric capacity and decreased gastric emptying. Providing nutrition through frequent feedings will help to increase body weight, increase subcutaneous fat, and provide glucose for energy to maintain body temperature.

Evaluation of Client Goal	• Temperature remains between 36.5°C and 37.4°C (97.7°F and 99.4°F) in open crib. • Skin pink in color with no signs of acrocyanosis or mottling.
Nursing Diagnosis #2	Imbalanced Nutrition: Less than Body Requirements related to increased glucose consumption secondary to metabolic effects of hypothermia and poor hepatic glycogen stores.
Client Goal	The newborn will maintain a glucose level above 45 mg/dL.
AEB:	• Glucose level remains above 45 mg/dL. • Weight will remain stable. • No signs of jitteriness or tremors are present.

Nursing Care Plan   For a Small-for-Gestational-Age Newborn *(Continued)*

NURSING INTERVENTIONS

1. Initiate early feedings.

2. Monitor glucose levels every 4 hours.

3. Monitor for signs of hypoglycemia.

4. Encourage on-demand feeding at least every 3 to 4 hours.

5. Offer supplemental feedings or additional glucose.

6. Maintain a neutral thermal environment.

RATIONALES

Rationale: Early feedings will help prevent a drop in blood glucose levels. If early formula and/or breastfeedings are initiated, and the feedings meet the fluid and caloric intake, the blood glucose concentration is likely to remain above hypoglycemic levels.

Rationale: Early identification of low blood glucose levels allows for immediate intervention and may minimize hypoglycemic effects on the newborn. Hypoglycemia is a result of increased utilization of glucose caused by increased oxygen consumption of the newborn, resulting in an increased metabolic rate caused by hypoglycemia.

Rationale: Glucose levels below 40 mg/dL may result in hypoglycemia. Signs and symptoms of hypoglycemia include lethargy, jitteriness, poor feeding, vomiting, pallor, apnea, hypothermia, irregular respirations, respiratory distress, tremors, seizure activity, jerkiness, and a high-pitched cry.

Rationale: Feeding the newborn at least every 3 to 4 hours will help the infant maintain glucose levels and help stabilize or regain lost weight.

Rationale: To prevent weight loss and prevent hypoglycemia. Small frequent feedings, high-calorie formula, or nutritional fortifiers may be added per physician orders to increase glucose and calorie intake.

Rationale: To meet the required energy needs of the newborn the metabolic rate will increase which in turn increases oxygen consumption and the utilization of glucose. This may result in hypoglycemia. Maintaining a neutral thermal environment will allow the newborn to conserve energy and maintain a normal glucose level thereby stabilizing weight.

Evaluation of Client Goal	• Glucose level remains above 45 mg/dL. • Weight is stabilized. • No signs of jitteriness or tremors are present.

CRITICAL THINKING QUESTIONS

1. What can the nurse do to prevent heat loss through convection when preparing the newborn for the open crib?

Answer: Wrap the newborn in a prewarmed blanket and place a stockinette hat on the newborn's head. A prewarmed blanket and stockinette hat will reduce heat loss through convection and assist the newborn to maintain body temperature. When newborns become chilled they increase their oxygen consumption and use glucose for physiologic processes.

2. What measure can the nurse take to reduce heat loss through evaporation and conduction? How many calories can a small infant lose through radiation?

Answer: To prevent heat loss through evaporation the nurse dries the newborn completely after birth and after the

bath. Wet linens are replaced with dry linens. To prevent heat loss through conduction the nurse warms any surfaces that come in contact with the newborn such as a cold X-ray plate, stethoscope, and scale. A small infant can lose 80 kcal/kg/day through radiation of body heat.

3. A mother of an SGA newborn asks the nurse when she should expect her infant to catch up in weight to normal-growth infants. What is the nurse's best response?

Answer: The nurse responds to the mother by explaining that a varied growth potential may be seen with the symmetric SGA infant but these infants tend not to catch up to their peers. Asymmetric IUGR infants can be expected to catch up in weight to normal infants by 3 to 6 months of age.

*For your reference, this care plan provides an example of how two nursing diagnoses might be addressed.

body length are in the upper limits of intrauterine growth. The exception to this rule is the infant of the diabetic mother, whose body weight increases while length and head circumference may remain in the normal range. Macrosomic infants have poor motor skills and have difficulty in regulating behavioral states. LGA infants tend to be more difficult to arouse to a quiet alert state. They may also have feeding difficulties.

Common Complications of the LGA Newborn

Complications of the LGA newborn can include the following:

- *Birth trauma caused by cephalopelvic disproportion (CPD).* Often LGA newborns have a biparietal diameter greater than 10 cm (4 in.) or are associated with a maternal fundal height measurement greater than 42 cm (16 in.) without the presence of polyhydramnios. Because of their excessive size, there are more breech presentations and shoulder dystocia. These complications may result in asphyxia, fractured clavicles, brachial palsy, facial paralysis, phrenic nerve palsy, depressed skull fractures, cephalhematoma, and intracranial hemorrhage caused by birth trauma.
- *Increased incidence of cesarean births and oxytocin-induced births* because of fetal size. Mothers and infants have all the risk factors associated with cesarean births.
- *Hypoglycemia, polycythemia, and hyperviscosity.* These disorders are most often seen in infants of diabetic mothers, infants with erythroblastosis fetalis, or infants with Beckwith-Wiedemann syndrome.

Nursing Care Management

The perinatal history, in conjunction with ultrasonic measurement of fetal skull (biparietal diameter) and gestational age testing, is important in identifying an at-risk LGA newborn. Nursing care is directed toward early identification and immediate treatment of the common disorders. Essential components of the nursing assessment are monitoring vital signs, screening for hypoglycemia and polycythemia, and observing for signs and symptoms related to birth trauma. The nurse should address parental concerns about the visual signs of birth trauma and the potential for continuation of the overweight pattern. The nurse helps parents learn to arouse and console their newborn and facilitate attachment behaviors. Mothers of LGA infants with facial or head bruising may be reluctant to interact with their newborns because they fear hurting their infants. The nursing care involved in the complications associated with LGA newborns is similar to the care needed by the infant of a diabetic mother and is discussed in the next section.

Care of the Infant of a Diabetic Mother

The **infant of a diabetic mother (IDM)** is considered at risk and requires close observation during the first few hours to the first few days of life. Mothers with severe diabetes or diabetes of long duration associated with vascular complications may give birth to SGA infants. However, the typical IDM, when the diabetes is poorly controlled or gestational, is LGA. The infant is macrosomic, ruddy in color, and has excessive adipose (fat) tissue (Figure 28–4 ■). The umbilical cord is thick and the placenta is large. There is a higher incidence of macrosomic infants born to certain ethnic groups (Native Americans, Mexican Americans, African Americans, Pacific Islanders).

IDMs have decreased total body water, particularly in the extracellular spaces, and are therefore not edematous. Their excessive weight is because of increased weight of the visceral organs, cardiomegaly (hypertrophy), and increased body fat. The only organ not affected is the brain.

The excessive fetal growth of the IDM is caused by exposure to high levels of maternal glucose, which readily crosses the placenta. The fetus responds to these high glucose levels with increased insulin production and hyperplasia of the pancreatic beta cells. The main action of the insulin is to facilitate the entry of glucose into muscle and fat cells. Once in the cells, glucose is converted to glycogen and stored. Insulin also inhibits the breakdown of fat to free fatty acids, thereby maintaining lipid synthesis; increases the uptake of amino acids; and promotes protein synthesis. Insulin is an important regulator of fetal metabolism and has a "growth hormone" effect that results in increased linear growth. Infants of diabetic mothers may be obese as children (Landon, Catalano, & Gabbe, 2008).

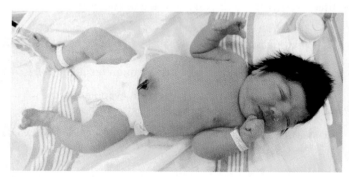

FIGURE 28–4 Macrosomic infant of a Class B insulin-dependent diabetic mother born at 38 weeks' gestation weighing 3402 grams.
Source: Courtesy of Carol Harrigan, RNC, MSN, NNP.

Common Complications of the IDM

Although IDMs are usually large, they have immature physiologic functions and exhibit many of the problems of the preterm (premature) infant. The complications most often seen in an IDM are as follows:

- *Hypoglycemia.* Hypoglycemia is defined as a blood sugar less than 40 mg/dL. Even though the high maternal blood supply is lost, the IDM continues to produce high levels of insulin, which deplete the infant's blood glucose within hours after birth. IDMs also have less ability to release glucagon and catecholamines, which normally stimulate glucagon breakdown and glucose release. The incidence of hypoglycemia in IDMs varies according to the degree of success in controlling the maternal diabetes, the maternal blood sugar level at the time of birth, the length of labor, the class of maternal diabetes, and early versus late feedings of the newborn. Signs and symptoms of hypoglycemia include tremors, cyanosis, apnea, temperature instability, poor feeding, and hypotonia. Seizures may occur in severe cases.

HINTS FOR PRACTICE

When beginning fluids on an IDM, it is sometimes best to start at a higher concentration of dextrose to avoid hypoglycemia episodes.

- *Hypocalcemia.* Tremors are the obvious clinical sign of hypocalcemia. They may be caused by the IDM's increased incidence of prematurity and by the stresses of difficult pregnancy, labor, and birth. Diabetic women tend to have decreased serum magnesium levels at term secondary to increased urinary calcium excretion, which causes secondary hypoparathyroidism in their infants. Other factors may include vitamin D antagonism, which results from elevated cortisol levels, hypophosphatemia from tissue catabolism, and decreased serum magnesium levels.
- *Hyperbilirubinemia.* This condition may be seen at 48 to 72 hours after birth. It may be caused by slightly decreased extracellular fluid volume, which increases the hematocrit level. This elevation facilitates an increase in red blood cell breakdown thereby increasing bilirubin levels. The presence of hepatic immaturity may impair bilirubin conjugation. Enclosed hemorrhages resulting from complicated vaginal birth may also cause hyperbilirubinemia.
- *Birth trauma.* Because most IDMs are macrosomic, trauma may occur during labor and birth from shoulder dystocia.
- *Polycythemia.* Fetal hyperglycemia and hyperinsulinism result in increased oxygen consumption, which

can lead to fetal hypoxia (Landon et al., 2008). Hemoglobin A_{1c} binds to oxygen, decreasing the oxygen available to the fetal tissues. This tissue hypoxia stimulates increased erythropoietin production, which increases both the hematocrit level and the potential for hyperbilirubinemia. See Chapter 15 ∞ for discussion of hemoglobin A_{1c}.

- *Respiratory distress syndrome (RDS).* This complication occurs especially in newborns of diabetic mothers in White's classes A to C who are not well controlled (Cloherty et al., 2008). Insulin antagonizes the cortisol-induced stimulation of lecithin synthesis that is necessary for lung maturation. Therefore, IDMs may have less mature lungs than expected for their gestational age. There is also a decrease in the phospholipid phosphatidylglycerol (PG), which stabilizes surfactant. The insufficiency of PG increases the incidence of RDS. Therefore, it is important to test for the presence of PG in the amniotic fluid before birth.

  RDS does not appear to be a problem for infants born of diabetic mothers in White's classes D to F; instead, the stresses of poor uterine blood supply may lead to increased production of steroids, which accelerates lung maturation. IDMs may also have a delay in closure of the ductus arteriosus and decreases in postnatal pulmonary artery pressure (Cloherty et al., 2008).

- *Congenital birth defects.* These may include congenital heart defects (transposition of the great vessels, ventricular septal defect, patent ductus arteriosus), small left colon syndrome, renal anomalies, neural tube defects, and sacral agenesis (caudal regression) (Cloherty et al., 2008). Early close control of maternal glucose levels before and during pregnancy decreases the risk of birth defects. See Chapter 15 ∞ .

Clinical Therapy

Prenatal management is directed toward controlling maternal glucose levels, which minimizes the common complications of IDMs. Because the onset of hypoglycemia occurs between 1 and 3 hours after birth in IDMs (with a spontaneous rise to normal levels by 4 to 6 hours), blood glucose determinations should be done on cord blood or by heel stick hourly during the first 4 hours after birth and then at 4-hour intervals until the risk period (about 48 hours) has passed or per agency protocol.

IDMs whose serum glucose level falls below 40 mg/dL should have early feedings with formula or breast milk (colostrum). If normal glucose levels cannot be maintained with oral feedings an intravenous (IV) infusion of glucose will be necessary. An infusion of $D_{10}W$ usually maintains normoglycemia in the IDM. If higher glucose concentrations are needed to maintain normal serum glucose levels, a central line will be placed to minimize tissue extravasation.

Newborns with refractory hypoglycemia may benefit from the administration of intravenous corticosteroids. Once the blood glucose level has been stable for 24 hours, the infusion rate can be decreased as oral feedings are increased. The newborn's blood glucose levels must be carefully monitored. Repeat dextrose as bolus infusion is contraindicated because it may lead to severe rebound hypoglycemia following an initial brief increase in glucose level.

Nursing Care Management

Nursing Assessment and Diagnosis

The nurse should not be lulled into thinking that a big baby is a mature baby. In almost every case, because of the infant's large size, the IDM will appear older than gestational age scoring indicates. The nurse must consider both the gestational age and whether the baby is AGA or LGA in planning and providing safe care. In caring for the IDM, the nurse assesses for signs of respiratory distress, hyperbilirubinemia, birth trauma, and congenital anomalies.

Nursing diagnoses that may apply to IDMs include the following:

- *Altered Nutrition: Less than Body Requirements* related to increased glucose metabolism secondary to hyperinsulinemia
- *Impaired Gas Exchange* related to respiratory distress secondary to impaired production of surfactant
- *Alteration in Calcium Homeostasis* related to inappropriate parathyroid response
- *Increased Incidence of Congenital Anomalies* related to poor maternal metabolic control
- *Ineffective Family Coping: Compromise* related to the illness of the baby

Nursing Plan and Implementation

Nursing care of the IDM is directed toward early detection and ongoing monitoring of hypoglycemia (by performing glucose tests) and polycythemia (by obtaining central hematocrits), RDS, and hyperbilirubinemia. (These conditions are presented in Chapter 29 ∞.) The nurse also assesses for signs of birth trauma and congenital anomalies.

Parent teaching is directed toward preventing macrosomia and the resulting fetal-neonatal problems by instituting early and ongoing diabetic control. Parents are advised that with early identification and care, most IDMs' neonatal problems have no significant sequelae.

Evaluation

Expected outcomes of nursing care include the following:

- The IDM's respiratory distress and metabolic problems are minimized.

- The parents understand the effects of maternal diabetes on the baby's health and preventive steps they can initiate to decrease its impact on subsequent pregnancies.
- The parents verbalize their concerns about their baby's health problems and understand the rationale behind management of their newborn.

Care of the Postterm Newborn

The **postterm newborn** is any newborn born after 42 completed weeks of gestation. Postterm or prolonged pregnancy occurs in less than 12% of all pregnancies (Cloherty et al., 2008). The cause of postterm pregnancy is not completely understood, but several factors are known to be associated with it. (See Chapter 21 ∞ for discussion of maternal factors.) Many pregnancies classified as prolonged are thought to be a result of inaccurate estimates of date of birth (EDB). Postterm pregnancy is more common in Australian, Greek, and Italian ethnic groups.

Most babies born as a result of prolonged pregnancy are of normal size and health; some continue growing and are over 4000 g at birth, which supports the contention that the postterm fetus can remain well nourished. Potential intrapartal problems for these healthy but large fetuses are cephalopelvic disproportion (CPD) and shoulder dystocia. See Chapter 22 ∞ for discussion of the necessary assessments and interventions for CPD and shoulder dystocia.

Common Complications of the Newborn with Postmaturity Syndrome

The term **postmaturity** applies only to the infant who is born after 42 completed weeks of gestation and also demonstrates characteristics of *postmaturity syndrome*. Only about 5% of postterm newborns show signs of postmaturity syndrome.

The truly postmature newborn is at high risk for morbidity and has a mortality rate two to three times greater than that of term infants. Although today the percentages are extremely low, the majority of postmature fetal deaths occur during labor, because the fetus uses up necessary body reserves.

Postmaturity syndrome is characterized by decreased placental function, which impairs nutrition transport and oxygenation, leaving the fetus prone to hypoglycemia and asphyxia when the stresses of labor begin. The following are common disorders of the postmature newborn:

- Hypoglycemia, from nutritional deprivation and depleted glycogen stores

- Meconium aspiration in response to in utero hypoxia (The presence of oligohydramnios increases the danger of aspirating thick meconium. Severe meconium aspiration syndrome increases the baby's chance of developing persistent pulmonary hypertension, pneumothorax, and pneumonia. See detailed discussion of meconium aspiration in Chapter 29 ∞.)
- Polycythemia caused by increased production of red blood cells (RBCs) in response to hypoxia
- Congenital anomalies of unknown cause
- Seizure activity because of hypoxic insult
- Cold stress because of loss or poor development of subcutaneous fat

The long-term effects of postmaturity syndrome are unclear. At present, studies do not agree on the effect of postmaturity syndrome on weight gain and IQ scores (Divon, 2007).

Prolonged pregnancy itself is not solely responsible for the postmaturity syndrome. The characteristics of postmature newborns are primarily caused by a combination of advanced gestational age, placental aging and subsequent insufficiency, and continued exposure to amniotic fluid.

Clinical Therapy

The aim of antenatal management is to differentiate the fetus who has postmaturity syndrome from the fetus who at birth is large, well nourished, alert, and tolerating the prolonged (postterm) pregnancy. Antenatal tests that are done to evaluate fetal status and determine obstetric management and their use in postterm pregnancy are discussed in more depth in Chapters 15 and 21 ∞. If the amniotic fluid is meconium stained, an amnioinfusion may be done during labor. This procedure dilutes the meconium by directly infusing either normal saline or Ringer's lactate into the uterus, decreasing the risk of meconium aspiration syndrome. (For detailed discussion of clinical management and care of the newborn at risk for meconium aspiration, see Chapter 29 ∞.)

Hypoglycemia is monitored by serial glucose determinations per agency protocols. The baby may be placed on glucose infusions or given early feedings if respiratory distress is not present, but these measures must be instituted with caution because of the frequency of asphyxia in the first 24 hours. Postmature newborns are often voracious eaters.

For the SGA infant who is postmature, peripheral and central hematocrits are tested to determine the presence of polycythemia. Fluid resuscitation can be initiated. In extreme cases a partial exchange transfusion may be necessary to prevent polycythemia and adverse sequelae such as hyperviscosity. Oxygen is provided for respiratory distress. In addition, temperature instability and excessive loss of heat can result from decreased liver glycogen stores. (See Chapter 29 ∞ for thermoregulation techniques.)

Nursing Care Management

Nursing Assessment and Diagnosis

The newborn with postmaturity syndrome appears alert. This wide-eyed, alert appearance is not necessarily a positive sign because it may indicate chronic intrauterine hypoxia. The infant typically has dry, cracking, parchmentlike skin without vernix or lanugo (Figure 28–5 ■). Fingernails are long, and scalp hair is profuse. The infant's body appears long and thin. The wasting involves depletion of previously stored subcutaneous tissue, causing the skin to be loose. Fat layers are almost nonexistent.

Postmature newborns frequently have meconium staining, which colors the nails, skin, and umbilical cord. The varying shades (yellow to green) of meconium staining can give some clue as to whether the expulsion of meconium in utero was a recent or chronic problem. Green coloring indicates a more recent event.

Nursing diagnoses that may apply to the postmature newborn include the following:

- *Hypothermia* related to decreased liver glycogen and brown fat stores
- *Altered Nutrition: Less than Body Requirements* related to increased use of glucose secondary to in utero stress and decreased placenta perfusion
- *Impaired Gas Exchange in the Lungs and at the Cellular Level* related to airway obstruction from meconium aspiration
- *Risk for Altered Tissue Perfusion* related to increased blood viscosity caused by polycythemia

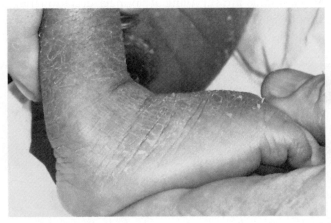

FIGURE 28–5 Postterm infant demonstrates deep cracking and peeling of skin.
Source: Dubowitz, L., & Dubowitz, V. (1977). *The gestational age of the newborn.* Redwood City, CA: Addison-Wesley. Reprinted by permission of V. Dubowitz, MD, Hammersmith Hospital, London, England.

Nursing Plan and Implementation

Nursing interventions are primarily supportive measures. The nurse needs to do the following:

- Monitor cardiopulmonary status because the stresses of labor are poorly tolerated and can result in hypoxemia in utero and possible asphyxia at birth.
- Provide warmth to counterbalance the infant's poor response to cold stress and decreased liver glycogen and brown fat stores.
- Frequently monitor blood glucose and initiate early feeding (at 1 or 2 hours of age) or intravenous glucose per physician order.
- Obtain a central line hematocrit to determine accurately the presence of polycythemia.

The nurse encourages parents to express their feelings and fears about the newborn's condition and potential long-term problems. The nurse gives careful explanations of procedures, includes the parents in the development of care plans for their baby, and encourages follow-up care as needed.

Evaluation

Expected outcomes of nursing care include the following:

- The postterm newborn establishes effective respiratory function.
- The postmature baby is free of metabolic alterations (hypoglycemia) and maintains a stable temperature.

Care of the Preterm (Premature) Newborn

A **preterm infant** is any infant born at 36 6/7 or less weeks' gestation (Figure 28–6 ■). With the help of modern technology, infants are surviving at younger gestational ages, but not without significant morbidity. The incidence of all preterm births in the United States is approximately 12%.

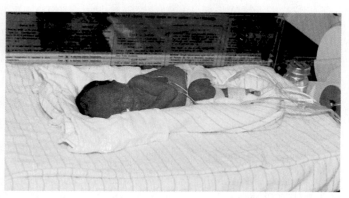

FIGURE 28–6 A 6-day-old, 28-week gestational age, 960 g preterm infant.
Source: Courtesy of Carol Harrigan, RNC, MSN, NNP.

In addition, 18% of African American newborns are preterm (Vargo & Trottter, 2007). The rise in multiple birth rates has markedly influenced overall rates of low-birth-weight (LBW) infants. Prematurity and low birth weight are common in single women and adolescents. (See Chapter 16 ∞ for a discussion of preterm labor.)

The major problem of the preterm newborn is the variable immaturity of all systems. The degree of immaturity depends on the length of gestation. The preterm newborn must traverse the same complex, interconnected pathways from intrauterine to extrauterine life as the term newborn. Because of immaturity, the premature newborn is ill equipped to make this transition smoothly. Maintenance of the preterm newborn falls within narrow physiologic parameters.

Alteration in Respiratory and Cardiac Physiology

The preterm newborn is at risk for respiratory problems because the lungs are not fully mature and not fully ready to take over the process of oxygen and carbon dioxide exchange without assistance until 37 to 38 weeks' gestation. Critical factors in the development of respiratory distress include the following:

1. The preterm infant is unable to produce adequate amounts of surfactant. (See Chapter 24 ∞ for discussion of respiratory adaptation and development.) Inadequate surfactant lessens compliance (ability of the lung to fill with air easily), thereby increasing the inspiratory pressure needed to expand the lungs with air. The collapsed (or atelectatic) alveoli will not facilitate an exchange of oxygen and carbon dioxide. As a result, the infant becomes hypoxic, pulmonary blood flow is inefficient, and the preterm newborn's available energy is depleted.

2. The muscular coat of pulmonary blood vessels is incompletely developed. Because of this, the pulmonary arterioles do not constrict as well in response to decreased oxygen levels. This lowered pulmonary vascular resistance leads to left-to-right shunting of blood through the ductus arteriosus, which increases the blood flow back into the lungs.

3. Normally the ductus arteriosus responds to increasing oxygen levels and prostaglandin E levels by vasoconstriction; in the preterm infant, who is more susceptible to hypoxia, the ductus may remain open. A patent ductus increases the blood volume to the lungs, causing pulmonary congestion, increased respiratory effort, carbon dioxide retention, and bounding femoral pulses.

The common complications of the cardiopulmonary system in preterm infants are discussed later in this chapter and in Chapter 29 ∞.

Alteration in Thermoregulation

Heat loss is a major problem in preterm newborns that the nurse can do much to prevent. Two factors limiting heat production, however, are the availability of glycogen in the liver and the amount of brown fat available for heat production. Both of these limiting factors appear in the third trimester. In the cold-stressed baby, norepinephine is released which in turn stimulates the metabolism of brown fat for heat production. As a complicating factor, the hypoxic newborn cannot increase oxygen consumption in response to cold stress because of the already limited reserves and thereby becomes progressively colder. Because the muscle mass is small in preterm infants, and muscular activity is diminished (they are unable to shiver), heat production is further limited.

Five physiologic and anatomic factors increase heat loss in the preterm infant:

1. The preterm baby has a higher ratio of body surface to body weight. This means that the baby's ability to produce heat (based on body weight) is much less than the potential for losing heat (based on surface area). The loss of heat in a preterm infant weighing 1500 g is five times greater per unit of body weight than in an adult.
2. The preterm baby has very little subcutaneous fat, which is the human body's insulation. Without adequate insulation, heat is easily conducted from the core of the body (warmer temperature) to the surface of the body (cooler temperature). Heat is lost from the body as the blood vessels, which lie close to the skin surface in the preterm infant, transport blood from the body core to the subcutaneous tissues.
3. The preterm baby has thinner, more permeable skin than the term infant. This increased permeability contributes to a greater insensible water loss as well as to heat loss.
4. The posture of the preterm baby influences heat loss. Flexion of the extremities decreases the amount of surface area exposed to the environment. Extension increases the surface area exposed to the environment and thus increases heat loss. The gestational age of the infant influences the amount of flexion, from completely hypotonic and extended at 28 weeks to strong flexion displayed by 36 weeks.
5. The preterm baby has a decreased ability to vasoconstrict superficial blood vessels and conserve heat in the body core.

In summary, gestational age is directly proportional to the ability to maintain thermoregulation; thus the more preterm the newborn, the less able the infant is to maintain heat balance. Preventing heat loss by providing a neutral thermal environment is one of the most important considerations in nursing management of the preterm infant (see Maintenance of Neutral Thermal Environment later in the chapter). Cold stress, with its accompanying severe complications, can be prevented (see Chapter 29 ∞).

Alteration in Gastrointestinal Physiology

The basic structure of the gastrointestinal (GI) tract is formed early in gestation. Maturation of the digestive and absorptive process is more variable, however, and occurs later in gestation. As a result of GI immaturity, the preterm newborn has the following ingestion, digestive, and absorption problems:

- A marked danger of aspiration and its associated complications because of the infant's poorly developed gag reflex, incompetent esophageal cardiac sphincter, and poor sucking and swallowing reflexes.
- Difficulty in meeting high caloric and fluid needs for growth because of small stomach capacity.
- Limited ability to convert certain essential amino acids to nonessential amino acids. Certain amino acids, such as histidine, taurine, and cysteine, are essential to the preterm infant but not to the term infant.
- Inability to handle the increased osmolarity of formula protein because of kidney immaturity. The preterm infant requires a higher concentration of whey protein than of casein.
- Difficulty absorbing saturated fats because of decreased bile salts and pancreatic lipase. Severe illness of the newborn may also prevent intake of adequate nutrients.
- Difficulty with lactose digestion initially because processes may not be fully functional during the first few days of a preterm infant's life. The preterm newborn can digest and absorb most simple sugars.
- Deficiency of calcium and phosphorus may exist because two-thirds of these minerals are deposited in the last trimester. Rickets and significant bone demineralization caused by deficiency of calcium and phosphorus, which are deposited primarily in the last trimester, are also problems.
- Increased basal metabolic rate and increased oxygen requirements caused by fatigue associated with sucking.
- Feeding intolerance and necrotizing enterocolitis (NEC) as a result of diminished blood flow and tissue perfusion to the intestinal tract because of prolonged hypoxia and hypoxemia at birth.

Alteration in Renal Physiology

The kidneys of the preterm infant are immature compared with those of the full-term infant, which poses clinical problems in the management of fluid and electrolyte balance. Specific characteristics of the preterm infant include the following:

- The glomerular filtration rate (GFR) is lower because of decreased renal blood flow. The GFR is directly related to lower gestational age, so the more preterm the newborn, the lower the GFR. The GFR is also decreased in the presence of diseases or conditions that decrease the renal blood flow and perfusion, such as severe respiratory distress, hypotension, and asphyxia. Anuria and oliguria may also be observed.
- The preterm infant's kidneys are limited in their ability to concentrate urine or to excrete excess amounts of fluid. This means that if excess fluid is administered, the infant is at risk for fluid retention and overhydration. If too little is administered, the infant will become dehydrated because of the inability to retain adequate fluid.
- The kidneys of the preterm infant begin excreting glucose (glycosuria) at a lower serum glucose level than those of the term infant. Therefore, glycosuria with hyperglycemia can lead to osmotic diuresis and polyuria.
- The buffering capacity of the kidney is reduced, predisposing the infant to metabolic acidosis. Bicarbonate is excreted at a lower serum level, and acid is excreted more slowly. Therefore, after periods of hypoxia or insult, the preterm infant's kidneys require a longer time to excrete the lactic acid that accumulates. Sodium bicarbonate is frequently required to treat the metabolic acidosis.
- The immaturity of the renal system affects the preterm infant's ability to excrete drugs. Because excretion time is longer, many drugs are given over longer intervals (i.e., every 24 hours instead of every 12 hours). Urine output must be carefully monitored when the infant is receiving nephrotoxic drugs such as gentamicin and vancomycin. In the event that urine output is poor, drugs can become toxic in the infant much more quickly than in the adult.

Alteration in Immunologic Physiology

The preterm infant is at a much greater risk for infection than the term infant. This increased susceptibility may be the result of an infection acquired in utero which may have precipitated preterm labor and birth. However, all preterm infants have immature specific and nonspecific immunity.

In utero the fetus receives passive immunity against a variety of infections from maternal IgG immunoglobulins, which cross the placenta (see Chapter 29 ∞). Because most of this immunity is acquired in the last trimester of pregnancy, the preterm infant has few antibodies at birth. These provide less protection and become depleted earlier than in a full-term infant. This may be a contributing factor in the higher incidence of recurrent bacterial infection during the first year of life as well as in the immediate neonatal period.

The other immunoglobulin significant for the preterm infant is secretory IgA, which does not cross the placenta but is found in breast milk in significant concentrations. Breast milk's secretory IgA provides immunity to the mucosal surfaces of the GI tract, protecting the newborn from enteric infections such as those caused by *Escherichia coli* and *Shigella*.

Another altered defense against infection in the preterm infant is the skin surface. In very small infants the skin is easily excoriated, and this factor, coupled with many invasive procedures, places the infant at great risk for nosocomial infections. It is vital to use good handwashing techniques in the care of these infants to prevent unnecessary infection.

HINTS FOR PRACTICE

The sudden onset of apnea and bradycardia, coupled with metabolic acidosis in an otherwise healthy, growing premature infant, may be suggestive of bacterial sepsis, especially if there is a central line present.

Alteration in Neurologic Physiology

The general shape of the brain is formed during the first 6 weeks of gestation. Between the second and fourth months of gestation the brain's total complement of neurons proliferate; these neurons migrate to specific sites throughout the central nervous system, and nerve impulse pathways organize. The final step in neurologic development is the covering of these nerves with myelin, which begins in the second trimester of gestation and continues into adult life (Volpe, 2008).

Because the period of most rapid brain growth and development occurs during the third trimester of pregnancy, the closer to term an infant is born, the better the neurologic prognosis. A common interruption of neurologic development in the preterm infant is caused by intraventricular hemorrhage (IVH) and intracranial hemorrhage (ICH). Hydrocephalus may develop as a consequence of an IVH caused by the obstruction at the cerebral aqueduct.

Alteration in Reactivity Periods and Behavioral States

The newborn infant's response to extrauterine life is characterized by two periods of reactivity (see Chapter 24 ∞). The preterm infant's periods of reactivity are delayed. In the very ill infant, these periods of reactivity may not be observed at all because the infant may be hypotonic and unreactive for several days after birth. As the preterm newborn grows and the condition stabilizes, identifying behavioral states and traits unique to each infant becomes increasingly possible. In general, stable preterm infants do not demonstrate the same behavioral states as term infants. Preterm infants tend to be more disorganized in their sleep-wake cycles and are unable to attend as well to the human face and objects in the environment. Neurologically, their responses (sucking, muscle tone, states of arousal) are weaker than full-term infants' responses.

By observing each infant's patterns of behavior and responses, especially the sleep-wake states, the parent and nurse can plan nursing care around the times when the infant is alert and best able to attend. In addition, the more knowledge parents have about the meaning of their infant's responses and behaviors, the better prepared they will be to meet their newborn's needs and to form a positive attachment with their child. See discussion of developmental care for the preterm newborn later in this section.

TEACHINGTIP

After observing an infant's pattern of behavior and responses, especially the sleep-wake states, the nurse uses the time when the infant is alert and best able to attend to help parents learn about and provide newborn care.

Management of Nutrition and Fluid Requirements

Early feedings are extremely valuable in maintaining normal metabolism and lowering the possibility of such complications as hypoglycemia, hyperbilirubinemia, and azotemia. However, the preterm infant is at risk for complications that may develop because of immaturity of the digestive system.

Nutritional Requirements

Oral (enteral) caloric intake necessary for growth in a healthy preterm newborn is 95 to 130 kcal/kg/day (Blackburn, 2007). In addition to these relatively high caloric needs, the preterm newborn requires more protein than the full-term infant. To meet these needs, many institutions use breast milk or special preterm formulas.

Whether breast milk or formula is used, feeding regimens are established based on the infant's weight and estimated stomach capacity (Table 28–1). Initial formula feedings are gradually increased as the infant tolerates them. It may be necessary to supplement oral feedings with parenteral fluids to maintain adequate hydration and caloric intake until the baby is on full oral feedings. Preterm infants who cannot tolerate any oral (enteral) feedings are given nutrition by total parenteral nutrition (TPN).

In addition to a higher calorie and protein formula, preterm infants should receive supplemental multivitamins, including vitamin A, D, and E, iron, and trace minerals. A diet high in polyunsaturated fats (which preterm infants tolerate best) increases the requirement for vitamin E. Preterm infants fed iron-fortified formulas have higher red cell hemolysis and lower vitamin E concentrations and thus require additional vitamin E. Preterm formulas also need to contain medium-chain triglycerides (MCT) and additional amino acids such as cysteine, as well as calcium, phosphorus, and vitamin D supplements to increase mineralization of bones. Rickets and significant bone demineralization have been documented in very-low-birth-weight infants and otherwise healthy preterm infants.

TABLE 28–1	Suggested Feeding Guidelines for the Preterm Infant			
Weight (g)	Feeding Interval	Beginning Volume (mL/kg/d)	Feeding Increments (mL/kg/d)	Days to Full Feedings[†]
< 1000	q 3 hour	10 to 20	10 to 20	16 to 13
1000 to 1500	q 3 hour	10 to 20	15 to 20	10 to 7
1501 to 1800 sick[‡]	q 3 hour	10 to 20	20 to 30	7 to 5
1501 to 1800 healthy[‡]	q 3 hour	20 to 40	30 to 50	5 to 3
> 1800 sick[‡]	q 3 hour	20 to 40	30 to 75	5 to 2

[†]Full feedings are defined as 120 kcal/kg/day of a 24 kcal/oz formula or human milk.

[‡]*Sick* refers to infants who have had symptoms of any medical or surgical condition, other than uncomplicated prematurity.
Healthy refers to term or preterm infants who have had no symptomatic medical or surgical conditions.

1. Advancement of feedings should occur only as the infant demonstrates tolerance of enteral feedings. Clinical signs of feeding intolerance or illness dictate discontinuing or holding the advancement of feedings.
2. Infants are started on either full-strength human milk or 24 kcal/oz premature infant formula.
3. At 100 to 120 mL/kg, fortifier is added to human milk.
4. Iron supplements are added at 2 to 4 mg/kg/day for the human milk fed infant at full feeds.

Source: Neonatal nutrition survival guide for the practitioner by Lisa R. Vanatta, MS, RD, CSP, Clinical Nutrition Services, Phoenix Children's Hospital; adapted from a similar table by Diane Anderson in "Nutrition for Premature Infants," from *Handbook of Pediatric Nutrition.* Jones & Bartlett Publishers, Sudbury, MA. www.jbpub.com. Reprinted with permission.

Nutritional intake is considered adequate when there is consistent weight gain of 20 to 30 g/day. Initially, no weight gain may be noted for several days, but total weight loss should not exceed 15% of the total birth weight or more than 1% to 2% per day. Some institutions add the criteria of head circumference growth and increase in body length of 1 cm (0.4 in.) per week, once the newborn is stable.

Methods of Feeding

The preterm infant is fed by various methods depending on the infant's gestational age, health and physical condition, and neurologic status. The three most common oral feeding methods are bottle, breast, and gavage.

BOTTLE-FEEDING   Preterm infants who have a coordinated as well as rhythmic suck-swallow-breathing pattern are usually between 35 and 36 weeks' postconceptual age and may be fed by bottle. Oral readiness to feed is best described by the following behaviors: remaining engaged in the feeding, organizing oral-motor functioning, coordinating the suck-swallow-breath skill, and maintaining physiological stability (Thoyre, Shaker, & Pridham, 2005).

Those premature infants who root when their cheek is stroked and actively search for the nipple are neurodevelopmentally ready to initiate oral feeding. To avoid excessive expenditure of energy, a soft, yellow, single-hole nipple is usually used (milk flow is less rapid). The infant is fed in a semisitting position and burped gently after each $1/2$ to 1 oz. The feeding should take no longer than 15 to 20 minutes (nippling requires more energy than other methods). Premature infants who are progressing from gavage feedings to bottle-feeding should start with one session of bottle-feeding a day and slowly increase the number of times a day a bottle is given until the baby tolerates all feedings from a bottle.

The nurse also assesses the infant's ability to suck. Sucking may be affected by age, asphyxia, sepsis, intraventricular hemorrhage, or other neurologic insult. Before initiating nipple feeding, the nurse observes for signs of stress, such as tachypnea (more than 60 respirations per minute), respiratory distress, or hypothermia, which may increase the risk of aspiration. During the feeding the nurse observes the infant for signs of feeding difficulty (tachypnea, cyanosis, bradycardia, lethargy, uncoordinated suck and swallow). Difficulty in bottle feeding is often associated with a milk bolus that is too large for the infant's oral cavity that can lead to aspiration. Demand feeding protocols, based on the infant's hunger cues, should be considered for a growing premature infant only when there is sufficient caloric intake to promote consistent weight gain (Kenner & Lott, 2007).

BREASTFEEDING   Mothers who wish to breastfeed their preterm infants are given the opportunity to put

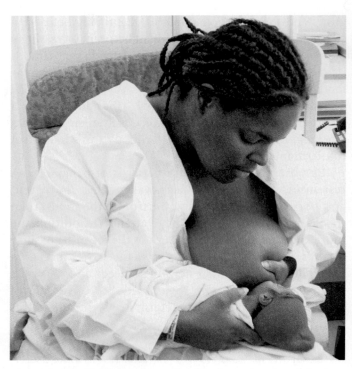

FIGURE 28–7 Mother breastfeeding her premature infant.

the infant to the breast as soon as the infant has demonstrated a coordinated suck and swallow reflex, is showing consistent weight gain, and can control body temperature outside of the incubator, regardless of weight. Preterm infants tolerate breastfeeding with higher transcutaneous oxygen pressures and better maintenance of body temperature than during bottle-feeding. Besides breast milk's many benefits for the infant, it allows the mother to contribute actively to the infant's well-being (Figure 28–7 ■). The nurse should encourage mothers to breastfeed if they choose to do so. It is important for the nurse to be aware of the advantages of breastfeeding, as well as the possible disadvantages of breast milk as the sole source of food for the preterm infant (see Chapter 27 ∞). Even if the infant cannot be put to the breast, mothers can pump their breasts, and the breast milk can be given via gavage. Use of the double-pumping system produces higher levels of prolactin than sequential pumping of the breasts.

By initiating skin-to-skin holding of premature infants in the early intensive care phase, mothers can significantly increase milk volume, thereby overcoming lactation problems (Turnage-Carrier, 2004). The infant is placed at the mother's breast. It has been suggested that the football hold is a convenient position for breastfeeding preterm babies. Feeding may take up to 45 minutes, and babies should be burped as they alternate breasts. The length of feeding time is monitored so that the preterm infant does not burn too many calories.

The nurse should coordinate a flexible feeding schedule so babies can nurse during alert times and be allowed to set their own pace. Feedings should be on demand, but a maximum number of hours between feedings should be set. A similar regimen should be used for the baby who is progressing from gavage feeding to breastfeeding. The mother begins with one feeding at the breast and then gradually increases the number of times during the day that the baby breastfeeds. When breastfeeding is not possible because the infant is too small or too weak to suck at the breast, an option for the mother may be to express her breast milk into a cup. The milk touches the infant's lips and is lapped by the protruding motions of the tongue.

HINTS FOR PRACTICE

For an otherwise healthy, growing premature infant who is receiving total enteral intake and has started to experience apnea and bradycardia, one differential diagnosis to think about is reflux rather than sepsis, although sepsis may need to be ruled out.

GAVAGE FEEDING The gavage feeding method is used with preterm infants (less than 34 weeks' gestation) who lack or have a poorly coordinated suck and swallow reflex or are ill and ventilator dependent. Gavage feeding may be used as an adjunct to nipple feeding if the infant tires easily or as an alternative if an infant is losing weight because of the energy expenditure required for nippling (see Clinical Skill: Performing Gavage Feeding). Gavage feedings are administered by either the nasogastric or orogastric route and by intermittent bolus or continuous drip method. Bolus feedings may be preferred because it is thought to be more like normal feedings than the continuous feeding method and enhances the release of certain GI hormones that are necessary for gut development (Kenner & Lott, 2007). Currently, there are no conclusive studies supporting one method over the other. In common practice, bolus feedings are usually initiated, but if intolerance occurs, then the feedings are changed to continuous.

Early initiation of minimal enteral nutrition (MEN) via gavage is now advocated as a supplement to parenteral nutrition. MEN refers to small-volume feedings of formula or human milk (usually less than 24 mL/kg/day) which are designed to "prime" the intestinal tract, thereby stimulating many of its hormonal and enzymatic functions (AAP & ACOG, 2007; Kenner & Lott, 2007). Benefits of early feeding (as early as 24 to 72 hours of life) include the following: no increased incidence in NEC; fewer days on TPN, thereby decreasing the incidence of cholestatic jaundice; increased weight gain; increased muscle maturation of the gut function which can lead to improved feeding tolerance; lower risk of osteopenia; and a possible decrease in the total number of hospital days in the NICU (Kenner & Lott, 2007).

HINTS FOR PRACTICE

Orogastric gavage catheter placement is preferable to nasogastric because most infants are obligatory nose breathers. If nasogastric is used, a #5 French catheter should be used to minimize airway obstruction.

TOTAL PARENTERAL NUTRITION TPN is used in situations that do not allow feeding the infant through the GI tract. The TPN method provides complete nutrition to the infant intravenously. TPN uses hyperalimentation to provide calories, vitamins, minerals, protein, and glucose, and uses intralipids to provide essential fatty acids.

Fluid Requirements

The calculation of fluid requirements must take into account the infant's weight and postnatal age. Recommendations for fluid therapy in the preterm infant are approximately 80 to 100 mL/kg/day for day 1, 100 to 120 mL/kg/day for day 2, and 120 to 150 mL/kg/day by day 3 of life. These amounts may be increased up to 200 mL/kg/day if the infant is very small, receiving phototherapy, or under a radiant warmer because of the increased insensible water losses. Fluid losses can be minimized through the use of heat shields and added humidification in the incubator. Daily weights, and sometimes twice-a-day weights, are the best indicator of fluid status in the preterm infant. The expected weight loss during the first 3 to 5 days of life in a preterm infant is 15% to 20% of birth weight. Premature infants who are being treated for complications such as respiratory distress syndrome or patent ductus arteriosus may be on diuretics that can influence their fluid requirements.

Common Complications of Preterm Newborns and Their Clinical Management

The goals of medical and nursing care are to meet the preterm infant's growth and development needs and to anticipate and manage the complications associated with prematurity. The most common complications associated with prematurity are as follows:

1. *Apnea of prematurity.* Apnea of prematurity refers to cessation of breathing for 20 seconds or longer or for less than 20 seconds when associated with cyanosis, pallor, and bradycardia. Apnea is a common problem in the preterm infant presenting between day 2 and day 7 of life. The etiology of apnea is multifactorial but is thought to be primarily a result of neuronal immaturity, a factor that contributes to the preterm infant's irregular breathing patterns (central apnea). Obstructive apnea can occur when there is cessation of airflow associated with blockage of the upper airway (small airway diameter, increased

Clinical Skill Performing Gavage Feeding

NURSING ACTION	RATIONALE

Preparation

1. When choosing the catheter size, consider the size of the infant, the area of insertion (oral or nasal), and the desired rate of flow.

2. Explain the procedure to the parents.

3. Elevate the head of the bed and position the infant on the back or side to allow easy passage of the tube.

4. Measure the distance from the tip of the ear to the nose to the xiphoid process, and mark the point with a small piece of paper tape (Figure 28–8 ■) to ensure enough tubing to enter the stomach.

The size of the catheter will influence the rate of flow.

The very small infant (less than 1600 g) requires a 5 Fr. feeding tube; an infant greater than 1600 g may tolerate a larger tube. The size of the catheter will also influence the rate of flow.

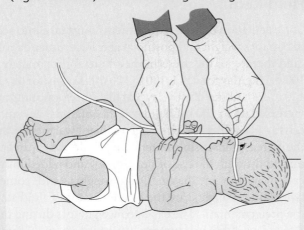

FIGURE 28–8 Measuring gavage tube length.

Equipment and Supplies

- No. 5 or no. 8 Fr. feeding tube
- 3 to 5 mL syringe, for aspirating stomach contents
- 1/4 in. paper tape, to mark the tube for insertion depth and to secure the catheter during feeding
- Stethoscope, for auscultating the rush of air into the stomach when testing the tube placement
- Appropriate formula
- Small cup of sterile water to test for tube placement and to act as lubricant

Orogastric insertion is preferable to nasogastric because most infants are obligatory nose breathers. If nasogastric is used, a #5 Fr. catheter should be used to minimize airway obstruction.

Procedure: Clean Gloves

Inserting and Checking Placement of Tube

1. If inserting the tube nasally, lubricate the tip in a cup of sterile water. Use water instead of an oil-based lubricant, in case the tube is inadvertently passed into a lung. Shake any excess drops to prevent aspiration.

2. If inserting the tube orally, the oral secretions are enough to lubricate the tube adequately.

3. Stabilize the infant's head with one hand and pass the tube via the mouth (or nose) into the stomach to the point previously marked. If the infant begins coughing or choking or becomes cyanotic or phonic, remove the tube immediately as the tube has probably entered the trachea.

Clinical Skill Performing Gavage Feeding (Continued)

NURSING ACTION	RATIONALE

4. If no respiratory distress is apparent, lightly tape the tube in position, draw up 0.5 to 1 mL of air into the syringe, and connect the syringe to the tubing. Place the stethoscope over the epigastrium and briskly inject the air (Figure 28–9 ■). You will hear a sudden rush as the air enters the stomach.

5. Aspirate the stomach contents with the syringe, and note the amount, color, and consistency to evaluate the infant's feeding tolerance. Return the residual to the stomach unless you are asked to discard it. It is usually not discarded because of the potential for electrolyte imbalance.

6. If the aspirated contents contain only a clear fluid or mucus and if it is unclear whether or not the tube is in the stomach, test the aspirate for pH. Stomach aspirate has a pH between 1 and 3.

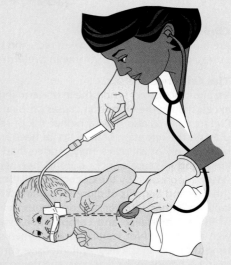

FIGURE 28–9 Auscultation for placement of gavage tube.

Administering the Feeding

1. Hold the infant for feeding, or position the infant on the right side.

This position decreases the risk of aspiration in case of emesis during feeding.

2. Separate the syringe from the tube, remove the plunger from the barrel, reconnect the barrel to the tube, and pour the formula into the syringe.

3. Elevate the syringe 6 to 8 in. over the infant's head, and allow the formula to flow by gravity at a slow, even rate. You may need to initiate the flow of formula by inserting the plunger of the syringe into the barrel just until you see formula enter the feeding tube. Do not use pressure.

4. Regulate the rate to prevent sudden stomach distention leading to vomiting and aspiration. Continue adding formula to the syringe until the infant has absorbed the desired volume.

Clearing and Removing the Tube

1. Clear the tubing with 2 to 3 mL sterile water or with air.

This ensures that the infant has received all of the formula. If the tube is going to be left in place, clearing it will decrease the risk of clogging and bacterial growth in the tube.

2. To remove the tube, loosen the tape, fold the tube over on itself, and quickly withdraw the tube in one smooth motion to minimize the potential for fluid aspiration as the tube passes the epiglottis. If the tube is to be left in, position it so that the infant is unable to remove it. Replace the tube per hospital policy.

Maximize the Feeding Pleasure of the Infant

1. Whenever possible, hold the infant during gavage feeding. If it is too awkward to hold the infant during feeding, be sure to take time for holding after the feeding.

Feeding time is important to the infant's tactile sensory input.
Sucking during feeding comforts and relaxes the infant, making the formula flow more easily. Infants can lose their sucking reflexes when fed by gavage for long periods.

2. Offer a pacifier to the infant during the feeding.

EVIDENCE-BASED PRACTICE

Diuretics for Respiratory Distress Syndrome in Preterm Infants

Clinical Question
Are diuretics safe and effective in reducing the complications of respiratory distress syndrome in preterm infants?

The Evidence
Respiratory distress syndrome in preterm infants may result in excess fluid in the lungs that causes problems with breathing. Preterm babies also have a higher risk of reduced urine output and the retention of fluid. It has been suggested that administration of diuretics may reduce fluid retention in the lungs and increase urinary output. Two separate systematic reviews sponsored by the Cochrane Collaboration focused on the risks and benefits of diuretics administered to preterm infants in either intravenous or aerosolized forms. Physical measures, mortality, and complications were examined, as well as the need for ventilation or oxygen supplementation. Length of stay in the neonatal intensive care unit, number of hospitalizations in the first year, and neurodevelopment were also documented. Two systematic reviews of multiple studies that meet the rigorous standards of the Cochrane Register are the strongest form of evidence.

What Is Effective?
The administration of a diuretic—specifically furosemide—in either intravenous or aerosol form had a transient therapeutic effect in reducing fluid retention. Pulmonary mechanics were improved after a single dose of furosemide. There were, however, no long-term benefits identified. These reviewers

cannot recommend a care standard that includes routine diuretic use in these babies. Elective administration should be a decision based on the risk of serious complications occasionally associated with the drug—specifically an increased risk for patent ductus arteriosus and for hemodynamic instability. There are other drugs that can improve pulmonary mechanics with fewer side effects. In addition, simple restriction of water intake to minimal levels may reduce fluid retention without pharmacological intervention.

What Is Inconclusive?
The effects of long-term administration of diuretics were not examined; more research is needed before it can be addressed. The specific amount of water restriction was not recommended.

Best Practice
Even though diuretics provide short-term relief from pulmonary edema for preterm babies and infants with chronic lung disease, the benefits are not long-term and are outweighed by the risks. You can support the fluid balance of the baby by restricting water intake to minimal levels.

References
Brion, L., & Soll, R. (2008). Diuretics for respiratory distress syndrome in preterm infants. *Cochrane Database of Systematic Reviews*, Issue 2.

Brion, L., Primhak, R., & Yong, W. (2007). Aerosolized diuretics for preterm infants with (or developing) chronic lung disease. *Cochrane Database of Systematic Reviews*, Issue 4.

---

pharyngeal secretions, altered body alignment and positioning). Gastroesophageal reflux (GER) is defined as a movement of gastric contents into the lower esophagus caused by poor esophageal sphincter tone, causing laryngospasm, which leads to bradycardia and apnea. Apnea of prematurity is then a diagnosis of exclusion.

2. *Patent ductus arteriosus (PDA).* The ductus arteriosus fails to close because of decreased pulmonary arteriole musculature and hypoxemia. Symptomatic PDA is often seen around the time when premature infants are recovering from RDS. Patent ductus arteriosus often prolongs the course of illness in a preterm newborn and leads to chronic pulmonary dysfunction.

HINTS FOR PRACTICE

A growing premature infant showing clinical signs of worsening respiratory status (i.e., increased oxygen needs, increased ventilatory settings), acidosis, and hypotension may be exhibiting signs and symptoms of a PDA.

---

3. *Respiratory distress syndrome (RDS).* Respiratory distress results from inadequate surfactant production (see Chapter 29 ∞).

4. *Intraventricular hemorrhage (IVH).* Intraventricular hemorrhage is the most common type of intracranial hemorrhage in small preterm infants, especially those weighing less than 1500 g or of less than 34 weeks' gestation. Up to 34 weeks' gestation the preterm's brain ventricles are lined by the germinal matrix, which is highly susceptible to hypoxic events such as respiratory distress, birth trauma, and birth asphyxia. The germinal matrix is highly vascular, and these blood vessels rupture in the presence of hypoxia.

HINTS FOR PRACTICE

An extreme premature, low-birth-weight infant who presents with a sudden drop in hemoglobin along with the onset of severe metabolic acidosis, a "waxy" color, and hypotension may have experienced an intracranial hemorrhage.

---

5. *Anemia of prematurity.* The preterm infant is at risk for anemia because of the rapid rate of growth required, shorter red blood cell life, excessive blood sampling, decreased iron stores, and deficiency of vitamin E. The hemoglobin usually reaches its lowest level by 3 to 12 weeks and remains low for 3 to 6 months.

Other common problems of preterm infants such as NEC are briefly discussed earlier in the physiologic sections. (For an in-depth discussion of RDS, hyperbilirubinemia, hypoglycemia, and sepsis, see Chapter 29 ∞.)

Long-Term Needs and Outcome

The care of preterm infants and their families does not stop on discharge from the nursery. Follow-up care is extremely important because many developmental problems are not noted until an infant is older and begins to demonstrate motor delays or sensory disability.

Within the first year of life, low-birth-weight preterm infants face higher mortality rates than term infants. Causes of death include sudden infant death syndrome (SIDS)—which occurs about five times more frequently in the preterm infant—respiratory infections, and neurologic defects. Morbidity is also much higher among preterm infants, with those weighing less than 1500 g at highest risk for long-term complications.

The most common long-term needs observed in preterm infants include the following:

- *Retinopathy of prematurity (ROP).* Premature newborns are particularly susceptible to characteristic retinal changes, known as ROP, which can result in visual impairment. The disease is now viewed as multifactorial in origin. Increased survival of very-low-birth-weight (VLBW) infants may be the most important factor in the increased incidence of ROP.
- *Bronchopulmonary dysplasia (BPD).* Long-term lung disease is a result of damage to the alveolar epithelium secondary to positive pressure respirator therapy and high oxygen concentration. These infants have long-term dependence on oxygen therapy and an increased incidence of respiratory infection during their first few years of life.
- *Speech defects.* The most frequently observed speech defects involve delayed development of receptive and expressive ability that may persist into the school-age years.
- *Neurologic defects.* The most common neurologic defects include cerebral palsy, hydrocephalus, seizure disorders, lower IQ, and learning disabilities. However, the socioeconomic climate and family support systems are extremely important influences on the child's ultimate school performance in the absence of major neurologic defects. Families can be reminded that risk does not equal injury, injury does not equal damage, and description of damage does not allow a precise prediction about recovery or outcome.
- *Auditory defects.* Preterm infants have a 1% to 4% incidence of moderate to profound hearing loss and should have a formal audiologic exam before discharge and at 3 to 6 months (corrected age). Tests currently used to measure hearing functions of the newborn are the evoked otoacoustic emissions (EOAE) or the automated auditory brain response (AABR) test. Any infant with repeated abnormal results should be referred to speech-and-language specialists.

When evaluating the infant's abilities and disabilities, parents must understand that developmental progress must be evaluated based on chronological age from the expected date of birth, not from the actual date of birth (corrected age). In addition, the parents need the consistent support of healthcare professionals in the long-term management of their infants. Many new and ongoing concerns arise as the high-risk infant grows and develops; the goal is to promote the highest quality of life possible.

Nursing Care Management

Nursing Assessment and Diagnosis

The nurse needs to assess the physical characteristics and gestational age of the preterm newborn accurately to anticipate the special needs and problems of the baby. Physical characteristics vary greatly depending on gestational age, but the following characteristics are frequently present:

- *Color* is usually pink or ruddy but may show acrocyanosis. (Cyanosis, jaundice, and pallor are abnormal and should be noted.)
- *Skin* is reddened and translucent, blood vessels are readily apparent, there is little subcutaneous fat.
- *Lanugo* is plentiful and widely distributed.
- *Head size* appears large in relation to the body.
- *Skull bones* are pliable; fontanelle is smooth and flat.
- *Ears* have minimal cartilage and are pliable, folded over.
- *Nails* are soft, short.
- *Genitals* are small; testes may not be descended and scrotum nonrugated; clitoris and labia minora are prominent.
- *Resting position* is flaccid, froglike.
- *Cry* is weak, feeble.
- *Reflexes* (sucking, swallowing, gag) are poor.
- *Activity* consists of jerky, generalized movements. (Seizure activity is abnormal.)

Determining gestational age in preterm newborns requires knowledge and experience in administering gestational assessment tools. The tool used should be specific, reliable, and valid. (For a discussion of gestational age assessment tools, see Chapter 25 ∞.)

Nursing diagnoses that may apply to the preterm newborn include the following:

- *Impaired Gas Exchange* related to immature pulmonary vasculature and inadequate surfactant production

- *Ineffective Breathing Pattern* related to immature central nervous system
- *Alteration in Cardiovascular Status* related to hypotension related to decreased tissue perfusion secondary to PDA
- *Alteration in Tissue Perfusion* related to anemia of prematurity
- *Altered Nutrition: Less than Body Requirements* related to weak suck and swallow reflexes and decreased ability to absorb nutrients
- *Ineffective Thermoregulation* related to hypothermia secondary to decreased glycogen and brown fat stores
- *Fluid Volume Deficit* related to high insensible water losses and inability of kidneys to concentrate urine
- *Ineffective Family Coping* related to anger or guilt at having given birth to a premature baby

Nursing Plan and Implementation

Maintenance of Respiratory Function

There is increased danger of respiratory obstruction in preterm newborns because their bronchi and trachea are so narrow that mucus can obstruct the airway. The nurse must maintain patency through judicious suctioning, but only on an as-needed basis.

Positioning can also affect respiratory function. If the baby is in the supine position, the nurse should slightly elevate the infant's head to maintain the airway, being careful to avoid hyperextension of the neck because the trachea will collapse. Also, because the newborn has weak neck muscles and cannot control head movement, the nurse should ensure that this head position is maintained by placing a small roll under the shoulders. Because the prone position splints the chest wall and decreases the amount of respiratory effort used to move the chest wall, it facilitates chest expansion and improves air entry and oxygenation. Weak or absent cough or gag reflexes increase the chance of aspiration in the premature newborn. The nurse should ensure that the infant's position facilitates drainage of mucus or regurgitated formula.

The nurse monitors heart and respiratory rates with cardiorespiratory monitors and observes the newborn to identify alterations in cardiopulmonary status. Signs of respiratory distress include the following:

- Cyanosis (serious sign when generalized)
- Tachypnea (sustained respiratory rate greater than 60/minute after first 4 hours of life)
- Retractions
- Expiratory grunting
- Nasal flaring
- Apneic episodes
- Presence of rales or rhonchi on auscultation
- Diminished air entry

If respiratory distress occurs, the nurse administers oxygen per physician or nurse practitioner order to relieve hypoxemia. If hypoxemia is not treated immediately, it may result in patent ductus arteriosus or metabolic acidosis. If oxygen is administered to the newborn, the nurse monitors the oxygen concentration with devices such as the transcutaneous oxygen monitor ($tcPO_2$) or the pulse oximeter. Periodic arterial blood gas sampling to monitor oxygen concentration in the baby's blood is essential because hyperoxemia may lead to ROP.

The nurse also needs to consider respiratory function before initiation of feedings as well as during feeding. To prevent aspiration as well as increased energy expenditure and oxygen consumption, the nurse must ensure that the infant's gag and suck reflexes are intact before starting oral feedings.

Maintenance of Neutral Thermal Environment

Providing a neutral thermal environment minimizes the oxygen consumption required to maintain a normal core temperature; it also prevents cold stress and facilitates growth by decreasing the calories needed to maintain body temperature. The preterm infant's immature central nervous system, as well as small brown fat stores, provides poor temperature control. A small infant (>1200 g) can lose 80 kcal/kg/day through radiation of body heat. The nurse implements all the usual thermoregulation measures discussed in Chapter 26 ∞.

In addition, to minimize heat loss and temperature instability for preterm and LBW newborns, the nurse should do the following:

1. Allow skin-to-skin contact between mother and newborn to maintain warmth and faster security (see kangaroo care, described later).
2. Warm and humidify oxygen to minimize evaporative heat loss and decrease oxygen consumption.
3. Place the baby in a double-walled incubator or use a Plexiglas heat shield over small preterm infants in single-walled incubators to avoid radiative heat losses. Some institutions use radiant warmers and plastic wrap over the baby and pipe in humidity (swamping). Do not use Plexiglas shields on radiant warmer beds because they block the infrared heat.
4. Avoid placing the baby on cold surfaces such as metal treatment tables and cold X-ray plates (conductive heat loss). Pad cold surfaces with diapers and use radiant warmers during procedures, place the preterm infant on prewarmed mattresses, and warm hands before handling the baby to prevent heat transfer via conduction.
5. Use warmed ambient humidity. Humidity can decrease insensible and transdermal water loss especially in VLBW infants (Blackburn, 2007).

6. Keep the skin dry (evaporative heat loss) and place a cap on the baby's head. The head makes up 25% of the total body size.
7. Keep radiant warmers, incubators, and cribs away from windows and cold external walls (radiative heat loss) and out of drafts (conductive heat loss).
8. Open incubator portholes and doors only when necessary, and use plastic sleeves on portholes to decrease convective heat loss.
9. Use a skin probe to monitor the baby's skin temperature. Correlate ambient temperatures with the skin probe in the incubator using the servocontrol rather than the manual mode. The temperature should be 36°C to 37°C (96.8°F to 98.6°F). Temperature fluctuations indicate hypothermia or hyperthermia. Be careful not to place skin temperature probes over bony prominences, areas of brown fat, poorly vasoreactive areas such as extremities, or excoriated areas.
10. Warm formula or stored breast milk before feeding.
11. Use reflector patch over the skin temperature probe when using a radiant warmer bed so that the probe does not sense the higher infrared temperature as the baby's skin temperature and therefore decrease the heater output.

Once preterm infants are medically stable, they can be clothed with a double-thickness cap, cotton shirt, and diaper and, if possible, swaddled in a blanket. The nurse begins the process of weaning to a crib when the premature infant is medically stable, does not require assisted ventilation, weighs approximately 1500 g, has 5 days of consistent weight gain, and is taking oral feedings and when apnea and bradycardia episodes have stabilized. The nurse should be familiar with the individual institution's protocol for weaning preterm infants to a crib.

Maintenance of Fluid and Electrolyte Status

The nurse maintains hydration by providing adequate intake based on the newborn's weight, gestational age, chronologic age, and volume of sensible and insensible water losses. Adequate fluid intake should compensate for increased insensible losses and the amount needed for renal excretion of metabolic products. Insensible water losses can be minimized by providing high ambient humidity, humidifying oxygen, using heat shields, covering the skin with plastic wrap, and placing the infant in a double-walled incubator.

The nurse evaluates the hydration status of the baby by assessing and recording signs of dehydration. Signs of dehydration include the following:

- Sunken fontanelle
- Loss of weight
- Poor skin turgor (skin returns to position slowly when squeezed gently)
- Dry oral mucous membranes

- Decreased urine output
- Increased specific gravity (greater than 1.013)

The nurse must also identify signs of overhydration by observing the newborn for edema or excessive weight gain and by comparing urine output with fluid intake.

The nurse weighs the preterm infant at least once daily at the same time each day. *Weight change is one of the most sensitive indicators of fluid balance.* Weighing diapers is also important for accurate input and output measurement (1 mL = 1 g). A comparison of intake and output measurements over an 8- or 24-hour period provides important information about renal function and fluid balance. Assessment of patterns and whether they show a net gain or loss over several days is also essential to fluid management. In addition, the nurse monitors blood serum levels and pH to evaluate for electrolyte imbalances.

Accurate hourly intake calculations are needed when administering intravenous fluids. Because the preterm infant is unable to excrete excess fluid, it is essential that the nurse maintain the correct amount of IV fluid to prevent overload. Accuracy can be ensured by using neonatal or pediatric infusion pumps. To prevent electrolyte imbalance and dehydration, the nurse takes care to give the correct intravenous (IV) solutions, as well as the correct volumes and concentrations of formulas. Urine-specific gravity and pH are obtained periodically. Urine osmolality provides an indication of hydration, although this factor must be correlated with other assessments (e.g., serum sodium). Hydration is considered adequate when the urine output is 1 to 3 mL/kg/hr.

Provision of Adequate Nutrition and Prevention of Fatigue During Feeding

The feeding method depends on the preterm newborn's feeding abilities and health status. Both nipple and gavage methods are initially supplemented with intravenous therapy until oral intake is sufficient to support growth (110 to 130 kcal/kg/day). Early, small-volume enteral feedings called *minimal enteral nutrition via gavage* have proved to be of benefit to the very-low-birth-weight infant (see Methods of Feeding earlier in the chapter). GI priming with these small-volume feedings is not intended to contribute to the total nutritional intake but rather to enhance gut metabolism. Trophic feedings may also help encourage earlier advancement to full feedings, thereby decreasing the development of NEC and the complications of parenteral nutrition. Formula or breast milk (with or without fortifiers to increase caloric content) is incorporated into the feedings slowly. This is done to avoid overtaxing the digestive capacity of the preterm newborn. The nurse should carefully watch for any signs of feeding intolerance, including:

- Increasing gastric residuals
- Abdominal distention (measured routinely before feedings) with visible bowel loops

- Guaiac-positive stools (occult blood in stools)
- Lactose in stools (reducing substance in the stools)
- Vomiting
- Diarrhea
- Water-loss stools

Before each feeding, the nurse measures abdominal girth and auscultates the abdomen to determine the presence and quality of bowel sounds. Such assessments permit early detection of abdominal distention, visible bowel loops, and decreased peristaltic activity, which may indicate necrotizing enterocolitis (NEC) or paralytic ileus. The nurse also checks for residual formula in the stomach before feeding when the newborn is fed by gavage. This procedure also can be performed when the nipple-fed newborn presents with abdominal distention. The presence of increasing residual formula is an indication of intolerance to the type or amount of feeding or the increase in amount of feeding.

HINTS FOR PRACTICE

Residual feeding may indicate early NEC and should be called to the attention of the clinician.

Preterm newborns who are ill or who fatigue easily with nipple feedings are usually fed by gavage. The infant is essentially passive with these methods, thus conserving energy and calories. As the baby matures, gavage feedings are replaced with nipple (breast or formula) feedings to assist in strengthening the sucking reflex and in meeting oral and emotional needs. Signs that indicate readiness for oral feedings are a strong gag reflex, presence of nonnutritive sucking, and rooting behavior. Both low-birth-weight and preterm infants nipple-feed more effectively in a quiet state. The nurse establishes a gradual nipple-feeding program, such as one nipple feeding per day, then one nipple feeding per shift, and then a nipple feeding every other feeding. Daily weights are monitored because often there is a small weight loss when nipple feedings are started. After feedings, the nurse places the baby on the right side (with support to maintain this position) or on the abdomen. These positions facilitate gastric emptying and decrease the chance of aspiration if regurgitation occurs. Gastroesophageal reflux is not uncommon in preterm newborns. Long-term gavage feeding may create nipple aversion that will require developmental occupational therapy interventions.

The nurse involves the parents in feeding their preterm baby (Figure 28–10 ■). This is essential to the development of attachment between parents and infant. In addition, it increases parental knowledge about the care of their infant and helps them cope with the situation.

Prevention of Infection

The nurse is responsible for minimizing the preterm newborn's exposure to pathogenic organisms. The preterm

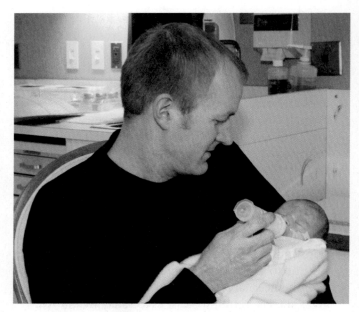

FIGURE 28–10 Father participating in feeding experience with his premature infant.

newborn is susceptible to infection because of an immature immune system and thin and permeable skin. Invasive procedures, techniques such as umbilical catheterization and mechanical ventilation, and prolonged hospitalization place the infant at greater risk for infection.

Strict handwashing and use of separate equipment for each infant help minimize the preterm newborn's exposure to infectious agents. Most nurseries have adopted the Centers for Disease Control and Prevention (CDC) standard precautions of isolating every baby and the Joint Commission on Accreditation of Healthcare Organization (JCAHO) requirement that staff members have short-trimmed nails and no artificial nails. Staff members are required to complete a 2- to 3-minute scrub using iodine-containing antibacterial solutions, which inhibit growth of gram-positive cocci and gram-negative rod organisms. Other specific nursing interventions include limiting visitors; requiring visitors to wash their hands, maintaining strict aseptic practices when changing IV tubing and solutions (IV solutions and tubing should be changed every 24 hours or per agency protocols), administering parenteral fluids, and assisting with sterile procedures. Incubators and radiant warmers should be changed weekly. The nurse prevents pressure-area breakdown by changing the baby's position regularly, doing range of motion exercises, and using water-bed pillows or an air mattress. To avoid skin tears, a protective transparent covering can be applied over vulnerable joints; however, this method is used sparingly (Blackburn, 2007). Chemical skin preps and tape may cause skin trauma and should be avoided as much as possible.

If infection (sepsis) occurs in the preterm newborn, the nurse may be the first to identify its subtle clinical signs, such as lethargy and increased episodes of apnea and bradycardia. The nurse informs the clinician of the findings immediately and implements the treatment plan per clinician orders in the presence of infection. (For specific nursing care required for the newborn with an infection, see Chapter 29 ∞).

Promotion of Parent-Infant Attachment

Preterm newborns can be separated from their parents for prolonged periods after illness or complications that are detected in the first few hours or days following birth. The resultant interruption in parent-newborn bonding necessitates intervention to ensure successful attachment.

Nurses need to take measures to promote positive parental feelings toward the preterm newborn. They can give photographs of the baby to parents to take home. These can also be given to the mother if she is in a different hospital or too ill to come to the nursery and visit. The infant's first name is placed on the incubator as soon as it is known to help the parents feel that their infant is a unique and special person. Parents are given a weekly card with the baby's footprint, weight, and length promote bonding. They are also given the telephone number of the nursery or intensive care unit and the names of staff members so that they have access to information about their baby at any time of the day or night. The nurse encourages visits from siblings and grandparents to foster attachment.

Early involvement in the care of and decisions about their baby provides the parents with realistic expectations for their baby. The individual personality characteristics of the infant and the parents influence the bonding and contribute to the interactive process for the family. By observing each infant's patterns of behavior and responses, especially sleep-wake states, the nurse can teach parents optimal times for interacting with their infants. Parents need education to develop caregiving skills and to understand the premature infant's behavioral characteristics. Their daily participation (if possible) is encouraged, as are early and frequent visits. The nurse should provide opportunities for parents to touch, hold, talk to, and care for the baby. Skin-to-skin holding *(kangaroo care)* helps parents feel close to their small infant (Figure 28–11 ■). Kangaroo care has been shown to improve sleep periods and parents' perception of their caregiving ability (Turnage-Carrier, 2004).

The parents and nurse can plan nursing care around the times when the infant is alert and best able to attend. The more knowledge parents have about the meaning of their infant's responses, behaviors, and cues for interaction, the better prepared they will be able to meet their newborn's needs and form a positive attachment with their child. Parental involvement in difficult care decisions is essential and discussed in greater detail in Chapter 29 ∞.

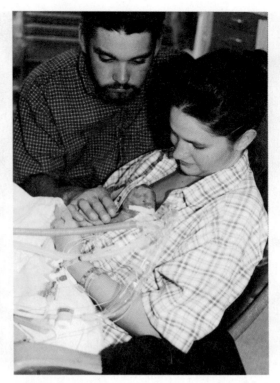

FIGURE 28–11 Kangaroo (skin-to-skin) care facilitates closeness and attachment between parents and their premature infant.
Source: Courtesy of Carol Harrigan, RNC, MSM, NNP.

Some parents may progress easily to touching and cuddling their infant; however, others will not. Parents need to know that their feelings are normal and that the progression of acquaintanceship is slow. Rooming-in can provide another opportunity for the stable preterm infant and family to get acquainted; it offers both privacy and readily available help (Figure 28–12 ■).

Promotion of Developmentally Supportive Care

Prolonged separation and the NICU environment necessitate individualized baby sensory stimulation programs. The nurse plays a key role in determining the appropriate type and amount of visual, tactile, and auditory stimulation.

Some preterm infants are not developmentally able to deal with more than one sensory input at a time. The Assessment of Preterm Infant Behavior (APIB) scale identifies individual preterm newborn behaviors according to five areas of development (Als, Lester, Tronick et al., 1982). The preterm baby's behavioral reactions to stimulation are observed, and developmental interventions are then based on reducing detrimental environmental stimuli to the lowest possible level and providing appropriate opportunities for development (Blackburn, 2007).

Providing developmentally supportive, as well as family-centered, care has been proven to improve the outcomes of the critically ill newborn (Bowie, Hall, Faulkner et al., 2003). With this in mind, specially designed NICUs

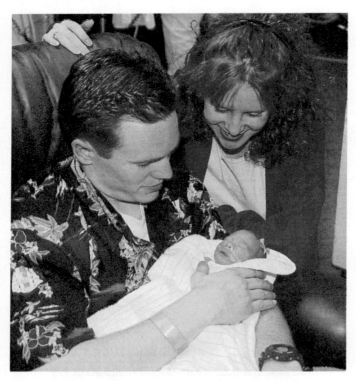

FIGURE 28–12 Family bonding occurs when parents have opportunities to spend time with their infant.
Source: Courtesy of Carol Harrigan, RNC, MSM, NNP.

with the single-room care concept are being developed to minimize lighting and noise as well as to provide privacy for the parents of the convalescing newborn.

The NICU environment contains many detrimental stimuli that the nurse can help reduce. Noise levels can be lowered by replacing alarms with lights. In addition, silencing alarms quickly and keeping conversations away from the baby's bedside can help. Dimmer switches should be used to shield the baby's eyes from bright lights, and blankets may be placed over the top portion of the incubator. Dimming the lights may encourage infants to open their eyes and be more responsive to their parents. Nursing care should be planned to decrease the number of times the baby is disturbed. Signs (e.g., "Quiet Please") can be placed near the bedside to allow the baby some periods of uninterrupted sleep (Blackburn, 2007). Some other suggested developmentally supportive interventions include the following:

- Facilitate handling by using containment measures when turning or moving the infant or doing procedures such as suctioning. Use the hands to hold the infant's arms and legs flexed close to the midline of the body. This helps stabilize the infant's motor and physiologic subsystems during stressful activities.
- Touch the infant gently and avoid sudden postural changes.
- Promote self-consoling and soothing activities, such as placing blanket rolls or approved manufactured

devices next to the infant's sides and against the feet to provide "nesting." Swaddle the infant to maintain extremities in a flexed position while ensuring that the hands can reach the face. This permits the infant to do hand-to-mouth activities, which can be consoling (Figure 28–13 ■).
- Simulate the kinesthetic advantages of the intrauterine environment by using sheepskin and approved water beds. Water bed and pillow use has been reported to improve sleep and decrease motor activity as well as lead to more mature motor behavior, fewer state changes, and a decreased heart rate.
- Provide opportunities for nonnutritive sucking with a pacifier. This improves transcutaneous oxygen saturation; decreases body movements; improves sleep, especially after feedings; and increases weight gain.
- Provide objects for the infant to grasp (e.g., a piece of blanket, oxygen tubing, a finger) during caregiving. Grasping may comfort the baby.

Teaching the parents to read behavioral cues will help them move at their infant's own pace when providing stimulation. Parents are ideally equipped to meet the baby's need for stimulation. Stroking, rocking, cuddling, quiet singing, and talking to the baby can all be integral parts of the baby's care. Visual stimulation in the form of *en face* interaction with caregivers and mobiles is also important.

Preparation for Home Care

Parents are often anxious when their premature infant is transferred out of the NICU or is discharged home. Parents of preterm babies should receive the same postpartal teaching as any parent taking a new infant home. In

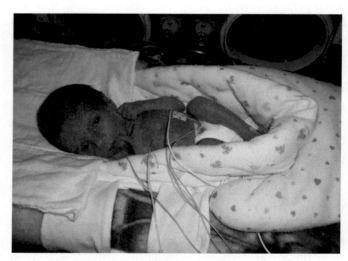

FIGURE 28–13 An 8-day-old, 30 weeks' gestational age, 860-gram IUGR infant is "nested." Hand-to-mouth behavior facilitates self-consoling and soothing activities.
Source: Courtesy of Carol Harnigan, RNC, MSN, NNP.

COMPLEMENTARY AND ALTERNATIVE THERAPIES

Complementary and Alternative Medicine (CAM) in the NICU

As NICUs are becoming more and more "developmentally" friendly, complementary and alternative medicine (CAM) has become an adjunct to that nurturing environment. This holistic approach in caring for the low-birth-weight infant attempts not only to mimic the intrauterine environment, but also to foster parent-infant bonding by simultaneously caring for the body, spirit, and mind.

Aromatherapy is the use of scent to alter mood or behavior to produce a calming and sedating effect. There is an enhanced bonding process between mothers and newborns associated with the natural body odor emitted from the mother (Jones, Kassity, & Duncan, 2001). Aromatherapy is utilized in the NICU by placing an article of clothing belonging to the mother next to the infant to produce a soothing and consoling effect on the infant in her absence. Researchers are also investigating other aromatherapies, including peppermint as a respiratory stimulant, chamomile as a method to regulate sleep-wake cycles, Brazilian guava for its analgesic effects, and lavendar sitz baths for management of diaper rash.

Skin-to-skin (kangaroo) care is becoming more prevalent in NICUs across the United States. It was first practiced in Bogota, Colombia, in the early 1980s because of the fear of the spread of infection from sharing incubators. Skin-to-skin care is defined as the practice of holding infants skin-to-skin next to their parents. The infant is usually naked, except for a diaper, and placed on his/her parent's bare chest. They are then both covered with a blanket. Benefits of skin-to-skin care as a developmental intervention include the following: improved oxygenation as evidenced by an increase in transcutaneous oxygen levels, enhanced temperature regulation, a decline in the episodes of apnea and bradycardia, increased periods of quiet sleep, stabilization of vital signs, positive interaction between parent and infant which enhances attachment and bonding, increased growth parameters, and early discharge (Kledzik, 2005). Limi-

tations to skin-to-skin care may be because of staff uneasiness when moving the infant while attached to multiple IV lines, monitor leads, and a ventilator. The limited confines of the nursery may be another limiting factor.

Music therapy as a noninvasive auditory stimulus has been shown to be advantageous in full-term infants but is not well studied in the premature infant (Gardner & Goldson, 2006). The music used in NICUs includes primarily lullabies and soft acoustical pieces which are pleasant, soothing, and calming. Such music has been shown to effect newborn physiologic responses, such as improving oxygenation and increasing weight gain. It also has behavioral effects, leading to enhanced parental bonding and increased intervals of nonnutritive sucking periods. Language development is also enhanced if the music is live and sung by the mother or another female, which is preferential to the infant (Gardner & Goldson, 2006). However, the overall noise level in the NICU needs to be considered before including any extra auditory stimulation, including music therapy.

Infant massage and gentle touch have been practiced for many centuries. The types of stimulation include massage with stroking, gentle touch without stroking, and therapeutic touch or "hands on" containment. Practitioners report such physiologic benefits as stimulating blood and lymphatic flow, promoting weight gain in premature infants, and regulating sleep patterns (Gardner & Goldson, 2006). Many emotional and behavioral benefits are also cited by practitioners. Classes are available to teach parents how to perform massage on their infants. Massage demonstrates compassion while increasing the parent's empathy and understanding of the baby. It helps parents learn to interpret their baby's behavioral cues such as facial expression, various crying patterns, and other body language. At the same time it helps infants learn about their various body parts and boundaries and feel how they integrate into the whole. Therapeutic touch reduces motor activity and energy expenditure by the infant and also promotes comfort.

---

preparing for discharge, the nurse encourages the parents to spend time caring directly for their baby. This familiarizes them with their baby's behavior patterns and helps them establish realistic expectations about the infant. Some hospitals have a special room near the nursery where parents can spend the night with their baby before discharge.

Discharge instruction includes breastfeeding and formula-feeding techniques, formula preparation, and vitamin administration. If the mother wishes to breastfeed, the nurse teaches her to pump her breasts to keep the milk flowing and provide milk even before discharge. The nurse gives information on bathing, diapering, hygiene, and normal elimination patterns and prepares the parents to expect changes in the color of the baby's stool, number of bowel movements, and timing of elimination when the infant is switched from formula-feeding to breastfeeding. This information can prevent unnecessary concern by the parents. The nurse also discusses normal growth and de-

velopment patterns, reflexes, and activity for preterm infants. In these discussions, the nurse should emphasize ways to promote bonding behaviors and deal with newborn crying. Care of the preterm infant with complications, preventing infections, recognizing signs of a sick baby, and the need for continued medical follow-up are other key issues.

Families with preterm infants usually do not need to be referred to community agencies, such as visiting nurse assistance. However, referral may be necessary if the infant has severe congenital abnormalities, feeding problems, or complications with infections or respiratory problems or if the parents seem unable to cope with an at-risk baby. Parents of preterm infants can benefit from meeting with others in a similar situation to share common experiences and concerns. Nurses should refer parents to support groups sponsored by the hospital or by others in the community and make connections for parents with early education intervention centers.

Preterm and low-birth-weight infants are at greater risk of increased morbidity from vaccine-preventable diseases (AAP & ACOG, 2007). The optimal timing to initiate hepatitis B in preterm infants weighing less than 2000 g whose mothers are hepatitis B surface antigen (HBsAg) negative has not been determined. Preterm infants who weigh less than 2000 g that are medically stable and thriving do show consistently high rates of seroconversion following the first dose of hepatitis B vaccine even when the first dose is given as early as 1 month after birth (AAP & ACOG, 2007). The medically stable preterm infant and LBW infant should receive full doses of diphtheria, tetanus, acellular pertussis, *Haemophilus influenzae* type b, poliovirus, and pneumococcal conjugate vaccines at a chronologic age consistent with the schedule recommended for full-term infants (AAP & ACOG, 2007). The influenza vaccine should be administered at 6 months of age before the beginning of and during the influenza season. Palivizumab for respiratory syncytial (RSV) should be administered during the local RSV season and before hospital discharge to preterm newborns born at less than 35 weeks of gestation as well as those with BPD or congenital heart disease (AAP & ACOG, 2007). Immunoprophylaxis should be continued on a monthly basis until the local RSV season ends.

Evaluation

Expected outcomes of nursing care include the following:

- The preterm newborn is free of respiratory distress and establishes effective respiratory function.
- The preterm newborn gains weight and shows no signs of fatigue or aspiration during feedings.
- The preterm newborn demonstrates a serial head circumference growth rate of 1 cm (0.4 in.) per week.
- The parents are able to verbalize their anger and guilt feelings about the birth of a preterm baby and show attachment behavior such as frequent visits and growing confidence in their participatory care activities.

Care of the Newborn with Congenital Anomalies

The birth of a baby with a congenital defect places both newborn and family at risk. Many congenital anomalies can be life threatening if not corrected within hours after birth; others are very visible and cause the families emotional distress. When one congenital anomaly is found, healthcare providers should look for others, particularly in body systems that develop at the same time during gestation. Table 28–2 identifies common anomalies and their early management and nursing care in the newborn period.

Care of the Infant of a Substance-Abusing Mother

An **infant of a substance-abusing mother (ISAM)** may also be alcohol or drug dependent. After birth, when an infant's connection with the maternal blood supply is severed, the newborn may suffer withdrawal. In addition, the drugs ingested by the mother may be teratogenic, resulting in congenital anomalies or in developmental problems.

Alcohol Dependence

The **fetal alcohol syndrome (FAS)**, a leading cause of mental retardation that is potentially preventable, includes a group of physical, behavioral, and cognitive abnormalities frequently found in infants exposed to alcohol in utero. It is estimated that complete FAS occurs in up to 1000 to 6000 live births (Kenner & Lott, 2007). FAS rates are higher among Native Americans, Alaska natives, African Americans, and women of low socioeconomic status. Children exposed to binge drinking are 1.7 times more likely to have mental retardation and 2.5 times more likely to demonstrate delinquent behavior than unexposed children (Wisner, Sit, Reynolds, Altemus, Bogen, Sunder, Misra, & Perel, 2007).

The National Center on Birth Defects and Developmental Disabilities at the CDC, in collaboration with the National Task Force on Fetal Alcohol Syndrome (FAS) and Fetal Alcohol Effects (FAE), have developed a new set of guidelines for diagnosis and referral of infants and children with FAS (Stokowski, 2004). The term *fetal alcohol effects* (FAE) was used to describe children who had some, but not all, of the characteristics of FAS; however, it was vague. Recently the term **fetal alcohol spectrum disorder (FASD)** has been used to include all categories of prenatal alcohol exposure, including FAS. FASD, however, is an umbrella term and not meant to be used as a clinical diagnosis (Kenner & Lott, 2007).

Alcohol-related birth defects (ARBD) are usually determined only by a positive maternal drinking history. They present with one or more birth defects including malformations and dysplasias of the heart, bone, kidney, vision, or hearing sytems and do not exhibit the classic facial dysmorphology (Moran, 2004). Another term applied to these children is *alcohol related neurodevelopmental disorder (ARND)*. These children have CNS neurodevelopmental abnormalities and complex behavior and cognitive abnormalities (Moran, 2004). ARBD and ARND can both occur together. The new diagnostic categories for FAS take into consideration the various clinical manifestations of FAS, the social and family environment, and, if available, the maternal alcohol history.

MyNursingKit | Partnership to Prevent Fetal Alcohol Spectrum Disorders

TABLE 28–2 Congenital Anomalies: Identification and Care in Newborn Period

Congenital Anomaly	Nursing Assessments	Nursing Goals and Interventions
Congenital Hydrocephalus (Enlarged head)	Enlarged or full fontanelles Split or widened sutures "Setting sun" eyes Head circumference greater than 90% on growth chart	Assess presence of hydrocephalus; Measure and plot occipital-frontal baseline measurements; then measure head circumference once a day. Check fontanelle for bulging and sutures for widening. Assist with head ultrasound and transillumination. Maintain skin integrity: Change position frequently. Clean skin creases after feeding or vomiting. Use sheepskin pillow under head. Postoperatively, position head off operative site. Watch for signs of infection.
Choanal Atresia (Occlusion of posterior nares)	Cyanosis and retractions at rest Noisy respirations Difficulty breathing during feeding Obstruction by thick mucus	Assess patency of nares: Listen for breath sounds while holding baby's mouth closed and alternately compressing each nostril. Assist with passing feeding tube to confirm diagnosis. Maintain respiratory function: Assist with taping airway in mouth to prevent respiratory distress. Position with head elevated to improve air exchange.
Cleft Lip (Unilateral or bilateral visible defect)	May involve external nares, nasal cartilage, nasal septum, and alveolar process Flattening or depression of midfacial contour 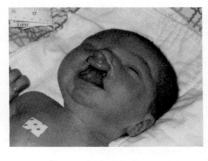	Provide nutrition: Feed with special nipple. Burp frequently (increased tendency to swallow air and reflex vomiting). Clean cleft with sterile water (to prevent crusting on cleft before repair). Support parental coping: Assist parents with grief over loss of idealized baby. Encourage verbalization of their feelings about visible defect. Provide role model in interacting with infant: Parents internalize others' responses to their newborn. (At left) Bilateral cleft lip with cleft abnormality involving both hard and soft palates. *Source:* Courtesy of Carol Harrigan, RNC, MSN, NNP.
Cleft Palate (Fissure connecting oral and nasal cavity)	May involve uvula and soft palate May extend forward to nostril involving hard palate and maxillary alveolar ridge Difficulty in sucking Expulsion of formula through nose	Prevent aspiration/infection: Place prone or in side-lying position to facilitate drainage. Suction nasopharyngeal cavity (to prevent aspiration or airway obstruction). During newborn period feed in upright position with head and chest tilted slightly backward (to aid swallowing and discourage aspiration). Provide nutrition: Feed with special nipple that fills cleft and allows sucking. Also decreases chance of aspiration through nasal cavity. Clean mouth with water after feedings. Burp after each ounce (tend to swallow large amounts of air). Thicken formula to provide extra calories. Plot weight gain patterns to assess adequacy of diet. Provide parental support: Refer parents to community agencies and support groups. Encourage verbalization of frustrations because feeding process is long and frustrating. Praise all parental efforts. Encourage parents to seek prompt treatment for upper respiratory infection (URI) and teach them ways to decrease URI.

(Continued)

TABLE 28–2 Congenital Anomalies: Identification and Care in Newborn Period *(Continued)*

Congenital Anomaly	Nursing Assessments	Nursing Goals and Interventions
Tracheoesophageal Fistula (type 3) (Connection between trachea and esophagus)	History of maternal polyhydramnios	Maintain respiratory status and prevent aspiration.
	Excessive oral secretions	Withhold feeding until esophageal patency is determined.
	Constant drooling	Quickly assess patency before putting to breast in birth area.
	Abdominal distention beginning soon after birth	Place on low intermittent suction to control saliva and mucus (to prevent aspiration pneumonia).
	Periodic choking and cyanotic episodes	Place in warmed, humidified incubator (liquefies secretions, facilitating removal).
	Immediate regurgitation of feeding	Elevate head of bed 20–40 degrees (to prevent reflux of gastric juices).
	Clinical symptoms of aspiration pneumonia (tachypnea, retractions, rhonchi, decreased breath sounds, cyanotic spells)	Keep quiet (crying causes air to pass through fistula and to distend intestines, causing respiratory embarrassment).
	Inability to pass nasogastric tube	Maintain fluid and electrolyte balance. Give fluids to replace esophageal drainage and maintain hydration.
		Provide parent education: Explain staged repair—provision of gastrostomy and ligation of fistula, then repair of atresia.
		Keep parents informed; clarify and reinforce physician's explanations regarding malformation, surgical repair, pre- and postoperative care, and prognosis (knowledge is ego strengthening).
		Involve parents in care of infant and in planning for future; facilitate touch and eye contact (to dispel feelings of inadequacy, increase self-esteem and self-worth, and promote incorporation of infant into family).

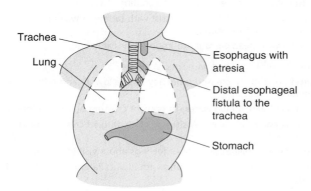

Labels: Trachea, Lung, Esophagus with atresia, Distal esophageal fistula to the trachea, Stomach

(At left) The most frequently seen type of congenital tracheoesophageal fistula and esophageal atresia.
Source: Courtesy Nancy Houck, RNC, BSN, NNP.

Congenital Anomaly	Nursing Assessments	Nursing Goals and Interventions
Diaphragmatic Hernia (Portion of intestines in the thoracic cavity through abnormal opening in diaphragm).	Difficulty initiating respirations	Nurse should never ventilate with bag and mask O_2 because the stomach will inflate, further compressing the lungs.
	Gasping respirations with nasal flaring and chest retraction	Maintain respiratory status: Immediately administer oxygen.
	Barrel chest and scaphoid abdomen	Initiate gastric decompression.
	Asymmetric chest expansion	Place in high semi-Fowler's position (to use gravity to keep abdominal organs' pressure off diaphragm).
	Breath sounds may be absent, usually on left side	Turn to affected side to allow unaffected lung expansion.
	Heart sounds displaced to right	Carry out interventions to alleviate respiratory and metabolic acidosis.
	Spasmodic attacks of cyanosis and difficulty in feeding	Assess for increased secretions around suction tube (denotes possible obstruction).
	Bowel sounds may be heard in thoracic cavity	Aspirate and irrigate tube with air or sterile water.

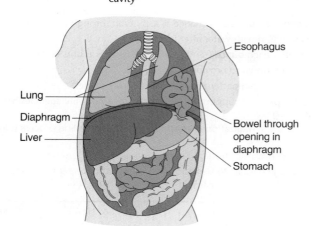

Labels: Esophagus, Lung, Diaphragm, Liver, Bowel through opening in diaphragm, Stomach

(At left) Diaphragmatic hernia. Note compression of the lung by the intestine on the affected side.
Source: Courtesy Nancy Houck, RNC, BSN, NNP.

TABLE 28–2 Congenital Anomalies: Identification and Care in Newborn Period *(Continued)*

Congenital Anomaly	Nursing Assessments	Nursing Goals and Interventions
Omphalocele (Herniation of abdominal contents into base of umbilical cord)	May have an enclosed transparent sac covering	Maintain hydration and temperature. Provide D₅LR and albumin for hypovolemia. Place infant in sterile bag up to and covering defect. Initiate gastric decompression by insertion of nasogastric tube attached to low suction (to prevent distention of lower bowel and impairment of blood flow). Prevent infection and trauma to defect. Position to prevent trauma to defect. Administer broad-spectrum antibiotics.

Maintain hydration and temperature.

Provide D_5LR and albumin for hypovolemia.

Place infant in sterile bag up to and covering defect.

Initiate gastric decompression by insertion of nasogastric tube attached to low suction (to prevent distention of lower bowel and impairment of blood flow).

Prevent infection and trauma to defect.

Position to prevent trauma to defect.

Administer broad-spectrum antibiotics.

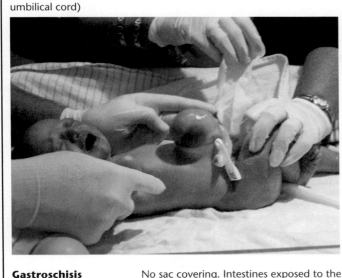

(At left) Newborn with omphalocele.
Source: Courtesy of Carol Harrigan, RNC, MSN, NNP.

Gastroschisis
(Full-thickness defect in abdominal wall allowing viscera outside the body to the right of an intact umbilical cord.)

No sac covering. Intestines exposed to the caustic amniotic fluid.
Associated with intestinal atresia, malrotation

Maintain hydration and temperature.

Prevent trauma and infection to defect.

Provide D_5LR normal saline, and/or albumin for hypovolemia.

Place infant in sterile bag up to axilla.

Initiate gastric decompression by insertion of nasogastric tube attached to low suction.

Administer broad-spectrum antibiotics.

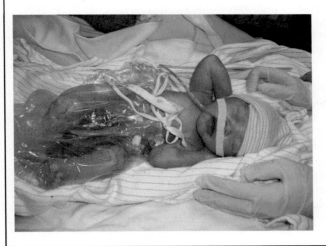

Term newborn with gastroschisis. Note the externalized loops of bowel visible through the bag.
Source: Courtesy of of Carol Harrigan, RNC, MSN, NNP.

(Continued)

TABLE 28–2	Congenital Anomalies: Identification and Care in Newborn Period *(Continued)*	
Congenital Anomaly	**Nursing Assessments**	**Nursing Goals and Interventions**
Prune Belly Syndrome (Congenital absence of one or more layers of abdominal muscles)	Oligohydramnious leading to pulmonary hypoplasia common Deficiency of the abdominal wall musculature causing the abdomen to be shapeless Skin hangs loosely and is wrinkled in appearance Associated with urinary abnormalities (urethral obstruction) In males, cryptorchidism is common; rarely occurs in females 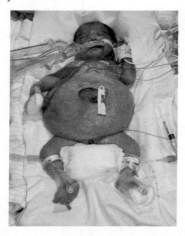	Maintain respiratory status: May need to be immediately intubated and ventilated. Prevent trauma and infection. Administer broad-spectrum antibiotics. Place a urinary catheter and monitor urinary output. Carry out interventions to alleviate respiratory and metabolic acidosis. Keep parents updated and informed about prognosis. Prune belly syndrome. Courtesy of Carol Harrigan, RNC, MSN, NNP.
Myelomeningocele (Saclike cyst containing meninges, spinal cord, and nerve roots in thoracic and/or lumbar area)	Myelomeningocele directly connects to subarachnoid space so hydrocephalus often associated No response or varying response to sensation below level of sac May have constant dribbling of urine Incontinence or retention of stool Anal wink may or may not be present 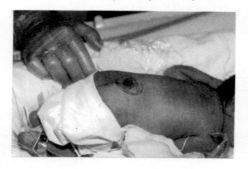	Prevent trauma and infection. Position on abdomen or on side and restrain (to prevent pressure and trauma to sac). Meticulously clean buttocks and genitals after each voiding and defecation (to prevent contamination of sac and decrease possibility of infection). May put protective covering over sac (to prevent rupture and drying). Observe sac for oozing of fluid. Credé bladder (apply downward pressure on bladder with thumbs, moving urine toward the urethra) as ordered to prevent urinary stasis. Assess amount of sensation and movement below defect. Observe for complications. Obtain occipital-frontal circumference baseline measurements; then measure head circumference once a day (to detect hydrocephalus). Check fontanelle for fullness and bulging. Newborn with lumbar myelomeningocele. *Source:* Courtesy of Carole Harrigan, RNC, MSN, NNP.
Imperforate Anus, Congenital Dislocated Hip, and Clubfoot	See discussion in Chapter 25 ∞, Anus and Extremities	Identify defect and initiate appropriate referral early.

Although it is known that ethanol freely crosses the placenta to the fetus, it is still not known whether the alcohol alone or the breakdown products of alcohol cause the damage. (Chapter 15 ∞ discusses alcohol abuse in pregnancy.) The effects of other substances often combined with alcohol, such as nicotine, diazepam (Valium), marijuana, and caffeine, as well as poor diet, enhance the likelihood of FAS.

Long-Term Complications for the Infant with FAS

The long-term prognosis for the FAS newborn is less than favorable. Because of the failure-to-thrive appearance, many FAS infants are often evaluated for deficiencies in organic and inorganic amino acids. These infants have a delay in oral feeding development but have a normal progression of oral motor function. Many FAS infants nurse poorly and have persistent vomiting until 6 to 7 months of age. They have difficulty adjusting to solid foods and show little spontaneous interest in food.

CNS dysfunctions are the most common and serious problem associated with FAS. Hypotonicity and increased placidity are seen in these infants. They also have a decreased ability to block out repetitive stimuli. Children exhibiting FAS can have either severe mental retardation or normal intelligence. The degree of mental retardation is directly proportional to the severity of the dysmorphic findings, meaning the more abnormal the facial features, the lower the IQ scores will be (Jones, 2003). Often there is little improvement in intelligence (as measured by IQ) despite positive environmental and educational factors (Moran, 2004). These children show impulsivity, cognitive impairment, and speech and language abnormalities indicative of CNS involvement (Moran, 2004). As they progress through the adolescent years, they change from a very thin and underweight child to one who is overweight and often obese. Short stature and microcephaly persist.

Nursing Care Management

Nursing Assessment and Diagnosis

Newborns with FAS show the following characteristics:

- *Abnormal structural development and CNS dysfunction.* This includes mental retardation, microcephaly, and hyperactivity.
- *Growth deficiencies.* The growth of infants with FAS is often restricted in regard to weight, length, and head circumference. These infants continue to show a persistent postnatal growth deficiency, with head circumference and linear growth most affected.
- *Distinctive facial abnormalities.* These include short palpebral fissures; epicanthal folds; broad nasal bridge;

flattened midfacies; short, upturned, or beaklike nose; micrognathia (abnormally small lower jaw); hypoplastic maxilla; thin upper lip or vermilion border; and smooth philtrum (groove on upper lip) (Kenner & Lott, 2007).
- *Associated anomalies.* Abnormalities affecting the heart (primarily septal and valvular defects), eyes (optic nerve hypoplasia), ears (conductive and sensorineural hearing loss), kidneys, and skeleton (especially involving joints, such as congenital dislocated hips) systems are often noted.

An alcohol-exposed newborn in the first week of life may show symptoms that include sleeplessness, excessive arousal states, unconsolable crying, abnormal reflexes, hyperactivity with little ability to maintain alertness and attentiveness to environment, jitteriness, abdominal distention, and exaggerated mouthing behaviors such as hyperactive rooting and increased nonnutritive sucking. Seizures may be common. These symptoms commonly persist throughout the first month of life but may continue longer. Alcohol dependence in the infant is physiologic, not psychologic. Signs and symptoms of withdrawal often appear within 6 to 12 hours and at least within the first 3 days of life. Seizures after the neonatal period are rare.

Nursing diagnoses that may apply to the FAS include the following:

- *Altered Nutrition: Less than Body Requirements* related to decreased food intake and hyperirritability
- *Alteration in Neurodevelopmental Status* related to central nervous system involvement secondary to maternal alcohol use
- *Ineffective Coping* related to dysfunctional family dynamics and substance-dependent mother
- *Altered Physical Appearance* related to facial dysmorphology secondary to FAS

Nursing Plan and Implementation

Hospital-Based Nursing Care

Nursing care of the FAS newborn is aimed at avoiding heat loss, providing adequate nutrition, and reducing environmental stimuli. The FAS baby is most comfortable in a quiet, dimly lit environment. Because of their feeding problems, these infants require extra time and patience during feedings. It is important to provide consistency in the staff working with the baby and parents and to keep personnel and visitors to a minimum at any one time.

The nurse should inform the alcohol-dependent mother that breastfeeding is not contraindicated but that excessive alcohol consumption may intoxicate the newborn

MyNursingKit | Fetal Alcohol Syndrome Fact Sheet

and inhibit the letdown reflex. The nurse should monitor the newborn's vital signs closely and observe for evidence of seizure activity and respiratory distress.

Community-Based Nursing Care

Infants affected by maternal alcohol abuse are also at risk psychologically. Restlessness, sleeplessness, agitation, resistance to cuddling or holding, and frequent crying can be frustrating to parents because their efforts to relieve the distress are unrewarded. Feeding difficulties can also result in frustrations for the caregiver and digestive upsets for the infant. Frustration may cause the parents to punish the baby or result in the unconscious desire to stay away from the infant. Either outcome may create an unstable family environment and result in failure to thrive.

The nurse should focus on providing support for the parents and reinforcing positive parenting activity. Before discharge, parents should be given opportunities to provide baby care so that they can feel confident in their interpretations of their baby's cues and ability to meet the baby's needs. Referring the family to social services and visiting nurse or public health nurse associations is essential for the well-being of the infant. Follow-up care and teaching can strengthen the parents' skill and coping abilities and help them create a stable, healthy environment for their family. The infant with FAS should be involved in intervention programs that monitor the child's developmental progress, health, and home environment.

Evaluation

Expected outcomes of nursing care include the following:

- The FAS newborn is able to tolerate feedings and gain weight.
- The FAS infant's hyperirritability or seizures are controlled, and the baby has suffered no physical injuries.
- The parents are able to identify the special needs of their newborn and accept outside assistance as needed.

Drug Dependency

Drugs of abuse by the pregnant woman can include the following substances, used singularly or in combination: tobacco, cocaine, phencyclidine (PCP), methamphetamines, inhalants, marijuana, heroin, and methadone. Patterns of abuse of alcohol, marijuana, and heroin in childbearing women have changed very little in the past few years. Although the incidence of cocaine (especially "crack") use has stabilized, oxycontin use has risen dramatically (see Substances Commonly Abused During

Pregnancy in Chapter 15 ∞ for more discussion of maternal substance abuse). Marijuana, alcohol, and nicotine are sometimes used in conjunction with cocaine.

Intrauterine drug-exposed infants are predisposed to a number of problems. Because almost all narcotic drugs cross the placenta and enter the fetal circulatory system, the fetus can develop problems in utero or soon after birth. The effects of polydrug use on the newborn must always be taken into consideration.

The greatest risks to the fetus of the drug-abusing mother are as follows:

- *Intrauterine asphyxia.* Asphyxia is often a direct result of fetal withdrawal secondary to maternal withdrawal. Fetal withdrawal is accompanied by hyperactivity, with increased oxygen consumption. Insufficiency of oxygen can lead to fetal asphyxia. Moreover, women addicted to narcotics tend to have a higher incidence of preeclampsia, abruptio placentae, and placenta previa, resulting in placental insufficiency and fetal asphyxia.
- *Intrauterine infection.* Sexually transmitted infection, HIV infection, and hepatitis are often connected with the pregnant addict's lifestyle. Such infections can involve the fetus.
- *Alterations in birth weight.* These alterations may depend on the type of drug the mother uses. Women using predominantly heroin have infants of lower birth weight who are SGA. Women maintained on methadone have higher-birth-weight infants, some of whom are LGA.
- *Low Apgar scores.* Low scores may be related to the intrauterine asphyxia or the medication the woman received during labor. The use of a narcotic antagonist (nalorphine or naloxone) to reverse respiratory depression is contraindicated because it may precipitate acute withdrawal in the infant.

Common Complications of the Drug-Exposed Newborn

The newborn of a woman who abused drugs during her pregnancy is predisposed to the following problems:

- *Respiratory distress.* The heroin-addicted newborn frequently suffers respiratory stress, mainly meconium-aspiration pneumonia and transient tachypnea. Meconium aspiration is usually secondary to increased oxygen consumption and activity experienced by the fetus during intrauterine withdrawal. Transient tachypnea may develop secondary to the inhibitory effects of narcotics on the reflex responsible for clearing the lungs. Respiratory distress syndrome, however, occurs less often in heroin-addicted newborns, even in those who are premature, because they have tissue-oxygen-unloading capabilities comparable to those of a 6-week-old term infant. In addition, heroin stimulates production of glucocorticoids via the anterior pituitary gland.

- *Jaundice.* Newborns of methadone-addicted women may develop jaundice because of prematurity. By contrast, infants of mothers addicted to heroin or cocaine have a lower incidence of hyperbilirubinemia because these substances contribute to early maturity of the liver.
- *Congenital anomalies and growth restriction.* The incidence of anomalies of the genitourinary and cardiovascular systems is slightly increased in infants of heroin- and cocaine-addicted mothers. Infants of cocaine-addicted mothers exhibit congenital malformations involving bony skull defects, such as microcephaly, and symmetric intrauterine growth restriction, cardiac defects, and genitourinary defects. In addition, there is a higher incidence of SIDS. Congenital anomalies, however, are rare. Infants exposed to methamphetamines during gestation may show a higher incidence of cleft lip and palate, cardiac anomalies, microcephaly, and LBW (Kenner & Lott, 2007).
- *Behavioral abnormalities.* Babies exposed to cocaine have poor state organization. They exhibit decreased interactive behaviors when tested with the Brazelton Neonatal Behavioral Assessment Scale. These infants also have difficulty moving through the various sleep and wake states and have problems attending to and actively engaging in auditory and visual stimuli.
- *Withdrawal.* The most significant postnatal problem of the drug-exposed newborn is opiate withdrawal (usually from heroin or methadone). The onset of the withdrawal manifestations often occurs after discharge, especially with short birthing-unit stays. See Table 28–3 for a discussion of withdrawal symptoms.

Long-Term Effects

During the first 2 years of life, many cocaine-exposed infants demonstrate susceptibility to behavior lability and the inability to express strong feelings such as pleasure, anger, or distress, or even a strong reaction to being separated from their parents. Cocaine-exposed infants are at higher risk for motor development problems, delays in expressive language skills, and feeding difficulties because of swallowing problems (Kenner & Lott, 2007). Behavioral state control is poorly developed in drug-exposed infants, who tend to rapidly progress from sleep to the awake state of crying without a smooth transition from one state to the next. As a result, these infants have poor social interaction skills; cannot habituate to external stimuli; and become easily overstimulated, having difficulty sleeping.

Infants of drug-addicted mothers often demonstrate a higher incidence of gastrointestinal and respiratory illnesses. These illnesses can be related not to drug exposure but to the mother's lack of education regarding proper infant care, feeding, and hygiene. After birth the infant born to a drug-dependent mother may also be subject to neglect or abuse, or both.

Clinical Therapy

For optimal fetal and neonatal outcome, the heroin-addicted woman should receive complete prenatal care as early as possible to reduce maternal morbidity and mortality rates and to promote fetal stability and growth (Kenner & Lott, 2007). For those women dependent on narcotics, the woman should not be withdrawn completely while pregnant because it induces fetal withdrawal with poor newborn outcomes. Unfortunately, however, pregnant women may be denied access to programs for substance abusers (Lester & Twomey, 2008).

TABLE 28-3 Clinical Manifestations: Newborn Withdrawal

Central Nervous System Signs
- Hyperactivity
- Hyperirritability (persistent shrill cry)
- Increased muscle tone
- Exaggerated reflexes
- Tremors and myoclonic jerks
- Sneezing, hiccups, yawning
- Short, unquiet sleep
- Fever (accompanies the increased neuromuscular activities)

Respiratory Signs
- Tachypnea (greater than 60 breaths per minute when quiet)
- Excessive secretions

Gastrointestinal Signs
- Disorganized, vigorous suck
- Vomiting
- Drooling
- Sensitive gag reflex
- Hyperphagia
- Diarrhea
- Poor feeding (less than 15 mL on first day of life; takes longer than 30 minutes per feeding)

Vasomotor Signs
- Stuffy nose, yawning, sneezing
- Flushing
- Sweating
- Sudden, circumoral pallor

Cutaneous Signs
- Excoriated buttocks, knees, elbows
- Facial scratches
- Pressure-point abrasions

Newborn treatment may include management of complications; serologic tests for syphilis, HIV, and hepatitis B; urine drug screen and meconium analysis; and social service referral (Beauman, 2005). Screening of meconium provides a more comprehensive and accurate indication of exposure over a longer gestational period than does screening of neonatal urine (AAP & ACOG, 2007). Drugs used to control withdrawal symptoms vary and may be regionally based. They include phenobarbital, paregoric, tincture of opium, oral morphine sulfate solution, oral methadone, and diazepam (Beauman, 2005). Nutritional support is important in light of the increase in energy expenditure that withdrawal may entail.

Nursing Care Management

Nursing Assessment and Diagnosis

Early identification of the newborn needing clinical or pharmacologic interventions decreases the incidence of neonatal mortality and morbidity. The identification of substance-exposed newborns is determined primarily by clinical indicators in the prenatal period including maternal presentation, history of substance use or abuse, medical history, or toxicology results. During the newborn period, nursing assessment focuses on the following:

- Discovering the mother's last drug intake and dosage level. This is accomplished through the perinatal history and laboratory tests. Women may be reluctant to disclose this information; therefore, a nonjudgmental interview technique is essential (AAP & ACOG, 2007).
- Assessing for congenital malformations and the complications related to intrauterine withdrawal such as SGA, asphyxia, meconium aspiration, and prematurity.
- Identifying the signs and symptoms of newborn withdrawal or neonatal abstinence syndrome (see Table 28–3).

Although many of the signs and symptoms of drug withdrawal are similar to those seen with hypoglycemia and hypocalcemia, glucose and calcium values are reported to be within normal limits.

Neonatal abstinence syndrome includes both physiologic and behavioral responses. Nursery nurses need to be competent in recognition of signs of neonatal withdrawal. A number of useful systematic scoring systems are available for assessing severity (AAP & ACOG, 2007). The severity of withdrawal can be assessed by a scoring system such as the Finnegan scale that is based on observations and measurement of the responses to neonatal abstinence.

It evaluates the infant on potentially life-threatening signs such as vomiting, diarrhea, weight loss, irritability, tremors, and tachypnea (Table 28–4).

Nursing diagnoses that may apply to drug-dependent newborns include the following:

- *High Risk for Infant CNS Injury* related to perinatal substance abuse
- *Risk for Ineffective Airway Clearance* related to suppression of respiratory system
- *Altered Nutrition: Less than Body Requirements* related to vomiting and diarrhea, uncoordinated suck and swallow reflex, and hypertonia secondary to withdrawal
- *Impaired Skin Integrity* related to constant activity, diarrhea
- *Sleep Pattern Disturbance* related to CNS excitation secondary to drug withdrawal
- *Altered Parenting* related to hyperirritable behavior of the infant and lack of knowledge of infant care
- *Ineffective Family Coping: Disabling* related to drug-dependent parent

Nursing Plan and Implementation
Hospital-Based Nursing Care

Care of the drug-dependent newborn is based on reducing withdrawal symptoms and promoting adequate respiration, temperature, and nutrition. See Nursing Care Plan for a Newborn of a Substance-Abusing Mother on pages 735–737 for specific nursing measures. Some general nursery care measures include the following:

- Performing neonatal abstinence scoring per hospital protocol
- Monitoring temperature for hypothermia
- Carefully monitoring pulse and respirations every 15 minutes until stable; stimulation if apnea occurs
- Providing small, frequent feedings, especially in the presence of vomiting, regurgitation, and diarrhea
- Administering intravenous therapy as needed
- Administering medications as ordered, such as oral morphine, phenobarbital, and tincture of opium
- Proper positioning on the right side-lying or semi-Fowler's to avoid possible aspiration of vomitus or secretions
- Monitoring frequency of diarrhea and vomiting, and weighing infant every 8 hours during withdrawal
- Observing for problems of SGA or LGA newborns
- Swaddling with hands near mouth to minimize injury and help achieve a more organized behavioral state. (Offer a pacifier for nonnutritive, excessive sucking. Gentle, vertical rocking can be successful

TABLE 28–4	Neonatal Abstinence Score Sheet						

		Neonatal Abstinence Scoring System					
System	Signs and Symptoms	Score		Am		Pm	Comments
Central Nervous System Disturbances	Excessive high-pitched (or other) cry	2					Daily weight
	Continuous high-pitched (or other) cry	3					
	Sleeps < 1 hour after feeding	3					
	Sleeps < 2 hours after feeding	2					
	Sleeps < 3 hours after feeding	1					
	Hyperactive Moro reflex	2					
	Markedly hyperactive Moro reflex	3					
	Mild tremors disturbed	1					
	Moderate-severe tremors disturbed	2					
	Mild tremors undisturbed	3					
	Moderate-severe tremors undisturbed	4					
	Increased muscle tone	2					
	Excoriation (specific area)	1					
	Myoclonic jerks	3					
	Generalized convulsions	5					
Metabolic/Vasomotor/ Respiratory Disturbances	Sweating	1					
	Fever < 101 (37.2°C to 38.2°C/99°F to 100.8°F)	1					
	Fever > 101 (38.4°C [101.1°F] and higher)	2					
	Frequent yawning (> 3 to 4 times/interval)	1					
	Mottling	1					
	Nasal stuffiness	1					
	Sneezing (> 3 to 4 times/interval)	1					
	Nasal flaring	2					
	Respiratory rate > 60/min	1					
	Respiratory rate > 60/min with retractions	2					
Gastrointestinal Disturbances	Excessive sucking	1					
	Poor feeding	2					
	Regurgitation	2					
	Projectile vomiting	3					
	Loose stools	2					
	Watery stools	3					
	Total Score						
	Initials of Scorer						

Source: Finnegan, L. P. (1990). Neonatal abstinence syndrome. In N. Nelson (Ed.), *Current therapy in neonatal-perinatal medicine* (2nd ed.). Ontario: BC Decker.

in calming an infant who is out of control.) (See Figure 28–14 ■.)

- Protecting face and extremities from excoriation by using mittens, and soft sheets or sheepskin
- Applying protective skin emollient to the groin area with each diaper change
- Placing the newborn in a quiet, dimly lit area of the nursery

Community-Based Nursing Care

Parents need assistance to prepare for what they can expect for the first few months at home. At the time of discharge, the mother should be instructed to anticipate mild jitteriness and irritability in the newborn, which may persist from 6 days to 8 weeks, depending on the initial severity of the withdrawal (Blackburn, 2007). Infants with neonatal abstinence syndrome are at significantly higher risk for SIDS when the mother used heroin or cocaine. The infant should sleep supine and home apnea monitoring should be implemented. The nurse should help the mother learn feeding techniques, comforting measures, how to recognize newborn cues, and appropriate parenting responses. Parents are to be counseled regarding available resources, such as support groups, as well as signs and symptoms that indicate the need for further care. Ongoing evaluation is necessary because of the potential for long-term problems. Follow-up on missed appointments can bring parents back into the healthcare system, thereby

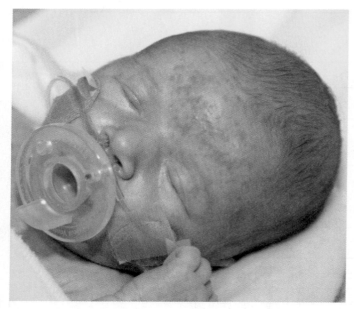

FIGURE 28–14 Nonnutritive sucking on a pacifier has a calming effect on newborn.

improving parent and infant outcomes and promoting a positive, interactive environment after birth (AAP & ACOG, 2007).

Evaluation

Expected outcomes of nursing care include the following:

- The newborn tolerates feedings, gains weight, and has a decreased number of stools.
- The parents learn innovative ways to comfort their newborn.
- The parents are able to cope with their frustrations and begin to use outside resources as needed.

Infants of Mothers Who Are Tobacco Dependent

Despite increased knowledge about the dangers to the fetus and newborn of smoking mothers, 15% to 25% of women continue to smoke during pregnancy. The common consequence of tobacco use is addiction to nicotine. Most smokers report true enjoyment, associated with a sense of relaxation during stress, especially with the first cigarette of the day (CDC, 2005). The tobacco-induced hazards on the pregnant woman and her developing fetus may be one of the most underrated health issues, at least in public opinion.

Preconceptual cigarette smoking has been found to increase infertility. Fortunately, the reduction in fertility is reversible if the woman stops smoking. Smoking during pregnancy has been associated with spontaneous abortion, placenta previa, and abruptio placentae. See Tobacco in Chapter 11 ∞ for discussion of maternal care.

Risks of Tobacco to the Fetus and Newborn

The most studied compound found in cigarette smoking that can adversely affect the intrauterine environment is carbon monoxide. Carbon monoxide binds hemoglobin to form carboxyhemoglobin which reduces the oxygen-carrying capacity of the blood. It also increases the binding of hemoglobin to oxygen, which impairs the release of oxygen to the tissues. Therefore the fetus can experience intrauterine hypoxia and ischemia. Mothers who smoke during pregnancy are nearly twice as likely to have a LBW infant, and smoking during pregnancy is linked to an increase in preterm and LBW infants (ACOG, 2005). These infants typically weigh 150 to 250 g or less than infants of nonsmokers (Cloherty et al., 2008). The nicotine in cigarettes acts as a neuroteratogen that interferes with fetal development, specifically the developing nervous system. The greatest risks to the fetus and newborn of the mother who smokes include the following (Barron, 2008):

- *Intrauterine growth restriction and/or prematurity* secondary to cigarette metabolites crossing the placenta causing vasoconstriction and decreased placental blood flow
- *Intrauterine distress* presenting as meconium staining and low Apgar scores
- *Neonatal neurobehavioral abnormalities* such as impaired habituation, orientation, consolability, orientation to sound
- *Hypertonia or hypotonia, increase in tremors, increased Moro reflex*
- *Signs of nicotine toxicity* (tachycardia, irritability, poor feeding)
- Sudden infant death syndrome

Clinical Therapy

Prevention is always the best intervention. Inquiry into tobacco and smoke exposure should be a routine part of the prenatal history. Preconception and prenatal counseling about the effects of cigarette smoking on pregnancy and the fetus should occur. An estimated 5% reduction in perinatal mortality would occur if smoking during pregnancy were eliminated (AAP & ACOG, 2007).

Cotinine, a metabolite of nicotine, has been found in fetal body fluids. There is also a positive correlation between the number of cigarettes smoked per day and the concentration of cotinine in maternal urine. Other factors that influence fetal and maternal serum cotinine concentrations are nicotine content of the cigarette and the time elapsed between the last cigarette smoked and the sampling. These findings indicate that cotinine may be used as a marker of maternal-fetal tobacco exposure during pregnancy (Kenner & Lott, 2007).

Nursing Care Plan   For a Newborn of a Substance-Abusing Mother

CLIENT SCENARIO

Samuel is a 38 weeks' gestation newborn, weighing 6 lb 4 oz. Apgars were 5, 7 and 8 at 1, 5 and 10 minutes. He was admitted to the nursery 12 hours ago. His mother, age 21, has a long history of drug and alcohol abuse. The drug and alcohol abuse continued throughout pregnancy but the mother states that she has not had any alcohol or cocaine since 3 days before labor. During the course of her pregnancy she has gained 22 lb and her prenatal care has been inconsistent. On admission to the nursery, the nurse drew blood for serum electrolytes and checked glucose levels. Formula-feeding has been initiated and Samuel is swaddled tightly in a side-lying position in an area of the nursery with decreased stimuli.

ASSESSMENT

Subjective: N/A

Objective: Weight 6 lb, 4 oz (2835 g), head circumference 30 cm (11.8 in.), length 45.7 cm (18 in.), vomited three times, formula intake 45 mL last 12 hours, exaggerated mouthing behaviors, watery stools, jitteriness, hypertonicity, and glucose level of 50 mg/dL.

Nursing Diagnosis #1	Imbalanced Nutrition: Less than Body Requirements related to decreased food intake, diarrhea, and weak sucking reflex.*
Client Goal	The newborn will tolerate feedings.
AEB:	• Increased birth weight • Improved sucking reflex • Decreased episodes of vomiting and diarrhea

NURSING INTERVENTIONS

1. Monitor weight every 8 hours.

2. Monitor vital signs every 4 hours.

3. Observe and document intake and output every 8 hours.

4. Administer IV fluids.

5. Assess glucose levels.

6. Provide small, frequent feedings every 3 to 4 hours.

7. Assess abdominal distention and gastric residual.

8. Encourage breastfeeding as ordered by physician.

RATIONALES

Rationale: Poor sucking reflex, vomiting and diarrhea, sensitive gag reflex, and a prolonged feeding time contribute to poor weight gain in the first few days of life.

Rationale: Newborn may experience tachypnea (> 60 breaths/minute), secondary to the inhibitory effects of narcotics on the reflex responsible for clearing the lungs. Temperature may be elevated. The newborn expends energy with the increase in temperature and respirations that in turn burns calories. Weight will decrease with the extra expenditure of calories.

Rationale: Assess for fluid loss and dehydration caused by vomiting and diarrhea secondary to CNS excitation.

Rationale: Nutritional support and replacement of fluids and electrolytes may be needed to correct deficiencies. Medications may also be given intravenously to control withdrawal symptoms in the newborn. Withdrawal symptoms include hyperactivity, jitteriness, hyperirritability, seizure activity, exaggerated reflexes, tremors, sleep disturbance, tachypnea, disorganization, vigorous suck, and stuffy nose.

Rationale: Newborn signs of narcotic withdrawal are similar to signs of hypoglycemia and hypocalcemia. To differentiate withdrawal signs from hypoglycemia and hypocalcemia in the newborn, glucose and calcium levels are drawn. Nutritional supplements of glucose may be needed if the newborn is hypoglycemic.

Rationale: These newborns are not able to tolerate large feedings because of gastrointestinal problems (poor suck, vomiting, diarrhea) and fatigue with feeding. As these problems subside feeding volume can be increased (if tolerated) and hyperactivity can decrease.

Rationale: Digestion and gastric motility may be impaired. Abdominal girth measurements will allow the nurse to assess for abdominal distention and feeding intolerance. Gastric residuals assess for the effectiveness of stomach emptying after feedings.

Rationale: Breastfeeding is not contraindicated in the newborn with fetal alcohol syndrome, but the mother must abstain from alcohol use during breastfeeding. Alcohol will affect letdown of breast milk. Supplement with breast milk only when medically indicated. Perform a toxicology screen of breast milk per agency protocol.

(Continued on next page)

Nursing Care Plan   For a Newborn of a Substance-Abusing Mother   *(Continued)*

NURSING INTERVENTIONS

9. Allow extended time to feed the newborn.

10. Maintain side-lying or semi-Fowler's position after feedings.

11. Place newborn in radiant warmer or swaddle in open crib to maintain temperature.

12. Obtain urine specimen and meconium analysis.

RATIONALES

Rationale: Because of disorganized, vigorous sucking, jitteriness, irritability, excessive rooting, and abdominal distention, feeding experience is difficult, very time consuming, and requires patience and extra feeding time.

Rationale: Vomiting is a common problem in newborns who are experiencing gastrointestinal problems caused by drug dependency. Side-lying or semi-Fowler's position will help to avoid aspiration.

Rationale: Newborns with fetal alcohol syndrome are prone to heat loss. Heat loss may cause shivering and thus burn more calories and affect weight gain.

Rationale: To identify drug substances in the newborn. Test results will help to direct treatment for possible drug dependency. Drug dependency and treatment measures may affect nutritional status.

Evaluation of Client Goal	• Newborn returns to birth weight in 1 week. • Improved nutritive sucking and able to complete feedings within a timely manner. • No episodes of vomiting or diarrhea documented.
Nursing Diagnosis #2	Disturbed Sleep Pattern related to CNS excitation secondary to drug withdrawal.
Client Goal	Organized sleep-wake cycles will be established.
AEB:	• An organized behavioral state of the newborn is established. • Periods of sleep are increased.

NURSING INTERVENTIONS

1. Monitor vital signs every 4 hours.

2. Assess altered sleep-wake cycle and rhythm every 24 to 48 hours.

3. Administer medications for withdrawal.

4. Swaddle newborn tightly in open crib.

5. Place newborn in quiet, dimly lit area of nursery.

6. Hold, rock, and cuddle infant.

7. Provide pacifier or position baby with hands near mouth.

8. Cluster care to meet newborn's sleep-wake schedule.

RATIONALES

Rationale: Tachypnea (> 60 breaths/minute), tachycardia (> 160 bpm), temperature instability along with stuffy nose may be present. The newborn expends energy when the vital signs are altered; therefore, rest is more difficult.

Rationale: Withdrawal symptoms such as hyperactivity, jitteriness, hyperirritability, seizure activity, exaggerated reflexes, tremors, and sleep disturbances interfere with sleep-wake cycles. Over 24 to 48 hours a trend may be evaluated to assess whether pharmacologic and nonpharmacologic treatments are effective. Treatments may include medications therapy to minimize withdrawal symptoms and swaddling for comfort to promote a more organized behavioral state.

Rationale: Administering medications for withdrawal will alleviate signs and symptoms of withdrawal, allow the newborn to rest, and improve nutritional status. Medications include phenobarbital, paregoric, oral morphine sulfate, and diazepam.

Rationale: To provide warmth and promote calming behaviors. Swaddle with newborn hands near mouth to minimize injury and help achieve a more organized behavioral state.

Rationale: This helps avoid overstimulation of the newborn. Newborns of substance-abusing mothers are more difficult to console which decreases the ability to rest and sleep.

Rationale: To decrease irritability and promote comfort. Use infant snuggly for closeness and carrying infant.

Rationale: Hand-to-mouth activity or pacifier helps organize baby's suck and satisfies increased need to suck during withdrawal.

Rationale: To decrease stimulation of newborn. Limiting personnel and visitors to a minimum at any one time will also promote rest and sleep.

Nursing Care Plan   For a Newborn of a Substance-Abusing Mother   *(Continued)*

NURSING INTERVENTIONS	RATIONALES
9. Provide consistency of staff members assigned to newborn.	*Rationale:* Allows staff to assess for subtle changes in newborn behaviors and decreases overstimulation. Staff is able to develop a trusting relationship with the parents and reinforce positive parenting activities.
Evaluation of Client Goal	• Sleep-wake states become more organized. • Periods of sleep increased.

CRITICAL THINKING QUESTIONS

1. The nurse is caring for two newborns experiencing signs and symptoms of drug withdrawal. One of the mothers is a methadone addict and the other mother is a heroin and cocaine addict. Which mother would most likely have a baby with hyperbilirubinemia?

Answer: Liver maturity is reached earlier in a newborn whose mother has a heroin or cocaine addiction, because of substances in the drug. Therefore the heroin or cocaine newborn has no greater chance for hyperbilirubinemia than the normal newborn population. Newborns of mothers who are addicted to methadone are more likely to develop hyperbilirubinemia.

2. The nurse is providing discharge instructions to two mothers who have substance abuse. One mother abuses alcohol and the other is a heroin addict. Which mother will the nurse provide with instructions on feeding problems of the newborn and which mother will the nurse educate on the prevention of SIDS?

Answer: Newborns of mothers who abuse alcohol may develop fetal alcohol syndrome. These newborns may experience failure to thrive and have feeding difficulties such as a delay in oral feeding development, nurse poorly, and have persistent vomiting until 6 to 7 months of age. The newborns of heroin-addicted mothers show a higher incidence of SIDS compared with the normal population. The nurse should instruct the mother to place the newborn in a supine position for sleep and get a home apnea monitor.

*For your reference, this care plan is an example of how two nursing diagnosis might be addressed.

Nursing Care Management

Mothers should be counseled that eliminating or reducing smoking even late in pregnancy can improve fetal growth. The use of nicotine patches (instead of smoking) reduces the absorption of nicotine and thereby may increase the birth weight of the fetus. See Tobacco in Chapter 11 ∞ for further discussion of prenatal smoking cessation and other intervention programs.. Newborns of mothers who are tobacco dependent may be screened with the NICU Network Neurobehavioral Scale (NNNS) to assess their neurological, behavioral, and stress/abstinence neurobehavioral function (Kenner & Lott, 2007).

The potential for long-term respiratory problems such as asthma, as well as cognitive and receptive language delays that may persist into school age, should be evaluated.

Care of the Newborn Exposed to HIV/AIDS

An increasing number of newborns are being born infected with HIV or at risk for acquiring it in the newborn period or early infancy. More than 90% of transmissions during the perinatal and neonatal periods can occur across the placenta or through breast milk or contaminated blood (Cloherty et al., 2008). The risk of vertical transmission can be decreased in mothers taking antiretroviral drug regimens during gestation to a rate of less than 2% (American Academy of Pediatrics [AAP] and American College of Obstetricians and Gynecologists [ACOG], 2007). (For discussion of maternal and fetal HIV/AIDS, see Chapter 11 ∞). Pregnant women should be universally tested (with client notification) for HIV infection as part of the routine battery of prenatal blood tests unless they decline the test (i.e., opt-out approach) as permitted by local and state regulations (AAP & ACOG, 2007). Refusal of testing should be documented.

Opportunistic diseases such as gram negative sepsis and problems associated with prematurity are the primary causes of mortality in HIV-infected babies. Some infants infected by maternal-fetal transmission suffer from severe immunodeficiency, with HIV disease progressing more rapidly during the first year of life.

Early identification of babies with or at risk for HIV/AIDS is essential during the newborn period. However, the currently available HIV serologic tests (ELISA and Western blot test) cannot distinguish between maternal and infant antibodies; therefore, they are inappropriate for infants up to 18 months of age. It may take up to 18 months for infected infants to form their own antibodies to the HIV (Read & Committee on Pediatric AIDS, 2007). Testing by HIV deoxyribonucleic acid (DNA) polymerase chain reaction (PCR) is the preferred test. Results can be made available within 24 hours (Venkatesh et al., 2006). A viral culture may also be performed at birth but it is more expensive. The first DNA PCR test should be performed on the newborn born to HIV-infected women during the first 48 hours of age. Umbilical cord blood should not be used for HIV testing because of possible contamination with maternal blood (AAP & ACOG, 2007). If PCR and viral culture are unavailable, the acid-dissociated p24 antigen may be used to assess HIV infection status in infants older than 1 month (Bernstein, 2007; Cloherty et al., 2008). A second test should be performed at 1 to 2 months of age. A third test is recommended at 2 to 4 months of age. An infant is considered infected if two separate samples are positive (AAP & ACOG, 2007). Most clinicians confirm the absence of HIV-1 infection with a negative HIV-1 antibody assay result at 12 to 18 months of age (Read & Committee on Pediatric AIDS, 2007). For term infants, AZT (zidovudine [ZDV]) is started prophylactically 2 mg/kg/dose PO every 6 hours (Nash & Smith, 2008). If the infant is confirmed to be HIV positive, ZDV is changed to a multidrug antiretroviral regimen.

Nursing Care Management

Nursing Assessment and Diagnosis

Many newborns exposed to HIV/AIDS are premature or SGA, or both, and show evidence of failure to thrive during neonatal and infant periods. They can show signs and symptoms of disease within days of birth. Signs that may be seen in the early infancy period include enlarged spleen and liver, swollen glands, recurrent respiratory infections, rhinorrhea, interstitial pneumonia (rarely seen in adults), recurrent GI (diarrhea and weight loss) and urinary system infections, persistent or recurrent oral candidiasis infections, and loss of achieved developmental milestones (Venkatesh et al., 2006). There is also a high risk of acquiring *Pneumocystis carnii* pneumonia.

Nursing diagnoses that may apply to an infant exposed to HIV/AIDS include the following:

- *Altered Nutrition: Less than Body Requirements* related to formula intolerance and inadequate intake
- *Risk for Impaired Skin Integrity* related to chronic diarrhea
- *Risk for Infection* related to perinatal exposure and immunoregulation suppression secondary to HIV/AIDS
- *Impaired Physical Mobility* related to decreased neuromuscular development

- *Altered Growth and Development* related to lack of attachment and stimulation
- *Altered Parenting* related to diagnosis of HIV/AIDS and fear of future outcome

Nursing Plan and Implementation

Hospital-Based Nursing Care

Nursing care of the newborn exposed to HIV/AIDS includes all the care normally given to any newborn in a nursery. In addition, the nurse must include care for a newborn suspected of having a blood-borne infection, as with hepatitis B. Standard precautions should be used when caring for the newborn immediately after birth and when obtaining blood samples via vein puncture or heel stick. (The blood of all newborns must be considered potentially infectious because the status of the infant's blood is often not known until after the infant is discharged. There is a window of time before seroconversion occurs when the baby is still considered infectious.)

Nursing care involves providing for comfort; keeping the newborn well nourished and protected from opportunistic infections; good skin care to prevent skin rashes; and facilitating growth, development, and attachment. Most institutions recommend that their caregivers wear gloves during all diaper changes and examination of babies. Disposable gloves are worn when changing diapers or cleaning the diaper area, especially in the presence of diarrhea, because blood may be in the stool and should be considered part of standard precautions for hospital personnel (AAP & ACOG, 2007). See Table 28–5.

Community-Based Nursing Care

Handwashing is crucial when caring for newborns at risk for AIDS. Parents should be taught proper handwashing technique. Nutrition is essential because failure to thrive and weight loss are common. Small, frequent feedings and food supplementation are helpful. The nurse discusses with parents sanitary techniques for preparing formula. The nurse also informs the parents that the baby should not be put to bed with juice or formula because of potential bacterial growth. Parents need to be alert to the signs of feeding intolerance, such as increasing regurgitation, abdominal distention, and loose stools. The newborn is weighed three times a week.

CRITICAL THINKING

Mrs. Jean Corrigan, a 23-year-old GIPI positive for HIV, has just given birth to a 7 lb, 1 oz baby girl. As she watches you assessing her daughter in the birthing room, she asks why you are wearing gloves and whether her daughter will have to be in isolation. What will your response be?

Answers can be found in Appendix F ∞.

TABLE 28–5	Issues for Caregivers of Infants at Risk for HIV/AIDS
Resuscitation	For suctioning use a bulb syringe, mucus extractor, or meconium aspirator with wall suction on low setting. Use masks, goggles, and gloves.
Admission care	To remove blood from baby's skin, give warm water-mild soap bath using gloves as soon as possible after admission.
Handwashing	Thorough handwashing is indicated before and after caring for infant. Hands must be washed immediately if contaminated with blood or body fluids. Wash hands after removal of gloves.
Gloves	Gloves are indicated with touching blood or other high-risk fluids. Gloves should also be worn when handling newborns before and during their initial baths, cord care, eye prophylactics, and vitamin K administration.
Mask, goggle, and gown	Not routinely needed unless coming in contact with placenta or the blood and amniotic fluid on the skin of the newborn.
Needles and syringes	Used needles should not be recapped or bent; they should be disposed of in a puncture-resistant plastic container belonging specifically to that baby. After the newborn is discharged the container is discarded.
Specimens	Blood and other specimens should be double-bagged and/or sealed in an impervious container and labeled according to agency protocol.
Equipment and linen	Articles contaminated with blood or body fluids should be discarded or bagged according to isolation or institution protocol.
Body fluid spills	Blood and body fluids should be cleaned promptly with a solution of 5.25% sodium hypochlorite (household bleach) diluted 1:10 with water. Apply for at least 30 seconds then wipe after the minimum contact time.
Education and support	Provide education and psychologic support for family and staff. Caregivers who avoid contact with a baby at risk or who overdress in unnecessary isolation garb subtly exacerbate an already difficult family situation. Information resources include the National AIDS Hotline (1-800-342-2437) and HIV/AIDS Treatment Enforcement Service Website http://www.hevatis.org
Exempted personnel	Immunologically compromised staff (pregnant women may be included in this group) and possibly infectious staff members should not care for these infants.

Source: Adapted from American Academy of Pediatrics, Committee on Pediatric AIDS and Committee on Infectious Diseases. (1999). Issues related to human immunodeficiency transmission in schools, child care, medical settings, the home, and community. *Pediatrics, 104* (2), 318–324; Mendez, H., & Jule, J. E. (1990). Care of the infant born exposed to AIDS. *Obstetric and Gynecologic Clinics of North America, 17* (3), 637; Krist, A. H., & Crawford-Faucher, A. (2002). Management of newborns exposed to maternal HIV infection. *American Family Physician, 65* (10), 2049–2056.

The baby has his or her own skin care items, towels, and washcloths. Most clothing and linens can be washed with other household laundry. Linen that is visibly soiled with blood or body fluids should be kept and washed separately in hot, sudsy water with household bleach. Prompt diaper changing and perineal care can prevent or minimize diaper rash and promote comfort. Soiled diapers should be placed in plastic bags, sealed, and disposed of daily. Diaper-changing areas should be cleaned with a 1:10 dilution of household bleach after each diaper change. Toys should be kept as clean as possible, not shared with other children, and checked for sharp edges to prevent scratches.

The nurse instructs the parents about signs of infection to be alert to and when to call their healthcare provider. The inability to feed without pain may indicate esophageal yeast infection and may require administration of nystatin (Mycostatin) for the oral thrush. Topical Mycostatin or Desitin ointment is used for diaper rashes. If diarrhea occurs, the baby needs frequent perineal care as well as fluid replacements. Antidiarrheal medications are often ineffective. Irritability may be the first sign of fever. Fluids, antipyretics, and sponging with tepid water are of use in managing fever. Preventive care for exposed infants is the same as for other infants and includes routine immunizations, except that the live polio vaccine should be avoided. If the infant is exposed to varicella, the parents should notify their healthcare professional because the baby may need varicella zoster immune globulin (VZIG) within 96 hours of exposure or if exposed to measles (may need vaccination within 72 hours of exposure).

Parents and family members need to be reassured that there are no documented cases of people contracting HIV/AIDS from routine care of infected babies. Emotional support for family members is essential because of the stress and social isolation they may face. Because of these stresses, parents may not bond with the baby or they may fail to provide the baby with enough sensory and tactile stimulation. The nurse encourages the parents to hold the baby during feedings because the infant benefits from frequent, gentle touch. Auditory stimulation may also be provided by using music or tapes of parents' voices. The nurse offers families information about support groups, available counseling, and information resources. Current therapeutic information about HIV is available to both healthcare providers and families through the AIDS Clinical Trials Information Service (1-800-TRIALS-A). The CDC recommends that HIV-infected women in developed countries not breastfeed because HIV can be transmitted via breast milk. Therefore, if there is a viable alternative feeding method, it should be used (Vankatesh et al., 2006).

Infants of infected mothers should be given antiretroviral drug therapy such as zidovudine (AZT) beginning at 8 to 12 hours of life and continuing for 6 weeks

(Nash & Smith, 2008). All infants born to HIV-positive mothers require regular clinical, immunologic, and virologic monitoring. At 1 month of age the baby's physical exam should include a developmental assessment and complete blood count, including differential blood count, CD4+ count, and platelet count. Prophylaxis for *Pneumocystis carinii* pneumonia (PCP) for all infants born to HIV-1-infected women should be begun after completion of the ZDV prophylaxis regimen (Nash & Smith, 2008). Pediatric HIV disease raises many healthcare issues for the family. The parents, depending on their health status, may or may not be able to care for their infant, and they must deal with many psychosocial and economic issues.

Evaluation

Expected outcomes of nursing care include the following:

- The parents are able to bond with their infant and have realistic expectations about the baby.
- Potential opportunistic infections are identified early and treated promptly.
- The parents verbalize their concerns about their baby's existing and potential health problems and long-term care needs and accept outside assistance as needed.

Care of the Newborn with Congenital Heart Defect

Congenital heart defects occur in 3% to 8% of live births (depending on the severity of structural defects). Because accurate diagnosis and surgical treatment are now available, many deaths can be prevented (Cloherty et al., 2008). Corrective cardiac surgery is being done at earlier ages; for example, more than half the children undergoing surgery are less than 1 year of age, and one-fourth are less than 1 month old. It is crucial for the nurse to have comprehensive knowledge of congenital heart disease to detect deviations from normal and initiate interventions.

Overview of Congenital Heart Defects

In the majority of cases of congenital heart malformations, the cause is multifactorial with no specific trigger. Other factors that might influence development of congenital heart malformation can be classified as environmental or genetic. Infections of the pregnant woman, such as rubella, cytomegalovirus, coxsackie B, and influenza, have been implicated. Steroids, alcohol, lithium, and some anticonvulsants have been shown to cause malformations of the heart. Seasonal spraying of pesticides has also been linked to an increase in congenital heart defects. Clinicians are also beginning to see cardiac defects in infants of mothers with PKU who do not follow their diets. Infants with Down syndrome, Turner syndrome, and Holt-Oram syndrome; as well as trisomy 13 and trisomy 18, frequently have heart lesions. Increased incidence and risk of recurrence of specific defects occur in families.

Congenital malformations of the heart have historically been described as either acyanotic (those that do not present with cyanosis) or cyanotic (those that present with cyanosis). If an opening exists between the right and left sides of the heart, blood will normally flow from the area of greater pressure (left side) to the area of lesser pressure (right side). This process, known as *left-to-right shunt*, increases blood flow to the lungs but does not produce cyanosis because oxygenated blood is still being pumped out to the systemic circulation. If pressure in the right side of the heart, caused by obstruction of normal flow, exceeds that in the left side, unoxygenated blood bypasses the lungs and will flow from the right side to the left side of the heart and out into the systemic circulation. This *right-to-left shunt* causes cyanosis. If the opening is large, there may be a *bidirectional shunt* with mixing of blood in both sides of the heart, which also produces cyanosis. Now cardiac malformations are also grouped based on the presence of cyanosis and whether there is obstruction to the outflow of blood from the heart.

The most common cardiac defects seen in the first 6 days of life are left ventricular outflow obstructions (mitral stenosis, aortic stenosis or atresia), hypoplastic left heart, coarctation of the aorta, patent ductus arteriosus (PDA, the most common defect in premature infants), transposition of the great vessels, tetralogy of Fallot, and large ventricular septal defect or atrial septal defects. Many cardiac defects may not manifest themselves until after discharge from the birthing unit.

HINTS FOR PRACTICE

When cyanosis occurs in an otherwise healthy 12- to 24-hour-old newborn displaying no respiratory distress and is not resolved with oxygen, think about cardiac issues, especially a ductal-dependent lesion.

Nursing Care Management

The primary goal of the neonatal nurse is to identify cardiac defects early and initiate referral to the physician. The three most common manifestations of cardiac defect are cyanosis, detectable heart murmur, and congestive heart failure signs (tachycardia, tachypnea, diaphoresis, hepatomegaly, cardiomegaly). Table 28–6 presents the clinical manifestations and medical-surgical management of

TABLE 28–6 Cardiac Defects of the Early Newborn Period

Congenital Heart Defect	Clinical Findings	Medical/Surgical Management
Acyanotic		
Increased Pulmonary Blood Flow		
Patent Ductus Arteriosus (PDA) ↑ in females, maternal rubella, RDS, less than 1500 g preterm newborns, high-altitude births 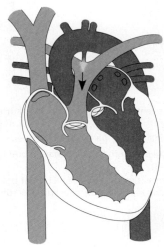	Harsh grade 2 to 3 machinery murmur upper left sternal border (LSB) just beneath clavicle ↑ difference between systolic and diastolic pulse pressure Can lead to right heart failure and pulmonary congestion ↑ left atrial (LA) and left ventricular (LV) enlargement, dilated ascending aorta ↑ pulmonary vascularity	Indomethacin—0.2 mg/kg IV (prostaglandin inhibitor) 3 doses, one every 12 hours Surgical ligation, occlusion coil Use of O_2 therapy and blood transfusion to improve tissue oxygenation and perfusion Fluid restriction and diuretics
	Congenital heart. The patent ductus arteriosus is a vascular connection that, during fetal life, short-circuits the pulmonary vascular bed and directs blood from the pulmonary artery to the aorta. Postnatally, blood shunts through the ductus from the aorta to the pulmonary artery.	
Atrial Septal Defect (ASD) ↑ in females and Down syndrome	Initially frequently asymptomatic Systolic murmur second left intercostal space (LICS) With large ASD, diastolic rumbling murmur lower left sternal (LLS) border Failure to thrive, upper respiratory infection (URI), poor exercise tolerance	Surgical closure with patch or suture Umbrella occluder
Ventricular Septal Defect (VSD) ↑ in males	Initially asymptomatic until end of first month or large enough to cause pulmonary edema Loud, blowing systolic murmur between the third and fourth intercostal space (ICS) pulmonary blood flow Right ventricular hypertrophy Rapid respirations, growth failure, feeding difficulties Congestive right heart failure at 6 weeks to 2 months of age	Follow medically—some spontaneously close Use of Lanoxin and diuretics in congestive heart failure (CHF) Surgical closure with Dacron patch or umbrella occluder
Obstruction to Systemic Blood Flow **Coarctation of Aorta** Can be preductal or postductal 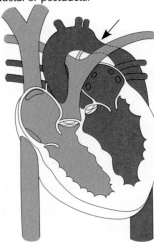	Absent or diminished femoral pulses Increased brachial pulses Late systolic murmur left intrascapular area Systolic BP in lower extremities Enlarged left ventricle Can present in CHF at 7 to 21 days of life	Surgical resection of narrowed portion of aorta Prostaglandin E_1 to maintain peripheral perfusion No afterload reducer drugs
	Coarctation of the aorta is characterized by a narrowed aortic lumen. The lesion produces an obstruction to the flow of blood through the aorta, causing an increased left ventricular pressure and workload.	

(Continued)

TABLE 28–6 Cardiac Defects of the Early Newborn Period *(Continued)*

Congenital Heart Defect	Clinical Findings	Medical/Surgical Management
Hypoplastic Left Heart Syndrome	Normal at birth—cyanosis and shocklike congestive heart failure develop within a few hours to days	PGE₁ until decision made
	Soft systolic murmur just left of the sternum	Norwood procedure Transplant
	Diminished pulses	
	Aortic and/or mitral atresia	
	Tiny, thick-walled left ventricle	
	Large, dilated, hypertrophied right ventricle	
	X-ray examination: cardiac enlargement and pulmonary venous congestion	

Cyanotic

Decreased Pulmonary Blood Flow

Tetralogy of Fallot	May be cyanotic at birth or within first few months of life	Prevention of dehydration, intercurrent infections
(Most common cyanotic heart defect)	Harsh systolic murmur LSB	Alleviation of paroxysmal dyspneic attacks
Pulmonary stenosis	Crying or feeding increases cyanosis and respiratory distress	Palliative surgery to increase blood flow to the lungs
Ventricular septal defect (VSD)	X-ray: boot-shaped appearance secondary to small pulmonary artery	Corrective surgery—resection of pulmonic stenosis, closure of VSD with Dacron patch
Overriding aorta	Right ventricular enlargement	
Right ventricular hypertrophy		

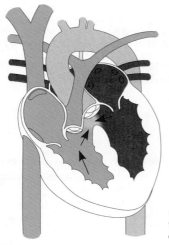

In tetralogy of Fallot, the severity of symptoms depends on the degree of pulmonary stenosis, the size of the ventricular septal defect, and the degree to which the aorta overrides the septal defect.

Mixed Defects*	Cyanosis at birth or within 3 days	Prostaglandin E to vasodilate ductus to keep it open
Transposition of Great Vessels (TGA)	Possible pulmonic stenosis murmur	
(↑ females, IDMs, LGAs)	Right ventricular hypertrophy	Initial surgery to create opening between right and left side of heart if none exists
	Polycythemia	Total surgical repair—usually the arterial switch procedure—done within first few days of life
	"Egg on its side" X-ray finding	

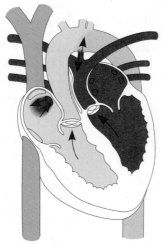

Complete transposition of great vessels is an embryologic defect caused by a straight division of the bulbar trunk without normal spiraling. As a result, the aorta originates from the right ventricle, and the pulmonary artery from the left ventricle. An abnormal communication between the two circulations must be present to sustain life.

Note: Mixed defects-postnatal survival is dependent upon mixing of systemic and pulmonary blood flow.

Source: All illustrations from *Congenital Heart Abnormalities*. Clinical Education Aid No. 7, Ross Laboratories, Columbus, OH.

these specific cardiac defects. Initial repair of heart defects in the newborn period is becoming more commonplace. The NICU staff is now involved in both the preoperative and postoperative care of newborns. The benefits for the cardiac infant of being cared for by NICU staff include the staff's knowledge of neonatal anatomy and physiology, experience in supporting the family, and an awareness of the newborn's developmental needs.

After the baby is stabilized, decisions are made about ongoing care. The parents need careful and complete explanations and the opportunity to take part in decision making. They also require ongoing emotional support. Families with a baby born with any congenital anomaly also need genetic counseling about future conception. Parents need opportunities to verbalize their concerns about their baby's health maintenance and their understanding of the rationale for follow-up care.

Care of the Newborn with an Inborn Error of Metabolism

Inborn errors of metabolism (IEM) are a group of hereditary disorders transmitted by mutant genes. Each causes an enzyme defect that blocks a metabolic pathway and leads to an accumulation of toxic metabolites. Most of the disorders are transmitted by an autosomal recessive gene, requiring two heterozygous parents to produce a homozygous infant with the disorder. Heterozygous parents carrying some inborn errors of metabolism disorders can be identified by special tests, and some inborn errors of metabolism can be detected and treated in utero. Some of the inborn errors of metabolism (especially those associated with mental retardation) are now detected neonatally through newborn screening programs. With new laboratory technology and the introduction of tandem mass spectrometry (MS/MS), a spot of blood from a newborn can detect more than 40 inborn errors of metabolism (Kenner & Lott, 2007). For discussion of other newborn screening tests such as cystic fibrosis (CF), see Chapter 26 ∞.

Types of Inborn Errors of Metabolism

Phenylketonuria (PKU) is the most common of the amino acid disorders. Newborn screenings have set its incidence to be about 1 in 12,000 live births in the United States; however, the incidence varies considerably among ethnic groups (Kenner & Lott, 2007). The highest incidence is noted in white populations from northern Europe and the United States. It is rarely observed in people of African, Hispanic, Chinese, or Japanese descent (Kaye & Committee on Genetics, 2006).

Phenylalanine is an essential amino acid (found in dietary protein) used by the body for growth. In the normal individual any excess is converted to tyrosine. The newborn with PKU lacks this converting ability, which results in an accumulation of phenylalanine in the blood. Phenylalanine produces two abnormal metabolites, phenylpyruvic acid and phenylacetic acid. These are eliminated in the urine, producing a musty odor (Kenner & Lott, 2007). Excessive accumulation of phenylalanine and its abnormal metabolites in the brain tissue leads to progressive mental retardation.

The Guthrie blood test for PKU, required for all newborns before discharge, uses a drop of blood collected from a heel stick and placed on filter paper. Because phenylalanine metabolites begin to build up in the PKU baby once milk feedings are initiated, the test is done at least 24 hours after the initiation of feedings containing the usual amounts of breast milk or formula. At-risk newborns should receive a 60% milk intake, with no more than 40% of their total intake from nonprotein intravenous fluids. The PKU testing of at-risk newborns should be deferred for at least 48 hours after hyperalimentation is initiated. It is vital that the parents understand the need for the screening procedure; a follow-up check is necessary to confirm that the test was done.

Maple syrup urine disease (MSUD) is an inborn error of metabolism that, when untreated, is a rapidly progressing and often fatal disease caused by an enzymatic defect in the metabolism of the branched-chain amino acids leucine, isoleucine, and alloisoleucine. Diagnosis of MSUD is made by analyzing blood levels of leucine, isoleucine, and alloisoleucine. Confirmation of the diagnosis depends on plasma amino acid assay.

Homocystinuria is a disorder caused by a deficiency of the enzyme cystathionine beta-synthase (CBS), which causes an elevated excretion of homocystine and methionine. Screening is done by a bacterial inhibition assay (BIA) to detect increased blood methionine (Kaye & Committee on Genetics, 2006). No symptoms are usually seen in the newborn period.

Galactosemia is an inborn error of carbohydrate metabolism in which the body is unable to use the sugars galactose and lactose. Enzyme pathways in liver cells normally convert galactose and lactose to glucose. In galactosemia, one step in that conversion pathway is absent, either because of the lack of the enzyme galactose 1-phosphate uridyl transferase or because of the lack of the enzyme galactokinase. High levels of unusable galactose circulate in the blood, which cause cataracts, brain damage, and liver damage. There appear to be ethnic differences in age at onset of symptoms and in severity of course. Caucasians have more severe symptoms and earlier onset (3 to 14 days) than people of African descent (14 to 28 days).

Another disorder frequently included in mandatory newborn screening blood tests is *congenital hypothyroidism (CH)*. An inborn enzymatic defect, lack of maternal dietary iodine, or maternal ingestion of drugs that depress or destroy thyroid tissue can cause CH. Congenital hypothyroidism occurs more often in Hispanic and American Indian/Alaska Native people. Infants with Down syndrome are also at increased risk of having CH (Kaye & Committee on Genetics, 2006).

The incidence of metabolic errors is relatively low, but for affected infants and their families these disorders pose a threat to the infant's survival. If they survive, these infants frequently require lifelong treatment.

Clinical Therapy

All states require screening of newborns for PKU and CH (Cloherty et al., 2008; Kayton, 2007). Mandatory newborn screening for other inborn errors of metabolism varies among states and often includes MSUD, homocystinuria, cystic fibrosis, sickle cell anemia, and congenital adrenal hypoplasia. In several states newborn screening includes an enzyme assay for galactose 1-phosphate uridyltransferase; however, this test does not detect galactosemia if it is caused by a deficiency of the enzyme galactokinase.

Identification via newborn screening and early clinical intervention for some inborn errors of metabolism becomes more difficult with the advent of early discharge of newborns. If the initial specimen is obtained before the newborn is 24 hours of age, then a second specimen should be obtained before 5 days of age, although few states currently require the second test (Kaye & Committee on Genetics, 2006). Early collection of specimens may yield false-positive results for certain metabolic disorders. Conversely, certain metabolic disorders may go undetected. Newborns in the NICU who require interhospital transfers as well as early-discharged healthy newborns are at risk for nonscreening. Newborn screen specimens are always collected before a blood transfusion.

Nursing Care Management

The nurse assesses the newborn for signs of inborn errors of metabolism and carries out state-mandated newborn screening tests. Parents of affected newborns should be referred to support groups. The nurse should also ensure that parents are informed about centers that can provide them with information about biochemical genetics and dietary management.

Infant with PKU

Typically, a PKU baby is a normal-appearing newborn, most often with blond hair, blue eyes, and fair complexion. Decreased pigmentation may be related to the competition

between phenylalanine and tyrosine for the available enzyme tyrosinase. Tyrosine is needed for the formation of melanin pigment and the hormones epinephrine and thyroxine. Without treatment, the infant fails to thrive and develops vomiting and eczematous rashes. By about 6 months of age, the infant exhibits behaviors indicative of mental retardation and other CNS involvement, including seizures and abnormal electroencephalogram (EEG) patterns.

The nurse advises parents that once identified, an afflicted PKU infant can be treated by a special diet that limits ingestion of phenylalanine. Special formulas low in phenylalanine, such as Lofenalac, Minafen, and Albumaid XP, are available. Special food lists are helpful for parents of a PKU child. If treatment is begun before 1 month of age, CNS damage can be minimized. There is an increased risk of producing a child with mental retardation if the mother with PKU is not on a low-phenylalanine diet during pregnancy. It is recommended that the woman reinstate her low-phenylalanine diet before becoming pregnant (Blackburn, 2007).

Infant with MSUD

Newborns with MSUD have feeding problems, weight loss, and neurologic signs (seizures, spasticity, opisthotonos) during the first week of life. A maple syrup, burnt sugar, or curry odor of the urine is noted, and when ferric chloride is added to the urine, its color changes to gray-green. An ear swab within 6 to 12 hours after birth has a similar smell. Diagnosis is confirmed with plasma amino acid analysis.

Newborns with MSUD must be given a formula that is low in the branched-chain amino acids leucine, isoleucine, and valine, which is continued indefinitely. Dietary treatment initiated before 12 days of life has been reported to result in normal intelligence.

Infant with Homocystinuria

Homocystinuria varies in its presentation, but the more common characteristics are skeletal abnormalities, dislocation of ocular lenses, intravascular thromboses, and mental retardation. Abnormalities occur because of the toxic effects of the accumulation of methionine and the metabolite homocystine in the blood.

Infants with homocystinuria are placed on a diet that is low in methionine but supplemented with cystine and pyridoxine (vitamin B_6). With early diagnosis and careful management, mental retardation may be prevented.

Infant with Galactosemia

Clinical manifestations of galactosemia include vomiting soon after ingestion of milk-based formula or breast milk, diarrhea, poor weight gain, excessive bleeding with venipunctures, jaundice, and mental retardation. The condition is frequently associated with anemia, sepsis, and cataracts in the neonatal period (Kaye & Committee on Genetics, 2006). Except for cataracts and mental retardation, those findings are reversible when galactose is excluded from the diet. Mental retardation can be prevented by early diagnosis and careful dietary management.

A baby with galactosemia is placed on a galactose-free diet. Galactose-free formulas include Nutramigen (a protein hydrolysate process formula), meat-based formulas, and soybean formulas. As the infant grows, parents must be educated to avoid giving their child milk and milk products, to read all labels carefully, and to avoid any foods containing dry milk products. Even with early treatment, children may have learning disabilities, speech problems, and ovarian failure (Kaye & Committee on Genetics, 2006).

Infant with CH

Approximately 5% of these infants, generally those who are more severely affected, have recognizable features at birth, including a large tongue, umbilical hernia, cool and mottled skin, low hairline, hypotonia, and large fontanelles (especially the posterior fontanelle in term infants) (Kaye & Committee on Genetics, 2006). Early symptoms include prolonged neonatal jaundice, poor feeding, constipation, low-pitched cry, poor weight gain, inactivity, early sleeping through the night, and delayed motor development. In addition, premature infants of less than 30 weeks' gestation frequently have lower T_4 values than those of term infants. This difference may reflect the premature infant's inability to bind thyroid and a risk for hypothyroidism.

Babies with congenital hypothyroidism need frequent follow-up laboratory monitoring and adjustment of thyroid medication to accommodate the child's growth and development. With adequate treatment, children remain free of symptoms, but if the condition is left untreated, stunted growth (slowed linear growth) and mental retardation occur.

Evaluation

Expected outcomes of nursing care include the following:

- Newborns at risk for inborn errors of metabolism are promptly identified and receive early intervention.
- The parents verbalize their concerns about their baby's nutritional status, health problems, long-term care needs, and potential outcomes.
- The parents are aware of available community health resources and use them as indicated.

CHAPTER HIGHLIGHTS

- Early identification of potential high-risk fetuses through assessment of preconception, prenatal, and intrapartal factors facilitates strategically timed nursing observations and interventions.
- High-risk newborns, whether they are premature, SGA, LGA, postterm, or infants of a diabetic or substance-abusing mother, have many similar problems, although their problems are based on different physiologic processes.
- SGA newborns are at risk for perinatal asphyxia and resulting aspiration syndrome, hypothermia, hypoglycemia, hypocalcemia, polycythemia, congenital anomalies, and intrauterine infections. Long-term problems include continued growth and learning difficulties.
- LGA newborns are at risk for birth trauma as a result of cephalopelvic disproportion, hypoglycemia, polycythemia, and hyperviscosity.
- IDMs are at risk for hypoglycemia, hypocalcemia, hyperbilirubinemia, polycythemia, and respiratory distress caused by delayed maturation of their lungs.
- Postterm newborns often encounter intrapartal problems such as CPD (shoulder dystocia) and birth traumas, hypoglycemia, polycythemia, meconium aspiration, cold stress, and possible seizure activity. Long-term complications may involve poor weight gain and low IQ scores.
- The common problems of the preterm newborn are a result of the baby's immature body systems. Potential problems include RDS, patent ductus arteriosus, hypothermia and cold stress, feeding difficulties and NEC, marked insensible water loss and loss of buffering agents through the kidneys, infection, anemia of prematurity, apnea, intraventricular hemorrhage, retinopathy of prematurity, and behavioral state disorganization. Long-term needs and problems include bronchopulmonary dysplasia, speech defects, sensorineural hearing loss, and neurologic defects.

- Newborns of alcohol-dependent mothers are at risk for physical characteristic alterations and the long-term complications of feeding problems; CNS dysfunction, including low IQ, hyperactivity, and language abnormalities; and congenital anomalies.
- Newborns of drug-dependent mothers experience drug withdrawal as well as respiratory distress, jaundice, congenital anomalies, and behavioral abnormalities. With early recognition and intervention, the potential long-term physiologic and emotional consequences of these difficulties can be avoided or at least lessened in severity.
- Newborns of mothers with AIDS require early recognition and treatment so that the physiologic and emotional consequences may be lessened in severity and CDC guidelines implemented.
- Cardiac defects are a significant cause of morbidity and mortality in the newborn period. Early identification and nursing and medical care of newborns with cardiac defects are essential to improve the outcome of these infants. Care is directed toward lessening the workload of the heart and decreasing oxygen and energy consumption.

- Inborn errors of metabolism such as galactosemia, PKU, homocystinuria, and MSUD are usually included in a newborn screening program designed to prevent mental retardation through dietary management and medication.
- The nursing care of the newborn with special problems involves the understanding of normal physiology, the pathophysiology of the disease process, clinical manifestations, and supportive or corrective therapies. Only with this theoretical background can the nurse make appropriate observations about responses to therapy and development of complications.
- The nurse facilitates interdisciplinary communication with the parents. Parents of at-risk newborns need support from nurses and healthcare providers to understand the special needs of their baby and feel confident in their ability to care for their baby at home.

EXPLORE PEARSON **mynursingkit**™

MyNursingKit is your one stop for online chapter review materials and resources. Prepare for success with additional NCLEX®-style practice questions, interactive assignments and activities, web links, animations and videos, and more!

Register your access code from the front of your book at
www.mynursingkit.com

CHAPTER REFERENCES

Als, H., Lester, B. M., Tronick, E., & Brazelton, T. B. (1982). Assessment of preterm infant behavior (APIB). In B. M. Fitzgerald Lester & M. W. Yogman (Eds.), *Theory and research in behavioral pediatrics* (Vol. 1). New York: Plenum.

American Academy of Pediatrics (AAP) Committee on Fetus and Newborn & American College of Obstetricians and Gynecologists (ACOG) Committee on Obstetrics. (2007). *Guidelines for perinatal care* (6th ed.). Elk Grove Village, IL: Author.

American College of Obstetricians and Gynecologists. (2005). Smoking cessation during pregnancy (Committee Opinion No. 316). Washington, DC: Author.

Barron, M. L. (2008). Antenatal care. In K. R. Simpson & P. A. Creehan, *AWHONN perinatal nursing* (3rd ed., pp. 88–124). Philadelphia: Lippincott Williams & Wilkins.

Baschat, A. A., Galan, H. L., Ross, M. G., & Gabbe, S. G. (2007). Intrauterine growth restriction. In S. G. Gabbe, J. R. Niebyl & J. L. Simpson (Eds.), *Obstetrics: Normal and problem pregnancies* (5th ed., pp. 771–814). Philadelphia: Churchill Livingstone/Elsevier.

Beauman, S. (2005). Identification and management of neonatal abstinence syndrome. *Journal of Infusion Nursing, 28* (3), 159–167.

Bernstein, H. (2007). Maternal and perinatal infection—viral. In S. G. Gabbe, J. R. Niebyl, & J. L. Simpson (Eds.), *Obstetrics: Normal and problem pregnancies* (5th ed., pp. 1203–1232). Philadelphia: Churchill Livingstone/Elsevier.

Blackburn, S. (2007). *Maternal-fetal-neonatal physiology: A clinical perspective* (3rd ed.). Philadelphia: Saunders.

Bowie, B., Hall, R., Faulkner, J., & Anderson, B. (2003). Single-room infant care: Future trends in special care nursery planning and design. *Neonatal Network, 22* (3), 27–34.

Centers for Disease Control and Prevention (CDC), National Center for Chronic Disease Prevention and Health Promotion. (2005). Pattern of tobacco use among women and girls: Fact sheet. Retrieved January 31, 2005, from www.cdc.gov/tobacco/sgr_forwomen/factsheet

Cloherty, J. R., Eichenwald, E. C., & Stark, A. R. (2008). *Manual of neonatal care.* Philadelphia: Lippincott Williams & Wilkins.

Divon, M. Y. (2007). Prolonged pregnancy. In S. G. Gabbe, J. R. Niebyl, & J. L. Simpson (Eds.), *Obstetrics: Normal and problem pregnancies* (5th ed., pp. 846–860). Philadelphia: Churchill Livingstone/Elsevier.

Gardner, S., & Goldson, E. (2006). The neonate and the environment: Impact on development. In G. B. Merenstein & S. L. Gardner (Eds.), *Handbook of neonatal intensive care* (6th ed., pp. 273–349). St. Louis, MO: Mosby.

Jones, J., Kassity, N., & Duncan, K. (2001). Complementary care: Alternatives for the neonatal intensive care unit. *Newborn and Infant Nursing Reviews, 1* (4), 207–210.

Jones, M. (2003). Fetal alcohol syndrome. *Neonatal Network, 22* (3), 63–69.

Kahn, B. F., Hobbins, J. C., & Galan, H. L. (2008). Intrauterine growth restriction. In R. S. Gibbs, B. Y. Karlan, A. F. Haney, & I. Nygaard, *Danforth's obstetrics and gynecology* (10th ed., pp. 198–219). Philadelphia: Lippincott Williams & Wilkins.

Kaye, C. I., & Committee on Genetics. (2006). Newborn screening facts sheets. *Pediatrics, 118*(3), 934–963.

Kayton, A. (2007). Newborn screening: A literature review. *Neonatal Network, 26*(2), 85–95.

Kenner, C., & Lott, J. W. (2007). *Comprehensive neonatal care: An interdisciplinary approach* (4th ed.). St. Louis: Saunders/Elsevier.

Kledzik, T. (2005). Holding the very low birth weight infant: Skin-to-skin techniques. *Neonatal Network, 24*(1), 7–14.

Landon, M. B., Catalano, P. M., & Gabbe, S. G. (2008). Diabetes mellitus complicating pregnancy. In R. S. Gibbs, B. Y. Karlan, A. F. Haney, & I. Nygaard, *Danforth's obstetrics and gynecology* (10th ed., pp. 976–1010). Philadelphia: Lippincott Williams & Wilkins.

Lester, B. M., & Twomey, J. E. (2008). Treatment of substance abuse during pregnancy. *Women's Health, 4*(1), 67–77.

Martin, G. L., & Hankins, G. D. (2006). The Apgar score. *Advances in Neonatal Care, 6*(4), 220–223.

Moran, B. A. (2004). Substance abuse in pregnancy. In S. Mattson & J. E. Smith (Eds.), *Core curriculum for maternal-newborn nursing* (3rd ed., pp. 750–770). St. Louis: Elsevier Saunders.

Nash, P., & Smith, J. R. (2008). Common neonatal complications. In K. R. Simpson & P. A. Creehan, *AWHONN perinatal nursing* (3rd ed., pp. 612–646). Philadelphia: Lippincott Williams & Wilkins.

Read, J. S., & Committee on Pediatrics AIDS. (2007). Diagnosis of HIV-1 infection in children younger than 18 months in the United States. *Pediatrics, 120*(6), e1547–e1562.

Stokowski, L. A. (2004). Fetal alcohol syndrome: New guidelines for referral and diagnosis. *Advances in neonatal care, 4*(6), 324.

Thoyre, S. M., Shaker, C. S., & Pridham, K. F. (2005). The early feeding skills assessment for preterm infants. *Neonatal Network, 24*(3), 7–14.

Turnage-Carrier, C. S. (2004). Caregiving and the environment. In C. Kenner & J. M. McGrath (Eds.), *Developmental care of newborns & infants: A guide for health professionals.* St. Louis: Elsevier Mosby.

Venkatesh, M., Merestein, G. B., Adams, K. M., & Weisman, L. E. (2006). Infection in the neonate. In G. B. Merenstein & S. L. Gardner (Eds.), *Handbook of neonatal intensive care* (6th ed., pp. 569–593). St. Louis, MO: Mosby.

Vargo, L. E., & Trotter, C. W. (2007). *The premature infant: Nursing assessment and management* (2nd ed.). White Plains, NY: March of Dimes Foundation.

Volpe, J. J. (2008). *Neurology of the newborn* (5th ed.). Philadelphia: Saunders.

Wisner, K. L., Sit, D., Reynolds, S. K., Altemus, M., Bogen, D. L., Sunder, K. R., Misra, D., & Perel, J. M. (2007). Psychiatric disorders. In S. G. Gabbe, J. R. Niebyl, & J. L. Simpson (Eds.), *Obstetrics: Normal and problem pregnancies* (5th ed., pp. 1249–1288). Philadelphia: Churchill Livingstone/Elsevier.

CHAPTER 29

The Newborn at Risk: Birth-Related Stressors

I work primarily in what our system calls the "high-risk transition nursery." When I am called to attend a birth it is usually because the labor and delivery team has detected a potential problem and they think the newborn will need some additional care at birth. The neonatal nurse practitioner (NNP) and I work together to anticipate and respond to whatever is needed at the time. Each situation is unique and deserves our complete attention. But it is also essential that the parents be kept informed and comforted as much as possible. With each infant that I care for, I ask myself, "If this were my baby, how would I be feeling right now, and what would I want to know?"

—High-Risk Nursery Nurse

LEARNING OUTCOMES

29-1. Describe how to identify infants in need of resuscitation and the appropriate method of resuscitation based on the antepartal/labor record and physiologic indicators seen at birth in the nursing care management of the infant at risk because of asphyxiation.

29-2. Based on clinical manifestations, differentiate among the various types of respiratory distress (respiratory distress syndrome, transient tachypnea of the newborn, and meconium aspiration syndrome) in the newborn and the nursing care related to each type.

29-3. Explain the causes, effects, and the nursing care management of newborns with selected metabolic abnormalities (including cold stress and hypoglycemia).

29-4. Differentiate between physiologic and pathologic jaundice according to timing of onset (in hours), cause, possible sequelae, and specific management.

29-5. Explain how Rh incompatibility or ABO incompatibility can lead to the development of hyperbilirubinemia.

29-6. Identify nursing responsibilities and rationale in caring for the newborn receiving phototherapy.

29-7. Describe the causes and nursing care management of infants with anemia and polycythemia.

29-8. Describe the nursing assessments that would lead the nurse to suspect newborn sepsis.

29-9. Relate the expected assessment findings of selected maternally transmitted infections, such as maternal syphilis, gonorrhea, herpesviridae family (HSV or CMV), and chlamydia, to the nursing care management for each of the infants in the neonatal period.

29-10. Identify parental responses, developmental consequences, and nursing care for the at-risk infant.

29-11. Identify the special initial and long-term needs of parents of at-risk infants.

Bilirubin encephalopathy **771**
Cold stress **765**
Erythroblastosis fetalis **771**
Hemolytic disease of the newborn **771**
Hydrops fetalis **771**
Hyperbilirubinemia **771**

Hypoglycemia **766**
Jaundice **770**
Kernicterus **771**
Meconium aspiration syndrome
 (MAS) **760**
Phototherapy **773**

Physiologic anemia of infancy **781**
Polycythemia **782**
Respiratory distress syndrome
 (RDS) **753**
Sepsis neonatorum **783**

Marked homeostatic changes occur during the infant's transition from fetal to neonatal life. Because the most rapid anatomic and physiologic changes occur in the cardiopulmonary system, most major problems of the newborn are usually related to this system. These problems include asphyxia, respiratory distress system (RDS), cold stress, jaundice, hemolytic disease, and anemia. Ideally, most problems are anticipated and identified prenatally. Some treatment may be initiated in the prenatal period, whereas other intervention measures are begun at or immediately after birth.

Care of the Newborn at Risk Because of Asphyxia

Neonatal asphyxia occurs in 1% to 1.5% of live births, and the incidence increases as the gestational age decreases (Cloherty, Eichenwald, & Stark, 2008). Neonatal asphyxia results in circulatory, respiratory, and biochemical changes. Circulatory patterns that accompany asphyxia indicate an inability of the newborn to make the transition to extrauterine circulation—in effect, a return to fetal circulatory patterns. Failure of lung expansion and establishment of respiration rapidly produces serious biochemical changes, including hypoxemia (decreased oxygen in the blood), metabolic acidosis (increased acidity of blood reflected by low pH), and hypercarbia (excess levels of carbon dioxide in the blood).

These biochemical changes result in pulmonary vasoconstriction and high pulmonary vascular resistance in relation to lower systemic vascular resistance (following birth the pulmonary vascular resistance should be markedly lower than the systemic vascular resistance), hypoperfusion of the lungs, and a large right-to-left shunt through the ductus arteriosus, bypassing the lungs and impeding oxygenation of the blood. As right atrial pressure exceeds left atrial pressure, the foramen ovale reopens, allowing blood to flow from right to left. (See Chapter 24 ∞ for a review of normal newborn cardiopulmonary adaptation.)

However, the most serious biochemical abnormality is a change from aerobic to anaerobic metabolism in the presence of hypoxia. This change results in the buildup of lactate, which combines with hydrogen to form lactic acid,

and the development of metabolic acidosis. Lactic acidosis can develop after prolonged tissue hypoxia (oxygen starvation) as active cells rely on anaerobic metabolism.

Simultaneous respiratory acidosis may also occur because of a rapid increase in carbon dioxide (PCO_2) during asphyxia. In response to hypoxia and anaerobic metabolism, the amounts of free fatty acids (FFAs) and glycerol in the blood increase. Glycogen stores are also mobilized to provide a continuous glucose source for the brain. Hepatic and cardiac stores of glycogen may be used up rapidly during an asphyxial incident.

The newborn is supplied with several protective mechanisms against hypoxic insults. These include a relatively immature brain and a resting metabolic rate lower than that of adults, an ability to mobilize substances within the body for anaerobic metabolism and to use energy more efficiently, and an intact circulatory system able to redistribute lactate and hydrogen ions in tissues still being perfused. Severe prolonged hypoxia overcomes these protective mechanisms, resulting in brain damage or death of the newborn. The newborn suffering apnea requires immediate resuscitative efforts. The need for resuscitation can be anticipated if specific risk factors are present during the pregnancy or labor and birth period.

Risk Factors Predisposing to Asphyxia

The need for resuscitation may be anticipated if the mother demonstrates the antepartal and intrapartal risk factors described in Tables 10–1 and 18–1 ∞. Fetal-neonatal risk factors for resuscitation are as follows (Cloherty et al., 2008; Dildy, 2005; Thureen, Deacon, Hernandez, & Hall, 2005):

• Nonreassuring fetal heart rate (FHR) pattern/sustained bradycardia
• Difficult birth, prolonged labor
• Fetal scalp/capillary blood sample—acidosis pH less than 7.2
• History of meconium in amniotic fluid
• Significant intrapartum bleeding
• Maternal infection/sepsis with cardiovascular collapse
• Male infant
• Prematurity
• Small for gestational age

- Multiple births
- Structural lung abnormality/oligohydramnios (congenital diaphragmatic hernia, lung hypoplasia)
- Gastrointestinal obstruction/polyhydramnios
- Congenital heart disease
- Narcotic use in labor
- Infant of a diabetic mother
- Anemia: isoimmunization, fetal-maternal hemorrhage, parovirus

At times no risk factors may be apparent prenatally. Particular attention must be paid to all at-risk pregnancies during the intrapartal period. Certain aspects of labor and birth challenge the oxygen supply to the fetus, and often the at-risk fetus has less tolerance for the stress of labor (indicated by decelerations or lack of variability of the FHR) and birth.

Clinical Therapy

The initial goal of clinical management is to identify the fetus at risk for asphyxia, so that resuscitative efforts can begin at birth.

Fetal biophysical assessment (see Chapter 14 ∞), combined with monitoring of fetal pH, FHRs, and fetal oximeter if available during the intrapartal period, may help identify the presence of nonreassuring fetal status. If nonreassuring fetal status is present, appropriate measures can be taken to deliver the fetus immediately, before major damage occurs, and to treat the asphyxiated newborn.

The fetal biophysical profile enhances the ability to predict an abnormal perinatal outcome. In addition to the fetal biophysical profile, fetal scalp blood sampling may indicate asphyxic insult and the degree of fetal acidosis, when considered in relation to the stage of labor, uterine contractions, and the presence of nonreassuring FHR patterns. The stress of labor causes an intermittent decrease in exchange of gases in the placental intervillous space, which causes the fall in pH and fetal acidosis. The acidosis is primarily metabolic.

During labor, a fetal pH of 7.25 or higher is considered normal (nonacidemia). A pH value of 7.20 or less is considered an ominous sign of intrauterine asphyxia (acidemia), whereas a pH of less than 7 is considered pathologic acidemia (Cloherty et al., 2008). However, low fetal pH without associated hypoxia can be caused by maternal acidosis secondary to prolonged labor, dehydration, and maternal lactate production.

Assessment of the newborn's need for resuscitation begins at the time of birth. The nurse should note the time of the first gasp, first cry, and onset of sustained respirations in the order of occurrence. The Apgar score (see Chapter 19 ∞) may be helpful in describing the status of the newborn at birth and his or her subsequent adaptation to the extrauterine environment but should not be used to determine if certain steps need to be taken during resusci-

tation (AAP & ACOG, 2007). If indicated, resuscitation should be started before the 1-minute Apgar score is obtained. The AAP Committee on Fetus and Newborn has recommended the use of an assisted Apgar scoring system that documents the assistance the infant is receiving at the time his or her score is assigned (AAP & ACOG, 2007).

As many as 10% of all newborns require some assistance at birth (Cloherty et al., 2008). The AAP and ACOG (2007, pg. 207) recommend identification of newborns who *do not* require resuscitation by carrying out a rapid assessment of these four characteristics:

1. Is the baby full term?
2. Is the amniotic fluid clear of meconium and evidence of infection?
3. Is the baby breathing or crying?
4. Does the baby have good muscle tone?

If the answer to these questions is "yes" then the baby does not need resuscitation and should not be separated from the mother. If the answer to *any* of the previous questions is "no," the infant should receive resuscitative assistance. The infant should receive one or more of the following categories of action: initial steps in stabilization (warmth, positioning, clearing the airway as necessary, drying, stimulating, and repositioning); oxygen administration; positive pressure ventilation; chest compressions, and administration of epinephrine, volume expansion, or both (AAP & ACOG, 2007). In the birthing room exposure to blood or other body fluids is inevitable. Standard precautions must be practiced by wearing caps, goggles or glasses, gloves, and impervious gowns until the cord is cut and the newborn is dried and wrapped (Cloherty et al., 2008).

Resuscitation Management

The goals of resuscitation are to provide an adequate airway with expansion of the lungs, to decrease the P_{CO_2} and increase the P_{O_2}, to support adequate cardiac output, and to minimize oxygen consumption by reducing heat loss and ensuring proper positioning.

Suctioning (clearing airway) is always performed before resuscitation measures are started so that mucus, blood, or meconium is not aspirated into the lungs. Caregivers should keep the infant in a head-down position to avoid aspiration of oropharyngeal secretions and suction the oropharynx and nasopharynx immediately. Clearing the nasal and oral passages of obstructive fluid, with a bulb syringe or suction catheter attached to low continuous suction, establishes a patent airway. Vigorous suctioning of the posterior pharynx should be avoided because it can produce significant reflex bradycardia and damage the oral mucosa. Although clear mucus routinely is suctioned from the mouth in most birthing units, there is no evidence to support the value of this practice (AAP & ACOG, 2007).

Breathing is established by employing the simplest form of resuscitative measures initially, with progression to more complicated methods as required; for example:

1. Position and clear the airway only as necessary. Simple stimulation is provided by rubbing the newborn's back with a blanket or towel, while simultaneously drying the baby.

2. If respirations have not been initiated or are inadequate (gasping or occasional respirations), the lungs must be inflated with positive pressure. The proper size mask is positioned securely on the face (over nose and mouth, avoiding the eyes), with the infant's head in a "sniffing" or neutral position (Figure 29–1 ■). Hyperextension of the infant's neck obstructs the trachea and must be avoided. An airtight connection is made between the baby's face and the mask (thus allowing the bag to inflate). The lungs are inflated rhythmically by squeezing the bag. Oxygen can be delivered at 100% with an anesthesia bag or modified self-inflating bag with reservoir and adequate liter flow of at least 8 L/min. The self-inflating (Ambu or Hope) bag delivers only 40% oxygen unless it has been adapted with an attached oxygen reservoir (Cloherty et al., 2008). It may not be possible to maintain adequate inspiratory pressure with self-inflating bags. In a crisis situation, it is crucial that 100% oxygen be delivered with adequate pressure.

3. Chest movement is observed for proper ventilation. Air entry and heart rate are checked by auscultation; heart rate may be quickly checked by palpating the base of the umbilical cord stump and counting the pulsations for 6 seconds and then multiplying by 10. Manual resusci-

tation is coordinated with any voluntary efforts. During positive pressure ventilation, the nurse should squeeze the resuscitation bag just enough to improve heart rate, color, and muscle tone. The rate of ventilation should be between 40 and 60 breaths per minute. Pressure should be adequate to move the chest wall. The pressure gauge (manometer) must be in place to avoid overdistention of the newborn's lungs and other problems such as pneumothorax or abdominal distention. Increasing the positive to 30 cm H_2O or greater is occasionally necessary if there is no improvement in these parameters (heart rate, color, muscle tone) (American Academy of Pediatrics [AAP] & American Heart Association [AHA], 2006). If ventilation is adequate, the chest moves with each inspiration, bilateral breath sounds are audible, and the lips and mucous membranes become pink. Distention of the stomach is controlled by inserting a nasogastric tube for decompression.

4. Endotracheal intubation may be needed. However, most newborns, except for very-low-birth-weight (VLBW) (<1500 g) infants, can be resuscitated by bag and mask ventilation. With preterm newborns, positive end-expiratory pressure (PEEP) is often required to help prevent alveolar collapse during exhalation. If the baby is intubated and the color and heart rate fail to respond to ventilatory efforts, poor or improper placement of an endotracheal tube may be the cause. If the baby is intubated improperly, pneumothorax, diaphragmatic hernia, or hypoplastic lungs (Potter's association) may exist. An increasing HR and CO_2 detection are the primary methods for confirming endotracheal tube placement.

Once breathing has been established, the heart rate should increase to over 100 beats per minute. If the heart rate is absent or the heart rate remains less than 60 beats per minute after 30 seconds of effective positive pressure ventilation with 100% oxygen, external cardiac massage (chest compression) is begun. Chest compressions are started immediately if there is no detectable heartbeat. The following procedure is used for performing chest compressions:

1. The infant is positioned properly on a firm surface.
2. The resuscitator stands at the foot or head of the infant and places both thumbs over the lower third of the sternum (just below an imaginary line drawn between the nipples), with the fingers wrapped around and supporting the back (Figure 29–2A ■). Alternatively, the resuscitator can use two fingers instead of thumbs (Figure 29–2B). The two-thumb method is preferred because it may provide better coronary perfusion pressure; however, it decreases thoracic expansion during ventilation and makes access to the umbilical cord for medication administration more difficult (Cloherty et al., 2008).

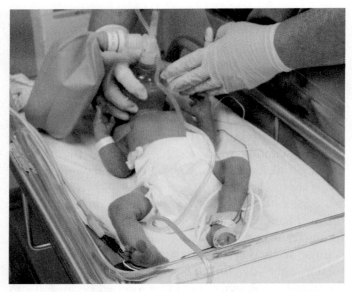

FIGURE 29–1 Demonstration of resuscitation of a newborn with bag and mask. Note that the mask covers the nose and mouth, and the head is in a neutral "sniff" position. The resuscitating bag is placed to the side of the baby so that chest movement can be seen.

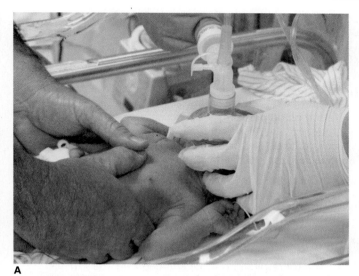

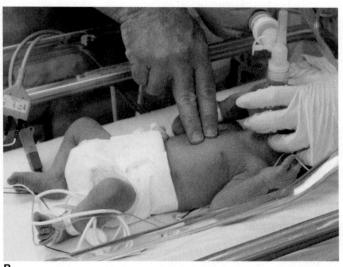

FIGURE 29–2 External cardiac massage. The lower third of the sternum is compressed with two fingertips or thumbs at a rate of 90 beats per minute. *A,* In the thumb method, the fingers support the infant's back and both thumbs compress the sternum. *B,* In the two-fingers method, the tips of two fingers of one hand compress the sternum, and the other hand or a firm surface supports the infant's back.

3. The sternum is depressed to sufficient depth to generate a palpable pulse or approximately one-third of the anterior-posterior diameter of the chest at a rate of 90 compressions per minute (AAP & AHA, 2006; Cloherty et al., 2008). Nurses use a 3:1 ratio of heartbeat to assisted ventilation.

Drugs that should be available in the birthing area include those needed in the treatment of shock, cardiac arrest, and narcosis. Oxygen, because of its effective use in ventilation, is the drug most often used. After 30 seconds of ventilation and cardiac compression, the nurse will reassess the newborn's cardiopulmonary status by palpating the umbilical cord for a pulse. If the newborn has not responded with spontaneous respirations and a heart rate above 60 beats per minute, resuscitative medications are necessary (Cloherty et al., 2008). The most accessible route for administering medications is the umbilical vein (give intravenously [IV]). When the heart rate remains below 60 beats per minute despite 30 seconds of assisted ventilation followed by another 30 seconds of coordinated chest compression, then epinephrine, a cardiac stimulant, is indicated (AAP & AHA, 2006). If bradycardia is present, an intravenous dose of epinephrine (0.1 to 0.3 mL/kg [up to 1.0 mL] of a 1:10,000 solution) is given through the umbilical vein catheter as rapidly as possible. Endotracheal administration may be considered while IV access is being established. When epinephrine is administered by endotracheal tube, consider a higher dose (0.3 to 1 mL/kg). The endotracheal route is associated with unreliable absorption and may not be effective at the lower dose (AAP & AHA, 2006). *Sodium bicarbonate is rarely given in the birthing room.* Sodium bicarbonate is given only to correct metabolic acidosis that results from lactic acid buildup caused by insufficient tissue oxygenation and after effective ventilation is established. Dextrose (2 mL/kg) is given to prevent progression of hypoglycemia. A 10% dextrose in water intravenous solution is usually sufficient to prevent or treat hypoglycemia in the birthing area. Naloxone hydrochloride (0.1 mg/kg), a narcotic antagonist, is used to reverse known iatrogenic narcotic depression (AAP & AHA, 2006). (See Drug Guide: Naloxone Hydrochloride [Narcan].)

If shock develops (low blood pressure, pallor, or poor peripheral perfusion), the baby may be given a volume expander such as normal saline or lactated Ringer's in a dose of 10 mL/kg via umbilical vein route. If there is a known fetal hemorrhage or fetal anemia, whole blood (O Rh-negative crossmatched against the mother's blood) and packed red blood cells (RBCs) given over a 5- to 10-minute period can also be used for volume expansion and treatment of hypovolemic shock. In some instances of prolonged resuscitation associated with shock and poor response to resuscitation, dopamine (5 mcg/kg/min) may be necessary.

Nursing Care Management

Nursing Assessment and Diagnosis

Communication between the obstetric office or clinic and the birthing area nurse facilitates the identification of newborns who may need resuscitation. When the woman arrives in the birthing area, the nurse should have the antepartal record, note any contributory perinatal history factors, and assess present fetal status. As labor progresses, nursing assessments include ongoing monitoring of fetal heartbeat and its response to contractions, assisting with fetal scalp blood sampling, and observing for the presence of meconium in the amniotic fluid to assess for fetal asphyxia. In addition, the nurse should alert the resuscitation

Drug Guide   Naloxone Hydrochloride (Narcan)

Overview of Neonatal Action   Naloxone hydrochloride (Narcan) is used to reverse respiratory depression caused by acute narcotic toxicity when the mother received a narcotic within 4 hours of birth. It displaces morphine-like drugs from receptor sites on the neurons; therefore the narcotics can no longer exert their depressive effects. It is essentially a pure opioid antagonist. Naloxone reverses narcotic-induced respiratory depression, analgesia, sedation, hypotension, and pupillary constriction.

Route, Dosage, Frequency   Intravenous dose is 0.1 mg/kg (0.25 mL/kg of 0.4 mg/mL concentration) at birth, including for premature infants. This drug is usually given through the umbilical vein or endotracheal tube (ET), although naloxone can be given intramuscularly (delays onset of action) if adequate perfusion exists. For IV push, infuse over at least 1 minute; for ET administration dilute in 1 to 2 milliliters of normal saline (NS).

Reversal of drug depression occurs within 1 to 2 minutes after IV administration and within 15 minutes of IM administration. The duration of action is variable (minutes to hours) and depends on the amount of the drug present and the rate of excretion. Duration of narcotic action often exceeds that of the naloxone. The dose may be repeated in 3 to 5 minutes. If there is no improvement after two or three doses, discontinue naloxone administration. If the initial reversal occurs, repeat the dose as needed (Young & Mangum, 2007).

Neonatal Contraindications   Naloxone should not be administered to infants of mothers who chronically use narcotics or those on methadone maintenance because it may precipitate acute withdrawal syndrome (increased heart rate and blood pressure, vomiting, seizures, tremors).

Respiratory depression may result from nonmorphine drugs, such as sedatives, hypnotics, anesthetics, or other nonnarcotic central nervous system (CNS) depressants.

Neonatal Side Effects   Excessive doses may result in irritability, increased crying, and possible prolongation of partial thromboplastin time (PTT).

Tachycardia may occur.

Nursing Considerations

- Monitor respirations—rate and depth—closely for improved respiratory effort.
- Assess for return of respiratory depression when naloxone effects wear off and effects of longer-acting narcotics reappear.
- Assess continued respiratory depression after positive-pressure ventilation has restored normal heart rate and color.
- Have resuscitative equipment, O_2, and ventilatory equipment available.
- Note that naloxone is incompatible with alkaline solutions such as sodium bicarbonate.
- Store at room temperature and protect from light.
- Remember that naloxone is compatible with heparin.

---

team and the practitioner responsible for care of the newborn of any potential high-risk laboring women.

Nursing diagnoses that may apply to the newborn with asphyxia and the newborn's parents include:

- *Ineffective Breathing Pattern* related to lack of spontaneous respirations at birth secondary to in utero asphyxia
- *Decreased Cardiac Output* related to impaired oxygenation
- *Ineffective Family Coping: Compromised* related to baby's lack of spontaneous respirations at birth and fear of losing their newborn

Nursing Plan and Implementation

Hospital-Based Nursing Care

Following identification of possible high-risk situations, the next step in effective resuscitation is assembling the necessary equipment and ensuring proper functioning.

In the high-risk nursery, resuscitation may be needed at any time. The reliability of the equipment must be maintained before an emergency arises, and the equipment must be restocked immediately after use and rechecked before every birth. The nurse inspects all equipment—bag and mask, oxygen and flowmeter, laryngoscope, and suction machine—for damaged or nonfunctioning parts before a birth or when setting up an admission bed. A systematic check of the emergency cart and equipment is a routine responsibility of each shift. In addition, resuscitative equipment in the birthing room must be sterilized after each use. It is desirable to assemble equipment for pH and blood gas determination as well.

During resuscitation, it is essential that the nurse keep the newborn warm. The nurse dries the newborn quickly with warmed towels or blankets and places a hat to prevent evaporative heat loss, then places him or her under a prewarmed radiant warmer with servocontrol set at 36.5°C (97.7°F). This device provides an overhead radiant heat source. (A thermostatic mechanism that is secured to the infant's abdomen, over a solid organ like the liver, triggers the radiant warmer to turn on or off to maintain a constant temperature.) An open bed is necessary for easy access to the newborn.

Training and knowledge about resuscitation are vital to personnel in the birth setting for both normal and at-risk births. Resuscitation is at least a two-person effort and the nurse should call for additional support as needed. One member must have the skill to perform airway management and ventilation. Resuscitative efforts are recorded on the newborn's chart so that all members of the healthcare team have access to the information.

Parent Teaching

The new CPR guidelines favor family members being present during resuscitation in the birthing room and in the neonatal intensive care unit (NICU), but nurses should be aware that the procedure is particularly distressing for parents. If the need for resuscitation is anticipated, the parents should be assured that a team will be present at the birth to care specifically for their newborn. Nurses should advise parents that a support person will be available for them as well if resuscitation is necessary. As soon as the infant's condition has stabilized, a member of the interdisciplinary team needs to discuss the newborn's condition with the parents. The parents may have many fears about the reasons for resuscitation and the condition of their baby following resuscitation.

Evaluation

Expected outcomes of nursing care include the following:

- The newborn requiring resuscitation is promptly identified, and intervention is started early.
- The newborn's metabolic and physiologic processes are stabilized, and recovery is proceeding without complications.
- The parents can verbalize the reason for resuscitation and what was done to resuscitate their newborn.
- The parents can verbalize their fears about the resuscitation process and potential implications for their baby's future.

Care of the Newborn with Respiratory Distress

One of the severest conditions to which the newborn may fall victim is respiratory distress—an inappropriate respiratory adaptation to extrauterine life. The nurse caring for a baby with respiratory distress needs to understand the normal pulmonary and circulatory physiology (Chapter 24 ∞), the pathophysiology of the disease process, clinical manifestations, and supportive and corrective therapies. Only with this knowledge can the nurse make appropriate observations about responses to therapy and development of complications. Unlike the verbalizing adult client, the newborn communicates needs only by behavior or physiologic parameters that must be interpreted by the NICU nurse. The neonatal

nurse interprets this behavior as clues about the individual baby's condition. This section discusses respiratory distress syndrome, transient tachypnea of the newborn, and meconium aspiration syndrome.

Respiratory Distress Syndrome

Respiratory distress syndrome (RDS), also referred to as *hyaline membrane disease (HMD)*, is the result of a primary absence, deficiency, or alteration in the production of pulmonary surfactant. It is a complex disease that affects approximately 24,000 infants a year in the United States, most of whom are preterm (Nash & Smith, 2008). The syndrome occurs more frequently in premature Caucasian infants than in infants of African or Hispanic descent and almost twice as often in males as in females.

All the factors precipitating the pathologic changes of RDS have not been determined, but the main factors associated with its development include:

1. *Prematurity.* All preterm newborns—whether AGA, SGA, or LGA—and especially infants of diabetic mothers (IDM) are at risk for RDS. The incidence of RDS increases with the degree of prematurity, and most deaths occur in newborns weighing less than 1500 g. The maternal and fetal factors resulting in preterm labor and birth, complications of pregnancy, cesarean birth (and its indications), and familial tendency are all associated with RDS.
2. *Surfactant deficiency disease.* Normal pulmonary adaptation requires adequate surfactant, a lipoprotein that coats the inner surfaces of the alveoli. Surfactant provides alveolar stability by decreasing the alveoli's surface tension and tendency to collapse. Surfactant is produced by type II alveolar cells starting at about 24 weeks' gestation. In the normal or mature newborn lung, it is continuously synthesized, oxidized during breathing, and replenished. Adequate surfactant levels lead to better lung compliance and permit breathing with less work. RDS is caused by alterations in surfactant quantity, composition, function, or production.

TEACHING TIP

You can help parents understand their baby's respiratory distress by having them think of the air sacs (alveoli) of the lungs as tiny balloons filled with water and no air. When the tiny balloon (alveoli) is emptied (as in expiration), water droplets can remain inside the balloon and the sides of the balloons stick together (increasing the surface tension between the sides of the balloon). This increased surface tension makes the next reinflation very difficult and requires an increased amount of energy.

Development of RDS indicates a failure to synthesize surfactant, which is required to maintain alveolar stability (see Factors Opposing the First Breath in Chapter 24 ∞).

MyNursingKit | Respiratory Distress in the Newborn

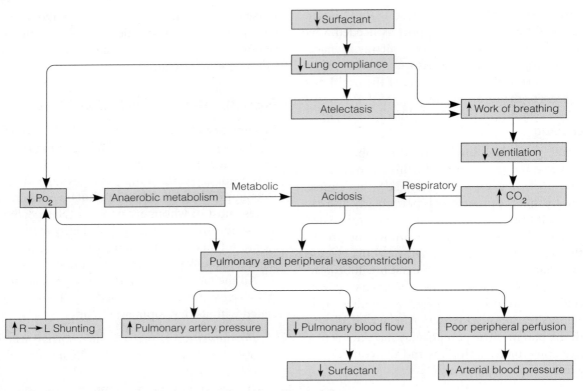

FIGURE 29–3 Cycle of events of RDS leading to eventual respiratory failure.
Source: Modified from Gluck, L., & Kulovich, M. V. (1973). Fetal lung development. *Pediatric Clinics of North America, 20,* 375.

Upon expiration this instability increases atelectasis, which causes hypoxia and acidosis because of the lack of gas exchange. These conditions further inhibit surfactant production and cause pulmonary vasoconstriction. The resulting lung instability causes the biochemical problems of hypoxemia (decreased Po_2), hypercarbia (increased Pco_2), and acidemia (decreased pH), primarily metabolic, which further increase pulmonary vasoconstriction and hypoperfusion; alveolar endothelial and epithelial damage; and subsequent protein-rich interstitial and alveolar edema (Nash & Smith, 2008). The cycle of events of RDS leading to eventual respiratory failure is diagrammed in Figure 29–3 ■.

Because of these pathophysiologic conditions, the newborn must expend increasing amounts of energy to reopen the collapsed alveoli with every breath, so that each breath becomes more difficult than the last. The progressive expiratory atelectasis upsets the physiologic homeostasis of the pulmonary and cardiovascular systems and prevents adequate gas exchange (Cole, Nogee, & Hamvas, 2006). Breathing becomes progressively harder as lung compliance decreases, which makes it more difficult to inflate the lungs and breathe.

The physiologic alterations of RDS produce the following complications.

1. *Hypoxia.* As a result of hypoxia, the pulmonary vasculature constricts, pulmonary vascular resistance increases, and pulmonary blood flow is reduced. Increased pulmonary vascular resistance may precipitate a return to fetal circulation as the ductus opens and blood flow is shunted around the lungs in a right-to-left blood flow. This shunting increases the hypoxia and further decreases pulmonary perfusion. Hypoxia also causes impairment or absence of metabolic response to cold; reversion to anaerobic metabolism, resulting in lactate accumulation (acidosis); and impaired cardiac output, which decreases perfusion to vital organs.

2. *Respiratory acidosis.* Increased Pco_2 and decreased pH are results of alveolar hypoventilation. A persistent rise in Pco_2 is a poor prognostic sign of pulmonary function and adequacy because the increased Pco_2 and decreased pH are results of alveolar hypoventilation.

3. *Metabolic acidosis.* Because of the lack of oxygen at the cellular level, the newborn begins an anaerobic pathway of metabolism, with an increase in lactate levels and a resulting base deficit (loss of bicarbonate). As the lactate levels increase, the pH decreases in an attempt to maintain acid-base homeostasis.

The classic radiologic picture of RDS is diffuse bilateral reticulogranular (ground glass appearance) density, with portions of the air-filled tracheobronchial tree (air bronchogram) outlined by the opaque ("white-out") lungs with widespread atelectasis, potentially obliterating the heart borders (Cloherty et al., 2008; Thureen, Deacon, Hernandez et al., 2005) (Figure 29–4 ■). The progression

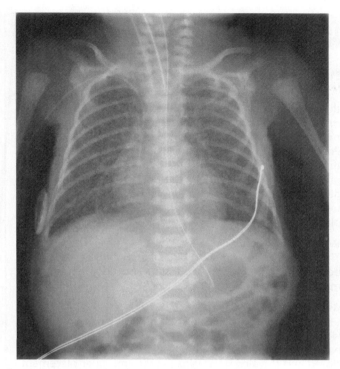

FIGURE 29–4 RDS chest X-ray. Chest radiograph of respiratory distress syndrome characterized by a reticulogranular pattern with areas of microatelectasis of uniform opacity and air bronchograms.
Source: Courtesy of Carol Harrigan, RNC, MSN, NNP.

of X-ray findings parallels the pattern of resolution, which usually occurs in 7 to 10 days, and the time of surfactant reappearance, unless surfactant replacement therapy has been used (Blackburn, 2007). Echocardiography is a valuable tool in diagnosing vascular shunts that move blood either away from or toward the lungs.

Clinical Therapy

The primary goal of prenatal management is to prevent preterm birth through early assessment of fetal lung maturity, aggressive treatment of preterm labor, and administration of glucocorticoids to enhance fetal lung development (see Chapter 16 ∞). Antenatal steroids reduce the incidence and severity of RDS and improve survivability of the 24 to 34 weeks' gestation and extremely low-birth-weight newborn (less than 1250 grams) (Cloherty et al., 2008). The goals of postnatal therapy are to maintain adequate oxygenation and ventilation, correct acid-base imbalance, and provide the supportive care required to maintain homeostasis.

Surfactant replacement therapy is available for infants to decrease the severity of RDS in low-birth-weight newborns. This is one of the best studied therapies in newborns. Surfactant replacement therapy is delivered through an endotracheal tube and may be given in either the birthing room or the nursery as indicated by the severity of RDS. Repeat doses

are often required. The most frequent reported response to treatment is rapidly improved oxygenation and decreased need for ventilatory support (AAP & ACOG, 2007).

Supportive medical management consists of ventilation therapy, transcutaneous oxygen and carbon dioxide monitoring, blood gas monitoring, correction of acid-base imbalance, environmental temperature regulation, adequate nutrition, and protection from infection. Ventilation therapy is directed toward preventing hypoventilation and hypoxia. Mild cases of RDS may require only increased humidified oxygen concentrations. Use of continuous positive airway pressure (CPAP) may be required in moderately afflicted infants. Babies with severe RDS require mechanical ventilatory assistance from a respirator (Figure 29–5 ■).

High-frequency ventilation (HFV) can be tried when conventional ventilator therapy has not been successful, and it sometimes can be the primary mode of ventilation to minimize lung injury in very small and/or sick infants (Cloherty et al., 2008). In some institutions, morphine or fentanyl is used for its analgesic and sedative effects. Sedation may be indicated for infants who have air leak respiratory problems. Using pancuronium (Pavulon) for muscle relaxation in infants with RDS is controversial.

HINTS FOR PRACTICE

In babies with RDS who are on ventilators, increased diuresis or urination (determined by weighing diapers) may be an early clue that the baby's condition is improving. As fluid moves out of the lungs into the bloodstream, alveoli open and kidney perfusion increases; this results in increased voiding. At this point, the nurse must monitor chest expansion closely. If chest expansion is increasing, pulmonary compliance is improving and ventilator settings may have to be decreased, sometimes quite soon after surfactant dosing. Too high a ventilator setting may "blow the lung," resulting in pneumothorax.

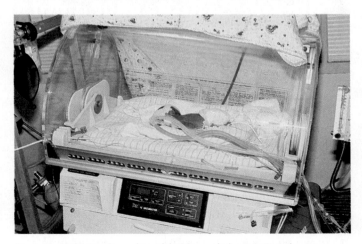

FIGURE 29–5 One-day-old, 29 weeks' gestational age, 1450 g baby on respirator and in isolette.
Source: Courtesy of Carol Harrigan, RNC, MSN, NNP.

EVIDENCE-BASED PRACTICE

Nursing Care of the Newborn with NCPAP

Clinical Questions

What nursing interventions support the most effective delivery of nasal continuous positive airway pressure (NCPAP)? How can the nurse avoid complications of NCPAP?

The Evidence

NCPAP has been used to support preterm infants with respiratory distress by increasing lung volume and supporting ventilation. It is an effective alternative to intubation because it is considered a gentler mode of ventilation associated with decreased pulmonary damage. A challenge in achieving effective NCPAP is obtaining a good fit with the NCPAP delivery device. Improperly fitted prongs or the baby's open mouth can allow the pressure in the system to drop below therapeutic levels. Furthermore, the nurse is challenged with preventing skin complications from the drying effects of oxygen and mechanical contact with the nasal prongs. The National Association of Neonatal Nurses sponsored the development of a practice guideline for the nursing care of newborns receiving NCPAP. An additional systematic review was conducted through the Cochrane Collaborative, focusing on appropriate devices for optimal administration of NCPAP. A practice guideline that integrates scientific evidence with content expertise, combined with a systematic review that meets the rigorous standards of the Cochrane Review, is the strongest evidence for nursing practice.

What Is Effective?

Short binasal prong devices are more effective than single prongs in improving ventilation and reducing the rate of intubation. The binasal prongs were more effective than both single nasal and nasopharyngeal prongs, as it appears short binasal prong devices decrease resistance while pressure is delivered to both nares. A key point for successful NCPAP therapy is obtained by using an appropriate fitting hat and mask. Nasal prongs should be placed so that there are no pressure points that might cause nasal and septum damage. Positioning the newborn so the infant's hand is tucked under the chin helps keep the mouth closed and maintains proper pressure. Using a roll under the neck or chest facilitates a patent airway. Vigilance for signs of skin damage and early intervention when redness is detected prevent long-term complications from skin breakdown.

What Is Inconclusive?

The choice of a specific short binasal prong device remains to be determined; several were tested and none emerged as most effective.

Best Practice

CPAP is most effectively delivered through binasal prong devices that are properly placed in the nares of a newborn that has been positioned so that the infant's mouth remains closed and the airway remains patent. Improper placement of the nasal device can cause skin breakdown of the nares and/or septum, so you should be vigilant for pressure points and signs of early skin breakdown. Use comfort measures, such as swaddling or a pacifier, to avoid dislodgement from excessive movement.

References

DePaoli, A., Davis, P., Faber, B., & Morley, C. (2008). Devices and pressure sources for administration of nasal continuous positive airway pressure (NCPAP) in preterm neonates. *Cochrane Database of Systematic Reviews,* Issue 1.

McCoskey, L. (2008). Nursing care guidelines for prevention of nasal breakdown in neonates receiving nasal CPAP. *Advances in Neonatal Care, 8*(2), 116–124.

Nursing Care Management

Nursing Assessment and Diagnosis

The nurse should look for characteristics of RDS such as increasing cyanosis, tachypnea (greater than 60 respirations per minute), grunting respirations, nasal flaring, significant retractions, and apnea. Table 29–1 reviews clinical findings associated with respiratory distress in general. The Silverman-Andersen index (Figure 29–6 ■) may be helpful in evaluating the signs of respiratory distress used in the birthing area.

Nursing diagnoses that may apply to the newborn with RDS include the following:

- *Impaired Gas Exchange* related to inadequate lung surfactant
- *Ineffective Thermoregulation* related to increased respiratory effort
- *Altered Nutrition: Less than Body Requirements* related to increased metabolic needs of the stressed infant
- *Risk for Fluid Volume Deficit* related to increased insensible water losses
- *Risk for Infection* related to invasive procedures

Nursing Plan and Implementation

Based on clinical parameters, the neonatal nurse implements therapeutic approaches to maintain physiologic homeostasis and provides supportive care to the newborn with RDS. (See Nursing Care Plan: Care of Newborn with Respiratory Distress, on pages 761–763.)

Nursing interventions and criteria for instituting mechanical ventilation depend on institutional protocol. Noninvasive oxygen monitoring provides real time trend information that is particularly useful in infants showing frequent swings in PaO$_2$ and oxygen saturation.

TABLE 29–1 Clinical Assessments Associated with Respiratory Distress

Clinical Picture	Significance
Skin Color	
Pallor or mottling	These represent poor peripheral circulation caused by systemic hypotension and vasoconstriction and pooling of independent areas (usually in conjunction with severe hypoxia).
Cyanosis (bluish tint)	Depending on hemoglobin concentration, peripheral circulation, intensity and quality of viewing light, and acuity of observer's color vision, this is frankly visible in advanced hypoxia. Central cyanosis is most easily detected by examination of mucous membranes and tongue.
Jaundice (yellow discoloration of skin and mucous membranes caused by presence of unconjugated [indirect] bilirubin)	Metabolic alterations (acidosis, hypercarbia, asphyxia) of respiratory distress predispose a newborn to dissociation of bilirubin from albumin-binding sites and deposition in the skin and central nervous system.
Edema (presents as slick, shiny taut skin)	This is characteristic of preterm infants because their total protein concentration is low, with a decrease in colloidal osmotic pressure and transudation of fluid. Edema of hands and feet is frequently seen within first 24 hours and resolved by fifth day in infants with severe RDS.
Respiratory System	
Tachypnea (normal respiratory rate [RR] 30 to 60/minute, sustained, elevated respiratory rate 60+/minute)	Increased respiratory rate is the easiest detectable sign of respiratory distress after birth. Because of the premature infant's very compliant chest wall, it is more energy efficient to increase the respiratory rate than the depth of respirations. This compensatory mechanism attempts to increase respiratory dead space to maintain alveolar ventilation and gas exchange in the face of an increase in mechanical resistance. As a decompensatory mechanism it increases workload and energy output by increasing respiratory rate, which causes increased metabolic demand for oxygen and thus increases alveolar ventilation on an already overstressed system. During shallow, rapid respirations, there is an increase in dead space ventilation, thus decreasing alveolar ventilation.
Apnea (episode of nonbreathing for more than 20 seconds) Periodic breathing, a common "normal" occurrence in preterm infants, is defined as apnea of 5 to 10 seconds alternating with 10 to 15 seconds of ventilation	This poor prognostic sign indicates cardiorespiratory disease, CNS disease, metabolic alterations, intracranial hemorrhage, sepsis, or immaturity. Physiologic alterations include decreased oxygen saturation, respiratory acidosis, and bradycardia.
Chest	
	Inspection of the thoracic cage includes shape, size, and symmetry of movement. Respiratory movements should be symmetrical and diaphragmatic; asymmetry reflects pathology (pneumothorax, diaphragmatic hernia). Increased anteroposterior diameter indicates air trapping (meconium aspiration syndrome).
Labored respirations (Silverman-Andersen index in Figure 29–6 indicates severity of retractions, grunting, and nasal flaring, which are signs of labored respirations)	Indicates marked increase in the work of breathing.
Retractions (inward pulling of soft parts of the chest cage—suprasternal (above the sterum), substernal (below xiphoid process), intercostals (between the ribs)—at inspiration)	These reflect the significant increase in negative intrathoracic pressure necessary to inflate stiff, noncompliant lungs. Infants attempt to increase lung compliance by using accessory muscles. Lung expansion markedly decreases. Seesaw respirations are seen when the chest flattens with inspiration and the abdomen bulges. Retractions increase the work of breathing and O_2 need. As a result, assisted ventilation may be necessary because of exhaustion.
Nasal flaring (inspiratory dilation of nostrils)	This compensatory mechanism attempts to lessen the resistance of the narrow nasal passage and increase the inflow of air.
Expiratory grunt (Valsalva maneuver in which the infant exhales against a partially closed glottis, thus producing an audible moan)	This increases intrapulmonary pressure, which decreases or prevents atelectasis, thus improving oxygenation and alveolar ventilation. It allows more time for the passage of oxygen into the circulatory system. Intubation should not be attempted unless the infant's condition is rapidly deteriorating, because it prevents this maneuver and allows the alveoli to collapse.
Rhythmic body movement with labored respirations (chin tug, head bobbing, retractions of anal area)	This is a result of using abdominal and other respiratory accessory muscles during prolonged forced respirations.
Auscultation of chest reveals decreased air exchange, with harsh breath sounds or fine inspiratory rales; rhonchi may be present	Decrease in breath sounds and distant quality may indicate interstitial or intrapleural air or fluid.
Cardiovascular System	
Continuous systolic murmur may be audible	Patent ductus arteriosus is a common occurrence with hypoxia, pulmonary vasoconstriction, right-to-left shunting, and congestive heart failure.
Heart rate usually within normal limits (fixed heart rate may occur with a rate of 110 to 120/minute)	A fixed heart rate indicates a decrease in vagal control.
Point of maximal impulse usually located at fourth to fifth intercostal space, left sternal border	Displacement may reflect dextrocardia, pneumothorax, or diaphragmatic hernia.

(Continued)

TABLE 29–1	Clinical Assessments Associated with Respiratory Distress *(Continued)*
Clinical Picture	**Significance**
Hypothermia	This is inadequate functioning of metabolic processes that require oxygen to produce necessary body heat.
Muscle Tone Flaccid, hypotonic, unresponsive to stimuli Hypertonia and/or seizure activity	These may indicate deterioration in the newborn's condition and possible CNS damage caused by hypoxia, acidemia, or hemorrhage.

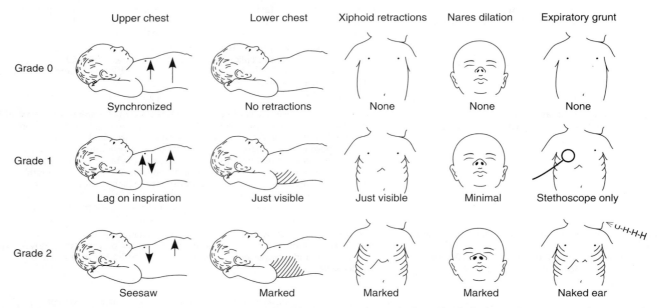

FIGURE 29–6 Evaluation of respiratory status using the Silverman-Andersen index. The baby's respiratory status is assessed. A grade of 0, 1, or 2 is determined for each area, and a total score is charted in the baby's record or on a copy of this tool and placed in the chart.
Source: Used with permission: Clinical Education Series No. 2: Columbus, Ohio: Ross Products Division, Abbott Laboratories.

These methods (pulse oximetry, transcutaneous oxygen monitor) can also reduce the frequency of blood gas sampling. Methods of noninvasive oxygen monitoring and nursing interventions are included in Table 29–2. (The nursing care of infants on ventilators or with umbilical artery catheters is not discussed here. These infants have severe respiratory distress and are cared for in neonatal intensive care units by nurses with advanced knowledge and training.) Ventilatory assistance with high-frequency ventilators shows positive results. The parents of a baby with respiratory distress should be provided with a very supportive environment (Figure 29–7 ■).

Evaluation

Expected outcomes of nursing care include the following:

- The newborn at risk for RDS is promptly identified and early intervention is initiated.
- The newborn is free of respiratory distress and metabolic alterations.

- The parents verbalize their concerns about their baby's health problem and survival and understand the rationale behind the management of their newborn.

CRITICAL THINKING

You are caring for baby girl Linn, who is a 39-week, AGA female born by repeat cesarean birth to a 34-year-old G3, now P3 mother. Baby Linn's Apgar scores were 7 at 1 minute and 9 at 5 minutes. At 2 hours of age, you note an elevated respiratory rate of 70 to 80 and mild cyanosis. The infant is now receiving 30% oxygen and has a respiratory rate of 100 to 120. The baby's clinical course, chest X-ray examination, and lab work are all consistent with transient tachypnea of the newborn. Her mother calls you to ask about her baby. She tells you that her last child was born at 30 weeks' gestation, had respiratory distress syndrome requiring ventilator support, and was hospitalized for 6 weeks. She asks you, "Is this the same respiratory distress?" What will you tell her?

Answers can be found in Appendix F ∞.

TABLE 29–2 Oxygen Monitors

Type	Function and Rationale	Nursing Interventions
Pulse Oximetry—SPo_2		
Estimates beat-to-beat arterial oxygen saturation.	Calibration is automatic.	Understand and use oxyhemoglobin dissociation curve.
Microprocessor measures saturation by the absorption of red and infrared light as it passes through tissue.	Less dependent on perfusion than TcPo_2 and TcPco_2, however, functions poorly if peripheral perfusion is decreased due to low cardiac output.	Monitor trends over time and correlate with arterial blood gases. Check disposable sensor at least q8h.
Changes in absorption related to blood pulsation through vessel determine saturation and pulse rate.	Much more rapid response time than TcPo_2—offers real-time readings.	Use disposable cuffs (reusable cuffs allow too much ambient light to enter, and readings may be inaccurate).
	Can be located on extremity, digit, or palm of hand, leaving chest free; not affected by skin characteristics.	
	Requires understanding of oxyhemoglobin dissociation curve.	
	Pulse oximeter reading of 85% to 95% reflects clinically safe range of saturation.	
	Extreme sensitivity to movement; decreases if average of 7th or 14th beat is selected rather than beat to beat.	
	Poor correlation with extreme hyperoxia.	
Transcutaneous Oxygen Monitor—TcPo_2		
Measures oxygen diffusion across the skin.	When transcutaneous monitors are properly calibrated and electrodes are appropriately positioned, they will provide reliable, continuous, noninvasive measurements of Po_2, Pco_2, and oxygen saturation.	Use TcPo_2 to monitor trends of oxygenation with routine nursing care procedures.
Clark electrode is heated to 43°C (preterm) or 44°C (term) to warm the skin beneath the electrode and promote diffusion of oxygen across the skin surface. Po_2 is measured when oxygen diffuses across the capillary membrane, skin, and electrode membrane.	Readings vary when skin perfusion is decreased.	Clean electrode surface to remove electrolyte deposits; change solution and membrane once a week.
	Reliable as trend monitor.	Allow machine to stabilize before drawing arterial gases; note reading when gases are drawn and use values to correlate.
	Frequent calibration necessary to overcome mechanical drift.	Ensure airtight seal between skin surface and electrode; place electrodes on clean, dry skin on upper chest, abdomen, or inner aspect of thigh; avoid bony prominences.
	Following membrane change, machine must "warm up" 1 hour prior to initial calibration; otherwise, after turning it on, it must equilibrate for 30 minutes prior to calibration.	
	When placed on infant, values will be low until skin is heated; approximately 15 minutes required to stabilize.	
	Second-degree burns are rare but can occur if electrodes remain in place too long.	Change skin site and recalibrate at least every 4 hours; inspect skin for burns; if burns occur, use lowest temperature setting and change position of electrode more frequently.
	Decreased correlations noted with older infants (related to skin thickness), with infants with low cardiac output (decreased skin perfusion), and with hyperoxic infants.	
	The adhesive that attaches the electrode may abrade the fragile skin of the preterm infant.	Adhesive disks may be cut to a smaller size, or skin prep may be used under the adhesive circle only; allow membrane to touch skin surface at center.
	May be used for both preductal and postductal monitoring of oxygenation for observations of shunting.	

Transient Tachypnea of the Newborn

Some newborns, primarily LGA and late preterm infants, may develop progressive respiratory distress that clinically can resemble RDS. They may have had intrauterine or intrapartal asphyxia caused by maternal oversedation, maternal bleeding, prolapsed cord, breech birth, or maternal diabetes. The newborn then fails to clear the airway of lung fluid, mucus, and other debris or an excess of fluid in the lungs caused by aspiration of amniotic or tracheal fluid. Transient tachypnea of the newborn (TTN), which occurs in 11 per 1000 live births (Nash & Smith, 2008), is also more prevalent in cesarean-birth newborns who have not had the thoracic squeeze that occurs during vaginal birth and removes some of the lung fluid (Blackburn, 2007).

Usually the newborn experiences little or no difficulty at the onset of breathing. However, shortly after birth, expiratory grunting, flaring of the nares, and mild cyanosis

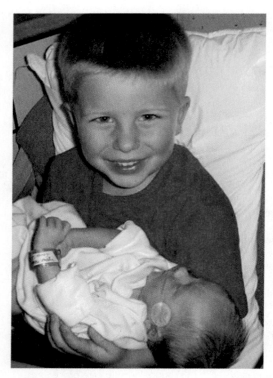

FIGURE 29–7 This baby born at 36 weeks' gestational age had severe RDS. He has ongoing oxygen needs provided by a nasal cannula but still can be held by his proud big brother.
Source: Courtesy of Lisa Smith-Pedersen, RNC, MSN, NNP.

may be noted in the newborn breathing room air. Air will become trapped and an increase in the anterior/posterior diameter of the chest will be observed (Blackburn, 2007). Tachypnea is usually present by 6 hours of age, with respiratory rates consistently greater than 60 breaths per minute. Mild respiratory and metabolic acidosis may be present at 2 to 6 hours. These clinical signs usually persist for 12 to 24 hours. In mild TTN, the signs can improve within 24 hours but may continue for 48 to 72 hours when more severe (Cloherty et al., 2008).

Clinical Therapy

Initial X-ray findings may be identical to those showing RDS within the first 3 hours. However, radiographs of infants with transient tachypnea usually reveal a generalized overexpansion of the lungs (hyperaeration of alveoli), which is identified principally by flattened contours of the diaphragm. Dense streaks (increased vascularity) radiate from the hilar region and represent engorgement of the lymphatic vessels, which clear alveolar fluid on initiation of air breathing. Within 48 to 72 hours, the chest X-ray examination is normal (Cloherty et al., 2008).

Ambient oxygen concentrations of less than 40%, usually under an oxyhood, may be required to correct the hypoxemia (Cloherty et al., 2008) (Figure 29–8 ■). Fluid and

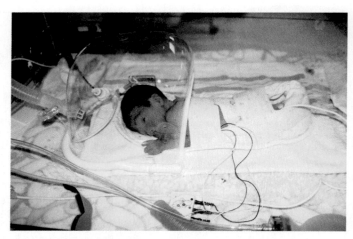

FIGURE 29–8 Premature infant under oxygen hood. Infant is nested and has a nonnutritive sucking pacifier.
Source: Courtesy of Lisa Smith-Pedersen, RNC, MSN, NNP.

electrolyte requirements should be met with IV during the acute phase of the disease. Oral feedings are contraindicated because of rapid respiratory rates and the subsequent risk of aspiration.

When hypoxemia is severe and tachypnea continues, persistent pulmonary hypertension must be considered and treatment measures initiated. If pneumonia is suspected initially, antibiotics may be administered prophylactically.

Nursing Care Management

For nursing actions, see the Nursing Care Plan of a Newborn with Respiratory Distress on pages 761–768.

Care of the Newborn with Meconium Aspiration Syndrome

Because the body's physiologic response to asphyxia is increased intestinal peristalsis, relaxation of the anal sphincter and presence of meconium in the amniotic fluid indicates that the fetus may be suffering from asphyxia. However, if the fetus is in a breech position, the presence of meconium in the amniotic fluid *does not necessarily* indicate asphyxia.

Approximately 8% to 15% of all live-born, late preterm or term infants are born through meconium-stained amniotic fluid (MSAF). Of the newborns born through MSAF, an average of 5% develop **meconium aspiration syndrome (MAS)** (Cloherty et al., 2008). This fluid may be aspirated into the tracheobronchial tree in utero or during the first few breaths taken by the newborn. This syndrome primarily affects term, SGA, and postterm newborns and those who have experienced a long labor.

Nursing Care Plan   Care of Newborn with Respiratory Distress

CLIENT SCENARIO

Baby boy Ryan, 3 hours old, born at 36 weeks' gestation weighs 6 lb, 12 oz. Ryan was born by cesarean section to a 26-year-old G1P0 mother. Apgars at birth were 6 at 1 min and 7 at 5 min. (normal range 7–10). On admission to the nursery Ryan's respirations were 80 breaths per minute with noticeable expiratory grunting and suprasternal retractions. The skin was pale and slightly cyanotic. Arterial blood gases showed a PaO_2 of 40 mm Hg and a PCO_2 of 70 mm Hg. Assessment data are consistent with respiratory distress syndrome (RDS). The nurse administers surfactant via endotracheal tube. Ryan was placed under an oxygen hood and continues to remain in the radiant warmer.

ASSESSMENT

Subjective: N/A

Objective: Respirations 80, expiratory grunting, cyanosis, nasal flaring, visible suprasternal retractions, oxygenation saturation 84%, ABGs: PaO_2 of 40 mm Hg and a PCO_2 of 70 mm Hg

Nursing Diagnosis #1	Impaired Gas Exchange related to inadequate lung surfactant*
Client Goal	The client will maintain adequate oxygenation and ventilation.
AEB:	• Vital signs within normal limits • No signs of suprasternal retractions, expiratory grunting, or nasal flaring

NURSING INTERVENTIONS

1. Administer surfactant replacement therapy as ordered.

2. Monitor respiratory rate every 2 hours and prn.

3. Assess chest wall movement.

4. Observe newborn for labored respirations.

5. Administer warmed, humidified oxygen to newborn as ordered.

6. Monitor arterial blood gases every 8 hours and prn.

RATIONALES

Rationale: Surfactant improves lung compliance; therefore the need for ventilatory support may be decreased. Surfactant provides alveolar stability by decreasing the alveoli's surface tension and tendency to collapse. Alterations in surfactant quantity, composition, function, or production results in respiratory distress syndrome. Surfactant replacement therapy may be administered via endotracheal tube either in the birthing room or in the nursery.

Rationale: Normal newborn respiratory rate is 30 to 60 breaths per minute. Elevations above 60 breaths per minute may be indicative of respiratory distress. The most frequent and easily detectable sign of respiratory distress is an increased respiratory rate.

Rationale: Respiratory movements that are asymmetrical may reflect pathology such as a pneumothorax or diaphragmatic hernia. Inspection of the chest wall for breathing effort should reflect symmetrical and diaphragmatic respiratory movements.

Rationale: The Silverman-Andersen index may be used to evaluate respiratory distress. Retractions, nasal flaring, and grunting indicate an increase in breathing effort. The Silverman-Andersen index grades retractions, nasal flaring, and grunting according to severity.

Rationale: Oxygenation and ventilatory therapy may prevent hypoventilation and hypoxia. Mild cases of respiratory distress may only require increased humidified oxygen concentrations whereas more severe cases may require continuous positive airway pressure. The nurse may administer oxygen to the newborn experiencing mild respiratory distress via nasal cannula or oxygen hood. With severe respiratory distress mechanical ventilatory assistance from a respirator may be necessary.

Rationale: A failure to synthesize surfactant increases atelectasis which causes hypoxia and acidosis caused by lack of gas exchange. Lung compliance will deteriorate and result in difficulty of inflation, labored respirations, and increased work of breathing. Progressive hypoxia may be seen when arterial blood gas levels are compared and evaluated.

(Continued on next page)

Nursing Care Plan Care of Newborn with Respiratory Distress *(Continued)*

NURSING INTERVENTIONS	RATIONALES
7. Monitor oxygen saturation every 4 hours and prn.	*Rationale:* Attach pulse oximeter to infant's extremity to measure tissue oxygenation. Oxygen saturation should be kept approximately 88% to 92% (Nash & Smith, 2008). Avoid excessive oxygenation which can increase the risk of developing chronic lung disease and retinopathy of prematurity.
8. Cluster newborn care procedures.	*Rationale:* Clustering newborn care procedures will allow the newborn to recover between procedures and avoid overstimulation. Combining care procedures helps to decrease energy expenditure of the newborn, thereby preventing a decrease in oxygen saturation.
9. Maintain a neutral thermal environment.	*Rationale:* Hypothermia places added metabolic demands on the already compromised newborn. Keeping the newborn warm will reduce the need for increased oxygen. The risk of cold stress is minimized when the newborn remains in a neutral thermal environment. Infants with RDS should receive care under a radiant warmer or in an incubator.

Evaluation of Client Goal	• Vital signs within normal limits. • No signs of suprasternal retractions, expiratory grunting, or nasal flaring.
Nursing Diagnosis #2	Altered Nutrition: Less than Body Requirements related to immaturity and increased metabolic needs associated with RDS
Client Goal	The newborn will maintain an adequate intake of calories to meet the needs for metabolism.
AEB:	• Weight will remain stable. • Newborn will tolerate feedings.

NURSING INTERVENTIONS	RATIONALES
1. Provide total parenteral nutrition as ordered.	*Rationale:* The newborn with respiratory distress syndrome is too exhausted to suck; therefore nutrition is provided via other routes.
2. Advance nutritional intake as tolerated.	*Rationale:* Once the newborn is able to suck without compromising oxygen demands, feedings may be advanced from parenteral to gastrointestinal feedings. Gavage or nipple feed if possible. When oral intake is sufficient IV fluids can be discontinued. Supplement breastfeeding only when medically indicated and ordered by MD/NP.
3. Provide gavage feedings as needed.	*Rationale:* Additional nutrients are necessary for the newborn to maintain or stabilize weight. Increases in calories are required to support the extra energy expenditure that is associated with RDS of the newborn.
4. Maintain IV rate via infusion pump as ordered.	*Rationale:* Usually 60 to 80 mL/kg/day may be offered depending on gestational age and organ efficiency. IV fluids provide supplemental glucose and electrolytes which support metabolism during the early neonatal period. Monitor for hypoglycemia that may occur from respiratory distress and increased metabolic demands.
5. Monitor hourly output.	*Rationale:* As fluid moves out of the lungs into the bloodstream, alveoli open and kidney perfusion increases, resulting in increased urination. For newborns with RDS and who are on ventilators, an increase in urination may be an early sign that the newborn's condition is improving. Urinary output should be 1 to 3 mL/kg/hour.

Nursing Care Plan Care of Newborn with Respiratory Distress (Continued)

CRITICAL THINKING QUESTIONS

1. What is the role of surfactant in the mature newborn? How are newborns affected when there is a failure to synthesize surfactant?

Answer: Surfactant, a lipoprotein, coats the inner surface of the alveoli and provides alveolar stability by decreasing the alveoli's surface tension and tendency to collapse. Surfactant is continuously synthesized, oxidized during breathing, and replenished in the normal or mature newborn lung. Newborns may present with RDS if there are alterations in the surfactant's quantity, composition, function, or in its production.

2. The nurse is assessing a newborn on admission to the nursery. The nurse hears a grunting sound on expiration while auscultating the lungs. What is causing a grunting sound on expiration? What is the significance of grunting in the newborn? Should the nurse intubate the newborn?

Answer: The grunting sound is caused by the Valsalva maneuver. As the newborn exhales against a closed glottis an audible moan can be heard. This increases intrapulmonary pressure, which also decreases or prevents atelectasis. Unless the newborn's condition is deteriorating, the nurse should not attempt to intubate the newborn because it could prevent the Valsalva maneuver and cause the alveoli to collapse.

*For your reference, this care plan is an example of how two nursing diagnoses might be addressed.

Presence of meconium in the lungs produces:

- Mechanical obstruction of airways: ball-valve action (air is allowed in but not exhaled), so that alveoli overdistend.
- Chemical pneumonitis; with oxygen and carbon dioxide trapping and hyperinflation, air leaks such as pneumothorax are common, occurring in 15% to 33% of babies with MAS; secondary bacterial pneumonia can occur.
- Vasoconstriction of pulmonary vessels; allowing development of persistent hypertension (PPHN).
- Inactivation of natural surfactant (Cloherty et al., 2008).

Clinical Manifestations of MAS

Clinical manifestations of MAS include (1) fetal hypoxia in utero a few days or a few minutes before birth, indicated by a sudden increase in fetal activity followed by diminished activity, slowing of FHR or weak and irregular heartbeat, loss of beat-to-beat variability, and meconium staining of amniotic fluid or particulate meconium; and (2) presence of signs of distress at birth, such as pallor, cyanosis, apnea, slow heartbeat, and low Apgar scores (below 6) at 1 and 5 minutes. Newborns with intrauterine asphyxia, meconium-stained newborns, or newborns who have aspirated particulate meconium often have respiratory depression at birth and require resuscitation to establish adequate respiratory effort.

After the initial assessment and stabilization, the severity of the ongoing clinical symptoms correlate with the extent of aspiration. Many infants require mechanical ventilation at

birth because of immediate signs of distress (generalized cyanosis, tachypnea, and severe retractions). An overdistended, barrel-shaped chest with increased anteroposterior diameter is common. Auscultation reveals diminished air movement, with prominent rales and rhonchi. Abdominal palpation may reveal a displaced liver caused by diaphragmatic depression resulting from the overexpansion of the lungs. Yellowish/pale green staining of the skin, nails, and umbilical cord is usually present, especially if the incident occurred some time before birth.

The chest X-ray film for newborns with MAS reveals asymmetric, coarse, patchy densities and possible hyperinflation (9 to 11 rib expansion), which may predispose the newborn to air leak syndrome such as pneumothorax or pneumomediastinum (Cloherty et al., 2008). Evidence of pulmonary air leak is frequently present. These infants have serious biochemical alterations, which include (1) extreme metabolic acidosis resulting from the cardiopulmonary shunting and hypoperfusion; (2) extreme respiratory acidosis caused by shunting and alveolar hypoventilation; and (3) extreme hypoxia, even in 100% O_2 concentration and with ventilatory assistance. Extreme hypoxia is also caused by the cardiopulmonary shunting and resultant failure to oxygenate and can lead to PPHN.

EVIDENCE IN ACTION
Suctioning of the oropharynx and nasopharynx before the delivery of the shoulders in the incidence of a meconium-stained amniotic fluid is no longer recommended.
(Organization Guidelines) (American Academy of Pediatrics (AAP), Committee on Fetus and Newborn, & American College of Obstetricians and Gynecolgists (ACOG), Committee on Obstetrics, 2007)

Clinical Therapy

The combined efforts of the maternity and pediatric team are needed to prevent MAS. Previously the most effective form of preventive management was intrapartum suctioning after the head of the newborn was delivered but the shoulders and chest were still in the birth canal. Current evidence does not support this practice, as routine intrapartum oropharyngeal and nasopharyngeal suctioning does not prevent or alter the course of MAS (AAP & ACOG, 2007; Wiedemann, Saugstad, Barnes-Powell, & Duran, 2008).

If the infant is vigorous even if there is meconium-stained amniotic fluid, no subsequent special resuscitation such as tracheal suctioning is indicated. Injury to the vocal cords is also more likely to occur during attempts to intubate a vigorous newborn.

If the infant has absent or depressed respirations, heart rate less than 100 beats per minute, or poor muscle tone, direct tracheal suctioning by specially trained personnel such as a neonatal nurse practitioner, an experienced NICU nurse trained in those skills, a respiratory therapist, or a nurse anesthetist is recommended. The glottis is visualized and the trachea suctioned to remove meconium or other aspirated material from beneath the glottis with use of a DeLee attached to wall suction. (This is also done with a cesarean birth.) To decrease the possibility of human immunodeficiency virus (HIV) transmission, low-pressure wall suction is used. When using mechanical suction, the suction pressure should be set so that negative pressure does not exceed 100 mm Hg.

Further resuscitative efforts are undertaken as indicated, following the same principles of clinical therapy used for asphyxia (discussed earlier in this chapter). Resuscitated newborns should be transferred immediately to the nursery for closer observation. The infant should be maintained in a neutral thermal environment and tactile stimulation should be minimized. An umbilical arterial line may be used for direct monitoring of arterial blood pressures, as well as blood sampling for pH and blood gases. An umbilical venous catheter may be placed for infusion of IV fluids, blood, or medications.

Treatment usually involves delivery of high levels of oxygen and high-pressure ventilation. Low positive end-expiratory pressures (PEEPs) are preferred to avoid air leaks such as pneumothorax. Unfortunately, high pressures may be needed to cause sufficient expiratory expansion of obstructed terminal airways or to stabilize airways that are weakened by inflammation so that the most distal atelectatic alveoli are ventilated.

Naturally occurring surfactant may be inactivated by the presence of meconium and the subsequent inflammatory response that occurs. Surfactant replacement therapy is most effective when used prophylactically. It improves oxygenation and decreases the incidence of air leaks (Cloherty et al., 2008). Systemic blood pressure and pulmonary blood flow must be maintained. Dopamine or dobutamine and/or volume expanders may be used to maintain systemic blood pressure.

Newborns with respiratory failure who are not responding to conventional ventilator therapy may require treatment with high-frequency ventilation and/or nitric oxide therapy or extracorporeal membrane oxygenation (ECMO) if the baby is greater than 2 kg (Cloherty et al., 2008). Inhaled nitric oxide has proven successful for newborns with meconium aspiration, pneumonia, and PPHN who are not responding to traditional treatment modalities, and it avoids the need for ECMO.

Treatment includes chest physiotherapy (chest percussion, vibration, and drainage) to remove debris. Prophylactic intravenous antibiotics are frequently given. Continuous infusion of bicarbonate to correct metabolic acidosis may be necessary for several days for severely ill newborns. Mortality in term or postterm infants is very high because the cycle of hypoxemia and acidemia is difficult to break.

Nursing Care Management

Nursing Assessment and Diagnosis

During the intrapartal period, the nurse should observe for signs of fetal hypoxia and meconium staining of amniotic fluid. At birth, the nurse assesses the newborn for signs of distress. During the ongoing assessment of the newborn, the nurse carefully observes for complications such as pulmonary air leaks; anoxic cerebral injury manifested by seizure and/or convulsions; myocardial injury evidenced by congestive heart failure or cardiomegaly; disseminated intravascular coagulation (DIC) resulting from hypoxic hepatic damage with depression of liver-dependent clotting factors; anoxic renal damage demonstrated by hematuria, oliguria, or anuria; fluid overload; sepsis secondary to bacterial pneumonia; and any signs of intestinal necrosis from ischemia, including GI obstruction or hemorrhage.

Nursing diagnoses that may apply to the newborn with MAS and the infants' parents include the following:

- *Ineffective Gas Exchange* related to aspiration of meconium and amniotic fluid during birth
- *Altered Nutrition: Less than Body Requirements* related to respiratory distress and increased energy requirements
- *Ineffective Family Coping: Compromised* related to life-threatening illness in term newborn

Nursing Plan and Implementation

Hospital-Based Nursing Care

Initial interventions are aimed at early identification of meconium aspiration. When significant aspiration occurs, therapy is supportive with the primary goals of maintaining appropriate gas exchange and minimizing complications. Nursing interventions after resuscitation should include maintaining adequate oxygenation and ventilation, regulating temperature, performing glucose testing by glucometer to check for hypoglycemia, observing IV fluid administration, calculating necessary fluids (which may be restricted in the first 48 to 72 hours because of cerebral edema), providing caloric requirements with TPN, and monitoring IV antibiotic therapy.

Evaluation

Expected outcomes of nursing care include the following:

- The newborn at risk for MAS is promptly identified and early intervention is initiated.
- The newborn is free of respiratory distress and metabolic alterations.
- The parents verbalize their concerns about their baby's health problem and survival and understand the rationale behind the management of their newborn.

Care of the Newborn with Cold Stress

Cold stress is excessive heat loss resulting in the use of compensatory mechanisms (such as increased respirations and nonshivering thermogenesis/use of brown fat stores) to maintain core body temperature. Heat loss that results in cold stress occurs in the newborn through the mechanisms of evaporation, convection, conduction, and radiation. (See Chapter 24 ∞ for types of thermoregulation.)

Heat loss at birth that leads to cold stress can play a significant role in the severity of RDS and the ultimate outcome for the infant. Both preterm and SGA newborns are at risk for cold stress because they have decreased adipose tissue, brown fat stores, and glycogen available for metabolism.

As discussed in Chapter 24 ∞, the newborn infant's major source of heat production in nonshivering thermogenesis (NST) is brown fat metabolism. The ability of an infant to respond to cold stress by NST is impaired in the presence of several conditions:

- Hypoxemia (PO_2 less than 50 torr)
- Intracranial hemorrhage or any CNS abnormality
- Hypoglycemia (blood glucose level less than 40 mg/dL)

When these conditions occur, the infant's temperature should be monitored more closely and the neutral thermal environment conscientiously maintained. The nurse must recognize these conditions and treat them as soon as possible. The metabolic consequences of cold stress can be devastating and potentially fatal to an infant. Oxygen requirements rise; even before noting a change in temperature, glucose use increases, acids are released into the bloodstream, and surfactant production decreases (Blackburn, 2007). The effects are graphically depicted in Figure 29–9 ■.

Nursing Care Management

The amount of heat an infant loses depends to a large extent on the actions of the nurse or caregiver. During the transfer of an NICU newborn from one bed to another, a transient (although not significant) decrease in temperature may be noted for up to 1 hour. Prevention of heat loss is especially critical in the very-low-birth-weight (VLBW) infant. Placing the VLBW newborn in a polyethylene wrapping immediately following birth can decrease the postnatal fall in temperature that normally occurs. Using head coverings made of insulated fabrics, wool, polyolefin, or lined with Gamgee can significantly decrease heat loss after childbirth (Blackburn, 2007). Convective, radiant, and evaporative heat loss can all be

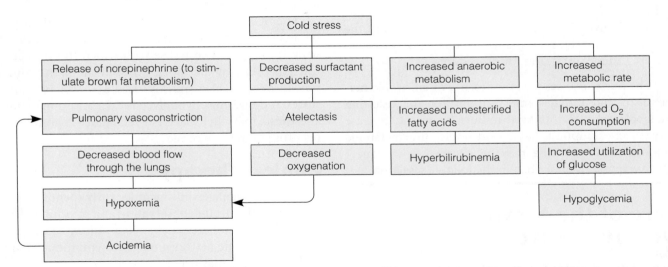

FIGURE 29–9 Cold stress chain of events. The hypothermic, or cold-stressed, newborn attempts to compensate by conserving heat and increasing heat production. These physiologic compensatory mechanisms initiate a series of metabolic events that result in hypoxemia and altered surfactant production, metabolic acidosis, hypoglycemia, and hyperbilirubinemia.

reduced (Blackburn, 2007). Swaddling and nesting maintain flexion, which reduces exposed surface area and thus convective and radiant losses.

The nurse observes all newborns for signs of cold stress, including increased movement and respirations, decreased skin temperature and peripheral perfusion, development of hypoglycemia, and possibly development of metabolic acidosis.

Vasoconstriction is the initial response to cold stress; because it initially decreases skin temperature, the nurse should monitor and assess skin temperature instead of rectal temperature. A decrease in rectal temperature means that the infant has long-standing cold stress. By monitoring skin temperature, a possible decrease will become apparent before the infant's core temperature is affected.

If a decrease in skin temperature is noted, the nurse determines whether hypoglycemia is present. Hypoglycemia is a result of the metabolic effects of cold stress and is suggested by glucometer values below 40 mg/dL, tremors, irritability or lethargy, apnea, or seizure activity.

If hypothermia occurs, the following nursing interventions should be initiated (Blackburn, 2007; Cloherty et al., 2008):

- Maintain a neutral thermal environment (NTE); adjust based on the gestational age and postnatal age.
- Warm the newborn slowly because rapid temperature elevation may cause hypotension and apnea.
- Increase the air temperature in hourly increments of 1°C (33.8°F) until the infant's temperature is stable.
- Monitor skin temperature every 15 to 30 minutes to determine if the newborn's temperature is increasing.
- Remove plastic wrap, caps, and heat shields while rewarming the infant so that cool air as well as warm air is not trapped.
- Warm IV fluids before infusion.
- Initiate efforts to block heat loss by evaporation, radiation, convection, and conduction and maintain the newborn in NTE such as a heated incubator for transport and radiant heater for procedures.

The nurse assesses for the presence of anaerobic metabolism and initiates interventions for the resulting metabolic acidosis. Attempts to burn brown fat increase oxygen consumption, lactic acid levels, and metabolic acidosis. Hypoglycemia may be reversed by adequate glucose intake, as described in the following section.

Care of the Newborn with Hypoglycemia

An operational threshold for intervention in newborn **hypoglycemia** is a plasma glucose concentration of less than 40 mg/dL at any time in any newborn. It requires follow-up

glucose measurement to document normal values (Cloherty et al., 2008). Within the first hours of life, normal asymptomatic newborns may have a transient glucose level in the 30s (mg/dL) that will increase either spontaneously or with feedings. Plasma glucose values less than 20 to 25 mg/dL should be treated with parenteral glucose $D_{10}W$, regardless of the age or gestation to raise plasma glucose to greater than 45 mg/dL. There is no absolute threshold which can be applied to all babies. Glucose concentrations must be looked at in conjunction with clinical manifestations. Follow-up studies have indicated developmental delay and seizures in term infants with symptomatic hypoglycemia; and studies in high risk infants suggest adverse neurodevelopmental outcomes in infants with a history of symptomatic hypoglycemia (McGowan & Perlman, 2006).

Hypoglycemia is the most common metabolic disorder occurring in IDMs, SGA infants, the smaller of twins, infants born to mothers with preeclampsia, male infants, and preterm AGA infants. The pathophysiology of hypoglycemia differs for each classification.

AGA preterm infants have not been in utero a sufficient time to store glycogen and fat. As a result, they have decreased ability to carry out gluconeogenesis. This situation is further aggravated by increased use of glucose by the tissues (especially the brain and heart) during stress and illness (chilling, asphyxia, sepsis, RDS).

Infants of White's classes A–C or type 1 diabetic mothers have increased stores of glycogen and fat (see Chapter 28 ∞). Circulating insulin and insulin responsiveness are also higher when compared with other newborns. Because the high glucose loads present in utero stop at birth, the newborn experiences rapid and profound hypoglycemia (Blackburn, 2007). Infants with recurrent episodes of hypoglycemia resulting from congenital hyperinsulinism showed that 50% have long-term neurological deficits (Nash & Smith, 2008).

The SGA infant has used up glycogen and fat stores because of intrauterine malnutrition and has a blunted hepatic enzymatic response with which to produce and use glucose. Any newborn stressed at birth from asphyxia or cold also quickly uses up available glucose stores and becomes hypoglycemic. In addition, epidural anesthesia may alter maternal-fetal glucose homeostasis, resulting in hypoglycemia.

Clinical Therapy

The goal of management includes early identification of hypoglycemia through observation and screening of newborns at risk (Cloherty et al., 2008; Mileic, 2008; Nash & Smith, 2008). The newborn may be asymptomatic, or any of the following may occur:

- Lethargy, apathy, and limpness
- Poor feeding, poor sucking, vomiting

- Pallor, cyanosis
- Hypothermia in LBW infants
- Apnea, irregular respirations, respiratory distress
- Hypotonia, possible loss of swallowing reflex
- Tremors, jerkiness, jitteriness, seizure activity
- High-pitched or weak cry
- Exaggerated Moro reflex

Aggressive treatment is recommended after a single low blood glucose value if the infant shows any of these symptoms. In at-risk infants, routine screening should be done frequently during the first 4 hours of life and then at 4-hour intervals until the risk period has passed.

Differential diagnosis of a newborn with nonspecific hypoglycemic symptoms includes determining if the newborn has any of the following:

- Sepsis
- CNS disease
- Metabolic aberrations (hypocalcemia, hyponatremia or hypernatremia, hypomagnesium)
- Polycythemia
- Congenital heart disease
- Drug withdrawal
- Temperature instability

Hypoglycemia may also be defined as a *glucose oxidase reagent strip with reflectance meter* below 40 mg/dL, but only when corroborated with laboratory plasma glucose testing (see Clinical Skill: Performing a Heel Stick on a Newborn). Common bedside methods use whole blood, an enzymatic reagent strip, and a reflectance meter or color chart. Bedside glucose oxidase strip tests may be used for screening for hypoglycemia, but laboratory determinations *must confirm* the results before a diagnosis of hypoglycemia can be made. Glucose reagent strips should not be used by themselves to screen for and diagnose hypoglycemia, because their results depend on the baby's hematocrit (they react to the glucose in the plasma, not the red blood cells) and there is a wide variance (5 to 15 mg/dL) when compared with laboratory plasma determinations.

Blood glucose sampling techniques can significantly affect the accuracy of the blood glucose value. It is important to note that whole blood glucose concentrations are 10% to 15% lower than plasma glucose concentrations (Cloherty et al., 2008). The higher the hematocrit, the greater the difference between whole blood and plasma values. Also, venous blood glucose concentrations are approximately 15% to 19% lower than arterial blood glucose concentrations because the tissues extract some glucose before the blood enters the venous system. Newer point of care techniques, such as using a glucose oxidase analyzer or an optical bedside glucose analyzer, are more reliable

---

EVIDENCE IN ACTION

There is not significant evidence to support the use of heel warmers preceding a capillary heelstick of an infant and no evidence of an increased yield of blood with the use of heel warmers.
(National Association of Neonatal Nurses' Guidelines)
(Folk, 2007)

---

for bedside screening but must also be validated with laboratory chemical analysis.

HINTS FOR PRACTICE

Blood samples for the laboratory should be placed on ice and analyzed within 30 minutes of drawing to prevent the RBCs from continuing to metabolize glucose and giving a falsely low reading.

Adequate caloric intake is important. Early formula-feeding or breastfeeding is one of the major preventive approaches. If early feeding or IV glucose is started to meet the recommended fluid and caloric needs, the blood glucose concentration is likely to remain above the hypoglycemic level. During the first hours after birth, asymptomatic newborns may also be given oral glucose contained in formula or breast milk (glucose water should not be used because it causes a rapid increase in glucose followed by an abrupt decrease), and then another plasma glucose measurement is obtained within 30 to 60 minutes after feeding.

IV infusions of a dextrose solution D_5W to $D_{10}W$ (5% to 10%) begun immediately after birth should prevent hypoglycemia. Plasma glucose levels are obtained when the parenteral infusion is started. However, in the very small AGA infant, infusions of 10% dextrose solution may cause hyperglycemia to develop, requiring an alteration in the glucose concentration. Infants require 6 to 8 mg/kg/min of glucose to maintain normal glucose concentrations. Therefore, an IV glucose solution should be calculated based on the infant's body weight and fluid requirements and correlated with blood glucose tests to determine adequacy of the infusion treatment.

A rapid infusion of greater than 25% dextrose or the use of glucose water in place of formula is contraindicated because it may lead to profound rebound hypoglycemia following an initial brief increase. In more severe cases of hypoglycemia, corticosteroids may be administered. It is thought that steroids enhance gluconeogenesis from non-carbohydrate protein sources and reduce peripheral glucose use (Cloherty et al., 2008).

Nursing Care Management

Nursing Assessment and Diagnosis

The objectives of nursing assessment are to identify newborns at risk and to screen symptomatic infants. For newborns diagnosed with hypoglycemia, assessment is ongoing and includes careful monitoring of glucose values. Glucose strips, urine dipstick, and urine volume tests

Clinical Skill Performing a Heel Stick on a Newborn

NURSING ACTION	RATIONALE

Preparation

- Explain to parents what will be done.
- Select a clear, previously unpunctured site.
- The infant's lateral heel is the site of choice because it precludes damaging the posterior tibial nerve and artery, plantar artery, and the important longitudinally oriented fat pad of the heel, which in later years could impede walking (Figure 29–10 ■). This is especially important for infants undergoing multiple heel stick procedures. Toes are acceptable sites if necessary.

Equipment and Supplies

- Microlancet (do not use a needle)
- Alcohol swabs
- 2 × 2 sterile gauze squares
- Small bandage
- Transfer pipette or capillary tubes
- Glucose reagent strips and reflectance meters
- Gloves

Procedure

1. Apply gloves.
2. May try warm wet wrap or specially designed chemical heat pad to warm the infant's heel for 5 to 10 seconds to facilitate blood flow.

Performing the Heel Stick

1. Grasp the infant's lower leg and foot so as to impede venous return slightly. This will facilitate extraction of the blood sample (Figure 29–11 ■).

The selection of a previously unpunctured site minimizes the risk of infection and excessive scar formation.

A needle may nick the periosteum.

Gloves are used to implement standard precautions and prevent nosocomial infections.

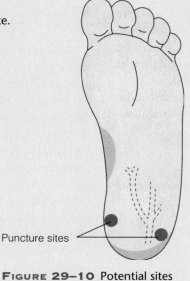

Puncture sites

FIGURE 29–10 Potential sites for heel sticks. Avoid shaded areas to prevent injury to arteries and nerves in the foot.

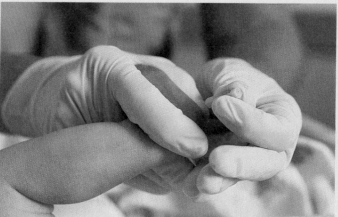

FIGURE 29–11 Heel stick.

Clinical Skill Performing a Heel Stick on a Newborn *(Continued)*

NURSING ACTION	RATIONALE
2. Clean the site by rubbing vigorously with 70% isopropyl alcohol swab.	*Friction produces local heat, which aids vasodilation.*
3. Blot the site dry completely with a dry gauze square before lancing.	*Alcohol is irritating to injured tissue and it may also produce hemolysis.*
4. With a quick, piercing motion, puncture the lateral heel with a microlancet. Be careful not to puncture too deeply. Optimal penetration is 4 mm.	
5. Wipe the first drop of blood away with the gauze.	*The first drop may be contaminated by skin contact and the blood cells may have been traumatized during the stick. Blood glucose may be lowered by residual alcohol.*

Collecting the Blood Sample

1. Use transfer pipette to place a drop of blood on the glucose reflectance meter.
2. Use the capillary tube for hematocrit testing.

Prevent Excessive Bleeding

1. Apply a folded gauze square to the puncture site and secure it firmly with a bandage.
2. Check the puncture site frequently for the first hour after sampling.

Documentation

Record the findings and interventions taken on the infant's chart. Document the confirmatory laboratory-determined glucose level if hypoglycemia is suspected.

(monitor only if above 1 to 3 mL/kg/hr) may be evaluated frequently for osmotic diuresis and glycosuria.

Nursing diagnoses that may apply to the newborn with hypoglycemia include the following:

- *Altered Nutrition: Less than Body Requirements* related to increased glucose use secondary to physiologic stress
- *Ineffective Breathing Pattern* related to tachypnea and apnea
- *Acute Pain* related to frequent heel sticks secondary to glucose monitoring

Nursing Plan and Implementation

Infants in at-risk groups should be monitored within 30 to 60 minutes after birth and before feedings or whenever there are abnormal clinical manifestations (Nash & Smith, 2008). The IDM should be monitored within 30 minutes of birth. Once an at-risk infant's blood sugar level is stable, glucose testing every 2 to 4 hours (or per agency protocol), or before feedings, adequately monitors glucose levels. See Clinical Skill: Performing a Heel Stick on a Newborn.

Calculating glucose requirements and maintaining IV glucose levels are necessary for any symptomatic infant with low serum glucose levels. The method of feeding greatly influences glucose and energy requirements; thus careful attention to glucose monitoring is again required during the transition from IV to oral feedings. Titration of IV glucose may be required until the infant is able to take adequate amounts of formula or breast milk to maintain a normal blood sugar level. Titrate by decreasing the concentration of parenteral glucose gradually to 5% (D_5W), then reducing the rate of infusion (mg/kg/min) and slowly discontinuing it over 4 to 6 hours. Enteral feedings are increased to maintain an adequate glucose and caloric intake.

The therapeutic nursing measure of nonnutritive sucking during gavage feedings has been reported to increase the baby's daily weight gain and lead to earlier formula-feeding or breastfeeding and discharge. Nonnutritive sucking may also lower activity levels, which allows newborns to conserve their energy stores. Hypothermia and activity can increase energy requirements; crying alone can double the baby's metabolic rate.

Evaluation

Expected outcomes of nursing care include the following:

- The newborn at risk for hypoglycemia is identified, and prompt intervention is started.
- The newborn's glucose level is stabilized, and recovery is proceeding without sequelae.

COMPLEMENTARY AND ALTERNATIVE THERAPIES

Pain Relief in the NICU

The newborn relies on the nurse's observational, assessment, and interventional skills for anticipation and prevention of pain if possible and then prompt, safe, and effective pain relief. It is vital that the nurse assist infants to cope with and recover from necessary painful clinical procedures (Saniski, 2005). A variety of nonpharmacologic pain-prevention and relief techniques have been shown to be effective in reducing pain from minor procedures in newborns.

Pain can be managed effectively by limiting or avoiding noxious stimuli and by providing analgesia. Any unnecessary stimuli (i.e., noise, visual, tactile, and vestibular) of the newborn should be avoided, if possible (AAP & ACOG, 2007). Developmental care, which includes limiting environmental stimuli, lateral positioning, the use of supportive bedding, and attention to behavioral cues, assists the newborn to cope with painful procedures (AAP & CPS, 2006).

Containment with swaddling or facilitated tucking (holding the arms and legs in a flexed position) is effective in reducing excessive immature motor responses. Swaddling also may provide comfort through other senses, such as thermal, tactile, and proprioceptive senses. Breastfeeding and skin-to-skin contact with the mother during the painful procedure may help to relieve pain. Nonnutritive sucking (NNS) refers to the provision of a pacifier into the infant's mouth to promote sucking without the provision of breast milk or for-mula for nutrition. NNS is thought to produce analgesia through stimulation of orotactile and mechanoreceptors when the pacifier is placed into the infant's mouth. Allowing nonnutritive sucking with a pacifier aids in the reduction of procedural pain and stress. Unfortunately a rebound in distress occurs when the NNS pacifier is removed from the infant's mouth (Walden, 2007).

A wide range of oral sucrose doses have been used for procedural pain relief (heel sticks, venipuncture, IM injections); but no optimal dose has been established (AAP & CPS, 2006). The sweetness of the sucrose, a disaccharide, elevates the pain threshold through endogenous opioid release in the CNS and produces a calming effect (AAP & CPS, 2006). A range of 0.05 to 0.5 mL of 24% sucrose is administered on the anterior part of the tongue via a syringe or nipple approximately 2 minutes before the procedure (Walden & Jorgensen, 2004). Some authors have suggested that multiple doses, such as giving a dose 2 minutes before and 1 to 2 minutes after a procedure, is more effective. It is important to be careful with repeated doses of sucrose, as the concern for hyperglycemia may arise. Also, repeated use of sucrose analgesia in preterm infants may affect their neurologic development and behavioral outcomes. Until further research is done, repeated doses of sucrose are not recommended (AAP & CPS, 2006). Because oral sucrose reduces but does not eliminate pain, it should be used with other non-pharmacologic measures to enhance effectiveness.

Care of the Newborn with Jaundice

The most common abnormal physical finding in newborns is jaundice *(icterus neonatorum)*. Some degree of jaundice, resulting from elevated unconjugated bilirubinemia, occurs in approximately 50% of term infants and 80% of preterm infants (Madan, MacMahon, & Stevenson, 2005). **Jaundice** is a yellowish coloration of the skin and sclera of the eyes that develops from deposit of the yellow pigment bilirubin in lipid/fat containing tissues as described in Chapter 24 ∞. Fetal unconjugated (indirect) bilirubin is normally cleared by the placenta in utero, so total bilirubin at birth is usually less than 3 mg/dL unless an abnormal hemolytic process has been present. Postnatally, the infant must conjugate bilirubin (convert a lipid-soluble pigment into a water-soluble pigment) in the liver.

The rate and amount of conjugation of bilirubin depend on the rate of hemolysis, the bilirubin load, the maturity of the liver, and the presence of albumin-binding sites. (See Chapter 24 ∞ for discussion of conjugation of bilirubin.) The liver of a normal, healthy term infant is usually mature enough and producing enough glucuronyl transferase that the total serum bilirubin does not reach a pathologic level.

Physiologic Jaundice

Physiologic or *neonatal jaundice* is a normal process that occurs during transition from intrauterine to extrauterine life and appears after 24 hours of life. It is caused by the newborn's shortened red blood cell lifespan (90 days as compared with 120 days in the adult), slower uptake by the liver, lack of intestinal bacteria, and/or poorly established hydration from initial breastfeeding (Gennaro, Schwoebel, Hall, & Bhutani, 2006).

Lab tests reveal a predominance of unconjugated bilirubin. The average level of unconjugated bilirubin in cord blood is approximately 2 mg/dL at birth. This level rises to an average level of 5 to 6 mg/dL between the third and fifth days of life. The jaundice is usually not visible after 14 days. The pattern of physiologic jaundice differs between breastfed and formula-fed newborns (for further discussion of physiologic jaundice, see Chapter 24 ∞). Physiologic jaundice remains a common problem for the term newborn and may require treatment with phototherapy.

Pathophysiology of Hyperbilirubinemia

Serum albumin-binding sites are usually sufficient to conjugate enough bilirubin to meet the normal demands of the newborn. However, certain conditions tend to decrease the sites available. Fetal or neonatal asphyxia and neonatal drugs such as indomethacin decrease the binding affinity of bilirubin to albumin, because acidosis impairs the capacity of albumin to hold bilirubin. Hypothermia and hypoglycemia release free fatty acids that dislocate bilirubin from albumin. Maternal medications such as sulfa drugs and salicylates compete with bilirubin for these sites. Finally, premature infants have less albumin available for binding with bilirubin. Neurotoxicity is possible because unconjugated bilirubin has a high affinity for extravascular tissue, such as fatty tissue (subcutaneous tissue) and cerebral tissue.

Bilirubin not bound to albumin can cross the blood-brain barrier, damage cells of the CNS, and produce kernicterus or acute **bilirubin encephalopathy** (ABE) (Gennaro et al., 2006; Juretschke, 2005). **Kernicterus** (meaning "yellow nucleus") refers to the deposition of indirect or unconjugated bilirubin in the basal ganglia of the brain and to the permanent neurologic sequelae of untreated **hyperbilirubinemia** (elevation of bilirubin level) (Cloherty et al., 2008).

The classic acute bilirubin encephalopathy of kernicterus most commonly found with Rh and ABO blood group incompatibility is less common today because of aggressive treatment with phototherapy and exchange transfusions. But cases of kernicterus are reappearing as a result of early discharge and the increased incidence of dehydration (as a result of discharge before the mother's milk is established). Current therapy can reduce the incidence of kernicterus encephalopathy but cannot distinguish all infants who are at risk.

Causes of Hyperbilirubinemia

A primary cause of hyperbilirubinemia is **hemolytic disease of the newborn**. All pregnant women who are Rh negative or who have blood type O (possible ABO blood incompatibility) should be asked about outcomes of any previous pregnancies and history of blood transfusion. Prenatal amniocentesis with spectrophotographic examination may be indicated in some cases. Cord blood from newborns is evaluated for bilirubin level, which normally does not exceed 5 mg/dL. Newborns of Rh-negative and O blood type mothers are carefully assessed for appearance of jaundice and levels of serum bilirubin.

Alloimmune hemolytic disease, also known as **erythroblastosis fetalis**, occurs when an Rh-negative mother is pregnant with an Rh-positive fetus and maternal antibodies cross the placenta. Maternal antibodies enter the fetal circulation, then attach to and destroy the fetal RBCs. The fetal system responds by increasing RBC production. Jaundice, anemia, and compensatory erythropoiesis result. A marked increase in immature RBCs (erythroblasts) also occurs, hence the designation erythroblastosis fetalis. Because of the widespread use of Rh immune globulin (RhoGAM), the incidence of erythroblastosis fetalis has dropped dramatically.

Hydrops fetalis, the most severe form of erythroblastosis fetalis, occurs when maternal antibodies attach to the Rh site on the fetal RBCs, making them susceptible to destruction; severe anemia and multiorgan system failure result. Cardiomegaly with severe cardiac decompensation and hepatosplenomegaly occurs. Severe generalized massive edema (anasarca) and generalized fluid effusion into the pleural cavity (hydrothorax), pericardial sac, and peritoneal cavity (ascites) develops. Jaundice is not present until the newborn period because the bilirubin pigments are excreted through the placenta into the maternal circulation. The hydropic hemolytic disease process is also characterized by hyperplasia of the pancreatic islets, which predisposes the infant to neonatal hypoglycemia similar to that of IDMs. These infants have increased bleeding tendencies because of associated thrombocytopenia and hypoxic damage to the capillaries. Hydrops is a frequent cause of intrauterine death among infants with Rh disease.

ABO incompatibility (the mother is blood type O and the baby is blood type A or B) may result in jaundice, although it rarely results in hemolytic disease severe enough to be clinically diagnosed and treated. Hepatosplenomegaly may be found occasionally in newborns with ABO incompatibility, but hydrops fetalis and stillbirth are rare.

Certain prenatal and perinatal factors predispose the newborn to hyperbilirubinemia. During pregnancy, maternal conditions that predispose the fetus to neonatal hyperbilirubinemia include hereditary spherocytosis, diabetes, intrauterine infections, and gram-negative bacilli infections that stimulate production of maternal alloimmune antibodies, drug ingestion (such as sulfas, salicylates, novobiocin, diazepam), and oxytocin administration. Early prenatal identification of the fetus at risk for Rh or ABO incompatibility allows prompt treatment.

In addition to Rh or ABO incompatibility, other newborn conditions can predispose to hyperbilirubinemia: polycythemia (central hematocrit 65% or more), pyloric stenosis, obstruction or atresia of the biliary duct or of the lower bowel, low-grade urinary tract infection, sepsis, hypothyroidism, enclosed hemorrhage (cephalohematoma, large bruises), asphyxia neonatorum, hypothermia, acidemia, and hypoglycemia. Neonatal hepatitis, atresia of the bile ducts, and GI atresia all can alter bilirubin metabolism and excretion. Table 29–3 presents risk factors for development of severe hyperbilirubinemia in their approximate order of importance.

The prognosis for a newborn with hyperbilirubinemia depends on the extent of the hemolytic process and the underlying cause. Severe hemolytic disease results in fetal and early neonatal death from the effects of severe

| **TABLE 29–3** | Risk Factors for Development of Severe Hyperbilirubinemia in Infants of 35 or More Weeks' Gestation (in Approximate Order of Importance) |

Major Risk Factors

- Predischarge TSB or TcB level in the high-risk zone
- Jaundice observed in the first 24 h
- Blood group incompatibility with positive direct antiglobulin test, other known hemolytic disease (e.g., G6PD deficiency), elevated ETCO$_c$
- Gestational age 35 to 36 wk
- Previous sibling received phototherapy
- Cephalohematoma or significant bruising
- Exclusive breastfeeding, particularly if nursing is not going well and weight loss is excessive
- East Asian race*

Minor Risk Factors

- Predischarge TSB or TcB level in the high intermediate-risk zone
- Gestational age 37 to 38 weeks
- Jaundice observed before discharge
- Previous sibling with jaundice
- Macrosomic infant of a diabetic mother
- Maternal age greater than or equal to 25 years
- Male gender

Decreased Risk (these factors are associated with decreased risk of significant jaundice, listed in order of decreasing importance)

- TSB or TcB level in the low-risk zone
- Gestational age greater than or equal to 41 weeks
- Exclusive formula-feeding
- Black race*
- Discharge from hospital after 72 hours

* Race as defined by mother's description.

Source: From American Academy of Pediatrics Subcommittee on Hyperbilirubinemia. (2004). Management of hyperbilirubinemia in the newborn infant 35 or more weeks of gestation. *Pediatrics, 114*(1), 297–316 (Table 2, p. 301).

anemia—cardiac decompensation, edema, ascites, and hydrothorax. Hyperbilirubinemia that is not aggressively treated may lead to kernicterus. The resultant neurologic damage is responsible for death, cerebral palsy, possible mental retardation, or hearing loss or, to a lesser degree, perceptual impairment, delayed speech development, hyperactivity, muscle incoordination, or learning difficulties.

Clinical Therapy

Laboratory and Diagnostic Assessments

The best treatment for hemolytic disease is prevention by early recognition of prenatal risk factors such as Rh and ABO incompatibility (see Chapter 16 ∞ for discussion of in utero management of this condition); and then

neonatal conditions. Neonatal hyperbilirubinemia can be considered pathologic and requires further investigation if any of the following criteria are met (Bhutani, Johnson, & Keren, 2004; Gennaro et al., 2006):

1. Clinically evident jaundice appearing before 24 hours of life or if jaundice seems excessive for the newborn's age in hours
2. Serum bilirubin concentration rising by more than 0.2 mg/dL per hour
3. Total serum bilirubin concentration exceeding the 95th percentile on the nomogram
4. Conjugated bilirubin concentrations greater than 2 mg/dL or more than 20% of the total serum bilirubin concentration
5. Clinical jaundice persisting for more than 2 weeks in a term newborn

Initial diagnostic procedures are aimed at differentiating jaundice resulting from increased bilirubin production, impaired conjugation or excretion, increased intestinal reabsorption, or a combination of these factors.

Transcutaneous bilirubin (TcB) measurements are a non-invasive method of assessing bilirubin levels and may be used for pre-discharge risk assessment. A TcB can be performed quickly and painlessly, and repeated measures are easily obtained. TcB can quantify the amount of bilirubin pigment in the infant's skin. Nurses need to measure bilirubin levels to confirm the presence, absence, or suspicion of jaundice. However, it is important to remember that total serum bilirubin levels remain the standard of care for confirmation or diagnosis of hyperbilirubinemia (Gennaro et al., 2006).

HINTS FOR PRACTICE

Because of exposure to sunlight, sternal area TcB measurements may be more accurate than those taken on the forehead. The sternum, in a dressed infant, is less likely to be affected by the influence of ambient light (such as sunlight) on the skin.

Because of the shorter lifespan of red blood cells in the newborn, a significant bilirubin load is produced. When bilirubin breaks down, carbon monoxide (CO) is released. This production of carbon monoxide is being investigated as a marker in the study of bilirubin production. Measuring end-tidal CO (ETCO) has been shown to provide results similar to laboratory bilirubin; however, devices to measure CO are not widely available (Gennaro et al., 2006; Madan et al., 2005).

Essential laboratory evaluations are Coombs' test, serum bilirubin levels (direct and total), hemoglobin, reticulocyte percentage, white cell count, and positive smear for cellular morphology.

The Coombs' test is performed to determine whether jaundice is because of Rh or ABO incompatibility. The indirect Coombs' test measures the amount of Rh-positive antibodies in the mother's blood. Rh-positive red blood cells are added to the maternal blood sample. If the mother's serum contains antibodies, the Rh-positive red blood cells will agglutinate (clump) when rabbit immune antiglobulin is added, which is a positive test result.

The direct Coombs' test reveals the presence of antibody-coated (sensitized) Rh-positive red blood cells in the newborn. Rabbit immune antiglobulin is added to the specimen of neonatal blood cells. If the neonatal red blood cells agglutinate, they have been coated with maternal antibodies, a positive result.

If the hemolytic process is caused by Rh sensitization, laboratory findings reveal the following: (1) an Rh-positive newborn with a positive Coombs' test; (2) increased erythropoiesis with many immature circulating red blood cells (nucleated blastocysts); (3) anemia, in most cases; (4) elevated levels (5 mg/dL or more) of bilirubin in cord blood; and (5) a reduction in albumin-binding capacity. Maternal data may include an elevated anti-Rh titer and spectrophotometric evidence of a fetal hemolytic process.

If the hemolytic process is caused by ABO incompatibility, laboratory findings reveal an increase in reticulocytes. The resulting anemia is usually not significant during the newborn period and is rare later on. The direct Coombs' test may be negative or mildly positive, whereas the indirect Coombs' test may be strongly positive. Infants with a positive direct Coombs' test have increased incidence of jaundice, with bilirubin levels in excess of 10 mg/dL. Increased numbers of spherocytes (spherical, plump, mature erythrocytes) are seen on a peripheral blood smear. Increased numbers of spherocytes are not seen on blood smears from Rh disease infants.

Therapeutic Management

Whatever the cause of hyperbilirubinemia, management of these infants is directed toward alleviating anemia, removing maternal antibodies and sensitized erythrocytes, increasing serum albumin levels, reducing serum bilirubin levels, and minimizing the consequences of hyperbilirubinemia. Early discharge of newborns from birthing centers has significantly influenced the diagnosis and management of neonatal jaundice, increasing the emphasis on outpatient and home care management.

If hemolytic disease is present, it may be treated with phototherapy, exchange transfusion, and drug therapy. When determining the appropriate management of hyperbilirubinemia caused by hemolytic disease, the three relevant variables are the newborn's (1) serum bilirubin level, (2) birth weight, and (3) age in hours. If a newborn has hemolysis with an unconjugated bilirubin level of 14 mg/dL, weighs less than 2500 g (birth weight), and is 24 hours old or less, an exchange transfusion may be the best management. However, if that same newborn is over 24 hours of age, which is past the time during which an increase in bilirubin would occur because of pathologic causes, phototherapy may be the treatment of choice to prevent the possible complication of kernicterus.

Phototherapy

Phototherapy is the exposure of the newborn to high-intensity light. It may be used alone or in conjunction with exchange transfusion to reduce serum bilirubin levels. Exposure of the newborn to high-intensity light (a bank of fluorescent light bulbs or bulbs in the blue-light spectrum) decreases serum bilirubin levels in the skin by facilitating biliary excretion of unconjugated bilirubin. Phototherapy decreases serum bilirubin levels by changing bilirubin from the nonwater-soluble (lipophilic) form to water-soluble by-products that can then be excreted via urine and bile. Photoisomerization occurs when the natural form of bilirubin is exposed to light at a certain wavelength and the bilirubin is converted to a less toxic form. The new isomer, photobilirubin, is created rapidly but is quite unstable. The photobilirubin is bound to albumin, transported to the liver, and incorporated into bile. If it is not quickly eliminated from the bowel, then it can convert back to its original form and return to the bloodstream. In addition, the photodegradation products formed when light oxidizes bilirubin can be excreted in the urine.

Phototherapy is an intervention that is used to prevent hyperbilirubinemia in order to halt bilirubin levels from climbing dangerously high. The decision to start phototherapy is based on two factors: gestational age and age in hours. Phototherapy is the most effective in the first 24 to 48 hours of usage; frequently the light can be discontinued during or immediately after this time frame. Phototherapy does not alter the underlying cause of jaundice, and hemolysis may continue to produce anemia. Many authors have recommended initiating phototherapy "prophylactically" in the first 24 hours of life in high-risk, VLBW, or severely bruised infants. Figure 29–12 ■ shows guidelines for the use of phototherapy.

Phototherapy can be provided by halogen spotlights (although these are not widely used because of the risk of thermal burns), conventional banks of fluorescent tube phototherapy lights, a fiberoptic blanket attached to a halogen light source around the trunk of the newborn, by a fiberoptic mattress placed under the baby, or by a combination of these delivery methods. Bank of fluorescent bilirubin lights utilize light in the blue spectrum. This is the most effective source available but can mask cyanosis and causes dizziness and nausea in the staff. With the fiberoptic

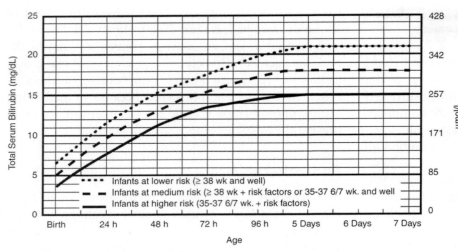

• Use total bilirubin. Do not subtract direct reacting or conjugated bilirubin.
• Risk factors = isoimmune hemolytic disease, G6PD deficiency, asphyxia, significant lethargy, temperature instability, sepsis, acidosis, or albumin < 3.0 g/dL (if measured)
• For well infants 35 to 37 6/7 wk can adjust TSB levels for intervention around the medium risk line. It is an option to intervene at lower TSB levels for infants closer to 35 wks and at higher TSB levels for those closer to 37 6/7 wk.
• It is an option to provide conventional phototherapy in hospital or at home at TSB levels 2 to 3 mg/dL (35 to 50 mmol/L) below those shown but home phototherapy should not be used in any infant with risk factors.

FIGURE 29–12 Guidelines for phototherapy in hospitalized infants of 35 or more weeks' gestation.
Note: These guidelines are based on limited evidence and the levels shown are approximations. The guidelines refer to the use of intensive phototherapy, which should be used when the TSB (total serum bilirubin) exceeds the line indicated for each category. Infants are designated as "higher risk" because of the potential negative effects of the conditions listed on albumin binding of bilirubin, the blood-brain barrier, and the susceptibility of the brain cells to damage by bilirubin.
Source: From American Academy of Pediatrics Subcommittee on Hyperbilirubinemia. (2004). Management of hyperbilirubinemia in the newborn infant 35 or more weeks of gestation. *Pediatrics, 114*(1), 297–316, Fig. 3, p. 304.

blanket, the light stays on at all times, and the newborn is accessible for care, feeding, and diaper changes; greater surface area is exposed and there are no thermoregulation issues. The eyes are not covered. The babies do not get overheated, and fluid and weight loss are not complications of this system. Furthermore, it makes the infant accessible to the parents and is less alarming to parents than standard phototherapy. Many institutions and pediatricians use fiberoptic blankets for home care. A combination of a fiberoptic light source in the mattress under or around the baby and a standard light source above has also been recommended (Gennaro et al., 2006; Thureen et al., 2005). This is termed *intensive phototherapy*. Intensive phototherapy should show a drop in total serum bilirubin (TSB) within 4 to 8 hours. Levels should continue to decline when phototherapy covers a wider surface area. If a drop in bilirubin levels is not reached then an exchange transfusion should be considered. Most phototherapy units provide the desired level of irradiance with the infant 45 to 50 cm below the lamps. The nurse uses a photometer to measure and maintain desired irradiance levels. The nurse keeps track of the number of hours each lamp is used so that each can be replaced before its effectiveness is lost.

Exchange Transfusion

Exchange transfusion is the withdrawal and replacement of the newborn's blood with donor blood. It is used to treat anemia with red blood cells that are susceptible to maternal antibodies, remove sensitized red blood cells that would soon be lysed, remove serum bilirubin, and provide bilirubin-free albumin and increase the binding sites for bilirubin. Concerns about exchange transfusion are related to the use of blood products and associated potential for HIV infection and hepatitis. If the TSB is at or approaching the exchange level, send blood for immediate type and crossmatch. Blood for exchange transfusion is modified whole blood (red cells and plasma) crossmatched against the mother and compatible with the infant.

Nursing Care Management

Nursing Assessment and Diagnosis

Assessment is aimed at identifying prenatal and perinatal factors that predispose the newborn to the development of jaundice and at recognizing the jaundice as soon as it is apparent. Clinically, ABO incompatibility presents as jaundice and occasionally as hepatosplenomegaly. Fetal hydrops or erythroblastosis is rare (see Chapter 16 ∞). Hemolytic disease of the newborn is suspected if the placenta is enlarged; if the newborn is edematous, with pleural and pericardial effusion plus ascites; if pallor or jaundice is noted during the first 24 to 36 hours; if hemolytic anemia is diagnosed; or if the spleen and liver are enlarged. The nurse carefully notes changes in behavior and observes for evidence of bleeding. If laboratory tests indicate elevated bilirubin levels, the nurse checks the newborn for jaundice about every 2 hours and records observations.

To check for jaundice in lighter skinned babies, the nurse blanches the skin over a bony prominence (forehead, nose, sternum) by pressing firmly with the thumb. After pressure is released, if jaundice is present, the area

Clinical Skill Infant Receiving Phototherapy

NURSING ACTION	RATIONALE

Preparation

- Explain the purpose of phototherapy, the procedure itself (including the need to use eye patches), and possible side effects such as dehydration and skin breakdown from more frequent stooling.

- Note evidence of jaundice in skin, sclera, and mucous membranes (in infants with darkly pigmented skin). Be sure that recent serum bilirubin levels are available.

The decision to use phototherapy is based on a careful assessment of the newborn's condition over a period of time. The most recent results before starting therapy serve as a baseline to evaluate the effectiveness of therapy.

Equipment and Supplies

- Bank of phototherapy lights
- Eye patches
- Small scale to weigh diapers

Procedure

1. Obtain vital signs including axillary temperature.

   Provides baseline data.

2. Remove all of the infant's clothing except the diaper.

   Exposure of the newborn to high-intensity light (a bank of fluorescent light bulbs or bulbs in the blue-white spectrum) decreases serum bilirubin levels in the skin by aiding biliary excretion of unconjugated bilirubin. Because the tissue absorbs the light, best results are obtained when there is maximum skin surface exposure.

3. Apply eye coverings (eye patches or a bili mask) to the infant according to agency policy (see Figure 29–13 ■).

   Eye coverings are used because it is not known if phototherapy injures delicate eye structures, particularly the retina.

4. Place the infant in an open crib or incubator (more commonly used in preterm infants and infants who are sicker) about 45 to 50 cm below the bank of phototherapy lights.

   Reposition every 2 hours.

   The incubator helps the infant maintain his or her temperature while undressed.

   Repositioning exposes different areas of skin to the lights, prevents the development of pressure areas on the skin, and varies the stimulation the infant receives.

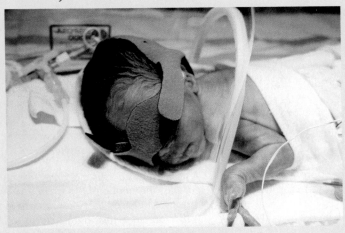

Figure 29–13 Infant receiving phototherapy. The phototherapy light is positioned over the incubator. Bilateral eye patches are always used during photo light therapy to protect the baby's eyes.
Source: Courtesy of Lisa Smith-Pedersen, RNC, MSN, NNP.

(Continued on next page)

Clinical Skill Infant Receiving Phototherapy (Continued)

NURSING ACTION	RATIONALE
5. Monitor vital signs every 4 hours with axillary temperatures.	*Temperature assessment is indicated to detect hypothermia or hyperthermia. Deviation in pulse and respirations may indicate developing complications.*
6. Cluster care activities.	*Care activities are clustered to help ensure that the newborn has maximum time under the lights.*
7. Discontinue phototherapy and remove eye patches at least every 2 to 3 hours when feeding the infant and when the parents visit.	*Eye patches are removed to assess for signs of complications such as excessive pressure, discharge, or conjunctivitis. Patches are also removed to provide some social stimulation and to promote parental attachment.*
8. Maintain adequate fluid intake. Evaluate need for IV fluids.	
9. Monitor intake and output carefully. Weigh diapers before discarding. Record quantity and characteristics of each stool.	*Infants undergoing phototherapy treatment have increased water loss through skin and loose stools. Loose stools and increased urine output are a result of bilirubin excretion. This increases their risk of dehydration.*
10. Assess specific gravity with each voiding. Weigh newborn daily.	*Specific gravity provides one measure of urine concentration. Highly concentrated urine is associated with a dehydrated state. Weight loss is also a sign of developing dehydration in the newborn.*
11. Observe the infant for signs of perianal excoriation and institute therapy if it develops.	*Perianal excoriation may develop because of the irritating effect of diarrhea stools.*
12. Ensure that serum bilirubin levels are drawn regularly according to orders or agency policy. Turn the phototherapy lights off while the blood is drawn.	*Serum bilirubin levels provide the most accurate indication of the effectiveness of phototherapy. They are generally drawn every 12 hours, but at least once daily. The phototherapy lights are turned off to ensure accurate serum bilirubin levels.*
13. Examine the newborn's skin regularly for signs of developing pressure areas, bronzing, maculopapular rash, and changes in degree of jaundice.	*Pressure areas may develop if the infant lies in one position for an extended period. A benign, transient bronze discoloration of the skin may occur with phototherapy when the infant has elevated direct serum bilirubin levels or liver disease. A maculopapular rash is another transient side effect of phototherapy that develops occasionally.*
14. Avoid using lotion or ointment on the exposed skin.	*Lotion and ointments on a newborn receiving phototherapy may cause skin burns.*
15. Provide parents with opportunities to hold the newborn and assist in the infant's care. Answer their questions accurately and keep them informed of developments or changes.	*A sick infant is a source of great anxiety for parents. Information helps them deal with their anxiety. Moreover, they have a right to be kept well informed of their baby's status so that they are able to make informed decisions as needed.*

Clinical Skill Infant Receiving Phototherapy (Continued)

NURSING ACTION	RATIONALE
16. May also provide phototherapy using lightweight, fiberoptic blankets ("bili blankets"). The baby is wrapped in the blanket, which is plugged into an outlet (see Figure 29–14 ■).	*With fiberoptic blankets the newborn is readily accessible for care, feedings, and diaper changes. The baby does not get overheated, and fluid and weight loss are not complications of this system. The procedure seems less alarming to parents than standard phototherapy.*

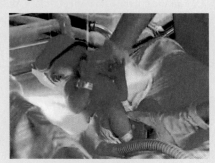

FIGURE 29–14 Newborn on fiberoptic "bili" mattress and under phototherapy lights. A combination of fiberoptic light source mattress and standard phototherapy light source above may also be used.
Note: The color is distorted because of the reflection of the bililight mattress.

appears yellow before normal color returns. The nurse checks oral mucosa and the posterior portion of the hard palate and conjunctival sacs for yellow pigmentation in darker skinned babies. Jaundice progresses in a cephalocaudal direction from the face to the trunk and then to the lower extremities. The overall progression of jaundice should be noted. Assessment in daylight gives the best results, because pink walls and surroundings may mask yellowish tints and yellow light makes differentiation of jaundice difficult. The time at onset of jaundice is recorded and reported. If jaundice appears, careful observation of the increase in depth of color and of the newborn's behavior is mandatory. In addition to visual inspection, reflectance photometers that measure transcutaneous bilirubin (TcB) should be used to screen and monitor neonatal jaundice. Some hospitals have developed a mandatory screening policy for all newborns before discharge using the TcB monitor. If the level comes back elevated then a follow-up TSB will be performed. Another portable screening tool is the analysis for end-tidal carbon monoxide (ETCO). This analysis allows for rapid identification of newborns with significant hemolytic disease who may be at risk for the sequelae of unconjugated hyperbilirubinemia (American Academy of Pediatrics Subcommittee on Hyperbilirubinemia, 2004).

The nurse assesses the newborn's behavior for neurologic signs associated with hyperbilirubinemia, which are rare but may include hypotonia, diminished reflexes, lethargy, or seizures.

CULTURAL PERSPECTIVES

Ethnic Variations and Jaundice

East Asian infants (Japanese, Chinese, and Filipino ethnic groups) have a higher occurrence of hyperbilirubinemia than Caucasian infants. In addition, infants with Asian fathers and Caucasian mothers have a higher incidence of jaundice than if both parents are Caucasian. Other ethnic groups at risk for increased bilirubinemia are Navajo, Eskimo, and Sioux Native American newborns; Greek newborns; Sephardic-Jewish (oriental ancestry) newborns; and some Hispanic newborns.

Nursing diagnoses that may apply to care of a newborn with jaundice include the following:

- *Risk for Fluid Volume Deficit* related to increased insensible water loss and frequent loose stools
- *Potential for Injury* related to use of phototherapy
- *Sensory-Perceptual Alterations* related to neurologic damage secondary to kernicterus
- *Risk for Altered Parenting* related to deficient knowledge of infant care and prolonged separation of infant and parents secondary to illness

Nursing Plan and Implementation

Hospital-Based Nursing Care

Hospital-based care is described in the Nursing Care Plan: For a Newborn with Hyperbilirubinemia, on pages 779–780.

If phototherapy lights are used, the nurse exposes the entire skin surface of the newborn to the light. Minimal covering may be applied over the genitals and buttocks to expose maximum skin surface while still protecting the bedding from soiling. Phototherapy success is measured every 12 hours or with daily serum bilirubin levels (more frequently if there is hemolysis or a higher level before initiation of phototherapy). The nurse must turn lights off while blood is drawn to ensure accurate serum bilirubin levels. Because it is not known if phototherapy injures the delicate eye structures, particularly the retina, the nurse applies eye patches over the newborn's closed eyes during exposure to banks of phototherapy lights (see Figure 29–13 in Clinical Skill: Infant Receiving Phototherapy). Conventional phototherapy is discontinued and the eye patches are removed at least once per shift to assess the eyes for conjunctivitis. Patches are also removed to allow eye contact during feeding (social stimulation) or when parents are visiting (to promote parental attachment).

HINTS FOR PRACTICE

If the area of jaundice around the eyes begins to disappear, it is probable that the eye patches are allowing light to enter and better eye protection is needed.

To parents, the terms *jaundice, hyperbilirubinemia, exchange transfusion,* and *phototherapy* may sound frightening and threatening. Some parents may feel guilty about their baby's condition and think they have caused the problem. Under stress, parents may not be able to understand the physician's first explanations. The nurse must expect that the parents will need explanations repeated and clarified and that they may need help in voicing their questions and fears. Eye and tactile contact with the newborn is encouraged. The nurse can coach parents when they visit with the baby. After the mother's discharge, parents are kept informed of their infant's condition and are encouraged to return to the hospital or telephone at any time so that they can be fully involved in the care of their infant. Parents are advised that after discontinuation of phototherapy, a rebound of 1 to 2 mg/dL can be expected and a follow-up bilirubin test may be done (Cloherty et al., 2008).

While the mother is still hospitalized, phototherapy can also be carried out in the parents' room if the only problem is hyperbilirubinemia. The parents must be willing to keep the baby in the room for 24 hours a day, be able to take emergency action (e.g., for choking) if necessary, and complete instruction checklists. Some institutions require that parents sign a consent form. The nurse instructs the parents but also continues to monitor the infant's temperature, activity, intake and output, and positioning of eye patches (if conventional light banks are used) at regular intervals (Table 29–4).

TABLE 29–4 Instructional Checklist for In-Room Phototherapy

Explain and demonstrate the placement of eye patches and explain that they must be in place when the infant is under the lights.

Explain the clothing to be worn (diaper under lights, dress and wrap when away from the lights).

Explain the importance of taking the infant's temperature regularly.

Explain the importance of adequate fluid intake.

Explain the charting flow sheet (intake, output, eyes covered).

Explain how to position the lights at a proper distance.

Explain the need to keep the infant under phototherapy except during feeding and diaper changes.

Community-Based Nursing Care

Some studies have shown that the early discharge of newborns and their mothers comes with an increase in hospital readmission and elevated risk of pathologic hyperbilirubinemia. Home phototherapy use is recommended only if the bilirubin level is plotted on the nomogram and found to be in the "optional phototherapy" range. Any newborn with a level in the higher range should be hospitalized for continual phototherapy and serum bilirubin levels closely monitored on a regular schedule (Bhutani et al., 2004).

Jaundice and its treatment can be disturbing to parents and may generate feelings of guilt and fear. Reassurance and support are vital especially for the breastfeeding mother, who may question her ability to adequately nourish her newborn. The parent's perception of and/or misconceptions about jaundice can affect parent-infant interactions. The nurse should explain the causes of jaundice and emphasize that it is usually a transient problem and one to which all infants must adapt after birth. It is essential that the impact of cultural beliefs be considered. Some Latina women believe that showing strong maternal emotions during pregnancy and breastfeeding can be detrimental. "Bilis" associated with anger may be blamed by some Latina women for jaundice. Cultural beliefs lead mothers to interpret illness within their cultural framework, especially when left without clear and understood explanations. Maternal reactions can be lessened by careful explanations to the mothers about the diagnosis, prognosis, duration, and management options for jaundice and about the possibility of its recurrence.

If the baby is to receive phototherapy at home, the nurse teaches the parents to record the infant's temperature, weight, fluid intake and output, stools, and feedings and to use the phototherapy equipment. In addition, if phototherapy lights are being used, parents must agree that the baby will be exposed to the lights for long periods of time; that they will hold the baby for only short periods for feeding, comforting, and cleansing of the perineal area; and that the room temperature will be regulated to minimize heat loss. Fiberoptic phototherapy blankets eliminate the

Nursing Care Plan For a Newborn with Hyperbilirubinemia

CLIENT SCENARIO

A nurse is caring for Alex, who is 36 hours old, born to a G1P1 mother at 38 weeks' gestation. Alex's mother is Rh negative. Alex has a unilateral cephalohematoma. During a routine assessment the nurse blanches the skin over the sternum and documents yellow discoloration of the skin. The sclera also appears yellow. During the assessment the newborn is very lethargic. Alex's lab test reveals a serum bilirubin level of 16 mg/dL, hematocrit 55%, and positive direct Coombs' test. Alex is diagnosed with hemolytic disease secondary to Rh incompatibility.

ASSESSMENT

Subjective: N/A

Objective: Skin over sternum blanches yellow, lethargic, total bilirubin level of 16 mg/dL, urine specific gravity of 1.015, positive direct Coombs' test, hematocrit 55%

Nursing Diagnosis #1 Fluid Volume Deficit related to increased insensible water loss and frequent loose stools*

Client Goal The newborn will not experience dehydration.

AEB:
- Stool characteristics within normal limits
- Urine specific gravity within normal limits
- Weight remains stable

NURSING INTERVENTIONS

1. Initiate early feedings.

2. Offer IV fluids between feedings as ordered.

3. Monitor intake and output every 8 hours.

4. Monitor urine specific gravity with each void.

5. Administer fluid intake that is 25% above normal requirements.

6. Monitor daily weights.

7. Assess quantity and characteristics of each stool.

RATIONALES

Rationale: To increase intestinal motility and promote the excretion of unconjugated bilirubin through the clearance of stools. Breastfeeding or formula-feeding can be offered every 2 to 4 hours while under phototherapy to decrease the potential for dehydration.

Rationale: IV fluids offered between feedings will provide extra nourishment and decrease the risk for dehydration.

Rationale: Strict monitoring of fluid intake and output will assess for dehydration. Increased urine output is the result of increased bilirubin excretion, therefore placing the newborn at risk for dehydration. Diapers should be weighed before discarding.

Rationale: Urine specific gravity can be an indicator of dehydration. Dehydration and fluid volume deficit will show an elevation in the urine specific gravity. If urine specific gravity is greater than 1.015 the physician should be notified.

Rationale: Additional fluids will help compensate for the increased water that is lost through the skin and in the stools.

Rationale: Increased fluid excretion in the stools and a decrease in fluid intake may put the newborn at risk for weight loss. Daily weights provide accurate determination of fluid intake and insensible water loss that is caused by phototherapy.

Rationale: Stools are usually loose and green. Loose stools indicate fluid loss which may lead to a fluid volume deficit. With an increase in the number of stools per day dehydration is a possibility. The stools may be green in color because of the excretion of bilirubin.

Evaluation of Client Goal
- Stools within normal limits
- Urine specific gravity within normal limits
- Weight remains stable

Nursing Diagnosis #2 Impaired Skin Integrity related to disruption of skin surfaces secondary to phototherapy

Client Goal The newborn's skin will remain intact without signs of breakdown, corneal irritation, or drainage.

AEB:
- No signs of skin breakdown
- No signs of corneal irritation

(Continued on next page)

Nursing Care Plan For a Newborn with Hyperbilirubinemia (Continued)

NURSING INTERVENTIONS	RATIONALES
1. Cover newborn's eyes with patches while under phototherapy lights.	**Rationale:** High-intensity lights may cause retinal injury and corneal burns. If patches are removed for feeding or other treatments then phototherapy lights should be turned off.
2. Assess eyes every 8 hours for pressure areas, corneal abrasions, and conjunctivitis.	**Rationale:** Eye patches may be irritating and should be removed to assess for signs of complications such as pressure areas, corneal abrasions, drainage, and conjunctivitis. Eye patches should be replaced every 24 hours to prevent complications. Label eye patches so they are placed on the same eye each time. This will help prevent cross-contamination.
3. Change newborn position every 2 hours.	**Rationale:** Newborn position changes will allow exposure of the phototherapy lights to all areas of the body that are uncovered. Pressure areas may develop if the newborn lies in one position for an extended period of time.
4. Monitor skin for rashes and bronzing every 8 hours.	**Rationale:** The newborn may develop a maculopapular rash which is a transient side effect of phototherapy. If the newborn has an elevated direct serum bilirubin or liver disease, a benign bronzing discoloration of the skin may appear. Parents need to know that the discoloration will fade with time.
5. Inspect perianal area after each diaper change for signs of skin breakdown.	**Rationale:** Newborns under phototherapy lights will have increased loose green acidic stools which can be irritating to the skin. The diaper area should be thoroughly cleaned after each soiled diaper to prevent skin breakdown.
6. Avoid using lotions or ointments on the newborn's skin while infant is receiving phototherapy.	**Rationale:** Lotions and ointments may cause skin to burn if applied to exposed areas during phototherapy.
7. Provide a fiberoptic blanket as ordered.	**Rationale:** Fiberoptic phototherapy blankets eliminate the need for eye patches and decrease heat loss because the newborn is clothed. The fiberoptic light source stays on at all times and the newborn is accessible for care, feeding, and diaper changes without interruption to phototherapy. Fluid and weight loss are not complications of this system.

Evaluation of Client Goal
- Skin intact with no signs of breakdown
- No signs of corneal irritation

CRITICAL THINKING QUESTIONS

1. Describe two assessment techniques used for assessing jaundice in the newborn.

Answer: Visual inspection of the skin and mucous membranes is one way to assess for signs of jaundice. To assess color of skin, observe the skin in the daylight or use white fluorescent lights. For light-skinned newborns blanch skin over bony prominence to remove capillary coloration and then assess degree of yellow discoloration. For dark-skinned newborns assess oral mucosa and conjunctival sac. Another method to assess for jaundice is to review serum bilirubin lab results. Serum bilirubin levels that increase 5 mg/dL/day or more than 0.5 mg/hr indicate severe hemolysis or a pathologic process.

2. Janice is being discharged with her 3-day-old newborn. The newborn is jaundiced and will continue with phototherapy at home. The nurse provides a fiberoptic blanket for the newborn. Janice questions the nurse about the benefits of the fiberoptic blanket versus phototherapy lights. What should the nurse include in her discharge teaching regarding the fiberoptic blanket?

Answer: Newborns who are discharged home with phototherapy require ongoing monitoring. The fiberoptic blanket provides continued phototherapy while allowing the newborn to be more accessible to the parents for care, feeding, holding, and diapering. Fiberoptic phototherapy blankets also eliminate the need for eye patches and allow the newborn to be fully clothed which decreases heat loss.

*For your reference, this care plan is an example of how two nursing diagnoses might be addressed.

need for eye patches, decrease heat loss because the baby is clothed, and provide more opportunities for interaction between the baby and parents. The best method of home phototherapy depends on the cause of the hyperbilirubinemia and the rate of progression of the jaundice. A combination of phototherapy lights and fiberoptic mattress may be used. (See Figure 29–14 in the accompanying Clinical Skill.) Ongoing monitoring of bilirubin levels is essential with home phototherapy and can be carried out in the home, in the follow-up clinic, or in the clinician's office.

Evaluation

Expected outcomes of nursing care include the following:

- The newborn at risk for development of hyperbilirubinemia is identified, and action is taken to minimize the potential impact of hyperbilirubinemia.
- The baby does not have any corneal irritation or drainage, skin breakdown, or major fluctuations in temperature.
- Parents understand the rationale for, goal of, and expected outcome of therapy.
- Parents verbalize concerns about their baby's condition and identify how they can facilitate their baby's improvement.

Care of the Newborn with Anemia

Neonatal anemia is often difficult to recognize by clinical evaluation alone. The hemoglobin concentration in a term newborn is 14 to 20 g/dL, slightly higher than that in premature newborns. Infants with hemoglobin values of less than 14 g/dL (term) and less than 12 g/dL (preterm) are usually considered anemic. The most common causes of neonatal anemia are blood loss, hemolysis/erythrocyte destruction, and impaired red blood cell production (Aher, Malwatkar, & Kadam, 2008; Rosenberg, 2007).

Blood loss (hypovolemia) occurs in utero from placental bleeding (placenta previa or abruptio placentae). Intrapartal blood loss may be fetomaternal, fetofetal, or the result of umbilical cord bleeding. Birth trauma to abdominal organs (adrenal hemorrhage) or the cranium (subgaleal bleed) may produce significant blood loss, and cerebral bleeding may occur because of hypoxia.

Excessive hemolysis of red blood cells is usually a result of blood group incompatibilities but may be caused by infections. The most common cause of impaired red blood cell production is a genetically transmitted deficiency in glucose-6-phosphate dehydrogenase (G-6-PD). Anemia and jaundice are the presenting signs.

A condition known as **physiologic anemia of infancy** exists as a result of the normal gradual drop in hemoglo-

bin for the first 6 to 12 weeks of life or corresponds with the decline in fetal hemoglobin. Theoretically, the bone marrow stops production of RBCs in response to higher oxygen levels that result from breathing changes after birth. When the amount of hemoglobin decreases, reaching levels of 10 to 11 g/dL at about 6 to 12 weeks of age (the average is 70 days) in term infants, the bone marrow begins production of RBCs again, and the anemia disappears.

Anemia in preterm newborns is seen earlier than in term newborns, and increased production of red blood cells does not start until hemoglobin is 7 to 9 g/dL. The preterm baby's hemoglobin reaches a low sooner (by 4 to 8 weeks after birth) than does a term newborn's (6 to 12 weeks) because a preterm infant's red blood cell survival time is shorter than that of a term newborn (Cloherty et al., 2008). This difference is because of several factors: the preterm infant's rapid growth rate, decreased iron stores, and an inadequate production of erythropoietin (EPO).

Clinical Therapy

Hematologic problems can be anticipated based on the pregnancy history and clinical manifestations. The age at which anemia is first noted is also of diagnostic value. Clinically, light-skinned anemic infants are very pale in the absence of other symptoms of shock and usually have abnormally low red blood cell counts. In acute blood loss, symptoms of shock such as pallor, low arterial blood pressure, and a decreasing hematocrit value may be present.

The initial laboratory workup should include hemoglobin and hematocrit measurements, reticulocyte count, ferritin concentrations, examination of peripheral blood smear, bilirubin determinations, direct Coombs' test of infant's blood, and examination of maternal blood smear for fetal erythrocytes (Kleihauer-Betke test). Clinical management depends on the severity of the anemia and on whether blood loss is acute or chronic. The baby should be placed on constant cardiac and respiratory monitoring. Mild or slow chronic anemia may be treated adequately with iron supplements alone or with iron-fortified formulas. Frequent determinations of hemoglobin, hematocrit, and bilirubin levels (in hemolytic disease) are essential. In severe cases of anemia, transfusions with 0-negative or typed and crossmatched irradiated packed red cells are the treatment of choice. The nurse should try to prevent iron deficiency by limiting phlebotomy losses and starting iron therapy at 2 weeks of postnatal age (Aher, Malwatkar, & Kadam, 2008). Management of anemia of prematurity includes treating the causative factor (i.e., antibiotics/antivirals used for infection, steroid therapy for disorders of erythrocyte production) and supplemental iron. Blood transfusions (dedicated units of blood) are kept to a minimum. Evidence supports use of recombinant human erythropoietin (rEPO) in only selected cases. For example, infants in whom it is desirable to maintain a relatively high hematocrit such as infants with bronchopulmonary dysplasia (Cloherty et al., 2008).

Nursing Care Management

The nurse assesses the newborn for symptoms of anemia (pallor). If the blood loss is acute, the baby may exhibit signs of shock (a capillary filling time greater than 3 seconds, decreased pulses, tachycardia, low blood pressure). Continued observation is necessary to identify physiologic anemia as the preterm newborn grows. Signs of compromise include poor weight gain, tachycardia, tachypnea, and apneic episodes. The nurse promptly reports any symptoms indicating shock. The amount of blood drawn for all laboratory tests is recorded in tenths of a milliliter, so that total blood removed can be assessed and replaced by transfusion when necessary. If the newborn exhibits signs of shock, the nurse may need to initiate interventions.

Care of the Newborn with Polycythemia

Polycythemia, a condition in which blood volume and hematocrit values are increased, is more common in intrauterine growth restricted (IUGR), full-term, or late preterm infants; newborns with placental transfusion caused by delayed cord clamping or cord stripping; infants receiving maternal-fetal and twin-to-twin transfusions; infants who have been exposed to intrauterine hypoxia; and babies of mothers who smoke; suffer from asphyxia, diabetes (IDM), or hypertension; or take propranolol during pregnancy. Other conditions that present with polycythemia are chromosomal anomalies such as trisomies 21, 18, and 13; endocrine disorders such as hypoglycemia and hypocalcemia; and births at altitudes over 5000 feet. The incidence ranges from 1.5% to 4%, and the condition is uncommon in newborns less than 34 weeks' gestation (Rosenberg, 2007). An infant is considered polycythemic when the central venous hematocrit value is greater than 65% (Cloherty et al., 2008). A potential complication of polycythemia is hyperviscosity which results in impaired perfusion of the capillary vessels (Rosenberg, 2007).

Clinical Therapy

The goal of therapy is to reduce the peripheral venous hematocrit value to a range of 55% to 60% in symptomatic infants. To decrease the red blood cell mass, the symptomatic infant receives a partial exchange transfusion in which blood is removed from the infant and replaced millimeter for millimeter with fresh frozen plasma

or 5% albumin, or crystalloids such as isotonic saline. The preference is to use crystalloids because of decreased promotion of infection, incidence of necrotizing enterocolitis (NEC), and their hypoallergenic properties. Supportive treatment of presenting symptoms is required until resolution, which usually occurs spontaneously following the partial exchange transfusion.

Nursing Care Management

The nurse assesses for, records, and reports symptoms of polycythemia. The nurse also does an initial screening of the newborn's hematocrit value on admission to the nursery. The peak of term newborn's hematocrit will occur at 2 hours of age and begin to drop slowly by 12 to 18 hours. If a capillary hematocrit is done, warming the heel before obtaining the blood helps to decrease falsely high values (see Clinical Skill: Performing a Heel Stick on a Newborn); however, peripheral free-flowing venous hematocrit samples are usually obtained from the antecubital fossa for confirmation.

Many infants are asymptomatic, but as symptoms develop, they are related to the increased blood volume, hyperviscosity (thickness) of the blood, and decreased deformability of red blood cells, all of which result in poor perfusion of tissues. The infants have a characteristic plethoric (ruddy) appearance. The most common symptoms observed include the following:

- *Cardiopulmonary.* Tachycardia and congestive heart failure caused by the increased blood volume
- *Respiratory.* Respiratory distress with grunting, tachypnea, and cyanosis; increased oxygen need; or respiratory hemorrhage caused by pulmonary venous congestion, edema, and hypoxemia
- *Hematologic.* Hyperbilirubinemia caused by increased numbers of RBCs breaking down; thrombocytopenia; or elevated reticulocytes and nucleated RBCs
- *Gastrointestinal.* Feeding intolerance, poor feeding, vomiting, or NEC
- *Renal.* Renal vein thrombosis with decreased urine output, hematuria, or proteinuria caused by thromboembolism; or renal tubular damage
- *Central nervous system.* Jitteriness, irritability, decreased activity and tone, lethargy, stroke (rare), or seizures caused by decreased perfusion of the brain and increased vascular resistance secondary to sluggish blood flow, which can result in neurologic or developmental problems
- *Endocrine.* Hypoglycemia or hypocalcemia

The nurse observes closely for the signs of distress or change in vital signs during the partial exchange. The nurse assesses carefully for potential complications resulting from partial exchange transfusion, such as transfusion overload (which may result in congestive heart failure), irregular cardiac rhythm, bacterial infection, hypovolemia, and anemia. Parents need specific explanations about polycythemia and its treatment. The newborn needs to be reunited with the parents as soon as the baby's status permits.

Care of the Newborn with Infection

Newborns up to 1 month of age are particularly susceptible to an infection, referred to as **sepsis neonatorum**, caused by organisms that do not cause significant disease in older children. Once any infection occurs in the newborn, it can spread rapidly through the bloodstream, regardless of its primary site. The incidence of primary neonatal sepsis is 1 to 5 per 1000 live births (0.1% to 0.5%) (Nash & Smith, 2008). The risk of mortality is 5% to 15% in this population. Nosocomial infection frequency is less in normal newborn infants and increases in infants in the neonatal intensive care unit (NICU).

Prematurity and low birth weight are associated with nosocomial infection rates up to 15 times higher than average. The general debilitation and underlying illnesses often associated with prematurity necessitate invasive procedures such as umbilical catheterization, intubation, resuscitation, ventilator support, monitoring, parenteral alimentation (especially lipid emulsions), and prior broad-spectrum antibiotic therapy.

However, even full-term infants are susceptible, because their immunologic systems are immature. They lack the complex factors involved in effective phagocytosis and the ability to localize infection or to respond with a well-defined, recognizable inflammatory response. In addition, all newborns lack IgM immunoglobin, which is necessary to protect against bacteria, because it does not cross the placenta (refer to Chapter 24 ∞ for immunologic adaptations in the newborn period).

Most nosocomial infections in the NICU present as bacteremia/sepsis, urinary tract infections, meningitis, or pneumonia. Maternal antepartal infections such as rubella, toxoplasmosis, cytomegalic inclusion disease, and herpes may cause congenital infections and resulting disorders in the newborn. Intrapartal maternal infections, such as amnionitis and those resulting from premature rupture of membranes (PROM) and precipitous birth, are sources of neonatal infection (see Chapter 16 ∞ for more detailed information). Passage through the birth canal and contact with the vaginal flora (β-hemolytic streptococci, herpes, *Listeria,* gonococci) expose the infant to infection (Table 29–5). With infection anywhere in the fetus or newborn, the adjacent tissues or organs are easily penetrated, and the blood-brain barrier is ineffective. Sep-

ticemia is more common in males, except for infections caused by group B β-hemolytic streptococcus.

Gram-negative organisms (especially *Escherichia coli, Enterobacter, Proteus,* and *Klebsiella*) and the gram-positive organism β-hemolytic streptococcus are the most common causative agents. *Pseudomonas* is a common fomite contaminant of ventilator support and oxygen therapy equipment. Gram-positive bacteria, especially coagulase-negative staphylococci, are common pathogens in nosocomial bacteremias, pneumonias, and urinary tract infections. Other gram-positive bacteria frequently isolated are enterococci and *Staphylococcus aureus* (Vargo & Trotter, 2007).

Protection of the newborn from infections starts prenatally and continues throughout pregnancy and birth. Prenatal prevention should include maternal screening for sexually transmitted infections and monitoring of rubella titers in women who test negative. Intrapartally, sterile technique is essential. Smears from genital lesions are taken, and placenta and amniotic fluid cultures are obtained if amnionitis is suspected. If genital herpes is present toward term, cesarean birth may be indicated. All newborns' eyes should be treated with an antibiotic ophthalmic ointment to prevent damage from gonococcal (occurring 3 days following birth) infection. Prophylactic antibiotic therapy, for asymptomatic women who test positive for group B streptococcus (GBS) during the intrapartum period, helps prevent early-onset sepsis (Nash & Smith, 2008).

Clinical Therapy

Cultures should be taken as soon after birth as possible for infants with a history of possible exposure to infection in utero (e.g., PROM more than 24 hours before birth or questionable maternal history of infection, maternal fever/chorioamnionitis, or high-risk behavior (such as multiple sexual partners or illicit drug use). Cultures are obtained before antibiotic therapy is begun.

1. Anaerobic and aerobic blood cultures are taken from a peripheral site rather than an umbilical vessel, because catheters have yielded false-positive results caused by contamination. The skin is prepared by cleaning with a unit antiseptic solution and allowed to dry; the specimen is obtained with a sterile needle and syringe to lessen the likelihood of contamination.
2. Spinal fluid culture is done following a spinal tap/ lumbar puncture if there are concerns about CNS symptoms/pathology.
3. The specimen for urine culture is best obtained by a suprapubic bladder aspiration or sterile catheterization.
4. Skin cultures are taken of any lesions or drainage from lesions or reddened areas.
5. Tracheal aspirate cultures, if intubated, may be obtained.

TABLE 29–5	Maternally Transmitted Newborn Infections	
Infection	**Nursing Assessment**	**Nursing Plan and Implementation**

Group B Streptococcus

1% to 2% colonized with 1 in 10 developing disease. Early onset—usually within hours of birth or within first week. Late onset—1 week to 3 months (Nash & Smith, 2008).	Severe respiratory distress (grunting and cyanosis). May become apneic or demonstrate symptoms of shock. Meconium-stained amniotic fluid seen at birth.	Early assessment of clinical signs necessary. Assist with X-ray examination—shows aspiration pneumonia or respiratory distress syndrome. Immediately obtain blood, gastric aspirate, external ear canal, and nasopharynx cultures. Administer antibiotics, usually aqueous penicillin or ampicillin combined with gentamicin, as soon as cultures are obtained. Early assessment and intervention are essential to survival.

Congenital Syphilis

Spirochetes (*Treponema pallidum*) cross placenta after 16th to 18th week of gestation. The more recent the maternal infection the more likelihood of transmission. Most are asymptomatic at birth but develop symptoms within first 3 months of life.	Check perinatal history for positive maternal serology. Assess infant using screening nontreponemal titer (RPR or VDRL) tests; then use treponemal (FTA-ABS or TP-PA) tests on infant serum to confirm diagnosis (AAP & ACOG, 2007). Rhinitis (sniffles). Fissures on mouth corners and excoriated upper lip. Red rash around mouth and anus. Copper-colored rash over face, palms, and soles. Irritability; generalized edema, particularly over joints; bone lesions; painful extremities, hepatosplenomegaly, jaundice, congenital cataracts, SGA, and failure to thrive.	Initiate standard precautions until infants have been on antibiotics for at least 24 hours. Administer penicillin. Initiate referral to evaluate for blindness, deafness, learning or behavioral problems. Provide emotional support for parents because of their feelings about mode of transmission and potential long-term sequelae.

Gonorrhea

Approximately 30% to 35% of newborns born vaginally to infected mothers acquire the infection.	Assess for Ophthalmia neonatorum (conjunctivitis). Purulent discharge and corneal ulcerations. Neonatal sepsis with temperature instability, poor feeding response, and/or hypotonia, jaundice.	Administer prophylaxis ophthalmic antibiotic ointment (see Drug Guide: Erythromycin [Ilotycin] Ophthalmic Ointment in Chapter 26 ∞) or tetracycline. If positive maternal test, single dose systemic antibiotic therapy (AAP & ACOG, 2007). Initiate follow-up referral to evaluate any loss of vision.

Herpes Type 2

Usually transmitted during vaginal birth; a few cases of in utero transmission have been reported.	Check perinatal history for active herpes genital lesions. Small cluster vesicular skin lesions over all the body about 6 to 9 days of life. Disseminated form—Pneumonia, DIC, hepatitis with jaundice, hepatosplenomegaly, and neurologic abnormalities. Without skin lesions, assess for fever or subnormal temperature, respiratory congestion, tachypnea, and tachycardia.	Carry out careful handwashing and contact precautions (gown and glove isolation with linen precautions) (AAP & ACOG, 2007). Obtain throat, conjunctiva, urine, stool, and lesion cultures to identify herpesvirus type 2 antibiotics in serum IgM fraction. Cultures positive in 24 to 48 hours after birth. Administer intravenous acyclovir (Zovirax). Make a follow-up referral to evaluate potential sequelae of microcephaly, spasticity, seizures, deafness, or blindness. Encourage parental rooming-in and touching of their newborn. Show parents appropriate handwashing procedures and precautions to be used at home if mother's lesions are active.

Cytomegalovirus (CMV)

Most common cause of congenital infection in the United States—approximately 1% of all newborn infants (AAP & ACOG, 2007). Transmission occurs in utero, during labor, or may happen postnatally through breast milk.	Congenital CMV disease, including intrauterine growth restriction, jaundice, hepatosplenomegaly, petechiae or purpura (blueberry muffin spots), thrombocytopenia, and pneumonia. CNS manifestations are very common and include lethargy and poor feeding, hypertonia or hypotonia, microcephaly, intracranial calcifications, chorioretinitis, and sensorineural deafness.	Diagnosis of congenital CMV infection is established by isolating virus from urine, saliva, or tissue obtained during the first 3 weeks of life. All infants in whom the diagnosis is suspected should have a viral culture performed; a CT scan of the brain is particularly important to document the extent of CNS involvement; eye exam and hearing test; close long-term follow-up evaluating for developmental effects.

TABLE 29–5 Maternally Transmitted Newborn Infections *(Continued)*		
Infection	Nursing Assessment	Nursing Plan and Implementation
Oral Candidal Infection (Thrush)		
Acquired during passage through birth canal.	Assess newborn's buccal mucosa, tongue, gums, and inside the cheeks for white plaques (seen 5 to 7 days of age).	Differentiate white plaque areas from milk curds by using cotton tip applicator (if it is thrush, removal of white areas causes raw, bleeding areas).
	Check diaper area for bright red, well-demarcated eruptions.	Maintain cleanliness of hands, linen, clothing, diapers, and feeding apparatus.
	Assess for thrush periodically when newborn is on long-term antibiotic therapy.	Instruct breastfeeding mothers on treating their nipples with nystatin.
		Administer nystatin swabbed on oral lesions 1 hour after feeding or nystatin instilled in baby's oral cavity and on mucosa.
		Swab skin lesions with topical nystatin.
		Discuss with parents that gentian violet stains mouth and clothing.
		Avoid placing gentian violet on normal mucosa; it causes irritation.
Chlamydia Trachomatis		
Acquired during passage through birth canal.	Assess for perinatal history of preterm birth.	Instillation of prophylactic ophthalmic erythromycin is controversial (AAP & ACOG, 2007).
	Symptomatic newborns present with conjunctivitis and pneumonia. Chlamydial conjunctivitis presents with inflammation, yellow discharge, and eyelid swelling 5 to 14 days after birth.	Treat chlamydial conjunctivitis or pneumonia with oral erythromycin for 14 days. Monitor for hypertrophic pyloric stenosis.
	Chronic follicular conjunctivitis (corneal neovascularization and conjunctival scarring).	Initiate follow-up referral for eye complications and late development of pneumonia at 4 to 11 weeks postnatally.

Other laboratory investigations include a complete blood count, C-reactive protein (CRP), chest X-ray examination, serology, and Gram stains of cerebrospinal fluid, urine, skin exudate, and umbilicus. White blood cell (WBC) count with differential may indicate the presence or absence of sepsis. A level of 30,000 to 40,000 mm^3 WBCs may be normal in the first 24 hours of life, whereas low WBC (less than 5000 to 7500/mm^3) may be indicative of sepsis. A low neutrophil count and a high band (immature white blood cells) count indicate that an infection is present. Stomach aspirate should be sent for culture and smear if a gonococcal infection or amnionitis is suspected. The C-reactive protein, an acute-phase reactant protein synthesized in response to inflammation, may or may not be elevated. Other inflammatory responses may cause an elevation in the CRP, so it should not be used as the only indicator of infection (Hawk, 2008; Nash & Smith, 2008). The CRP may be helpful in watching for improvement once antibiotic therapy is initiated.

Serum IgM levels are elevated (normal level less than 20 mg/dL) in response to transplacental infections (Blackburn, 2007). If available, counterimmunoelectrophoresis tests for specific bacterial antigens are performed. In the future repetitive sequence-based polymerase chain reactions (rep-PCR) will be used to identify specific infectious organisms within hours instead of days (Cloherty et al., 2008). Evidence of congenital infections may be seen on skull X-ray films for cerebral calcifications (cytomegalovirus, toxoplasmosis), on bone X-ray films (syphilis, cytomegalovirus), and in serum-specific IgM levels (rubella). Cytomegalovirus infection is best diagnosed by urine culture.

Because neonatal infection causes high mortality, therapy is instituted before results of the septic workup are obtained. A combination of two broad-spectrum antibiotics, such as ampicillin and gentamicin, is given in large doses until a culture with sensitivities is obtained.

After the pathogen and its sensitivities are determined, appropriate specific antibiotic therapy is begun. Combinations of penicillin or ampicillin and kanamycin have been used in the past, but new kanamycin-resistant enterobacteria and penicillin-resistant staphylococcus necessitate increasing use of gentamicin. Rotating aminoglycosides has been suggested to prevent development of resistance. Use of cephalosporins and, in particular, cefotaxime has emerged as an alternative to aminoglycoside therapy in the treatment of neonatal infections. Duration of therapy varies from 7 to 14 days (Table 29–6). If cultures are negative and symptoms subside, antibiotics may be discontinued after 2 days/48 hours of negative blood cultures. Supportive physiologic care may be required to maintain respiratory, hemodynamic, nutritional, and metabolic homeostasis.

TABLE 29–6 Neonatal Sepsis Antibiotic Therapy

Drug	Dose (mg/kg) Total Daily Dose	Schedule for Divided Doses	Route	Comments
Acyclovir (Zovirax)	20 mg/kg	Every 8 hours	IV	Length of treatment is 14 days for skin/eye/mouth (SEM) or 21 days for CNS and disseminated disease: *Herpes*.
Ampicillin	50 to 100 mg/kg	Every 12 hours* Every 8 hours†	IM or IV	Effective against gram-positive microorganisms, *Haemophilus influenzae*, and most *Escherichia coli* strains. Higher doses indicated for meningitis. Used with aminoglycoside for synergy.
Cefotaxime	50 mg/kg 100 to 150 mg/kg/day	Every 12 hours* Every 8 hours†	IM or IV	Active against most major pathogens in infants; effective against aminoglycoside-resistant organisms; achieves CSF bactericidal activity; lack of ototoxicity and nephrotoxicity; wide therapeutic index (levels not required); resistant organisms can develop rapidly if used extensively; ineffective against *Pseudomonas, Listeria*.
Gentamicin	2.5 to 3 mg/kg 5 to 7.5 mg/kg/day 4 to 5 mg/kg/dose (first week of life)	Every 12 to 24 hours*‡ Every 8 to 24 hours† Every 24 to 48 hours	IM or IV	Effective against gram-negative rods and staphylococci; may be used instead of kanamycin against penicillin-resistant staphylococci and *E. coli* strains and *Pseudomonas aeruginosa*. May cause ototoxicity and nephrotoxicity. Need to follow serum levels. Must never be given as IV push. Must be given over at least 30 to 60 minutes. In presence of oliguria or anuria, dose must be decreased or discontinued. In infants less than 1000 g or 29 weeks, lower dosage 2.5 to 3 mg/kg/day. Monitor serum levels before administration of second dose. Peak 5 to 12 mcg/mL Trough 0.5 to 1 mcg/mL
Nafcillin	25 to 50 mg/kg dependent on age	Every 8 to 12 hours* Every 6 to 8 hours†	IM or IV	Effective against penicillinase-resistant staphylococci aureus. Avoid IM if possible. Monitor CBC, UA, LFTs. Caution in presence of jaundice.
Penicillin G (aqueous crystalline)	25,000 to 50,000 units/kg 50,000 to 125,000 units/kg/day Up to 400,000 units/kg/day for group β strep. meningitis	Every 12 hours* Every 8 hours†	IM or IV	Initial sepsis therapy effective against most gram-positive microorganisms except resistant staphylococci; can cause heart block in infants.
Vancomycin	10 to 20 mg/kg 30 mg/kg/day	Every 12 to 24 hours*‡ Every 8 hours†	IV	Effective for methicillin-resistant strains (*Staphylococcus epidermis*); must be administered by slow intravenous infusion to avoid prolonged cutaneous eruption. For smaller infants, < 1200 g, < 29 weeks, smaller dosages and longer intervals between doses. Nephrotoxic, especially in combination with aminoglycosides. Slow IV infusion over at least 60 minutes. Peak 25 to 40 mcg/mL Trough 5 to 10 mcg/mL

*Up to 7 days of age. †Greater than 7 days of age. ‡Dependent on GA.

Nursing Care Management

Nursing Assessment and Diagnosis

Symptoms of infection are most often noticed by the nurse during daily care of the newborn. The infant may deteriorate rapidly in the first 12 to 24 hours after birth if β-hemolytic streptococcal infection is present, with signs and symptoms mimicking RDS. In other cases, the onset of sepsis may be gradual, with more subtle signs and symptoms (Nash & Smith, 2008). The most common signs observed include the following:

1. Subtle behavioral changes; the infant "is not doing well" and is often lethargic or irritable (especially after the first 24 hours) and hypotonic; color changes may include pallor, duskiness, cyanosis, or a "shocky" appearance; skin is cool and clammy

2. Temperature instability, manifested by either hypothermia (recognized by a decrease in skin temperature) or, rarely in newborns, hyperthermia (elevation of skin temperature) necessitating a corresponding increase or decrease in incubator temperature to maintain a neutral thermal environment

3. Feeding intolerance, as evidenced by a decrease in total intake, abdominal distention, vomiting, poor sucking, lack of interest in feeding, and diarrhea
4. Hyperbilirubinemia
5. Tachycardia initially, followed by spells of apnea or bradycardia

Signs and symptoms may suggest CNS disease (jitteriness, tremors, seizure activity), respiratory system disease (tachypnea, labored respirations, apnea, cyanosis), hematologic disease (jaundice, petechial hemorrhages, hepatosplenomegaly), or gastrointestinal disease (diarrhea, vomiting, bile-stained aspirate, hepatomegaly). A differential diagnosis is necessary because of the similarity of symptoms to other more specific conditions.

Nursing diagnoses that may apply to the infant with sepsis neonatorum and the family include the following:

- *Risk for Infection* related to newborn's immature immunologic system
- *Deficient Fluid Volume* related to feeding intolerance
- *Ineffective Family Coping: Compromised* related to present illness resulting in prolonged hospital stay for the newborn

Nursing Plan and Implementation

In the nursery, environmental control and prevention of acquired infection are the responsibilities of the neonatal nurse. An infected newborn can be isolated effectively in an isolette and receive close observation. The nurse must promote strict handwashing technique for all who enter the nursery, including nursing colleagues; physicians; laboratory, X-ray, and respiratory therapists; and parents. Visits to the nursery area by unnecessary personnel should be discouraged. The nurse must be prepared to assist in the aseptic collection of specimens for laboratory investigations. Scrupulous care of equipment—changing and cleaning of incubators at least every 7 days, removing and sterilizing wet equipment every 24 hours, preventing cross use of linen and equipment, cleaning sinkside equipment such as soap containers periodically, and taking special care with the open radiant warmers (access without prior handwashing is much more likely than with the closed incubator)—will prevent contamination.

Provision of Antibiotic Therapy

The nurse administers antibiotics as ordered by the nurse practitioner or physician. It is the nurse's responsibility to be knowledgeable about the following:

- The proper dose to be administered, based on the weight of the newborn and desired peak and trough levels
- The appropriate route of administration, because some antibiotics cannot be given intravenously

- Admixture incompatibilities, because some antibiotics are precipitated by intravenous solutions or by other antibiotics
- Side effects and toxicity

In the case of term infants who are being treated for infections, neonatal home infusion of antibiotics should be considered as a viable alternative to continued hospitalization. The infusion of antibiotics at home by skilled RNs facilitates parent-infant bonding while meeting the infant's ongoing healthcare needs.

Provision of Supportive Care

In addition to antibiotic therapy, physiologic supportive care is essential in caring for a septic infant. The nurse should carry out the following:

- Observe for resolution of symptoms or development of other symptoms of sepsis
- Maintain neutral thermal environment with accurate regulation of humidity and oxygen administration
- Provide respiratory support: administer oxygen and observe and monitor respiratory effort
- Provide cardiovascular support: observe and monitor pulse and blood pressure; observe for hyperbilirubinemia, anemia, and hemorrhagic symptoms
- Provide adequate calories, because oral feedings may be discontinued because of increased mucus, abdominal distention, vomiting, and aspiration
- Provide fluids and electrolytes to maintain homeostasis; monitor weight changes, urine output, and urine specific gravity
- Observe for the development of hypoglycemia, hyperglycemia, acidosis, hyponatremia, and hypocalcemia

Restricting parental visits has not been shown to have any effect on the rate of infection and may be harmful for the newborn's psychologic development. With instruction and guidance from the nurse, both parents should be allowed to handle the baby and participate in daily care. Support of the parents is crucial. They need to be informed of the newborn's prognosis as treatment continues and to be involved in care as much as possible. They also need to understand how infection is transmitted.

Evaluation

Expected outcomes of nursing care include the following:

- The risks for development of sepsis are identified early, and immediate action is taken to minimize the development of the illness.
- Appropriate use of aseptic technique protects the newborn from further exposure to illness.
- The baby's symptoms are relieved, and the infection is treated.

> • The parents verbalize concerns about their baby's illness and understand the rationale behind the management of their newborn.

Care of Family with Birth of an At-Risk Newborn

The birth of a preterm or ill infant or an infant with a congenital anomaly is a serious crisis for a family. Throughout the pregnancy, both parents, together and separately, have felt excitement, experienced thoughts of acceptance, and pictured what their baby would look like. Both parents have wished for a perfect baby and feared an unhealthy one. Each parent and family member must accept and adjust when the fantasized fears become reality.

Parental Responses

Family members have acute grief reactions to the loss of the idealized baby they have envisioned. In a preterm birth, the mother is denied the last few weeks of pregnancy that seem to prepare her psychologically for the stress of birth and the attachment process. Attachment at this time is fragile, and interruption of the process by separation can affect the future mother-child relationship. Parents express grief as shock and disbelief, denial of reality, anger toward self and others, guilt, blame, and concern for the future. Self-esteem and feelings of self-worth are jeopardized.

Feelings of guilt and failure often plague mothers of preterm newborns. They may question themselves: "Why did labor start?" or "What did I do (or not do)?" A woman may have guilt fantasies and wonder what she may have done to cause the early labor: "Was it because I had sexual intercourse with my husband (a week, 3 days, a day) ago?" "Was it because I carried three loads of wash up from the basement?" or "Am I being punished for something done in the past—even in childhood?"

The period of waiting between suspicion and confirmation of abnormality or dysfunction is a very anxious one for parents because it is difficult, if not impossible, to begin attachment to the infant if the newborn's future is questionable. During the knowing period, parents need support and acknowledgment that this is an anxious time. They must be kept informed about tests and efforts to gather additional data, as well as efforts to improve their baby's outcome. It is helpful to tell both parents about the problem at the same time, with the baby present. An honest discussion of the problem and anticipatory management at the earliest possible time by health professionals help the parents (1) maintain trust in the physician and nurse, (2) appreciate the reality of the situation by dispelling fantasy and misconception, (3) begin the grieving process, and (4) mobilize internal and external support.

Nurses need to be aware that anger is a universal response by parents to a preterm birth. It is best that the parents direct it outward because holding it in check requires great energy which is then diverted away from grieving and physical recovery from pregnancy and giving birth. Anger may be directed at the physician and/or nurse, at the food, at nursing care, or at hospital regulations and routines. Parents rarely show anger with the baby; such responses can precipitate guilt feelings.

Although reactions and steps of attachment are altered by the birth of at-risk infants, a healthy parent-child relationship can occur. Kaplan and Mason (1974) have identified four psychologic tasks as essential for coping with the stress of an at-risk newborn and for providing a basis for the maternal-infant relationship:

1. Anticipatory grief as a psychologic preparation for possible loss of the child while still hoping for his or her survival
2. Acknowledgment of maternal failure to produce a term or perfect newborn expressed as anticipatory grief and depression and lasting until the chances of survival seem secure
3. Resumption of the process of relating to the infant, which was interrupted by the threat of nonsurvival; this task may be impaired by continuous threat of death or abnormality, and the mother may be slow in her response of hope for the infant's survival
4. Understanding of the special needs and growth patterns of the at-risk newborn, which are temporary and yield to normal patterns

Solnit and Stark (1961) postulate that grief and mourning over the loss of the loved object—the idealized child—mark parental reactions to a child with abnormalities. *Grief work*, the emotional reaction to a significant loss, must occur before adequate attachment to the actual child is possible. Parental detachment precedes parental attachment. The parents must first grieve the loss of the wished-for-perfect child, and then must adopt the imperfect child as the new love object.

Parental responses to a child with health problems may be viewed as a five-stage process (Klaus & Kennell, 1982):

1. *Shock* is felt at the reality of the birth of this child. This stage may be characterized by forgetfulness, amnesia about the situation, and a feeling of desperation.
2. There is *disbelief (denial)* of the reality of the situation, characterized by a refusal to believe the child is defective. This stage is exemplified by assertions that "It didn't really happen!" or "There has been a mistake; it's someone else's baby."
3. *Depression* over the reality of the situation and a corresponding grief reaction follows acceptance of the situation. This stage is characterized by much crying and sadness. Anger may also emerge at this stage. A projec-

tion of blame on others or on self and feelings of "not me" are characteristic of this stage.

4. *Equilibrium and acceptance* are characteristic of a decrease in the emotional reactions of the parents. This stage is variable and may be prolonged by a continuing threat to the infant's survival. Some parents experience chronic sorrow in relation to their child.

5. *Reorganization* of the family is necessary to deal with the child's problems. Mutual support of the parents facilitates this process, but the crisis of the situation may precipitate alienation between the mother and father.

Postpartal depression occurs in new mothers from 5% to 25% of the time, and stressful events can exaggerate the problem (Currie & Rademacher, 2004). Fathers also may suffer from depression both before and after the birth of their child, adding to the discord in the family unit and compounding the perceived stress experienced by the mother.

Developmental Consequences

The baby who is born prematurely, is ill, or has a malformation or disorder is at risk for emotional, intellectual, and cognitive development delays. The risk is directly proportional to the seriousness of the problem and the length of treatment. The necessary physical separation of family and infant and the tremendous emotional and financial burdens may adversely affect the parent-child relationship. The recent trends to involve the parents with their newborn early, repeatedly, and over protracted periods of time has done much to facilitate positive parent-child relationships.

Parents must have a clear picture of the reality of the handicap and the types of developmental hurdles ahead. Unexpected behaviors and responses from the baby because of his or her defect or disorder can be upsetting and frightening. The demands of care for the child and disputes regarding management or behavior stress family relationships. The entire multidisciplinary team may need to pool their resources and expertise to help parents of children born with problems or disorders so that both parents and children can thrive.

A variety of behavioral patterns may occur. For example, one or more members of the family may make a scapegoat of the child. Another may become the youngster's champion to the exclusion of others. One or the other spouse may feel pushed aside or denied attention, and thus may withdraw or leave the family unit. Parents or siblings may feel that their own needs (schooling, material goods, freedom of movement) are being set aside whereas all assets (financial and other) go to support the one child's needs. There may also be an increase in child abuse.

Nursing Care Management

Nursing Assessment and Diagnosis

A positive nurse-family relationship helps information gathering in areas of concern. A concurrent illness of the mother or other family members or other concurrent stress (lack of hospitalization insurance, loss of job, age of parents) may alter the family response to the baby. Feelings of apprehension, guilt, failure, and grief expressed verbally or nonverbally are important aspects of the nursing history. These observations enable all professionals to be aware of the parental state, coping behaviors, and readiness for attachment, bonding, and caretaking. Appropriate nursing observations during interviewing and relating to the family include the following:

1. *Level of understanding.* Observations concerning the family's ability to assimilate the information given and to ask appropriate questions; the need for constant repetition of information

2. *Behavioral responses.* Appropriateness of behavior in relation to information given; lack of response; flat affect

3. *Difficulties with communication.* Deafness (reads lips only); blindness; dysphasia; understanding only a non-English language

4. *Paternal and maternal education level.* Parents unable to read or write; parents with eighth-grade-level education; parents with a graduate-level degree or healthcare background

Documentation of such information, gathered through continuing contact and development of a therapeutic family relationship, lets all professionals understand and use the nursing history to provide continuous individual care.

Visiting and caregiving patterns indicate the level or lack of parental attachment. A record of visits, caretaking procedures, affect (in relating to the newborn), and telephone calls is essential. Serial observations, rather than just isolated observations that cause concern, must be obtained. Grant (1978) has developed a conceptual framework depicting adaptive and maladaptive responses to parenting of an infant with an actual or potential problem (Figure 29–15 ■).

If a pattern of distancing behaviors evolves, the nurse should institute appropriate interventions. Follow-up studies have found that a statistically significant number of preterm, sick, and congenitally defective infants suffer from failure to thrive, battering, or other parenting disorders. Early detection and intervention will prevent these aberrations in parenting behaviors from leading to irreparable damage or death.

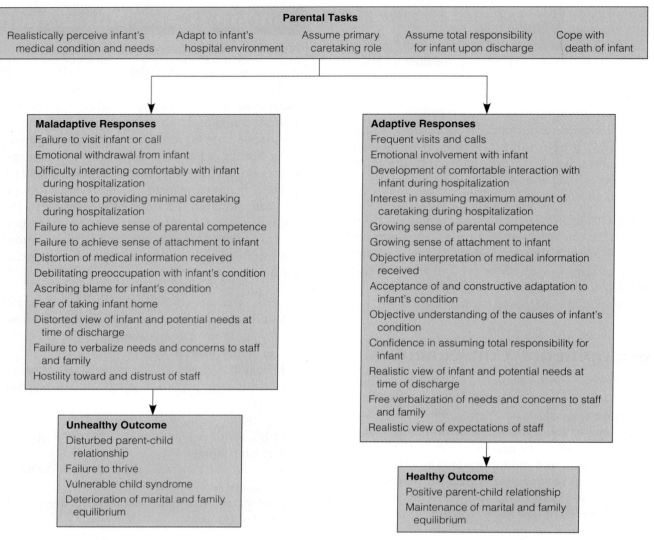

FIGURE 29–15 Maladaptive and adaptive parental responses during crisis period, showing unhealthy and healthy outcomes.
Source: Grant, P. (1978). Psychological needs of families of high-risk infants. *Family and Community Health, 11,* 93, Fig. 1. Philadelphia: Lippincott Williams & Wilkins.

Nursing diagnoses that may apply to the family of a newborn at risk include the following:

- *Dysfunctional Grieving* related to loss of idealized newborn
- *Fear* related to emotional involvement with an at-risk newborn
- *Altered Parenting* related to impaired bonding secondary to feelings of inadequacy about caretaking activities

Nursing Plan and Implementation

Hospital-Based Nursing Care

In their sensitive and vulnerable state, parents are acutely perceptive of others' responses and reactions (particularly nonverbal) to the child. Parents can be expected to identify with the responses of others. Therefore, it is impera-

tive that medical and nursing staff be fully aware of and come to terms with their own feelings so they are comfortable and at ease with the baby and grieving family.

Nurses may feel uncomfortable, may not know what to say to parents, or may fear confronting their own feelings as well as those of the parents. Each nurse must work out personal reactions with instructors, peers, clergy, parents, or significant others. It is helpful to have a stockpile of therapeutic questions and statements to initiate meaningful dialogue with parents. Opening statements might include the following: "You must be wondering what could have caused this," "Are you thinking that you (or someone else) may have done something?" "How can I help?" and "Are you wondering how you are going to manage?" Avoid statements such as: "It could have been worse," "It's God's will," "You have other children," "You are still young and can have more," and "I understand how you feel." This child is important now.

SUPPORT OF PARENTS FOR INITIAL VIEWING OF THE NEWBORN   Before parents see their child, the nurse must prepare them for the visit. It is important to maintain a positive, realistic attitude regarding the infant. An overly negative, fatalistic attitude further alienates the parents from their infant and retards attachment behaviors. Instead of beginning to bond with their child, the parents will anticipate their loss and begin the process of grieving. Once started, the grieving process is difficult to reverse.

Before preparing parents for the first view of their infant, the nurse should observe the baby. All infants exhibit strengths as well as deficiencies; prepare the parents to see both the deviations and the normal aspects of their infant. The nurse may say, "Your baby is small, about the length of my two hands. She weighs 2 lb, 3 oz, but is very active and cries when we disturb her. She is having some difficulty breathing but is breathing without assistance. Her breathing is in only 35% oxygen and room air is 21%."

The equipment being used for the at-risk newborn and its purpose should be described before the parents enter the intensive care unit. Many NICUs have booklets for parents to read before entering the units. Through explanations and pictures, the parents are better prepared to deal with the feelings they may experience when they see their infant for the first time (Figure 29–16 ■).

Upon entering the unit, parents may be overwhelmed by the sounds of monitors, alarms, and respirators, as well as by the unfamiliar language and "foreign" atmosphere. Preparing the parents by having the same healthcare professionals accompany them to the unit can be reassuring. The primary nurse and physician caring for the newborn need to be with the parents when they first visit their baby.

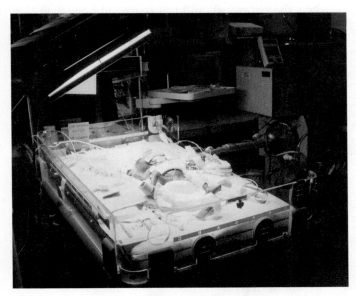

Figure 29–16 This 25 weeks' gestational age infant with respiratory distress syndrome may be frightening for her parents to see for the first time because of the technology that is attached to her.
Source: Courtesy of Lisa Smith-Pedersen, RNC, MSN, NNP.

Parental reactions vary, but initially there is usually an element of shock. Providing chairs and time to regain composure assists the parents. Slow, complete, and simple explanations—first about the infant and then about the equipment—allay fear and anxiety.

As parents attempt to deal with the initial stages of shock and grief, they may fail to grasp new information. They may need repeated explanations to accept the reality of the situation, procedures, equipment, and the infant's condition on subsequent visits.

Concern about the infant's physical appearance is common yet may remain unvoiced. Parents may express such concerns as: "He looks so small and red—like a drowned rat," "Why do her genitals look so abnormal?" and "Will that awful-looking mouth [cleft lip and palate] ever be normal?" The nurse needs to anticipate and address such questions. As just noted, use of pictures, such as of an infant after cleft lip repair, may be reassuring to doubting parents. Knowledge of the development of a "normal" preterm infant allows the nurse to make reassuring statements such as, "The baby's skin may look very red and transparent with lots of visible veins, but it is normal for her maturity. As she grows, subcutaneous fat will be laid down, and these superficial veins will begin to disappear."

The nursing staff set the tone of the NICU. Nurses foster the development of a safe, trusting environment by viewing the parents as essential caregivers, not as visitors or nuisances in the unit. It is important to provide parents privacy when needed and easy access to staff and facilities. An uncrowded and welcoming atmosphere lets parents know, "You are welcome there." However, even in crowded physical surroundings, the nurses can convey an attitude of openness and trust.

A trusting relationship is essential for collaborative efforts in caring for the infant. Nurses need to therapeutically use their own responses to relate to the parents on a one-to-one basis. Each individual has different needs, different ways of adapting to crisis, and different means of support. Nurses can use techniques that are real and spontaneous to them and avoid words or actions that are foreign to them. Nurses must also gauge their interventions so that they match the parents' pace and needs.

Nurses show concern and support by planning time to spend with the parents, by being psychologically as well as physically present, by encouraging open discussion and grieving, by repetitive explanations (as necessary), by providing privacy as needed, and by encouraging contact with the newborn. Identifying and clarifying feelings and fears decrease distortions in perception, thinking, and feeling. Nurses invest the baby with value in the eyes of the parents when they provide meticulous care to the newborn, talk and coo (especially in the face-to-face position) while holding or providing care to the newborn, refer to the child by gender or name, and relate the newborn's activities ("He took a whole ounce of formula," "She took hold of the blanket and just wouldn't let go"). Nurses should note the "normal" characteristics and capabilities of each newborn as well as the newborn's needs. The nurse should also learn the baby's name and refer to him or her by name.

FACILITATION OF ATTACHMENT IF NEONATAL TRANSPORT OCCURS Transport to a regional referral center some distance from the parents may be necessary. It is essential that the mother see and touch her infant before the infant is transported. Bring the mother to the nursery or take the infant in a warmed transport incubator to the mother's bedside to allow her to see the infant before transportation to the center. When the infant reaches the referral center, a staff member should call the parents with information about the infant's condition during transport, safe arrival at the center, and present condition.

Support of parents, with explanations from the professional staff, is crucial. Occasionally the mother may be unable to see the infant before transport (e.g., if she is still under general anesthesia or experiencing complications such as shock, hemorrhage, or seizures). In these cases, the infant should be photographed before transport. The picture should be given to the mother, along with an explanation of the infant's condition, present problems, and a detailed description of the infant's characteristics, to facilitate the attachment process until the mother can visit. An additional photograph is also helpful for the father to share with siblings or extended family. With the increased attention on improved fetal outcome, prenatal maternal transports, rather than neonatal transports, are occurring more frequently. This practice gives the mother of an at-risk infant the opportunity to visit and care for her infant during the early postpartal period.

PROMOTION OF TOUCHING AND PARENTAL CARETAKING Parents visiting a small or sick infant may need several visits to become comfortable and confident in their ability to touch the infant without injuring her or him. Barriers such as incubators, incisions, monitor electrodes, and tubes may delay the mother's development of comfort in touching the newborn. Knowledge of this normal delay in touching behavior will help the nurse understand parental behavior.

Klaus and Kennell (1982) have demonstrated a significant difference in the amount of eye contact and touching behaviors of mothers of normal newborns and mothers of preterm infants. Whereas mothers of normal newborns progress within minutes to palm contact of the infant's trunk, mothers of preterm infants are slower to progress from fingertip to palm contact and from the extremities to the trunk. The progression to palm contact with the infant's trunk may take several visits to the nursery.

Through support, reassurance, and encouragement, the nurse can facilitate the mother's positive feelings about

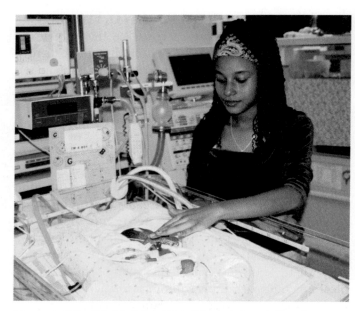

FIGURE 29–17 Mother of this 26 weeks' gestational age 600 g baby begins attachment through fingertip touch. *Source:* Courtesy of Lisa Smith-Pedersen, RNC, MSN, NNP.

her ability and her importance to her infant. Touching facilitates "getting to know" the infant and thus establishes a bond with the infant. Touching and seeing the infant help the mother realize the "normals" and potential of her baby (Figure 29–17 ■).

The nurse can also encourage parents to meet their newborn's need for stimulation. Stroking, rocking, cuddling, singing, and talking should be an integral part of the parents' caretaking responsibilities. Bonding can be facilitated by encouraging parents to visit and become involved in their baby's care (Figure 29–18 ■). When visiting is impossible, the parents should feel free to phone when they wish to receive information about their baby. A nurse's warm, receptive attitude provides support. Nurses can also facilitate parenting by personalizing a baby to the parents,

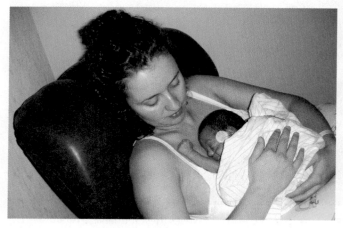

FIGURE 29–18 This mother of a 31 weeks' gestational age infant with respiratory distress syndrome is spending time with her newborn and meeting the baby's need for cuddling. *Source:* Courtesy of Lisa Smith-Pedersen, RNC, MSN, NNP.

by referring to the infant by name, or relating personal behavioral characteristics. Remarks such as "Jenny loves her pacifier" help make the infant seem individual and unique.

The variety of equipment needed for life support is hardly conducive to anxiety-free caretaking by the parents. However, even the sickest infant may be cared for, if only in a small way, by the parents. As a facilitator of parental caretaking, the nurse can promote the parents' success. Demonstration and explanation, followed by support of the parents in initial caretaking behaviors, positively reinforce this behavior. Changing their infant's diaper, providing skin or oral care, or helping the nurse turn the infant may at first provoke anxiety, but the parents will become more comfortable and confident in caretaking and feel satisfied by the baby's reactions and their ability "to do something." Complimenting the parents' competence in caretaking also increases their self-esteem, which has received recent "blows" of guilt and failure. *It is vitally important that the nurse never give the parents a task that they might not be able to accomplish.* Cues that the parents are ready to become involved with the child's care include their reference to the baby by name and their questioning as to amount of feeding taken, sleeping patterns, appearance today, and the like (Loo, Espinosa, Tyler et al., 2003).

The nurse should accept this behavior, but continue to remind the parents that it is okay and natural to feel disappointment, a sense of failure, helplessness, or anger. The overprotectiveness and overoptimism are defense mechanisms. To deny the negative feelings only entrenches them further, delays their resolution, and delays realistic planning.

Often parents of high-risk infants have ambivalent feelings toward the nurse. These feelings may take the form of criticism of the care of the infant, manipulation of staff, or personal guilt. Instead of fostering (by silence) these inferiority feelings of parents, nurses need to recognize that such feelings are needed to intervene appropriately to enhance parent-infant attachment. The nurse needs to deal with ambivalent feelings that contribute to a competitive atmosphere. For example, the nurse should avoid making unfavorable comparisons between the baby's responses to parental and nursing caretaking. During a quiet time it may help for the nurse to encourage the parents to talk about their hopes and fears and to facilitate their involvement in parent groups. Parents are also often anxious when their baby is transferred from the NICU to the "regular nursery." They may feel that their infant is not being cared for as proficiently because the nurses are not at the infant's bedside as often as they were in the NICU. Verbalizations that improve parental self-esteem are essential and easily shared. The nurse can point out that, in addition to physiologic use, breast milk is important because of the emotional investment of the mother. Pumping, storing, labeling, and delivering quantities of breast milk is a time-consuming "labor of love" for mothers. Positive remarks about breast milk reinforce the maternal behavior of caretaking and providing for her infant: "Breast milk is something that only you can give your baby," "You really have brought a lot of milk today," "Look how rich this breast milk is," or "Even small amounts of milk are important, and look how rich it is."

If the infant begins to gain weight while being fed breast milk, it is important that the nurse point this correlation out to the mother. Parents should also be advised that initial weight loss with beginning nipple feedings is common because of the increased energy expended when the infant begins active rather than passive nutritional intake.

Encourage parents to provide care for their infant even if the baby is very sick and likely to die. Detachment is easier after attachment, because the parents are comforted by the knowledge that they did all they could for their child while he or she was alive.

FACILITATION OF FAMILY ADJUSTMENT During crisis, it is difficult to maintain interpersonal relationships. Yet in a newborn intensive care area, the parents are expected to relate to many different care providers. It is important that parents have as few professionals as possible relaying information to them. A primary nurse should coordinate care and provide continuity for parents. Care providers are individuals and thus will use different terms, inflections, and attitudes. These subtle differences are monumental to parents and may confuse, confound, and produce anxiety. The transfer of the baby from NICU to a step-down unit or transport back to the home hospital provokes parental anxiety because they must now deal with new healthcare professionals. The nurse not only functions as a liaison between the parents and the various professionals interacting with the infant and parents but also offers clarification, explanation, interpretation of information, and support to the parents.

The nurse encourages parents to deal with the crisis with help from their support system. The support system attempts to meet the emotional needs and to provide support for the family members in crisis and stress situations. Biologic kinship is not the only valid criterion for a support system; an emotional kinship is the most important factor. In our mobile society of isolated nuclear families, the support system may be a next-door neighbor, a best friend, or perhaps a schoolmate. The nurse needs to search out the significant others in the lives of the parents and help them understand the problems so that they can be a constant parental support.

The impact of the crisis on the family is individual and varied. The nurse obtains information about the family's ability to adapt to the situation through interaction with the family. To institute appropriate interventions, the nurse should view the birth of the infant (normal newborn, preterm infant, infant with congenital anomaly) as defined by the family.

It is important for the nurse to encourage open intrafamily communication. The nurse should discourage the family from keeping secrets from one another, especially between spouses, because secrets undermine the trust of relationships. Well-meaning rationales such as "I want to protect her," "I don't want him to worry about it," and so on can be destructive to open communication and to the basic element of a relationship—trust.

Open communication is especially important when the mother is hospitalized apart from the infant. The first person to visit the infant relays information regarding the infant's care and condition to the mother and family. In this situation, the mother has had minimal contact, if any, with her infant. Because of her anxiety and isolation, she may mistrust all those who provide information (the father, nurse, physician, or extended family) until she sees the infant for herself. This can put tremendous stress on the relationship between spouses. The parents (and family) should be given information together. This practice helps overcome misunderstandings and misinterpretations and promotes cooperative "working through" of problems.

The nurse should encourage the entire family—siblings as well as other relatives—to visit and obtain information about the baby. Methods of intervention in helping the family cope with the situation include providing support, confronting the crisis, and understanding the reality. Support, explanations, and the helping role must extend to the kin network, as well as to the nuclear family, to aid the extended family in communication and support ties with the nuclear family.

The needs of siblings should not be overlooked. Siblings have been looking forward to the new baby, and they, too, suffer a degree of loss. Young children may react with hostility and older ones with shame at the birth of an infant with an anomaly. Both reactions may make siblings feel guilty. Parents, who may be preoccupied with working through their own feelings, often cannot give the other children the attention and support they need. Sometimes another child becomes the focus of family tension. Anxiety thus directed can take the form of finding fault or of overconcern. This is a form of denial; the parents cannot face the real worry—the infant at risk. After assessing the situation, the observant nurse can ensure that another family member or friend steps in to support the siblings of the affected baby.

The nurse must respect and seek to meet the desires and needs of the individuals involved and understand that differences can exist side by side. The nurse can often elicit the parents' feelings about the experience by asking "How are you doing?" The emphasis is on you, and the interest must be sincere.

Parents from minority cultures must deal with language barriers and cultural differences that can make feelings of isolation and uncertainty more acute. Healthcare providers have the professional responsibility to be aware of cultural needs of all clients and to ensure their needs are met. Feelings of isolation and uncertainty influence not only the parent's emotional responses to the ill newborn, but also the utilization of services and their interaction with health professionals. Hospital cultural interpreter programs can assist families with interactions with staff, as well as provide translation during family meetings, multidisciplinary family conferences, and parent support groups (Lipson & Dibble, 2008).

Families with children in the NICU may become friends and support one another. To encourage the development of these friendships and to provide support, many units have established parent groups. The core of the groups consists of parents whose infants were once in the intensive care unit. Most groups make contact with families within a day or two of the infant's admission to the unit, through either phone calls or visits to the hospital. Early one-on-one parent contacts are more effective than discussion groups in helping families work through their feelings. This personalized method gives the grieving parents an opportunity to express personal feelings about the pregnancy, labor, and birth and their "different from expected" infant with others who have experienced the same feelings and with whom they can identify.

Community-Based Nursing Care

Predischarge planning begins once the infant's condition becomes stable and it seems likely the newborn will survive. Discharge preparation and care conferences should involve a multidisciplinary team approach (Hummel & Cronin, 2004). NICU nursing staff is the fulcrum for aiding in the transition of high-risk infants from the intensive care unit to the home. Effective open communication with the families during the entire discharge-planning phase of care empowers the families to assume the role of primary caregiver for their children.

Adequate predischarge teaching helps parents transform any feelings of inadequacy they may have into feelings of self-assurance and attachment. From the beginning the parents should be taught about their infant's special needs and growth patterns. This teaching and involvement are best facilitated by a nurse who is familiar with the infant and his or her family over a period of time and who has developed a comfortable and supportive relationship with them.

Cobedding of twins is often used in the NICU to provide comfort, decrease stress to the co-multiples and provide a form of developmentally supportive care. Cobedding is also a strategy to maximize the synchronization of sleep-wake cycles (Bowers, Curran, Freda, Krening et al., 2008). Parents of multiples may desire cobedding at home to allow for clustering of care and to facilitate the parents' ability to spend time with both of their children (Figure 29–19 ■). If twins or other multiples experienced cobedding in the NICU, the nurse needs to discuss the advantages and disad-

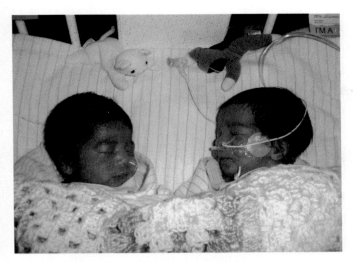

FIGURE 29–19 Cobedding of twins facilitates delivery of care and parent interaction with healthcare members. These twins were born at 33 weeks' gestation and required oxygen and gavage feeding while in the NICU.
Source: Courtesy of Lisa Smith-Pedersen, RNC, MSN, NNP.

vantages of continuing the practice at home. Currently, there is no evidence to establish cobedding of multiples outside the NICU as a safe or unsafe sleep practice. (Gromada & Bowers, 2005). The high incidence of prematurity and LBW in multiple birth infants and the corresponding risks for SIDS should be considered. As with all families at discharge, parents of multiples should be taught SIDS risk-reduction practices. SIDS reduction practices include supine positioning, babies sleeping in parents' room, firm bedding surface, no loose coverings/items and no barriers between infants (Bowers et al., 2008).

The nurse's responsibility is to provide home care instructions in an optimal environment for parental learning. Learning should take place over time, to avoid bombarding the parents with instructions in the day or hour before discharge. Parents often enjoy performing minimal caretaking tasks, with gradual expansion of their role.

Many NICUs provide facilities for parents to room in with their infants for a few days before discharge. This allows parents a degree of independence in the care of their infant with the security of nursing help nearby. This practice is particularly helpful for anxious parents, parents who have not had the opportunity to spend extended time with their infant, or parents who will be giving complex physical care at home, such as gastrostomy feeding and care (Collins, Makrides, & McPhee, 2008).

The families are able to interact with staff while gradually transitioning to sole caretakers of their medically complex high-risk infant. When discharging a medically fragile infant to home, schedule a predischarge home visit by a public health nurse or home health agency. This discharge visit evaluates the home for any possible issues that may complicate the parents' ability to care for their at-risk infant, especially if there are multiple monitoring equipment needs.

The basic elements of discharge and home care instruction are as follows:

1. Teach the parents routine well-baby care, such as bathing, taking a temperature, preparing formula, and breastfeeding.
2. Help parents learn to do special procedures as needed by the newborn, such as gavage or gastrostomy feedings, tracheostomy or enterostomy care, medication administration, CPR, and operation of the apnea monitor. Before discharge, the parents should be as comfortable as possible with these tasks and should demonstrate independence. Written tools and instructions are useful for parents to refer to once they are home with the infant, but they should not replace actual participation in the infant's care.
3. Make sure that all applicable screening (metabolic, vision, hearing) tests, immunizations, and respiratory syncytial virus (RSV) prophylaxis are done before discharge and that all records are given to the primary care provider and parents.
4. Refer parents to community health and support organizations. The Visiting Nurse Association, public health nurses, or social services can assist the parents in the stressful transition from hospital to home by providing the necessary home teaching and support. Some NICUs have their own parent support groups to help bridge the gap between hospital and home care. Parents can also find support from a variety of community organizations, such as mothers-of-twins groups, March of Dimes Birth Defects Foundation, handicapped children services, and teen mother and child programs. Each community has numerous agencies capable of assisting the family in adapting emotionally, physically, and financially to the chronically ill infant. The nurse should be familiar with community resources and help the parents identify which agencies may benefit them.
5. Help parents recognize the growth and development needs of their infant. A development program begun in the hospital can be continued at home, or parents may be referred to an infant development program in the community.
6. Arrange medical follow-up care before discharge. The infant will need to be followed up by a family pediatrician, a well-baby clinic, or a specialty clinic. The first appointment should be made before the infant is discharged from the hospital.
7. Evaluate the need for special equipment for infant care (such as a respirator, oxygen, apnea monitor, feeding pump) in the home. Any equipment or supplies should be placed in the home before the infant's discharge.
8. Arrange for neonatal hospice for parents of the medically fragile infant as needed.

Further evaluation after the infant has gone home is useful in determining whether the crisis has been resolved satisfactorily. The parents are usually given the intensive care nursery's telephone number to call for support and advice. The staff can follow up with each family with visits or telephone calls at intervals for several weeks to assess and evaluate the infant's (and parents') progress (Fig. 29–20 ■).

Evaluation

Expected outcomes of nursing care include the following:

- The parents are able to verbalize their feelings of grief and loss.
- The parents verbalize their concerns about their baby's health problems, care needs, and potential outcome.
- The parents are able to participate in their infant's care and show attachment behaviors.

Considerations for the Nurse Who Works with At-Risk Newborns

The birth of a baby with a problem is a traumatic event with the potential for either disruption or growth of the involved family. The NICU staff nurses may never see the long-term results of the specialized sensitive care they give to parents and their newborns. Their only immediate evidence of effective care may be the beginning resolution of parental grief; discharge of a recovered, thriving infant to the care of happy parents; and the beginning of reintegration of family life.

Nurses cannot provide support unless they themselves are supported. Working in an emotional environment of "lots of living and lots of dying" takes its toll on staff. NICUs are among the most stressful areas in health care for patients, families, and nurses. Nurses bear most of the stress and largely determine the atmosphere of the NICU.

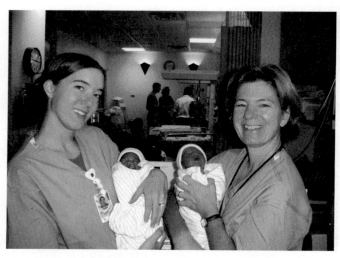

FIGURE 29–20 These 33 weeks' gestational age twins are being held by staff in the NICU on the happy day of discharge. This is what is so rewarding about working in the NICU: Healthy babies going home to their families.
Source: Courtesy of Lisa Smith-Pedersen, RNC, MSN, NNP.

The nurse's ability to cope with stress is the key to creating an emotionally healthy environment and a positive working atmosphere. The emotional needs and feelings of the staff must be recognized and dealt with so that staff can support the parents. An environment of openness to feelings and support in dealing with their human needs and emotions is essential for staff.

As caregivers, nurses may be unaware of their need to grieve for their own losses in the NICU. Nurses must also go through the grief work that parents experience. Techniques such as group meetings, individual support, and primary care nursing may assist in maintaining staff mental health. Reunions in some nurseries are beneficial for the families and healthcare professionals so they are able to see the children after discharge.

CHAPTER HIGHLIGHTS

- The sick newborn—whether preterm, term, or postterm—must be managed within narrow physiologic parameters.
- These parameters (respiratory, cardiovascular, and thermal regulation) maintain physiologic homeostasis and prevent introduction of iatrogenic stress to the already stressed infant.
- The nursing care of the newborn with special problems involves the understanding of normal physiology, the pathophysiology of the disease process, clinical manifestations, and supportive or corrective therapies. Only with this knowledge can the nurse caring for newborns make appropriate observations concerning responses to therapy and development of complications.
- Asphyxia results in significant circulatory, respiratory, and biochemical changes in the newborn that make the successful transition to extrauterine life difficult. Asphyxia requires early identification and resuscitative management.

- Newborn conditions that commonly present with respiratory distress and require oxygen and ventilator assistance are respiratory distress syndrome, transient tachypnea of the newborn, and meconium aspiration syndrome.
- Cold stress sets up the chain of physiologic events of hypoglycemia, pulmonary vasoconstriction, hyperbilirubinemia, respiratory distress, and metabolic acidosis.
- Nurses are responsible for early detection and initiation of treatment for hypoglycemia.
- Differentiation between pathologic and physiologic jaundice is the key to early and successful intervention.
- Anemia (decreased red blood cell volume) and polycythemia (excess amount) place the newborn at risk for alterations in blood flow and the oxygen-carrying capacity of the blood.

- Nursing assessment of the septic newborn involves identification of very subtle clinical signs that are also seen in other clinical disease states.
- The nurse is the facilitator for interdisciplinary communication with the parents and identifies an understanding of their infant's care and their needs for emotional support.

- Parents of at-risk newborns need support from nurses and healthcare providers to understand the special needs of their baby and to feel comfortable in an overwhelming and often unfamiliar environment.

CHAPTER REFERENCES

Aher, S., Malwatkar, K., & Kadam, S. (2008). Neonatal anemia. *Seminars in fetal & neonatal medicine 13*, 239–247.

American Academy of Pediatrics [AAP] & American Heart Association [AHA]. (2006). *Neonatal resuscitation: Instructor manual* (5th ed.). Evanston, IL: Author.

American Academy of Pediatrics (AAP) & Canadian Paediatric Society. (2006). Prevention and management of pain in the neonate: An update. *Pediatrics, 118*(5), 2231–2241.

American Academy of Pediatrics (AAP), Committee on Fetus and Newborn, & American College of Obstetricians and Gynecologists (ACOG), Committee on Obstetrics. (2007). *Guidelines for perinatal care* (6th ed.). Evanston, IL: Author.

American Academy of Pediatrics Subcommittee on Hyperbilirubinemia. (2004). Management of hyperbilirubinemia in the newborn infant 35 or more weeks of gestation. *Pediatrics, 114*(1), 297–316.

Bhutani, V. K., Johnson, L. H., & Keren, R. (2004). Diagnosis and management of hyperbilirubinemia in the term neonate: For a safer first week. *Pediatric Clinics of North America, 51*(4), 843–861.

Blackburn, S. T. (2007). *Maternal, fetal, & neonatal physiology: A clinical perspective* (3rd ed.). St. Louis: Saunders.

Bowers, N. A., Curran, C. A., Freda, M. C., Poole, J. H., Slocum, J. & Sosa, M. E. (2008). High-risk pregancy. In K. R. Simpson & P. A. Creehan, *AWHONN perinatal nursing* (3rd ed., pp. 125–299). Philadelphia, PA.: Lippincott Williams & Wilkins.

Cloherty, J. P., Eichenwald, E. C., & Stark, A. R. (2008). *Manual of neonatal care* (6th ed.). Philadelphia: Lippincott Williams & Wilkins.

Cole, F. S., Nogee, L. M., & Hamvas, A. (2006). Defects in surfactant synthesis: Clinical implications. *Pediatrics Clinics of North America, 53*(5), 911–927.

Collins, C. T., Makrides, M. E., & McPhee, A. J. (2008). Early discharge with home support of gavage feeding for stable preterm infants who have not established full oral feeds. *Cochrane database of systematic reviews. 2*, ID #CD003743.

Currie, M. L., & Rademacher, R. (2004). The pediatrician's role in recognizing and intervening in postpartum depression. *Pediatric Clinics of North America, 51*(3), 785–801.

Dildy, G. A. (2005). Intrapartum assessment of the fetus: Historical and evidence-based practice. *Obstetrics and Gynecology Clinics of North America, 32*(2), 225–271.

Folk, L. A. (2007). Guide to capillary heelstick blood sampling in infants. *Advances in Neonatal Care, 7*(4), 171–178.

Gennaro, S., Schwoebel, A., Hall, J. Y., & Bhutani, V. K. (2006). *Hyperbilirubinemia: Identification and management in the healthy term and near-term newborn* (2nd ed.). Washington, DC: Association of Women's Health, Obstetric, and Neonatal Nurses.

Grant, P. (1978). Psychological needs of families of high-risk infants. *Family and Community Health, 11*(3), 93–97.

Gromada, K. K., & Bowers, N. A. (2005). Care of the multiple-birth family: *Postpartum through infancy* (Nursing Module). New York: March of Dimes Birth Defects Foundation.

Hawk, M. (2008). C-Reactive protein in neonatal sepsis. *Neonatal Network, 27*(2), 117–123.

Hummel, P., & Cronin, J. (2004). Home care of the high-risk infant. *Advances in Neonatal Care, 4*(6), 354–364.

Juretschke, L. J. (2005). Kernicterus: Still a concern. *Neonatal Network, 24*(2), 7–19.

Kaplan, D. M., & Mason, E. A. (1974). Maternal reactions to premature birth viewed as an acute emotional disorder. In H. J. Parad (Ed.), *Crisis intervention* (Ch. 9, pp. 118–128). New York: Family Services Association of America.

Klaus, M. H., & Kennell, J. H. (1982). *Maternal-infant bonding* (2nd ed.). St. Louis: Mosby.

Lipson, J. G., & Dibble, S. L. (2008). Culture & clinical care. (7th ed.). San Francisco, CA: The Regents, University of California.

Loo, K. K., Espinosa, M., Tyler, R., & Howard, J. (2003). Using knowledge to cope with stress in the NICU: How parents integrate learning to read the physiologic and behavioral cues of the infant. *Neonatal Network, 22*(1), 31–37.

Madan, A., MacMahon, J. R., & Stevenson, D. K. (2005). Neonatal hyperbilirubinemia. In H. W.

Taeusch, R. A. Ballard, & C. A. Gleason (Eds.), *Avery's diseases of the newborn* (8th ed., pp. 1226–1257). Philadelphia, PA: Elsevier Saunders.

McGowan, J. E., & Perlman, J. M. (2006). Glucose management during and after intensive delivery room resuscitation. *Clinics in Perinatology, 33*(4), 184–196.

Mileic, T. L. (2008). Neonatal glucose homeostasis. *Neonatal Network, 27*(3), 203–207.

Nash, P., & Smith, J. R. (2008). Common neonatal complications. In K. R. Simpson & P. A. Creehan, *AWHONN perinatal nursing* (3rd ed., pp. 612–646). Philadelphia, PA.: Lippincott Williams & Wilkins.

Rosenberg, A. A. (2007). The neonate. In S. G. Gabbe, J. R. Niebyl, & J. L. Simpson (Eds.), *Obstetrics: Normal and problem pregnancies* (5th ed., pp. 523–565). Philadelphia, PA: Churchill Livingstone/Elsevier.

Saniski, D. (2005). Neonatal pain relief protocols in their infancy. *Nurse Week News*. Retrieved November 3, 2005, from www.nurseweek.com/news/features/05-02/Clinical_Baby pain

Solnit, A., & Stark, M. (1961). Mourning and the birth of a defective child. *Psychoanalytic Study of the Child, 16*, 505.

Thureen, P. J., Deacon, J., Hernandez, J. A., & Hall, D. M. (2005). *Assessment and care of the well newborn* (2nd ed.). St. Louis: Elsevier Saunders.

Vargo, L. E., & Trotter, C. W. (2007). The premature infant: Nursing assessment and management. (2nd ed.). White Plains, NY: March of Dimes.

Walden, M. (2007). Pain in the newborn and infant. In C. Kenner & J. W. Lott. *Comprehensive neonatal care: An interdisciplinary approach* (4th ed., pp. 350–371). St. Louis: Elsevier Saunders.

Watson, R. L. (2004). Gastrointestinal disorders. In M. T. Verklan & M. Walden (Eds.), *Core curriculum for neonatal intensive care nursing* (3rd ed., pp. 643–702). St. Louis: Elsevier Saunders.

Wiedemann, J. R., Saugstad, A. M., Barnes-Powell, L., & Duran, K. (2008). Meconium aspiration syndrome. *Neonatal Network, 27*(2), 81–87.

Young, T. E., & Mangum, O. B. (2007). *Neofax®: A manual of drugs used in neonatal care* (20th ed.). Raleigh, NC: Acorn.

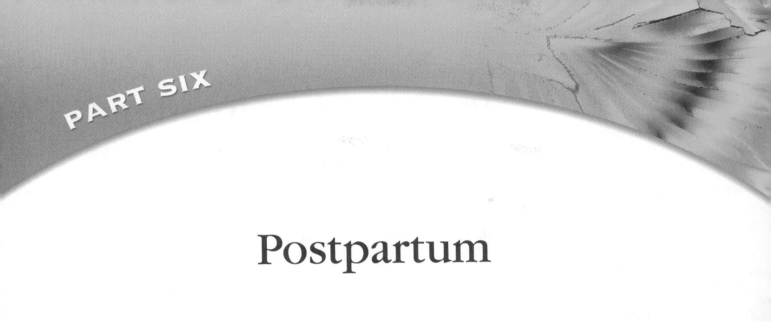

PART SIX

Postpartum

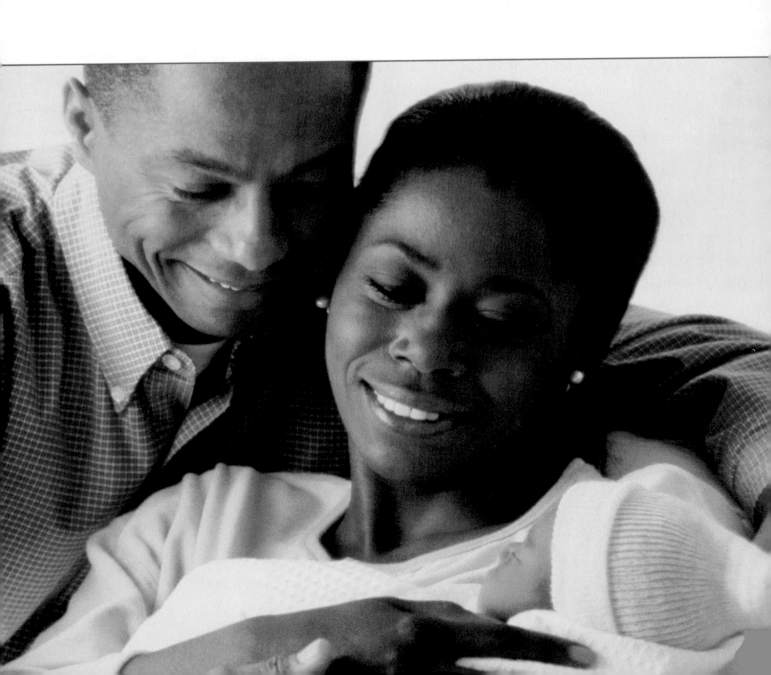

CHAPTER 30

Postpartal Adaptation and Nursing Assessment

My position as a postpartal nurse involves helping the new family get to know one another. The real challenge is to balance the introduction of new skills and information with the time and space needed for the family to recover, both physically and mentally, from the birth experience. I want the families I care for to regard me as a resource, not an authority.

—Postpartum Nurse

LEARNING OUTCOMES

30-1. Describe the basic physiologic changes that occur in the postpartal period as a woman's body returns to its prepregnant state and the related nursing care.

30-2. Describe the psychologic adjustments that normally occur during the postpartal period and the related nursing care and support.

30-3. Explain the impact of cultural influence on providing nursing care during the postpartal period.

30-4. Explain the components and methods of a systematic postpartal assessment.

30-5. Describe the normal characteristics and common concerns of the mother considered in a postpartal assessment.

30-6. Compare abnormal findings in a postpartal assessment to possible causes and nursing responses.

30-7. Examine the physical and developmental tasks that the mother must accomplish during the postpartal period.

30-8. Explain the factors that influence the development of parent-infant attachment in the nursing assessment of early attachment.

KEY TERMS

Afterpains **807**
Boggy uterus (uterine atony) **801**
Diastasis recti abdominis **804**
En face **809**
Engrossment **810**
Fundus **801**
Involution **801**
Lochia **802**
Lochia alba **803**
Lochia rubra **802**
Lochia serosa **802**
Maternal role attainment **807**
Postpartum blues **808**
Puerperium **801**
Reciprocity **810**
Subinvolution **802**

During the **puerperium**, or postpartal period, the woman readjusts, physically and psychologically, from pregnancy and birth. The period begins immediately after birth and continues for approximately 6 weeks, or until the body has returned to a near prepregnant state.

This chapter describes the physiologic and psychologic changes that occur postpartally and the basic aspects of a thorough postpartal assessment.

Postpartal Physical Adaptations

Comprehensive nursing assessment is based on a sound understanding of the normal anatomic and physiologic processes of the puerperium. These processes involve the reproductive organs and other major body systems.

Reproductive System

Involution of the Uterus

The term **involution** is used to describe the rapid reduction in size and the return of the uterus to a nonpregnant state. Following separation of the placenta, the decidua of the uterus is irregular, jagged, and varied in thickness. The spongy layer of the decidua is cast off as lochia, and the basal layer of the decidua remains in the uterus to become differentiated into two layers. This occurs within the first 48 to 72 hours after birth. The outermost layer becomes necrotic and is sloughed off in the lochia. The layer closest to the myometrium contains the fundi of the uterine endometrial glands, and these glands lay the foundation for the new endometrium. Except at the placental site, this process is completed in approximately 3 weeks. Healing at the placenta site occurs gradually over 6 weeks, at which point the site is completely healed (Blackburn, 2007). Bleeding from the larger uterine vessels of the placenta site is controlled by compression of the retracted uterine muscle fibers. The clotted blood is gradually absorbed by the body. Some of these vessels are eventually obliterated and replaced by new vessels with smaller lumens.

The placenta site heals by a process of exfoliation and growth of endometrial tissue. This occurs with upward endometrial growth in the decidua basalis under the placental site, with simultaneous growth of endometrial tissue from the margins of the site. The infarcted superficial tissue then becomes necrotic and is sloughed off (Blackburn, 2007). *Exfoliation* is a very important aspect of involution; if healing of the placenta site leaves a fibrous scar, the area available for future implantation is limited, as is the number of possible pregnancies.

With the dramatic decrease in the levels of circulating estrogen and progesterone following placental separation, the uterine cells atrophy, and the hyperplasia of pregnancy

TABLE 30–1	Factors that Retard Uterine Involution
Factor	**Rationale**
Prolonged labor	Muscles relax because of prolonged time of contraction during labor.
Anesthesia	Muscles relax.
Difficult birth	The uterus is manipulated excessively.
Grand multiparity	Repeated distention of uterus during pregnancy and labor leads to muscle stretching, diminished tone, and muscle relaxation.
Full bladder	As the uterus is pushed up and usually to the right, pressure on it interferes with effective uterine contraction.
Incomplete expulsion of placenta or membranes	The presence of even small amounts of tissue interferes with the ability of the uterus to remain firmly contracted.
Infection	Inflammation interferes with the uterine muscle's ability to contract effectively.
Overdistention of uterus	Overstretching of uterine muscles with conditions such as multiple gestation, hydramnios, or a very large baby may set the stage for slower uterine involution.

begins to reverse. Proteolytic enzymes are released, and macrophages migrate to the uterus to promote autolysis (self-digestion). Protein material in the uterine wall is broken down and absorbed. Factors that enhance involution include an uncomplicated labor and birth, complete expulsion of the placenta or membranes, breastfeeding, manual removal of the placenta during a cesarean birth, and early ambulation. Factors that slow uterine involution and rationale for each factor are listed in Table 30–1.

Changes in Fundal Position

The **fundus** (top portion of the uterus) is situated in the midline midway between the symphysis pubis and the umbilicus (Figure 30–1 ■). Immediately following the birth of the placenta, the uterus contracts to the size of a large grapefruit. The walls of the contracted uterus are in close proximity, and the uterine blood vessels are firmly compressed by the myometrium. Within 6 to 12 hours after birth, the fundus of the uterus rises to the level of the umbilicus because of blood and clots that remain within the uterus and changes in support of the uterus by the ligaments. A fundus that is above the umbilicus and boggy (feels soft and spongy rather than firm and well contracted) is associated with excessive uterine bleeding. As blood collects and forms clots within the uterus, the fundus rises; firm contractions of the uterus are interrupted, causing a **boggy uterus (uterine atony)**. When the fundus is higher than expected on palpation and is not in the midline (usually deviated to the right), distention of the bladder should be suspected; the bladder should be emptied

MyNursingKit | Video: Fourth Stage

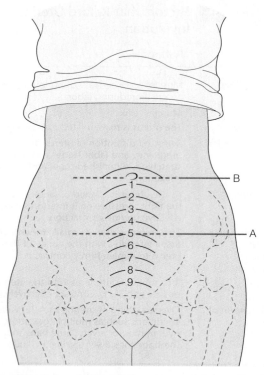

FIGURE 30–1 Involution of the uterus. *A,* Immediately after delivery of the placenta, the top of the fundus is in the midline and approximately halfway between the symphysis pubis and the umbilicus. About 6 to 12 hours after birth, the fundus is at the level of the umbilicus. *B,* The height of the fundus then decreases about one finger breadth (approximately 1 cm) each day.

immediately and the uterus remeasured (Figure 30–2 ■). If the woman is unable to void, in-and-out catheterization of the bladder may be required. In the immediate postpartum period many women may not be aware of a full bladder. Because the uterine ligaments are still stretched, a full bladder can move the uterus. By the end of the puerperium these ligaments have regained their nonpregnant length and tension.

After birth the top of the fundus remains at the level of the umbilicus for about half a day. On the first postpartum day, the top of the fundus is located about 1 cm below the umbilicus. The top of the fundus descends approximately one finger breadth (width of index, second, or third finger), or 1 cm, per day until it descends into the pelvis on about the 10th day.

CRITICAL THINKING

You have completed your assessment of Patty Clark, a 24-year-old, G2P2 woman who is 24 hours past childbirth. The fundus is just above the umbilicus and slightly to the right. Lochia rubra is present, and a pad is soaked every 2 hours. What would you do?

Answers can be found in Appendix F ∞.

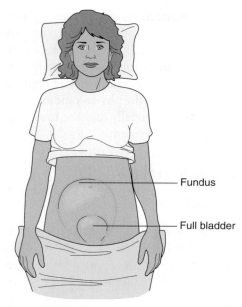

FIGURE 30–2 The uterus becomes displaced and deviated to the right when the bladder is full.

If the mother is breastfeeding, the release of endogenous oxytocin from the posterior pituitary in response to suckling hastens involution of the uterus. Barring complications, such as infection or retained placental fragments, the uterus approaches its prepregnant size and location by 5 to 6 weeks. In women who had an oversized uterus during the pregnancy (because of hydramnios, birth of a large-for-gestational-age {LGA} infant, or multiple gestation), the time frame for an immediate uterine involution process is lengthened. If intrauterine infection is present, in addition to foul-smelling lochia or vaginal discharge, the uterine fundus descends much more slowly. When infection is suspected, other clinical signs such as fever and tachycardia in addition to delay in involution must be assessed. Any slowing of descent is called **subinvolution** (for further discussion of subinvolution, see Chapter 33 ∞).

Lochia

The uterus rids itself of the debris remaining after birth through a discharge called **lochia**, which is classified according to its appearance and contents. **Lochia rubra** is dark red. It occurs for the first 2 to 3 days and contains epithelial cells, erythrocytes, leukocytes, shreds of decidua, and occasionally fetal meconium, lanugo, and vernix. Clotting is often the result of pooling of blood in the upper portion of the vagina. A few small clots (no larger than a nickel) are common, particularly in the first few days after birth. However, lochia should not contain large (plum-size) clots; if it does the cause should be investigated without delay. **Lochia serosa** is a pinkish color. It follows from about day 3 until day 10. Lochia serosa is composed of serous exudate (hence the name), shreds of degenerating decidua, erythrocytes, leukocytes, cervical mucus, and numerous microorganisms (Blackburn, 2007).

The red blood cell (RBC) component decreases gradually, and a creamy or yellowish discharge persists for an additional week or two. This final discharge, termed **lochia alba** from the Latin word for *white*, is composed primarily of leukocytes, decidual cells, epithelial cells, fat, cervical mucus, cholesterol crystals, and bacteria. Recent studies examining lochia patterns have found that the lochia rubra phase lasts longer than generally assumed and that it varies according to breastfeeding practice and parity (Blackburn, 2007). Variation in the duration of lochia discharge is not uncommon; however, the trend should be toward a lighter amount of flow and a lighter color of discharge. When the lochia flow stops, the cervix is considered closed, and chances of infection ascending from the vagina to the uterus decrease.

Like menstrual discharge, lochia flow has a musty, stale odor that is not offensive. Microorganisms are always present in the vaginal lochia, and by the second day following birth the uterus is contaminated with the vaginal bacteria. It is thought that an infection does not develop because the organisms involved are relatively nonvirulent. Any foul smell to the lochia or used peripad suggests infection and the need for prompt additional assessment, such as white blood cell (WBC) count and differential and assessment for uterine tenderness and fever.

The total average volume of lochia is about 225 mL, and the daily volume gradually decreases (Blackburn, 2007). Discharge is greater in the morning because of pooling in the vagina and uterus while the mother lies sleeping. The amount of lochia may also be increased by exertion or breastfeeding. Multiparous women usually have more lochia than first-time mothers. Women who undergo a cesarean birth typically have less lochia than women who give birth vaginally (Blackburn, 2007).

Evaluation of lochia is necessary not only to determine the presence of hemorrhage but also to assess uterine involution. The type, amount, and consistency of lochia determines the stage of healing of the placenta site, and a progressive change from bright red at birth to dark red to pink to white or clear discharge should be observed. Persistent discharge of lochia rubra or a return to lochia rubra indicates subinvolution or late postpartal hemorrhage (see Chapter 33 ∞).

The nurse should exercise caution in evaluating bleeding immediately after birth. The continuous seepage of blood is more consistent with cervical or vaginal lacerations and may be effectively diagnosed when the bleeding is evaluated in conjunction with the consistency of the uterus. Lacerations should be suspected if the uterus is firm and of expected size and if no clots can be expressed.

Cervical Changes

Following birth the cervix is flabby, formless, and may appear bruised. The lateral aspects of the external os are frequently lacerated during the birth process (Cunningham et al., 2005). The external os is markedly irregular and closes slowly. It admits two fingers for a few days following birth, but by the end of the first week it admits only a fingertip.

The shape of the external os is permanently changed by the first childbearing. The characteristic dimplelike os of the nullipara changes to the transverse slit (fish-mouth) os of the multipara (Blackburn, 2007). After significant cervical laceration or several lacerations, the cervix may appear lopsided. Because of the slight change in the size of the cervix, a diaphragm or cervical cap will need to be refitted if the woman is using one of these methods of contraception.

Vaginal Changes

Following birth the vagina appears edematous and may be bruised. Small superficial lacerations may be evident, and the rugae are obliterated. The apparent bruising is caused by pelvic congestion and trauma and will quickly disappear. The hymen, torn and jagged, heals irregularly, leaving small tags called *carunculae myrtiformes*.

The size of the vagina decreases and rugae return within 3 to 4 weeks (Blackburn, 2007). This facilitates the gradual return to smaller, although not nulliparous, dimensions. By 6 weeks the nonbreastfeeding woman's vagina usually appears normal. The lactating woman is in a hypoestrogenic state because of ovarian suppression, and her vaginal mucosa may be pale and without rugae; the effects of the lowered estrogen level may lead to dyspareunia (painful intercourse), which may be reduced by the addition of a water-soluble personal lubricant. Tone and contractility of the vaginal orifice may be improved by perineal tightening exercises such as Kegel exercises (see Chapter 11 ∞), which may begin soon after birth. The labia majora and labia minora are more flaccid in the woman who has borne a child than in the nullipara.

Perineal Changes

During the early postpartal period the soft tissue in and around the perineum may appear edematous, with some bruising. If an episiotomy or a laceration is present, the edges should be drawn together. Occasionally, ecchymosis occurs, and this may delay healing. Initial healing of the episiotomy or laceration occurs in 2 to 3 weeks after the birth, although complete healing may take up to 4 to 6 months (Blackburn, 2007). Perineal discomfort may be present during this time.

Recurrence of Ovulation and Menstruation

The return of ovulation and menstruation varies for each postpartal woman. In nonbreastfeeding mothers, menstruation generally returns between 4 and 6 weeks after birth. The first postpartum menstrual cycles may be anovulatory, although up to 25% of these cycles are preceded by ovulation (Blackburn, 2007). The return of ovulation is directly associated with a rise in the serum progesterone level. In nonlactating mothers the average time to first ovulation can be as early as 27 days with a mean time of 70 to 75 days (Lipscomb & Novy, 2007).

The return of ovulation and menstruation in breastfeeding mothers is usually prolonged and is associated with the length of time the woman breastfeeds and whether formula supplements are used. If a mother breastfeeds for less than 1 month, the return of menstruation and ovulation is similar to that of the nonbreastfeeding mother. In women who exclusively breastfeed, menstruation is usually delayed for at least 3 months. Suckling by the infant typically results in alterations in the gonadotropin releasing hormone (GnRH) production, which is thought to be the cause of amenorrhea (Blackburn, 2007). Although exclusive breastfeeding helps to reduce the risk of pregnancy for the first 6 months after birth, it should be relied upon only temporarily and if it meets the observed criteria for lactational amenorrhea method (LAM). Furthermore, because ovulation precedes menstruation and women often supplement breastfeeding with bottles and pacifiers, breastfeeding is not considered a reliable means of contraception.

Abdomen

The uterine ligaments (notably the round and broad ligaments) are stretched and require the length of the puerperium to recover. Although the stretched abdominal wall appears loose and flabby, it responds to exercise within 2 to 3 months. However, the abdomen may fail to regain good tone and will remain flabby in the grand multipara, in the woman whose abdomen is overdistended, or in the woman with poor muscle tone before pregnancy. **Diastasis recti abdominis**, a separation of the abdominal muscle, may occur with pregnancy, especially in women with poor abdominal muscle tone (Figure 30–3 ■). If diastasis occurs, part of the abdominal wall has no muscular support but is formed only by skin, subcutaneous fat, fascia, and peritoneum. This may be especially pronounced in women who have undergone a cesarean section, as the rectus abdominis muscles are manually separated to access the uterine muscle. Improvement depends on the physical condition of the mother, the total number of pregnancies, pregnancy spacing, and the type and amount of physical exercise. This may result in a pendulous abdomen and increased maternal backache. Fortunately, diastasis responds well to exercise, and abdominal muscle tone can improve significantly.

The striae (stretch marks), which occurred as a result of stretching and rupture of the elastic fibers of the skin,

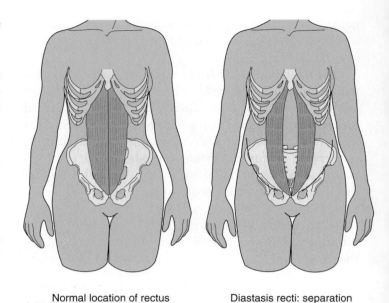

Normal location of rectus muscles of the abdomen

Diastasis recti: separation of the rectus muscles

FIGURE 30–3 Diastasis recti abdominis, a separation of the abdominal musculature, commonly occurs after pregnancy.

take on different colors based on the mother's skin color. The striae of Caucasian mothers are red to purple at the time of birth and gradually fade to silver or white. The striae of mothers with darker skin, in contrast, are darker than the surrounding skin and remain darker. These marks gradually fade after a time but remain visible.

Lactation

During pregnancy, breast development in preparation for lactation results from the influence of both estrogen and progesterone. After birth, the interplay of maternal hormones leads to milk production. (For further details, see the section on breastfeeding in Chapter 27 ∞).

Gastrointestinal System

Hunger following birth is common, and the mother may enjoy eating a light meal. Frequently, she is quite thirsty and will drink large amounts of fluid. Drinking fluids helps replace fluids lost during labor, in the urine, and through perspiration.

The bowels tend to be sluggish following birth because of the lingering effects of progesterone, decreased abdominal muscle tone, and bowel evacuation associated with the labor and birth process. Women who have had an episiotomy, lacerations, or hemorrhoids may tend to delay elimination for fear of increasing their pain or because they believe their stitches will be torn if they bear down. In refusing or delaying the bowel movement, the woman may cause increased constipation and more pain when bowel elimination finally occurs.

The woman with a cesarean birth may receive clear liquids shortly after surgery; once bowel sounds are present, her diet is quickly advanced to solid food. In addition, the woman may experience some initial discomfort from flatulence, which is relieved by early ambulation and use of antiflatulent medications. Chamomile tea and peppermint tea may also be helpful in reducing discomfort from flatulence. It may take a few days for the bowel to regain its tone, especially if general anesthesia was used. The woman who has had a cesarean or a difficult birth may benefit from stool softeners.

Urinary Tract

The postpartal woman has an increased bladder capacity, swelling and bruising of the tissue around the urethra, decreased sensitivity to fluid pressure, and a decreased sensation of bladder filling. Consequently, she is at risk for overdistention, incomplete bladder emptying, and a buildup of residual urine. Women who have had an anesthetic block have inhibited neural functioning of the bladder and are more susceptible to bladder distention, difficulty voiding, and bladder infections. In addition, immediate postpartal use of oxytocin to facilitate uterine contractions following expulsion of the placenta has an antidiuretic effect. Following cessation of the oxytocin the woman will experience rapid bladder filling (Cunningham et al., 2005).

Urinary output increases during the early postpartal period (first 12 to 24 hours) because of *puerperal diuresis*. The kidneys must eliminate an estimated 2000 to 3000 mL of extracellular fluid with the normal pregnancy, which causes rapid filling of the bladder. Thus adequate bladder elimination is an immediate concern. Women with preeclampsia, chronic hypertension, and diabetes experience greater fluid retention than other women, and postpartal diuresis is increased accordingly.

If urine stasis exists, chances for urinary tract infection increase because of bacteriuria and the presence of dilated ureters and renal pelves, which persist for about 6 weeks after birth. A full bladder may also increase the tendency of the uterus to relax by displacing the uterus and interfering with its contractility, leading to hemorrhage. In the absence of infection, the dilated ureters and renal pelves return to prepregnant size by the end of the sixth week.

Vital Signs

During the postpartal period, with the exception of the first 24 hours, the woman should be afebrile. Epidural anesthesia for labor, which can interfere with heat dissipation, has a direct effect on maternal temperature but rarely results in overt fever (Alexander, 2005). A maternal temperature of up to 38°C (100.4°F) may occur after childbirth as a result of the exertion and dehydration of labor. An increase in temperature to between 37.8°C and 39°C (100°F to 102.2°F) may also occur during the first 24 hours after the mother's milk comes in (Cunningham et al., 2005). However, in women not meeting these criteria, infection must be considered in the presence of an increased temperature (see discussion in Chapter 33 ∞).

Immediately following childbirth, many women experience a transient rise in both systolic and diastolic blood pressure, which spontaneously returns to the prepregnancy baseline over the next few days (Varney et al., 2004). A decrease may indicate physiologic readjustment to decreased intrapelvic pressure, or it may be related to uterine hemorrhage. Orthostatic hypotension, as indicated by feelings of faintness or dizziness immediately after standing up, can develop in the first 48 hours as a result of abdominal engorgement that may occur after birth. A low or decreasing blood pressure may reflect hypovolemia secondary to hemorrhage, but it is a late sign. Blood pressure elevations may result from excessive use of oxytocin or vasopressor medications. Because preeclampsia can persist into or occur first in the postpartum period, routine evaluation of blood pressure is needed. If a woman complains of headache, hypertension must be ruled out before analgesics are administered.

Puerperal bradycardia with rates of 50 to 70 beats per minute (bpm) commonly occurs during the first 6 to 10 days of the postpartal period. It may be related to decreased cardiac effort, the decreased blood volume following placental separation and contraction of the uterus, and increased stroke volume. A pulse rate greater than 100 bpm may be indicative of hypovolemia, infection, fear, or pain and requires further assessment.

Blood Values

Blood values should return to the prepregnant state by the end of the postpartal period. Pregnancy-associated activation of coagulation factors may continue for variable amounts of time after birth. This condition, in conjunction with trauma, immobility, or sepsis, predisposes the woman to the development of thromboembolism. The incidence of thromboembolism is reduced by early mobilization.

Nonpathologic leukocytosis often occurs during labor and in the immediate postpartum period, with white blood cell counts of 25,000 to 30,000/mm³ (James, 2008). WBC values typically return to normal levels by the end of the first postpartum week. Leukocytosis combined with the normal increase in erythrocyte sedimentation rate may obscure the diagnosis of acute infection at this time (James, 2008).

Hemoglobin and hematocrit levels may be difficult to interpret in the first 2 days after birth because of the changing blood volume. This loss in blood in the first 24 hours accounts for half of the RBC volume gained during the course of the pregnancy. Blood loss averages 400 mL with a vaginal birth and nearly 1000 mL with a cesarean birth (Lipscomb & Novy, 2007). Lochia constitutes less than 25% of this blood loss (Varney, Kriebs, & Gegor, 2004). As extracellular fluid is excreted, hemoconcentration occurs, with a concomitant rise in hematocrit. A drop in values indicates an abnormal blood loss. The following is a convenient rule to remember: A two to three percentage point drop in hematocrit equals a blood loss of 500 mL (James, 2008). After 3 to 4 days, mobilization of interstitial fluid leads to a slight increase in plasma volume. This hemodilution leads to a decrease in hemoglobin, hematocrit, and plasma protein by the end of the first postpartum week. Decreases in plasma volume reach nonpregnant levels by 4 to 6 weeks postpartum (Blackburn, 2007).

Platelet levels typically fall as a result of placental separation. They then begin to increase by the third to fourth postpartum day, gradually returning to normal by the sixth postpartum week. Fibrinolytic activity typically returns to normal during the hours following birth. The hemostatic system as a whole reaches its normal prepregnant status by 3 to 4 weeks postpartum; however, the diameter of deep veins can take up to 6 weeks to return to prepregnant levels (Blackburn, 2007). This is why there is a prolonged risk of thromboembolism in the first 6 weeks following birth.

Cardiovascular Changes

The cardiovascular system undergoes dramatic changes during the birth that can result in cardiovascular instability because of an increase in the cardiac output. The cardiac output typically stabilizes and returns to pregnancy levels within an hour following birth. Maternal hypervolemia acts to protect the mother from excessive blood loss. Cardiac output declines by 30% in the first 2 weeks and reaches normal levels by 6 to 12 weeks (Blackburn, 2007). For a more detailed description of cardiovascular changes that occur immediately following birth, consult a perinatal physiology text. Diuresis in the first 2 to 5 days assists to decrease the extracellular fluid and results in a weight loss of 3 kg (James, 2008). Failure to diuresis in the immediate postpartum period can lead to pulmonary edema and subsequent cardiac problems. This is seen more commonly in women with a history of preeclampsia or preexisting cardiac problems (Cunningham et al., 2005; James, 2008).

Neurologic and Immunologic Changes

Neurologic problems and disorders can predispose women to higher rates of morbidity and mortality during pregnancy and in the postpartum period. Headaches are the most common neurologic symptoms encountered by postpartum women. Headaches may result from fluid shifts in the first week after birth, leakage of cerebrospinal fluid into the extradural space during spinal anesthesia, gestational hypertension, or stress (James, 2008). Migraine headaches, although less frequent during pregnancy, tend to resume in the postpartum period. Women with epilepsy are at a 1% to 2% risk of having a seizure in the immediate postpartum period (Tatum, Liporace, Benbadis et al., 2004). It is nine times more likely that a woman will have a seizure during labor or in the first 24 hours after birth than it is during the pregnancy (Shehata & Okosun, 2004). Women with epilepsy also have more feeding difficulties, irritability, and lethargy. Women with MS or Guillain-Barré syndrome are more likely to have symptoms in the postpartum period than during pregnancy (Samuels & Niebyl, 2007). Myasthenia gravis is an autoimmune disease that affects the neuromuscular junctions. The exacerbation of symptoms during pregnancy is variable; however, the first month of pregnancy and the first month of the postpartal period is the most critical (Kalayjian & Goodwin, 2007).

Weight Loss

An initial weight loss of about 10 to 12 lb occurs as a result of the birth of the infant, placenta, and amniotic fluid. Diuresis accounts for the loss of an additional 5 lb during the early puerperium. By the sixth to eighth week after birth, many women have returned to approximately prepregnant weight if they gained the average 25 to 30 lb. For others, a return to prepregnant weight may take longer. Women often express concern about the slow pace of their postpartum weight loss. Multiparas tend to be more positive than primiparas, probably because the multipara's previous experience has prepared her for the fact that the body does not immediately return to a prepregnant state.

Postpartal Chill

Frequently the mother experiences intense tremors that resemble shivering from a chill immediately after birth. Several theories have been offered to explain this shivering: It is the result of sudden release of pressure on the pelvic nerves after birth, a response to a fetus-to-mother transfusion that occurred during placental separation, a reaction to maternal adrenaline production during labor and birth, or a reaction to epidural anesthesia. If not followed by fever, this chill is of no clinical concern, but it is uncomfortable for the woman. The nurse can increase the woman's comfort by covering her with a warmed blanket and reassuring her that the shivering is a common, self-limiting situation. If she allows herself to go with the shaking, the shivering will last only a short time. Some women may also find a warm beverage helpful. Later in the puerperium, chill and fever indicate infection and require further evaluation.

Postpartal Diaphoresis

The elimination of excess fluid and waste products via the skin during the puerperium produces increased perspiration. Diaphoretic (sweating) episodes frequently occur at night, and the woman may awaken drenched with perspiration. This perspiration is not significant clinically, but the mother should be protected from chilling.

Afterpains

Afterpains are more common in multiparas than in primiparas and are caused by intermittent uterine contractions. Although the uterus of the primipara usually remains consistently contracted, the lost tone of the multiparous uterus results in alternate contraction and relaxation. This phenomenon also occurs if the uterus has been markedly distended, as with a multiple-gestation pregnancy or hydramnios, or if clots or placental fragments were retained. These afterpains may cause the mother severe discomfort for 2 to 3 days after birth. The administration of oxytocic agents (intravenous infusion with Pitocin or oral administration of Methergine) stimulates uterine contraction and increases the discomfort of the afterpains. Because endogenous oxytocin is released when the infant suckles, breastfeeding also increases the frequency and severity of the afterpains. A warm water bottle placed against the lower abdomen may reduce the discomfort of afterpains. In addition, the breastfeeding mother may find it helpful to take a mild analgesic agent approximately 1 hour before feeding her infant. (See the Teaching Card on postpartal comfort measures in the center of this text.) The nurse can assure the nursing mother that the prescribed analgesics are not harmful to the newborn and help improve the quality of the breastfeeding experience. An analgesic is also helpful at bedtime if the afterpains interfere with the mother's rest.

Postpartal Psychologic Adaptations

The postpartal period is a time of readjustment and adaptation for the entire childbearing family, but especially for the mother. The woman experiences a variety of responses as she adjusts to a new family member, postpartal discomforts, changes in her body image, and the reality that she is no longer pregnant.

Taking-In and Taking-Hold

During the first day or two after birth, the woman tends to be passive and somewhat dependent. She follows suggestions, hesitates to make decisions, and is still rather preoccupied with her needs. She may have a great need to talk about her perceptions of her labor and birth. This helps her work through the process, sort out the reality from her fantasized experience, and clarify anything that she did not understand. Food and sleep are major needs. In her early work, Rubin (1961) labeled this the *taking-in* period.

By the second or third day after birth, the new mother was observed to be ready to resume control of her body, her mothering, and her life in general. Rubin (1961) labeled this the *taking-hold* period. If she is breastfeeding, she may worry about her technique or the quality of her milk. If her baby spits up after a feeding, she may view it as a personal failure. She may also feel demoralized by the fact that the nurse or an older family member handles her baby proficiently while she feels unsure and tentative. She requires assurance that she is doing well as a mother. Today's mothers seem to be more independent and adjust more rapidly, exhibiting behaviors of "taking-in" and "taking-hold" in shorter time periods than those previously identified.

Maternal Role Attainment

Maternal role attainment is the process by which a woman learns mothering behaviors and becomes comfortable with her identity as a mother. Formation of a maternal identity occurs with each child a woman bears. As the mother grows to know this child and forms a relationship, the mother's maternal identity gradually and systematically evolves and she "binds in" to the infant (Rubin, 1984).

Maternal role attainment often occurs in four stages (Mercer, 1995):

1. The *anticipatory stage* occurs during pregnancy. The woman looks to role models, especially her own mother, for examples of how to mother.
2. The *formal stage* begins when the child is born. The woman is still influenced by the guidance of others and tries to act as she believes others expect her to act.
3. The *informal stage* begins when the mother begins to make her own choices about mothering. The woman begins to develop her own style of mothering and finds ways of functioning that work well for her.
4. The *personal stage* is the final stage of maternal role attainment. When the woman reaches this stage, she is comfortable with the notion of herself as "mother."

In most cases, maternal role attainment occurs within 3 to 10 months after birth. Social support, the woman's age and personality traits, the marital relationship, the presence of underlying anxiety or depression, the woman's previous childcare skills, the temperament of her infant, and the family's socioeconomic status all influence the woman's success in attaining the maternal role. The postpartum woman faces a number of challenges as she adjusts to her new role (Mercer, 1995):

- For many women, finding time for themselves is one of the greatest challenges. It is often difficult for the new mother to find time to read a book, talk to her partner, or even eat a meal without interruption.
- Women also report feelings of incompetence because they have not mastered all aspects of the mothering role. Often they are unsure of what to do in a given situation.
- The next greatest challenge involves fatigue resulting from sleep deprivation. The demands of nighttime care are tremendously draining, especially if the woman has other children.
- Another challenge faced by the new mother involves the feeling of responsibility that having a child brings. Women experience a sense of lost freedom, an awareness that they will never again be quite as carefree as they were before becoming mothers.
- For women with older children, finding time for them is a challenge. Many women feel guilty because the new baby takes up so much of their time. Sibling rivalry or ill feelings about the baby from other children can put additional stress on the mother.
- Mothers sometimes cite the infant's behavior as a challenge, especially when the child is about 8 months old. Stranger anxiety develops, the infant begins crawling and getting into things, teething may cause fussiness, and the baby's tendency to put everything in his or her mouth requires constant vigilance by the parent.

In 2004, Mercer proposed replacing the term *maternal role attainment* (MRA) with the term *becoming a mother* (BAM). She stated that BAM "more accurately encompasses the dynamic transformation and evolution of a woman's persona than does MRA, and the term MRA should be discontinued" (p. 226) (Mercer, 2004). BAM more accurately reflects the transition process of becoming a mother that changes throughout the maternal-child relationship.

Postpartal nurses need to be aware of the long-term adjustments and stresses that the childbearing family faces as its members adjust to new and different roles. They can help by providing anticipatory guidance about the realities of being a parent, and by giving the postpartal family parenting literature for reference at home. Ongoing parenting groups give parents an opportunity to discuss problems and become comfortable in new roles.

Postpartum Blues

The **postpartum blues** consist of a transient period of depression that occurs during the first few days of the puerperium in 70% of all postpartal women (Varney et al., 2004). It may be manifested by mood swings, anger, weepiness, anorexia, difficulty sleeping, and a feeling of letdown. This mood change frequently occurs while the woman is still hospitalized, but it may occur at home as well. Changing hormone levels are certainly a factor; psychologic adjustments, an unsupportive environment, and insecurity also have been identified as potential causes. In addition, fatigue, discomfort, and overstimulation may play a role. The postpartum blues usually resolve naturally within 10 to 14 days, but if they persist or symptoms worsen, the woman may need evaluation for postpartum depression (see Chapter 33 ∞). Ideally a depression assessment should be completed each trimester to update a pregnant woman's risk status (Beck, 2002). If not done previously, the nurse assesses the woman for predisposing factors during labor and the postpartum stay. Several depression scales are available for assessing postpartum depression. The routine use of a screening tool such as the Edinburgh Postnatal Depression Scale or Postpartum Depression. Predictors Inventory-Revised in a matter-of-fact approach significantly increases the diagnosis (Beck, 2008).

Importance of Social Support

The psychologic outcomes of the postpartal period are far more positive when the parents have access to a support network. Women and their partners may find that family relationships become increasingly important, but the increased family interaction can be a source of stress. The new parents may also have increasing contact with other parents of small children although contact with coworkers declines. Of great concern are women and their partners who have no family or friends with whom to form a social network. Isolation at a time when the woman feels an increased need for support can result in tremendous stress and is often a contributing factor in situations of postpartum depression, child neglect, or abuse. New mother support groups are helpful for women who lack a social support system. The attention that their infant receives from family members is a source of satisfaction to the new parents. In many cases, the ties to the woman's family become especially good. Fathers may report that their relationships with their in-laws become far more positive and supportive. However, the increased family interaction can be a source of stress, especially for the new mother, who tends to have more contact with the families. Postpartum doulas are professionals trained to help the new mother after the birth of the baby. As a "mother helper," postpartum doula services are tailored to help the new mother feel as rested as possible and well-

CULTURAL PERSPECTIVES

Middle East Initial Postpartum Experience

In many countries in the Middle East that follow a patriarchal system, the new mother and her infant stay with the husband's family following the birth of the infant. Frequent visits from the woman's family are discouraged and may even be viewed as burdensome by the husband's family. Typically, only women visit the new mother during the postpartum period. For the birth of the first baby, the wife's parents are expected to purchase all of the baby's supplies and clothing.

nourished, and to place her household in good order so that she can focus her energy on her new baby.

Development of Family Attachment

A mother's first interaction with her infant is influenced by many factors, including her involvement with her family of origin, her relationships, the stability of her home environment, the communication patterns she developed, and the degree of nurturing she received as a child. These factors have shaped the person she has become. The following personal characteristics are also important.

- *Level of trust.* What level of trust has this mother developed in response to her life experiences? What is her philosophy of childrearing? Will she be able to treat her infant as a unique individual with changing needs that should be met as much as possible?
- *Level of self-esteem.* How much does she value herself as a woman and as a mother? Does she feel generally able to cope with the adjustments of life?
- *Capacity for enjoying herself.* Is the mother able to find pleasure in everyday activities and human relationships?
- *Adequacy of knowledge about childbearing and childrearing.* What beliefs about the course of pregnancy, the capabilities of newborns, previous experiences with infants/children, and the nature of her emotions may influence her behavior at first contact with her infant and later?
- *Prevailing mood or usual feeling tone.* Is the woman predominantly content, angry, depressed, or anxious? Is she sensitive to her own feelings and those of others? Will she be able to accept her own needs and to obtain support in meeting them?
- *Reactions to the present pregnancy.* Was the pregnancy planned? Did it go smoothly? Were there ongoing life events that enhanced her pregnancy or depleted her reserves of energy? How have other life roles changed because of her pregnancy and motherhood?

By the time of birth each mother has developed an emotional orientation of some kind to the baby based on these factors.

Initial Maternal Attachment Behavior

After labor and birth, a new mother will demonstrate a fairly regular pattern of maternal behaviors as she continues to familiarize herself with her newborn. In a progression of touching activities, the mother proceeds from fingertip exploration of the newborn's extremities toward palmar contact with larger body areas and finally to enfolding the infant with the whole hand and arm. The time taken to accomplish these steps varies from minutes to days. The mother increases the proportion of time spent in the **en face** position (Figure 30–4 ■). She arranges herself or the newborn so that she has direct face-to-face and eye-to-eye contact. There is an intense interest in having the infant's eyes open. When the infant's eyes are open, the mother characteristically greets the newborn and talks in high-pitched tones to him or her.

In most instances the mother relies heavily on her senses of sight, touch, and hearing in getting to know what her baby is really like. She tends also to respond verbally to any sounds emitted by the newborn, such as cries, coughs, sneezes, and grunts. The sense of smell may be involved as well.

HINTS FOR PRACTICE

Newborns are sometimes taken from their parents immediately after birth and placed in a special care or intensive care nursery. This separation can interfere with the normal attachment process. If this occurs, parents should be brought to the nursery as soon as possible to interact with their infants, and should be allowed to hold and care for their infant as much as possible. If the infant is in an incubator and cannot be held, encourage the parents to stroke the infant's hand, foot, or cheek. Provide reassurance that this will not hurt the infant and is in fact beneficial.

While interacting with her newborn, the mother may be experiencing shock, disbelief, or denial. She may state, "I can't believe she's finally here" or "I feel like he is a stranger." On the other hand, feelings of connectedness between the newborn and the rest of the family can be expressed in positive or negative terms: "She's got your cute nose, Daddy" or "Oh, no! He looks just like Matthew, and he was an impossible baby." A mother's facial expressions or the frequency and content of her questions may demonstrate concerns about the infant's general condition or normality, especially if her pregnancy was complicated or if a previous baby was not healthy.

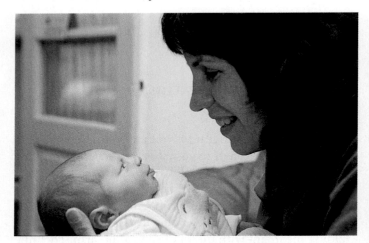

FIGURE 30–4 The mother has direct face-to-face and eye-to-eye contact in the *en face* position.
Source: © Stella Johnson (www.stellajohnson.com).

During the first few days after her child's birth, the new mother applies herself to the task of getting to know her baby. This is termed the *acquaintance phase.* If the infant gives clear behavioral cues about needs the infant's responses to mothering will be predictable, which will make the mother feel effective and competent. Other behaviors that make an infant more attractive to caretakers are smiling, grasping a finger, nursing eagerly, and being easy to console.

During this time the newborn is also becoming acquainted. Within a few days after birth, infants show signs of recognizing recurrent situations and responding to changes in routine. To the extent that their mother is their world, it can be said that they are actively acquainting themselves with her.

During the *phase of mutual regulation,* mother and infant seek to determine the degree of control each partner in their relationship will exert. In this phase of adjustment, a balance is sought between the needs of the mother and the needs of the infant. The most important consideration is that each should obtain a good measure of enjoyment from the interaction. During this phase, negative maternal feelings are likely to surface or intensify. Because "everyone knows that mothers love their babies," these negative feelings often go unexpressed and are allowed to build up. If they are expressed, the response of friends, relatives, or healthcare personnel is often to deny the feelings to the mother: "You don't mean that." Some negative feelings are normal in the first few days after birth, and the nurse should be supportive when the mother vocalizes these feelings.

When mutual regulation arrives at the point where both mother and infant primarily enjoy each other's company, reciprocity has been achieved. **Reciprocity** is an interactional cycle that occurs simultaneously between mother and infant. It involves mutual cuing behaviors, expectancy, rhythmicity, and synchrony. The mother develops a new relationship with an individual who has a unique character

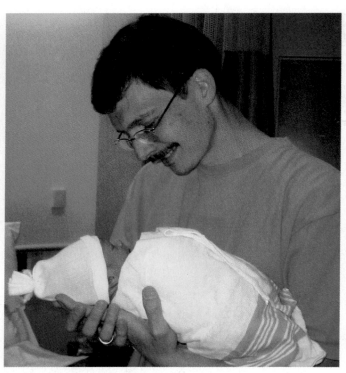

FIGURE 30–5 The father experiences strong feelings of attraction during engrossment.

and evokes a response entirely different from the fantasy response of pregnancy. When reciprocity is synchronous, the interaction between mother and infant is mutually gratifying and is sought and initiated by both partners.

Father-Infant Interactions

In Western cultures, commitment to family-centered maternity care has fostered interest in understanding the feelings and experiences of the new father. Evidence suggests that the father has a strong attraction to his newborn and that the feelings he experiences are similar to the mother's feelings of attachment (Figure 30–5 ■). The characteristic sense of absorption, preoccupation, and interest in the infant demonstrated by fathers during early contact is termed **engrossment**. Differences in involvement still exist among fathers in Western culture and may be influenced by factors other than culture (e.g., previous experience with paternal role or exposure to male/father role models).

> **CULTURAL PERSPECTIVES**
> **Muslim Paternal Attachment**
> In some cultures, there may be little involvement of the father in newborn care. In the Muslim culture, for example, emphasis on childrearing and infant care activities is on the mother and extended female family members. Nurses need to be aware of cultural differences when evaluating a father's interaction with his newborn.

Siblings and Others

Infants are capable of maintaining a number of strong attachments without loss of quality. These attachments may include siblings, grandparents, aunts, and uncles. The social setting and personality of the individual seem to be significant factors in the development of multiple attachments. Birth centers are especially geared toward the inclusion of the family in the birth process. In the hospital setting, the advent of open visiting hours and rooming-in permits siblings and others to participate in the attachment process.

Cultural Influences in the Postpartal Period

Whereas Western culture places primary emphasis on the events of birth, many other cultures place greater emphasis on the postpartum period. For women not of the dominant American culture, the new mother's culture and personal values influence her beliefs about her postpartal care. Her expectations about food, fluids, rest, hygiene, medications and relief measures, support, and counsel—as well as other aspects of her life—will be influenced by the beliefs and values of her family and cultural group. Sometimes, a new mother's wishes will differ from the expectations of the certified nurse-midwife (CNM), physician, or nurse. (See Chapter 2 ∞ for an in-depth discussion.)

Nurses belong to a particular ethnoculture and also share in the culture of health care. Thus their nursing care may include practices that support the general beliefs of these groups, such as offering food and fluids in the recovery period after birth, expecting the woman to ambulate as soon as possible, and assuming the woman will want to shower and perhaps wash her hair soon after giving birth. It is important for nurses to recognize that they are approaching their client's care from their own perspective and that, to individualize care for each mother, they need to assess the woman's preferences, her level of acculturation and assimilation to Western culture, her linguistic abilities, and her educational level (Kim-Goodwin, 2005). In addition, the nurse should have the mother exercise her choices when possible, and support those choices, with the help of cultural awareness and a sound knowledge base.

Although describing particular practices of differing cultural groups always involves some generalization, it is helpful for nurses to understand some of the possible differences in beliefs and practices. The woman of European heritage may expect to eat a full meal and have large amounts of iced fluids after the birth, in the belief that the food restores energy and the fluids help replace fluid lost during the labor. She may want to ambulate shortly after the birth, shower, wash her hair, and put on a fresh gown. She may expect a short stay in the hospital and may or may not be interested in educational classes. Women of the Islamic faith may have specific modesty requirements; the woman must be completely covered, with only her feet and hands exposed, and no man, other than the husband or a family member, may be alone with her (Al-Oballi Kridli, 2002; Lauderdale, 2008).

Some cultures emphasize certain postpartal routines or rituals for mother and baby that are designed to restore the hot-cold balance of the body. Some women of Hispanic, African, and Asian cultures may avoid cold after birth. This prohibition includes cold air, wind, and all water (even if heated). On the other hand, some women of traditional Mexican descent may avoid eating "hot" foods such as pork just after the birth of a baby (considered a "hot" experience). It is important to note that each individual or cultural group may define hot and cold conditions and foods differently. The nurse should ask each woman what she can eat and what foods she thinks would be helpful for healing. The nurse may encourage family members to bring preferred foods and drinks for the mother. For more detailed discussion of the hot-cold balance concept see Cultural Influences Affecting the Family in Chapter 2 ∞.

In many cultures, the extended family plays an essential role during the puerperium. The grandmother is often the primary helper to the mother and newborn. She brings wisdom and experience, allowing the new mother time to rest and giving her ready access to someone who can help with problems and concerns as they arise. It is important to ensure access of all family members to the mother and newborn. Visiting hours may be waived to allow family members or authority figures access to the mother and newborn. These practices show respect and foster a blending of old and new behaviors to meet the goals of all concerned (Purnell & Paulanka, 2008). African American mothers model their mothering skills after their older female relatives. In addition, these same older female relatives usually provide child care as needed (Purnell & Paulanka, 2008). People of Jewish faith observe a Sabbath from sundown Friday to sundown Saturday. During this time, Orthodox Jews do not perform any manual labor; for the postpartal woman, this includes turning on or off the lights, pressing the call bell, or raising/lowering the head of the bed (De Sovo, 1997). Jewish clients may also request a kosher diet. Some traditional Jewish couples avoid physical contact while the woman is experiencing any vaginal discharge; unfortunately the man following this custom may be viewed as unsupportive by the staff during the postpartal period (D'Avanzo & Geissler, 2008).

Postpartal Nursing Assessment

Comprehensive care is based on a thorough assessment that identifies individual needs or potential problems. See the accompanying Assessment Guide: Postpartal—First 24 Hours After Birth.

Physical Assessment/ Normal Findings	Alterations and Possible Causes*	Nursing Responses to Data†
Vital Signs		
Blood pressure (BP): Should remain consistent with baseline BP during pregnancy.	High BP (preeclampsia, essential hypertension, renal disease, anxiety). Drop in BP (may be normal; uterine hemorrhage).	Evaluate history of preexisting disorders and check for other signs of preeclampsia (edema, proteinuria). Assess for other signs of hemorrhage (↑ pulse, cool clammy skin).
Pulse: 50 to 90 beats/minute. May be bradycardia of 50 to 70 beats/minute.	Tachycardia (difficult labor and birth, hemorrhage).	Evaluate for other signs of hemorrhage (↓ BP, cool clammy skin).
Respirations: 16 to 24/minute.	Marked tachypnea (respiratory disease).	Assess for other signs of respiratory disease.
Temperature: 36.6°C to 38°C (98°F to 100.4°F).	After first 24 hours temperature of 38°C (100.4°F) or above suggests infection.	Assess for other signs of infection; notify physician/certified nurse-midwife.
Breasts		
General appearance: Smooth, even pigmentation, changes of pregnancy still apparent; one may appear larger.	Reddened area (mastitis).	Assess further for signs of infection.
Palpation: Depending on postpartal day, may be soft, filling, full, or engorged.	Palpable mass (caked breast, mastitis). Engorgement (venous stasis). Tenderness, heat, edema (engorgement, caked breast, mastitis).	Assess for other signs of infection: If blocked duct, consider heat, massage, position change for breastfeeding. Assess for further signs. Report mastitis to physician/certified nurse-midwife.
Nipples: Supple, pigmented, intact; become erect when stimulated.	Fissures, cracks, soreness (problems with breastfeeding), not erectile with stimulation (inverted nipples).	Reassess technique; recommend appropriate interventions.
Lungs		
Sounds: clear to bases bilaterally.	Diminished (fluid overload, asthma, pulmonary embolus, pulmonary edema).	Assess for other signs of respiratory distress.
Abdomen		
Musculature: Abdomen may be soft, have a "doughy" texture; rectus muscle intact.	Separation in musculature (diastasis recti abdominis).	Evaluate size of diastasis; teach appropriate exercises for decreasing the separation.
Fundus: Firm, midline; following expected process of involution.	Boggy (full bladder, uterine bleeding).	Massage until firm; assess bladder and have woman void if needed; attempt to express clots when firm. If bogginess remains or recurs, report to physician/certified nurse-midwife.
May be tender when palpated.	Constant tenderness (infection).	Assess for evidence of endometritis.
Cesarean section incision dressing; dry and intact.	Moderate to large amount of blood or serosanguinous drainage on dressing.	Assess for hemorrhage. Reinforce dressing and notify healthcare provider.
Lochia		
Scant to moderate amount, earthy odor; no clots.	Large amount, clots (hemorrhage).	Assess for firmness, express additional clots; begin peripad count.
	Foul-smelling lochia (infection).	Assess for other signs of infection; report to physician/certified nurse-midwife.
Normal progression: First 1 to 3 days: rubra.	Failure to progress normally or return to rubra from serosa (subinvolution).	Report to physician/certified nurse-midwife.
Following rubra: Days 3 to 10: serosa (alba seldom seen in hospital).		

Alba = white discharge from 11-14 days.

*Possible causes of alterations are identified in parentheses.

†This column provides guidelines for further assessment and initial nursing actions.

Physical Assessment/ Normal Findings	Alterations and Possible Causes*	Nursing Responses to Data[†]
Perineum		
Slight edema and bruising in intact perineum.	Marked fullness, bruising, pain (vulvar hematoma).	Assess size; apply ice glove or ice pack; report to physician/certified nurse-midwife.
Episiotomy: No redness, edema, ecchymosis, or discharge; edges well approximated.	Redness, edema, ecchymosis, discharge, or gaping stitches (infection).	Encourage sitz baths; review perineal care, appropriate wiping techniques.
Hemorrhoids: None present; if present, should be small and nontender.	Full, tender, inflamed hemorrhoids.	Encourage sitz baths, side-lying position; Tucks pads, anesthetic ointments, manual replacement of hemorrhoids, stool softeners, increased fluid intake.
Costovertebral Angle (CVA) Tenderness		
None.	Present (kidney infection).	Assess for other symptoms of urinary tract infection (UTI); obtain clean-catch urine; report to physician/certified nurse-midwife.
Lower Extremities		
No pain with palpation; negative Homans' sign.	Positive findings (thrombophlebitis).	Report to physician/certified nurse-midwife.
Elimination		
Urinary output: Voiding in sufficient quantities at least every 4 to 6 hours; bladder not palpable.	Inability to void (urinary retention). Symptoms of urgency, frequency, dysuria (UTI).	Employ nursing interventions to promote voiding; if not successful, obtain order for catheterization. Report symptoms of UTI to physician/certified nurse-midwife.
Bowel elimination: Should have normal bowel movement by second or third day after birth.	Inability to pass feces (constipation caused by fear of pain from episiotomy, hemorrhoids, perineal trauma).	Encourage fluids, ambulation, roughage in diet; sitz baths to promote healing of perineum; obtain order for stool softener.

Cultural Assessment[‡]	Variations to Consider*	Nursing Responses to Data[†]
Determine customs and practices regarding postpartum care. Ask the mother whether she would like fluids, and ask what temperature she prefers.	Individual preference may include: Room-temperature or warmed fluids rather than iced drinks.	Provide for specific request if possible. If woman is unable to provide specific information, the nurse may draw from general information regarding cultural variation.
Ask the mother what foods or fluids she would like.	Special foods or fluids to hasten healing after childbirth.	Mexican women may want food and fluids that restore hot-cold balance to the body. Women of European background may ask for iced fluids.
Ask the mother whether she would prefer to be alone during breastfeeding.	Some women may be hesitant to have someone with them when their breast is exposed.	Provide privacy as desired by mother.

Psychosocial Assessment/ Normal Findings	Variations to Consider*	Nursing Responses to Data[†]
Psychologic Adaptation		
During first 24 hours: Passive; preoccupied with own needs; may talk about her labor and birth experience; may be talkative, elated, or very quiet.	Very quiet and passive; sleeps frequently (fatigue from long labor; feelings of disappointment about some aspect of the experience; may be following cultural expectation).	Provide opportunities for adequate rest; provide nutritious meals and snacks that are consistent with what the woman desires to eat and drink; provide opportunities to discuss birth experience in nonjudgmental atmosphere if the woman desires to do so.
[‡]These are only a few suggestions. It is not our intent to imply this is a comprehensive cultural assessment.	*Possible causes of alterations are identified in parentheses.	[†]This column provides guidelines for further assessment and initial nursing actions.

(Continued on next page)

ASSESSMENT GUIDE   POSTPARTAL—FIRST 24 HOURS AFTER BIRTH *(Continued)*

Psychosocial Assessment/ Normal Findings	Variations to Consider*	Nursing Responses to Data†
Usually by 12 hours: Beginning to assume responsibility; some women eager to learn; easily feels overwhelmed.	Excessive weepiness, mood swings, pronounced irritability (postpartum blues; feelings of inadequacy; culturally proscribed behavior).	Explain postpartum blues; provide supportive atmosphere; determine support available for mother; consider referral for evidence of profound depression.
Attachment *En face* position; holds baby close; cuddles and soothes; calls by name; identifies characteristics of family members in infant; may be awkward in providing care. Initially may express disappointment over sex or appearance of infant but within 1 to 2 days demonstrates attachment behaviors.	Continued expressions of disappointment in sex, appearance of infant; refusal to care for infant; derogatory comments; lack of bonding behaviors (difficulty in attachment, following expectations of cultural/ethnic group).	Provide reinforcement and support for infant caretaking behaviors; maintain nonjudgmental approach and gather more information if caretaking behaviors are not evident.
Client Education Has basic understanding of self-care activities and infant care needs; can identify signs of complications that should be reported.	Unable to demonstrate basic self-care and infant care activities (knowledge deficit; postpartum blues; following prescribed cultural behavior and will be cared for by grandmother or other family member).	Identify predominate learning style. Determine whether woman understands English and provide interpreter if needed; provide reinforcement of information through conversation and through written material (remember that some women and their families may not be able to understand written materials because of language difficulties or inability to read); provide information regarding infant care skills that are culturally consistent; give woman opportunity to express her feelings; consider social service home referral for women who have no family or other support, are unable to take in information about self-care and infant care, and demonstrate no caretaking activities.
	*Possible causes of alterations are identified in parentheses.	†This column provides guidelines for further assessment and initial nursing actions.

Risk Factors

Ongoing assessment and client education during the puerperium is designed to meet the needs of the childbearing family and to detect and treat possible complications. Table 30–2 identifies factors that may place the new mother at risk during the postpartal period. The nurse uses this knowledge during the assessment and is particularly alert for possible complications associated with identified risk factors. (See the Teaching Card: Teaching Postpartum Warning Signs in the center of this text.)

Physical Assessment

The nurse should remember the following principles in preparing for and completing the assessment of the postpartal woman.

- Select a time that will provide the most accurate data. Palpating the fundus when the woman has a full bladder, for example, may give false information about the progress of involution. Ask the woman to void before assessment.

TABLE 30-2

Preeclampsia	↑ Blood pressure ↑ CNS irritability ↑ Need for bed rest → ↑ risk thrombophlebitis
Diabetes	Need for insulin regulation Episodes of hypoglycemia or hyperglycemia ↓ Healing
Cardiac disease	↑ Maternal exhaustion
Cesarean birth	↑ Healing needs ↑ Pain from incision ↑ Risk of infection ↑ Length of hospitalization
Overdistention of uterus (multiple gestation, hydramnios)	↑ Risk of hemorrhage ↑ Risk of thrombophlebitis (C/S risk) ↑ Risk of anemia ↑ Risk of breastfeeding problems (C/S risk) ↑ Stretching of abdominal muscles ↑ Incidence and severity of afterpains
Abruptio placentae, placenta previa	Hemorrhage → anemia ↓ Uterine contractility after birth → ↑ infection risk
Precipitous labor (less than 3 hours)	↑ Risk of lacerations to birth canal → hemorrhage
Prolonged labor (greater than 24 hours)	Exhaustion ↑ Risk of hemorrhage Nutritional and fluid depletion ↑ Bladder atony and/or trauma
Difficult birth	Exhaustion ↑ Risk of perineal lacerations ↑ Risk of hematomas ↑ Risk of hemorrhage → anemia
Extended period of time in stirrups at birth	↑ Risk of thrombophlebitis
Retained placenta	↑ Risk of hemorrhage ↑ Risk of infection

KEY FACTS TO REMEMBER

Common Postpartal Concerns

Several postpartal occurrences cause special concern for mothers. The nurse will frequently be asked about the following events.

SOURCE OF CONCERN	EXPLANATION
Gush of blood that sometimes occurs when she first arises	Because of normal pooling of blood in the vagina when the woman lies down to rest or sleep. Gravity causes blood to flow out when she stands.
Passing clots	Blood pools at the top of the vagina and forms clots that are passed upon rising or sitting on the toilet.
Night sweats	Normal physiologic occurrence that results as the body attempts to eliminate excess fluids that were present during pregnancy. May be aggravated by a plastic mattress pad.
Afterpains	More common in multiparas. Caused by contractions and relaxation of uterus. Increased by oxytocin, breastfeeding. Relieved with mild analgesics and time.
"Large stomach" after birth and failure to lose all weight gained during pregnancy	The baby, amniotic fluid, and placenta account for only a portion of the weight gained during pregnancy. The remainder takes approximately 6 weeks to lose. Abdomen also appears large because of decreased muscle tone. Postpartal exercises will help.

• Explain the purpose of regular assessment.

• Ensure that the woman is relaxed before starting; perform the procedures as gently as possible to avoid unnecessary discomfort.

• Record and report the results as clearly as possible.

• Take appropriate precautions to prevent exposure to body fluids.

While performing the physical assessment, the nurse should also be teaching the woman. For example, when assessing the breasts of a lactating woman, the nurse can discuss breast care, breast milk production, the letdown reflex, and breast self-examination. A new mother may be very receptive to instruction on postpartal abdominal tightening exercises when the nurse assesses the woman's fundal height and diastasis. The assessment also provides an excellent time to provide information about the body's postpartal physical and anatomic changes as well as danger signs to report. (See Key Facts to Remember: Common Postpartal Concerns.) Because the time new mothers spend in the postpartum unit is limited, nurses need to use every available opportunity for client education about self-care. To assist nurses in recognizing these opportuni-

ties, examples of client teaching during the assessment are provided throughout the following discussion.

Vital Signs

The nurse may choose to organize the physical assessment in a variety of ways. Many nurses begin by assessing vital signs because the findings are more accurate when they are obtained with the woman at rest. In addition, establishing whether the vital signs are within the expected normal range will assist the nurse in determining if other assessments are needed. For instance, if the temperature is elevated, the nurse considers the time since birth and gathers information to determine whether the woman is dehydrated or whether an infection is developing.

Temperature elevations (less than 38°C [100.4°F]) caused by normal processes should last for only 24 hours. The nurse evaluates any elevation of temperature in light of associated signs and symptoms and carefully reviews the woman's history to identify other factors, such as premature rupture of membranes (PROM) or prolonged labor that might increase the incidence of infection in the genital tract.

Alterations in vital signs may indicate complications, so the nurse assesses them at regular intervals. After an immediate, transient rise after birth, the blood pressure should remain stable. The pulse often shows a characteristic slowness that is no cause for alarm. Pulse rates return to prepregnant norms very quickly unless complications arise.

The nurse informs the woman of her vital signs and provides information about the normal changes in blood pressure and pulse. This may be an opportunity to determine whether the mother knows how to assess her own and her infant's temperature, how to read a thermometer, and how to select a thermometer from the wide variety now available.

HINTS FOR PRACTICE

During the first few hours after birth, the woman may have some orthostatic hypotension. This will cause her to have a lower blood pressure reading in a sitting position. For the most accurate reading, measure her blood pressure with her in the same position each time, preferably lying on her back with her arm at her side. Because of the propensity for hypotension, the nurse should assist the mother the first few times she attempts to ambulate after childbirth.

Auscultation of Lungs

The breath sounds should be clear. Women who have been treated for preterm labor or preeclampsia are at higher risk for pulmonary edema (see Care of the Woman with a Hypertensive Disorder in Chapter 16 ∞ for further discussion).

HINTS FOR PRACTICE

An easy way to remember the components specific to the postpartal examination is to remember the term BUBBLEHE: B-breast, U-uterus, B-bladder, B-bowel, L-lochia, E-episiotomy/laceration/edema, H-Homans'/hemorrhoids, E-emotional.

Breasts

Before examining the breasts, the nurse dons gloves and then assesses the fit and support provided by the woman's bra and, if appropriate, offers information about how to select a supportive bra. A properly fitting bra supports the breasts and helps maintain breast shape by limiting stretching of supporting ligaments and connective tissue. If the mother is breastfeeding, the straps of the bra should be cloth, not elastic (because cloth has less stretch and provides more support), and easily adjustable. The back should be wide and have at least three rows of hooks to adjust for fit. Traditional nursing bras have a fixed inner cup and a separate half cup that can be unhooked for breastfeeding while the cup continues to support the breast. Purchasing a nursing bra one size larger than the prepregnant size will usually result in a good fit because the breasts increase in size with milk production.

The nurse can then ask the woman to remove her bra so the breasts can be examined. The nurse notes the size and shape of the breasts and any abnormalities, reddened or hot areas, or engorgement. The breasts are also lightly palpated for softness, slight firmness associated with filling, firmness associated with engorgement, warmth, and tenderness. The nipples are assessed for fissures, cracks, soreness, and inversion. The nurse teaches the woman the characteristics of the breast and explains how to recognize problems such as fissures and cracks in the nipples.

The nonbreastfeeding mother is assessed for evidence of breast discomfort, and relief measures are instituted if necessary. (See discussion of lactation suppression in the nonbreastfeeding mother in Chapter 31 ∞.) Breast assessment findings for a nonbreastfeeding woman may be recorded as follows: "Breasts soft, filling, no evidence of nipple tenderness or cracking, nipples everted."

Abdomen and Fundus

Before examination of the abdomen, the woman should void. This practice ensures that a full bladder is not displacing the uterus or causing any uterine atony; if atony is present, other causes (such as uterine relaxation associated with a regional block, overstretched uterus, or distended bladder) must be investigated.

The nurse determines the relationship of the fundus to the umbilicus and also assesses the firmness of the fundus. (See the Teaching Card: Teaching Initial Postpartum Care in the center of this text.) The top of the fundus is measured in finger breaths above, below, or at the umbilicus. The nurse notes whether the fundus is in the midline or displaced to either side of the abdomen. If not midline, the uterus position should be located. The most common cause of displacement is a full bladder; this finding requires further assessment. If the fundus is in midline but higher than expected, it is usually associated with clots within the uterus. The nurse should then record the results of the assessment (see Clinical Skill: Assessing the Status of the Uterine Fundus After Birth).

While completing the assessment, the nurse teaches the woman about fundal position and how to determine firmness. The mother can be taught to massage her fundus gently if it is not firm.

TEACHING TIP

Assessing the status of the uterine fundus may be uncomfortable. In addition to explaining the importance of the assessment to the mother, you can show her how to perform frequent light massage of the fundus herself to promote uterine involution. Involving her in her own care encourages her participation. In addition, having her massage her own uterus may lessen bleeding and reduce the need for more thorough massage.

In the woman who has had a cesarean birth, the abdominal incision is extremely tender. The nurse should palpate the fundus with extreme care and inspect the abdominal incision for signs of healing, such as approximation (edges of incision appear "glued" together), bleeding,

Clinical Skill Assessing the Status of the Uterine Fundus After Birth

NURSING ACTION	RATIONALE
Preparation	

1. Explain the procedure, the information it provides, and what it might feel like.

2. Ask the woman to void.

A full bladder can cause uterine atony.

3. Have the woman lie flat in bed with her head on a pillow. If the procedure is uncomfortable, she may find that it helps to flex her legs.

The supine position prevents falsely high assessment of fundal height. Flexing the legs relaxes the abdominal muscles.

Equipment and Supplies

Gloves may be put on before assessing the abdomen and fundus or when you are ready to assess the perineum and lochia.

• A clean perineal pad (see Clinical Skill: Evaluating Lochia)

Clinical Tip

Procedure

1. Gently place one hand on the lower segment of the uterus. Using the side of the other hand, palpate the abdomen until you locate the top of the fundus.

One hand stabilizes the uterus while the other hand locates the top of the fundus. (Support of the uterus prevents stretching of the ligaments that support the uterus.)

2. Determine whether the fundus is firm. If it is, it will feel like a hard round object (similar to a grapefruit) in the abdomen. If it is not firm, massage the abdomen lightly until the fundus is firm.

A firm fundus indicates that the uterine muscles are contracted and bleeding will not occur.

3. Measure the top of the fundus in finger breadths above, below, or at the fundus. See Figure 30–6 ▪.

Fundal height gives information about the progress of involution.

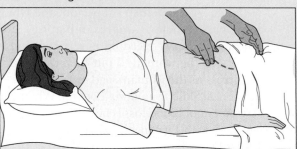

FIGURE 30–6 Measurement of descent of fundus for the woman with vaginal birth. The fundus is located two finger breadths below the umbilicus.

4. Determine the position of the fundus in relation to the midline of the body. If it is not in the midline, locate it and then evaluate the bladder for distention.

The fundus may deviate from the midline when the bladder is full because the enlarged bladder pushes the uterus aside.

5. If the bladder is distended, use nursing measures to help the woman void. If she is not able to void after a specified period of time, catheterization may be necessary.

6. Measure urine output for the next few hours until normal elimination is established.

During the postpartum as diuresis occurs; the bladder may fill far more rapidly than normal, putting the woman at risk for uterine atony and hemorrhage. (Diminished tone of the uterus may cause loss of the urge to void.)

7. Assess the lochia (see Clinical Skill: Evaluating Lochia).

(Continued on next page)

Clinical Skill Assessing the Status of the Uterine Fundus After Birth (Continued)

8. During the first few hours postpartum, if the fundus becomes boggy frequently or is located high above the umbilicus and the woman's bladder is empty, the uterine cavity may be filled with clots of blood. In this case, do the following:
   • Release the front of the perineal pad and lay it back so that you can see the perineum and the pad laying between the woman's legs.
   • Massage the uterine fundus until it is firm.
   • Keep one hand in position stabilizing the lower portion of the uterus. With the hand you used to massage the fundus, put steady pressure on the top of the now-firm fundus and see if you are able to express any clots. (Watch the pad between her legs for clots to pass from the vagina.)

9. If measurement of the blood loss is needed, the perineal pads and Chux can be weighed (see Clinical Skill: Evaluating Lochia).

10. Provide the woman with a clean perineal pad.

11. Record findings. Fundal height is recorded in finger breadths (e.g., "2 FB ↓ U" or "1 FB ↑ U"). If fundal massage was necessary, note that fact: "Uterus boggy → firm with light massage."

12. Communicate bogginess or heavy flow to primary provider.

If the woman's uterus is filled with blood, it acts as an irritant and the uterus will not remain contracted. When the muscle fibers relax, bleeding results, further aggravating the problem. Pushing on a uterus that is not firm is dangerous because it is possible to cause the uterus to invert, which is a true emergency.

and any signs of infection, including drainage, foul odor, or redness. The nurse should document whether internal sutures, steri-strips, or staples are intact. The nurse can also review characteristics of normal healing, incision care, and discuss signs of infection.

Lochia

The nurse then evaluates the lochia, including character, amount, odor, and the presence of clots. Nurses must wear disposable gloves when assessing the perineum and lochia. Nurses may put on the gloves before beginning the assessment, just before assessing the abdomen and fundus, or when they are ready to assess the perineum and lochia. During the first 1 to 3 days the lochia should be rubra. A few small clots are normal and occur as a result of blood pooling in the vagina. However, the passage of numerous or large clots is abnormal, and the cause should be investigated immediately. After 2 to 3 days, the lochia flow becomes serosa.

Lochia should never exceed a moderate amount, such as that needed to partially saturate perineal pads daily, with an average of six. However, because this number is influenced by an individual woman's pad-changing practices, as well as the absorbency of the pad, the nurse needs to question her about the length of time the current pad has been in use, whether the amount is normal compared with her typical menstrual period, and whether any clots were passed before this examination, such as during voiding. If heavy bleeding is reported but not seen, the nurse asks the woman to put on a clean perineal pad and then reassess the woman's pad in 1 hour (see Figure 30–7 ■ in Clinical Skill: Evaluating Lochia). When a more accurate assessment of blood loss is needed, the perineal pads can be weighed, with 1 g considered the approximate equivalent of 1 mL of blood.

Clots and heavy bleeding may be caused by uterine relaxation (atony), retained placental fragments, or rarely, an unknown cervical laceration, seen as heavy bleeding but with firm fundus, that may require further assessment (Table 30–3). Because of the evacuation of the uterine cavity during cesarean birth, women with

TABLE 30–3	Changes in Lochia That Cause Concern	
Change	Possible Problem	Nursing Action
Presence of clots	Inadequate uterine contractions that allow bleeding from vessels at the placental site.	Assess location and firmness of fundus. Assess voiding pattern. Record and report findings.
Persistent lochia rubra	Inadequate uterine contractions; retained placental fragments; infection; undetected cervical laceration.	Assess location and firmness of fundus. Assess activity pattern. Assess for signs of infection. Record and report findings.

Clinical Skill Evaluating Lochia

NURSING ACTION	RATIONALE

Preparation

1. Explain why lochia occurs, why it is assessed, how it is assessed, and how it changes during the postpartum.

2. Ask the woman to void.

A full bladder can cause uterine atony and increase the amount of lochia.

3. Complete the assessment of uterine fundal height and firmness.

In almost all cases, fundal height and firmness are evaluated with an assessment of lochia. This practice provides a more thorough assessment.

4. If she has not already done so for the fundal assessment, ask the woman to flex her legs. Then ask her to spread her legs apart. Use the bed sheet as a drape to preserve her modesty.

This position allows you to see the perineum and the perineal pad more effectively.

Equipment and Supplies

Note: Gloves are put on before assessing the perineum and lochia.

- Gloves
- Clean perineal pad

Scant amount
Blood only on tissue when wiped or less than 1-inch stain on peripad within 1 hour

Procedures: Clean Gloves

1. Don gloves.

2. Lower the perineal pad and observe the amount of lochia on the pad. Because women's pad-changing practices vary, ask her about the length of time the current pad has been in use, whether the amount is normal, and whether any clots were passed before this examination, such as during voiding.

Light amount
Less than 4-inch stain on peripad within 1 hour

During the first 1 to 3 days the woman's lochia should be rubra, which is dark red in color. A few small clots are normal and occur as a result of pooling of blood in the vagina when the woman is lying down. The passage of large clots is abnormal and the cause should be investigated immediately.

Clinical Tip

If blood loss exceeds the guidelines given in this chapter, weigh the perineal pads and the Chux pads to estimate the blood loss more accurately. Typically, 1g = 1mL blood. Because blood can pool below the woman on the Chux pad, the pads are included in your assessment.

Moderate amount
Less than 6-inch stain on peripad within 1 hour

3. If the woman reports heavy bleeding or clots, ask her to put on a clean perineal pad and then reassess the pad in 1 hour. Also ask her to call you before flushing any clots she passes into the toilet during voiding.

Heavy amount
Saturated peripad within 1 hour

4. When the uterine fundus is firm and stabilized with the nondominant hand, press down on it with the dominant hand while watching to see if any clots are expelled. (See Clinical Skill: Assessing the Status of the Uterine Fundus After Birth, step 8.)

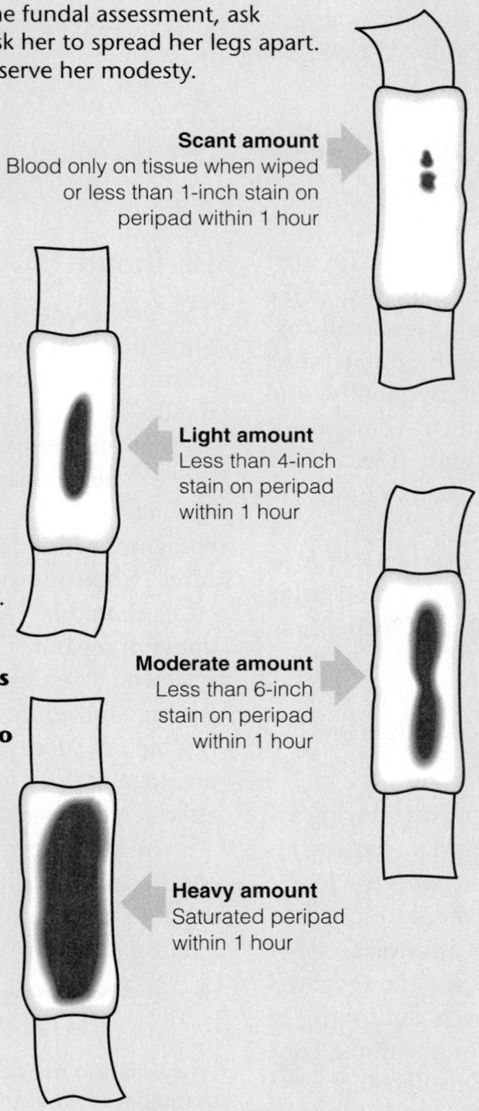

FIGURE 30–7 Suggested guideline for assessing lochia volume.
Source: Jacobson, H. (1985, May–June). A standard for assessing lochia volume. *Maternal-Child Nursing.*

(Continued on next page)

Clinical Skill Evaluating Lochia *(Continued)*

NURSING ACTION	RATIONALE
5. Determine the amount of lochia, using the following guide (see Figure 30–7 ■):	*Lochia should never exceed a moderate amount such as 4 to 8 partially saturated perineal pads daily. Using a consistent standard for measuring lochia improves the accuracy of the information charted and conveyed to others.*
• Heavy amount—Perineal pad has a stain larger than 6 inches in length within 1 hour; 30 to 80 mL lochia.	
• Moderate amount—Perineal pad has a stain less than 6 inches in length within 1 hour; 25 to 50 mL lochia.	
• Small (light) amount—Perineal pad has a stain less than 4 inches in length after 1 hour; 10 to 25 mL lochia.	
• Scant amount—Perineal pad has a stain less than 1 inch in length after 1 hour or lochia is only on tissue when the woman wipes.	
6. In most cases, a woman is discharged while her lochia is still rubra. Provide her with information about lochia serosa and lochia alba.	*Accurate discharge information enables the woman to assess herself more accurately and enables her to judge better when to contact her caregiver.*
7. Record the findings specifically. For example, "Uterus firm, 1FB ↓ U, Lochia: moderate rubra, no clots passed."	

such surgery usually have less lochia after the first 24 hours than mothers who give birth vaginally. If the woman is at increased risk for bleeding, or is actually experiencing heavy flow of lochia rubra, her blood pressure, pulse, and uterus need to be assessed frequently, and the physician/CNM may prescribe oxytocin (Pitocin) or methylergonovine maleate (Methergine). (See Drug Guide: Methylergonovine Maleate [Methergine], in Chapter 31 ∞.)

The odor of the lochia is nonoffensive and never foul. If a foul odor is present, so is an infection. When using narrative nursing notes, chart the amount of lochia first, followed by character. For example:

- Lochia: moderate rubra
- Lochia: small rubra/serosa

Client teaching that the nurse may address during assessment of the lochia may center on normal changes, effect of position changes, or what can be expected in the amount and color of the flow. Hygienic measures, such as wiping the perineum from front to back and washing her hands after toileting and changing pads, may be reviewed if appropriate. The nurse should approach the timing of teaching hygienic practices delicately, along with the content to be included. By establishing positive goals for the teaching—promoting comfort, enhancing tissue healing, and preventing infection—the nurse can avoid value-laden statements regarding personal beliefs about the need for cleanliness or control of body odor. The nurse should review with the mother the need to notify a healthcare professional if there is regression in the lochia flow pattern (i.e., color or amount).

Perineum

The perineum is inspected with the woman lying in a Sims' position (see Clinical Skill: Postpartum Perineal Assessment). The nurse lifts the buttock to expose the perineum and anus.

If an episiotomy was done or a laceration required suturing, the nurse assesses the wound. To evaluate the state of healing, the nurse inspects the wound for redness, edema, ecchymosis, drainage, and approximation (REEDA scale). After 24 hours some edema may still be present, but the skin edges should be well approximated so that gentle pressure does not separate them. Gentle palpation should elicit minimal tenderness, and there should be no hardened areas suggesting infection. Ecchymosis interferes with normal healing, as does infection. Foul odors associated with drainage indicate infection. Hematomas sometimes occur, although these are considered abnormal.

The nurse next assesses whether hemorrhoids are present around the anus. If present, they are assessed for size, number, and pain or tenderness. (See Figure 30–8 ■ in Clinical Skill: Postpartum Perineal Assessment.)

HINTS FOR PRACTICE

In evaluating the perineum, use the REEDA scale as a quick reminder of what to assess. Specifically:

R = redness
E = edema or swelling
E = ecchymosis or bruising
D = discharge
A = approximation (how well the edges of an incision—the episiotomy—or a repaired laceration seem to be holding together)

Clinical Skill Postpartum Perineal Assessment

NURSING ACTION	RATIONALE

Preparation

1. Explain the purpose and the procedure for assessing the perineum during the postpartum period.

2. Complete the assessment of fundal height and lochia as described in Clinical Skill: Assessing the Status of the Uterine Fundus After Birth and Clinical Skill: Evaluating Lochia.

Typically, perineal assessment is the final step of the postpartum assessment.

3. At this point in a postpartal assessment, the woman is lying on her back with her knees flexed. Her perineal pad has already been lifted away from her perineum to permit inspection of the lochia. If an episiotomy was performed or if the birth was difficult, the woman may be using an ice pack on her perineum to reduce swelling. The ice pack would also have been removed for inspection of the lochia.

4. Ask her to turn onto her side with her upper knee drawn forward and resting on the bed (Sims' position).

When the woman is supine, even with her knees flexed, it is very difficult to expose the posterior portion of the perineum. Thus, Sims' position makes it easiest to inspect the perineum and anal area.

Equipment and Supplies

- Clean perineal pad, clean ice pack if desired/needed
- Small light source such as a penlight may be necessary

Procedures: Clean Gloves

1. Use a systematic approach to assessment.

A systematic approach helps ensure that you don't overlook a significant finding.

2. In evaluating the perineum, begin by asking the woman's perceptions. How does she describe her discomfort? Does it seem excessive to her? Has it become worse since the birth? Does it seem more severe than you would expect?

   (Note: Pain that seems disproportionately severe may indicate that the woman is developing a vulvar hematoma.)

Information from the client herself often helps identify developing problems.

3. After talking with the woman, assess the condition of the tissue. To allow for full visualization, it may be helpful to ask the woman to lift the knee of her upper leg to expose her perineum more fully. In some cases it may help to use the nondominant hand to lift the buttocks and tissue. Note any swelling (edema) and bruising (ecchymosis).

The tissue is often traumatized by the birth and mild bruising is not unusual. However, excessive bruising may indicate that a hematoma is developing.

4. Evaluate the episiotomy, if there is one, or any repaired laceration for its state of healing. Is it reddened? Note the edges of the incision. Are they well approximated? Tell the woman that you are going to palpate the incision gently, then do so. Note any areas of hardness. Note whether the incision is warmer to the touch than the surrounding tissue.

Gentle palpation should elicit minimal tenderness and there should be no redness, warmth, or areas of hardness, which suggest infection. Both bruising and infection interfere with normal healing. Typically, within 24 hours the edges of the incision should be "glued" together (well approximated).

5. During the assessment be alert for odors. Typically the lochia has an earthy, but not unpleasant, smell that is easily identifiable.

A foul odor associated with drainage often indicates infection.

(Continued on next page)

Clinical Skill Postpartum Perineal Assessment *(Continued)*

6. Finally, assess for hemorrhoids. To visualize the anal area, lift the upper buttocks to fully expose the anal area (see Figure 30–8 ■). If hemorrhoids are present, note the size, number, and pain or tenderness.

Hemorrhoids often develop during pregnancy or labor and can cause considerable discomfort. If hemorrhoids are present, the woman may benefit from available comfort measures.

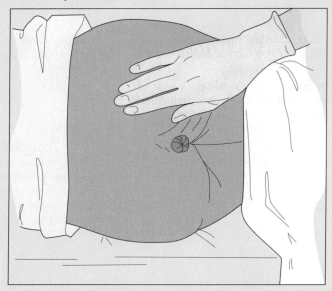

FIGURE 30–8 Intact perineum with hemorrhoids.

7. During the assessment, talk to the woman about the effectiveness of comfort measures being used. Provide teaching about care of the episiotomy, hemorrhoids, and the like.

Health teaching is an important part of nursing care. Many women have concerns about the episiotomy and may not know, for example, that the suture used is dissolvable. This is an excellent time to provide information about good healthcare practices in both the short and long term.

8. Provide the woman with a clean perineal pad. Replenish the ice pack if necessary.

9. Record findings. For example: "Midline episiotomy; no edema, ecchymosis, tenderness or discharge. Skin edges well approximated. Woman reports pain relief measures are controlling discomfort." or "Perineal repair is approximated, minimal edema, no ecchymosis or tenderness; ice pack to perineum relieves pain."

During the assessment, the nurse talks with the woman to determine the effectiveness of comfort measures that have been used. The nurse provides teaching about the episiotomy or perineal laceration. Some women do not thoroughly understand what and where an episiotomy is, and they may believe that the stitches must be removed as with other types of surgery. Frequently, when women fear that the stitches must be removed manually, they are afraid to ask about them. While explaining the findings of the assessment, the nurse provides information about the episiotomy, its location, and the signs that are being assessed. In addition, the nurse can casually add that the sutures are special and will dissolve slowly over the next few weeks as the tissues heal. By the time the sutures are dissolved the tissues are strong and the incision edges will not separate. This is also an opportunity to teach comfort measures that may be used and reinforce the need to consult with the healthcare provider before using over-the-counter (OTC) medications/supplements if breastfeeding (see Relief of Perineal Discomfort in Chapter 31 ∞).

An example of documenting a perineal assessment might read: "Midline episiotomy; no edema, tenderness, or ecchymosis present. Skin edges well approximated"; or, if a perineal laceration repair, "Skin edges intact, no edema, tenderness, or ecchymosis, pain meds helpful. Woman reports sitz bath and Tucks pads or pain relief measures are controlling discomfort."

MyNursingKit | Care After a Cesarean Birth

COMPLEMENTARY AND ALTERNATIVE THERAPIES

Lysine, an essential amino acid, has been identified as a supplement that decreases the incidence of pain following an episiotomy. Lysine is available as a supplement. The recommended adult dosage is 12 mg/kg of body weight per day. It is also present in dietary sources including meat, cheese, fish, eggs, soybeans, and nuts.

Lower Extremities

Postpartal women are at increased risk for *thrombophlebitis*, thrombus formation, and inflammation involving a vein (see Chapter 33 ∞). The most likely site of thrombophlebitis is in the woman's legs. Conditions that predispose a client for thrombophlebitis are hypercoagulability, severe anemia, obesity, and traumatic childbirth. To assess for thrombophlebitis, the nurse should have the woman stretch her legs out with the knees slightly flexed and the legs relaxed. The nurse then grasps the woman's foot and sharply dorsiflexes it. The second leg is assessed in the same way. No discomfort or pain should be present. If pain is elicited, the nurse notifies the physician/CNM that the woman has a positive Homans' sign (Figure 30–9 ■). The pain is caused by inflammation of the vessel. The nurse also evaluates the legs for edema by comparing both legs, because usually only one leg is involved. Any areas of redness, tenderness, and increased skin temperature are also noted.

Some facilities have discontinued performing a Homans' sign in the nursing assessment, stating it is not diagnostic and could lead to an emboli if the clot is dislodged during assessment. Although assessment of the Homans' sign is not diagnostic, supporters advocate its use as a screening tool. There are no published reports of an emboli occurring as a result of performing a Homans' sign. In the event of a positive Homans' sign, diagnosis is

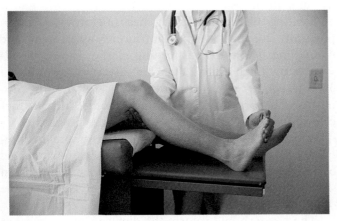

FIGURE 30–9 Homans' sign: With the woman's knee flexed, the nurse dorsiflexes the foot. Pain in the foot or leg is a positive Homans' sign.
Source: Photographer: Elena Dorfman.

made by compression or duplex ultrasonography. Heparin therapy is used in postpartum women who do develop a deep vein thrombosis.

Early ambulation is an important aspect in the prevention of thrombophlebitis. Most women are able to be up shortly after birth or once they have fully recovered from the effects of regional anesthetic agents, if one has been used. The mother's legs should be assessed for return of sensation following regional anesthesia. The cesarean birth client requires range of motion exercises until she is ambulating more freely.

Client teaching associated with assessment of the lower extremities focuses on the signs and symptoms of thrombophlebitis. In addition, the nurse may review self-care measures to promote circulation and measures to prevent thrombophlebitis, such as leg exercises that may be performed in bed, dorsiflexion on an hourly basis while on bed rest, ambulation, and avoiding pressure behind the knees and crossing the legs.

Usually, the nurse records the results of the assessment on a flowsheet or a summary nursing note. If tenderness and warmth have been noted, they might be recorded as follows: "Tenderness, warmth, slight edema, and slight redness noted on posterior aspect of left calf—positive Homans' sign. Woman advised to avoid pressure to this area; lower leg elevated and moist heat applied per agency protocol. Call placed to Dr. Garcia to report findings."

Elimination

During the hours after birth the nurse carefully monitors a new mother's bladder status. A boggy uterus, a displaced uterus, or a palpable bladder are signs of bladder distention and require nursing intervention.

Following birth, the postpartal woman should be encouraged to void every 4 to 6 hours. The nurse should assess the bladder for distention until the woman demonstrates complete emptying of the bladder with each voiding. The nurse may employ techniques to facilitate voiding, such as helping the woman out of bed to void or pouring warm water on the vulva, running water in the sink, and encouraging the woman to relax and take deep breaths. The physician will order catheterization when the bladder is distended and the woman cannot void, when she is voiding small amounts (less than 100 mL) frequently, or when no voiding has occurred in 8 hours. Although many physicians or CNMs write orders stating that the woman can be catheterized in 8 hours if she has not voided, the nurse needs to assess the bladder and any voiding pattern frequently before the end of the 8-hour period. Some women require catheterization sooner. The cesarean birth mother may have an indwelling catheter inserted prophylactically.

The same assessments should be made in evaluating bladder emptying once the catheter is removed.

During the physical assessment, the nurse elicits information from the woman about the adequacy of her fluid intake, whether she feels she is emptying her bladder completely when she voids, and any signs of urinary tract infection (UTI) she may be experiencing.

In the same way, the nurse obtains information about the new mother's intestinal elimination and any concerns she may have about it. Many mothers fear that the first bowel movement will be painful and possibly even damaging if an episiotomy has been done. Often, women have defecated during labor or childbirth; therefore, bowel movements normally return within 2 to 3 days after a vaginal childbirth. Stool softeners may be ordered to increase bulk and moisture in the fecal material and to allow more comfortable and complete evacuation. Constipation is avoided to prevent pressure on sutures and increase discomfort and therefore should be prevented. To enhance bowel elimination and help the woman reestablish her normal bowel pattern, the nurse can encourage ambulation, increased fluid intake (up to 2000 mL/day or more), and additional fresh fruits and roughage in her diet.

During the assessment, the nurse may provide information about postpartal diuresis and explain why the woman may be emptying her bladder so frequently. Information about the need for additional fluid intake, with suggestions of specific amounts, may be helpful. The woman should drink at least eight (8 oz) glasses of water or juice in addition to other fluids. Breastfeeding mothers will have a higher requirement. The nurse discusses signs of urinary retention and overflow voiding and may review symptoms of UTI if it seems an appropriate moment for teaching. The nurse can also review methods of assisting bowel elimination and provide opportunities for the woman to ask questions.

Rest and Sleep Status

Physical fatigue often affects other adjustments and functions of the new mother. The mother requires energy to make the psychologic adjustments to a new infant and to assume new roles. Fatigue is often a highly significant factor in a new mother's apparent disinterest in her newborn. Frequently the woman is so tired from a long labor and birth that everything seems to be an effort. To avoid inadvertently classifying a very tired mother as one with a potential attachment problem, the nurse should do a psychologic assessment on more than one occasion. After a nap the new mother is often far more receptive to her baby and her surroundings. During the postpartal assessment, the nurse evaluates the amount of rest a new mother is getting. If the woman reports difficulty sleeping at night, the nurse should try to determine the cause. If it is simply the strange environment, a warm drink and backrub may prove helpful. Ap-

> ### CULTURAL PERSPECTIVES
>
> Rest, seclusion, and dietary restraint practices in many traditional non-Western cultures (African, traditional Mexico, Chinese, Japanese, South Asian groups) are designed to assist the woman and her baby during postpartum vulnerable periods. The period of postpartum vulnerability and seclusion varies between 7 and 40 days. In Ghana, new mothers are relieved from all chores, told to abstain from sex, and not allowed to leave the home (Holtz & Grisdale, 2008; Lauderdale, 2008). Decreased activity and seclusion practices are designed to decrease the influence of spirits or of spreading evil and misfortune. The time of seclusion coincides with the period of lochial flow or postpartum bleeding.

propriate nursing measures are indicated if the woman is bothered by normal postpartal discomforts such as afterpains, diaphoresis, or episiotomy or hemorrhoidal pain. The impact of rooming-in on the mother's ability to rest should be assessed. See Chapter 31 ∞ for more detailed discussion of comfort/pain relief measures.

The nurse should encourage a daily rest period and schedule hospital activities to allow time for napping. The nurse can also provide information about the fatigue a new mother experiences, strategies to promote rest/sleep at home, and the impact it can have on a woman's emotions and sense of control.

Nutritional Status

Determination of postpartal nutritional status is based primarily on information provided by the mother and on direct assessment. During pregnancy the daily recommended dietary allowances call for increases in calories, protein, and most vitamins and minerals. After birth, the nonbreastfeeding mother's dietary requirements return to prepregnancy levels, whereas the nursing mother's requirements increase.

Visiting the mother during mealtime provides an opportunity for unobtrusive nutritional assessment and counseling. The nonbreastfeeding mother should be advised about the need to reduce her caloric intake by about 300 kcal and to return to prepregnancy levels for other nutrients. The breastfeeding mother should increase her caloric intake by about 200 kcal over the pregnancy requirements, or a total of 500 kcal over the nonpregnant requirement. Basic discussion often proves helpful, followed by referral as needed. In all cases, literature on nutrition should be provided, so that the woman will have a source of information after discharge.

The nurse should inform the dietician of any mother who is a vegetarian, has food allergies or lactose intolerance, or whose cultural or religious beliefs require specific foods. Appropriate meals can then be prepared for her.

TABLE 30–4	Daily Eating to Encourage Healthful Nutrition During the Postpartal Period

2 to 3 servings of milk, yogurt, and cheese group
2 to 3 servings of meat or protein group
3 to 5 servings of vegetable group
4 servings of whole grain
2 to 4 servings of fruit group
6 to 11 servings of bread, cereal, rice, and pasta group
Fats, oils, and sweets sparingly

Many women, especially those who gained more than the recommended number of pounds, are interested in losing weight after birth. The dietician can design weight-reduction diets to meet nutritional needs and food preferences. The nurse may also refer women with unusual eating habits or numerous questions about good nutrition to the dietician.

New mothers are advised that it is common practice to prescribe iron supplements for 3 months after birth. The hemoglobin and hematocrit values are then checked at the postpartal visit to detect any anemia.

As a part of the nutritional assessment, the nurse can provide teaching about the nutritional needs of the woman during the postpartal period. See Table 30–4 as well as the discussion in Chapter 12 ∞ .

Psychologic Assessment

During the first several postpartal weeks, the woman must accomplish certain physical and developmental tasks:

- Restoring physical condition
- Developing competence in caring for and meeting the needs of her infant
- Establishing a relationship with her new child
- Adapting to altered lifestyles and family structure resulting from the addition of a new member

Adequate assessment of the mother's psychologic adjustment is an integral part of postpartal evaluation. This assessment focuses on the mother's general attitude, feelings of competence, available support systems, and caregiving skills. It also evaluates her fatigue level, sense of satisfaction, and ability to accomplish her developmental tasks.

Some new mothers have little or no experience with newborns and may feel totally overwhelmed. They may show these feelings by asking questions and reading all available material or by becoming passive and quiet because they simply cannot deal with their feelings of inadequacy. Unless a nurse questions the woman about her plans and previous experience in a supportive, nonjudgmental way, the nurse might conclude that the woman is disinterested, withdrawn, or depressed. Clues indicating adjustment difficulties include excessive continued fatigue, marked depression, excessive preoccupation with physical status or discomfort, evidence of low self-esteem, lack of support systems, marital problems, inability to care for or nurture the newborn, and current family crises (illness or unemployment). These characteristics frequently indicate a potential for maladaptive parenting, which may lead to child abuse or neglect (physical, emotional, intellectual) and cannot be ignored. Referrals to public health nurses or other available community resources may provide greatly needed assistance and alleviate potentially dangerous situations.

Assessment of Early Attachment

A nurse in any of the various postpartal settings can periodically observe and note progress toward attachment. The assessment should include both parents when possible; however, in this section, these behaviors focus primarily on the mother's attachment process. As discussed previously, research shows that fathers experience similar attachment feelings to those experienced by mothers. The following questions can be addressed in the course of nurse-client interaction:

- Is the mother attracted to her newborn? To what extent does she seek face-to-face contact and eye contact? Has she progressed from fingertip touch, to palmar contact, to enfolding the infant close to her own body? Is attraction increasing or decreasing? If the mother does not exhibit increasing attraction, why not? Do the reasons lie primarily within her, in the baby, or in the environment?
- Is the mother inclined to nurture her infant? Is she progressing in her interactions with her infant?
- Does the mother act consistently? If not, is the source of unpredictability within her or her infant?
- Is her mothering consistently carried out? Does she seek information and evaluate it objectively? Does she develop solutions based on adequate knowledge of valid data? Does she evaluate the effectiveness of her maternal care and adjust appropriately?
- Is she sensitive to the newborn's needs as they arise? How quickly does she interpret her infant's behavior and react to cues? Does she seem happy and satisfied with the infant's responses to her efforts? Is she pleased with feeding behaviors? How much of this ability and willingness to respond is related to the baby's nature and how much to her own?
- Does she seem pleased with her baby's appearance and sex? Is she experiencing pleasure in interaction with her infant? What interferes with the enjoyment? Does she speak to the baby frequently and affectionately? Does she call him or her by name? Does she point out family traits or characteristics she sees in the newborn?

- Are there any cultural factors that might modify the mother's response? For instance, is it customary for the grandmother to assume most of the childcare responsibilities while the mother recovers from childbirth?

When the nurse has addressed these questions and assembled the facts, the nurse's intuition and knowledge should combine to answer three more questions: Is there a problem in attachment? What is the problem? What is its source? The nurse can then devise a creative approach to the problem as it presents itself in the context of a unique, developing mother-infant relationship.

Discharge Assessment and Follow-Up

The final discharge assessment should include a physical examination and appropriate discharge teaching that includes both maternal and newborn care guidelines. The mother's laboratory values are examined. If the mother was nonimmune to rubella, a rubella vaccine is administered before discharge. Rh-negative mothers whose infants are Rh positive need RhoGAM before they go home. If either is given, the nurse should document this in the mother's chart. If referrals, such as social service programs, support groups, lactation consultant, or a pediatrician, are needed, they should be provided before the family leaves the facility.

Some obstetricians, certified nurse-midwives, and nurse practitioners see postpartal women 1 to 2 weeks after birth in addition to the routine 6-week checkup. These visits provide an opportunity for physical assessment as well as evaluation of the mother's psychologic and informational needs and needs of the family. The routine physical assessment, which can be made rapidly, focuses on the woman's general appearance, breasts, reproductive tract, bladder and bowel elimination, and any specific problems or complaints. In addition, the nurse should talk with the mother about her diet, fatigue level, family adjustment, and psychologic status. The nurse explores any problems with child care and refers the mother to a pediatric nurse practitioner or pediatrician if needed. Available community resources, including public health department follow-up visits, are mentioned when appropriate. If not already discussed, teaching about family planning is appropriate at this time, and the nurse provides information regarding birth control methods. Women who gave birth vaginally tend to abstain from resuming sexual intercourse for a longer period of time than those who had a cesarean birth. Women who breastfed resumed sexual relations later than those who did not breastfeed.

Postdischarge care for the postpartal woman may also be accomplished by home visits, follow-up phone calls, or both. The optimal time for a home visit or follow-up phone call is between 3 to 4 days after birth; this provides opportunities for further assessment of mothers and their infants and teaching. (See Assessment Guide: Postpartal—First Home Visit and Anticipated Progress at 6 Weeks in Chapter 32 ∞). During this time period, infections, poor infant feeding, excessive weight loss, jaundice, and other problems become apparent (Simpson & James, 2005). The follow-up telephone call is often initiated by a nurse from the postpartal unit of the agency where the mother gave birth. It is made soon after discharge and is designed to provide assessment and care if necessary, to reinforce knowledge and provide additional teaching, and to make referrals if indicated. Alternatively, a follow-up phone call from a nurse at the physician's or nurse-midwife's office can provide new mothers with a source of support and an opportunity to ask questions. Women who appear to be having adjustment problems should be scheduled for an appointment for further evaluation.

In ideal situations, a family approach involving the father, infant, other siblings, and grandparents permits a total evaluation and provides an opportunity for all family members to ask questions and express concerns. In addition, a family approach can sometimes enable the nurse to identify disturbed family patterns more readily and suggest, or even institute, therapeutic measures to prevent future problems of neglect or abuse.

CHAPTER HIGHLIGHTS

- The uterus involutes rapidly, primarily through a reduction in cell size.
- Involution is assessed by measuring fundal height. The fundus is at the level of the umbilicus within a few hours after childbirth and should decrease by approximately one finger breadth per day.
- The placental site heals by a process of exfoliation, so no scar formation occurs.
- Lochia progresses from rubra to serosa to alba and is assessed in terms of type, quantity, and characteristics.

- The abdomen may have decreased muscle tone (flabby consistency) initially. The nurse should assess for diastasis recti abdominis, separation of the rectus abdominis muscles.
- Constipation may develop postpartally because of decreased tone, limited diet, and denial of the urge to defecate because of fear of pain.
- Decreased bladder sensitivity, increased capacity, and postpartal diuresis may lead to problems with bladder elimination. Frequent assessment and prompt intervention are indicated. A fundus that is boggy but does not respond to

massage, is higher than expected, or deviates to the side usually indicates a full bladder.

- Postpartally a healthy woman should be normotensive and afebrile. Bradycardia is common.
- Postpartally the white blood cell (WBC) count is often elevated. Activation of clotting factors predisposes the woman to thrombus formation.
- Psychologic adaptations of the postpartal woman are traditionally described as "taking-in" and "taking-hold."
- In consideration of the client's background, the nurse should recognize and respect cultural variations and individual preferences.

- Postpartal assessment should be completed in a systematic way, usually from head to toe and should include assessment of rest and sleep, nutrition, and attachment. The assessment provides opportunities for informal client teaching.
- In the weeks following birth, the woman's physical condition returns to a nonpregnant state and she gains competence and confidence in herself as a parent.
- Postdischarge assessment may be accomplished via an outpatient visit 1 to 2 weeks postpartum, a home care visit, or telephone follow-up. A 6-week postpartum visit with the physician/CNM is standard practice.

EXPLORE PEARSON **mynursingkit**™

MyNursingKit is your one stop for online chapter review materials and resources. Prepare for success with additional NCLEX®-style practice questions, interactive assignments and activities, web links, animations and videos, and more!

Register your access code from the front of your book at
www.mynursingkit.com

CHAPTER REFERENCES

Alexander, J. M. (2005). Epidural anesthesia for labor pain and its relationship to fever. *Clinics in Perinatology, 32*(3), 777–787.

Al-Oballi Kridli, S. (2002). Health beliefs and practices among Arab women. *American Journal of Maternal Child Nursing, 27*(3), 178–182.

Beck, C. T. (2002). Revision of the postpartum depression predictors inventory. *Journal of Obstetric, Gynecologic, and Neonatal Nursing, 31*(4), 394–402.

Beck, C. T. (2008). *Postpartum mood and anxiety disorders: Case studies, research, and nursing care* (2nd ed.). Washington, DC: Association of Women's Health, Obstetric and Neonatal Nurses.

Blackburn, S. T. (2007). *Maternal, fetal, & neonatal physiology: A clinical perspective* (3rd ed.). St. Louis, MO: Saunders.

Cunningham, F. G., Leveno, K. J., Bloom, S. L., Hauth, J. C., Gilstrap, L. C., & Wenstrom, K. D. (2005). *Williams obstetrics* (22nd ed.). New York: McGraw-Hill.

D'Avanzo, C. E., & Geissler, E. M. (2008). *Cultural health assessment* (4th ed.). St. Louis, MO: Mosby.

De Sovo, M. R. (1997, August). Keeping the faith: Jewish traditions in pregnancy and childbirth. *Lifelines, 1*(4), 46–49.

Holtz, C., & Grisdale, S. (2008). Global health in reproduction and infants. In C. Holtz, *Global health care: Issues and policies* (1st ed., pp. 437–476). Boston, MA: Jones & Bartlett.

James, D. C. (2008). Postpartum care. In K. R. Simpson & P. A. Creehan, *Perinatal nursing* (3rd ed., pp. 473–526). Philadelphia: Lippincott Williams & Wilkins.

Kalayjian, L., & Goodwin, T. M. (2007). Nervous system & autoimmune disorders in pregnancy. . In A. H. Decherney, L. Nathan, T. M Goodwin, & N. Laufer (Eds.), *Current diagnosis and treatment: Obstetrics & gynecology* (10th ed.). Boston: McGraw Hill.

Kim-Goodwin, Y. S. (2005). Postpartum beliefs & practices among non-Western cultures. *American Journal of Maternal-Child Nursing, 28*(2), 75–80.

Lauderdale, J. (2008). Transcultural perspectives in childbearing. In M. M. Andrews & J. S. Boyle, *Transcultural concepts in nursing care* (5th ed.). Philadelphia: Lippincott Williams & Wilkins.

Lipscomb, K., & Novy, M. J. (2007). The normal puerperium. In A. H. DeCherney, L. Nathan, T. M. Goodwin, & N. Laufer (Eds.), *Current diagnosis and treatment: Obstetrics & gynecology* (10th ed.). Boston: McGraw Hill.

Mercer, R. T. (1995). *Becoming a mother*. New York: Springer.

Mercer, R. T. (2004). Becoming a mother versus maternal role attainment. *Journal of Nursing Scholarship, 36*(3), 226–232.

Purnell, L. D., & Paulanka, B. J. (2008). *Transcultural health care: A culturally competent approach* (3rd ed.). Philadelphia: F. A. Davis.

Rubin, R. (1961). Puerperal change. *Nursing Outlook, 9*, 753.

Rubin, R. (1984). *Maternal identity and the maternal experience*. New York: Springer.

Samuels, P., & Niebyl, J. R. (2007). Neurologic disorders. In S. G. Gabbe, J. R. Niebyl, & J. L. Simpson (Eds.), *Obstetrics: Normal and problem pregnancies* (5th ed., pp. 1132–1152). Philadelphia, PA: Churchill Livingstone/ Elsevier.

Shehata, H. A., & Okosun, H. (2004). Neurological disorders in pregnancy. *Current Opinion in Obstetrics & Gynecology, 16*(2), 117–122.

Simpson, K. R., & James, D. C. (2005). *Postpartum care: Continuing education for registered nurses and certified nurse-midwives*. White Plains, NY: March of Dimes.

Tatum, W., Liporace, J., Benbadis, S., & Kaplan, P. (2004). Updates on the treatment of epilepsy in women. *Archives of Internal Medicine, 164*(2), 137–145.

Varney, H., Kriebs, J. M., & Gegor, C. L. (2004). *Varney's midwifery* (4th ed.). Sudbury, MA: Jones & Bartlett.

CHAPTER 31

The Postpartal Family: Needs and Care

I truly believe I have the best job there is in the nursing profession. I look forward to work each day, and I return home feeling satisfied that I have given my best. I'm using my nursing education to the fullest, as a hands-on caregiver, an educator, and a client advocate. There are plenty of challenges to keep me on my toes and plenty of new directions to explore. I know it may sound corny, but I love what I do!

—A Postpartum Staff Nurse

LEARNING OUTCOMES

31-1. Formulate nursing diagnoses and nursing care based on the findings of the "normal" postpartum assessment.

31-2. Delineate strategies for promoting family learning during the early postpartal period.

31-3. Formulate nursing interventions and client teaching that promote postpartum maternal comfort and well-being.

31-4. Describe the nurse's role in promoting maternal rest and helping the mother gradually resume an appropriate level of activity.

31-5. Explain factors that affect postpartal family wellness in the provision of nursing care and client teaching.

31-6. Compare the postpartal nursing needs of the woman who experienced a cesarean birth with the needs of a woman who gave birth vaginally.

31-7. Examine the nursing needs of the childbearing adolescent during the postpartal period.

31-8. Describe possible approaches to sensitive, holistic nursing care for the woman who relinquishes her newborn.

31-9. Identify teaching topics related to postpartum discharge.

31-10. Evaluate the mother and newborn's progress toward identified outcomes before discharge.

KEY TERMS

Continuous epidural infusion (CEI) **846**
Couplet care **841**
Family-centered care **829**
Mother-baby care **841**
Patient-controlled analgesia (PCA) **846**

Certain premises form the basis of effective nursing care during the postpartal period:

- The best postpartal care is **family-centered care** which incorporates the family's needs, desires, and values as much as possible; and disrupts the family unit as little as possible while providing optimal health care to the mother and baby in the acute care setting. This approach uses the family's resources to support an early and smooth adjustment to the newborn by all family members.

- Knowledge of the range of normal physiologic and psychologic adaptations occurring during the postpartal period allows the nurse to recognize alterations and initiate interventions early. Communicating information about postpartal adaptations to the family members facilitates adjustment to their situation.

- Nursing care is aimed at accomplishing specific goals that are intended to meet individual and family needs. These goals are formulated after careful assessment, consultation with the woman and her family, and consideration of factors that could influence the outcome of care, such as cultural or economic considerations.

Chapter 30 ∞ provides a thorough discussion of postpartal assessment. This chapter describes how the nurse can use the remaining steps of the nursing process effectively to plan and provide care. Specific nursing responses to the mother's physical needs and the family's psychosocial needs are described at length. A Clinical Pathway for the Postpartal Period begins on page 830.

Nursing Care During the Early Postpartal Period

For most postpartal women, physical recovery goes smoothly and is considered a healthy process. Because of this perception, caregivers too often assume that the woman and her family have no real needs and that no care plan is needed. Nothing could be further from the truth. Every member of the family has needs, although the needs may not be obvious, especially if they are psychologic or educational.

Nursing Diagnosis

The postpartal family's needs, which should be identified during assessment, are the basis for developing nursing diagnoses. Many nurses have suggested that nursing diagnoses are difficult to make in a wellness setting because of their emphasis on "problems." Nurses involved in the effort to formulate standardized diagnoses recognize this difficulty and continue working to develop nursing diagnoses that are more congruent with wellness settings.

Many agencies that use nursing diagnoses prefer to use only the NANDA list. Consequently, physiologic alter-

ations form the basis of many postpartal diagnoses. Examples of such diagnoses include:

- *Impaired Urinary Elimination* related to dysuria
- *Ineffective Breastfeeding* related to postpartal pain from a cesarean birth or maternal fatigue
- *Constipation* related to fear of tearing stitches or pain
- *Acute Pain* related to perineal trauma secondary to episiotomy or birth

Diagnoses related to family coping or instructional needs are also used frequently. Examples of these diagnoses include:

- *Health-Seeking Behaviors: Information About Infant Care* related to an expressed desire to improve parenting skills
- *Anxiety* related to self and infant care secondary to lack of knowledge of appropriate care practices
- *Readiness* for enhanced family coping related to successful adjustment to new baby

Nursing Plan and Implementation

An important component of postpartal nursing care is client teaching, which must be individualized to the learning capability and readiness of the parent(s). Many mothers and family members take childbirth education classes in preparation for the labor and birth which should include relevant postpartum teaching. This is an ideal time to introduce postpartum teaching because families are less distracted with a new baby, fatigue, and stress. As part of the teaching role, the nurse discusses desired outcomes and goals with the mother and family members as soon as possible following the birth. Interventions can then be designed to achieve optimal health promotion. Strategies for promoting effective parent learning are discussed shortly, and specific teaching content is provided throughout the rest of this chapter.

Following discharge, various services are available in most communities to meet the needs of the postpartal family. These services range from educational, such as classes on nutrition, exercise, infant care, and parenting, to specific healthcare programs, such as well-baby checks, immunization clinics, family-planning services, new mother support groups, and more. Some are offered by private caregivers, whereas others are the domain of city, county, state, or federal agencies. In all cases, the goal is to help ensure that all family members have the opportunity to meet healthcare needs, regardless of their resources.

Home health care is an important form of community-based nursing care offered to postpartal families. Home care visits and phone contacts help ensure that new parents have the necessary skills and resources to care for their infant. (Home care is discussed in depth in Chapter 32 ∞.)

Clinical Pathway FOR THE POSTPARTAL PERIOD

	FIRST 4 HOURS	4 TO 8 HOURS PAST BIRTH	8 TO 24 HOURS PAST BIRTH
REFERRAL	Report from labor nurse if not continuing in an LDR room	Lactation consultation as needed	Home nursing, WIC referral if indicated **Expected Outcomes** Referrals made

ASSESSMENTS

FIRST 4 HOURS	4 TO 8 HOURS PAST BIRTH	8 TO 24 HOURS PAST BIRTH
Postpartum assessments q30min × 2, q1h × 2, then q4h. Includes: • Fundus firm, midline, at or below umbilicus • Lochia rubra less than 1 pad/h; no free flow or passage of clots with massage • Bladder: voids large amounts of urine spontaneously; bladder not palpable following voiding • Perineum: sutures intact; no bulging or marked swelling; no c/o severe pain. Minimal bruising may be present. If hemorrhoids present, no tenseness or marked engorgement; less than 2 cm diameter • Breasts: soft, colostrum present Vital Signs: • BP WNL; no hypotension; not greater than 30 mm systolic or 15 mm diastolic over baseline • Temperature: less than 38°C (100.4°F) • Pulse: bradycardia normal, consistent with baseline • Respirations: 16 to 24/min; quiet, easy • Comfort level: less than 3 on scale of 1 to 10	Continue postpartum assessment q4h × 2, then q8h Breast: evaluate nipple status; should be no evidence of cracks or bruising Observe feeding technique with newborn Vital signs assessment q8h; all WNL; report temperature greater than 38°C (100.4°F) Assess Homans' sign q8h Continue assessment of comfort level	Continue postpartum assessment q8h Breasts: nipples should remain free of cracks, fissures, bruising Feeding technique with newborn: should be good or improving Vital signs assessment q8h; all WNL; report temperature greater than 38°C (100.4°F) Continue assessment of comfort level **Expected Outcomes** Vital signs medically acceptable, voids qs, postpartum assessment WNL; comfort level: less than 3 on 1 to 10 scale, involution of uterus in process, demonstrates and verbalizes appropriate newborn feeding techniques

TEACHING/PSYCHOSOCIAL

FIRST 4 HOURS	4 TO 8 HOURS PAST BIRTH	8 TO 24 HOURS PAST BIRTH
Explain postpartum assessments Teach self-massage of fundus and expected findings; rationale for fundal massage Instruct to call for assistance first time OOB and PRN Demonstrate pericare, surgigator, sitz bath PRN Explain comfort measures Begin newborn teaching; bulb suctioning, positioning, feeding, diaper change, cord care Orient to room if transferred from LDR room Provide information on early postpartal period Assess mother-infant attachment	Discuss psychologic changes of postpartum period; facilitate transition through tasks of taking on maternal role Discuss pericare/hygiene; encourage use of supportive brassiere for formula- or breastfeeding Stress need for frequent rest periods Continue newborn teaching: soothing/comforting techniques, swaddling; return demonstrations indicate woman's understanding Provide opportunities for questions and review; reinforce previous teaching Breastfeeding: nipple care: air-drying, lanolin; proper latch-on technique; tea bags Formula-feeding: supportive bra, ice bags, breast binder Assess mother-infant attachment	Reinforce previous teaching, complete teaching evaluation Discuss involution; anticipated physical changes in first 2 weeks postpartum; postpartal exercises; need to limit visitors Discuss postpartal nutrition; balanced diet Breastfeeding: • Increase calories by 500 kcal over nonpregnant state (200 kcal over pregnant intake) • Explain milk production, letdown reflex, use of supplements, breast pumping, and milk storage Formula feeding: • Return to nonpregnant caloric intake • Explain formula preparation and storage Discuss birth control options, sexuality Discuss sibling rivalry and plan for supporting siblings at home Discuss pets; suggestions for improving acceptance of infant by pets **Expected Outcomes** Mother verbalizes teaching comprehension Positive bonding and emotional behaviors observed

Clinical Pathway   FOR THE POSTPARTAL PERIOD *(Continued)*

FIRST 4 HOURS	4 TO 8 HOURS PAST BIRTH	8 TO 24 HOURS PAST BIRTH
NURSING CARE MANAGEMENT AND REPORTS		
Ice pack to perineum to decrease swelling and increase comfort Straight catheter PRN × 1 if distended or voiding small amounts If continues unable to void or voiding small amounts, insert Foley catheter and notify physician/CNM	Sitz baths PRN If woman Rh− and infant Rh+, RhoGAM workup; obtain consent; complete teaching Determine rubella status Obtain consent for rubella vaccine if indicated; explain purpose, procedure, implications of vaccine Obtain hematocrit	Continue sitz baths PRN May shower if ambulating without difficulty DC heparin lock if present Administer rubella vaccine as indicated **Expected Outcomes** Using sitz bath; voids qs; lab work WNL; performs ADL without sequelae
ACTIVITY		
Assistance when OOB first time, then PRN Ambulate ad lib Rests comfortably between assessments	Encourage rest periods Ambulate ad lib; may leave birthing unit after notifying staff of plan to ambulate off unit	Up ad lib **Expected Outcomes** Ambulates ad lib
COMFORT		
Institute comfort measures: • Perineal discomfort: pericare; sitz baths, topical analgesics • Hemorrhoids: sitz baths, topical analgesics, digital replacement of external hemorrhoids; side-lying or prone position • Afterpains: prone with small pillow under abdomen; warm shower or sitz baths; ambulation • Administer pain medication	Continue with pain management techniques Offer alternative pain management options: distraction with music, television, visitors; massage; warmed blankets or towels to affected area; using breathing techniques when infant latches on to breast and/or during cramping until medication's action is felt	Continue with pain management techniques **Expected Outcomes** Comfort level less than 3 on 1 to 10 scale Verbalizes alternative pain management options
NUTRITION		
Regular diet Fluid of 2000 mL per day or more	Continue diet and fluids	Continue diet and fluids **Expected Outcomes** Regular diet/fluids tolerated
ELIMINATION		
Voiding large amounts of straw-colored urine	Voiding large quantities May have bowel movement	Same **Expected Outcomes** Voiding qs; passing flatus or bowel movement
MEDICATIONS		
Pain medications as ordered Methergine 0.2 mg q4h PO if ordered Stool softener Tucks pad PRN, perineal analgesic spray	Continue meds Lanolin to nipples PRN; tea bags to nipples if tender; heparin flush to heparin lock (if present) q8h or as ordered May take own prenatal vitamins	Continue medications RhoGAM and rubella vaccine administered if indicated **Expected Outcomes** Vaccines administered; pain controlled

(Continued on next page)

Clinical Pathway FOR THE POSTPARTAL PERIOD (Continued)

	FIRST 4 HOURS	4 TO 8 HOURS PAST BIRTH	8 TO 24 HOURS PAST BIRTH
DISCHARGE PLANNING/HOME			
	Evaluate knowledge of normal postpartum and newborn care Evaluate support systems	Discuss typical newborn schedule; plan for periods of rest Birth certificate paperwork completed Evaluate plans for transporting newborn; car seat available	Review discharge instruction sheet/checklist Describe postpartum warning signs and when to call physician/CNM Provide prescriptions. Provide gift packs as appropriate for formula- or breastfeeding Arrangements for baby pictures as per agency protocol Postpartum and newborn visits scheduled **Expected Outcomes** Discharged home; mother verbalizes postpartum warning s/s, follow-up appointment times/dates
FAMILY INVOLVEMENT			
	Identify available support persons Assess family perceptions of birth experience Parenting: demonstrates culturally expected early parenting behaviors	Involve support persons in care, teaching; answer questions Evidence of parental bonding behaviors present	Continue to involve support persons in teaching, involve siblings as appropriate Plans made for providing support to mother following discharge **Expected Outcomes** Evidence of parental bonding behavior; support persons verbalize understanding of woman's need for rest, good nutrition, fluids, and emotional support
DATE			

Information is included for both vaginal birth (VB) and cesarean birth (CB). However, because many of the nursing care interventions are the same for either, specific interventions or suggestions related to vaginal birth are designated VB, and those specific to cesarean are designated CB.
ADL, activities of daily living; BP, blood pressure; CB, cesarean birth; CNM, certified nurse-midwife; c/o, complaints of; D/C, discharge; DC, discontinue; LDR, labor, delivery, and recovery; LOC, level of consciousness; LOS, level of sensation; OOB, out of bed; OR, operating room; PCA, patient-controlled analgesia; PP, postpartum; PRN, as needed; qs, quantity sufficient; s/s, signs and symptoms; TC & DB, turn-cough and deep breathe; VB, vaginal birth; VS, vital signs; WNL, within normal limits.

Promotion of Effective Parent Learning

Meeting the educational needs of the new mother and her family is a primary challenge facing the postpartum nurse. Each woman's educational needs vary based on her age, background, educational level, experience, and expectations. However, because the mother spends only a brief period of time in the postpartal area, identifying and addressing individual instructional needs can be difficult. Effective education provides the childbearing family with sufficient knowledge to meet many of their own health needs and to seek assistance if necessary.

The nurse first assesses the learning needs of the new mother through observation, sensitivity to nonverbal cues, and tactfully phrased questions. For example, "What plans have you made for handling things when you get home?" may elicit a response of several words and may provide the opportunity for some information sharing and guidance. Some agencies also use checklists of common concerns for new mothers. The woman can check the concerns that are of interest to her.

Teaching during the postpartum period is a continuous process in which the nurse takes opportunities throughout interactions with the new parents to identify learning opportunities and offer teaching interventions. The nurse can also plan and implement teaching in a logical, nonthreatening way based on knowledge and respect of the family's cultural values and beliefs. Unless the nurse believes a culturally related activity would be harmful, it can be supported and encouraged.

Nurses need to consider the mother's physical and psychosocial needs when conducting postpartum teaching. Initially, women may be exhausted from the birth experience and their concentration may be impaired. Later, the new mother may be preoccupied with visitors and phone calls. Information should be delivered a little at a time and repeated to make sure that the parents understand what the nurse has discussed with them. Repetition is a valuable tool in the postpartum environment. In addition, many women are discharged during the first 48 hours after birth, making postpartum education difficult (Bernstein, Spino, & Finch et al., 2007). When performing teaching sessions, the partner's schedule must also be considered. If the partner returns to work during the immediate postpartal period, there may be more convenient teaching sessions scheduled in the late afternoon or early evening (Figure 31–1 ■). In some cultures, such as the Hispanic culture, female relatives often assist the new mother and baby. It is important to include any care providers in the teaching session.

Postpartal units use a variety of instructional methods, including handouts, formal classes, videotapes, and individual interaction. Printed materials are helpful for new mothers to consult if questions arise at home. Some facilities offer a hotline service in which new mothers can call with questions or concerns. As the cultural diversity in the United States continues to grow, the need for culturally sensitive information is imperative. Along with culturally diverse material, teaching aid should be presented in the woman's native language when possible. Written materials should be available and translators or language lines should be utilized. Many clients are now accustomed to using the Internet and may prefer to use on-line support groups and access educational materials via the Internet. As technology expands, the nurse must remain current with the changing technology and the resources it creates. Evaluation of learning may also take several forms: return demonstrations, question-and-answer sessions, and even

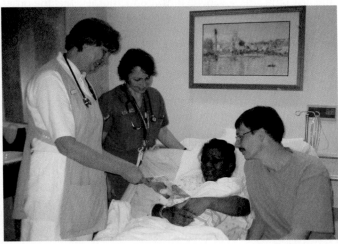

Figure 31–1 The nurse provides educational information to both parents.

formal evaluation tools. Follow-up phone calls after discharge provide additional evaluative information and continue the helping process for the family.

Teaching content should include information on role changes and psychologic adjustments as well as skills. Risk factors and signs of postpartum depression should be reviewed with all women. Information is also essential for women with specialized educational needs such as the mother who has had a cesarean birth, the parents of twins, the parents of an infant with congenital anomalies, parents with other young children, parents with a child that will require long-term hospitalization, and so on. Because more and more women with disabilities are now having children, they may require additional support and education. Anticipatory guidance can help prepare parents for the many changes they will experience with a new family member.

Promotion of Maternal Comfort and Well-Being

The nurse can promote and restore maternal physical well-being by monitoring uterine status, vital signs, cardiovascular status, elimination patterns, nutritional needs, sleep and rest, and learning needs. Some women also require medication to relieve pain, treat anemia, provide immunity to rubella, and prevent development of antibodies in the nonsensitized Rh-negative woman. Most postpartal women need nursing interventions to promote their comfort and relieve stress. These measures are discussed here and summarized in the Teaching Cards inserted in the center of this text.

Monitoring Uterine Status

The nurse completes an assessment of the uterus as discussed in Chapter 30 ∞. The assessment interval is usually every 15 minutes for the first hour after childbirth, every 30 minutes for the next hour, and then hourly for approximately 2 more hours. After that, the nurse monitors uterine status every 8 hours or more frequently if problems arise such as the following:

- Bogginess (uterus is not firm and is difficult to palpate because it lacks shape and consistency)
- Positioning out of midline
- Heavy lochia flow
- Presence of clots

Occasionally medications are needed to promote uterine contractions. These include oxytocin, discussed in Chapter 23 ∞, and methylergonovine maleate (see the accompanying Drug Guide: Methylergonovine Maleate [Methergine]). The nurse also monitors the amount, consistency, color, and odor of the lochia on an ongoing basis.

Drug Guide Methylergonovine Maleate (Methergine)

Overview of Action Methylergonovine maleate (Methergine) is an ergot alkaloid that stimulates smooth muscle tissue. Because the smooth muscle of the uterus is especially sensitive to this drug, it is used postpartally to stimulate the uterus to contract in order to decrease blood loss by clamping off uterine blood vessels and to promote the involution process. In addition, the drug has a vasoconstrictive effect on all blood vessels, especially the larger arteries. This may result in hypertension, particularly in a woman whose blood pressure is already elevated.

Route, Dosage, and Frequency Methergine has a rapid onset of action and may be given orally or intramuscularly.

Usual IM dose: 0.2 mg following expulsion of the placenta. The dose may be repeated every 2 to 4 hours if necessary.
Usual oral dose: 0.2 mg every 4 hours (six doses).

Maternal Contraindications Pregnancy, hepatic or renal disease, cardiac disease, hypertension, or preeclampsia contraindicate this drug's use. Methylergonovine maleate must be used with caution during lactation (Wilson, Shannon, & Shields, 2009).

Maternal Side Effects Hypertension, nausea, vomiting, headache, bradycardia, dizziness, tinnitus, abdominal cramps, palpitations, dyspnea, chest pain, and allergic reactions may be noted.

Effects on Fetus or Newborn Because Methergine has a long duration (3 hours [Wilson et al., 2009]) and action and can thus produce tetanic contractions, it *should never be used during pregnancy or in labor*, when it may result in a sustained uterine contraction that may cause amniotic fluid embolism (increased pressure in uterus may allow entry of amniotic fluid under the edge of the placenta and thus entry into the maternal venous system), uterine rupture, cervical and perineal lacerations (resulting from tetanic contractions and rapid birth of the baby), and hypoxia and intracranial hemorrhage in the baby (because of tetanic contractions, which severely decrease the maternal-placental-fetal blood flow, or uterine rupture, which causes cessation of blood flow to the unborn baby) (Wilson et al., 2009).

Nursing Considerations

- Monitor fundal height and consistency and the amount and character of the lochia.
- Assess the blood pressure before and routinely throughout drug administration.
- Observe for adverse effects or symptoms of ergot toxicity (ergotism) such as nausea and vomiting, headache, muscle pain, cold or numb fingers and toes, chest pain, and general weakness (Wilson et al., 2009).
- Provide client and family teaching regarding importance of not smoking during Methergine administration (nicotine from cigarettes leads to constricted vessels and may lead to hypertension) and signs of toxicity.

Continued assessment is warranted during the first 24 hours because early postpartum hemorrhage typically occurs in the 24 hours after birth and is most commonly related to uterine atony (AWHONN, 2006).

Relief of Perineal Discomfort

Many nursing interventions are available for the relief of perineal discomfort. Before selecting a method, the nurse needs to assess the perineum to determine the degree of edema and other problems. It is also important to ask the woman if she believes any special measures will be particularly effective and to offer her choices when possible. The nurse uses disposable gloves while applying all relief measures and washes hands before and after using the gloves. At all times it is essential for the nurse to remember hygienic practices, such as moving from the front of the perineum (area of the symphysis pubis) to the back (area around the anus). Avoiding contamination between the anal area and the urethral/vaginal area is vital to the prevention of infection. It is important to remember that in some cultures or religions, such as Orthodox Judaism, women are prohibited to touch or change their own perineal pads and will require the nurse or a family member to do so.

HINTS FOR PRACTICE

You may be surprised by how quickly the postpartal woman shows signs of bladder distention, possibly as soon as 1 to 2 hours after childbirth. This distention results because of normal postpartum diuresis. You can help prevent overdistention by palpating the woman's bladder frequently and encouraging her to void. When attempting to void for the first time after a vaginal birth, some mothers feel the urge to urinate but are unable to begin the flow of urine. Interventions that help many women in this situation include letting the mother hear running water by turning water on in the sink or tub, running warm water in the sink and having her place one hand in the water, and/or placing her feet in a basin of warm water.

Perineal Care

Perineal care after each elimination cleanses the perineum, prevents infection, and helps promote comfort. The woman should be instructed to wash her hands before and after changing peripads or performing pericare. The nurse demonstrates how to cleanse the perineum and assists the woman as necessary. Many agencies provide "peri bottles" that the woman can use to squirt warm tap water over her perineum following elimination. To cleanse her perineum, the woman should use moist antiseptic towelettes or toilet paper in a blotting (patting) motion and should be taught to start at the front (area just under the symphysis pubis) and proceed toward the back (area around the anus), to prevent contamination from the anal area. See the Teaching Card on Teaching Initial Postpartum Care in the center of this text.

Many women have never used perineal pads and will need teaching and assistance in using them during the postpartal period. To prevent contamination, the perineal pad should be applied from front to back (place the front portion against the perineum first) and changed when saturation occurs or after each perineal cleansing. The woman is advised to hold the pad on the sides to prevent contamination. The pad needs to be placed snugly against the perineum but should not produce pressure. If the pad is worn too loosely, it may rub back and forth, irritating perineal tissues and causing contamination between the anal and vaginal areas. The pad should be changed after urination and defecation. Women should be advised to cleanse the perineal area with soap and water at least one time per day in addition to using the peri bottle after each void or pad change (AWHONN, 2006). Advise the woman that the pad should be changed at least four times per day to prevent contamination from bacteria (AWHONN, 2006). Women should be advised that perineal pain is common and will decrease gradually each day. Most women note complete resolution within 8 weeks of birth (Andrews, Thakar, Sultan et al., 2007). (For information regarding the care of the perineum following an episiotomy, see Client Teaching: Episiotomy Care.)

Ice Pack

If an episiotomy is done at the time of birth, an ice pack is generally applied to the perineum to reduce edema and provide numbing of the tissues, which promotes comfort. In some agencies, chemical ice bags are used: These are usually activated by folding both ends toward the middle. The nurse can create inexpensive ice bags by filling a disposable glove with ice chips or crushed ice and then taping the top of the glove. To protect the perineum from burns caused by contact with such an ice pack, the glove needs to be rinsed under running water to remove any powder and then wrapped in an absorbent towel or washcloth before placing it against the perineum. To attain the maximum effect of this cold treatment, a pattern of applying the ice pack for approximately 20 minutes and then removing it for about 10 minutes should be followed. Usually ice packs are needed for the first 24 hours. Ice packs are used during the first two hours to reduce edema. Continued use of ice packs during the first 24 hours reduces pain (AWHONN, 2006). The nurse provides information about the purpose of the ice pack, as well as anticipated effects, benefits, and possible problems, and explains how to prepare an ice pack for home use if edema is present and early discharge is planned.

Sitz Bath

The warmth of the water in the sitz bath provides comfort, decreases pain, and promotes circulation to the tissues, which promotes healing and reduces the incidence of infection (Figure 31–2 ■). In some facilities, the use of the

MyNursingKit | Video: Types of Incisions

Client Teaching EPISIOTOMY CARE

Content

- Describe the process of wound healing, including the value of healing by first intention as opposed to a jagged tear. Discuss the risk of contamination of the episiotomy by bacteria from the anal area.
- Explain techniques that are used to keep the episiotomy clean and promote healing such as:
  - Sitz bath
  - Use of peri bottle following each voiding or defecation. Wash with soap and water at least once every 24 hours. Change peripads at least four times per day.
- Describe comfort measures:
  - Ice pack or glove immediately following birth
  - Sitz bath
  - Judicious use of analgesics or topical anesthetics
  - Tightening buttocks before sitting
- Identify signs of episiotomy infection. Advise the woman to contact her caregiver if infection develops.

Teaching Method

Many women do not consider the episiotomy a surgical incision.
Discussion helps them understand the importance of good wound care.
Focus on open discussion. Demonstrate correct use of the peri bottle or sitz bath if necessary.

Focus on discussion and provide an opportunity for questions.

Encourage discussion and provide printed handouts. Some of this content may also be covered during a small postpartum class.

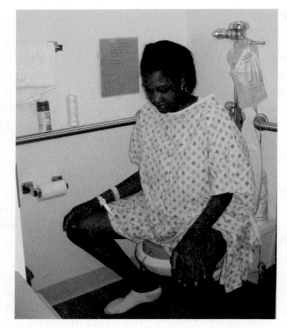

Figure 31–2 A sitz bath promotes healing and provides relief from perineal discomfort during the initial weeks following birth.

sitz bath has declined and is reserved only for women who have third- and fourth-degree lacerations, whereas in other facilities, it is offered to all women who have edema or a laceration following birth. Sitz baths may be ordered three times a day (TID) and as needed (PRN). The nurse prepares the sitz bath by cleaning the equipment and adding water at 38.9°C to 40.6°C (102°F to 105°F). The woman is encouraged to remain in the sitz bath for about 20 minutes. It is important for the woman to have a clean, unused towel to pat dry her perineum after the sitz bath and to have a clean perineal pad to apply. Care needs to be taken during the first sitz bath because the moist heat may cause the woman to faint. The nurse places a call bell well within reach and asks the woman to use it if she feels dizzy or lightheaded or develops difficulty hearing. The nurse also checks on the woman at frequent intervals.

Cool sitz baths have been used because they are effective in reducing perineal edema and reducing the response

COMPLEMENTARY AND ALTERNATIVE THERAPIES

For centuries, lavender oil has been infused into warm water for relief of perineal pain associated with childbirth. Lavender is grown in Africa, Russia, the Arabic peninsula, and the Mediterranean region. The fragrance of lavender is said to promote a calming effect. The anti-anxiety qualities, combined with its soothing properties when diffused in water, make it a popular alternative therapy modality for postpartum women. Lavender may also have some antibacterial effects that may prevent infection in postpartal women.

of nerve endings which cause perineal discomfort (Tejirian & Abbas, 2005). However, many women are reluctant and voice discomfort while sitting in a cool tub of water (Steen, Briggs, & King, 2006). Because women may find the practice uncomfortable, nurses should ask the woman if she would prefer a warm or cool sitz bath based on personal choice (Steen et al., 2006). In administering a cool sitz bath, have the woman start with the water at room temperature and add ice according to the woman's comfort. Because women may have different preferences, it is best to offer the woman a choice of either a warm or cold sitz bath.

The nurse provides information about the purpose and use of the sitz bath; anticipated effects, benefits, and possible problems; and safety measures to prevent overheating, scalds, chills, or injury from fainting or slipping while getting into or out of the tub. Home use of sitz baths may be recommended for the woman with an extensive episiotomy. The woman may use a portable sitz bath or her bathtub. It is important for the nurse to emphasize that in using a bathtub, the woman draws only 4 to 6 in of water, assesses the temperature, and uses the water only for the sitz and not for bathing. If the woman takes a sitz bath, she should release the water, have a helper clean the tub, and draw new water before bathing to prevent infection.

TEACHING TIP

After the mother completes the sitz bath, teach her to inspect the perineal area for burns (that could be related to using water that is too hot), edema, and approximation by using a handheld mirror. If the mother routinely inspects the area, she will be aware of changes that may indicate an infection, such as redness, poor approximation, drainage, or odor.

Topical Agents

Topical anesthetics such as Dermoplast© aerosol spray and Americaine© spray may be used to relieve perineal discomfort. The woman is advised to apply the anesthetic after a sitz bath or perineal care. Witch hazel compresses may be used to relieve perineal discomfort and edema. Nupercainal© ointment or Tucks© or witch hazel pads may be ordered for relief of both hemorrhoidal and perineal pain. The nurse should emphasize the need for the woman to wash her hands before and after using the topical treatments.

The nurse provides information about the anesthetic spray or topical agent. The woman needs to understand the purpose, use, anticipated effects and benefits, and possible problems associated with the product. The nurse can combine a demonstration of application with teaching. A return demonstration is a useful method of evaluating the woman's understanding.

Relief of Hemorrhoidal Discomfort

Some mothers experience hemorrhoidal pain after giving birth. Relief measures include the use of sitz baths, topical anesthetic ointments, rectal suppositories, or witch hazel pads applied directly to the anal area. The woman may be taught to digitally replace external hemorrhoids in her rectum. Handwashing to prevent contamination to the vagina is essential. She may also find it helpful to maintain a side-lying position when possible and to avoid prolonged sitting. The mother is encouraged to maintain an adequate fluid intake, and stool softeners are administered to ensure greater comfort with bowel movements. Mothers should be advised to avoid straining with bowel movements because this can increase the severity and discomfort associated with hemorrhoids. The hemorrhoids usually disappear a few weeks after birth if the woman did not have them before her pregnancy.

Relief of Afterpains

Afterpains are the result of intermittent uterine contractions. A primipara may not experience afterpains because her uterus is able to maintain a contracted state. However, multiparous women and those who have had a multiple-gestation pregnancy or hydramnios frequently experience discomfort from afterpains as the uterus contracts intermittently. Breastfeeding women are also more likely to experience afterpains than formula-feeding women because of the release of oxytocin when the infant suckles.

The nurse can suggest that the woman lie prone, with a small pillow under her lower abdomen, and explain that the discomfort may feel intensified for about 5 minutes but then diminishes greatly if not completely. The prone position applies pressure to the uterus and therefore stimulates contractions. When the uterus maintains a constant contraction, the afterpains cease. Additional nursing interventions include a sitz bath (for warmth), positioning, ambulation, or administration of an analgesic agent. For breastfeeding mothers, an analgesic administered 30 minutes to an hour before nursing helps promote comfort and enhances maternal-infant interaction (Table 31–1).

The nurse provides information about the cause of afterpains and methods to decrease discomfort. She or he explains any medications that are ordered, including their expected effect, benefits, and possible side effects, and any special considerations such as the possibility of dizziness or sleepiness with particular medications.

Relief of Discomfort from Immobility and Muscle Strain

Discomfort may be caused by immobility. The woman who has been in stirrups or has pulled back on her legs for an extended period of time may experience muscular aches from such extreme positioning. It is not unusual for women to experience joint pains and muscular pain in both arms and legs, depending on the effort they exerted during the second stage of labor.

Early ambulation is encouraged to help reduce the incidence of complications such as constipation and thrombophlebitis. It also helps promote a feeling of general well-being. The nurse provides information about ambulation and the importance of monitoring any signs of dizziness or weakness.

The nurse assists the woman the first few times she gets up during the postpartal period. Fatigue, effects of medications, loss of blood, and lack of food intake may cause feelings of dizziness or faintness when the woman stands up. Because this may be a problem during the woman's first shower, the nurse should remain in the room, check the woman frequently, and have a chair close by in case she becomes faint. During this first shower the nurse instructs the woman in the use of the emergency call button in the bathroom; she is advised that, if she becomes faint during a future shower, she should sit down and press the call button for assistance immediately.

MyNursingKit | Afterpains

TEACHING TIP

When assessing Homans' sign, many women will respond that the back of the leg is uncomfortable or that it hurts when performing the Homans' sign. If the discomfort is bilateral and there is no redness, warmth, or tenderness, question the woman further to determine if it is muscular in nature. Many women may indicate they have pain in the back of the calf indicating a positive Homans' sign. However, upon further questioning and clarification, the etiology is muscle strain.

Relief of Discomfort from Postpartal Diaphoresis

Postpartal diaphoresis (excessive perspiration) may cause discomfort for new mothers. The nurse can offer a fresh, dry gown and change bed linens to enhance the mother's comfort. Some women may feel refreshed by a shower. For women experiencing hot flashes as a result of changing hormones, a cool shower may be preferable over a warm or hot shower. It is necessary to consider cultural practices and realize that some Hispanic and Asian women prefer to delay showering. Nurses can offer these women a warm washcloth to increase comfort. The nurse provides information about the normal physiologic changes that cause diaphoresis and methods to increase comfort.

Because diaphoresis may also increase thirst, the nurse can offer fluids as the woman desires. Again, the nurse needs to ask the woman about her preferred beverage. Women of western European background may prefer iced drinks, whereas Asian women may prefer hot tea or water

TABLE 31–1 Essential Information for Common Postpartum Drugs

Tylenol No. 3 (300 mg acetaminophen and 30 mg codeine)

Drug Class:

Narcotic analgesic.

Dose/Route:

Usual adult dose: 1 to 2 tablets PO every 4 hours PRN.

Indication:

For relief of mild to moderate pain.

Adverse Effects:

Respiratory depression, apnea, lightheadedness, dizziness, nausea, sweating, dry mouth, constipation, facial flushing, suppression of cough reflex, ureteral spasm, urinary retention, pruritus, hepatotoxicity (overdose).

Nursing Implications:

Determine whether woman is sensitive to acetaminophen or codeine; has history of impaired hepatic or renal function. Monitor bowel sounds, respirations, urine output.

Administer with food or after meals if GI upset occurs; encourage woman to drink one full glass (240 mL) with the tablet to reduce the risk of the tablet lodging in the esophagus.

Client Teaching:

Inform client about name of drug, expected action, possible side effects, that it is secreted in breast milk (Note: Some physicians/certified nurse-midwives may avoid ordering this medication for breastfeeding mothers), and review safety measures (assess for dizziness, use side rails, call for assistance when getting out of bed and ambulating, report to nurse any signs of adverse effects); ask if she has any questions.

Nursing Diagnoses Related to Drug Therapy:

Health-Seeking Behavior related to information regarding drug therapy

Risk for Injury related to dizziness secondary to effect of drug

Constipation related to slowed gastrointestinal activity secondary to effects of medications.

Percocet (325 mg acetaminophen and 5 mg oxycodone)

Drug Class:

Narcotic analgesic.

Dose/Route:

1 to 2 tablets PO every 4 hours PRN.

Indication:

For moderate to moderately severe pain. Can be used in aspirin-sensitive women.

Adverse Effects:

Acetaminophen: Hepatotoxicity, headache, rash, hypoglycemia.

Oxycodone: Respiratory depression, apnea, circulatory depression, euphoria, facial flushing, constipation, suppression of cough reflex, ureteral spasm, urinary retention.

Nursing Implications:

Determine whether woman is sensitive to acetaminophen or codeine; has bronchial asthma, respiratory depression, convulsive disorder.

Observe woman carefully for respiratory depression if given with barbiturates or sedative/hypnotics. Consider that postcesarean-birth woman may have depressed cough reflex, so teaching and encouragement to deep breathe and cough are needed.

Monitor bowel sounds, urine and bowel elimination.

Client Teaching:

Teaching should include name of drug, expected effect, possible adverse effects, that drug is secreted in the breast milk, encouragement to report any signs of adverse effects immediately.

Nursing Diagnoses Related to Drug Therapy:

Ineffective Breathing Pattern related to respiratory depression

Constipation related to slowed gastrointestinal activity secondary to the effects of medications.

Rubella Virus Vaccine, Live (Meruvax 2)

Dose/Route:

Single-dose vial, inject subcutaneously in outer aspect of the upper arm.

Indication:

Stimulate active immunity against rubella virus.

Adverse Effects:

Burning or stinging at the injection site; about 2 to 4 weeks later may have rash, malaise, sore throat, or headache.

Nursing Implications:

Determine whether woman has sensitivity to neomycin (vaccine contains neomycin); is immunosuppressed, or has received blood transfusions (not to be administered within 28 days of blood transfusion, plasma transfusion, or serum immune globulin). To be given at discharge.

Client Teaching:

Name of drug, expected effect, possible adverse effects, possible comfort measures to use if adverse effects occur; rubella titer will be assessed in about 3 months. Instruct woman to AVOID PREGNANCY FOR 3 MONTHS following vaccination. Provide information regarding contraceptives and their use.

Nursing Diagnoses Related to Drug Therapy:

Deficient Knowledge regarding drug therapy

Health-Seeking Behavior related to information about postpartum contraception regarding an expressed desire to avoid pregnancy following rubella vaccination

Pain related to rash and malaise

| **TABLE 31–1** | Essential Information for Common Postpartum Drugs   *(Continued)* |

RhoGAM (Rh immune globulin specific for D antigen)

Dose/Route:

Postpartum: One vial IM within 72 hours of birth. Antepartal: One vial microdose RhoGAM IM at 28 weeks in Rh-negative women; after amniocentesis, spontaneous or therapeutic abortion, or ectopic pregnancy.

Indication:

Prevention of sensitization to the Rh factor in Rh-negative women and to prevent hemolytic disease in the newborn in subsequent pregnancies. Mother must be Rh negative, not previously sensitized to Rh factor. Infant must be Rh positive, direct antiglobulin negative.

Adverse Effects:

Soreness at injection site.

Nursing Implications:

Confirm criteria for administration are present. Ensure correct vial is used for the client (each vial is cross-matched to the specific woman and must be carefully checked).

Inject entire contents of vial.

Client Teaching:

Name of drug, expected action, possible side effects; report soreness at injection site to nurse; woman should carry information regarding Rh status and dates of RhoGAM injections with her at all times; explain use of RhoGAM with subsequent pregnancies.

Nursing Diagnoses Related to Drug Therapy:

Health-Seeking Behavior related to information about future need for Rh immune globulin regarding an expressed desire to understand the long-term implications of her Rh-negative status

Pain related to soreness at injection site

Ambien (Zolpidem tartrate)

Drug Class:

Hypnotic, sedative.

Dose/Route:

5 to 10 mg PO at bedtime.

Indication:

Promote sleep.

Adverse Effects:

Dizziness, daytime drowsiness, diarrhea, drugged feelings, amnesia.

Nursing Implications:

Determine if woman has compromised respiratory function. Monitor respirations, blood pressure, pulse. Modify environment to increase relaxation and promote sleep. Monitor for drug interaction if woman is taking other CNS depressants.

Client Teaching:

Name of drug, expected effect, possible adverse effects, safety measures (siderails, use call bell, ask for assistance when out of bed); medication is secreted in breast milk.

Nursing Diagnoses Related to Drug Therapy:

Risk for Injury related to possible ataxia or vertigo

Altered Thought Processes related to drug-induced confusion

Health-Seeking Behavior related to information regarding drug therapy

at room temperature. It is important to ascertain the woman's wishes rather than operate from one's own values or cultural beliefs.

Suppression of Lactation in the Non-Breastfeeding Mother

For the woman who chooses not to breastfeed, lactation may be suppressed by mechanical inhibition. Although signs of engorgement do not usually appear until the second or third postpartum day, engorgement is best prevented by beginning mechanical methods of lactation suppression as soon as possible after birth. Ideally, this involves having the woman begin wearing a supportive, well-fitting bra within 6 hours after birth. A tight fitting sports bra may be preferred by some women. The bra is worn continuously until lactation is suppressed (usually about 5 to 7 days) and is removed only for showers. The bra provides support and eases the discomfort that can occur with tension on the breasts because of fullness. Ice packs should be applied over the axillary area of each breast for 20 minutes four times daily.

This practice should also begin soon after birth. In addition, ice is useful in relieving discomfort if engorgement occurs.

The mother is advised to avoid any stimulation of her breasts by her baby, herself, breast pumps, or her sexual partner until the sensation of fullness has passed (usually about 5 to 7 days). Such stimulation increases milk production and delays the suppression process. Heat is avoided for the same reason; therefore, the mother is encouraged to let shower water flow over her back rather than her breasts.

Some mothers may inquire about suppression medications used in the past for non-nursing mothers. Women should be informed that, because of concerns related to side effects, these medications are no longer used. Mechanical, rather than pharmacologic, methods are now employed.

Pharmacologic Interventions

Pharmacologic preparations, including pain medications, vaccinations, and Rh immune globulin, are frequently administered in the postpartal period (see Table 31–1).

Rubella Vaccine

Women who have a rubella titer of less than 1:10, or test antibody negative or indeterminate on the enzyme-linked immunosorbent assay (ELISA), are usually given rubella vaccine in the postpartal period (Gabbe, Niebyl, & Simpson, 2007). The nurse needs to ensure that the woman understands the purpose of the vaccine and that she must avoid becoming pregnant in the next 28 days. To ensure that the woman understands, informed consent is obtained before administration. Because the avoidance of pregnancy is so important, counseling about contraception is suggested.

Rh Immune Globulin

All Rh-negative women who meet specific criteria should receive Rh immune globulin (RhoGAM) within 72 hours after childbirth to prevent sensitization from the fetomaternal transfusion of Rh-positive fetal red blood cells. (See discussion in Chapter 15 ∞.)

The Rh-negative woman needs to understand the implications of her Rh-negative status in future pregnancies. The nurse provides opportunities for questions.

Relief of Emotional Stress

The birth of a child, with the changes in role and the increased responsibilities it produces, is a time of emotional stress for the new mother. During the early postpartal period the mother may be emotionally labile, and mood swings and tearfulness are common. Initially the mother may repeatedly discuss her experiences of labor and birth. This allows the mother to integrate her experiences. If she believes that she did not cope well with labor, she may have feelings of inadequacy and may benefit from reassurance that she did well. Some women feel that they did not have any perception of time during the labor and birth and want to know how long it really lasted, or they may not remember the entire experience. In this case, it is helpful for the nurse to talk with the woman and provide the information that she is missing and desires.

During this time the new mother must also adjust to the loss of her fantasized child and accept the child she has borne. This task may be more difficult if the child is not of the desired sex or if he or she has birth defects (see Chapter 28 ∞). Women who gave birth prematurely may experience guilt or have feelings of inadequacy. Immediately after the birth (the taking-in period) the mother is focused on bodily concerns and may not be fully ready to learn about personal and infant care. Following the initial dependent period, the mother becomes very concerned about her ability to be a successful parent (the taking-hold period). During this time the mother requires reassurance that she is effective. She also tends to be receptive to teaching and demonstration designed to assist her in mothering successfully. The depression, weepiness, and "let-down feeling" that characterize the postpartum blues are often a surprise for the new mother. She requires reassurance that these feelings are normal, an explanation of why they occur, and a supportive environment that permits her to cry without feeling guilty.

Promotion of Maternal Rest and Activity

Following childbirth some women feel exhausted and in need of rest. Other women may be euphoric and full of psychic energy, ready to relive and recount the experience of birth repeatedly. The nurse can provide a period for airing of feelings and then encourage a period of rest. Nurses also promote rest by organizing their activities to avoid frequent interruptions for the woman.

Relief of Fatigue

Physical fatigue often affects other adjustments and functions of the new mother. For example, fatigue can reduce milk flow, thereby increasing problems with establishing breastfeeding. Energy is also needed to make the psychologic adjustments to a new infant and to assume new roles. It is helpful for the new mother to know that fatigue may persist for several weeks or even months. Persistent fatigue is especially common when mothers attempt to perform activities while the baby is napping, instead of resting themselves. Mothers who have other children may feel overwhelmed with trying to meet the needs of her other child(ren). As a result, spending time with them results in additional fatigue. The nurse teaches women that this practice can lead to chronic fatigue and should be avoided. Severe ongoing fatigue can also be a symptom of a thyroid disorder and should be evaluated by a clinician (Gabbe, Niebyl, & Simpson, 2007). Although most new mothers feel tired, if they have perceived the pregnancy and birth as a natural process, they tend to view themselves as healthy and well. Fatigue can also be a symptom of postpartum depression and should be discussed with the healthcare provider if symptoms continue or are accompanied by other signs of depression.

Most mothers view the postpartal period as a time for recuperation. In many non-Western cultures, the 40 days following the birth are a time of recovery when female relatives or friends assist the new mother in her daily activities (Lin, Wang, & Chang, 2007). In Northern Africa, for example, the 40-day period after birth is considered a time of transition for the mother. The mother and infant are not separated during this time. This practice is known to prevent postpartum psychosis and facilitate bonding (Jones, 2006). This is also the custom in India, where it is believed that the mother and new baby need protection from evil spirits as well as from exposure to illness, because they are both considered vulnerable during this time period (Jones, 2006).

In Mexico, this period is briefer, lasting only 20 days. During the first 7 days, nonhousehold members are not permitted to visit or enter the home. The mother gradually increases activity after the first week. The end of the postpartum period is marked by a *sobada*, a massage performed by the midwife on the 20th day after birth (Spector, 2009).

Specific groups of mothers are at a higher risk for postpartum fatigue. These include mothers of multiples, mothers with infants who are still hospitalized that engage in multiple trips to the hospital to visit their babies, mothers of infants with birth defects or special needs, mothers who lack social support, and mothers who return to work before the advised 6-week time period. A mother who has been on extended bedrest during the pregnancy may also be more at risk for fatigue. Because many families are now geographically separated and may be unable to come and spend time with the mother and new baby, fatigue may also be more common in these women when the mother is left to care for herself and baby in the early postpartum period.

Resumption of Activity

Ambulation and activity may gradually increase after birth. The new mother should avoid heavy lifting, excessive stair climbing, and strenuous activity. One or two daily naps are essential and are most easily achieved if the mother sleeps when her baby does. Women with older children often find it difficult to get adequate rest because they want to spend time with their older children when the infant is napping. The woman should be cautioned that fatigue and exhaustion can become a vicious cycle and should be avoided. Assistance in the household can help prevent this and can enable the mother to spend special time with older children while others take over household tasks.

By the second week at home, the woman may resume light housekeeping. Although it is customary to delay returning to work for 6 weeks, most women are physically able to resume practically all activities by 4 to 5 weeks. In some cases, if bleeding returns, it is often a sign that the mother is overdoing her activities and should decrease some activity. Delaying the return to work until after the final postpartal examination minimizes the possibility of problems.

Postpartal Exercises

The woman should be encouraged to begin simple exercises while in the birthing unit and to continue them at home. Kegel exercises should be reviewed and begun while the woman is still in the hospital. She is advised that increased lochia or pain means she should reevaluate her activity and make necessary alterations. Most agencies provide a booklet describing suggested postpartal exercises, such as those shown in Figure 31–3 ■. (Exercise routines vary for women undergoing cesarean birth or tubal ligation after childbirth.)

Exercise during the postpartum period has several health benefits for new mothers. Exercise can help maintain insulin and high-density lipoprotein (HDL) cholesterol levels, as well as improve aerobic fitness. The postpartal woman is more likely to have positive views of her well-being, more self-esteem, and less fatigue if she continues to do stretching and her own pattern of exercise after she is home. The addition of pelvic floor exercises can also decrease such problems as urinary leakage or urinary incontinence. Exercise also helps facilitate postpartum weight loss, reduces stress, and provides the mother with needed time alone.

Promotion of Family Wellness

A positive maternity experience is likely to have a positive effect on the entire family. The family that receives appropriate information and has adequate time to interact with its newest member in a supportive environment will feel more comfortable and secure at home.

Today most facilities support *family-centered care* that is focused on keeping the mother and baby together as much as the mother desires. This type of care is called **mother-baby care,** or **couplet care**, and provides increased opportunities for parent-child interaction because the newborn shares the mother's room and they are cared for together. Mother-baby care enables the mother to have time to bond with her baby and learn to care for her or him in a supportive environment. It is especially conducive to a hunger-demand feeding schedule for both breast- and formula-feeding babies. This arrangement also allows the father, siblings, grandparents, and others to participate in the care of the new baby. Women who give birth in a facility that offers mother-baby care are often more satisfied with their postpartum experience than women who are cared for under different care models. The World Health Organization (WHO) advocates for a "rooming-in" model of care where the mother and infant remain together as much as possible (WHO, 2007).

Mother-baby unit policies must be flexible enough to permit the mother to return the baby to the nursery if she finds it necessary because of fatigue or physical discomfort. Some mother-baby units also return the newborns to a central nursery at night so the mothers can get more rest.

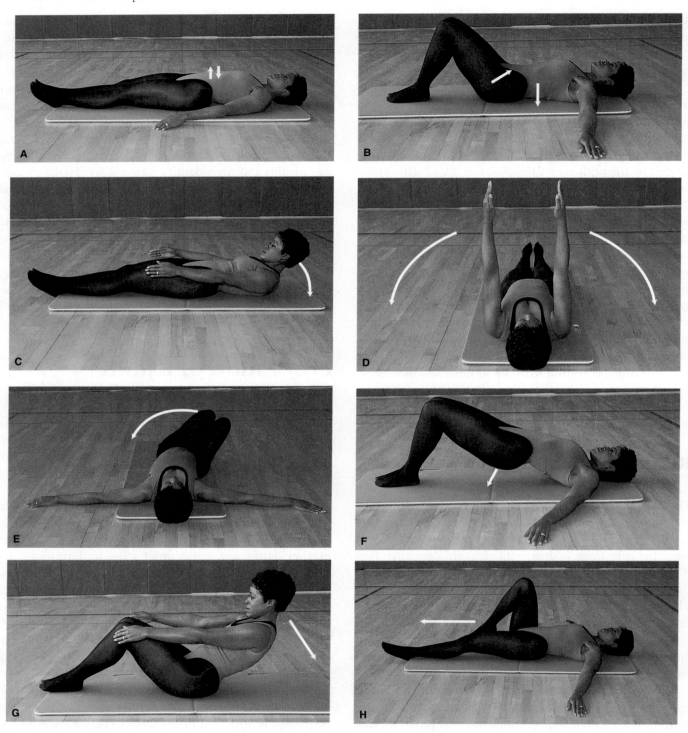

FIGURE 31-3 Postpartal exercises. Begin with five repetitions two or three times daily, and gradually increase to 10 repetitions. First day: *A,* Abdominal breathing. Lying supine, inhale deeply, using the abdominal muscles. The abdomen should expand. Then exhale slowly through pursed lips, tightening the abdominal muscles. *B,* Pelvic rocking. Lying supine with arms at sides, knees bent, and feet flat, tighten abdomen and buttocks, and attempt to flatten back on floor. Hold for a count of 10; then arch the back, causing the pelvis to "rock." On the second day, add *C,* Chin to chest. Lying supine with legs straight, raise head and attempt to touch chin to chest. Slowly lower head. *D,* Arm raises. Lying supine, arms extended at a 90-degree angle from body, raise arms so that they are perpendicular and hands touch. Lower slowly. On fourth day, add *E,* Knee rolls. Lying supine with knees bent, feet flat, arms extended to the side, roll knees slowly to one side, keeping shoulders flat. Return to original position, and roll to opposite side. *F,* Buttocks lift. Lying supine, arms at sides, knees bent, feet flat, slowly raise the buttocks, and arch the back. Return slowly to starting position. On sixth day, add *G,* Abdominal tighteners. Lying supine, knees bent, feet flat, slowly raise head toward knees. Arms should extend along either side of legs. Return slowly to original position. *H,* Knee to abdomen. Lying supine, arms at sides, bend one knee and thigh until foot touches buttocks. Straighten leg and lower it slowly. Repeat with other leg. After 2 to 3 weeks, more strenuous exercises, such as push-ups and side leg raises, may be added as tolerated. Kegel exercises, begun antepartally, should be done many times daily during postpartum to restore vaginal and perineal tone.

CULTURAL PERSPECTIVES

Postpartal clients may have culturally based beliefs about the types of foods and beverages that should be consumed in the postpartum period. For example, Asian clients may believe that a balance of yin and yang is necessary for optimal health. On the postpartal unit, these clients may wish to consume only hot fluids in an effort to restore their yin–yang balance. No matter her cultural background, always ask the woman if she prefers hot, warm, or cold fluids at her bedside. If the desired temperature is not accessible to the woman, fluid intake could be decreased.

Unless contraindicated, nurses should encourage all women to incorporate food preferences with strong cultural significance into their postpartal diet. Family members can bring these items to the hospital for consumption during the immediate recovery period.

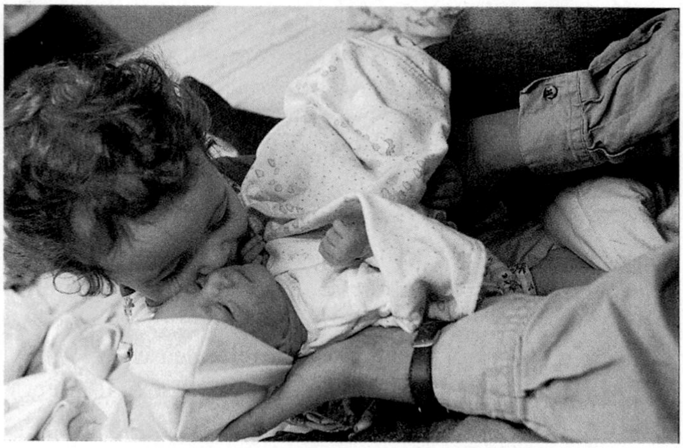

FIGURE 31–4 The sister of this newborn becomes acquainted with the new family member during a nursing assessment.
Source: © Stella Johnson (www.stellajohnson.com).

Reactions of Siblings

Mother-baby care provides excellent opportunities for family bonds to grow when the mother, father/partner, newborn, and siblings begin functioning as a family unit immediately after the birth. When mother-baby care is not available, liberal sibling visitation policies can meet the family's needs. A visit to the mother-baby unit reassures children that their mother is well and still loves them. It also provides an opportunity for the children to become familiar with the new baby. For the mother, the pangs of separation are lessened as she interacts with her children and introduces them to the newest family member (Figure 31–4 ■). Even infants who require intensive care nursery admissions should be allowed to have sibling visits whenever possible. Although there is a valid concern to prevent preemies and other infants who require intensive care services from infection, policies that involve taking the child's temperature before each visit and documenting the child's health status can provide a safeguard that still promotes family bonding. Some of these infants may be hospitalized for weeks or months. Sibling visitation allows the early incorporation of the infant into the family unit for siblings.

HINTS FOR PRACTICE

Because siblings may feel left out with the addition of a new family member, provide positive feedback to promote attachment. For example, pointing out to the older child that "Carlos is looking at you" or asking, "Do you think he knows you're his big sister?" can help make siblings feel accepted and valued. Also identify ways in which siblings can help the new mother, for example, by bringing her a cup of water or singing the baby a favorite lullaby.

Teach parents that, although they may have prepared their children for the presence of a new brother or sister, the actual arrival of the infant in the home requires some adjustments. Although it may be more chaotic for the parents, allowing the children to come to the hospital to pick up mom and the new baby can signify their importance in the family process. If small children are waiting at home, it is helpful if the father carries the baby inside. This practice keeps the mother's arms free to hug and touch her older children. Many mothers bring a doll home with them for an older child. Caring for the doll alongside the mother or father helps the child to identify with the parents. This identification helps decrease anger and the need to regress for attention.

Parents may also provide supervised times when older children can hold the new baby and perhaps even help with a feeding or diapering. Many parents may have concerns about the children "hurting" the new baby, but with proper supervision, the siblings are more likely to develop an attachment to their new sibling. The other children feel a sense of accomplishment and learn tenderness and caring. The nurse also suggests that parents spend one-to-one quality time with each of their older children each day. This may require some careful planning, but it confirms the parents' continuing love for the other children and promotes their acceptance of the newborn.

Sexual Activity and Contraception

Typically, postpartum couples resume sexual intercourse once the episiotomy is healed and the lochial flow has stopped (AWHONN, 2006). Because this usually occurs by the end of the third week, before the 6-week check, it is important that the woman and her partner have information about what to expect. The nurse may inform the couple that, because the vaginal vault is "dry" (lacking estrogen), some form of water-soluble lubrication such as K-Y© jelly or Astroglide© may be necessary during intercourse. The female-superior and side-lying coital positions may be preferable because they allow the woman to control the depth of penile penetration. Couples should be counseled that intercourse may be uncomfortable for the woman for some time and that patience is imperative.

Breastfeeding couples should be forewarned that during orgasm milk may spurt from the nipples because of the release of oxytocin. Some couples find this spurt pleasurable or amusing, but others choose to have the woman wear a bra during sexual activity. Nursing the baby before lovemaking reduces the chance of milk release.

Other factors may inhibit satisfactory sexual experiences: the baby's crying may "spoil the mood," the woman's changed body may seem unattractive to her or her partner, maternal sleep deprivation may reduce the woman's desire, and the woman's physiologic response to sexual stimulation may be altered because of hormonal changes. By 3 months postpartum, many couples have returned to prepregnant levels of sexual interest and activity; however, this is highly variable. It is not abnormal for women, especially when breastfeeding, to experience decreased libido for several months. Decreased libido can be associated with hormonal changes, fatigue, stress, and lack of time because of family and work demands.

With anticipatory guidance during the prenatal and postpartal periods, the couple can be forewarned of potential temporary problems. Anticipatory guidance is enhanced if the couple can discuss their feelings and reactions as they are experienced. (See Client Teaching: Resuming Sexual Activity After Childbirth and the Teaching Card summarizing this topic in the center of this text.)

Information on contraception is often provided as part of discharge teaching if it is permissible within the healthcare agency. The nurse can also be an important resource for the woman and her partner during postpartum follow-up. Couples typically choose to use contraception to control the number of children they will have or to determine the spacing of future children. However, some religious-based hospital facilities prohibit nurses and other healthcare providers from discussing contraception. If the nurse is discussing birth control, it is important to emphasize that in choosing a specific method, consistency of use is essential. The nurse needs to identify the advantages, disadvantages, risks, and contraindications of the various methods to help the couple, or the single mother, make an informed choice about the most practical and compatible method. (For a more detailed discussion of contraceptive methods, see Chapter 5 ∞.) Breastfeeding women are commonly concerned that a con-

---

Client Teaching RESUMING SEXUAL ACTIVITY AFTER CHILDBIRTH

Content

- Present information about changes that may affect sexual activity, including the following:
  - Tenderness of the vagina and perineum
  - Presence of lochia and the healing process
  - Dryness of the vagina
  - Breast engorgement and tenderness
  - Escape of milk during sexual activity

- Discuss healing at the placental site and stress that the presence of lochia indicates that healing is not yet complete. Point out that because the vagina is "hormone-poor" postpartally, vaginal dryness may pose a problem. This can be avoided by using a water-soluble lubricant. Explain that escape of milk during sexual activity can be minimized by breastfeeding the baby immediately beforehand.

- Discuss the importance of contraception during the early postpartal period. Provide information on the advantages and disadvantages of different methods. The woman's body needs adequate time to heal and recover from the stress of pregnancy and childbirth. Couples who are opposed to contraception may choose abstinence at this time.

- Discuss the impact of fatigue and the new baby's schedule on the woman's feelings of desire. Refer the couple to a physician/CNM for additional information if needed.

Teaching Method

Discussion is a logical approach. It may be useful to make a universal statement and link it with a question to determine a couple's initial level of knowledge. For example, "Many women experience vaginal dryness when they resume intercourse for the first several weeks after childbirth. Are you familiar with this change and the cause for it?" Use the information gained during this discussion to determine the depth to which to cover the material.

Provide printed information to clarify content and serve as a resource for the couple following discharge.

Provide samples of different types of contraceptives.
Provide literature on specific contraceptive methods.

traceptive method will interfere with their ability to breast-feed. Breastfeeding women should be given available options and choose the method that best fits their lifestyle, financial situation, and personal preference.

Parent-Infant Attachment

Nursing interventions to enhance the quality of parent-infant attachment should be designed to promote feelings of well-being, comfort, and satisfaction. Certain groups of women are at higher risk for alterations in parent-infant attachment. These include women who have less than a ninth-grade education; are unemployed, single, or unmarried; have a previous history of depression or psychologic problems, gave birth to a female infant, or had an infant admission into the neonatal intensive care nursery (Conde, Figueiredo, Costa, Pacheco, & Pais, 2008). These mothers warrant additional assessment and support from the nurse to ensure proper bonding is taking place.

Some parents may lack any expereince with babies and may feel overwhelmed by the infant. Bonding is a series of steps in which the mother and infant develop a realtionship. Although certain medical interruptions can delay bonding, such as when an extremely premature infant is hospitalized for a prolonged period of time, bonding still takes place.

Following are some suggestions for ways of promoting parent-infant attachment during the postpartal stay:

- Determine the parenting style and goals of the infant's mother and father/partner and adapt them when possible in planning nursing care for the family. This includes giving the parents choices about their initial time with their new infant.

- Provide time and as much privacy as possible for the new family to become acquainted. Allow siblings to visit throughout the postpartal stay if requested by the parents.
- Arrange the healthcare setting so that the individual nurse-client relationship can be developed. A primary nurse can develop rapport and assess the mother's strengths and needs.
- Use anticipatory guidance to prepare the parents for expected problems of adjustment. Model appropriate behaviors based on the infant's cues and behaviors.
- Include parents in any nursing intervention, planning, and evaluation. Give choices when possible.
- Initiate and support measures to alleviate fatigue in the parents.
- Help parents identify, understand, and accept both positive and negative feelings related to the overall parenting experience.
- Support and assist parents in determining the personality and unique needs of their infant.

The beginnings of parent-newborn attachment may be observed in the first few hours after birth. Continued assessments may occur during the postpartal stay and in home visits after discharge. As the nurse assesses attachment, it is important to remember that cultural values, beliefs, and practices will direct the childcare activities and self-care practices. For example, some women of Mexican American and Southeast Asian descent may deflect compliments directed toward their baby because of their belief that they may attract the attention of evil spirits. (See Table 31–2 for behaviors related to attachment.)

TABLE 31–2	Parent Attachment Behaviors	
Assessment Area	Attachment	Behavior Requiring Assessment and Information
Caretaking	Talks with baby. Demonstrates and seeks eye-to-eye contact. Touches and holds baby. Changes diapers when needed. Baby is clean. Clothing is appropriate for room temperature. Feeds baby as needed and baby is gaining weight. Positions baby comfortably and checks on baby.	Does not refer to baby. Completes activities without addressing the baby or looking at the baby. Lack of interaction. Does not recognize need for or demonstrate concern for baby's comfort or needs. Feeding occurs intermittently. Baby does not gain weight. Waits for baby to cry and then hesitates to respond.
Perception of the baby	Has knowledge of expected child development. Understands that the baby is dependent and cannot meet parent's needs. Accepts sex of child and characteristics.	Has unrealistic expectations of the baby's abilities and behaviors. Expects love and interaction from the baby. Believes that the baby will fulfill parent's needs. Is strongly distressed over sex of baby or feels that some aspect of the baby is unacceptable.
Support	Has friends who are available for support. Seems to be comfortable with being a parent. Has realistic beliefs of parenting role.	Is alone or isolated. Is on edge, tense, anxious, and hesitant with the baby. Demonstrates difficulty incorporating parenting with own wants and needs.

Note: These are a few of the behaviors that may be associated with attachment. It is vitally important for the nurse to observe the parents on more than one occasion and to take into consideration individual characteristics, values, beliefs, and customs.

MyNursingKit | Bonding with the Newborn

MyNursingKit | Bonding: Recent Observations That Alter Perinatal Care

Nursing Care Following Cesarean Birth

After a cesarean birth the new mother has postpartal needs similar to those of women who have given birth vaginally. Because she has undergone major abdominal surgery, however, the woman's nursing care needs are also similar to those of other surgical clients.

Promotion of Maternal Physical Well-Being After Cesarean Birth

The chances of pulmonary infection are increased because of immobility after the use of narcotics and sedatives and because of the altered immune response in postoperative clients. Therefore, the woman is encouraged to cough and deep breathe every 2 to 4 hours while awake until she is ambulating frequently.

Leg exercises are also encouraged every 2 hours until the woman is ambulating. These exercises increase circulation, help prevent thrombophlebitis, and also aid intestinal motility by tightening abdominal muscles.

Many of the historical complications of post-cesarean birth were related to postpartum care practices in which mothers were encouraged to stay in bed for prolonged periods of time. Early ambulation, eating a low roughage diet shortly after birth, and breastfeeding or infant feeding soon after birth all enhance the recovery of the mother and decrease complications in the postoperative period. Even though a cesarean birth is an operative procedure, most women giving birth are relatively healthy and therefore are less likely to experience postoperative complications when compared with other surgical clients.

The nurse monitors and manages the woman's pain experience during the postpartum period. Sources of pain include incisional pain, gas pain, referred shoulder pain, periodic uterine contractions (afterbirth pains), discomfort related to breastfeeding, and pain from voiding, defecation, or constipation.

Nursing interventions are oriented toward preventing or alleviating pain or helping the woman cope with pain. The nurse should undertake the following measures:

- Administer analgesics as needed, especially during the first 24 to 72 hours after childbirth. Use of analgesics relieves the woman's pain and enables her to be more mobile and active. Some facilities administer ibuprofen on a continuous basis in the early postpartum period to decrease swelling, reduce pain, and decrease the need for, or frequency of, narcotic agents.
- Promote comfort through proper positioning, frequent position changes, massage, back rubs, oral care, and the reduction of noxious stimuli such as noise and unpleasant odors.

- Encourage visits by significant others, including the newborn and older children. These visits distract the woman from the painful sensations and help reduce her fear and anxiety.
- Encourage the use of breathing, relaxation, guided imagery, and distraction (e.g., stimulation of cutaneous tissue) techniques taught in childbirth preparation class.

Epidural analgesia administered just after the cesarean birth is an effective method of pain relief for most women in the first 24 hours following birth (see Drug Guide: Postpartum Epidural Morphine).

The physician may order **patient-controlled analgesia (PCA)**. With this approach the woman is given a bolus of analgesia, usually morphine or fentanyl, at the beginning of therapy. Using a special intravenous (IV) pump system, the woman presses a button to self-administer small doses of the medication as needed. For safety, the pump is preset with a time lockout so that the woman cannot deliver another dose until a specified period of time has elapsed. The use of a PCA helps women feel a greater sense of control and less dependence on nursing staff. The frequent, smaller doses help the woman experience rapid pain relief without grogginess and avoid the discomfort associated with injections.

Another technique of pain control that is sometimes used is the **continuous epidural infusion (CEI)** technique, in which the epidural catheter is left in place following the cesarean birth and medication is continually administered via an electric pump. The device also has a button which the woman can depress if additional pain relief is needed. Fentanyl is the most commonly used drug because it tends to provide good pain relief (Viscusi, 2008). Nursing assessments are hourly for women with a CEI in place and include vital signs, level of pain, amount of drug received, and amount of self-administration. The tubing is inspected to ensure connections are maintained because movement by the woman in bed could disrupt the line. The epidural site should also be assessed to ensure the catheter has not been displaced.

Another technique used for pain control for post-cesarean birth is the use of a continuous peripheral nerve block that delivers a local anesthetic through a tiny catheter that is positioned directly into the wound site. An external balloon allows medication to be delivered at a steady rate up to 5 days after the birth and creates a numbing effect at the incision site. After a specified time period, the catheter is displaced by gently pulling it from the site. Additional surgical intervention is not required to remove the device. The use of one of these devices can reduce the amount of systemic analgesia that is needed in the postpartum period (Gucev, Yasui, Chang et al., 2008). Most recently, ultrasound guidance has been utilized to produce better pain relief results (Gucev et al., 2008). Although

Drug Guide Postpartum Epidural Morphine

Overview of Obstetric Action Epidural morphine is used to provide relief of pain associated with cesarean birth, extensive episiotomies (mediolaterals), or third- and fourth-degree lacerations. Epidural morphine pain relief results directly from its effect on the opiate receptors in the spinal cord (it depresses pain impulse transmission). Morphine binds opiate receptors, thereby altering both the perception of and emotional response to pain. Women experience little or no discomfort or pain during recovery and for up to 24 hours afterward. There is no motor or sympathetic block or associated hypotension. Onset of analgesia is slower, but duration is longer.

Route, Dosage, and Frequency Morphine (5 to 7.5 mg) is injected through a catheter into the epidural space, providing pain relief for about 24 hours (Wilson et al., 2009).

Maternal Contraindications Allergy to morphine, narcotic addiction, chronic debilitating respiratory disease, infection at the injection site, or administration of parenteral corticosteroids in past 14 days (Wilson et al., 2009).

Maternal Side Effects Late-onset respiratory depression (rare but may occur 8 to 12 hours after administration), nausea and vomiting (occurring between 4 and 7 hours after injection), itching (begins within 3 hours and lasts up to 10 hours), urinary retention, and rarely somnolence. Side effects can be managed with naloxone.

Neonatal Effects No adverse effects because medication is injected after the birth of the baby.

Nursing Considerations

- Obtain history: sensitivity (allergy) to morphine, presence of any contraindications (Wilson et al., 2009).

- Assess orientation, reflexes, skin color, texture, breath sounds, presence of lesions or infection over area of lumbar spine, voiding pattern, urinary output within normal limits (Wilson et al., 2009).
- Monitor and evaluate analgesic effect. Ask client about comfort level and notify anesthesiologist of inadequate pain relief.
- Check catheter for obvious knots, breaks, and leakage at insertion site and catheter hub.
- Assess for pruritus (scratching and rubbing, especially around face and neck).
- Administer comfort measures for narcotic-induced pruritus, such as lotion, backrubs, cool/warm packs, or diversional activities. If the itching can be tolerated, naloxone should be avoided, especially because it counteracts the pain relief.
- If allergic reaction (urticaria, edema, or respiratory difficulties) occurs, administer naloxone or diphenhydramine per physician order.
- Provide comfort measures for nausea/vomiting, such as frequent oral hygiene or gradual increase of activity; administer naloxone, trimethobenzamide (Tigan), or metoclopramide HCl per physician order.
- Assess postural blood pressure and heart rate before ambulation.
- Assist client with her first ambulation and then as needed.
- Assess respiratory function every hour for 24 hours, then q2–8 hr as needed. Also assess level of consciousness and mucous membrane color. May need to monitor client via apnea monitor for 24 hours.
- Monitor urinary output and assess bladder for distention. Assist client to void.

these devices are not widely used, they can be an option for a woman undergoing a cesarean birth.

Although the use of general anesthesia continues to decline, women who receive general anesthesia warrant additional assessments in the immediate postpartum period. Vital signs should be monitored continually until the woman has regained consciousness. Cardiopulmonary equipment should be in close range with cardiac monitoring available as needed. The pulse oximeter should be used to determine the woman's oxygen status.

If a general anesthetic was used, abdominal distention may produce marked discomfort for the woman during the first few postpartal days. Measures to prevent or minimize abdominal distention include leg exercises, abdominal tightening, ambulation, avoiding carbonated or very hot or cold beverages, and avoiding the use of straws. Women can be started on a low residue diet within 6 hours of birth (Göçmen, Göçmen, & Saraoğlu, 2002). Medical intervention for gas pain includes using rectal suppositories and enemas to stimulate passage of flatus and stool

and encouraging the woman to lie on her left side. Lying on the left side allows the gas to pass from the descending colon to the sigmoid colon so that it can be expelled more readily.

Many physicians also order a nonsteroidal anti-inflammatory drug (NSAID) in addition to the previously mentioned agents once the woman is tolerating oral fluids well. NSAIDs assist with decreasing inflammation and do not have the negative side effects associated with many narcotics, such as sedation and constipation. NSAIDs are often given in combination with narcotic agents in the immediate postpartum period and often result in a decreased intake of narcotic agents.

Sometimes women who have a cesarean birth have other discomforts that can be relieved with pharmacologic interventions. The nurse assesses the woman for other symptoms, such as nausea, itching (which is typically related to the morphine used in the epidural), and headache. If the woman is experiencing nausea, an antiemetic can be administered. Itching can also be relieved with pharmacologic interventions. NSAIDs are effective in managing headaches and other body aches.

The nurse can minimize discomfort and promote satisfaction as the mother assumes the activities of her new role. Instruction and assistance in assuming comfortable positions when holding or breastfeeding the infant will do much to increase the mother's sense of competence and comfort. The woman should be taught to splint her incision when she ambulates to decrease pulling on the incision and the discomfort created by contraction of the abdominal muscles.

Other measures are aimed at needs that are unique to the woman who has had an operative birth. These include the following (AWHONN, 2006):

- Assessing for the return of bowel sounds in all four quadrants every 4 hours. Assessing the consistency of the abdomen. Women with a firm, distended abdomen may be having difficulty passing flatus or stool.
- Assessing the intravenous (IV) site, flow rate, and patency of the IV tubing.
- Monitoring the condition of surgical dressings or the incision site using the REEDA scale (redness, edema, ecchymosis, discharge, and approximation of the suture line) along with skin temperature at and around the incision line.

The cesarean birth mother usually does extremely well postoperatively. Most women are ambulating by the day after the surgery. Usually by the second postpartal day the woman can shower, which seems to provide a mental as well as physical lift. Most women are discharged by the third day after birth.

Promotion of Parent-Infant Interaction After Cesarean Birth

Many factors associated with cesarean birth may hinder successful and frequent parent-infant interaction. These factors include the physical condition of the mother and newborn and maternal reactions to stress, anesthesia, and medications. The significant other may be concerned about the mother and preoccupied with her condition, resulting in less interaction with the newborn. The mother and her infant may be separated after birth because of birthing unit routines, prematurity, or neonatal complications or a birth defect. A healthy infant born by uncomplicated cesarean is no more fragile than one born vaginally.

In some cases, signs of depression, anger, or withdrawal may indicate a grief response to the loss of the fantasized birth experience. Fathers as well as mothers may experience feelings of "missing out," guilt, or even jealousy toward another couple who had a vaginal birth. The cesarean birth couple may need the opportunity to tell their story repeatedly to work through these feelings. The nurse can provide factual information about their situation and support the

couple's effective coping behaviors. The nurse should acknowledge their feelings while emphasizing the importance of a healthy birth outcome. Enhanced communication during the labor, birth, and in the immediate period along with specific teaching related to issues regarding a cesarean birth are associated with less maternal distress and improved satisfaction with the birth experience (Porter, van Teijlingen, Chi Ying Yip et al., 2007). It is also important to remember that some women may feel more comfortable with a cesarean birth and may have requested a primary or repeat cesarean birth (Wiklund, Edman, & Andolf, 2007). During the initial taking-in phase, the new parents are processing their new role and may be nurturing themselves and each other. This is normal and expected.

By the second or third day the cesarean birth mother moves into the "taking-hold" period and is usually receptive to learning how to care for herself and her infant. During this period, the focus shifts from the mother and father/partner to the baby. Vulnerability can occur during this period and the parents may feel overwhelmed. The need for nursing intervention to guide the new parents is essential. Special emphasis should be given to home management. The nurse can encourage the mother to let others assume responsibility for housekeeping and cooking. Fatigue not only prolongs recovery but also interferes with breastfeeding and mother-infant interaction, increases the risk of prolonged postpartum blues, and leads to feelings of being overwhelmed.

The presence of the father or significant other during the birth process positively influences the woman's perception of the birth event. The partner's presence reduces the woman's fears, enhances her sense of control, and enables the couple to share feelings and respond to each other with touch and eye contact. Later, they have the opportunity to relive the experience and fill in any gaps or missing pieces. The presence of the father or significant other is especially valuable if the mother has had general anesthesia. The partner can take pictures, hold the baby, and foster the discovery process by directing the mother's attention to the details of the newborn. Sometimes, during the taking-hold phase, the father/partner can feel neglected or excluded. This will soon pass as the letting-go stage begins. During this transition, the family incorporates the baby into the family unit and other family members, such as grandparents and siblings, get to know the baby and be included in the new family routine.

The infant born by cesarean is typically removed from the operating room before the mother is able to hold the newborn. Separation of the family unit is not medically necessary unless the infant needs to be stabilized or there is a complication occurring in the operating room. The practice is typically historical in nature. Agencies that embrace family centered care can advocate to keep the mother-baby couple together as much as possible. The nurse can play a crucial role in facilitating interaction by encouraging the father or support person to stand beside the warmer and interact with the infant. Often, the infant can be given to the father or support person to hold. The father or support person can hold the infant close to the mother and place the infant against the mother's cheek so direct eye contact can occur. The nurse can also arrange for the infant to stay with the parents in the recovery area in the immediate postoperative period. This gives the family time to interact when the infant is in an alert state.

Often new parents perceive the parenting role as an extension of the childbearing role. Inability to fulfill expected childbearing behavior (vaginal birth) may lead to parental feelings of role failure and frustration. If the parents' attitude is more positive than negative, successful resolution of subsequent stressful events is more likely. The nurse can help families alter their negative definitions of cesarean birth and bolster and encourage positive perceptions.

Nursing Care of the Postpartal Adolescent

The adolescent mother may have special postpartal needs, depending on her level of maturity and support system. The nurse needs to assess maternal-infant interaction, roles of support people, plans for discharge, knowledge of childrearing, and plans for follow-up care. It is imperative that a community health service contact the adolescent shortly after discharge.

Contraception counseling is an important part of teaching. The incidence of repeat pregnancies during adolescence is high. The younger the adolescent, the more likely she is to become pregnant again. Nurses should be aware of the state laws that govern their jurisdiction in order to determine if providing contraception without parental consent is allowed. In states where adolescents can obtain birth control without parental consent, it is often more comfortable for the adolescent to address these issues without others present (see Chapter 13 ∞). Adolescents may encounter obstacles when attempting to obtain contraceptives. These may include embarrassment about discussing the topic; concerns about confidentiality, such as not wanting their parents to know or having to give permission; and lack of knowledge regarding available methods (Lemay, Cashman, Elfenbein et al., 2007). Nurses can play a key role in overcoming these obstacles by providing teaching and referrals that address these barriers.

The nurse has many opportunities for teaching the adolescent about her newborn in the postpartal unit. Because the nurse is a role model, the manner in which she handles the newborn greatly influences the young mother. If he is present, the father should be included in as much of the teaching as possible. If the grandparents are going to take an active role in caring for the infant, they should also be included in teaching *if* desired by the new mother.

As with older parents, a newborn examination done at the bedside gives adolescents information about their baby's health and shows possible positions for handling the baby. The nurse can also use this time to provide information about newborn and infant behavior. Parents who have some idea of what to expect from their infant are less frustrated with the newborn's behavior.

The adolescent mother appreciates positive feedback about her newborn and her developing maternal responses. Praise and encouragement will increase her confidence and self-esteem. Young mothers with low self-esteem, family conflict, and few social supports are more likely to encounter postpartum depression (Reid & Meadows-Oliver, 2007). Careful assessment of these factors should be made during the postpartum so appropriate referrals can be provided before discharge.

Group classes for adolescent mothers should include information about infant care skills, such as taking the baby's temperature, clearing the nose and mouth, monitoring growth and development, feeding the infant, providing well-baby care, and identifying danger signals in the ill newborn. These classes can also address unique needs of teen mothers, such as peer relationships, added responsibilities, and goal setting.

Ideally, teenage mothers should visit adolescent clinics for assessment of themselves and their newborn for several years after birth. In this way, the adolescent's enrollment in classes on parenting, need for vocational guidance, and school attendance can be supported and followed closely. School systems' classes for young mothers are an excellent way of helping adolescents finish school and learn how to parent at the same time. Some public high schools have on-site childcare centers to assist with childcare needs and to provide an opportunity for adolescents to learn important child development principles and childcare tasks.

Nursing Care of the Woman Who Relinquishes Her Infant

Women who choose to give their infants up for adoption typically are single, white, never-married adolescents. It is much less common in blacks and Hispanic cultures to consider adoption. The majority of young women who relinquish their children have higher education and income levels, higher future educational or career goals, and mothers and fathers that favor adoption. The number of women, approximately 14,000 in the United States, who give their babies up voluntarily is shrinking because of an increase in acceptability of single motherhood and teenage parenting. Less than 1% of all births in the United States result in an adoption (Child Welfare Information Gateway, 2005). Still others may feel that they are not emotionally ready for the responsibilities of parenthood, or their partner may strongly disapprove of the pregnancy. These and many other reasons may prompt the woman to relinquish her baby.

Increasingly, mothers are forced to relinquish their infants because of lifestyle choices such as illicit drug use, past history of abusing children, and incarceration. The number of infants that are placed for adoption because of these circumstances is unknown. Many of these infants may be placed with relatives or in the foster care system. Several factors must be met including clear evidence that the parent is unfit and that severing the parental rights are in the best interest of the child (Child Welfare Information Gateway, 2007a).

In the 1990s, a number of infants were abandoned and left to die because the mothers did not want them and did not want others to know of their pregnancies. Starting in 1997, Infant Safe Haven Acts were enacted which provided a means for a mother to place her baby up for adoption anonymously. The legislation was enacted to protect newborns from death caused by abandonment. There are now 47 states with legislation in place to ensure relinquished babies are left with safe providers who can care for them and provide medical services. The relinquishing mother is protected from prosecution for neglect or abandonment under the law (Child Welfare Information Gateway, 2007b).

Surrogacy is also becoming more common in the United States, resulting in relinquishment agreements that may not show up in the adoption statistics. Even though the mother has entered a legal agreement to give up the child she is carrying, she still faces grief issues.

The mother who chooses to let her child be adopted usually experiences intense ambivalence. Several factors contribute to this ambivalence. First, there are social pressures against giving up one's child. Additionally, the woman has usually made considerable adjustments in her lifestyle to carry and give birth to this child, and may be unaware of the growing bond between her and her child. Her attachment feelings may peak upon seeing her baby. At the same time, she may not have told friends and relatives about the pregnancy and so may lack a support system to help her work through her feelings and support her decision making. After childbirth, the mother needs to complete a grieving process to work through her loss and its accompanying grief, loneliness, guilt, and other feelings. Mothers who relinquish their infants and have open adoptions experience less grief than those who have closed adoptions (Henney, Ayers-Lopez, McCoy et al., 2007). When the relinquishing mother is admitted to the birthing unit, the nurse should be informed about the mother's decision to relinquish the baby. The nurse needs to respect any special requests for the birth and encourage the woman to express her emotions. After the birth the

mother should have access to the baby; she will decide whether she wants to see the newborn. Seeing the newborn often aids the grieving process and provides an opportunity for the birthmother to say goodbye. When the mother sees her baby, she may feel strong attachment and love. The nurse needs to assure the woman that these feelings do not mean that her decision to relinquish the child is wrong; relinquishment is often a painful act of love (Henney et al., 2007).

Postpartal nursing care also includes arranging ongoing care for the relinquishing mother. Some mothers may request an early discharge or a transfer to another medical unit. When possible, the nurse supports these requests.

Preparation for Discharge

In 1998, the Newborns' and Mothers' Health Protection Act went into effect. This federal law ensures that all insurance companies cover a 48-hour stay for vaginal deliveries and a 96-hour stay for women who have undergone a cesarean birth (United States Department of Labor, 2007). Despite this legislation, a decade later, women are still being pressured to leave the hospital before the time frames allotted by federal law. In consideration of the risks associated with voluntary early discharge, more than half of all U.S. states have passed legislation mandating a home visit if the family was discharged before 48 hours. One study examining the use of home visits found that the new legislation increased length of stay and home visits for those women who were discharged early; however, the majority of mothers who were discharged early did not receive early follow-up (Madlon-Kay & DeFor, 2005).

In preparation for discharge, the nurse evaluates the mother and newborn's progress toward identified outcomes and provides discharge teaching. See the Teaching Cards on Postpartum Discharge Teaching in the center of this text.

Discharge Criteria

Before discharge, the nurse assesses the mother's physical and psychologic condition, the newborn's adjustment to extrauterine life, the family's overall adjustment, and the need for outside resources in the postpartal period. In general, the following criteria should be assessed and met before discharge:

- Normal vital signs
- Appropriate involution of the uterus
- Appropriate amount of lochia without evidence of infection
- Knowledge of signs of infection
- Episiotomy or laceration well approximated with a decrease in edema or bruising

- Ability to perform pericare and apply medications to perineal or anal area if ordered
- Ability to void and pass flatus (some facilities' criteria may include having a bowel movement before discharge)
- Ability to take fluids and foods without difficulty
- Ability to care for self and newborn
- Has received rubella vaccine or RhoGAM if indicated

In addition, the mother should perform the following activities:

- Reviews pamphlets, videos, or other teaching materials for self and baby care
- Demonstrates care for self and baby
- Displays appropriate interaction with baby
- Practices principles of infant safety
- Demonstrates proper breastfeeding and breast care or describes formula preparation, formula-feeding techniques, and breast care
- Identifies the symptoms of postpartum depression and available resources

Additional outcomes for the cesarean birth mother include the following:

- States in own words the reason for the cesarean birth
- Maintains desired pain control
- Maintains moderate mobility level

Ensuring that the woman has met the criteria before discharge decreases the incidence of complications or readmission in the postpartum period.

CRITICAL THINKING

You walk in and find Dana Sullivan, a 29-year-old G2P2, crying 48 hours after a repeat cesarean birth. She states, "I'm not ready to go home. With my first baby they made me go home after 2 days. Can they make me again?"

Answers can be found in Appendix F ∞.

Discharge Teaching

Ideally, preparation for discharge begins the moment a woman is admitted to the birthing unit. Nursing efforts should be directed toward assessing the parents' knowledge, expectations, and beliefs and then providing anticipatory guidance and teaching accordingly. Because teaching is one of the primary responsibilities of the postpartum nurse, many agencies have elaborate teaching programs and videos. Before the actual discharge the nurse should spend time with the parents to determine if they have any last-minute questions.

Table 31–3 is a sample discharge teaching checklist. In general, discharge teaching includes at least the following information.

KEY FACTS TO REMEMBER

When to Contact the Primary Care Provider

After discharge, a woman should contact her physician or CNM if any of the following develop:

- Sudden, persistent, or spiking fever
- Change in the character of the lochia—foul smell, return to bright-red bleeding, excessive amount, passage of large clots
- Pain at the site of a laceration, episiotomy, or abdominal incision
- Evidence of wound infection including redness, swelling, severe or worsening pain, or foul smelling discharge
- Evidence of mastitis, such as breast tenderness, reddened areas, malaise
- Evidence of thrombophlebitis, such as calf pain, tenderness, redness
- Evidence of urinary tract infection, such as urgency, frequency, burning on urination
- Continued severe or incapacitating postpartal depression
- Inability to care for self or baby for any physical or psychologic reason

1. Signs of possible complications (see Key Facts to Remember: When to Contact the Primary Care Provider) and encouragement for the woman to contact her caregiver if she develops any of them
2. Review of literature the woman has received that explains recommended postpartum exercises, the need for adequate rest, the need to avoid overexertion initially, and the recommendation to abstain from sexual intercourse until lochia has ceased (If the family desires information about birth control methods, the nurse can provide such information at this time.)
3. Phone number of the mother-baby unit or information hotline and encouragement to call if she has any questions or concerns
4. Information on local agencies and/or support groups, such as La Leche League, Mothers of Twins, adolescent groups, or new mother support groups, that might be of particular assistance to the family
5. Information geared to the specific nutritional needs of breastfeeding or formula-feeding mothers (If the mother has been receiving vitamins and/or iron supplements, the nurse encourages her to continue until the first postpartal examination.)
6. When to schedule the first appointment for her postpartal examination and for her newborn's first well-baby examination
7. Procedure for obtaining copies of her infant's birth certificate
8. How to provide basic care for the infant; when to anticipate that the cord will fall off; when the infant can

TABLE 31–3	Areas to Include in Postpartal Teaching				
			Teaching Method		
Knowledge and Skills to Be Taught		Video	Verbal Only	Verbally Reinforced	Demonstration
Care of the Mother					
Breast care					
Breastfeeding or lactation suppression					
Possible problems and care					
Involutional changes					
Position of fundus					
Afterpains					
Changes in lochia					
Signs of possible problems					
Bladder function					
Fluid needs					
Signs of possible problems					
Bowel function					
Normal patterns					
Dietary assistance					
Perineal care					
Expected healing changes in episiotomy					
Comfort measures (rinsing with warm water, use of ice packs, use of analgesic/anesthetic spray, sitz bath), home care					
Signs of possible problems					
Rest and activity					
Scheduling rest periods, handling fatigue					
Ambulation					
Watching for circulatory problems in legs					
Emotional changes					
Changes in mood, crying, depression					
Care of the Father/Partner					
Emotional changes					
Emotional changes and challenges that may occur					
Encouragement to seek support as needed					
Physiologic and psychologic changes to anticipate in the mother/newborn					
Infant care concerns					
Possible supportive measures for the new family					
Care of the Baby					
Observing the baby					
General appearance					
Senses					
Visual					
Hearing					
Touch					
Smell					
Taste					
Vital signs					
Normal parameters					
How to take a temperature					
Skin					
Coloring					
Normal rashes					
Diaper care					
Elimination cycles of stool/urine					
Normal characteristics					
Signs of diarrhea and treatment					
Signs of constipation and treatment					

TABLE 31-3 Areas to Include in Postpartal Teaching *(Continued)*

Knowledge and Skills to Be Taught	Video	Verbal Only	Verbally Reinforced	Demonstration
Emotional and comforting needs				
Protective reflexes				
Blinking				
Sneezing				
Swallowing				
Normal reflexes				
Moro				
Fencing				
Head lag				
Stepping				
Feeding the baby				
Schedule				
Breastfeeding				
Positioning, initiating, and ending feeding				
Infant cues for feeding				
Identifying problem areas and possible solutions				
Signs of dehydration				
Formula-feeding				
Positioning				
Preparation of bottles and formula				
Burping or bubbling the baby				
Holding, wrapping, and diapering the baby				
Various holds (cradle, football)				
Securing baby in blanket to provide warmth				
Diapering				
Comparison of reusable (cloth) and single use (paper)				
Methods of diapering and care of soiled diapers				
Perineal skin care				
Positioning the baby for sleep				
Bathing the baby				
Supplies				
Method				
Safety				
Use of bulb syringe and care if choking				
Positioning				
Car seat				
Health promotion				
When to call healthcare provider				
Temp				
Diarrhea				
Eating problems				
Malaise				
Protecting baby from infections				
Immunization schedule				
Aspects of Parenting				
Newborn cues and capacity for interaction				
Parenting needs				
Acquaintance with individual characteristics of their newborn and possible techniques to use				
Resources available				

have a tub bath; when the infant will need her or his first immunizations; and so on (Parents should also be comfortable feeding and handling the baby, and should be aware of basic safety considerations, including the need to use a car seat when the infant is in a car.)

9. Signs and symptoms that indicate possible problems in the infant and who the parents should contact about them

10. Plans for home care visits so that the parents know when to expect the visit and what it entails (see Chapter 32 ∞)

The nurse can also use this final opportunity to reassure the couple of their ability to be successful parents. The nurse can stress the infant's need to feel loved and secure and urge parents to talk to each other and work together to solve any problems that arise.

Evaluation

Anticipated outcomes of comprehensive nursing care of the postpartal family include the following:

- The mother is reasonably comfortable and has learned pain relief measures.
- The mother is rested and understands how to add more activity over the next few days and weeks.
- The mother's physiologic and psychologic well-being have been supported.
- The mother verbalizes her understanding of self-care measures.
- The new parents demonstrate how to care for their baby.
- The new parents have had opportunities to form attachment with their baby.

CHAPTER HIGHLIGHTS

- Nursing diagnoses can be used effectively in caring for women postpartally.
- Postpartum discomfort may be caused by a variety of factors, including engorged breasts, an edematous perineum, an episiotomy or laceration, engorged hemorrhoids, or hematoma formation. Various self-care approaches are helpful in promoting comfort.
- Lactation suppression may be accomplished by mechanical techniques.
- The new mother requires opportunities to discuss her childbirth experience with an empathetic listener.
- Mother-baby care provides the childbearing family with opportunities to interact with their new member during the first hours and days of life. It enables the family to develop some confidence and skill in a safe environment.
- Sexual intercourse may resume once the episiotomy/laceration has healed and lochia has ceased.
- After a cesarean birth, the woman has the nursing care needs of an abdominal surgical client in addition to her needs as a postpartum client. She may also require assis-

tance in working through her feelings if the cesarean birth was unexpected.

- Postpartally the nurse evaluates the adolescent mother in terms of her level of maturity, available support systems, cultural background, and existing knowledge and then plans care accordingly.
- The mother who decides to relinquish her baby needs emotional support. She should be able to decide whether to see and hold her baby, and any special requests regarding the birth should be honored.
- Before discharge the couple should be given any information necessary for the woman to provide appropriate self-care. Parents should have a beginning skill in caring for their newborn and should be familiar with warning signs of possible complications for mother or baby. Printed information is valuable in helping couples deal with questions that may arise at home.
- Because of the trend toward early discharge, follow-up care is more important than ever. Many approaches are used, especially home visits and telephone follow-up.

CHAPTER REFERENCES

Andrews, V., Thakar, R., Sultan, A. H., & Jones, P. W. (2007). Evaluation of postpartum perineal pain and dyspareunia: A prospective study. *European Journal of Obstetrics, Gynecology, & Reproductive Biology* (2007 Aug 1) [Epub ahead of print].

Association of Women's Health, Obstetrical, and Neonatal Nurses. (AWHONN). (2006). *Compendium of postpartum care.* Washington, DC: Author.

Bernstein, H. H., Spino, C., Finch, S., Wasserman, R., Slora, E., Lalama, C., Touloukian, C. L., Lilienfeld, H., & McCormick, M. C. (2007). Decision-making for postpartum discharge of 4300 mothers and their healthy infants: The Life Around Newborn Discharge study. *Pediatrics, 120*(2), e391-e400 [Epub 2007 Jul 16].

Child Welfare Information Gateway. (2005). Voluntary relinquishment for adoption. Retrieved May 19, 2008, from http://www.childwelfare.gov/pubs/s_place.cfm

Child Welfare Information Gateway. (2007a). Grounds for involuntary termination of parental rights. Retrieved May 19, 2008, from http://www.childwelfare.gov/systemwide/laws_policies/statutes/groundtermin.cfm

Child Welfare Information Gateway. (2007b). Infant safe haven laws. Retrieved May 19, 2008, from http://www.childwelfare.gov/systemwide/laws_policies/statutes/safehaven.cfm

Conde, A. A., Figueiredo, B., Costa, R., Pacheco, A., & Pais, A. (2008). Perception of the childbirth experience: continuity and changes over the postpartum period. *Journal of Reproductive and Infant Psychology, 26*(2), 139–154.

Gabbe, S. G., Niebyl, J. R., & Simpson, J. L. (2007). *Obstetrics: Normal and problem pregnancies* (5th ed.). Philadelphia: Churchill Livingstone.

Göçmen, A., Göçmen, M., & Saraoğlu, M. (2002). Early post-operative feeding after caesarean delivery. *Journal of Internal Medicine Research, 30*(5), 506–511.

Gucev, G., Yasui, G. M., Chang, T. Y., & Lee, J. (2008). Bilateral ultrasound-guided continuous ilioinguinal-iliohypogastric block for pain relief after cesarean delivery. *Anesthesia & Analgesia,106,* 1220–1222.

Henney, S. M., Ayers-Lopez, S., McCoy, R. G., & Grotevant, H. D. (2007). Evolution and revolution: Birthmothers' experiences with grief and loss at different levels of adoption openness. *Journal of Social and Personal Relationships, 24*(6), 875–889.

Jones, C. C. (2006). The functions of childbirth and postpartum henna traditions. Retrieved September 8, 2007, at http://www.hennapage.com/henna/encyclopedia/pregbirth/postpart.pdf

Lemay, C. A., Cashman, S. B., Elfenbein, D. S., & Felice, M. E. (2007). Adolescent mothers' attitudes toward contraceptive use before and after pregnancy. *Journal of Pediatric & Adolescent Gynecology, 20*(4), 233–240.

Lin, J. P., Wang, H. H., & Chang, H. H. (2007). "Doing the month" experiences of Vietnamese primipara in Taiwan. *Hu Li Za Zhi, 54*(2), 47–54.

Madlon-Kay, D. J., & DeFor, T. A. (2005). Maternal postpartum health care utilization and the effect of Minnesota early discharge legislation. *Journal of the American Board of Family Practice, 18,* 307–311.

Porter, M., van Teijlingen, E., Chi Ying Yip, L., & Bhattacharya, S. (2007). Satisfaction with cesarean section: Qualitative analysis of open-ended questions in a large postal survey. *Birth, 34*(2), 148–154.

Reid, V., & Meadows-Oliver, M. (2007). Postpartum depression in adolescent mothers: An integrative review of the literature. *Journal of Pediatric Health Care, 21*(5), 289–298.

Spector, R. E. (2009). Cultural diversity in health and illness (7th ed). Upper Saddle River, NJ: Prentice Hall Health.

Steen, M., Briggs, M., & King, D. (2006). Alleviating postpartal perineal trauma: Too cool or not too cool? *British Journal of Nurse Midwifery, 14*(5), 305–306.

Tejirian, T., & Abbas, M. A. (2005). Sitz bath: Where is the evidence? Scientific basis of a common practice. *Disorders of the Colon & Rectum, 48*(12), 2336–2340.

United States Department of Labor. (2007). Fact sheet: Newborn & mother's health protection act. Retrieved on September 11, 2007, at http://www.dol.gov/ebsa/newsroom/fsnmhafs.html

Viscusi, E. R. (2008). Patient-controlled drug delivery for acute postoperative pain management: A review of current and emerging technologies. *Regional Anesthesia Pain Medicine, 33*(2), 146–158.

Wiklund, I., Edman, G., & Andolf, E. (2007). Cesarean section on maternal request: Reasons for the request, self-estimated health, expectations, experience of birth and signs of depression among first-time mothers. *Acta Obstetrics & Gynecology Scandanavia, 86*(4), 451–456.

Wilson, B. A., Shannon, M. T., & Shields, K. M. (2009). *Nurse's drug guide 2009.* Upper Saddle River, NJ: Pearson Education.

World Health Organization. (2007). Pospartum care of the mother and newborn: A practical guide. Retrieved on September 8, 2007, at http://www.who.int/reproductive-health/publications/msm_98_3/msm_98_3_11.html

CHAPTER 32

Home Care of the Postpartal Family

When I first became a nurse I thought I would always practice maternity nursing in a hospital. I loved the pace, the excitement! I began making home visits at the request of my supervisor when our unit partnered with the local midwives and obstetricians to provide postpartum follow-up services. Now I can't imagine doing anything else. Each day is different as I am challenged to improvise and help families deal with issues that arise. I value the independence of this role and the feeling that I am making a difference.

—A Home Care Nurse Working with Postpartal Families

LEARNING OUTCOMES

32-1. Identify the main purposes and components of home visits during the postpartal period.

32-2. Examine strategies and actions a nurse should take to ensure personal safety during a home visit.

32-3. Identify the goals and nursing approaches to fostering a caring relationship in the home.

32-4. Describe the assessment and care of the newborn during postpartal home care.

32-5. Identify the goals for reinforcement of parent teaching in the home and appropriate interventions.

32-6. Describe the nursing care and teaching needs of the postpartal mother and family in the first home visit based on the assessment findings and possible causes of alterations.

32-7. Relate the anticipated progress at 6 weeks of the mother and family to the assessment, identification of possible alterations, and care of the mother and family in the home visit.

32-8. Identify the common concerns of breastfeeding mothers following discharge and corresponding remedies.

32-9. Describe the nursing care for mothers and newborns experiencing difficulty in breastfeeding following discharge based on assessment data and rationale.

32-10. Identify follow-up care available to postpartal families in addition to home visits.

Home care is an essential component of perinatal nursing care, particularly as caregivers struggle to find an appropriate balance between providing quality client care and managing escalating healthcare costs.

Role of Length of Stay in Postpartal Home Care

In the 1990s, in an effort to contain healthcare costs, many insurers mandated that following an uncomplicated vaginal birth, postpartal families be discharged within 48 hours. In practice, discharge within 24 hours of vaginal birth was not uncommon. Not surprisingly, these early discharges were associated with an increase in neonatal complications, and in 1996 legislation was passed to outlaw *mandatory* early discharge. This federal legislation, The Newborns' and Mothers' Health Protection Act, became effective in 1998. It prohibits insurance companies from mandating discharge of mothers and newborns before 48 hours if they delivered vaginally or before 96 hours if they had a cesarean birth (Paul, Lehman, Hollenbeak et al., 2006). Research has demonstrated that extending the length of stay does not increase costs when death rates and readmission costs are considered and indicates that the 1998 legislation was effective (Burgos, Schmitt, Stevenson et al., 2008).

Discharge before 48 hours now occurs only at the family's request. These early discharges present a challenge to nurses because the time available for nursing assessments and client teaching is greatly reduced. In addition, many conditions in the newborn, such as jaundice, ductal-dependent cardiac lesions, and gastrointestinal obstructions, may take longer than 2 days to develop, and identification of these problems depends on a skilled, experienced professional (AAP Committee on Fetus and Newborn, 2004). Other experts contend that breastfeeding may not be well established before 48 hours and discharge before this time can lead to increased rates of dehydration and poor breastfeeding outcomes (de Almeida & Draque, 2007).

Special emphasis has also been placed on the needs of **late preterm infants**, born between 34 and 37 weeks (Engle, Tomashek, Wallman, & Committee on Fetus & Newborn, 2007). These infants are at a greater risk for increases in mortality and morbidity because they are physically not mature and are more prone to have physiological and metabolic complications (Engle et al., 2007). Read-missions for infection and jaundice are more common in later preterm infants than in term infants (Engle et al., 2007). The American Academy of Pediatrics (AAP) has identified specific risk factors in late preterm infants that increase the likelihood of readmission and neonatal mortality. These include: being first born, breastfeeding at the time of discharge, having a mother who has had labor and childbirth complications, having public insurance as your source of payment, and being Asian/Pacific Islander (Engle et al., 2007). Special attention by the home health nurse is warranted for these infants to ensure a proper home transition and to identify possible early complications (Engle et al., 2007).

Early discharges also have implications for the mother. The risk of postpartum hemorrhage, difficulties with breastfeeding, and opportunities for the mother to become comfortable with her new baby may be compromised. The risk of postpartum depression commonly occurs in the first month following the birth. Women who receive some type of follow-up assessment from a nurse experience less depression than those who do not receive postpartum follow-up (Goulet, D'Amour, & Pineault, 2007). In addition, extended family members who live at a distance and have agreed to assist the new family in the first few weeks after birth may not have arrived yet. Furthermore, in the first 24 hours after childbirth, the mother may be too tired or may not be ready emotionally to participate in learning activities. In all cases of early discharge, a home visit by an experienced postpartal nurse can be invaluable.

Considerations for the Home Visit

The home setting provides an opportunity for the nurse and family to interact in a more relaxed environment in which the family has control. In some instances, the challenges of assessing and enhancing self-care and infant care may be unique in the home, and the nurse will have many opportunities to exercise critical thinking to develop creative options with the family.

The postpartal home visit usually occurs within 24 to 48 hours of discharge and is conducted by a registered nurse who is experienced in postpartal maternal and newborn care. Before the home visit, the nurse prepares by identifying the purpose of the home visit and gathering needed materials and equipment. A personal contact while the woman is still in the birth setting or a previsit telephone call is used to arrange the appointment with the woman and her family. During the previsit contact, it is important for the nurse to clearly identify the purpose and goals of the visit and to begin establishing rapport. The nurse should explain that, unlike community health visits, only one or two home visits are typically planned, and long-term follow-up by the postpartal nurse is not anticipated.

Purpose of the Home Visit

Postpartal home care is focused more on assessment, teaching, facilitating learning, and counseling than on physical care. First, it provides an opportunity to assess the status of the mother and infant after birth for signs of any complications. The established guidelines for discharge of the mother and baby (see Chapter 31 ∞) mean the nurse can expect certain levels of health and wellness. However, because the status of the mother and newborn can change, the nurse should stay alert for deviations from the norm and identify conditions that may warrant further medical evaluation or rehospitalization. The nurse can also complete follow-up blood work if needed.

In addition, the nurse assesses adaptation of the family to the new baby and adjustment of any siblings. The nurse also assesses the parents' skill in bathing, dressing, handling, and comforting their newborn, and the appropriateness and safety of the home environment.

Another purpose of the home visit is to ascertain current informational needs, and to offer requested information, in a more relaxed setting. Postpartal home care provides opportunities for enhancing self- and infant-care techniques initially presented in the birth setting. Many times, questions and concerns arise at home that were not identified in the hospital.

In addition, the nurse answers questions about breastfeeding, provides support and encouragement, and addresses the need for referrals to clinics, classes, or postpartal support groups. (See the Teaching Card on Home Care of the Postpartal Family in the center of this book.)

Fostering a Caring Relationship with the Family

Although the nurse in the birthing center strives to enhance family autonomy and control, the atmosphere of the institutional environment may cause the new mother and family to feel disempowered. It is important for the professional nurse to recognize that the parameters of the home visit are different. In the home, the family members have control of their environment and the nurse is an invited visitor. The nurse can rely on the same characteristics of a caring relationship that have been integral to hospital-based practice—regard for clients, genuineness, empathy, and establishment of trust and rapport—when providing care in the home setting (see Key Facts to Remember: Fostering a Caring Relationship).

◆

KEY FACTS TO REMEMBER
Fostering a Caring Relationship

Evidence of genuineness and empathy, coupled with the establishment of trust and rapport, form the foundation for a caring relationship.

DEMONSTRATED GOAL	APPROACHES TO ACHIEVE GOAL
Regard	Introduce yourself to the family. Call the family members by their surnames until you have been invited to use the given or a less formal name. Ask to be introduced to other members of the family who are present. Allow the mother or spokesperson to assume this role. Remember, in some cultures, it may be a male figure or a mother figure who assumes the primary role. Use active listening. Maintain objectivity. Ask permission before sitting.
Genuineness	Mean what you say. Make sure that your verbal and nonverbal messages are congruent. Be nonjudgmental. Do not make assumptions about individuals or settings. Always strive to demonstrate caring behaviors. Be prepared for the visit, honestly answer questions and provide information, and be truthful. If you do not know the answer to a question, tell the client you will find the information and report back.
Empathy	Listen to the mother and family "where they are" without judgment. Be attentive to what the birthing experience is for them so that you will understand from their perspective. Remember that empathy denotes understanding, not sympathy.
Trust and rapport	Do what you say you will do. Be prepared for the visit and be on time. Follow-up on any areas that are needed.

Maintaining Safety

In the past, nurses were perceived as a mainstay of communities and could move in most settings without fear or concern for safety. Today, some communities are not safe for visiting nurses. It is important for the nurse to follow basic safety rules when conducting a home visit. Obviously, the nurse needs to know the specific address and ask for directions during the previsit contact. If the area is not familiar, the nurse should trace out the route on a map or use an Internet program to provide directions before leaving for the visit and take a map along. Some vehicles are now equipped with a global positioning system (GPS). However, some newer areas may not be included or found within the system, so the nurse should always have a back-up plan in place. It is also wise for the nurse to wear a name tag and carry identification. The nurse should avoid wearing expensive jewelry or pins of a religious or political nature that might be seen as offensive. A fully charged cellular phone provides a means of contact and is advisable, as is a working flashlight, especially for night visits. In addition, the nurse should carry a phone card or sufficient change to call from a pay phone. The nurse should also notify an instructor or supervisor when leaving for a visit and check in as soon as the visit is completed.

Many agencies that provide home care services have established violence prevention programs to help ensure safety. Nurses in the community need to be aware of their environment and alert to environmental cues, whether overt or subtle. In addition, the following recommendations are important (McPhaul, Rosen, Bobb et al., 2007).

- Invest time in personal safety by driving around a neighborhood before making an initial visit to identify potential cues to violence. Avoid walking through a crowd or staying in an elevator with others if it makes you uneasy.
- In high-risk areas, visit the family during daylight hours. Inform the family when you plan to arrive and advise them to call a supervisor if you do not arrive within 15 minutes of the arranged time. Provide them with a contact name and phone number.
- Do not park in deserted or unlit areas. Make sure your car is in good working order and has gas. Keep doors locked and windows closed.
- Before leaving for the visit, lock personal belongings in the trunk of the car, out of sight. Do not carry a purse, medications, or other items.
- In accordance with agency policy, wear scrubs, a lab coat, or other uniform that identifies you as a nurse.
- Be aware of personal body language and how it might be interpreted. (For example, avoid crossing arms or shoving hands in pockets, which may suggest hostility; remain calm and convey a sense of respect at all times.)

- Pay attention to the body language of anyone present during the visit, not just the client.
- Be alert for signs that a person is becoming enraged (reddened neck and/or face, clenched fists, pacing). If any family member is violent, or if drug or alcohol abuse is occurring, leave the home and report the incident to your supervisor.
- Leave the home immediately if a gun or knife is visible. Do not confront the client or family member.
- If a situation arises that feels unsafe, or a "gut feeling" tells you something is not right, terminate the visit immediately.

If the visit is in an area that seems unsafe, it may be wise for two nurses to go together. Nurses should avoid entering areas where violence is in progress. In such cases, they should return to the car and contact the police or dial 911. (See the Teaching Card on Safety Considerations During Home Visits in the center of this book.)

Most people are more comfortable in familiar neighborhoods and have some hesitation when entering homes in other residential areas. First home visits may feel uncomfortable because they are unfamiliar, but with experience comfort increases (Figure 32–1 ■).

Carrying Out the Home Visit

When the door is answered, the nurse should introduce herself or himself and confirm that the location is correct. If a place to sit is not indicated, the nurse may inquire, "Where is the best place to sit so that we can talk for

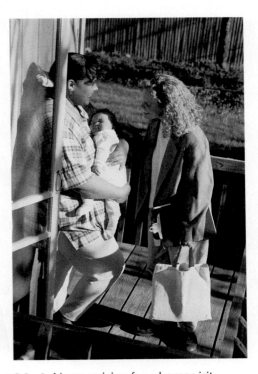

FIGURE 32–1 Nurse arriving for a home visit.

a while?" In some families, offering refreshments may be an important aspect of welcoming a visitor. In this case, it is beneficial to the relationship for the nurse to accept the refreshment graciously. Many cultures have strong ties to certain foods and beverages during the postpartum period. Accepting the food or beverage conveys acceptance of cultural norms. It is helpful for the nurse to be familiar with various cultural norms and traditions (Spector, 2009).

As discussed, the nurse completes planned assessments, provides direct care as necessary, carries out family and client teaching, makes necessary referrals to community agencies, and schedules an additional home visit or telephone contact. The nurse should report significant medical concerns to the physician/CNM immediately and plan for appropriate follow-up. The aspects assessed and addressed during the home visit are discussed in the following sections.

Home Care: The Newborn

In the home, a newborn physical examination is performed as described in Chapter 25 ∞. The nurse also assesses and reinforces knowledge related to infant care as detailed in the following paragraphs.

Positioning and Handling

The nurse demonstrates methods of positioning and handling the newborn as needed. As the family members provide care, the nurse can instill confidence by giving them positive feedback. If a family member encounters prob-

lems, the nurse can suggest alternatives and serve as a role model.

When holding the newborn, one of the following positions can be used (Figure 32–2 ■). The *cradle hold* is frequently used during feeding. It provides a sense of warmth and closeness, permits eye contact, frees one of the adult's hands, and provides security because the cradling protects the newborn's body. Extra security is provided by gripping the baby's thigh with the hand while the arm supports the newborn's body. This grip is important to use when the infant is being carried. The *upright position* provides security and a sense of closeness and is ideal for burping the infant. One hand should support the neck and shoulders, while the other hand holds the buttocks or is placed between the newborn's legs. The newborn may also be held upright in a cloth sling carrier that gently holds the baby against the parent's chest and frees the hands for other tasks. The *football hold* frees one of the caregiver's hands and permits eye contact. This hold is ideal for shampooing, carrying, or breastfeeding. It frees the caregiver to talk on the telephone, answer the door, or do the myriad tasks that await attention at this busy time.

The infant's position should be changed periodically throughout the early months of life, because skull bones are soft, and permanently flattened areas may develop if the newborn consistently lies in one position. The awake newborn is frequently positioned on her or his side with the dependent arm forward to provide support and to prevent rolling. The side-lying position aids drainage of mucus and allows air to circulate around the cord. It is also comfortable for the newly circumcised male. After

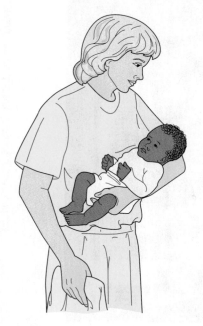
A

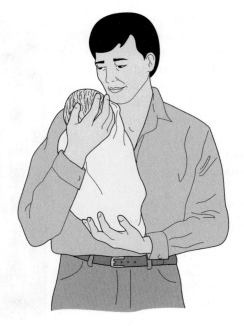
B

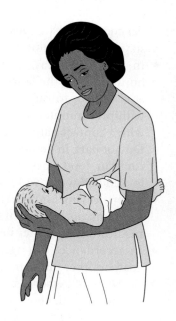
C

FIGURE 32–2 Various positions for holding an infant. *A,* Cradle hold. *B,* Upright position. *C,* Football hold.

Bathing

An actual bath demonstration is the best way for the nurse to provide information to parents. Because excess bathing and the use of soap remove natural skin oils and dry out the newborn's sensitive skin, bathing should be done every other day or twice a week. Sponge baths are recommended for the first 2 weeks or until the umbilical cord completely falls off and the umbilicus has healed. Some agencies use a tub bath for the bath demonstration.

Supplies can be kept in a plastic bag or some type of container to eliminate the necessity of hunting for them each time. For the baby's tub, the family may want to use a plastic dishpan, a clean kitchen or bathroom sink, or a large bowl. If using a sink, care should be taken to keep the infant away from faucets via which accidental burns could occur. Expensive baby tubs are not necessary, but some prefer to purchase them.

Before starting, if no one else is at home, the parent may want to take the phone off the hook and put a sign on the door to prevent being disturbed. Having someone home during the first few baths will be helpful, because that person can get forgotten items, attend to interruptions, and provide moral support. The room should be warm and free of drafts. (See Client Teaching: Newborn Bathing as well as the Teaching Card on the same topic in the center of this book.)

Sponge Baths

After the supplies are gathered, the tub (or any of the containers mentioned) is filled with water that is warm to the touch. Even though the newborn will not be placed in the tub, the bath giver carefully tests the water temperature with an elbow or forearm. Families may also choose to purchase a thermometer to help them determine when the bath water is at approximately 37.8°C (100°F) and safe to use. An unperfumed, mild soap such as Castile or Neutrogena should be used and kept on a soap dish or paper towel, not added to the water. Before the bath, the newborn should be wrapped in a blanket, with a T-shirt and diaper on, to keep her or him warm and secure.

To start the bath, the adult wraps a washcloth once around the index finger and wets it with water. *Soap is not used on the face.* Each eye is gently wiped from inner to outer corner. This direction prevents the potential for clogging the tear duct at the inner corner, where the eye naturally drains. A different portion of the washcloth is used for each eye to prevent cross contamination. Cotton balls can also be used for this purpose, a new one for each eye. Some swelling and drainage may be present the first few days after birth because of eye prophylaxis.

The bath giver washes the ears next by wrapping the washcloth once around an index finger and gently

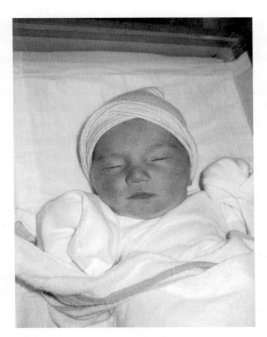

FIGURE 32–3 Infants should be placed on their backs when sleeping.

feeding, the newborn may be placed on the right side to aid digestion and to prevent aspiration of regurgitated feedings; this position also makes it easier to expel air bubbles from the stomach.

Although the side-lying position is appropriate when the infant is awake and under observation, infants should always sleep on their backs (Figure 32–3 ■). The American Academy of Pediatrics has recommended sleeping in non-prone positions since 1992 to reduce the risk of sudden infant death syndrome (SIDS). Since the initiation of the "Back to Sleep" campaign, there has been an increase in malformation of the skull caused by a decrease in tummy time. The syndrome is also known as *deformational plagiocephaly,* or positional plagiocephaly. These infants commonly have a flat spot on their skull, usually on the back or side, that is caused from continued placement in the same position. Prone positioning while awake, also known as **tummy time**, is important for all babies because it assists them with learning developmentally appropriate skills; builds muscle strength for their shoulders, neck, and back; and prevents the syndrome (National Institute of Child Health & Human Development, 2006). Infants who are not placed on their stomachs while awake at least three times daily are at risk for this skull malformation. Infants should only be placed on their tummies when they are under direct supervision of a parent or adult. Often these malformations will resolve on their own by one year of age, but sometimes infants need to wear a specially fitted helmet to correct the malformation (van Vlimmeren, van der Graaf, Boere-Boonekamp et al., 2007).

EVIDENCE IN ACTION

Newborns should be placed in the supine position during sleep to reduce the risk of SIDS.

(Organization Guidelines) (American Academy of Pediatrics: Task force on Sudden Infant Death Syndrome, 2005)

---

cleaning the external ear and behind the ear. Cotton swabs are never used in the ear canal because it is possible to put the swab too far into the ear and damage the ear drum. In addition, the swab may push any discharge farther down into the ear canal. The caregiver then wipes the remainder of the baby's face. Many babies start to cry at this point. The face should be washed every day and the mouth and chin wiped off after each feeding.

The neck is washed carefully but thoroughly with the washcloth. Soap may now be used. Formula or breast milk and lint collect in the skin folds of the neck, so it may be helpful to sit the newborn up, supporting the neck and shoulders with one hand while washing the neck with the other hand.

Next the bath giver unwraps the blanket, removes the T-shirt, and wets the chest, back, and arms with the washcloth. The bath giver may then lather the hands with soap and wash the baby's chest, back, and arms. Wetting the cord is avoided, if possible, because it delays drying. Soap is rinsed off with the wet washcloth, and the upper part of the body is dried with a towel or blanket. The newborn's upper body is then wrapped with a clean, dry blanket to prevent a chill.

The bath giver then unwraps the newborn's legs, wets them with the washcloth, and lathers, rinses, and dries them well. If the newborn has dry skin, a small amount of unscented lotion or ointment (petroleum jelly or A & D ointment) may be used. Ointments are thought to be better than lotions for dry, cracked feet and hands. Baby oil is not recommended, because it clogs skin pores. Powders are not currently recommended. Families should be warned that baby powder can cause serious respiratory problems if inhaled. If parents want to use powder, they should be advised to use one that is talc free. The powder should be shaken into the hand and then placed on the newborn rather than shaken directly onto the baby.

The genital area is cleansed with soap and water daily and with water after each wet or dirty diaper. Females are washed from the front of the genital area toward the rectum to prevent fecal contamination of the urethra and thus the bladder. Newborn females often have a thick, white mucous discharge or a slight bloody discharge from the vaginal area. This discharge is normal for the first 1 to 2 weeks after birth and should be wiped off with a damp cloth during diaper changes. The labia should be wiped, but the inner vagina should not be aggressively cleaned.

Parents of uncircumcised males should cleanse the penis daily. Even minimal retraction of the foreskin is not advised (see in-depth discussion of care of uncircumcised male babies in Chapter 26 ∞). Males who have been circumcised also need daily gentle cleansing. Squeeze warm water over the baby's penis, letting the warm water run over the circumcision site. The area is rinsed off with warm water and lightly patted dry. A small amount of petroleum jelly, A & D ointment, or bactericidal ointment may be put on the circumcised area until the healing is complete, but excessive amounts may block the meatus and should be avoided. It is important to avoid using ointments if a Plastibell is in place because use of ointments may cause the Plastibell ring to slip off the penis too early. The Plastibell usually falls off within 5 to 8 days. If it does not, the family needs to call the healthcare provider.

It is important to cleanse the diaper area with each diaper change to prevent diaper rash. Although this cleansing is done on a routine basis, a diaper rash may occasionally occur. Baby powder or cornstarch is not recommended for diaper rash. Baby powder may cake with urine and irritate the perineal area; cornstarch may promote fungal infection. Ointments that provide a barrier, such as zinc oxide, A & D ointment, and petroleum jelly, are more effective for diaper rash. If the ointment does not help the rash, families using single-use (disposable) diapers should try another brand. If they use cloth diapers, a different detergent or fabric softener, more thorough rinsing, and hanging them in the sun to dry may alleviate the problem. If the rash persists, parents should discuss the problem with their nurse practitioner or physician, because it may be caused by a fungal infection.

The umbilical cord should be kept clean and dry. The close proximity of the umbilical vessels makes the cord a possible entry area for infection. The cord stump generally falls off in 7 to 14 days. The diaper should be folded down to allow air to circulate around the cord. The parents should consult their healthcare provider if redness, bright-red bleeding, or puslike drainage with foul odor appears around the umbilicus or if the area remains unhealed 2 to 3 days after the cord stump has sloughed off.

The last step in bathing is washing the hair (a step some suggest doing first). The newborn is swaddled in a dry blanket, leaving only the head exposed, and held in the football hold with the head tilted slightly downward to prevent water from running into the eyes. Water should be brought to the head by a cupped hand. The infant should never be placed under running water because extreme changes in temperature can lead to burns. The hair is moistened and lathered with a small amount of mild shampoo. A very soft brush may be used to massage the shampoo over the entire head, including the fontanelles. The hair is then rinsed and toweled dry. Oils or lotions are not used on the newborn's head unless there is evidence of cradle cap. Moistening the scaly area with lotion or mineral oil half an hour or more before shampooing softens the crusts or scales and makes it easier to remove them with a soft brush during the shampoo.

Tub Baths

The baby may be put in a small tub after the cord has fallen off and the circumcision site is healed (approximately

Client Teaching NEWBORN BATHING

Content

Describe the proper timing and environment (including safety factors) for sponge and tub bathing for newborns.

Identify proper bathing supplies that are needed for both sponge and tub baths.

Demonstrate sponge bathing.

Discuss and demonstrate tub bathing using an infant model.

Explain the need for neutral pH, fragrance-free, and dye-free cleansing products for newborn use.

Teaching Method

Clarify information related to sponge bathing and the proper timing of tub baths for safe newborn bathing. Explain that the proper environment is needed for newborn safety and comfort.

Encourage the family to assemble supplies before beginning the newborn bath to avoid cold exposure and ensure that proper supplies are being used.

Demonstrate proper technique and encourage the family to ask questions as they arise. Help instill confidence in new parents.

Clarify the need for appropriate cleansing agents for newborns.

2 weeks) (Figure 32–4 ■). Newborns usually enjoy a tub bath more than a sponge bath, although some cry during either type. Only 3 or 4 inches of water is needed in the tub. To prevent slipping, a washcloth is placed in the bottom of the tub or sink. Some parents choose to bring the newborn into the tub with them.

The baby's face is washed in the same manner as for a sponge bath. The parent then places the newborn in the tub using the cradle hold and grasping the distal thigh. The neck is supported by the parent's elbow in the cradle position. An alternative hold is to support the newborn's head and neck with the forearm while grasping the distal shoulder and arm.

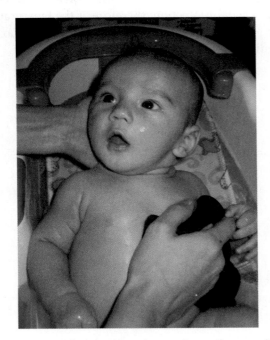

FIGURE 32–4 When bathing the newborn, the caregiver must support the head. Wet babies are very slippery.

Because wet newborns are slippery, some parents pull a cotton sock (with holes cut out for the fingers) over the supporting arm to provide a "nonskid" surface. The newborn's body may be washed with a soapy washcloth or hand. To wash the back, the bath giver places his or her noncradling hand on the newborn's chest with the thumb under the newborn's arm closest to the adult. Gently tipping the newborn forward onto the supporting hand frees the cradling arm to wash the back. After the bath, the newborn is lifted out of the tub in the cradle position, dried well, and wrapped in a dry blanket. The hair is then washed in the same way as for a sponge bath.

Nail Care

The nails of the newborn are seldom cut in the birthing center. During the first days of life, the nails may adhere to the skin of the fingers, and cutting is contraindicated. Within a week the nails separate from the skin and frequently break off. If the nails are long or if the newborn is scratching his or her face, the nails may be trimmed. Trimming is most easily done while the infant is asleep. Nails should be cut straight across using adult cuticle scissors or blunt-ended infant cuticle scissors. Infant nails may also be filed.

Dressing the Newborn

Newborns need to wear a T-shirt, diaper (diaper cover or plastic pants if using cloth diapers), and a sleeper. On a fairly cool day, they should be wrapped in a light blanket while being fed. Newborns should be covered with a blanket in air-conditioned buildings. The blanket should be unwrapped or removed when inside a warm building. At home, the amount of clothing the newborn wears is determined by the temperature. Families who maintain their home at 15.5°C to 18.3°C (60°F to 65°F) should dress the infant more warmly than those who maintain a temperature of 21.1°C to 23.9°C (70°F to 75°F).

Newborns should wear head coverings outdoors to protect their sensitive ears from drafts. A blanket can be wrapped around the baby, leaving one corner free to place over the head while outdoors or in crowds for added protection. The nurse must advise families about the ease with which a newborn's skin can burn when exposed to the sun. To prevent sunburn, the newborn should remain shaded, wear a light layer of clothing, or be protected with sunscreen specifically formulated for infants.

Diaper shapes vary and are subject to personal preference (Figure 32–5 ■). Prefolded and disposable diapers are usually rectangular. Cloth diapers may also be triangular or kite folded. Extra material is placed in front for males and toward the back for females to increase absorbency. Cloth diapers, some of which now use velcro and highly absorbant materials, have been used more frequently in recent years because of the environmental concerns related to disposible diapers.

Baby clothing should be laundered separately with a mild soap or detergent. Diapers may be presoaked before washing. All clothing should be rinsed twice to remove soap and residue and to decrease the possibility of rash. Some newborns may not tolerate clothing treated with fabric softeners added to the washer or dryer.

Temperature Assessment

As the nurse prepares to teach parents about taking their baby's temperature, it is important to provide opportunities for discussion and demonstration. Families often need a review of how to take the baby's temperature and when to call their primary healthcare provider.

The nurse discusses the different types of thermometers available for home use. It is important that parents understand the differences and how to select the appropriate one. Tympanic membrane (ear) thermometers use infrared temperature scanning techniques to determine the infant's temperature. Infrared forehead thermometers are also available, but these devices may be less accurate than internal monitoring techniques (Pusnik & Drnovsek, 2005). Other parents elect to use a digital thermometer. The nurse reviews the correct procedure for using the chosen thermometer. The same digital thermometers should not be used for both oral and rectal temperature taking. Parents should label the thermometer and only use it for one route.

HINTS FOR PRACTICE

Healthcare facilities no longer use glass thermometers because of the risks associated with resulting mercury spillage should one break. Parents should be advised not to use mercury thermometers and should be encouraged to discard them at a hazardous materials site specific to mercury thermometers. Before teaching families about temperature taking, you might find it helpful to visit a local pharmacy and review the types of thermometers available, the costs of the most commonly used methods, and the instructions provided. This will enable you to answer questions accurately when you work with parents or caregivers.

Parents need to take the newborn's temperature only when the signs of illness are present. They should call their pediatrician or pediatric nurse practitioner immediately if the temperature exceeds 38.4°C (101°F) rectally or 38°C (100.4°F) axillary. In premature infants, a low temperature may be a sign of infection; therefore, if the temperature is below 36.1°C (97°F) rectally or 36.6°C (97.8°F) axillary, the pediatrician should be notified.

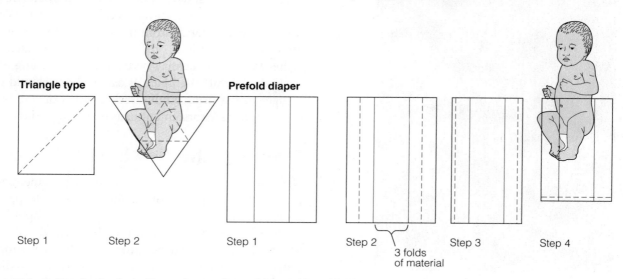

Triangle type   **Prefold diaper**

Step 1   Step 2   Step 1   Step 2   Step 3   Step 4

3 folds of material

FIGURE 32–5 Two basic cloth diaper shapes. Dotted lines indicate folds.

Parents should discuss management of flu, colds, teething, constipation, diarrhea, gas discomfort, and other common ailments with their clinician before they occur. When analgesic or antipyretic medication is needed, clinicians frequently recommend acetaminophen or ibuprofen drops. Parents should not give any form of aspirin for an illness unless specifically directed to do so by their healthcare provider; use of aspirin in viral illnesses has been linked to Reye's syndrome in children.

Stools and Urine

The appearance and frequency of a newborn's stools can cause concern for parents. The nurse prepares them by discussing and showing pictures of meconium stools and transitional stools and by describing the difference between breast-milk and formula stools. Although each baby develops his or her own stooling patterns, parents can expect the following (see Figure 24–9 ■).

- Breastfed newborns may have 6 to 10 small, semiliquid, yellow stools per day by the third or fourth day, when milk production is established, unless the mother is having problems with her milk supply. Once breastfeeding is well established, usually by 1 month, the newborn may have only one stool every few days because of the increased digestibility of breast milk. However, they may still have several daily. Constipation is unlikely to occur in newborns receiving only breast milk. Infrequent stooling in the first few weeks may indicate inadequate milk intake.
- Formula-fed babies may have only one or two stools a day; they are more formed and yellow or yellow-brown.

The parents may also be shown pictures of a constipated stool (small, pelletlike) and diarrhea (loose, green, or perhaps blood tinged). Families should understand that a green color is common in transitional stools, so that transitional stools are not confused with diarrhea during the first week of a newborn's life. Constipation may indicate that the newborn needs additional fluid intake. Parents may try offering additional water in an attempt to reverse the constipation. Parents should be counseled that each baby develops his or her own stooling pattern, and some babies may not pass a stool daily. As long as the infant appears comfortable and is not in distress, this can be normal for that infant and is not a cause for concern.

Babies normally void (urinate) five to eight times per day. Fewer than six to eight wet diapers a day may indicate that the newborn needs more fluids. Frequency of voiding is easy to assess with cloth diapers. Parents who use superabsorbent single-use disposable diapers may have difficulty determining voiding patterns because the surface of the diaper feels dry. The liquid pools inside the filling of the diaper.

Sleep and Activity

The newborn demonstrates several different sleep-wake states after the initial periods of reactivity described in Chapter 24 ∞. It is not uncommon for a newborn to sleep almost continuously for the first 2 to 3 days following birth, awakening only for feedings every few hours. Indeed, it is not uncommon to have difficulty feeding the infant during the first 24 to 48 hours because of this deep sleep. Some newborns bypass this stage and require only 12 to 16 hours of sleep. The parents need to know that this pattern is normal.

Six newborn sleep-wake states have been identified. **Quiet sleep**, also known as deep sleep, is characterized by regular breathing and no movement except for sudden body jerks. During this sleep state, normal household noise will not awaken the infant. In **active sleep**, also known as **light sleep**, the newborn has irregular breathing and fine muscular twitching. The newborn may cry out during sleep, but this does not mean he or she is uncomfortable or awake. Unusual household noise may awaken the newborn more easily in this state; however, he or she will quickly go back to sleep. In the **drowsy state**, newborns open and close their eyes, but the eyes appear glazed and the face is often still. Newborns return to sleep easily from this state, or awaken in response to stimuli.

In the **quiet alert state**, newborns are quietly involved with the environment. They watch a moving mobile, smile, and, as they age, discover and play with their hands and feet. When newborns become uncomfortable because of wet diapers, hunger, or cold, they enter the **active alert state** and **crying state**. In these states, parents should identify and eliminate the cause of the crying. Sometimes families are frustrated as they try to identify the external or internal stimuli that are causing the crying. Parents need to be told that the state may be changed from crying to quiet alert by moving the newborn toward an upright position where scanning and exploration are possible. (Table 32–1 identifies characteristics of the various states.)

Infants typically do not sleep through the night until they are at least 3 months of age or weigh 12 to 13 lb (5443 gms to 5897 gms). Some infants sleep through the night as early as 8 weeks whereas others do not sleep through the night until 6 months of age or beyond. It is estimated that two-thirds of infants sleep through the

TABLE 32–1 Infant Sleep and Awake States*

Infant States	Physical Characteristics	Body Activity	Eye Movements	Facial Movements	Breathing Pattern	Responses	Caregiver Implications
Sleep States							
Quiet sleep (also known as deep sleep)	Anabolic, restorative sleep, increased cell mitosis and replication, lowered oxygen consumption, release of growth hormone.	Typically still, may occasionally startle or twitch.	None	None or may have occasional sucking movements.	Slow and regular.	Only intense or disturbing stimuli will arouse infant, threshold to stimuli is high.	Difficult to arouse for feedings. Teach parents to time feedings when infant is in a more responsive state. Infant may arouse slightly if an attempt is made to awaken but typically returns to the quiet sleep state.
Active sleep (also known as light sleep or rapid eye movement [REM] state)	Processing and recording information. Often linked to learning. Is the highest proportion of sleep and precedes awakening.	Some body movements.	REM, eyelids flutter beneath closed eyelids.	May smile or make fussing or crying noises.	Irregular.	More responsive to internal stimuli (hunger) and external stimuli (such as being picked up by caregiver). When stimulated may arouse, return to quiet sleep, or remain in active sleep.	Inexperienced care providers may attempt to feed when infant makes normal crying sounds.
Awake States							
Drowsy	May return to sleep or awaken further.	Smooth movements with variable activity level. May experience mild startles intermittently.	Eyes may open and close. May appear heavy-lidded, or eyes may appear like slits.	May have no facial movements and appear still, or may have some facial movements.	Irregular.	Usually reacts to stimuli but may be slowed. May change to other states such as quiet alert, active alert, or crying.	To stimulate infant, provide verbal, sight, or oral stimulation. If left alone, infant may return to a sleep state.
Quiet alert	Attentive to environment, focus attention on stimuli.	Minimal	Eyes bright and wide.	Attentive appearance.	Regular.	Most attentive, focus attention on stimuli.	In the first hours after birth, may experience intense alertness before going into a long sleeping period. This state increases in intensity as the infant becomes older. Providing stimuli will help maintain an active alert state or a drowsy or active-alert state. Infant provides pleasure and positive feedback to care providers. Good time to feed infant.
Active alert	Infant's eyes are open, not as bright as in quiet alert. More body activity than in a quiet alert state.	Smooth movements may be interspersed with mild startles from time to time.	Eyes open with a gazed, dull appearance.	May be still with or without facial movements.	Irregular.	Reacts to stimuli with delayed responses to stimuli, or may change to quiet alert or crying state.	Infant may be fussy and become sensitive to stimuli, may become more and more active and start crying. If fatigue or caregiver interventions disturb this state, infant may return to a drowsy or sleep state.
Crying	Communication tool, response to unpleasant stimuli from environment or internal stimuli. Characterized by intense crying for more than 15 seconds.	Increased motor activity, skin color changes to darkened appearance, red, or ruddy.	Eyes may be tightly closed or open.	Grimaces	More irregular than in other states.	Very responsive to internal or external unpleasant stimuli.	Indicates that the infant's limits have been reached. May be able to console himself or herself and return to an alert or sleep state, or may need intervention from caregiver.

*A *state* is a group of characteristic behaviors and physiologic changes that occur together in a regular pattern.

Source: March of Dimes. (2003). *Understanding the behavior of term infants.* White Plains, NY: Author.

night by the age of 6 months. Although newborns typically sleep up to 16 hours per day, they do so in short time intervals. Some parents may be tempted to try home remedies, such as giving infants cereal in their bottles or other additives which are said to assist their children in sleeping through the night. Parents should be counseled that these remedies are not recommended.

Crying

For the newborn, crying is the only means of expressing needs vocally. Families learn to distinguish different tones and qualities of the newborn's cry. The amount of crying is highly individual. Some cry as little as 15 to 30 minutes in 24 hours, and others cry as long as 2 hours every 24 hours. When crying continues after causes such as discomfort and hunger are eliminated, the newborn may be comforted by swaddling or by rocking and other reassuring activities. There is some indication that newborns who are held more tend to be calmer and cry less when not being held. Some parents are afraid that holding may "spoil" the newborn and need reassurance that this is not the case. Picking babies up when they cry teaches them that adults are responsive to them. This helps build a sense of trust in humankind. Excessive crying should be noted and assessed, taking other factors into consideration. After the first 2 or 3 days, newborns settle into individual patterns.

Coping with prolonged crying may be a challenge for new parents, who may respond by withdrawing their affection from the newborn, providing routine care and feeding, but not becoming emotionally attached. Other parents may respond by neglecting, abandoning, or even hitting or shaking their newborn. Parents need to understand the serious, even life-threatening consequences of such behavior. For example, a neglected or abandoned newborn can quickly become dehydrated, and hitting can cause internal hemorrhage, bruising, and fractures. Shaking can cause brain hemorrhage, spinal cord injury, retinal hemorrhage or detachment, long-term developmental problems, mental retardation, or even death. This collection of symptoms that are caused by vigorously shaking an infant is known as **shaken baby injuries**. (For more information on child abuse, consult a pediatric nursing text.)

TEACHING TIP

Advise parents that if they become frustrated with a crying baby, they should put the baby in the crib or in a safe location and allow themselves time to calm down. Sometimes going outside the door, counting to 10, doing deep breathing, or calling a friend can help. Remind parents that crying never hurts a baby, but shaking can seriously injure the baby. Reassure parents that all new parents have times when they feel frustrated and do not know what to do. This is a normal part of parenting a newborn.

To increase parents' coping abilities, suggest that they initially respond to the baby's crying by checking for hunger, a wet or soiled diaper, excessive cold or heat, restrictive or chafing clothing or blankets, or other comfort concerns. If these are not present, suggest holding or rocking the infant as previously discussed. Other calming measures include burping the infant (which provides repetitive tactile stimulation and disperses air bubbles), placing the infant in a mechanized infant swing, or taking the infant for a ride in a stroller or car. Some infants are soothed by white noise such as the sound of a dryer or the static on an untuned radio, whereas others are soothed when bound "papoose style" on the mother's chest, swaddled, bathed, or massaged.

Crying can also be associated with gastrointestinal upset in infants. The parents should discuss concerns with the physician or nurse practitioner to ensure the crying is not associated with a physical cause, such as acid reflux, ear infections, or other physical conditions. In addition, it is not uncommon for infants to cry after feedings because of pain from a buildup of air bubbles in the stomach and an inability to pass flatus. Some practitioners recommend simethicone after each feeding to decrease the incidence of flatus pain. Placing the infant in a prone position across the lap while burping the infant can also aid in passing flatus.

Safety Considerations

Newborns should not have pillows or stuffed animals in the crib while they sleep; these items could cause suffocation. Mattresses should fit snugly in a crib to prevent entrapment and suffocation, and the crib should be inspected regularly to determine whether it is in safe working order. Crib slats should be no more than 2⅜ in. apart. Parents can be encouraged to attend infant cardiopulmonary resuscitation (CPR) classes, especially if there is a family history of SIDS or the infant requires special care.

Many families, especially breastfeeding families, practice **cosleeping**, in which the infant sleeps with the mother or both parents during the night. The American Academy of Pediatrics does not recommend the infant cosleeping with parents, as it is considered a risk factor for SIDS. Some families and cultures, however, may still participate in this practice and thus warrant appropriate teaching measures.

Cosleeping families should be counseled to follow these safety guidelines:

- Place the infant on a firm mattress, never on comforters, pillows, or a waterbed.
- Never sleep with your infant if you have been using drugs, or have become intoxicated.
- Ensure that the infant is protected from rolling off the bed or becoming entrapped in bed rails or a space between the frame and the mattress.
- As with crib sleeping, remove all decorative pillows, stuffed animals, toys, or blankets that could impair the

baby's breathing. Do not cover the baby with blankets, sheets, or down comforters.

- Make sure the baby is sleeping on his or her back.
- Ensure plenty of ventilation to the infant.
- Avoid overdressing the infant because the parent's body heat will reduce the need for excess clothing.
- Never smoke in bed with the infant. Family members should smoke outdoors and not in the household with the infant.
- If additional children are sleeping in the bed, make sure they are not sleeping directly next to the infant.

Smoking poses multiple risks to the newborn and any older children living in the household. Infants living in a household with a smoker have a higher rate of hospital admissions during the first year of life. They are more prone to ear infections, asthma, allergies, and other respiratory problems. As discussed earlier, the incidence of SIDS increases when the infant is exposed to smoke (AAP, 2005). Smoking also creates a fire hazard within the household. Smoking is the primary cause of household fires in the United States. The incidence of such fires increases dramatically when other intoxicating agents are ingested, such as alcohol or drugs. Parents should be counseled to smoke outdoors; use large, heavy ashtrays to avoid tipping; ensure that all cigarette butts are properly extinguished; never smoke in bed; and never smoke if other intoxicating agents have been used.

Other significant risk factors for SIDS related to cosleeping include being extremely overtired, sharing the bed with other young children, use of alcohol or drugs, sleeping with infants younger than 11 weeks, multiple bed sharers, and having the baby remain in the bed for the entire night (AAP, 2005). The American Academy of Pediatrics (2005) recommends that the safest place for the infant to sleep is in the same room with the infant in a crib in close proximity to the parents for the first 6 months of life. The use of pacifiers has also been associated with a reduction in SIDS deaths (AAP, 2005).

Newborn Screening and Immunization Program

Before the newborn and mother are discharged from the hospital, parents are informed about the normal screening tests for newborns and told when to return for further tests if needed (see Chapter 26 ∞ for discussion of initial newborn screening). Early newborn discharge puts infants at risk for delayed or even missed diagnosis of PKU and congenital hypothryroidism because of decreased sensitivity of screening before 24 hours of age. Newborns should be retested by 2 weeks of age if the first test was done before 24 hours of age. Nurses should stress that an abnormal test result is not diagnostic. More definitive tests must be

performed to verify the results. It is important to follow protocols that incorporate state laws about newborn testing. If additional tests are positive, treatment is initiated. These conditions may be treated by dietary means or by administration of missing hormones. The inborn conditions cannot be cured, but they can be treated. They are not contagious, but they may be inherited by other siblings.

Hearing screenings before discharge are now conducted in all 50 states. According to the National Center for Hearing Assessment & Management (2007), 95.7% of all infants obtained hearing screening in the United States. Sometimes infants fail to pass these tests for reasons other than hearing loss. Amniotic fluid in the ear canals is a frequent cause of suboptimal test results. In these cases, infants are retested in a week or two. Parents should be informed of the need for retesting and the importance of follow-up.

Immunization programs against the Hepatitis B virus during the newborn period and infancy are in place in many states. Newborns should receive the first dose of hepatitis B (hep B) vaccine at birth to 2 months of age. Parents need to be advised whether their birthing center provides newborn hepatitis vaccination so that an adequate follow-up program can be set in motion (AAP & ACOG, 2007). For more detailed discussion of newborn screening and immunization needs see Chapter 26 ∞.

TEACHING TIP

As many as 50% of parents whose infants failed the initial hearing test do not arrange for a rescreening. Many parents do not understand the importance of rescreening or how early diagnosis of hearing loss can impact early speech and development. Explain the importance of rescreening to the parents and encourage them to verbalize their questions. Few infants who are rescreened have actual hearing loss, but early detection can greatly improve the development of infants with hearing loss or those who are hard of hearing.

Home Care: The Mother and Family

During the first home visit, the nurse completes a physical assessment of the mother and a psychosocial assessment of the family. Teaching for self-care is commonly required for new mothers, especially breastfeeding mothers with nipple soreness, engorgement, and other concerns. Family teaching related to resumption of sexual activity and contraception may also be required, as discussed in Chapter 31 ∞.

Assessment of the Mother and Family

Before performing the physical assessment, the nurse should ensure the mother's privacy. The physical assessment focuses on maternal physical adaptation, which is assessed by focusing on vital signs, breasts, abdominal musculature, elimination patterns, reproductive tract, and laboratory values. The nurse also talks with the mother about her diet, fatigue level, ability to rest and sleep, pain management, and signs of postpartal complications. In addition, for breastfeeding mothers, the nurse assesses the woman's feeding technique and presents information about possible problems that may occur.

Many new mothers are concerned about weight loss. Women who have gained excess weight during the pregnancy are at risk for obesity in later life. Counseling the mother about proper diet and exercise is an effective strategy to lose weight in the postpartum period. Nursing women should be counseled that extreme weight loss strategies are not advised, but that healthy food choices and exercise can aid in weight reduction. There are also weight loss programs designed specifically for nursing mothers that can offer counseling, group support, and monitoring in the postpartum period.

The psychologic assessment focuses on attachment, adjustment to the parental role, sibling adjustment, her perception of her new role and coping, and educational needs. When appropriate, the nurse mentions available community resources, including public health department follow-up visits or new mother support groups. If not already discussed, teaching about family planning is appropriate at this time, and the nurse provides information about birth control methods.

In ideal situations a family approach involving the presence of the father and any siblings provides an opportunity to observe family interactions and opportunities for all family members to ask questions and express concerns. In addition, any questionable family interaction pattern such as one suggestive of abuse or neglect may be evident and further referral could be considered if needed. (See Assessment Guide: Postpartal—First Home Visit and Anticipated Progress at 6 Weeks.)

In addition, the nurse continues to provide teaching to the mother and her family as needed, including

EVIDENCE-BASED PRACTICE

Postpartum Weight Management

Clinical Questions
What are the most effective weight management interventions for postpartum women?

The Evidence
There is a high prevalence of obesity during childbearing. Excessive prepregnancy weight or weight gain during pregnancy, ethnicity, postpartum changes in roles, dietary changes during pregnancy, and changes in physical activity are all risk factors for weight retention after birth. The majority of women do not lose all of the weight gained during pregnancy, and this often contributes to later obesity. The nurse can advise postpartum mothers about ways they can manage their weight to achieve healthy prepregnancy levels. A team of expert advanced practice nurses, researchers, and a physician conducted a comprehensive, systematic review of published intervention studies to identify the best available evidence for guiding weight management interventions in postpartum women. Systematic reviews of multiple studies guided by content experts provide the highest level of evidence for practice.

What Is Effective?
Interventions should target women early in their childbearing years so that they have the most significant long-term impact. Multilevel strategies were found to be the most effective in helping women manage their weight in the postpartum period. A multilevel approach is one in which individual strategies are enhanced by interpersonal efforts and community-based support. At the individual level, mothers can be assured that physical activity and appropriate nutritional intake will have no adverse effects on lactation. Teaching mothers about physical activity and appropriate nutrition is effective, whether delivered at the individual or group level. Effective interpersonal level activities included social support through group participation and engaging the family in healthy eating habits. At the community level, locating safe places to walk and exercise in their neighborhoods and helping mothers map walking routes to parks, schools, and other safe destinations is effective in increasing physical activity.

What Is Inconclusive?
Most of the studies recruited only white women, so it is unknown how these interventions work with women of varied ethnic backgrounds. There was considerable variation in how nutrition and physical activity education was delivered to the mothers in these studies. Most commonly, both group- and individual-level interventions were used, and there was no distinction as to which method was best.

Best Practice
Helping new mothers manage their weight in the postpartum period can prevent long-term problems with obesity. Multilevel strategies are most effective, including individual, interpersonal, and community level services. All of the strategies focus on helping mothers increase physical activity and achieve healthy nutritional intake. You can reassure new mothers that physical activity and appropriate nutrition will not reduce lactation or negatively affect their newborn.

Reference
Keller, C., Records, K., Ainsworth, B., Permana, P., & Coonrod, D. (2008). Interventions for weight management in postpartum women. *JOGNN: The Journal of Obstetric, Gynecologic, and Neonatal Nursing, 37*, 71–79.

ASSESSMENT GUIDE

POSTPARTAL—FIRST HOME VISIT AND ANTICIPATED PROGRESS AT 6 WEEKS

Physical Assessment/ Normal Findings	Alterations and Possible Causes*	Nursing Responses to Data†
Vital Signs		
Blood pressure: Return to normal prepregnant level.	Elevated blood pressure (anxiety, essential hypertension, renal disease), preeclampsia (can occur postpartum).	Review history, evaluate normal baseline; refer to physician/CNM if necessary.
Pulse: 60 to 90 beats/min (or prepregnant normal rate).	Increased pulse rate, tachycardia, chest pain (excitement, anxiety, cardiac disorders).	Count pulse for full minute, note irregularities; marked tachycardia or beat irregularities require additional assessment and possible physician/CNM referral.
Respirations: 16 to 24/min.	Marked tachypnea or abnormal patterns (respiratory disorders).	Evaluate for respiratory disease; refer to physician/CNM if necessary.
Temperature: 36.6°C to 37.6°C (98°F to 99.6°F).	Increased temperature (infection).	Assess for signs and symptoms of infection or disease state.
Weight		
2 days: Possible weight loss of 12 to 20+ lb.	Minimal weight loss (fluid retention, preeclampsia).	Evaluate for fluid retention, edema, deep tendon reflexes, and blood pressure elevation.
6 weeks: Returning to normal prepregnant weight.	Retained weight (excessive caloric intake).	Determine amount of daily exercise. Provide dietary teaching. Refer to dietician if necessary for additional dietary counseling.
	Extreme weight loss (excessive dieting, inadequate caloric intake).	Discuss appropriate diets, refer to dietician for additional counseling if necessary.
Breasts		
Nonbreastfeeding: 2 days: May have mild to moderate tenderness; small amount of milk may be expressed. 6 weeks: Soft, with no tenderness; return to prepregnant size.	Some engorgement (incomplete suppression of lactation). Redness; marked tenderness (mastitis). Palpable mass (tumor).	Engorgement may be seen in nonbreastfeeding mothers. Advise client to wear a supportive, well-fitted bra; avoid very warm showers; avoid pumping or any stimulation of breasts; use ice packs for comfort; evaluate for signs and symptoms of mastitis (rare in nonbreastfeeding mothers). Parcooked cabbage leaves can be placed against the breast to relieve engorgement.
Breastfeeding: Full, with prominent nipples; lactation established.	Cracked, fissured nipples (feeding problems). Redness, marked tenderness, or even abscess formation (mastitis). Palpable mass (full milk duct, tumor).	Counsel about nipple care. Observe infant feeding. Evaluate client condition, evidence of fever, redness, or tender area, refer to physician/CNM for initiation of antibiotic therapy, if indicated.
		Opinion varies as to value of breast examination for breastfeeding mothers; some feel a breastfeeding mother should examine her breasts monthly, after feeding, when breasts are empty; if palpable mass is felt, refer to physician for further evaluation.
	*Possible causes of alterations are identified in parentheses.	†This column provides guidelines for further assessment and initial nursing intervention.

ASSESSMENT GUIDE

POSTPARTAL—FIRST HOME VISIT AND ANTICIPATED PROGRESS AT 6 WEEKS *(Continued)*

Physical Assessment/ Normal Findings	Alterations and Possible Causes*	Nursing Responses to Data†
Breasts *(Continued)*		For breast inflammation instruct the mother to: 1. Keep breast empty by frequent feeding. 2. Rest when possible. 3. Take prescribed pain relief med. 4. Force fluids. 5. Take antibiotics if ordered. If symptoms are accompanied by fever, flulike symptoms, or redness, instruct woman to call her physician/CNM and take an analgesic.
Abdominal Musculature 2 days: Improved firmness, although "bread dough" consistency is not unusual, especially in multipara. Striae pink and obvious.	Marked relaxation of muscles.	Evaluate exercise level; provide information on appropriate exercise program.
Cesarean incision healing.	Use the REEDA scoring system which includes: redness, ecchymosis, edema, discharge from incision site, and approximation. Assess for tenderness and pain.	Evaluate for infection; refer to physician/CNM if necessary.
6 weeks: Muscle tone continues to improve; striae may be beginning to fade, may not achieve a silvery appearance for several more weeks; linea nigra fading.		
Elimination Pattern **Urinary Tract:** Return to prepregnant urinary elimination routine.	Urinary incontinence, especially when lifting, coughing, laughing, and so on (urethral trauma, cystocele).	Assess for cystocele; instruct in appropriate muscle tightening exercises; refer to physician/CNM.
	Pain or burning when voiding, urgency and/or frequency, pus, blood, or white blood cells (WBC) in urine, pathogenic organisms in culture (urinary tract infection).	Evaluate for urinary tract infection; obtain clean-catch urine; refer to physician/CNM for treatment if indicated.
Routine urinalysis within normal limits (proteinuria disappeared).	Sugar or ketone in urine—may be some lactose present in urine of breastfeeding mothers (diabetes).	Evaluate diet; assess for signs and symptoms of diabetes; refer to physician/CNM.
Bowel Habits: 2 days: May be some discomfort with defecation, especially if client had severe hemorrhoids or third- or fourth-degree extension.	Severe constipation or pain when defecating (trauma or hemorrhoids).	Discuss dietary patterns; encourage fluids and high fiber diet, adequate roughage. Counsel on the effects of medications. Continue use of stool softener if necessary to prevent pain associated with straining; continue sitz baths, periods of rest for severe hemorrhoids; assess healing of episiotomy and/or lacerations; severe constipation may require administration of laxatives, stool softeners, and an enema if not contraindicated (check with physician/CNM).
*Possible causes of alterations are identified in parentheses.		†This column provides guidelines for further assessment and initial nursing intervention.

(Continued on next page)

Physical Assessment/ Normal Findings	Alterations and Possible Causes*	Nursing Responses to Data†
Elimination Pattern (Continued)	Marked constipation (inadequate fluid/fiber intake).	See previous discussed interventions.
6 weeks: Return to normal prepregnancy bowel elimination.	Fecal incontinence or constipation (rectocele).	Assess for evidence of rectocele; instruct in muscle tightening exercises; refer to physician/CNM.
Reproductive Tract		
Lochia: 2 days: Lochia rubra or lochia serosa, scant amounts, fleshy odor.	Excessive amounts and/or large clots (nonfirm uterus), foul odor (infection), passing tissue (possible retained placenta).	Assess for evidence of infection and/or failure of the uterus to decrease in size; refer to physician/CNM.
6 weeks: No lochia, or return to normal menstruation pattern.	See above.	See above.
Fundus and Perineum: 2 days: Fundus is at least two finger breadths below the umbilicus; uterine muscles still somewhat lax; introitus of vagina lacks tone—gapes when intra-abdominal pressure is increased by coughing or straining.	Uterus not decreasing in size appropriately (infection).	Assess fundus for firmness and/or signs of infection; refer to physician/CNM if indicated.
Episiotomy and/or lacerations healing; no signs of infection; may have some bruising and tenderness.	Evidence of redness, severe pain, poor tissue approximation in episiotomy and/or laceration (wound infection).	Utilize cool or warm sitz baths, topical medications.
6 weeks: Uterus almost returned to prepregnant size with almost completely restored muscle tone.	Continued flow of lochia, failure to decrease appropriately in size (subinvolution).	Assess for evidence of subinvolution and/or infection; refer to physician for further evaluation and treatment if necessary.
Hemoglobin and Hematocrit Levels		
6 weeks: Hemoglobin (Hb) 12 g/dL; Hematocrit (Hct) 37% ± 5%	Hb less than 12 g/dL; Hct 32% (anemia)	Assess nutritional status, assess for signs or symptoms of anemia, begin (or continue) supplemental iron; for marked anemia (Hb less than or equal to 9 g/dL) additional assessment and/or physician/CNM referral may be necessary.
Attachment		
Bonding process demonstrated by soothing, cuddling, and talking to infant; appropriate feeding techniques; eye-to-eye contact; calling infant by name.	Failure to bond demonstrated by lack of behaviors associated with bonding process, calling infant by nickname that promotes ridicule, inadequate infant weight gain, infant is dirty, hygienic measures are not being maintained, severe diaper rash, failure to obtain adequate supplies to provide infant care (malattachment).	Provide counseling; talk with the woman about her feelings regarding the infant; provide support for the caretaking activities that are being performed; refer to public health nurse for continued home visits; refer if abuse or neglect is suspected.
	*Possible causes of alterations are identified in parentheses.	†This column provides guidelines for further assessment and initial nursing intervention.

ASSESSMENT GUIDE

POSTPARTAL—FIRST HOME VISIT AND ANTICIPATED PROGRESS AT 6 WEEKS *(Continued)*

Physical Assessment/ Normal Findings	Alterations and Possible Causes*	Nursing Responses to Data†
Attachment *(Continued)*		
Parent interacts with infant and provides soothing, caretaking activities.	Parent is unable to respond to infant needs (inability to recognize needs, inadequate education and support, fear, family stress).	Provide support for caretaking activities observed; provide information regarding caretaking activities, such as responding to infant cry; methods of wrapping infant; methods of soothing the infant such as swaddling, rocking, increasing stimuli by singing to the infant or decreasing stimuli by putting infant to rest in quiet room; methods of holding the infant; differences in the cry. Identify support system such as friends, neighbors; provide information regarding community resources and support groups.
Parents express feelings of comfort and success with the parent role.	Evidence of stress and anxiety (difficulty moving into or dealing with the parent role).	Provide support and encouragement; provide information regarding progression into parent role and assist parents in talking through their feelings; refer to community resources and support groups.
Woman is in the informal or personal stage of maternal role attainment.	Woman is still greatly influenced by others, has not developed an image or style of her own (woman remains in the anticipatory stage).	Provide role modeling for the woman in working through problem solving with the infant, provide encouragement as she thinks through decisions and develops her sense of problem solving; encourage her to make decisions regarding infant care.
Adjustment to Parental Role		
Parents are coping with new roles in terms of division of labor, financial status, communication, readjustment of sexual relations, and adjusting to new daily tasks.	Inability to adjust to new roles (immaturity, inadequate education and preparation, ineffective communication patterns, inadequate support, current family crisis).	Provide counseling, refer to parent groups.
Education		
Mother understands self-care measures.	Inadequate knowledge of self-care (inadequate education).	Provide education and counseling.
Parents are knowledgeable regarding infant care.	Inadequate knowledge of infant care (inadequate education).	
Siblings are adjusting to new baby.	Excessive sibling rivalry.	
Parents have a method of contraception.	Birth control method not chosen.	
	*Possible causes of alterations are identified in parentheses.	†This column provides guidelines for further assessment and initial nursing intervention.

descriptions of relevant self-care measures. Generally the new mother has a final postpartum examination with her caregiver about 6 weeks after childbirth. However, if the nurse's assessment indicates a need, the nurse refers the woman to her healthcare provider for care before the 6-week check.

Breastfeeding Concerns Following Discharge

Because mothers are discharged from the birthing unit before breastfeeding is well established, they are frequently alone when they encounter changes in the breastfeeding process. Many women stop nursing if the situations they encounter seem problematic. For this reason, the nurse providing a home visit is in a unique position to positively impact the success of breastfeeding (Association of Women's Health, Obstetric and Neonatal Nurses [AWHONN], 2006). Table 32–2 summarizes self-care measures the nurse can suggest to a woman with a breastfeeding problem.

Newborn feeding is discussed in detail in Chapter 27 ∞. Regardless of feeding method, it is important for the nurse to assess the newborn's fluid and nutritional intake. As part of the physical assessment the newborn's nude weight is determined. If the weight loss since birth is 10% or more, the nurse assesses the baby for signs of dehydration such as loose skin with decreased skin turgor, dry mucous membranes, sunken anterior fontanelle, and decreased frequency and amount of voiding and stooling. Risk factors for suboptimal breastfeeding include maternal obesity, primiparity, young maternal age, use of formula supplementation, use of pacifiers, cesarean birth, second stage greater than 1 hour, low birth weight, breastfeeding difficulty, and flat or inverted nipples (Jevitt, Hernandez, & Groër, 2007; Walker, 2007).

Nipple Soreness

Some discomfort often occurs initially with breastfeeding; it peaks between day 3 and 6 and then recedes. Breastfeeding difficulty and nipple soreness are often causes for women to discontinue breastfeeding. The nurse should counsel the mother not to switch to formula-feeding or delay feedings because these measures cause engorgement and more soreness (Locke, Paul, & DiMatteo, 2006). Discomfort that lasts throughout the feeding or past the first week demands attention.

The baby's position at the breast is a critical factor in nipple soreness. The mother's hand should be off the areola, and the baby should be facing the mother's chest, with ear, shoulder, and hip aligned (see Figure 26–5 ■). Because the area of greatest stress to the nipple is in line

with the newborn's chin and nose, nipple soreness may be decreased by encouraging the mother to rotate positions when feeding the infant. Changing positions alters the focus of greatest stress and promotes more complete breast emptying.

Nipple soreness may also develop if the infant has faulty sucking habits. Nipples may have injured tips that are bruised, scabbed, or blistered from the nipple entering the baby's mouth at an upward angle and rubbing against the roof of the mouth or from poor latch-on (Locke et al., 2006). Soreness may also result from continuous negative pressure if the infant falls asleep with the breast in his or her mouth.

Chewed nipples, which result from improper positioning, are cracked or tender at or near the base. In these cases, the baby's jaws close only on the nipple instead of on the areola, or the baby's mouth is not opened wide enough or has slipped down to the nipple from the areola as a result of engorgement. Soreness on the underside of the nipple is caused by the infant nursing with her or his bottom lip tucked in rather than out, causing a friction burn. In such cases, even vigorous sucking produces little milk because the milk sinuses under the areola are not compressed. This situation results in a frustrated infant and marked soreness for the mother. The problem is overcome by manipulating the baby's bottom lip with a fingertip before beginning the feeding, positioning the infant with as much areola as possible in his or her mouth, and rotating the baby's positions at the breast.

Nipple soreness is especially pronounced during the first few minutes of a feeding. If the mother is not expecting this discomfort, she may become discouraged and quickly stop. The letdown reflex may take a few minutes to activate, and it may not occur if the mother stops nursing too quickly. The infant is unsatisfied, and the possibility of breast engorgement increases.

TEACHING TIP

If the mother continually has soreness because of a delay in letdown, encourage her to massage the breast in a circular pattern and apply warm compresses just before each breastfeeding session. These activities encourage letdown, increasing the chance that it will occur at the same time that the infant is placed on the breast.

Nipple soreness can also result from the vigorous feeding of an overeager infant. Thus the mother may find it helpful to nurse more frequently. Again, promoting letdown just before feeding may help. Other self-care measures include applying ice to the nipples and areola for a few minutes before feeding to promote nipple erectness and numb the tissue initially. To promote dryness, the mother may leave her bra flaps down for a few minutes

TABLE 32–2 Common Breastfeeding Problems and Remedies

Nipples Not Graspable

Flat or inverted nipples
- Use Hoffman technique to break adhesions.
- Wear breast shells to encourage nipples to protrude.
- Grasp nipples and roll gently between the fingers to increase protractility.
- Form the nipple before breastfeeding by hand shaping, ice, or wearing nipple shells a half-hour before feeding.
- Use a breast pump to draw nipples out so that the mother can then put the baby to the breast.

Engorged breasts
- Treat engorgement by feeding the baby more frequently.
- A hand or electric pump or manual emptying of the breast can be done if the baby is unable to grasp the nipple.

Large breasts
- Support breast with opposite hand, or use rolled towel under breast to bring nipple to the level of baby's mouth.
- Avoid having the nipple pointing downward because this makes latch-on more difficult.
- Use C-hold to make nipple accessible to baby.

Engorgement

Missed or infrequent feedings
- Breastfeed frequently (every 1 1/2 hours).
- Massage and hand express or pump to empty breasts completely when feedings are missed or when a full feeling develops in breasts and baby is not available or willing to feed.
- Avoid excessive stimulation or pumping between feedings because this will increase milk production.
- Place warm compresses on breast just before feeding to soften breast.
- Use cold applications between feedings to slow milk production (frozen bagged vegetables, ice packs, and par-cooked cabbage leaves (AWHONN, 2006)).

Breasts not emptied at feedings
- Massage breasts and use warm cloths before feedings.
- Breastfeed long enough to empty breasts (10 to 15 minutes on each side at each feeding).
- If baby will not feed long enough to empty breasts, hand express or pump after feeding.

Inadequate letdown
- Use relaxation techniques, massage, and warm compresses before breastfeeding.
- Relax in warm shower with water running from back over shoulders and breasts, hand expressing to relieve fullness.
- Use hand or electric pump before placing baby on breast to encourage letdown.
- Listen to soothing music, use visualization or breathing techniques.
- If caused by anxiety, try to eliminate the source of tension.

Baby sleepy or not eager to feed
- Use rousing techniques (e.g., hold baby upright, unwrap blanket, change diaper).
- Pre-express milk onto nipple or baby's lips to entice baby.
- Avoid use of bottles of water or formula; these will decrease baby's willingness to suckle.

Inadequate Letdown

Letdown not well established
- Give the baby ample time at the breast (at least 15 minutes per side) to allow for letdown and complete emptying.
- Breastfeed in a quiet spot away from distractions.

- Massage breasts and apply warm compresses before breastfeeding.
- Drink juice, water, or tea (no caffeine) before and during breastfeeding.
- Condition letdown by setting up a routine for beginning feedings.
- Use relaxation, visualization, and breathing techniques.
- Stimulate the nipple manually before breastfeeding.
- Concentrate thought on the baby and milk flow; turn on a faucet so that the sound of running water helps stimulate letdown.
- Take a warm shower before feedings.
- Use breast pump to stimulate the letdown.
- Avoid waiting to put baby to breast until the baby is famished because this may increase maternal anxiety.
- Assess for maternal pain, cold temperature, or anxiety before feeding.

Mother overtired or overextended
- Nap or rest when the baby rests.
- Limit distractions, limit visitors, focus on personal needs.
- Lie down to breastfeed.
- Simplify daily chores; set priorities.

Mother tense, pressured
- Identify the causes of tensions and eliminate or minimize them.
- Decrease fatigue.
- Have others assist with other household duties or tasks.
- Use relaxation, visualization, and breathing exercises to promote relaxation and comfort.

Mother caught in cycle of little milk, worry, less milk
- Try all the actions above.
- Counsel mother that most women do produce enough milk.
- Have infant weighed to ensure adequate weight gain which is a reflection of milk supply.
- Encourage frequent, uninterrupted feedings.
- Consult a lactation consultant as needed.

Cracked Nipples

All causes of sore nipples carried to extreme
- Refer to all actions for sore nipples.
- Ensure infant is properly positioned.
- Feed infant more frequently.
- Avoid soaps, perfumes, or other cleaning products that can dry out nipples and predispose them to cracking.
- Express milk post-feeding and rub into nipple allowing it to air dry.
- Use emollients or lanolin as directed by physician/CNM/lactation consultant.
- Consult doctor about using ibuprofen (Motrin), acetaminophen (Tylenol), or other painkiller.
- Improve nutritional status, increasing protein, vitamin C, zinc.

Local infection (baby with staph or other organism may have infected mother's nipples)
- Refer to physician.

Plugged Ducts

Poor positioning
- Try a variety of positions for complete emptying.
- Alternate positions so that different areas of the nipple have different compression pressure.
- Incomplete emptying of breast.
- Breastfeed at least 10 minutes per side after letdown.
- Alternate breastfeeding positions.
- If baby does not empty breasts, pump or express milk after feedings.

(Continued on next page)

TABLE 32–2	Common Breastfeeding Problems and Remedies *(Continued)*

External pressure on breast
- Use larger-size bra, insert bra extender, or go braless.
- Wear a sports bra instead of a traditional bra.
- Use nursing bra instead of pulling up conventional bra to breastfeed to avoid pressure on ducts.
- Avoid bunching up sweater or nightgown under arm during breastfeeding.

Sore Nipples

Poor positioning
- Alternate breastfeeding positions throughout the day.
- Bring the baby close to feed so the baby does not pull on the breast.
- Place the nipple and some of the areola in the baby's mouth.
- Check to ensure the baby is put on and off the breast properly.
- Check to ensure the nipple is back far enough in the baby's mouth.
- Hold the baby closely during feeding so the nipple is not constantly being pulled.
- Ensure that shoulder, hip, and knees are all properly aligned and facing the mother.

Baby chewing or nuzzling onto nipple
- Form the nipple for the baby.
- Set up a pattern of getting the baby onto the breast using the rooting reflex.

Baby sucking on end of nipple
- Ensure the nipple is way back in the baby's mouth by getting the baby properly onto the breast.
- Check for an inverted nipple.
- Check for engorgement.
- If baby is initially placed incorrectly on the end of the nipple, break the suction using a fish hook motion with your index finger and reposition baby on nipple properly.

- Do not allow baby to nurse on end of nipple, reposition immediately.

Baby chewing his or her way off the nipple (nipple being pulled out of baby's mouth at end of feeding)
- Remove the baby from the breast by placing a finger between the baby's gums to ensure suction is broken.
- End feeding when the baby's suckling slows, before he or she has a chance to chew on the nipple.

Baby overly eager to nurse
- Breastfeed more often.
- Pre-express milk to hasten letdown, avoiding vigorous suckling.

Dry colostrum or milk causing nipple to stick to bra or breast pads
- Moisten bra or pads before taking off so as not to remove keratin.
- Ensure that nipples are dry before replacing bra or clothing against nipples.

Nipples not allowed to dry
- Remove plastic liners from milk pads.
- Air dry breast completely after nursing.
- Change nursing pads frequently.
- Switch to cotton nursing pads.

Nipple skin not resistant to stress
- Improve diet, especially adding fresh fruits and vegetables and vitamin supplements.
- Eliminate or decrease use of sugary foods, alcohol, caffeine, cigarettes.
- Check use of cleansing or drying agents.

Natural oils removed or keratin layers broken down by drying agents (soap, alcohol, shampoo, deodorant)
- Eliminate irritants.
- Wash breasts with water only.

after feeding (Figure 32–6 ■) or expose her nipples to sunlight or ultraviolet light for 30 seconds at first, gradually increasing to 3 minutes. Drying the nipples with a hair dryer on a low heat setting also facilitates drying and promotes healing (Locke et al., 2006). The use of petroleum-based products such as Vaseline, A & D, cocoa butter, and baby oil to lubricate the nipples is discouraged because the petroleum interferes with skin respiration and may prolong soreness. Because of the risk of allergic reactions, Massé cream (risk of peanut allergy) is discouraged. For some women, the use of lanolin cream or peppermint gel may help prevent or aid in healing cracked nipples (Melli, Rashidi, Nokhoodchi et al., 2007). In addition, products that are washed off before breastfeeding are avoided because of the irritation that washing produces. During bathing, mothers should be advised to only rinse their nipples with water and to avoid soap because this can dry the nipple out and lead to soreness.

Current research as to the effectiveness of nipple lubricants is inconclusive. Thus many lactation experts recommend that the mother's own milk be applied to the nipples and allowed to air dry. Breast milk is high in fat, fights infection, and will not irritate the nipples. Moreover, it is

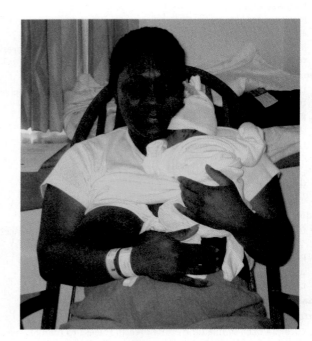

FIGURE 32–6 Mothers with sore nipples can leave bra flaps down after feedings to promote air drying and prevent chapping.

readily available at no cost to the mother. In cases of very dry or severely sore nipples, hypoallergenic medical-grade anhydrous lanolin or peppermint gel may be helpful (Melli et al., 2007). This product poses a low risk of allergy because the alcohols that contribute to the allergic response have been removed.

If the woman finds that her bra or clothing rubs against her nipples and adds to her discomfort, she may insert shells into her bra. Medela Shells relieve friction and promote air circulation. If a woman uses breast pads inside her bra to keep milk from leaking onto her clothes, she should change the pads frequently so the nipples remain dry. Some women may be sensitive to the plastic liner within the disposable pad, so the plastic can be removed or they can be encouraged to try cotton pads.

Older remedies for nipple soreness are receiving renewed acceptance. For instance, tea bags may be moistened in warm water and applied to the nipples. The tannic acid seems to help toughen the nipples, and the warmth is soothing and promotes healing. Tannic acid also has anti-inflammatory properties which can help relieve discomfort. Other therapies have included warm compresses and heat applications (Morland-Schultz & Hill, 2005).

If nipple soreness persists, the woman should be advised to consult a certified lactation consultant to determine the etiology of the soreness. Nipple dermatitis, which causes swollen, reddened, burning nipples, is most commonly caused by thrush or by allergic response to breast cream preparations. If the nipple soreness has a sudden onset and is accompanied by burning or itching, shooting pains through the breast, and a deep pink coloration of the nipple, it may be caused by a thrush infection transmitted from the infant to the mother. White patches or streaks in the infant's mouth indicate a need for treatment of the mouth and nipple infection. The infection can be treated with a variety of antifungal preparations and does not preclude breastfeeding. It is important for both the mother and the infant to receive treatment to prevent cross-transferring of the fungus.

Cracked Nipples

Nipple soreness is often coupled with cracked nipples. When a breastfeeding mother complains of soreness, the nurse carefully examines the nipples for fissures or cracks and observes the mother during breastfeeding to see whether the infant is correctly positioned at the breast. If the positioning is correct and cracks exist, interventions are necessary. All the interventions described for sore nipples may be used. It may also help the mother to begin nursing on the breast that is less sore. This approach allows the letdown reflex to occur in the affected breast and permits the infant to do more vigorous sucking on the less tender breast, which decreases trauma to the cracked nip-

ple. For the mother's comfort, analgesics may be taken approximately 1 hour before nursing.

Breast Engorgement

A distinction exists between breast fullness and engorgement. All lactating women experience a transitional fullness at first, initially caused by venous congestion and later caused by accumulating milk. However, this fullness generally lasts only 24 hours, the breasts remain soft enough for the newborn to suckle, and there is no pain. Engorged breasts are hard, painful, and warm and appear taut and shiny. The consistency is like gravel.

The infant should suckle for an average of 15 minutes per feeding and should feed at least 8 to 12 times in 24 hours (Lawrence & Lawrence, 2005). If the baby is unable to nurse more frequently, the mother may express some milk manually or with a pump, taking care to avoid traumatizing the breast tissue. As just noted, warm compresses before nursing stimulate letdown and soften the breast so that the infant can grasp the areola more easily. Cool compresses after nursing can help slow refilling of the breasts and provide comfort to the mother. Ice packs may also be used as a comfort measure. The mother should wear a well-fitted nursing bra 24 hours a day to support the breasts and prevent discomfort from tension. (See the Teaching Card on Breastfeeding in the center of this book.)

The use of fresh green cabbage leaves placed inside the bra to treat engorgement is a long-recognized home remedy that recently has sparked clinical interest. Although the exact action of the cabbage is not understood, it appears to reduce the edema of engorgement. The amount of relief women experience varies. Some women report relief in as little as 30 minutes, whereas other women require more continuous use to perceive an effect. It should be noted that prolonged use of cabbage can cause the milk to dry up, which may be helpful if sudden weaning is necessary. Analgesics such as acetaminophen and ibuprofen, alone or in combination with codeine, are appropriate. Mothers should be counseled that these medications will not harm their baby and are considered safe for breastfeeding mothers. For more information, see the accompanying Nursing Care Plan: For a Woman with Engorgement.

Plugged Ducts

Some mothers experience plugging of one or more ducts, especially in conjunction with or following engorgement. When breast milk pools within a duct and then dries, it forms a white, hardened plug that is typically visible at the outlet of the duct at the nipple surface. Because milk accumulates behind a plugged duct, women also experience an area of fullness, tenderness, and/or lumpiness in the associated region of the breast.

Nursing Care Plan For a Woman with Engorgement

CLIENT SCENARIO

Cathy McPhee delivered a healthy newborn girl, named Callie, 4 days ago. At the time of birth, she was able to put the newborn to breast within the first hour. Callie was very alert at birth, latching-on without difficulty. Cathy was able to breastfeed successfully during the remainder of her hospital stay.

Today, Cathy has returned to the clinic complaining of pain and swelling in both breasts and a low-grade fever. She has also had trouble getting Callie to latch-on.

ASSESSMENT

Subjective: Breast pain and tenderness, anxiety

Objective: Temperature 38°C (100.4°F). Breast tissue: firm, warm, and skin is shiny and taut. Swelling in axillary area and flattened nipples.

Nursing Diagnosis	Acute Pain related to increased breast fullness secondary to increased blood supply to breast tissue causing swelling of tissue around milk ducts*
Client Goal	Client will remain free of breast fullness and pain.
AEB:	• Decreased swelling of breast tissue • Decreased pain • No signs of breast tenderness or firmness

NURSING INTERVENTIONS

1. Instruct client to nurse frequently.

2. Instruct client to nurse at least 10 to 15 minutes on each breast per feeding.

3. Assist client to pre-express milk onto nipple or baby's lips.

4. Initiate pumping or manually express milk at the beginning of the feeding.

5. Instruct client to pump, hand express, or massage to empty breast when feedings are missed.

6. Administer analgesics before nursing.

7. Apply warm and/or cold compresses before nursing.

8. Apply fresh cabbage leaves to the breast between feedings.

RATIONALES

Rationale: Engorgement may be a result of infrequent or missed feedings. Frequent feedings will prevent the breast from becoming increasingly full which in turn decreases pain caused by engorgement. The newborn should be offered the breast at least eight to ten times in a 24-hour period.

Rationale: Hind milk may be brought forward when the newborn is able to suckle for 10 to 15 minutes per breast. This will allow the breast ducts to empty with each feeding.

Rationale: Engorgement may be the result of newborns who are too sleepy to suck at each feeding or not eager to nurse vigorously. Expressing some milk onto the nipple may entice the newborn to nurse more aggressively.

Rationale: Engorgement may be the result of the breast not emptying at each feeding. Pumping or manually expressing the breast will allow the breast to empty. Pumping or hand expressing the milk at the beginning of each feeding will help soften the breast so the newborn can latch-on to the nipple and facilitate letdown.

Rationale: If client develops a feeling of fullness in the breast, or the newborn has missed a feeding, then pumping or hand expressing the milk will help keep the milk ducts empty. When the milk ducts become backed up, milk production can be inhibited, eventually decreasing the milk supply. Pumping during engorgement should not affect the milk supply.

Rationale: Acetaminophen and ibuprofen alone or in combination with codeine may be administered just before nursing to relieve pain and discomfort. The medication will reach the milk within 30 minutes.

Rationale: Warm compresses may be applied before nursing to stimulate letdown or soften the breast. This will allow the newborn to grasp the areola. A proper latch-on will help prevent plugged ducts and assist in emptying the breast to reduce breast fullness and pain associated with engorgement. Relaxing in the shower with warm water running over the breast may have the same effect. Cold compresses may also be used to help reduce pain.

Rationale: Placing fresh cabbage leaves inside the bra is a home remedy that may relieve edema associated with engorgement, thereby reducing pain. Relief may be experienced within 30 minutes. Prolonged application of cabbage leaves may reduce the milk supply.

Nursing Care Plan For a Woman with Engorgement *(Continued)*

Evaluation of Client Goal
- No evidence of swelling found in breast tissue.
- Pain has decreased.
- Breast tissue is soft and without tenderness.

CRITICAL THINKING QUESTIONS

1. The nurse preparing Cathy for discharge notices that Callie nursed 3 hours ago but for only 3 to 4 minutes on each breast. Cathy states that the baby is very sleepy and has slept most of the day. She says she will wait to nurse again until she is home and more comfortable because her breasts hurt and are swollen. The nurse assesses the client's breasts and they are firm and tender with some swelling under the arm. What should the nurse instruct the client to do before discharge? What can Cathy do to minimize the breast fullness and discomfort?

Answer: Cathy is experiencing engorgement. Because it has been 3 hours since the last feeding, and the last feeding was brief, Callie is likely to be hungry, and Cathy should attempt to nurse her now, for at least 10 minutes on each breast. This will allow the breasts to empty and relieve Cathy's discomfort. Waiting until she gets home may increase her discomfort and Callie will likely become hungry and nurse more vigorously, which may be uncomfortable. When feedings are missed or the breasts are not emptied during feedings, Cathy should pump or manually express her breast milk. This will help relieve engorgement. The nurse can instruct Cathy to arouse Callie for feedings by holding her upright, unwrapping her blanket, or changing her diaper.

2. A postpartum nurse is teaching a breastfeeding class to new mothers. During the class one client states she had a problem with engorgement after the birth of her first child and wants to know what she can do differently this time to avoid the problem again. What strategies can the nurse suggest to help prevent engorgement?

Answer: The nurse explains that most women experience a feeling of fullness in the beginning because of venous congestion and accumulation of milk in the milk ducts. Usually it lasts only 24 hours. For some women this seems to occur around day 3 or 4 postpartum and is painful. Strategies to prevent engorgement may include: nurse frequently (every 3 hours or more frequently if needed); before nursing, massage or manually express milk to lubricate the nipple, use warm compresses to soften the breast for a better latch-on, and entice the baby to suck; apply a warm compress or cabbage leaves inside the bra for a short time to reduce swelling; and pump the breast if a feeding is missed.

*For your reference, this care plan is an example of how one nursing diagnosis might be addressed.

CRITICAL THINKING

Ann Nyembe calls you from home in tears on her third postpartum day. She states that, although breastfeeding was going well in the hospital, her breasts are now swollen, hard, and very painful, and her baby is refusing to suckle. Ann expresses extreme disappointment that "the breastfeeding didn't work" because she truly believes that breast milk is best for babies and she had enjoyed her breastfeeding experience in the hospital, especially nursing the baby immediately after birth. But she also states she has not been able to stop crying all day and can no longer tolerate her painful breasts. In addition she says that the baby "seems happier" with the bottle. What would you do?

Answers can be found in Appendix F ∞.

Self-care measures include the use of heat and massage. The nurse can encourage the mother to massage her breasts from her chest wall forward to the nipple while standing in a warm shower or following the application of moist heat to the breast. Warm compresses can be used and changed as temperature requires. The mother should then nurse her infant starting on the unaffected breast if the plugged breast is tender. Some lactation consultants advocate starting on the affected side because the more vigorous sucking may help dislodge the plug. A breast pump may also be effective in unplugging the duct.

Prevention of plugged ducts involves frequent nursing and the use of a variety of positions to ensure complete emptying. Some mothers discover that pressure from a shoulder strap on a purse, their infant sling, or a car seat belt causes recurring plugged ducts in the compressed area. Repositioning the device may help prevent plugged ducts in these women. Prevention and prompt correction of plugged ducts is important because it could lead to mastitis (discussed in Chapter 33 ∞).

Effect of Alcohol and Medications

Mothers may ask the home care nurse about the use of alcohol and medications when breastfeeding. According to the American Academy of Pediatrics (2005), alcohol consumption among breastfeeding women should be limited to occasional use. Breastfeeding mothers should not consume alcohol for at least 2 hours before nursing (O'Keefe, 2005). Alcohol levels in breast milk parallel those found in the maternal plasma, peaking 30 to 60 minutes after consumption. Mothers who do occasionally drink while lactating should be advised to consume the alcohol after breastfeeding rather than shortly before a feeding in order to minimize the amount the infant receives. Mothers with alcoholism who consume large quantities of alcohol daily may be advised not to breastfeed.

As discussed in Chapter 27 ∞, most medications pass into the breast milk. Women should consult their primary care provider or other practitioner before taking over-the-counter medications, prescription medications, or herbal supplements.

Breastfeeding and the Working Mother

The best preparation for maintaining lactation after returning to work is frequent, unlimited breastfeeding. Even when well planned, the first day back to work may be fraught with emotional and physical distress. Anticipatory guidance from the nurse may facilitate the transition from maternity leave to work. The earlier the breastfeeding mother returns to work, the more often she will need to pump her breasts to express the breast milk. Because milk production follows the principle of supply and demand, if breasts are not pumped, the milk supply will decrease.

An electric breast pump and double collection system are considered the optimal means of milk expression. However, this is not the only method; mechanical means may not suit some women. Sometimes a mother has a flexible schedule and can return home or have the baby brought to her to nurse at lunch time. If this is not possible, the infant may be fed expressed milk via bottle or spoon. (For proper storage of breast milk, see Bottle-Feeding Breast Milk in Chapter 27 ∞.) If the baby is 3 months or older, cup feeding is an option. The mother should wait until lactation is well established before introducing the bottle. Most babies adjust to the bottle within 7 to 10 days.

To maintain a milk supply, the working mother must pay special attention to her fluid intake. She can ensure adequate intake by drinking extra fluid at each break and when possible during the day. It is also helpful to nurse more on weekends, nurse during the night, eat a nutritionally sound diet, and continue manual expression or pumping when not nursing.

Night nursing presents a dilemma: It may help a working mother maintain her milk supply, but it may also contribute to fatigue. Some women choose to have the infant sleep nearby so that breastfeeding is more easily accomplished; other women find it difficult to sleep soundly when the infant is in close proximity. For the mother who works long hours or has a rigid work schedule, the best alternative may be to limit breastfeeding to morning and evening feedings, with supplemental feedings at other times. This choice allows her to maintain a close relationship with the infant and provides some of the unique benefits of breast milk.

Weaning

The decision to wean the baby from the breast may be made for a variety of reasons, including family or cultural pressures, changes in the home situation, pressure from the woman's partner, or a personal opinion about when weaning should occur. Some infants wean themselves spontaneously, despite the wishes of the mother. For the woman who is comfortable with breastfeeding and well informed about the process, the appropriate time to wean her infant will become evident if she is sensitive to the child's cues. Often weaning falls between periods of great developmental activity for the child. Thus weaning commonly occurs at 8 to 9 months, 12 to 14 months, 18 months, 2 years, and 3 years of age. The infant who is weaned before 12 months should be given iron-fortified infant formula, not cow's milk. The ACOG recommends breastfeeding for a duration of at least 6 months, longer if feasible (American College of Obstetricians and Gynecologists, 2007).

If weaning is timed to respond to the child's cues, and if the mother is comfortable with the timing, it can be accomplished with less difficulty than if the process begins before mother and child are ready emotionally. Nevertheless, weaning is a time of emotional separation for mother and baby; it may be difficult for them to give up the closeness of their nursing sessions. The nurse who is understanding about this possibility can help the mother see that her infant is growing up and plan other comforting, consoling, and play activities to replace breastfeeding. A gradual approach is the easiest and most comforting way to wean the child from breastfeedings.

During weaning, the mother should substitute one cup feeding or bottle feeding for one breastfeeding session over a few days to a week so that her breasts gradually produce less milk. Eliminating the breastfeedings associated with meals first facilitates the mother's ability to wean the infant, because satiation with food lessens the desire for milk. Over a period of several weeks she can substitute more cup feedings or bottle feedings for breastfeedings. The slow method of weaning prevents breast engorgement, allows infants to alter their eating methods at their own rates, and provides time for psychologic adjustment.

TEACHING TIP

Infants with special needs sometimes benefit from a longer duration of breastfeeding. Infants who are prone to allergies, gastrointestinal reflux, or impaired motility of the gastrointestinal tract may receive benefits from continued breastfeeding that the mother may be unaware of. These women should be counseled to discuss weaning with the pediatrician or infant specialist before weaning because the benefits of breastfeeding may influence the woman's choice of timing regarding weaning.

Other Types of Follow-Up Care

Other types of follow-up care may include return home visits, telephone follow-up, and postpartal classes and support groups.

Return Visits

If the mother, family, and physician/CNM have chosen discharge earlier than 48 hours after vaginal birth, in some states, the mother may request a total of three home visits. In such cases the nurse would schedule the first visit about 24 hours after discharge and then space out the other two visits over the next week. In other instances the nurse may schedule additional home visits based on the findings of the first home visit and the follow-up phone call.

Telephone Follow-Up

Telephone follow-up is offered to families before discharge, and a mutually agreed upon time is set for the call. Typically the call is made within 3 days after discharge or earlier if desired, lasts about 20 minutes, and is goal directed. To perform effective telephone assessment, the nurse must be able to listen skillfully, ask open-ended questions, and project an attitude of caring. If the assessment reveals any signs of a postpartum complication, the nurse refers the woman to her healthcare provider for further evaluation. The plan of care developed and implemented during a telephone conversation is limited to supportive counseling, teaching, and referral.

It is also fairly common for a home care nurse to make a telephone follow-up call to a family a few days after a home visit to provide additional information, address questions or areas of confusion, and make referrals if indicated. The mother may have multiple questions, and is generally at a high level of learning readiness. Some women may prefer a telephone-based follow-up because it requires less preparation and time than a home visit.

In addition to these scheduled follow-up telephone calls, nurses in birthing, newborn, and postpartum units, as well as clinic nurses, often receive phone calls from postpartal families seeking advice or care. These calls must be triaged immediately. Calls with urgent or life-threatening implications should be referred appropriately, either by initiating an immediate call to the practitioner or, in rare circumstances, calling 911.

Finally, many communities have established 24-hour help lines for new parents to call when they have questions or need support. In areas where help lines are not available, parents may be directed to call the birthing center. In either case, the nurse provides the number so that it is readily accessible for the family.

Postpartal Classes and Support Groups

Postpartal classes are becoming more common as caregivers recognize the continuing needs of the childbearing family. In many instances, classes are prepared to meet the specific needs of a variety of families so that, for example, single mothers and adolescent mothers can attend class with peers. A series of structured classes may focus on topics such as parenting, postpartal exercise, or nutrition, or there may be loosely structured group sessions that address mothers' concerns as they arise. Such classes offer chances for the new mother to socialize, share her concerns, and receive encouragement. Because baby-sitting arrangements may be difficult or expensive, it is desirable to provide child care for newborns and siblings; in some instances infants may remain with mothers in the class.

Many communities offer support groups through birthing centers, hospitals, or other facilities. La Leche League, an excellent support group for breastfeeding mothers, typically meets monthly and is open to all pregnant and breastfeeding mothers of infants and toddlers. Women who have children with special needs may need additional support. Referring them to peer counselors or support groups is an effective way to help them find both support and information. Once again, such groups provide an opportunity for parents to share information, advice, and experiences.

Many parents today look to the Internet for information on parenting and newborn care. Nurses have an opportunity to assist parents in evaluating the reliability of the information they find. Criteria that suggest that Internet information is reliable and of high quality include affiliation with a university medical or nursing school or a government agency; inclusion of authors' credentials, education, board certification, and affiliations; referencing of information; currency of information; similarity of information when compared with other sources; and easy accessibility.

CULTURAL PERSPECTIVES

In some cultures, extended family members such as grandmothers and aunts play a major role in the care of the postpartal woman and her family. Sometimes, these family members take full responsibility for running the household throughout the postpartum period. In other families, they concentrate entirely on the mother's or newborn's care. When culturally appropriate, include these extended family members in postpartum education sessions.

CHAPTER HIGHLIGHTS

- The Newborns' and Mothers' Health Protection Act provides for a guaranteed minimum stay of up to 48 hours following an uncomplicated vaginal birth and 96 hours following an uncomplicated cesarean birth. For women discharged earlier than the mandated time, more than half of all U.S. states require coverage for home care follow-up.

- The overall goal of postpartal home visits is to enhance opportunities for smooth transition of the new family. The home visit provides opportunities for assessment, teaching, and fostering a caring relationship with new families.

- Nurses need to act proactively to maintain their safety when making home visits by exercising reasonable caution and remaining alert to environmental cues.

- Teaching goals during home visits include reinforcement of daily newborn care, discussion of temperature assessment and maintenance of a neutral thermal environment, promotion of adequate hydration and nutrition, prevention of complications, promotion of safe and appropriate newborn sleeping, encouragement of newborn screenings and immunizations, and enhancement of family attachment and confidence in newborn care.

- The physician or pediatric nurse practitioner should be notified if there is evidence of redness around the umbilicus, bright-red bleeding or puslike drainage near the cord stump, or if the umbilicus remains unhealed.

- A primary risk factor for sudden infant death syndrome is sleeping in the prone position and smoking within the household. Cosleeping is also a risk factor for SIDS.

- Screening for galactosemia, hemocystinuria, hypothyroidism, phenylketonuria, and sickle cell anemia is done on all newborns in the first 1 to 3 days, with a second blood specimen drawn after 7 to 14 days.

- The primary focus of the maternal assessment includes a physical and psychologic assessment and identification of teaching needs for the new mother.

- To prevent nipple soreness, cracked nipples, engorgement, and plugged ducts, the nurse can encourage the breastfeeding mother to nurse frequently, to change the infant's position regularly, and to allow her nipples to air dry after breastfeeding.

- Return visits, telephone follow-up, classes, and support groups can provide valuable information and support to new mothers and their families.

EXPLORE 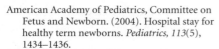 PEARSON

MyNursingKit is your one stop for online chapter review materials and resources. Prepare for success with additional NCLEX®-style practice questions, interactive assignments and activities, web links, animations and videos, and more!

Register your access code from the front of your book at
www.mynursingkit.com

CHAPTER REFERENCES

American Academy of Pediatrics, Committee on Fetus and Newborn. (2004). Hospital stay for healthy term newborns. *Pediatrics, 113*(5), 1434–1436.

American Academy of Pediatrics. (2005, November). Policy statement: The changing concept of sudden infant death syndrome: Diagnostic coding shifts, controversies regarding the sleeping environment, and new variables to consider in reducing risk. *Pediatrics, 116*(5), 1245–1255.

American Academy of Pediatrics (AAP), Committee on Fetus and Newborn & American College of Obstetricians and Gynecologists (ACOG) Committee on Obstetrics. (2007). *Guidelines for perinatal care* (6th ed.). Evanston, IL: Author.

American College of Obstetricians and Gynecologists. (2007). *Breastfeeding: Maternal and infant aspects* (ACOG Committee Opinion, No. 361). Washington, DC: Author.

Association of Women's Health, Obstetrical, and Neonatal Nurses (AWHONN). (2006). *The compendium of postpartum care.* Washington, DC: AWHONN.

Burgos, A. E., Schmitt, S. K., Stevenson, D. K., & Phibbs, C. S. (2008). Readmission for neonatal jaundice in California, 1991–2000: Trends and implications. *Pediatrics, 121*(4), e864–e869.

de Almeida, M. F. B., & Draque, C. M. (2007). Neonatal jaundice and breastfeeding. *Neonatal Reviews, 8*(7), e282. Retrieved May 8, 2008, from http://neoreviews.aappublications.org/cgi/content/short/8/7/e282

Engle, W. A., Tomashek, K. M., Wallman, C., & the Committee on Fetus & Newborn. (2007). Late preterm infants: A population at risk. *Pediatrics, 120*(6), 1390–1401.

Goulet, L., D'Amour, D., & Pineault, R. (2007). Type and timing of services following postnatal discharge: Do they make a difference? *Women's Health, 45*(4), 19–39.

Jevitt, C., Hernandez, I., & Groër, M. (2007). Lactation complicated by overweight and obesity: Supporting the mother and newborn. *Journal of Midwifery & Women's Health, 52*(6), 606–613.

Lawrence, R. A., & Lawrence, R. M. (2005). *Breastfeeding: A guide for the medical profession.* Philadelphia: Elsevier Mosby.

Locke, R. O., Paul, D., & DiMatteo, D. (2006). Breastfeeding continuation factors in a cohort of Delaware mothers. *Delaware Medical Journal, 78*(8), 295–300.

McPhaul, K. M., Rosen, J., Bobb, S., Okechukwu, C., Geiger-Brown, J., Kauffman, K., Johnson, J. V., & Lipscomb, J. (2007). An exploratory study of mandated safety measures for home visiting case managers. *Canadian Journal of Nursing Research, 39*(4), 173–189.

Melli, M. S., Rashidi, M. R., Nokhoodchi, A., Tagavi, S., Farzadi, L., Sadaghat, K., Tahmasebi, Z., & Sheshvan, M. K. (2007). A randomized trial of peppermint gel, lanolin ointment, and placebo gel to prevent nipple crack in primiparous breastfeeding women. *Medical Science Monitor, 13*(9), CR406–CR411.

Morland-Schultz, K., & Hill, P. D. (2005). Prevention of and therapies for nipple pain: A systematic review. *Journal of Obstetric, Gynecologic, & Neonatal Nursing, 34*(4), 428–437.

National Center for Hearing Assessment & Management (NCHAM). (2007). *State summary statistics: Universal newborn hearing screen.* Logan, UT: Source.

National Institute of Child Health & Human Development. (2006). Tummy time. Retrieved on May 8, 2008, at http://www.nichd.nih.gov/health/topics/tummy_time.cfm

O'Keffe, K. (2005). Expanded AAP breastfeeding policy calls for support of nursing moms. *AAP News, 26*, 1–10.

Paul, I. M., Lehman, E. B., Hollenback, C. S., & Maisels, M. J. (2006). Preventable newborn readmissions since passage of the Newborns' and Mothers' Health Protection Act. *Pediatrics, 118*(6), 2349–2358.

Pusnik, I., & Drnovsek, J. (2005). Infrared ear thermometers—parameters influencing their reading and accuracy. *Physiological Measurement, 26*(6), 1075–1084.

Spector, R. E. (2009). Cultural diversity in health and illness (7th ed.). Upper Saddle River, NJ: Pearson Prentice Hall.

van Vlimmeren, L. A., van der Graaf, Y., Boere-Boonekamp, M. M., L'Hoir, M. P., Helders, P. J., & Engelbert, R. H. (2007). Risk factors for deformational plagiocephaly at birth and at 7 weeks of age: A prospective cohort study. *Pediatrics, 119*(2), e408–e418.

Walker, M. (2007). International breastfeeding initiatives and their relevance to the current state of breastfeeding in the United States. *Journal of Nurse Midwifery & Women's Health, 52*(6), 549–555.

CHAPTER 33

The Postpartal Family at Risk

With hospital stays lasting only a couple of days, postpartum problems often develop after the family goes home. Fortunately, in my community, families receive a minimum of two postpartum visits, and more if a specific problem is identified. Whenever I encounter a family needing re-admission or referral, I wonder about the new moms, dads, and babies that don't have this type of follow-up care. It is so needed.

—Home Care/Postpartum Nurse

LEARNING OUTCOMES

33-1. Examine the nurse's impact in both the hospital and community-based settings in assessing predisposing factors of postpartum complications, implementing preventive care, and teaching for self-help.

33-2. Explain the causes, contributing factors, signs and symptoms, and clinical therapy of early postpartal hemorrhage, as well as the causes and treatment of late postpartal hemorrhage, in determining the hospital and community-based nursing care management of the woman with hemorrhage during the postpartal period.

33-3. Explain the causes, signs and symptoms, and clinical therapy in determining the hospital and community-based nursing care management of the woman with a reproductive tract infection or wound infection during the postpartal period.

33-4. Explain the causes, signs and symptoms, and clinical therapy in determining the hospital and community-based nursing management of the woman with a urinary tract infection during the postpartal period.

33-5. Explain the causes, contributing factors, signs and symptoms, and clinical therapy in determining the hospital and community-based nursing management of the woman with mastitis during the postpartal period.

33-6. Explain the causes, contributing factors, preventive measures, signs and symptoms, and clinical therapy in determining the hospital and community-based nursing management of the woman with thrombolytic disease during the postpartal period.

33-7. Explain the incidence, risk factors, signs and symptoms, use of screening tools, and clinical therapy in determining the hospital and community-based nursing management of the woman with postpartal psychiatric disorder.

33-8. Evaluate the woman's knowledge of self-care measures, signs of complications to be reported to the primary care provider, and measures to prevent recurrence of complications.

KEY TERMS

The postpartal period is typically viewed as a smooth, uneventful transition time—and often it is, even with the challenges of new parenthood and the integration of a new person into the family. However, it is equally important for the nurse to be aware of physical or emotional complications that may develop postpartally. The nurse should teach the family the signs of postpartal complications, findings to report to the physician or certified nurse-midwife (CNM), and preventive measures, if available.

Written instructions to supplement any discussion will be of great value in the early weeks at home with a newborn, when life can be chaotic and instructions may be forgotten. The family should have telephone numbers for postpartum follow-up services and other resources to answer questions. By communicating an attitude of willingness to answer questions and listen to concerns, the nurse enhances the parents' comfort in making calls later for what they might otherwise perceive as issues "too trivial to bother someone about."

When a telephone follow-up or an examination at the home visit provides evidence of a developing complication, the nurse shares these findings or impressions with the woman, and they mutually plan an appropriate next step. In the case of telephone follow-up, the nurse usually counsels the women to notify her physician or certified nurse-midwife, being prepared to schedule an appointment immediately if risk assessment indicates. The nurse who identifies a complication at the home visit will need to communicate the clinical findings to the certified nurse-midwife or physician and document them, as well as any interventions, for the permanent record. (See Chapter 32 ∞ for a more detailed discussion of home care for the postpartal family.)

Complications, by their very nature, suggest the need for immediate collaborative management and are inherently stressful. Postpartum complications sometimes necessitate readmission of the postpartum client to the hospital, thereby disrupting the family and adding concerns not only about her health but the way in which infant care will be managed. The most common complications of the postpartal period are hemorrhage, infection, thromboembolic disease, and postpartal psychiatric disorders. This chapter will focus on these issues.

Care of the Woman with Postpartal Hemorrhage

Hemorrhage in the postpartum period is described as either early (immediate or primary) or late (delayed or secondary). **Early (primary) postpartal hemorrhage** occurs in the first 24 hours after childbirth. **Late (secondary) postpartal hemorrhage** occurs from 24 hours to 6 weeks after birth. Postpartal hemorrhage continues to be a cause of significant maternal mortality and morbidity and accounts for approximately one-sixth of all maternal deaths attributed to pregnancy-related hemorrhage in the United States (Poggi, 2007).

The traditional definition of postpartal hemorrhage has been a blood loss of greater than 500 mL following childbirth. That definition is currently being questioned, however, because careful quantification indicates that the average blood loss in a vaginal birth is actually greater than 500 mL, the average blood loss after a cesarean childbirth exceeds 1000 mL, and the average blood loss is more than 1500 mL during repeat cesarean birth (James, 2008; Poggi, 2007). Clinical estimates of blood loss tend to underestimate actual loss by up to 50%. Some clinicians believe that postpartal hemorrhage can be objectively and reliably defined as a decrease in the hematocrit of 10% between the time of admission and the postbirth period. However, clinical estimation of blood loss at childbirth is difficult because blood mixes with amniotic fluid and is obscured as it oozes onto sterile drapes or is sponged away. Without vigilant watching, it may be difficult for the nurse to appreciate the significance of slow, steady blood loss over the next few hours. As the amount of blood loss increases, as in the case of hemorrhage, estimates are likely to be even less accurate. Moreover, postpartal hemorrhage may occur intra-abdominally, into the broad ligament, or into hematomas arising from genital tract trauma, wherein the blood loss is concealed. Given the increased blood volume of pregnancy, the clinical signs of hemorrhage—such as increasing pulse, decreased blood pressure, and decreasing urinary output—do not appear until as much as 1000 to 2000 mL has been lost, shortly before the woman becomes hemodynamically unstable (James, 2008).

Early (Primary) Postpartal Hemorrhage

At term, blood volume and cardiac output have increased so that 20% of cardiac output, or 600 mL per minute, perfuses the pregnant uterus, supporting the developing fetus. When the placenta separates from the uterine wall, the many uterine vessels that have carried blood to and from the placenta are severed abruptly. The normal mechanism for hemostasis after delivery of the placenta is contraction of the interlacing uterine muscles to occlude the open sinuses that previously brought blood into the placenta. Absence of prompt and sustained uterine contractions (uterine atony) can result in significant blood loss. Other causes of postpartal hemorrhage include laceration of the genital tract; episiotomy; retained placental fragments; vulvar, vaginal, or subperitoneal hematomas; uterine inversion; uterine rupture; problems of placental implantation; and coagulation disorders.

Uterine Atony

Uterine atony (relaxation of the uterus) is a common cause of early postpartal hemorrhage (Cunningham et al., 2005). As many as 1 in 20 new mothers will experience some degree of uterine atony. Although uterine atony can occur after any childbirth, its contributing factors include the following:

- Overdistention of the uterus caused by multiple gestation, hydramnios, or a large infant (macrosomia)
- Dysfunctional or prolonged labor, which indicates that the uterus is contracting abnormally
- Oxytocin augmentation or induction of labor
- Grand multiparity, because stretched uterine musculature contracts less vigorously
- Use of anesthesia (especially halothane) or other drugs, such as magnesium sulfate, calcium channel blockers such as nifedipine, or tocolytics like terbutaline (Brethine), any of which cause the uterus to relax
- Prolonged third stage of labor—more than 30 minutes
- Preeclampsia
- Asian or Hispanic heritage
- Operative birth (includes vacuum extraction or forceps-assisted births)
- Retained placental fragments
- Placenta previa

Hemorrhage from uterine atony may be slow and steady rather than sudden and massive. The blood may escape the vagina or collect in the uterus, evident as large clots. The uterine cavity may distend with up to 1000 mL or more blood although the perineal pad and linen protectors remain suspiciously dry. A treacherous feature of postpartal hemorrhage is that maternal vital signs may not change until significant blood loss has occurred because of the increased blood volume associated with pregnancy. The woman with preeclampsia is an exception to this finding because she does not have the normal hypervolemia of pregnancy and cannot tolerate even normal postchildbirth blood loss (Cunningham et al., 2005).

Ideally, postpartal hemorrhage is prevented, beginning with adequate prenatal care, good nutrition, avoidance of traumatic procedures, risk assessment, early recognition, and management of complications as they arise. Any woman at risk should be typed and crossmatched for blood and have intravenous (IV) lines in place with needles suitable for blood transfusion (18-gauge minimum). Excellent labor management and childbirth techniques are imperative.

After expulsion of the placenta, the fundus is palpated to ensure that it is firmly contracted. If it is not firm (if it is boggy), fundal massage is performed until the uterus contracts. Fundal massage is painful for the woman who has not received regional anesthesia; consequently, she will need explanation for why this procedure is necessary, and give verbal support as massage is initiated. If bleeding is excessive, the clinician will likely order intravenous (IV) oxytocin at a rapid infusion rate and may elect to do a bimanual massage (Figure 33–1A ■). Table 33–1 summarizes critical nursing information about the use of uterine stimulants. The need for intravenous fluid replacement and blood transfusion is determined on the basis of hemoglobin and hematocrit results as well as coagulation studies.

Conservative management includes uterine stimulants to contract the atonic musculature. Oxytocin, ergotamine, and prostaglandin are most often used. Misoprostol, best known to the obstetric community for its use in labor induction, is being used to prevent and treat uterine atony after failed attempts to control bleeding with oxytocics. Misoprostol used rectally is absorbed quickly and causes uterine contraction within minutes (Rebarker & Roman, 2003). When conservative measures do not successfully control bleeding, surgical intervention is required. In order of increasing invasiveness, surgical procedures include uterine balloon tamponade, selective radiographic-guided pelvic arterial embolization, uterine suturing techniques, ligation of the uterine or hypogastric arteries, and, as a last resort, hysterectomy, which clearly ends childbearing (AAP & ACOG, 2007; Poggi, 2007).

Uterine packing, common in the past for cases of postpartal hemorrhage, has been used less often out of concerns of concealed hemorrhage and uterine overdistention that might actually increase bleeding. Instead, physicians in many clinical settings are resorting to uterine balloon

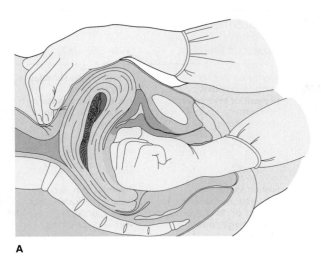

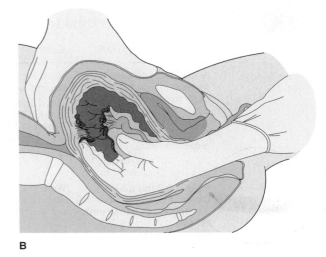

A **B**

FIGURE 33–1 *A,* Manual compression of the uterus and massage with the abdominal hand usually will effectively control hemorrhage from uterine atony. *B,* Manual removal of placenta. The fingers are alternately abducted, adducted, and advanced until the placenta is completely detached. Both procedures are performed only by the medical clinician.
Source: Adapted from Cunningham, F. G., MacDonald, P. C., & Gant, N. F. (Eds.). (1989). *Williams obstetrics* (18th ed., pp. 417–418). Norwalk, CT: Appleton & Lange.

tamponade, using large Foley catheters or Sengstaken-Blakemore tubes to control bleeding. Both of these tubes have open tops, which permit any continuous drainage from the uterus to be visualized even as pressure tamponade is effectively controlling bleeding.

Lacerations of the Genital Tract

Early postpartum hemorrhage is associated with lacerations of the perineum, vagina, or cervix. Several factors predispose women to higher risk of reproductive tract lacerations:

- Nulliparity
- Epidural anesthesia
- Precipitous childbirth (less than 3 hours)
- Forceps- or vacuum-assisted birth
- Macrosomia
  - Use of oxytocin

Thorough inspection of the genital tract by the birth attendant facilitates recognition and timely repair of most lacerations. Genital tract lacerations should be suspected when vaginal bleeding persists in the presence of a firmly contracted uterus. The nurse who suspects a laceration should notify the clinician so that the laceration can be immediately sutured to control the hemorrhage and restore the integrity of the reproductive tract (AAP & ACOG, 2007).

Episiotomy is an often underappreciated source of postpartal blood loss because of slow, steady bleeding. The risk for bleeding is increased with mediolateral episiotomies. (See discussion in Chapter 23 ∞.) Postpartal nurses are wise to appreciate that most deaths from postpartal hemorrhage are not caused by catastrophic bleeding episodes but by ineffective management of slow, steady blood loss.

Retained Placental Fragments

Retained placental fragments may be a cause of early postpartal hemorrhage and are also the most common cause of late hemorrhage. Retention of fragments is usually attributable to partial separation of the placenta during massage of the fundus before spontaneous placental separation. Therefore, this practice should be avoided.

Following birth, the placenta should always be inspected for intactness and for evidence of missing fragments or cotyledons on the maternal side and for vessels that transverse to the edge of the placenta outward along the membranes of the fetal side, which may indicate succenturiate placenta and a retained lobe. Uterine exploration may be required to remove missing fragments. This cause should be immediately suspected if bleeding persists and no lacerations are noted (Figure 33–1B). Sonography may be used to diagnose retained placental fragments. Curettage, formerly standard treatment, is now thought by some to traumatize the implantation site, thereby increasing bleeding and the potential for uterine adhesions. However, it may be necessitated by the degree of hemorrhage (Cunningham et al., 2005).

Vulvar, Vaginal, and Pelvic Hematomas

Hematomas occur as a result of injury to a blood vessel from birth trauma, often without noticeable trauma to the superficial tissue, or from inadequate hemostasis at the site of repair of an incision or laceration. The soft tissue in the area offers no resistance, and hematomas containing 250 to 500 mL of blood may develop rapidly. Signs and symptoms vary somewhat with the type of hematoma. Hematomas may be vulvar (involving branches of the pudendal artery),

TABLE 33–1 Uterine Stimulants Used to Prevent and Manage Uterine Atony

Drug	Dosing Information	Contraindications	Expected Effects	Side Effects
Oxytocin (Pitocin, Syntocinon)	IV use: 10 to 40 units in 500 to 1000 mL crystalloid fluid at 50 milliunits/min administration rate. Onset: immediate. Duration: 1 h. *IV bolus administration not recommended.* IM use: 10 units. Onset: 3 to 5 min. Duration: 2 to 3 h.	None for use in postpartum hemorrhage. Avoid undiluted rapid IV infusion which causes hypotension.	Rhythmic uterine contractions that help to prevent or reverse postpartal hemorrhage caused by uterine atony.	Uterine hyperstimulation, mild transient hypertension, water intoxication rare in postpartum use.
Methylergonovine maleate (Methergine)	IM use: 0.2 mg q2–4h. Onset: 2 to 5 min. Duration: 3 h (for 5 dose maximum). PO use: 0.2 mg q6–12h. Onset: 7 to 15 min. Duration: 3 h (for 1 week). *IV administration not recommended.*	Women with labile or high blood pressure, known sensitivity to drug, or cardiac disease.	Sustained uterine contractions that help to prevent or reverse postpartal hemorrhage caused by uterine atony; management of postpartal subinvolution.	Hypertension, dizziness, headache, flushing/hot flashes, tinnitus, nausea and vomiting, palpitations, chest pain. Overdose or hypersensitivity is recognized by seizures; tingling and numbness of fingers and toes from vasoconstrictive effect, leading rarely to gangrene; hypertension; weak pulse; chest pain.
Ergonovine maleate (Ergotrate Maleate)	IM use: 0.2 mg q2–4h. Onset: 7 min. Duration: 3 h (5 dose maximum). PO use: 0.2 mg q6–12h. Onset: 15 min. Duration: 3 h (for 2–7 days). *IV administration not recommended.*	Women with labile or high blood pressure or known sensitivity to drug.	Sustained uterine contractions that help to prevent or reverse postpartal hemorrhage caused by uterine atony; management of postpartal subinvolution.	Hypertension, dizziness, headache, nausea and vomiting, chest pain. Hypersensitivity is noted by systemic vasoconstrictive effects: seizure, chest pain, and tingling and numbness of fingers and toes that leads rarely to gangrene.
Prostaglandin (PGF$_{2\alpha}$ carboprost tromethamine [Hemabate], Prostin/15M)	IM use: 0.25 mg q15 to 90 minutes, repeated up to maximum 8 doses. Physician may elect to administer by direct intramyometrial injection.	Women with active cardiovascular, renal, liver disease, or asthma or with known hypersensitivity to drug.	Control of refractory cases of postpartal hemorrhage caused by uterine atony; generally used after failed attempts at control of hemorrhage with oxytocic agents.	Nausea, vomiting, diarrhea, headache, flushing, bradycardia, bronchospasm, wheezing, cough, chills, fever.
Misoprostol (Cytotec)	800 to 1000 microgram rectally.	History of allergies to prostaglandins.	Used to prevent and treat uterine atony after failed attempts to control bleeding with oxytocics.	Diarrhea, abdominal pain, headache.
Dinoprostone (Prostin E$_2$)	Suppository (vaginally or rectally) 20 microgram every 2 hours. Store frozen—must be thawed to room temperature.	Avoid if woman is hypotensive, or has asthma or acute inflammatory disease.	Stimulate uterine contractions.	Fever is common and occurs within 15 to 45 min of insertion; bleeding, abdominal cramps, N/V.

Implications for Nursing Management of the Postpartal Woman Receiving Uterine Stimulants

- Assess fundus for evidence of contraction and amount of uterine bleeding at least q10–15min × 1–2 h after administration, then q30–60 min until stable. *More frequent assessments are determined by the woman's condition or by orders of the physician/CNM.*
- Assess blood loss by hematocrit and hemoglobin levels.
- Monitor pulse and blood pressure q15min for at least 1 h after administration, then q30–60min until stable.
  - Apply pulse oximeter and administer oxygen according to agency protocol.
  - Weigh peripads or Chux dressing.
- Note expected duration of action of drug being administered, and take care to recheck fundus at that time.
- When the drug is ineffective, the fundus remains atonic (boggy or uncontracted), and bleeding continues, massage the fundus. If massage fails to cause sustained contraction, notify the physician/CNM immediately.
- Monitor woman for signs of known side effects of the drug; report to physician/CNM if side effects occur.

- Continuous EKG monitoring may be indicated for hypotension, continuous bleeding, tachycardia, or shock.
- Elevate the legs to a 20- to 30-degree angle to increase venous return.
- Remind the woman and her support person that uterine cramping is an expected result of these drugs and that medication is available for discomfort. Administer analgesic medications as needed for pain relief. Provide nonpharmacologic comfort measures. If analgesic medication ordered is insufficient for pain relief, notify the physician/CNM.

When Prostaglandin Is Used

- Check temperature q1–2h and/or after chill. Administer antipyretic medication as ordered for prostaglandin-induced fever.
- Auscultate breath sounds frequently for signs of adverse respiratory effects.
- Assess for nausea, vomiting, and diarrhea. Administer antiemetic and antidiarrheal medications as ordered. (In some settings, women are premedicated with these drugs.)

vaginal (especially in the area of the ischial spines), vulvovaginal, or subperitoneal. The latter are rare; however, they are the most dangerous because of the large amount of blood loss that can occur without clinical symptoms until the woman becomes hemodynamically unstable. Subperitoneal hematomas involve the uterine artery branches or vessels in the broad ligaments.

Risk factors for hematomas include preeclampsia, use of pudendal anesthesia, first full-term birth, precipitous labor, prolonged second stage of labor, macrosomia, forceps- or vacuum-assisted births, and history of vulvar varicosities. Hematomas less than 5 cm (2 in.) in size and nonexpanding are managed expectantly with ice packs and analgesia. They usually resolve over several days. For larger hematomas and those that expand, surgical management is usually required; the hematoma is evacuated, the bleeding vessel ligated, and the wound closed, with or without vaginal packing. An indwelling urinary catheter may be necessary because voiding may be impossible with packing in place.

The hematoma site is an ideal medium for the growth of flora normally present in the genital tract. Consequently, broad-spectrum antibiotics are usually ordered to prevent infection or abscess.

The nurse can decrease the risk of vulvar or vaginal hematoma by applying an ice pack to the woman's perineum during the first hour after birth and intermittently for the next 8 to 12 hours. If a small hematoma develops despite preventive measures, a sitz bath after the first 12 hours will aid fluid absorption once bleeding has stopped and will promote comfort, as will the judicious use of analgesic agents.

Uterine Inversion

Uterine inversion—a prolapse of the fundus to or through the cervix so that the uterus is, in effect, turned inside out after birth—is a rare but life threatening cause of postpartal hemorrhage. Although not always preventable, uterine inversion is often associated with factors such as: fundal implantation or abnormal adherence of the placenta, protracted labor, weakness of the uterine musculature, uterine relaxation secondary to anesthesia or drugs such as magnesium sulfate, and excess traction on the umbilical cord or vigorous manual removal of the placenta. Most cases of uterine inversion are managed by immediate repositioning of the uterus within the pelvis by the physician.

Late (Secondary) Postpartal Hemorrhage

Although early postpartal hemorrhage usually occurs within hours after birth, delayed hemorrhage generally occurs within 1 to 2 weeks after childbirth, most frequently as a result of **subinvolution** (failure to return to normal size) of the placental site or retention of placental fragments. Blood loss at this time may be excessive but rarely poses the same risk as that from immediate postpartal hemorrhage. Late postpartum hemorrhage is much less common but can be extremely stressful for the woman and her family who are at home by this time.

The site of placental implantation is always the last area of the uterus to regenerate after childbirth. In the case of subinvolution, adjacent endometrium and the decidua basalis fail to regenerate to cover the placental site. Deficiency of immunologic factors has been implicated as a cause. Faulty implantation in the less vascular lower uterine segment, retention of placental tissue, or infection may contribute to subinvolution. With subinvolution, the postpartum fundal height is greater than expected. In addition, lochia flow often fails to progress from rubra to serosa to alba normally. Lochia rubra that persists longer than 2 weeks postpartum is highly suggestive of subinvolution (Poggi, 2007). Some women report scant brown lochia or irregular heavy bleeding. Leukorrhea, backache, and foul lochia may occur if infection is a cause. There may be a history of heavy early postpartal bleeding or difficulty with expulsion of the placenta. When portions of the placenta have been retained in the uterus, bleeding continues because normal uterine contractions that constrict the bleeding site are prohibited. Presence of placental tissue within the uterus can be confirmed by pelvic ultrasound.

Subinvolution is most commonly diagnosed during the routine postpartal examination at 4 to 6 weeks. The woman may relate a history of irregular or excessive bleeding or describe the symptoms listed previously. An enlarged, softer-than-normal uterus palpated bimanually is an objective indication of subinvolution. Treatment includes oral administration of methylergonovine maleate 0.2 mg orally every 3 to 4 hours for 24 to 48 hours (see Drug Guide: Methylergonovine Maleate [Methergine] in Chapter 31 ∞). When uterine infection is present, antibiotics are also administered. The woman is reevaluated in 2 weeks. If retained placenta is suspected or other treatment is ineffective, curettage may be indicated (Poggi, 2007).

Nursing Care Management

Nursing Assessment and Diagnosis

Careful and ongoing assessment of the woman during labor and birth and evaluation of her prenatal history will help identify factors that put her at risk for postpartal hemorrhage. Following birth, periodic assessment for evidence of vaginal bleeding is a major nursing responsibility. Regular and frequent assessment of fundal height and evidence of uterine tone or contractility will alert the nurse to the possible development or recurrence of hemorrhage.

The nurse observes and documents vaginal bleeding to determine whether further medical intervention is needed. This assessment can be done visually, by pad counts, or by weighing the perineal pads. In cases of excessive bleeding, nurses should be alert for signs of impending hypovolemic shock and the development of coagulation problems, such as DIC.

When regional anesthesia is used, frequent assessment of the woman's perineum is important. Once the effects of anesthesia have subsided, vaginal and vulvar hematomas are generally associated with perineal pain. The pain is often intense, out of proportion or excessive, and usually from the woman's "stitches." If the hematoma is localized in the posterior vaginal area, rectal pressure may also be a presenting complaint. Hematomas that develop in the upper vagina may cause difficulty voiding because of pressure against the urinary meatus or urethra. Rather than automatically attributing complaints of perineal pain to the presence of an episiotomy, the nurse should examine the perineal area for signs of hematomas: ecchymosis; edema; tenseness of tissue overlying the hematomas; fluctuant, bulging mass at the introitus; and extreme tenderness to palpation. Estimating the size of the hematoma on first assessment of the perineum enables the nurse to better identify increases in size and the potential blood loss. The nurse notifies the physician/CNM if a hematoma is suspected.

Nursing diagnoses that may apply to a woman experiencing postpartal hemorrhage include the following:

- *Deficient Fluid Volume* related to blood loss secondary to uterine atony, lacerations, or retained placental fragments
- *Health-Seeking Behaviors* related to lack of information about signs of delayed postpartal hemorrhage

Nursing Plan and Implementation

Hospital-Based Nursing Care

If the nurse detects a soft, boggy uterus, it is massaged until firm. If the uterus is not contracting well and appears larger than anticipated, the nurse may express clots during fundal massage. Once clots are expressed, the uterus tends to contract more effectively.

If the woman seems to have a slow, steady, free flow of blood, the nurse should do pad counts and if possible begin to weigh the perineal pads (1 mL = 1 g) (James, 2008). The nurse monitors the woman's vital signs every 15 minutes, or more frequently if indicated. If the fundus is displaced upward or to one side because of a full bladder, the nurse encourages the woman to empty her bladder—or catheterizes her if she is unable to void—to allow for efficient uterine contractions.

When there are risk factors for postpartal hemorrhage or frequent fundal massage has been necessary to sustain uterine contractions, the nurse maintains any vascular access (IV) started during labor and anticipates the need for a second IV in case additional fluids, meds, or blood is necessary. Sometimes physicians and CNMs write orders that specify "discontinue IV after present bottle." The astute postpartum nurse will assess the consistency of the fundus and the presence of normal versus excessive lochia before discontinuing the infusion. If the assessments are not reassuring, the nurse continues the intravenous (IV) infusion and notifies the physician or CNM.

HINTS FOR PRACTICE

As you know, bogginess indicates that the uterus is not contracting well, which results in increased uterine bleeding. This blood may remain in the uterus and form clots or may result in increased flow. In assessing the amount of blood loss, first massage the uterus until it is firm and then express clots. Do not be misled by the fact that a woman has a firm uterus. Significant bleeding can occur from causes other than uterine atony. To accurately determine the amount of blood loss, it is not sufficient to assess only the peripads. You should also ask the woman to turn on her side so you can assess underneath her for pooling of blood.

The nurse reviews postpartum hemoglobin and hematocrit values when available, compares them to the admission baseline, and notifies the physician or CNM if the hematocrit has decreased by 10 percentage points or more. In cases where there is risk of postpartal hemorrhage (i.e., women with prenatal anemia or L/D complications) and blood has been crossmatched earlier, the nurse checks that blood is available in the blood bank.

The nurse assesses the woman for signs of anemia, such as fatigue, pallor, headache, thirst, and orthostatic changes in pulse or blood pressure, and reviews the results of all hematocrit determinations. All medical interventions, intravenous infusions, blood transfusions, oxygen therapy, and medications such as uterine stimulants are monitored as necessary and evaluated for effectiveness. The nurse also monitors urinary output to determine adequacy of fluid replacement and renal perfusion and reports amounts less than 30 mL/h to the physician (James, 2008). The nurse also helps the woman plan activities so that adequate rest is possible.

The woman who is experiencing anemia and fatigue related to hemorrhage may need assistance with self-care and progressive ambulation for several days. When she is able to be out of bed to shower, use of a shower chair permits independence while providing a measure of safety in case the woman experiences weakness or dizziness. The emergency call light should be easily accessible.

The mother may find it difficult to care for her baby because of the fatigue associated with blood loss. The nurse can often find ways to promote maternal-infant attachment while accommodating the mother's health needs. The mother may require additional assistance in caring for her infant. If she has intravenous lines in place, even carrying the newborn may be awkward. For the mother who feels compelled to do as much as possible, the nurse may also need to give the mother "permission" to return her infant to the nursery so she can have adequate periods of uninterrupted rest.

If the father of the child or partner is involved in the birth experience, including that person in the plan of care is a productive strategy. This person can support the mother's recovery by helping to meet her physical needs while encouraging her to rest. The mother is likely to feel less concern over her limited opportunities for the newborn's care if she can witness the father/partner interacting with and caring for the newborn. The extent to which the father/partner becomes involved with the care of the mother and baby must be carefully balanced with the need to be rested for the extra responsibilities the support person will assume when the mother and newborn child are discharged from the hospital.

Teaching for Self-Care

The woman and her family or other support persons should receive clear, preferably written, explanations of the normal postpartum course, including changes in the lochia and fundus and signs of abnormal bleeding. Instructions for the prevention of bleeding should include fundal massage, ways to assess the fundal height and consistency, and inspection of any episiotomy and lacerations, if present. The woman should receive instruction in perineal care (see discussion on perineal care in Chapter 31 ∞). The mother and her family are advised to contact her caregiver if any of the signs of postpartal hemorrhage occur. (See Key Facts to Remember: Signs of Postpartal Hemorrhage.) If iron supplementation is ordered, instructions for proper dosage should be provided along with client teaching to enhance absorption and avoid constipation and nausea (ACOG, 2006).

Community-Based Nursing Care

For postpartal women, the usual discharge instructions include advice such as: "You take care of your baby, and let someone else care for you, the family, and the household." Because of her fatigue and weakened condition, the woman who experienced postpartal hemorrhage may be unable even to care for her newborn unassisted. The caregivers at home need clear, concise explanations of her condition and needs for recovery. For example, they should understand the woman's need to rest and to be given extra time to rest after any necessary activity.

To ensure her safety, the woman should be advised to rise slowly to minimize the likelihood of orthostatic hypotension. Until she regains strength, she should be seated when holding the newborn.

KEY FACTS TO REMEMBER

Signs of Postpartal Hemorrhage

Excessive or bright-red bleeding (saturation of more than one pad per hour)
A boggy fundus that does not respond to massage
Abnormal clots
High temperature
Any unusual pelvic discomfort or backache
Persistent bleeding in the presence of a firmly contracted uterus
Rise in the level of the fundus of the uterus
Increased pulse or decreased BP
Hematoma formation or bulging/shiny skin in the perineal area
Decreased level of consciousness

The person who assumes responsibility for grocery shopping and meal preparation needs advice about the importance of including foods high in iron in the daily menus. Having the woman indicate her preferences from a list of such foods will promote cooperation with the diet. The nurse also explains the rationale for continuing medications containing iron.

The woman should continue to count perineal pads for several days so that she can recognize any recurring problems with excessive blood loss. The debilitated condition and anemia associated with hemorrhage increase the woman's risk of puerperal infection. She and her caregivers should use good handwashing and minimize exposure to infection in the home. The nurse should give the woman's caregiver a list of the signs of infection and ensure that she or he understands the importance of alerting the physician immediately if signs occur.

A sense of emergency often accompanies late postpartal hemorrhage. Because it commonly occurs 1 to 2 weeks after birth, the couple is generally at home, involved in the day-to-day activities demanded by their new roles, when the unexpected, excessive bleeding begins. Quick decisions about childcare arrangements must often be made so that the mother can return to the hospital. Both mother and father are likely to be alarmed by the excessive bleeding and concerned about her prognosis. There may be additional worries about separation from the newborn, especially when the mother is breastfeeding. The father may find himself torn between the needs of the mother and those of the newborn. Ideally, arrangements can be made to minimize separation of the family members.

In addition to meeting the woman's physical needs, the nurse assesses the couple's coping strategies and resources for dealing with the impending crisis. Providing realistic information, offering to call those in their support network, and exploring effective coping strategies can be of immeasurable value as the family tries to maintain a sense of balance in this situation.

Evaluation

Expected outcomes of nursing care include the following:

- Signs of postpartal hemorrhage are detected quickly and managed effectively.
- Maternal-infant attachment is maintained successfully.
- The woman is able to identify abnormal changes that might occur following discharge and understands the importance of notifying her caregiver if they develop.

Care of the Woman with a Reproductive Tract Infection or Wound Infection

Puerperal infection is an infection of the reproductive tract associated with childbirth that occurs any time up to 6 weeks postpartum. The most common postpartal infection is endometritis (metritis), which is infection limited to the uterine lining. Indeed, the cause of postpartal fever is presumed to be metritis until proven otherwise. However, infection can be spread by way of the lymphatic and circulatory systems to become a progressive disease resulting in parametrial cellulitis and peritonitis. The woman's prognosis is directly related to the stage of the disease at the time of diagnosis, the causative organism, and the state of her health and immune system.

The standard definition of **puerperal morbidity**, established by the Joint Committee on Maternal Welfare, is a temperature of 38°C (100.4°F) or higher, with the temperature occurring on any 2 of the first 10 postpartum days, exclusive of the first 24 hours, and when taken by mouth by standard technique at least four times a day. However, serious infections can occur in the first 24 hours or may cause only persistent low-grade temperatures. Therefore, careful assessment of all postpartum women with elevated temperatures is essential.

The vagina and cervix of approximately 70% of all healthy pregnant women contain pathogenic bacteria that, alone or in combination, are sufficiently virulent to cause excessive infection. Although the uterus is considered a sterile cavity before rupture of the fetal membranes, bacterial contamination of amniotic fluid with membranes still intact at term is more common than previously believed and may contribute to premature labor. Following rupture of membranes and during labor, contamination of the uterine cavity by vaginal or cervical bacteria can easily occur. Other factors must also be present for infection to occur such as the change to an alkaline pH of the vagina postpartally that favors growth of aerobes. Uterine infec-

tions are relatively uncommon following uncomplicated vaginal births, but they continue to be a major source of morbidity for women who give birth by cesarean.

Routine antibiotic prophylaxis for cesarean childbirth has significantly reduced infection rates (AAP & ACOG, 2007). Antibiotic therapy alone has not caused the decrease in overall postpartal morbidity and mortality that is seen today. Aseptic technique, fewer traumatic operative births, a better understanding of labor dystocia, improved surgical intervention, and a population that is generally at less risk from malnutrition and chronic debilitative disease have also contributed to this reduction.

Postpartal Uterine Infection

Postpartal uterine infection is known variously as *metritis and endometritis*. Because the infection involves the decidual lining of the uterus, the myometrium, and parametrial tissue, some authorities are proposing the terminology metritis with parametrial cellulitis (Cunningham et al., 2005). Risk factors for postpartal uterine infection include the following:

- Cesarean birth—the single most significant risk (10 times greater than in vaginal births) (James, 2008)
- Prolonged premature rupture of the amniotic membranes (PPROM)
- Prolonged labor preceding cesarean birth
- Multiple vaginal examinations during labor
- Compromised health status (low socioeconomic status, obesity, smoking, use of illicit drugs or alcohol, poor nutritional intake, and anemia)
- Use of fetal scalp electrode or intrauterine pressure catheter for internal monitoring during labor
- Obstetric trauma—episiotomy and lacerations of perineum, vagina, or cervix
- Chorioamnionitis
- Diabetes (four times more common than in nondiabetic mothers) (Davies & Gibbs, 2008)
- Preexisting bacterial vaginosis or *Chlamydia trachomatis* infection
- Instrument-assisted childbirth—vacuum or forceps
- Manual removal of the placenta
- Lapses in aseptic technique by surgical staff or prolonged duration of surgery

Endometritis (Metritis)

Endometritis (metritis), an inflammation of the endometrium portion of the uterine lining, may occur postpartally in 1% to 3% of women who give birth vaginally and ranges from 5% to 15% of those who give birth by cesarean (Duff, 2007). After expulsion of the placenta, the placental site provides an excellent culture medium for bacterial growth. The site in the contracted uterus is a round, dark red, elevated area of 4 cm (1.6 in.), with a nodular surface composed of numerous veins, many of which may become occluded because of clot formation. The remaining portion of the decidua is also susceptible to pathogenic bacteria because of its thinness (approximately 2 mm) and its large blood supply. The cervix presents a bacterial breeding ground because of the multiple small lacerations attending normal labor and spontaneous birth.

Both aerobic and anaerobic organisms cause metritis, which is often polymicrobial (Duff, 2007). See Table 33–2 for a list of common causative organisms. Clinical findings of metritis in the initial 24 to 36 hours postpartally tend to be related to group B streptococcus (GBS). Late-onset postpartal metritis is most commonly associated with genital mycoplasmas and *Chlamydia trachomatis.* These microbes have a longer replication time and latency period than other bacteria and are not consistently eradicated by antibiotics used for early postpartal infections.

In mild cases of metritis, the woman generally has vaginal discharge that is bloody, foul smelling, and either scant or profuse. In more severe cases, she also has uterine tenderness; sawtooth temperature spikes, usually between 38.3°C (101°F) and 40°C (104°F); tachycardia; and chills. Foul-smelling lochia is cited as a classic sign of endometritis; however, in the case of infection with β-hemolytic streptococcus the lochia may be scant, serosanguineous, and odorless (Gibbs et al., 2004).

Pelvic Cellulitis (Parametritis)

Pelvic cellulitis (parametritis) is infection involving the connective tissue of the broad ligament or, in more severe forms, the connective tissue of all the pelvic structures.

TABLE 33–2	Common Causative Organisms in Metritis
Aerobes	**Anaerobes**
• Group A, B, D streptococcus	• *Peptostreptococcus*
• Enterococcus	• *Clostridium* species
• *Staphylococcus* species	• *Bacteroides* species
• *Escherichia coli*	• *Chlamydia trachomatis*
• *Klebsiella pneumoniae*	• Genital *mycoplasma*
• *Proteus mirabilis*	

Source: Data from: Baxley, E. G. (2001). Postpartum biomedical concerns. Section B postpartum endometritis. In S. D. Ratcliffe, E. G. Baxley, J. E. Byrd, & E. L. Sakornbut (Eds.), *Family practice obstetrics* (2nd ed., pp. 602–607). Philadelphia: Hanley & Belfus; Duff, P. (2008). Maternal and perinatal infection—Bacterial. In S. G. Gabbe, J. R. Niebyl, & J. L. Simpson (Eds.), *Obstetrics: Normal and problem pregnancies* (5th ed., pp. 1233–1248). Philadelphia, PA: Churchill Livingstone/Elsevier; Gibbs, R. S., Sweet, R. L., & Duff, W. P. (2004). Maternal and fetal infectious disorders. In R. K. Creasy & R. Resnik (Eds.), *Maternal-fetal medicine: Principles and practice* (5th ed., pp. 741–800). Philadelphia: Saunders; James, D. C. (2008). Postpartum care. In K. R. Simpson & P. A. Creehan, *AWHONN perinatal nursing* (3rd ed., pp. 473–526). Philadelphia, PA: Lippincott Williams & Wilkins.

The infection generally ascends upward in the pelvis by way of the lymphatics in the uterine wall but may also occur if pathogenic organisms invade a cervical laceration that extends upward into the connective tissue of the broad ligament—a direct pathway into the pelvis. Infection involving the peritoneal cavity is **peritonitis**.

A pelvic abscess may form in the case of postpartal peritonitis and is most commonly found in the uterine ligaments, the cul-de-sac of Douglas, and the subdiaphragmatic space. Parametritis may be a secondary result of pelvic vein thrombophlebitis. This condition occurs when the clot, usually in the right ovarian vein, becomes infected and the wall of the vein breaks down from necrosis, spilling the infection into the connective tissues of the pelvis.

A woman suffering from parametritis may demonstrate a variety of symptoms, including marked high temperature (38.9°C to 40°C [102°F to 104°F]), chills, malaise, lethargy, abdominal pain, subinvolution of the uterus, tachycardia, and local and referred rebound tenderness. If peritonitis develops, the woman becomes acutely ill, with severe pain, marked anxiety, high fever, rapid and shallow respirations, pronounced tachycardia, excessive thirst, abdominal distention, nausea, and vomiting.

Perineal Wound Infections

Given the degree of bacterial contamination that occurs with normal vaginal birth, it is surprising that more women do not have infections of the episiotomy or repaired lacerations of the perineum, vagina, or vulva. Good aseptic technique is the likely rationale. When perineal wound infection occurs, it is recognized by the classic signs: redness, warmth, edema, purulent drainage, and, later, gaping of the wound that had previously been well approximated. Local pain may be severe. Infected perineal wounds, like other infected wounds, are treated by draining the purulent material. Sutures are removed, and the wound is left open. A regimen of broad-spectrum antibiotics is used. When the surface of the wound is free of infectious exudate and tissue granulation is evident, the mother returns for secondary closure of the wound under regional anesthesia.

Cesarean Wound Infections

The infection rate following cesarean births is 3% to 5%, with the highest rate occurring after emergency cesarean because there is more traumatization of the tissue (Duff, 2007). Predisposing factors to infection include obesity, diabetes mellitus, prolonged postpartal hospitalization, PROM, metritis, prolonged labor, anemia, steroid therapy, and immunosuppression. Signs of an abdominal wound infection, which may not be evident until after discharge, include erythema; warmth; skin discoloration; edema;

tenderness; purulent drainage, sometimes mixed with sanguineous fluid; or gaping of the wound edges. Fever, pain, malodorous lochia, and other systemic signs are also common. Abdominal distention and decreased bowel sounds may be noted. Culture of the wound drainage commonly reveals mixed pathogens.

Clinical Therapy

The infection site and causative organism are diagnosed by careful history and complete physical examination, blood tests, aerobic and anaerobic endometrial cultures (although cultures may be of limited value because multiple organisms are usually present), and urinalysis to rule out urinary tract infection (UTI). When a localized infection develops, it is treated with antibiotics, sitz baths, and analgesics as necessary for pain relief. If an abscess has developed or a stitch site is infected, the suture is removed and the area is allowed to drain. Packing the wound with saline gauze twice to three times daily, using aseptic technique, allows removal of necrotic debris when packing is removed. Broad-spectrum antibiotic coverage is used to treat postpartal wound infections. Cephalosporins, penicillinase-resistant penicillin, are commonly used with anaerobic coverage by clindamycin and gentamicin or ampicillin in refractory cases (Cunningham et al., 2005; James, 2008).

The incidence of metritis has been reduced by prophylactic administration of antibiotics to women undergoing cesarean childbirth. Metritis, once diagnosed, is treated by aggressive administration of antibiotics (Duff, 2007). With appropriate antibiotic coverage, improvement should occur within 48 to 72 hours (James, 2008). Antibiotics are generally continued until the woman is afebrile for 24 to 48 hours (James, 2008). The route and dosage are determined by the severity of the infection. Careful monitoring is also necessary to prevent the development of a more serious infection.

Parametritis and peritonitis are treated with intravenous antibiotics. Broad-spectrum antibiotics effective against the most commonly occurring causative organisms are chosen initially, until the results of culture and sensitivity reports are available. If multiple organisms are present, the approach to antibiotic therapy is continued unless no improvement is observed; then the antibiotic is changed. Antibiotics are generally continued until the woman has been afebrile for 48 hours. Oral antibiotics are rarely needed on discharge.

An abscess is frequently manifested by the development of a palpable mass and may be confirmed with ultrasound. It usually requires incision and drainage to avoid rupture into the peritoneal cavity and the possible development of peritonitis. After drainage of the abscess, the cavity may be packed with iodoform gauze to promote drainage and facilitate healing.

The woman with a severe systemic infection is acutely ill and may require care in an intensive care unit. Supportive therapy includes maintenance of adequate hydration with intravenous fluids, analgesic medications, ongoing assessment of the infection, and possibly continuous nasogastric suctioning if paralytic ileus develops.

Nursing Care Management

Nursing Assessment and Diagnosis

The nurse should inspect the woman's perineum every 8 to 12 hours for signs of early infection. The REEDA scale helps the nurse remember to consider *r*edness, *e*dema, *e*cchymosis, *d*ischarge, and *a*pproximation. The nurse immediately reports any degree of induration (hardening) to the clinician.

The nurse notes and reports the presence of fever, malaise, abdominal pain, foul-smelling lochia, larger than expected uterus, tachycardia, and other signs of infection so that treatment can begin. The white blood cell (WBC) count, a usual objective measure of infection, cannot be used reliably because of the normal increase in WBCs during the postpartum period; a WBC count of 14,000 to 16,000 mm^3 is not an unusual finding. An increase in WBC level of more than 30% in a 6-hour period, however, is indicative of infection.

Nursing diagnoses that may apply to the women with a puerperal infection include the following:

- *Risk for Injury* related to the spread of infection
- *Pain* related to the presence of infection
- *Risk for Impaired Parenting* related to delayed parent-infant attachment secondary to malaise and other symptoms of infection

Nursing Plan and Implementation

Hospital-Based Nursing Care

The nurse caring for a woman during the postpartal period is responsible for teaching the woman self-care measures that are helpful in preventing infection. The woman should understand the importance of perineal care, good hygiene practices to prevent contamination of the perineum (including wiping from front to back, changing perineal pads after voiding), and thorough handwashing. Careful attention to aseptic technique during labor, birth, and postpartum is essential. Once edema and perineal pain are under control, the nurse can also encourage sitz baths, which are cleansing and promote healing. Adequate fluid intake and a diet high in protein and vitamin C, which are necessary for wound healing, also help prevent infection (James, 2008).

If the woman has a draining wound or purulent lochia, it is especially important that those in contact with soiled items and linens practice good handwashing. Clear, concise instructions about wound care and how to discard soiled dressings appropriately must be provided to safeguard the woman and her caregivers. If the woman is seriously ill, ongoing assessment of urine-specific gravity, as well as intake and output, is necessary. The nurse also carefully administers antibiotics as ordered and regulates the intravenous fluid rate. Ongoing assessment of the woman's condition is vital to detect subtle changes in her health status. The nurse also addresses the woman's comfort needs related to hygiene, positioning, oral hygiene, and pain relief.

Promoting maternal-infant attachment can be difficult with the acutely ill woman. The nurse may provide pictures of the infant and keep the mother informed of the infant's well-being. Mementos, such as a footprint, a note written by the father "from the baby," or a videotape of the baby can be comforting to the mother during their separation. If she feels up to it, the new mother will also benefit from brief visits with her newborn. The woman who wishes to breastfeed when her condition allows can maintain lactation by pumping her breasts regularly. Understanding that the opportunity to breastfeed is simply delayed, not eliminated, by the infectious process may improve the woman's morale.

The partner of a seriously ill woman will be concerned about her condition and torn about spending time with her and with their newborn. Because maternal-infant bonding may be compromised, allow for privacy with limited interruptions to facilitate father-newborn bonding. See Nursing Care Plan for a Woman with a Puerperal Perineal Wound Infection for specific nursing care measures.

Community-Based Nursing Care

The woman with a puerperal infection needs assistance when she is discharged from the hospital. If the family cannot provide this home assistance, a referral to home care services is needed. Home care services should be contacted as soon as puerperal infection is diagnosed so that the nurse can meet with the woman for a family and home assessment and development of a home care plan.

The family needs instruction in the care of a newborn, including feeding, bathing, cord care, immunizations, and significant observations that should be reported. A well-baby appointment should be scheduled. The woman who wishes to breastfeed when her condition allows can maintain lactation by pumping her breasts regularly. Breastfeeding mothers receiving antibiotics should be instructed to inspect the infant's mouth for signs of thrush and to report the finding to their physician.

The mother should be instructed regarding activity, rest, medications, diet, and signs and symptoms of complications. She should also be scheduled for a return medical visit. She needs to know the importance of taking the entire course of prescribed antibiotics even though she may begin to feel better before the bottle is empty. She also

needs to be informed about the importance of pelvic rest; that is, she should not use tampons or douches nor have intercourse until she has been examined by the physician and told it is safe to resume those activities.

Evaluation

Expected outcomes of nursing care include the following:

- The infection is quickly identified and treated successfully, without further complications.
- The woman understands the infection and the purpose of therapy; she cooperates with ongoing antibiotic therapy after discharge.
- Maternal-infant attachment is maintained.

Care of the Woman with a Urinary Tract Infection

The postpartal woman is at increased risk of developing urinary tract problems caused by the normal postpartal diuresis, increased bladder capacity, decreased bladder sensitivity from stretching or trauma, and possible inhibited neural control of the bladder following the use of general or regional anesthesia and contamination from catheterization. The number of catheterizations performed during labor has increased. It is essential that the mother empty the bladder completely with each voiding.

Overdistention of the Bladder

Overdistention occurs postpartally when the woman is unable to empty her bladder, usually because of trauma or the effects of anesthesia. Women who have not sufficiently recovered from the effects of anesthesia cannot void spontaneously, and catheterization is necessary. After the effects of regional anesthesia have worn off, if the woman cannot void, postpartal urinary retention is highly indicative of UTI. Other risk factors for urinary retention after childbirth include nulliparity, instrumental childbirth, and prolonged labor (Yip, Shota, Pang et al., 2005).

Clinical Therapy

Overdistention in the early postpartal period is often managed by draining the bladder with a straight catheter as a one-time measure. If the overdistention recurs or is diagnosed later in the postpartal period, an indwelling catheter is generally ordered for 24 hours. An alternative urinary retention protocol involves bladder ultrasound scans with intervention based on the amount of urine volume. For example, if the volume is greater than 400 mL, the bladder is drained and the catheter removed, whereas if the volume is 400 mL or less, a spontaneous void is awaited for 1 hour after which another scan is performed (Yip et al., 2005).

Nursing Care Plan   For a Woman with a Puerperal Perineal Wound Infection

CLIENT SCENARIO

Terri, age 24, G1P1, gave birth to a healthy baby boy 36 hours ago. She had a midline episiotomy and a second-degree laceration of the perineum. Terri is complaining of increased pain of the perineum. It has become increasingly tender and swollen despite careful cleansing and good perineal care.

The nurse assesses Terri and documents a temperature of 38.6°C (101.6°F), pulse 110, respirations 16, and BP 128/72. The perineal area is red and edematous, and purulent drainage is noted coming from the suture site. The physician is notified and Terri is diagnosed with a perineal wound infection. The nurse administers antibiotics per physician order.

ASSESSMENT

Subjective: Chills, perineal tenderness, malaise, weakness, and pain

Objective: Temperature 38.6°C (101.6°F), pulse 110, respirations 16, BP 128/72, purulent drainage from episiotomy incision

Nursing Diagnosis	Risk for Infection related to decreased skin integrity of the perineal tissue secondary to episiotomy*
Client Goal	Client remains free of infection.
AEB:	• Vital signs within normal limits. • No signs of edema, redness, drainage, or tenderness of the perineal tissue.

NURSING INTERVENTIONS

1. Perform a routine complete postpartum history and physical exam.

2. Monitor vital signs every 4 hours; temperature every 2 hours if elevated

3. Assess perineum every 8 to 12 hours.

4. Remove episiotomy sutures at the site of infection per agency protocol.

5. Obtain wound culture and administer medications as ordered.

6. Instruct client on proper perineal care.

7. Encourage sitz bath if skin is intact and pain is under control.

8. Increase protein, vitamin C, and iron in diet.

RATIONALES

Rationale: To assess client for factors, signs, and symptoms that place the client at risk for infection. Baseline data may be used to compare further assessment findings and identify any deviation from the norm. See text for timing of and components of postpartum exams.

Rationale: Increases in temperature, pulse, and/or respirations may indicate signs of infection. Report temperature greater than 38°C (100.4°F) to the physician.

Rationale: The perineum should be assessed for signs of infection, including redness, edema, ecchymosis, purulent discharge, and a gaping wound that once was approximated.

Rationale: If a stitch site becomes infected or an abscess has developed then the sutures are removed and the area is left open and allowed to drain. Packing of the abscess area may be required twice a day using aseptic technique. This allows for the removal of necrotic debris when packing is removed. Once the surface of the wound is free of infectious exudates and tissue granulation is present, the wound is closed under regional anesthesia.

Rationale: Broad-spectrum antibiotics are used to treat postpartal wound infections until an organism-sensitive antibiotic can be started.

Rationale: To prevent contamination of the perineum and spread of infection instruct client to use good handwashing, wipe from front to back after each void, and frequently change pads.

Rationale: Promotes wound healing by increasing circulation and cleanses surrounding tissue.

Rationale: Protein, vitamin C, and iron aid in the promotion of wound healing.

Evaluation of Client Goal	• Vital signs are within normal limits. • No signs of edema, redness, drainage, or tenderness of the perineal tissue are noted.

(Continued on next page)

Nursing Care Plan

For a Woman with a Puerperal Perineal Wound Infection *(Continued)*

CRITICAL THINKING QUESTIONS

1. The nurse is preparing Terri for discharge. Terri states that her family lives too far away to visit at this time and her husband works long hours. Based on the nurse's assessment, Terri will require additional help at home during her recovery. What can be done for Terri before discharge?

Answer: The nurse may contact a referral service so Terri can receive care at home. A home care service should be contacted once a puerperal infection is diagnosed. This will allow the home care service to do a home assessment and develop a plan of care.

2. What should the nurse include in Terri's discharge teaching instructions?

Answer: The nurse should advise Terri to complete the full course of antibiotics, maintain pelvic rest (no tampons, intercourse, or douches), decrease activity level, encourage frequent rest periods, report signs and symptoms that might indicate a problem with recovery (elevated temperature, chills, malaise, change in blood flow, increased pain, any foul-smelling discharge), provide instructions on dressing and wound care, and advise her when she should return for a medical visit.

*For your reference, this care plan is an example of how one nursing diagnosis might be addressed.

Nursing Care Management

Nursing Assessment and Diagnosis

The overdistended bladder appears as a large mass, reaching sometimes to the umbilicus and displacing the uterine fundus upward. Increased vaginal bleeding occurs, the fundus is boggy, and the woman may complain of cramping as the uterus attempts to contract. Some women also experience backache and restlessness.

Nursing diagnoses that may apply when a woman has difficulties with overdistention of the bladder include the following:

- *Risk for Infection* related to urinary stasis secondary to overdistention
- *Urinary Retention* related to decreased bladder sensitivity and normal postpartal diuresis

HINTS FOR PRACTICE

Postpartum urinary retention is often defined as "the absence of spontaneous urination within 6 hours of a vaginal delivery or within 6 hours after removal of an indwelling catheter post-Cesarean delivery." The astute nurse will watch the woman's bladder for signs of retention—not the clock! As urinary retention promotes uterine atony and a subsequent increase in bleeding and also contributes to the possibility of UTI, timely intervention is crucial.

Nursing Plan and Implementation

Diligent monitoring of the bladder during the recovery period and preventive health measures greatly reduce the chances for overdistention of the bladder. Encouraging the mother to void spontaneously and helping her use the toilet, if possible, or the bedpan, if she has received conductive anesthesia, prevents overdistention in most cases. The nurse assists the woman to a normal position for voiding

(i.e., sitting with the legs and feet lower than the trunk) and provides privacy to encourage voiding. The woman should receive medication for whatever pain she may be having before she attempts to void because pain may cause a reflex spasm of the urethra. Applying perineal ice packs after childbirth helps minimize edema, which may interfere with voiding. Pouring warm water over the perineum or having the woman void in the sitz bath may also be effective.

If catheterization becomes necessary, careful, meticulous aseptic technique is employed during catheter insertion. The vagina and vulva are traumatized to some degree by vaginal birth, and edema is common. This edema may obscure the urinary meatus; therefore, the nurse needs to be extremely careful in cleansing the vulva and inserting the catheter. It is imperative to discard a catheter that has inadvertently been introduced into the vagina and thus contaminated. Catheterization is an uncomfortable procedure because of the postpartal trauma and edema of the tissue, so the nurse should be careful and gentle not only in inserting the catheter but also in handling and cleaning the perineal area.

If the amount of urine drained from the bladder reaches 900 to 1000 mL, the catheter is clamped and taped firmly to the woman's leg. The nurse takes the woman's vital signs before and after the procedure and notes the woman's responses. After an hour, the catheter may be unclamped and placed on gravity drainage. This technique protects the bladder and prevents rapid intra-abdominal decompression. When the indwelling catheter is removed, a urine specimen is often sent to the laboratory. The tip of the catheter may also be removed and sent for culture.

Evaluation

Expected outcomes of nursing care include the following:

- The woman voids adequately to meet the demands of the increased fluid shifts during the postpartal period.

MyNursingKit | Video: Nursing in Action: Massaging a Uterine Fundus

- The woman does not develop infection caused by stasis of urine.
- The woman actively incorporates self-care measures to decrease bladder overdistention.

Cystitis (Lower Urinary Tract Infection)

Retention of residual urine, bacteria introduced at the time of catheterization, and a bladder traumatized by birth combine to provide an excellent environment for the development of cystitis. *Escherichia coli* has been demonstrated to be the causative agent in most cases of postpartal cystitis and pyelonephritis (in both lower and upper UTI). Generally, the infection ascends the urinary tract from the urethra to the bladder and then to the kidneys because vesicoureteral reflux (backward flow of urine) forces contaminated urine into the renal pelvis.

Clinical Therapy

When cystitis is suspected, a clean-catch midstream urine sample is obtained for microscopic examination, culture, and sensitivity tests. The specimen may require collection by the nurse with the woman on a bedpan because few postpartal women can collect a true midstream, clean-catch specimen without contaminating the specimen with lochia. A catheterized specimen is avoided when possible because of the increased risk of infection. When the bacterial concentration is greater than 100,000 colonies of the same organism per milliliter of fresh urine, infection is generally present. Counts between 10,000 and 100,000 suggest infection, particularly if clinical symptoms are noted.

In the clinical setting, antibiotic therapy is often initiated before culture and sensitivity reports are available. Frequently used antibiotics include a preparation of trimethoprim-sulfamethoxazole—double strength (Bactrim DS, Septra DS), one of the short-acting sulfonamides, nitrofurantoin (Macrobid), and, in the case of sulfa allergy, ampicillin or amoxicillin–clavulanic acid (Augmentin). The antibiotic is changed later if indicated by the results of the sensitivity report (Gilbert, 2007; James, 2008). Antispasmodics or urinary analgesic agents, such as Pyridium, may be given to relieve discomfort.

Nursing Care Management

Nursing Assessment and Diagnosis

Symptoms of cystitis often appear 2 to 3 days after childbirth. The initial symptoms of cystitis may include frequency, urgency, dysuria, and nocturia. Hematuria and suprapubic pain may also be present. A slightly elevated temperature may occur, but systemic symptoms are often absent (James, 2008).

When a UTI progresses to pyelonephritis, systemic symptoms usually occur, and the woman becomes acutely ill. Symptoms include chills, high fever, flank pain (unilateral or bilateral), nausea, and vomiting, in addition to the signs of lower UTI. Costovertebral angle tenderness on palpation and pain may or may not be present. The nurse obtains a urine culture so that sensitivity can identify the causative organism.

Nursing diagnoses that may apply if a woman develops a postpartal UTI include the following:

- *Pain with Voiding* related to dysuria secondary to infection
- *Health-Seeking Behaviors* related to need for information about self-care measures to prevent UTI

Nursing Plan and Implementation

Screening for asymptomatic bacteriuria in pregnancy should be routine. The nurse needs to encourage frequent emptying of the bladder during labor and postpartum to prevent overdistention and trauma to the bladder. Catheterization technique and nursing actions to prevent overdistention (previously discussed) also apply. The woman with pyelonephritis must understand the importance of follow-up care after discharge to prevent recurrence or further complications.

Teaching for Self-Care

The nurse should advise the postpartal woman to continue good perineal hygiene after discharge. The nurse also advises the woman to maintain a good fluid intake (at least 8 to 10, 8-oz glasses daily), especially of water, and to empty her bladder whenever she feels the urge to void, but at least every 2 to 4 hours while awake. Once sexual intercourse is resumed, the new mother should void before (to prevent bladder trauma) and following intercourse (to wash contaminants from the vicinity of the urinary meatus). Wearing underwear with a cotton crotch to facilitate air circulation also reduces the risk of UTI.

Acidification of the urine is thought to aid in preventing and managing UTI. The nurse thus advises the woman to avoid carbonated beverages, which increase the alkalinity of urine, and to drink low sugar juices and take vitamin C or cranberry tablets, which increase the acidity of urine (Gilbert, 2007).

Evaluation

Expected outcomes of nursing care include the following:

- The woman identifies the signs of UTI and her condition is treated successfully.

- The woman incorporates self-care measures to prevent the recurrence of UTI as part of her personal hygiene routine.
- The woman cooperates with any long-term therapy or follow-up.
- Maternal-infant attachment is maintained and the woman is able to care for her newborn effectively.

Care of the Woman with Mastitis

Mastitis is an infection of the breast connective tissue that occurs primarily in lactating women. The incidence of sporadic mastitis is 2% to 10% of breastfeeding mothers and less than 1% in nonlactating mothers (Newton, 2007). The usual causative organisms are *Staphylococcus aureus*, *Haemophilus parainfluenzae*, *H. influenzae*, *Escherichia coli*, and *Streptococcus* species. Infectious mastitis is a more serious infection, with fever, chills, headache, flulike muscle aches and malaise, and a warm, reddened, painful area of the breast, often wedge shaped because of the connective tissue septal divisions of the breast (Figure 33–2 ■). Because symptoms seldom occur before the second to fourth week postpartum, birthing unit nurses often are not fully aware of how uncomfortable and acutely ill the woman can be; they must ensure that all breastfeeding women are taught preventive techniques, ways of recognizing it, and the appropriate response of immediate notification of their physician/CNM.

The infection usually begins when bacteria invade the breast tissue after it has been traumatized in some way

(see the factors commonly associated with mastitis in Table 33–3). Milk serves as a favorable medium for the invasive bacteria; thus milk stasis is another risk factor. The most common sources of pathogenic organisms are the infant's nose and throat, although other sources include the hands of the mother or birthing unit personnel and the woman's circulating blood. Infants of women with mastitis generally remain well.

In some cases, *Candida albicans* is the causative organism of mastitis, entering the breast through a small fissure or abrasion on the nipple; the baby will often have thrush, a candidal infection of the mouth. There may be a history of a recent course of antibiotics in the woman. Signs include late-onset nipple pain and burning pain of the nipple/areola, followed by stabbing pain of the breast during and between feedings, often radiating to the chest wall (Newton, 2007; Wiener, 2006). Eventually, the skin of the affected breast becomes pink, shiny, flaking, and pruritic (Wiener, 2006). Women may notice a yeasty odor to their milk. Unless the mother and her newborn are treated for *Candida*, recolonization will occur when breastfeeding is resumed. Pacifiers, bottles, and pump equipment in contact with

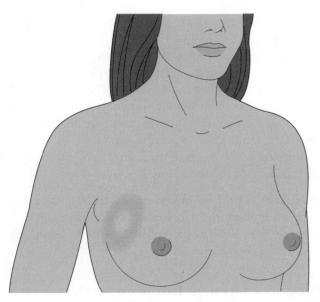

FIGURE 33–2 Mastitis. Erythema and swelling are present in the upper outer quadrant of the breast. Axillary lymph nodes are often enlarged and tender. The segmental anatomy of the breast accounts for the demarcated, often V-shaped wedge of inflammation.

TABLE 33–3	Factors Associated with Development of Mastitis

Milk Stasis
Failure to change infant position to allow emptying all lobes
Failure to alternate breasts at feedings
Poor suck
Poor letdown

Actions That Promote Access/Multiplication of Bacteria
Poor handwashing technique
Improper breast hygiene
Failure to air dry breasts after breastfeeding
Use of plastic-lined breast pads that trap moisture against nipple

Breast/Nipple Trauma
Incorrect positioning for breastfeeding
Poor latch-on
Failure to rotate position on nipple
Incorrect or aggressive pumping technique
Cracked nipples

Obstruction of Ducts
Restrictive clothing
Constricting bra
Underwire bra

Change in Number of Feedings/Failure to Empty Breasts
Attempted weaning
Missed feeding
Prolonged sleeping, including sleeping through night
Favoring side of nipple soreness

Lowered Maternal Defenses
Fatigue
Stress

Candida should be boiled for 20 minutes, and clothing in contact with the breast should be laundered in dilute bleach solution (Mass, 2004).

Clinical Therapy

Diagnosis is usually based on history and physical examination; a culture and sensitivity testing of breast milk obtained by a midstream-type collection process may be done. The nipple is washed first; then the first 3 mL of breast milk are manually expressed and discarded, after which the actual specimen is collected. A leukocyte count of 1 million/mL and a bacterial count of greater than 10,000/mL are diagnostic (Newton, 2007).

Treatment of mastitis involves bed rest for at least 24 hours; increased fluid intake (at least 2 to 2.5 L/day); a supportive bra; frequent breastfeeding; local application of warm, moist-heat compresses; and analgesics that are compatible with breastfeeding (James, 2008). Nonsteroidal anti-inflammatory agents are recommended to treat both fever and inflammation. Also, a course of 7 to 10 days of antibiotics is appropriate, usually with a penicillinase-resistant penicillin or cephalosporin (Newton, 2007).

Candidal infections can be especially stubborn. Initial treatment generally involves antifungal (Nystatin [Mycostatin]), miconazole (Monistat-Derm) or clotrimazole (Lotrimin) creams or ointments once or twice daily (Wiener, 2006). Treatment regimen must include the simultaneous treatment of the mother and baby dyad. Oral nystatin (Mycostatin Suspension) is the most common treatment for the baby, followed by oral fluconazole (Diflucan) (Weiner, 2006). Oral Diflucan for the mother is excreted in breast milk but is not considered toxic to the infant and can be used if other agents fail (Wiener, 2006).

COMPLEMENTARY AND ALTERNATIVE THERAPIES

Probiotics

Probiotics are a category of dietary supplements consisting of beneficial microorganisms (*pro* means "for" and *biotic* means "life" versus *antibiotic,* which literally means "against life"). Probiotics compete with disease-causing microorganisms in the gastrointestinal tract. When antibiotics are taken, they kill many of the beneficial bacteria that exist naturally in the digestive tract. Supplementing with probiotics after a course of antibiotics is frequently prescribed by nutritionists and complementary practitioners. Commonly used probiotics include *Lactobacillus acidophilus* and *Bifidobacterium bifidum;* there are other species of *Lactobacillus* and *Bifidobacterium* that have been shown to be effective in such conditions as diarrhea and vaginal infections (Reid & Bocking, 2003). Bifidobacterium also competes against *Candida albicans*. Probiotics can be taken in the form of powder, capsules, and suppositories, or in fermented milk products such as yogurt or *kefir.*

Women should be instructed to cleanse their nipples with warm water and allow air drying before application of the antifungal medication. For women who prefer to avoid medication, an alternative treatment is cleansing of the nipples with a solution of 1 tablespoon of vinegar in 1 cup of water or 1 teaspoon of baking soda in 1 cup of water, followed by air drying.

Improved outcome, decreased duration of symptoms, and decreased incidence of breast abscess result if the breasts continue to be emptied by either nursing or pumping. Thus continued breastfeeding is recommended in the presence of mastitis. The woman should be contacted within 24 hours of initiation of treatment to ensure that symptoms are subsiding.

Ten percent of cases will progress to abscess formation if mastitis remains untreated, treatment fails, or the infant is abruptly weaned. Early treatment may prevent the progression of milk stasis and noninfectious inflammation to mastitis. Abscess is more common when there is a lag of 24 hours or more between onset of symptoms and when the woman seeks care (Newton, 2007). Breast abscess may require incision and drainage done by percutaneous needle aspiration under ultrasound guidance or possible surgical incision, and intravenous antistaphylococcal antibiotics (Newton, 2007).

Nursing Care Management

Nursing Assessment and Diagnosis

Each day the nurse assesses the mother's breast consistency, skin color, surface temperature, nipple condition, and presence of pain to detect early signs of problems that may predispose her to mastitis. The mother should be observed breastfeeding her baby to ensure proper technique.

If an infection develops, the nurse assesses for contributing factors such as cracked nipples, poor hygiene, engorgement, supplemental feedings, change in routine or infant feeding pattern, abrupt weaning, and lack of proper breast support so that these factors can be corrected as part of the treatment plan.

Nursing diagnoses that may apply to the woman with mastitis include the following:

- *Health-Seeking Behaviors* related to lack of information about appropriate breastfeeding practices
- *Ineffective Breastfeeding* related to pain secondary to development of mastitis

Nursing Plan and Implementation

Preventing mastitis is far simpler than treating it. Ideally mothers are instructed in proper breastfeeding technique prenatally. The nurse assists the mother to breastfeed soon after childbirth and reviews correct technique. Comanagement of breastfeeding between the nurse and a certified lactation specialist is often possible. Nurses need to encourage new mothers, even those not breastfeeding, to wear a good supportive bra at all times to prevent milk stasis, especially in the lower lobes.

Meticulous handwashing by the breastfeeding mother and all personnel is the primary measure in preventing epidemic nursery infections and subsequent maternal mastitis. Prompt attention to mothers who have blocked milk ducts eliminates stagnant milk as a growth medium for bacteria. If the mother finds that one area of her breast feels distended, she can rotate the position of her infant for nursing, manually express milk remaining in the breast after feeding (usually necessary only if the infant is not sucking well), or massage the caked area toward the nipple as the infant nurses. Mothers who develop mastitis can apply warm, moist compresses to the affected area before and during breastfeeding. The nurse encourages the mother to breastfeed frequently, starting with the unaffected breast until letdown occurs in the affected breast, then switching to the affected breast until it is emptied completely (James, 2008). After nursing, the mother can leave a small amount of milk on each nipple to prevent cracking and allow nipples to air dry. Early identification of and intervention for sore nipples are also essential, as is prompt assessment of the breastfeeding mother's breast when thrush is discovered in her newborn's mouth.

Discharge Planning and Home Care Teaching

The nurse must stress to the breastfeeding woman the importance of adequate breast and nipple care to prevent the development of cracks and fissures, a common portal for bacterial entry. (For a detailed discussion of breastfeeding, see Chapter 27 ∞.)

The woman should be aware of the importance of regular, complete emptying of the breasts to prevent engorgement and stasis. She should also understand the role of letdown in successful breastfeeding, correct positioning of the infant on the nipple, proper latch-on, and the principle of supply and demand. If the mother is taking antibiotics, she needs to understand the importance of completing the full course of antibiotics, even if the infection seems to clear quickly. Infants tolerate the small amount of antibiotics in breast milk without difficulty. The infant should also be checked for possible colonization with the same bacteria present in the mother's breast. Breastfeeding mothers who are returning to work outside the home need information on how to do so successfully. Because mastitis tends to develop after discharge, it is important to include information about signs and symptoms in the discharge teaching and printed materials (Table 33–4). All flulike symptoms should be considered a sign of mastitis until proven otherwise. If symptoms develop, the woman should contact her caregiver immediately because prompt treatment helps to prevent abscess formation.

Community-Based Nursing Care

The home care nurse who suspects mastitis on the basis of assessment findings refers the woman to the physician. The nurse may be asked to obtain a sample of breast milk to be cultured for the causative organism.

If the mother feels too ill to breastfeed or develops an abscess that prevents nursing, the home care nurse can help the mother obtain a breast pump to help her maintain lactation and can provide opportunities for demonstration and return demonstration of pumping. The nurse can also assist the mother to deal with her feelings about temporarily being unable to breastfeed. Referral to a lactation consultant or to La Leche League can be invaluable to the woman's physical and emotional adjustment to mastitis.

Evaluation

Expected outcomes of nursing care include the following:

- The woman is aware of the signs and symptoms of mastitis.
- The woman reports the mastitis signs and symptoms early and is treated successfully.
- The woman resumes breastfeeding if she chooses.
- The woman understands self-care measures she can employ to prevent the recurrence of the mastitis.

TABLE 33–4	Comparison of Findings of Engorgement, Plugged Duct, and Mastitis		
Characteristics	Engorgement	Plugged Duct	Mastitis
Onset	Gradual, immediately postpartum	Gradual, after feedings	Sudden, after 10 days
Site	Bilateral	Unilateral	Usually unilateral
Swelling and heat	Generalized	May shift, little or no heat	Localized, red, hot, and swollen
Pain	Generalized	Mild but localized	Intense but localized
Body temperature	< 38.4°C (101.1°F)	< 38.4°C (101.1°F)	> 38.4°C (101.1°F)
Systemic symptoms	Feels well	Feels well	Flulike symptoms

Source: Lawrence, R. A., & Lawrence, R. M. (1999). *Breastfeeding: A guide for the medical profession* (5th ed., p. 276). Mosby Inc., with permission from Elsevier Science.

Care of the Woman with Postpartal Thromboembolic Disease

Thromboembolic disease may occur antepartally, but it is generally considered a postpartal complication. *Venous thrombosis* refers to blood clot (thrombus formation) at an area of impeded blood flow in a superficial or deep vein, usually in the legs. When the thrombus is formed in response to inflammation in the vein wall, it is termed **thrombophlebitis**. Pulmonary embolism, a rare, life-threatening condition, occurs when thrombi formed in the deep leg veins are carried to the pulmonary artery, obstructing pulmonary blood flow to one or both lungs. These vascular occlusive processes—venous thrombosis, thrombophlebitis, septic pelvic thrombophlebitis, and pulmonary thromboembolism—are known as thromboembolic diseases (Krakow, 2008).

Three major causes of thromboembolic disease are hypercoagulability of blood, venous stasis, and injury to the epithelium of the blood vessel. Changes in the woman's coagulation system in pregnancy contribute to hypercoagulability and compression of the common iliac vein by the gravid uterus, which leads to venous stasis. These factors increase the risk of thromboembolic disease in pregnant and postpartal women approximately 2 to 6 times (Poggi, 2007). Superficial vein thrombophlebitis complicates the general childbearing period for 1 in 500 to 750 women. In contrast, deep vein thrombosis (DVT), which is more serious, occurs most commonly in postpartum women between postpartum days 10 to 20. These types are discussed shortly.

Factors associated with increased risk of thromboembolic disease are identified in Table 33–5. Factors contributing directly to the development of thromboembolic disease postpartally include (1) increased amounts of certain blood-clotting factors; (2) postpartal thrombocytosis (increased quantity of circulating platelets and their increased adhesiveness); (3) release of thromboplastin substances from the tissue of the decidua, placenta, and fetal membranes; and (4) increased amounts of fibrinolysis inhibitors. Because all women are at risk for thromboembolic disease during the childbearing period, attention should be given to measures that might prevent this complication (Table 33–6).

Superficial Leg Vein Disease

Superficial thrombophlebitis is far more common postpartally than during pregnancy. Often the clot involves one of the saphenous veins. This disorder is more common in women with preexisting varices (enlarged veins), although it is not limited to these women. They may also occur as a sequelae to IV catheterization. Symptoms usu-

TABLE 33–5	Factors Associated with Increased Risk of Thromboembolic Disease

- Cesarean birth
- Immobility
- Obesity
- Cigarette smoking
- Previous thromboembolic disease
- Trauma to extremity (can include injury from incorrect positioning or prolonged interval in stirrups during labor)
- Varicose veins
- Diabetes mellitus
- Advanced maternal age
- Inherited coagulation disorders
- Multiparity
  - Exogenous hormone use (oral contraceptives, hormone replacement therapy)
  - Malignancy
- Anemia

TABLE 33–6	Measures to Decrease Risk of Thromboembolic Disease in Childbearing Women

Antepartum Measures	Intrapartum Measures	Postpartum Measures
Advise woman to avoid sedentary lifestyle and to exercise as possible (walking is ideal).	Encourage ambulation unless contraindicated in early labor. Later, encourage leg exercises.	Encourage early ambulation.
Recommend plenty of fluids to avoid dehydration.	Do not gatch bed or use pillows under knees.	For clients on bed rest, advise or assist with turning and leg exercises every 2 hours (woman may be encouraged to rotate ankles and to "write baby's name in the air with her toes").
Advise to quit smoking.	Pad stirrups.	
Teach to avoid prolonged standing or sitting in one position or sitting with legs crossed.	Ensure correct positioning in stirrups that minimizes pressure on the popliteal area.	Encourage fluids to avoid dehydration.
Encourage elevation of legs when sitting.	Limit time in stirrups as possible.	Advise no smoking.
Teach to avoid tight knee-high hose or other constrictive garments.	After cesarean birth, initiate leg/foot exercises as soon as possible (in recovery).	Use antiembolism stockings with those at risk, including after cesarean birth.
Encourage to take frequent breaks during long car trips to walk around, thereby preventing prolonged venous stasis.	Use antiembolism stockings for women at risk for DVT.	Advise against prolonged sitting and crossing legs.
		Encourage elevation of legs while sitting.

ally become apparent about postpartal day 3 or 4 and include tenderness in a portion of the vein, some local heat and redness, normal temperature or low-grade fever, and occasionally slight elevation of the pulse. A tender palpable cord may be noted along a portion of the veins. Treatment involves application of local heat, elevation of the affected limb, bed rest, analgesics, and the use of elastic support hose. Anticoagulants are usually not necessary unless complications develop. Pulmonary embolism is extremely rare.

Deep Vein Thrombosis

Deep vein thrombosis (DVT) is more frequently seen in women with a history of thrombosis. Certain obstetric complications, such as hydramnios, preeclampsia, and operative birth, are also associated with an increased incidence. After a clinical diagnosis of DVT, a woman's risk in a subsequent pregnancy increases.

Clinical manifestations may include edema of the ankle and leg and an initial low-grade fever often followed by high temperature and chills. Other findings include tenderness or pain, a palpable cord, changes in limb color, and difference in limb circumference of more than 2 cm (0.8 in.). Depending on the vein involved, the woman may complain of pain in the popliteal and lateral tibial areas (popliteal vein), pain in the entire lower leg and foot (anterior and posterior tibial veins), inguinal tenderness (femoral vein), or pain in the lower abdomen (iliofemoral vein). The Homans' sign (refer to Figure 30–9 ∞) may or may not be positive. A positive Homans' sign is a specific finding but has low sensitivity for helping diagnose DVT (Chelmow, Aronson, & Wosu, 2007). Most DVTs occur in the left leg. Because of reflex arterial spasm, sometimes the limb is pale and cool to the touch—the so-called milk leg or *phlegmasia alba dolens*—and peripheral pulses may be decreased.

Septic Pelvic Thrombophlebitis

Septic pelvic thrombophlebitis is a complication that develops in conjunction with infections of the reproductive tract and is more common in women who have had a cesarean birth. Infection ascends upward along the venous system, and thrombophlebitis develops in the uterine, ovarian, or hypogastric veins (Cunningham et al., 2005). This diagnosis is suspected with clinical findings resembling metritis that fails to respond to being treated with antibiotics. Abdominal or flank pain, or both, sometimes accompanied by guarding, occurs on the second or third day postpartum, along with fever and tachycardia. Bimanual examination may reveal a parametrial mass; the uterus is generally exquisitely tender. Treatment should consist of anticoagulation and broad-spectrum antibiotic therapy. Within 48 to 72 hours of initiation of heparin therapy, fever should resolve (Duff, 2007).

Clinical Therapy

Because cases of thromboembolic disease are seldom clear-cut, diagnosis involves a variety of approaches, such as client history and physical examination, occlusive cuff impedance plethysmography (IPG), Doppler ultrasonography, and contrast venography (increased circumference of affected extremity). In questionable cases, venography provides the most accurate diagnosis of DVT; however, it is not practical for multiple examinations or prospective screening and may itself induce phlebitis. Positive D-dimer has a high sensitivity in non-pregnant women but it is not a reliable marker because of the wide variation in normal lab valves in the pregnant population (Pettker & Lockwood, 2007).

Treatment involves the administration of intravenous heparin, using an infusion pump to permit continuous, accurate infusion of medication. Strict bed rest and elevation of the leg are required; analgesics are given as necessary to relieve discomfort. If fever is present, deep thrombophlebitis is suspected, and the woman is also given antibiotics. In most cases thrombectomy (surgical removal of the clot) is not necessary.

Once the symptoms have subsided (usually in several days), the woman may begin ambulation while wearing elastic support stockings. Intravenous heparin is continued until prothrombin time reaches 1.5 to 2, and treatment with sodium warfarin (Coumadin) is begun (James, 2008). The woman continues taking warfarin for 2 to 6 months at home. While taking warfarin, prothrombin times are assessed periodically to maintain correct dosage levels.

CRITICAL THINKING

Wanda Sugiyama, G1P1, had a cesarean birth after a prolonged labor and failure to progress. As she is walking in the hallway with her husband, you notice that Wanda is limping slightly, and you comment on that observation. Wanda responds that she is having pain in her right lower leg. She says, "Maybe I pulled a muscle during labor." What would you do?

Answers can be found in Appendix F ∞.

Nursing Care Management

Nursing Assessment and Diagnosis

The nurse carefully assesses the woman's history for factors predisposing her to development of thrombosis or thrombophlebitis. In addition, as part of regular postpartal assessment, the nurse is alert to any complaints of pain in the legs, inguinal area, or lower abdomen because such pain may indicate DVT. The nurse also assesses the woman's legs for evidence of edema, temperature change, or pain with palpation.

Nursing diagnoses that may apply to a postpartal woman with a thrombotic disease include the following:

- *Ineffective Tissue Perfusion in Periphery* related to obstructed venous return
- *Pain* related to tissue hypoxia and edema secondary to vascular obstruction
- *Risk for Impaired Parenting* related to decreased maternal-infant interaction secondary to bed rest and intravenous lines
- *Deficient Knowledge* related to self-care after discharge on anticoagulant therapy

Nursing Plan and Implementation

Hospital-Based Nursing Care

The need for support hose for women with varicosities is evaluated during labor and the postpartum period. Adequate fluid intake is necessary during labor to avoid dehydration. Because trauma is often a factor in the development of thrombophlebitis, the nurse avoids keeping the woman's legs elevated in stirrups for prolonged periods. If stirrups are used, they should be comfortably padded and adjusted to provide correct support and prevent pressure on popliteal vessels. Early ambulation is encouraged following birth, and the knee gatch on the bed should be avoided. Women confined to bed following a cesarean birth are encouraged to perform regular leg exercises to promote venous return.

Once DVT is diagnosed, the nurse maintains the heparin therapy, provides appropriate comfort measures, and monitors the woman closely for signs of pulmonary embolism. The nurse also assesses for evidence of bleeding related to heparin and keeps the antagonist for heparin, protamine sulfate, readily available.

Discharge Planning

At discharge, the nurse instructs the woman to avoid prolonged standing or sitting because these positions contribute to venous stasis. The nurse also advises the woman to avoid crossing her legs because of the pressure it causes. The nurse recommends that the woman take frequent breaks during car trips and while working if she sits most of the day. Walking is acceptable because it promotes venous return. The woman is reminded to mention her history of thrombosis or thrombophlebitis to her physician during subsequent pregnancies so that preventive measures can be instituted early (Crowther & McCourt, 2005).

Women discharged on warfarin should be taught about the drug and safety factors associated with its use. Clients need to be educated about foods high in vitamin K and the need to strive for consistent daily intake. When the dietary intake of these foods decreases significantly, there is a risk of bleeding (Table 33–7). Many multivitamins contain vitamin K; clients on warfarin may take them but should do so consistently. Vitamin C doses up to 500 mg per day and vitamin E doses up to 400 international units per day are considered safe; higher doses can affect coagulation. While taking anticoagulants, the woman will be asked to undergo frequent coagulant tests to guide dosing. Point-of-care testing is now available to decrease the inconvenience of going to the laboratory. Home self-testing involves a single capillary finger stick (Coaguchek, ProTime, Avocet) to test thromboplastin-mediated clotting expressed as prothrombin time (PT) or international normalized ratio (INR). The risk of bleeding increases significantly when the INR is greater than 4 (Pettker & Lockwood, 2007). Bleeding should be reported if it fails to stop within 10 minutes.

Women who are discharged on warfarin must understand the purpose of the medication and be alert for signs of bleeding such as bleeding gums, epistaxis, petechiae or ecchymosis, and evidence of blood in the urine or stool. Because careful monitoring is important, the woman should clearly understand the need to keep scheduled appointments for PT assessment. Certain medications such as aspirin and other nonsteroidal anti-inflammatory drugs increase anticoagulant activity and should be avoided; when she is taking warfarin the woman should check for possible medication interaction before taking *any* other medication. Binge alcohol use inhibits warfarin metabolism; however, an occasional alcoholic beverage does not affect coagulation adversely. Many herbals affect the efficacy of warfarin; for example, garlic, ginger, and ginkgo prolong prothrombin and should be avoided. The nurse should encourage the woman to carry a MedicAlert card in case of emergency and to inform all medical care providers, including dentists, that she is taking anticoagulants. She should also have vitamin K available in case bleeding occurs. (See Nursing Care Plan for a Woman with Deep Vein Thrombosis (DVT) for specific nursing care measures.)

TABLE 33–7	Foods High in Vitamin K
• Basil	• Kale
• Broccoli	• Lettuce
• Brussels sprouts	• Mint
• Cabbage	• Mustard greens
• Canola oil, soybean oil, mayonnaise	• Parsley
• Cauliflower	• Peppers
• Chives	• Spinach
• Collard greens	• Turnips
• Coriander	• Watercress
• Green and black tea	

Nursing Care Plan

For a Woman with Deep Vein Thrombosis (DVT)

CLIENT SCENARIO

Jamie, 26 years old, G2P2, had a repeat cesarean section 2 days ago because of complications of preeclampsia. This morning the nurse assisted Jamie to the bathroom and Jamie complained of pain in her lower left leg. The nurse's assessment reveals that Jamie has a low-grade fever, decreased peripheral pulse, and edema in the left leg. The physician is notified, a Doppler scan is ordered, and Jamie is placed on heparin therapy for deep vein thrombosis.

ASSESSMENT

Subjective: Chills, pain in lower left leg

Objective: Temperature 38°C (100.4°F), pulse 94, respirations 14, BP 130/82. Lower left leg: edematous, peripheral pulses weak, positive Homans' sign, painful but cool to touch, and pale in color

Nursing Diagnosis	Ineffective Tissue Perfusion, Peripheral related to obstructed venous return*
Client Goal	The client will have increased venous return from lower leg.
AEB:	• Decreased edema in lower leg • Negative Homans' sign • No pain or tenderness in lower leg

NURSING INTERVENTIONS

1. Monitor vital signs every 8 hours.

2. Assess leg for edema, peripheral pulse, temperature, color, and tenderness every 8 hours.

3. Assess Homans' sign every 8 hours.

4. Assist client to elevate leg.

5. Encourage strict bed rest during acute phase.

6. Initiate progressive ambulation following acute phase and apply elastic support stockings before ambulation.

7. Administer pain medication as needed.

RATIONALES

Rationale: Temperature may be low initially then rise with DVT. Peripheral pulses may be decreased or absent because of impaired venous flow. Peripheral pulses in both legs should be palpated for pulse rate and pulse strength to allow for comparison.

Rationale: Assessment provides baseline data that may be used to monitor success of treatment. Signs of edema/swelling, diminished or absent peripheral pulse, pallor, cool skin temperature, and tenderness are symptoms of DVT and indicate dysfunction of peripheral circulation in the lower extremities. A calf circumference difference of more than 2 cm (8 in.) is classified as leg swelling. Lower extremities that are pale and cool to the touch may be because of reflex arterial spasm.

Rationale: To assess for Homans' sign, the leg is stretched out straight with the knee flexed and the foot is sharply dorsiflexed. Both legs should be assessed. Normally there is no pain or discomfort associated with this procedure. Pain is caused by inflammation of the vessel. If pain is elicited, the nurse documents the response as a positive Homans' sign and reports findings to the physician.

Rationale: Elevating the leg will prevent venous stasis and promote venous return. The knee gatch on the bed should be avoided to reduce pressure behind the knees. Prolonged sitting, standing, and crossing legs should be avoided as these activities decrease venous return.

Rationale: Initial treatment involves strict bed rest to reduce the possibility of embolism. The client may begin to ambulate within a few days and when symptoms subside.

Rationale: To promote venous return and prevent venous stasis. Elastic stockings provide support and also help to promote venous return and prevent venous stasis.

Rationale: Pain is associated with DVT and can be treated with acetaminophen. Once the pain is decreased the client is more likely to ambulate which will help increase venous return and decrease edema. Increased anticoagulant activity is associated with aspirin and nonsteroidal anti-inflammatory drugs and therefore should be avoided.

(Continued on next page)

Nursing Care Plan For a Woman with Deep Vein Thrombosis (DVT) (Continued)

NURSING INTERVENTIONS	RATIONALES
8. Observe and report signs and symptoms of pulmonary embolism.	**Rationale:** A portion of the clot may break off resulting in a pulmonary embolism. This can be life threatening. Signs and symptoms include sudden onset of severe chest pain, often substernally; apprehension and a sense of impending catastrophe; cough, which may be accompanied by hemoptysis; tachycardia; fever; hypotension; diaphoresis; pallor; weakness; shortness of breath; neck engorgement; friction rub; and evidence of atelectasis upon auscultation.
9. Obtain baseline anticoagulation studies, then administer heparin per physician orders.	**Rationale:** International normalized ratio (INR) and partial thromboplastin time (PTT) tests provide basis for interpreting the degree of anticoagulation achieved with unfractionated heparin. Normal PTT for nonpregnant woman is 12 to 14 seconds but in normal pregnancy will be slightly decreased. Heparin may be given via a continuous infusion pump to prevent further thrombus formation and improve tissue perfusion. Heparin is continued until symptoms subside and warfarin (Coumadin) is begun.
10. Observe for signs of bleeding while on heparin.	**Rationale:** Heparin overdose may result in overanticoagulation and cause excessive bleeding or possible hemorrhage which may be life threatening. Inspect for hematuria, epistaxis, ecchymosis, and bleeding gums. Protamine sulfate, a heparin antagonist, should be readily available.
11. Administer oral warfarin (Coumadin) once heparin is discontinued and assess for signs of bleeding during therapy.	**Rationale:** The client is placed on warfarin (Coumadin) therapy for 2 to 6 months at home. Signs of bleeding associated with warfarin therapy are similar to those while on heparin with the addition of rectal bleeding.
12. Educate client regarding self-care with warfarin (Coumadin) therapy at home.	**Rationale:** Warfarin (Coumadin) is an anticoagulant and may cause side effects such as excessive bleeding. Instruct client to carry a MedicAlert card indicating she is on anticoagulant therapy and to routinely check body for bruising. The use of an electric razor and a soft toothbrush should be used to minimize the chance for bleeding. The client should avoid alcohol intake; certain herbs such as ginger, garlic, and ginkgo; and any other drugs without checking with a physician first. Discuss the need to have a consistent intake of foods high in vitamin K because these foods may affect the dose of warfarin and PT balance. To check for accurate dosage of warfarin (Coumadin) a prothrombin time (PT) should be taken periodically.

Evaluation of Client Goal	• No signs of edema or pain in lower extremities • Negative Homans' sign

CRITICAL THINKING QUESTIONS

1. The nurse is reviewing the prenatal medical history of a client who gave birth 3 days ago. The nurse finds a history of varices (enlarged veins) in the prenatal records. What would the nurse include in her assessment of this client? What treatment may be indicated?

Answer: The nurse would assess for superficial vein leg disease and inspect local tenderness in a portion of the vein, local heat, and redness. Vital signs may be altered; the client may have a normal to low-grade temperature and slight elevation in pulse that appears on day 3 or 4. Treatment may include application of local heat, elevation of the leg, bed rest, support stockings, and analgesics.

2. The nurse is providing discharge instructions to a breastfeeding mother who has been diagnosed with DVT. The nurse reviews the medication regime for DVT. The client asks why she is taking heparin. How will the nurse respond? Which anticoagulant is not recommended for breastfeeding?

Answer: Heparin is the better choice because it is not excreted in breast milk. Warfarin (Coumadin) is excreted in breast milk and may be a problem for the newborn; therefore, it is not recommended for breastfeeding mothers.

*For your reference, this care plan is an example of how one nursing diagnosis might be addressed.

Community-Based Nursing Care

Because the mother with postpartal thromboembolic disease will depend on others for much of her initial home care, it is helpful for the father of the newborn to be involved in preparations for discharge. The nurse should provide ample time to answer questions and clarify instructions, verbally and in writing. The nurse will evaluate the extent to which both the mother and father have understood instructions regarding the plan of care. It is especially important to assess the couple's plans to ensure complete bed rest for the mother. They might explore ways for her to maintain bed rest and still spend quality time with her newborn and any other children. For example, young children can sit on the bed for storytelling or play quiet games, and the newborn's crib can be placed next to the mother's bed.

The father/partner may be assuming multiple roles in these circumstances—household manager, parent, worker, and caregiver. Fatigue is inevitable. There may also be financial concerns as a result of prolonged health care or his extended time away from work to care for the family. Many concerns will not surface until the couple actually returns home and fully comprehends the reality of their situation. For that reason, it is valuable to provide them with an accessible resource person and to plan telephone or home visit follow-up care.

Signs of postpartum thrombophlebitis may not occur until after discharge from the birthing unit. Consequently all couples must be taught to recognize its signs and symptoms and appreciate the importance of reporting them immediately and not massaging the affected leg. If signs and symptoms occur after discharge, a short readmission may be required. In that case every effort is made to allow mother, father, and newborn to remain together.

Evaluation

Expected outcomes of nursing care include the following:

- The woman seeks treatment for her thrombophlebitis early and is managed successfully, without further complications.
- At discharge the woman is able to explain the purpose, dosage regimen, and necessary precautions associated with any prescribed medications such as anticoagulants.
- The woman can discuss the self-care measures and ongoing therapies (such as the use of elastic stockings) that are indicated.
- The woman has bonded successfully with her newborn and is able to care for her baby effectively.

Care of the Woman with a Postpartum Psychiatric Disorder

The relationship of affective disorders to childbirth is reflected in the fact that the rate of admission to a psychiatric hospital is greater during the year after childbirth than at any other time in a woman's life.

Types of Postpartum Psychiatric Disorders

The classification of postpartum psychiatric disorders is a subject of some controversy. The *Diagnostic and Statistical Manual of Mental Disorders* (APA, 2000) has added a postpartum onset specifier to the mood disorder diagnostic category of psychiatric disorders. It is proposed that postpartum psychiatric disorders be considered one diagnosable syndrome with three subclasses: (1) adjustment reaction with depressed mood, (2) postpartum psychosis, and (3) postpartum major mood disorder. The incidence, etiology, symptoms, treatment, and prognosis vary with each subclass.

Adjustment Reaction with Depressed Mood

Adjustment reaction with depressed mood is also known as **postpartum blues**, or as *maternal* or *"baby blues."* It occurs in as many as 50% to 80% of mothers and is characterized by mild depression interspersed with happier feelings (Beck, 2006). Postpartum blues typically occur within a few days after the baby's birth and are self-limiting, lasting from a few hours to 10 days or longer. The depression is more severe in primiparas than in multiparas and seems related to the rapid alteration of estrogen, progesterone, and prolactin levels after birth. New mothers experiencing postpartum blues commonly report feeling overwhelmed, unable to cope, fatigued, anxious, irritable, and oversensitive. A key feature is episodic tearfulness, often without an identifiable reason. Often, when the woman is asked why she is crying, she will respond that she does not know. Cunningham et al. (2005, p. 705) speculate that several factors contribute to the blues:

- Emotional letdown that follows labor and childbirth
- Physical discomfort typical in the early postpartum
- Fatigue
- Anxiety about caring for the newborn after discharge
- Fears about her physical attractiveness

Validating the existence of this phenomenon, labeling it as a real but normal adjustment reaction, and providing reassurance can offer a measure of relief. Assistance with self- and infant care, rest, good nutrition, information, and family support aids recovery. The partner should be encouraged to watch for and report signs that the new mother is not returning to a more normal mood but slipping into a deeper depression. Most affected women reported that they did not seek help because they felt their depression was caused by the stress of becoming a mother, thought it was a normal reaction, and/or feared that they would be labeled mentally ill and considered unfit mothers (Driscoll, 2008).

Postpartum Psychosis

Postpartum psychosis, which has an incidence of 1 to 2 per 1000, usually becomes evident within the first 1 to 3 months postpartum (Beck, 2006). Although relatively rare, new onset postpartum psychosis gains considerable national attention in the media when there is an incident of infanticide associated with it. Symptoms include agitation, hyperactivity, insomnia, mood lability, confusion, irrationality, difficulty remembering or concentrating, poor judgment, delusions, and hallucinations which tend to be related to the infant. With appropriate treatment, improvement is seen in 95% of women in 2 to 3 months. Surprisingly, it is not associated with depression during the antenatal period (Haessler & Rosenthal, 2007). Recurrence in subsequent pregnancies may be as high as 20% to 30%.

Postpartum psychosis is considered an emergency because of the risk of suicide and/or infanticide (Beck, 2006). The psychotic woman may experience delusions or hallucinations that support her perceptions that the infant should not be allowed to live. Illogical thinking or evidence of bonding difficulties may serve as cues to infanticide and suicide risk; however, this assessment is often challenging because of the lucidity seen in some psychotic clients.

Postpartum Major Mood Disorder

Postpartum major mood disorder, also known as **postpartum depression,** develops in about 3% to 30% of all postpartum women in North America (Beck & Driscoll, 2006). Although it may occur at any time during the first postpartum year, the periods of greatest risk occur around the fourth week, just before the initiation of menses, and upon weaning.

Risk factors for postpartum depression include the following:

- Primiparity
- Ambivalence about maintaining the pregnancy
- History of postpartum depression or bipolar illness
- Lack of social support
- Lack of a stable and supportive relationship with parents or partner
- Lack of a supportive relationship with her parents, especially her father, as a child

- The woman's dissatisfaction with herself, including body image problems and eating disorders

Women with postpartum depression are at risk for suicide, most prominently as they enter or exit the deeply depressed state. In a deep depression, the woman is unlikely to be able to plan and carry out suicide. For that reason, signs of improvement in depression should be celebrated with some caution. Whereas the woman with postpartal psychosis may attempt suicide because of illogical thought processes, the woman with major depression attempts suicide because her suffering is so great that dying seems a more favorable option than continuing to live in such pain. She may also attempt suicide to save her newborn from some perceived or real threat—including the possibility that she herself might harm the baby. The risk of suicide is greater in those who have attempted suicide previously, have a specific plan, and can access the means or weapon identified within the plan. The more specific the plan, the greater is the probability of an attempt.

Clinical Therapy

Women with a history of postpartum psychosis or depression or other risk factors should be referred to a mental health professional for counseling and biweekly visits between the second and sixth week postpartum for evaluation. Medication, individual or group psychotherapy, and practical assistance with child care and other demands of daily life are common treatment measures for both disorders; however, the specific therapies used may vary.

Treatment of postpartum depression is not unlike treatment of any significant depression: psychotherapy and antidepression medications, usually the selective serotonin reuptake inhibitors. Based on an expert consensus guideline for breastfeeding mothers, it is recommended that sertraline (e.g., Zoloft, Lustral) be the first-line treatment for PPD and paroxetine (e.g., Paxil, Seroxat, Deroxat) as an alternative first-line treatment (Beck, 2008). It is recommended that a combination of antidepressants and psychosocial interventions be used regardless of whether the woman is breastfeeding. It is important to realize that many of the drugs used in treating postpartum psychiatric conditions may be contraindicated in breastfeeding women. Fluoxetine (e.g., Prozac, Sarafem) is not recommended for lactating women because of its long half-life (Beck, 2008). Some of the antidepressive drugs have been linked to an increase in congenital defects so birth control use should also be emphasized. The woman and her partner should be reminded that antidepressants may take several weeks to have an effect. Providers may prefer to start antidepressants before the birth of the baby (usually started at 36 weeks of gestation) so that a therapeutic blood level is achieved before the birth of the baby.

Support groups have proved to be successful adjuncts to such treatment. Within a support group of postpartal women and their partners, a couple may feel consolation that they are not alone in their experience. Moreover, the group provides a forum for exchanging information about postpartum depression, learning stress reduction measures, and experiencing renewed self-esteem and support. The most effective support groups provide for safe child care to facilitate attendance. If a support group is not available locally, the woman and her family may be encouraged to contact Depression after Delivery (DAD), now a national Web-based support network that provides education and volunteers, or Postpartum Support International. The Mills Depression and Anxiety Symptom-Feeling Checklist is also available online.

Treatment of postpartum psychosis is directed at the specific type of psychotic symptoms displayed and may include lithium, antipsychotics, or electroconvulsive therapy in combination with psychotherapy, removal of the infant, and social support. It is important for the nurse to realize that many of the drugs used in treating postpartum psychiatric conditions are contraindicated in breastfeeding women.

Nursing Care Management

Nursing Assessment and Diagnosis

Assessment for factors predisposing a client to postpartal depression or psychosis should begin prenatally (Beck, 2002). Questions designed to detect problems can be included as part of the routine prenatal history interview or questionnaire. Women with a personal or family history of psychiatric disease, particularly postpartum depression or psychosis, need prenatal instructions on the signs and symptoms of depression and may need additional emotional support. Ideally a depression assessment should be completed each trimester to update a pregnant woman's risk status (Beck, 2002). If not done previously, the nurse assesses the woman for predisposing factors during labor and the postpartum stay. Several depression scales are available for assessing postpartum depression. The routine use of a screening tool in a matter-of-fact approach significantly increases the diagnosis. The Edinburgh Postnatal Depression Scale (Table 33–8) is the most widely used screening tool for postpartum depression in large populations of women. The tool has been validated, computerized, and used in telephone screening. Mothers who score above 12 on the Edinburgh Postpartum Depression Scale are likely to be suffering from postpartum depression. Another tool is Beck's (2002) revised Postpartum Depression Predictors Inventory (PDPI-revised). This tool is also a practical and simple screening checklist to use during routine care with all postpartum women to identify those who might be experiencing postpartum depression so that early management might be initiated (Table 33–9).

TABLE 33–8	Edinburgh Postnatal Depression Scale

In the past 7 days:

1. I have been able to laugh and see the funny side of things.
As much as I always could
Not quite so much now
Definitely not so much now
Not at all

2. I have looked forward with enjoyment of things.
As much as I ever did
Rather less than I used to
Definitely less than I used to
Hardly at all

***3.** I have blamed myself unnecessarily when things went wrong.
Yes, most of the time
Yes, some of the time
Not very often
No, never

4. I have been anxious or worried for no good reason.
No, not at all
Hardly ever
Yes, sometimes
Yes, very often

***5.** I have felt scared or panicky for no very good reason.
Yes, quite a lot
Yes, sometimes
No, not much
No, not at all

***6.** Things have been getting on top of me.
Yes, most of the time I haven't been able to cope at all
Yes, sometimes I haven't been coping as well as usual
No, I have been coping quite well
No, I have been coping as well as ever

***7.** I have been so unhappy that I have had difficulty sleeping.
Yes, most of the time
Yes, sometimes
Not very often
No, not at all

***8.** I have felt sad or miserable.
Yes, most of the time
Yes, quite often
Not very often
No, not at all

***9.** I have been so unhappy that I have been crying.
Yes, most of the time
Yes, quite often
Only occasionally
No, never

***10.** The thought of harming myself has occurred to me.
Yes, quite often
Sometimes
Hardly ever
Never

Note: Response categories are scored 0, 1, 2, and 3 according to increased severity of the symptoms. Items marked with an asterisk are reverse-scored (3, 2, 1,0). The total score is calculated by adding together the scores for each of the 10 items. A score above the threshold of 12 to 13 out of 30 indicates with 86% sensitivity that the woman is suffering from postpartum depression. *Source:* Cox, J. L., Holden, J. M., & Sagovsky, R. (1987). Detection of postnatal depression: Development of the 10-item Edinburgh Postnatal Depression Scale. *British Journal of Psychiatry, 150,* 782–786. Users may reproduce the scale without further permission provided they respect copyright by quoting the names of the authors, the title, and the source of the paper in all reproduced copies.

TABLE 33–9	Postpartum Depression Predictors Inventory (PDPI)—Revised and Guide Questions for Its Use

During Pregnancy

Marital status

	Check One
1. Single	o
2. Married/cohabitating	o
3. Separated	o
4. Divorced	o
5. Widowed	o
6. Partnered	o

Socioeconomic status

Low	o
Middle	o
High	o

Self-esteem

	Yes	No
Do you feel good about yourself as a person?	o	o
Do you feel worthwhile?	o	o
Do you feel you have a number of good qualities as a person?	o	o

Prenatal depression

	Yes	No
1. Have you felt depressed during your pregnancy?	o	o
If yes, when and how long have you been feeling this way?		
If yes, how mild or severe would you consider your depression?		

Prenatal anxiety

	Yes	No
Have you been feeling anxious during your pregnancy?	o	o
If yes, how long have you been feeling this way?		

Unplanned/unwanted pregnancy

	Yes	No
Was the pregnancy planned?	o	o
Is the pregnancy unwanted?	o	o

History of previous depression

	Yes	No
1. Before this pregnancy, have you ever been depressed?	o	o
If yes, when did you experience this depression?		
If yes, have you been under a physician's care for this past depression?	o	o
If yes, did the physician prescribe any medication for your depression?	o	o

Social support

	Yes	No
1. Do you feel you receive adequate emotional support from your partner?	o	o
2. Do you feel you receive adequate instrumental support from your partner (e.g., help with household chores or baby-sitting)?	o	o
3. Do you feel you can rely on your partner when you need help?	o	o
4. Do you feel you can confide in your partner? (repeat same questions for family and again for friends)	o	o

Marital satisfaction

	Yes	No
1. Are you satisfied with your marriage (or living arrangement)?	o	o
2. Are you currently experiencing any marital problems?	o	o
3. Are things going well between you and your partner?	o	o

Life stress

1. Are you currently experiencing any stressful events in your life such as:

	Yes	No
Financial problems	o	o
Marital problems	o	o
Death in the family	o	o
Serious illness in the family	o	o
Moving	o	o
Unemployment	o	o
Job change	o	o

TABLE 33–9	Postpartum Depression Predictors Inventory (PDPI)—Revised and Guide Questions for Its Use *(Continued)*		

After Delivery, Add the Following Items

Childcare stress	**Yes**	**No**
1. Is your infant experiencing any health problems?	o	o
2. Are you having problems with your baby feeding?	o	o
3. Are you having problems with your baby sleeping?	o	o

Infant temperament		
1. Would you consider your baby irritable or fussy?	o	o
2. Does your baby cry a lot?	o	o
3. Is your baby difficult to console or soothe?	o	o

Maternity blues		
1. Did you experience a brief period of tearfulness and mood swings during the 1st week after delivery?	o	o

Comments:

Source: AWHONN. (2002). Beck, C. T. Revision of the Postpartum Predictors Inventory. *Journal of Obstetric, Gynecologic, and Neonatal Nursing, 31*(4), 394–402 (Table 2 on PDPI, pp. 399–400). Washington, DC: Author. © 2002 by the Association of Women's Health, Obstetric and Neonatal Nurses. All rights reserved.

No matter what approach the nurse uses to assess for postpartum depression, enabling the woman's voice to be heard about her feelings of maternal role transition and how she is adjusting in this vulnerable time is of inestimable value (Beck, 2008). Listening to her story provides a critical emic (insider's) view of her circumstances as opposed to an etic (outsider's) view.

In providing daily care, the nurse observes the woman for objective signs of depression—anxiety, irritability, poor concentration, forgetfulness, sleep difficulties, appetite change, fatigue, and tearfulness—and listens for statements indicating feelings of failure and self-accusation. Severity and duration of symptoms should be noted. Behavior and verbalizations that are bizarre or seem to indicate a potential for violence against herself or others, including the infant, are reported as soon as possible for further evaluation.

The nurse needs to be aware that many normal physiologic changes of the puerperium are similar to symptoms of depression (lack of sexual interest, appetite change, fatigue). It is essential that observations be as specific and as objective as possible and that they are carefully documented. Beck and Indman (2005) found that anxiety was a prominent feature of illness for some women and suggested that women be assessed for their level of anxiety, particularly regarding infant care. Because of the strong association of interrupted sleep and postpartum depression and the finding that severe fatigue was an excellent predictor of postpartum depression (Corwin, Brownstead, Barton et al., 2005), assessing fatigue level at 2 weeks postpartum by telephone may be helpful in predicting depression risk early. Restorative sleep improves one's ability to cope and make decisions, thereby producing a sense of

better self-control. A central challenge for nursing is identifying women at risk of suicide. Family members of the depressed woman should also be alert to signals that she may be intent on self-harm; they must be advised that threats should always be taken seriously. Family members should be told to be especially vigilant for suicide when the woman seems to be feeling better.

Possible nursing diagnoses that may apply to a woman with a postpartum psychiatric disorder include the following:

- *Ineffective Individual Coping* related to postpartum depression
- *Risk for Altered Parenting* related to postpartal mental illness
- *Risk for Violence* against self (suicide), newborn, and other children related to depression

Nursing Plan and Implementation

Nurses working in antepartal settings or teaching childbirth classes play indispensable roles in helping prospective parents appreciate the lifestyle changes and role demands associated with parenthood. Offering realistic information and anticipatory guidance and debunking myths about the perfect mother or perfect newborn may help prevent postpartum depression. Social support teaching guides are available for nurses to help postpartum women explore their needs for postpartum support.

The nurse should alert the mother, spouse, and other family members to the possibility of postpartum blues in the early days after birth and reassure them of the short-term nature of the condition. Symptoms of postpartum

EVIDENCE-BASED PRACTICE

Prevention, Identification, and Intervention for Postpartum Depression

Clinical Questions

How can the risk of postpartum depression be identified early in a pregnancy? What is the most effective way to prevent postpartum depression? When it occurs, how can it be treated?

The Evidence

Postpartum depression is a serious condition that occurs in the first twelve weeks after birth; approximately 13% of new mothers will experience it. Untreated, the condition may have consequences for mothers, infants, and their families. It often goes undetected, as symptoms may be hidden or misinterpreted. A team of advanced practice nurses developed recommendations for AWHONN, the professional association for nurses practicing in women's and neonatal health. Their recommendations focused on identification and prevention of depression and were based on a systematic review of research and expert opinion. Other evidence included a meta-analysis of studies focused on effective treatment of postnatal depression. This type of integrative review provides the strongest evidence for practice.

What Is Effective?

The strongest evidence supported individualized, flexible postpartum care that focused on the identification of risk for depression and/or signs of depression early in the pregnancy. Routine screening for depression should be part of the prenatal and post-natal assessment. The best outcomes are achieved when early preventive strategies accompany depression screening. When depression symptoms appear, supportive weekly interactions and ongoing assessment focused on mental health needs should be part of the routine postnatal treatment plan. Peer support, via technology or group delivery, can help mediate depressive symptoms and encourage

problem solving. Standard instruments should be used to identify mothers who are at risk for depression so that they can be referred to their primary care physician or a specialist in mental health for treatment.

What Is Inconclusive?

The best screening tool for depression during the peri-natal period was not definitively recommended. Several tools were used in these studies to determine risk of depression. Although various methods were shown to be effective in treating postnatal depression, no one therapy emerged as a definitive treatment.

Best Practice

Nurses are in a particularly good position to screen mothers for depression during the prenatal period and for at least 12 weeks after birth. You should use a standard instrument for screening at each encounter, and increased risk of depression should be cause for referral to a medical provider. Early detection and prevention will produce better outcomes for the mother, baby, and family. Diverse treatments—both pharmaceutical and counseling-based—have been shown to be effective in mediating the symptoms of depression. The treatment program should be matched to the specific patient characteristics and needs.

References

Bledsoe, S., & Grote, N. (2006). Treating depression during pregnancy and the postpartum: A preliminary meta-analysis. *Research on Social Work Practice, 16*, 109–120.

McQueen, K., Montgomery, P., Lappan-Gracon, S., Evans, M., & Hunter, J. 2008. Evidence-based recommendations for depressive symptoms in postpartum women. *JOGNN: Journal of Obstetric, Gynecologic, and Neonatal Nursing, 37*, 127–136.

---

depression should be described and the mother encouraged to call her healthcare provider if symptoms become severe, if they fail to subside quickly, or if at any time she feels she is unable to function. Encouraging the mother to plan how she will manage at home and providing concrete suggestions on how to cope aid in her adjustment to motherhood. Table 33–10 provides suggestions that serve as primary prevention measures for postpartum depression.

Community-Based Nursing Care

Home visits, especially for early-discharge families, are essential to fostering positive adjustments for the new family constellation. Telephone follow-up at 2 to 3 weeks postpartum to ask whether the mother is experiencing difficulties is also helpful. If a mother calls with a seemingly innocuous question, she should be asked two or three open-ended questions about her general status (Katz, 2007). These questions allow the woman to open up if

there is an underlying depression that she is too guilty/afraid to express initially; for example:

1. How do you feel things are going?
2. How are things going?
3. Are you feeling like you expected?

Monitoring for signs of depression or performing brief screening at well-child follow-ups also can be valuable for early identification and timely intervention (Katz, 2007).

In all women, the presence of three symptoms of depression on one day or one symptom for 3 days may signal serious depression and requires immediate referral to a mental health professional. Immediate referral should also be made if rejection of the infant or threatened or actual aggression against the infant has occurred. In such cases the newborn is never left unattended with the mother. Depression does appear to interfere with optimal mothering; there is less interaction between mother and

TABLE 33–10 Primary Prevention Strategies for Postpartum Depression

1. Celebrate childbirth but appreciate that it is a life-changing transition that can be stressful—at times it can seem overwhelming. Share your feelings with each other and/or others.
2. Consider keeping a journal where you write down feelings. Not only is it emotionally cathartic, it provides a great memory book.
3. Appreciate that you do not have to know everything to be a good parent—it is okay to seek advice during this transition.
4. Connect to others who are parents—use them as a support and information network.
5. Set a daily schedule and follow it even if you do not feel like it. Structuring activity helps counteract inertia that comes with feeling sad or unsettled.
6. Prioritize daily tasks. Decide what must be done and what can wait. Try to get one major thing done every day. Remember, you do not always have to look like a magazine fashion model.
7. Remember that you do not have to entertain or care for everyone who drops by. Doing something for someone else, however, often tends to make you feel better.
8. If someone volunteers to help you with tasks or baby care, take him or her up on it. While your volunteer is in action, do something pleasurable or get some rest.
9. Maintain outside interests. Plan some time every day—even if it's just 15 minutes—to do something exclusively for "you" that is pleasurable.
10. Eat a healthful diet. Limit alcohol. Quit smoking. Get some exercise. (All of these can positively affect the immune system.)
11. Get as much sleep as possible. Rest whenever you can, such as when the baby is napping. If you have other young children, bring them onto your bed to read or play quietly while you lie down.
12. Limit major changes (moves, job changes, etc.) the first year insofar as possible.
13. Spend time with others.
14. If things get overwhelming, and you feel yourself slipping into depression, reach out to someone for help.
15. Attend a postpartum support group if one is available. Consider also an international program such as Postpartum Support International, 927 North Kellogg Avenue, Santa Barbara, CA 93111, 1-805-967-7636 or online at http://www.postpartum.net

child, an increased incidence of mood and cognitive development problems, and more visits to the doctor in these children (Beck, 2002).

A diagnosis of postpartum depression or other psychiatric disorder poses major problems for the family, especially the father. The symptoms of these disorders are difficult to witness and may be harder to understand than physical problems such as hemorrhage and infection. The father may feel hurt by his partner's hostility, worry that she is becoming insane, or be baffled by her mood swings and lack of concern about herself, the newborn, or household responsibilities. He may be troubled by their lack of intimacy or deteriorating communication. Certainly, he has cause for concern about how the newborn and any other children are being affected. Very real practical matters—running the household; managing the children, including the totally dependent newborn; and caring for the mother—may be added to his usual routines and work responsibilities. It is not surprising that, even in the most supportive families, relationships may suffer in response to these circumstances. It is often the father or another close family member who in desperation makes contact with the healthcare agency. This is especially difficult when the mother is reluctant to admit she is suffering emotional difficulty or is too ill to recognize her own needs. The integration of the newborn into the family and care of the new-born and other children can be further compromised by co-occurrent postpartum depression in fathers. An examination of research studies that cite incidences of paternal postpartum depression indicate 24% to 50% incidence of depression among men whose partners were experiencing postpartum depression (Goodman, 2004).

Information, emotional support, and assistance in providing or obtaining care for the infant may be needed. The nurse can assist family members by identifying community resources, making referrals to public health nursing services and social services, and providing a list of telephone numbers as well as emergency services that she may need. Postpartum follow-up is especially important, as well as visits from a psychiatric home health nurse.

Evaluation

Expected outcomes of nursing care include the following:

- The woman's signs of depression are identified and she receives therapy quickly.
- The newborn is cared for effectively by the father or another support person until the mother is able to provide care.
- The mother and newborn will remain safe.
- The newborn is integrated into the family.

CHAPTER HIGHLIGHTS

- Nursing assessment and intervention play a large role in preventing postpartal complications.
- The main causes of early postpartal hemorrhage are uterine atony, lacerations of the vagina and cervix, and retained placental fragments. Late postpartum hemorrhage most often originates from retained placental fragments and, though not usually as catastrophic as early hemorrhage, may require readmission.
- The most common postpartal infection is metritis, which is limited to the uterine cavity.
- A postpartal woman is at increased risk for developing urinary tract problems caused by normal postpartal diuresis, increased bladder capacity, decreased bladder sensitivity from stretching or trauma, and, possibly, inhibited neural control of the bladder following the use of anesthetic agents.
- Mastitis is an inflammation of the breast often caused by *Staphylococcus, Escherichia coli,* and *Streptococcus species.* Mastitis is primarily seen in breastfeeding women. Symptoms seldom occur before the second to fourth week after birth. Continuation of breastfeeding is recommended as part of the treatment.

- Thromboembolic disease originating in the veins of the leg, thigh, or pelvis may occur in the antepartum or postpartum periods and carries with it the potential for creating a life-threatening pulmonary embolus.
- Although many different types of psychiatric problems may be encountered in the postpartal period, postpartum blues is the most common. Postpartum blues episodes occur frequently in the week after childbirth and are typically transient.
- Risk factors for postpartum depression and postpartum psychosis should be screened for each trimester during pregnancy and during the immediate postpartal period. Nurses should be alert to the risk of suicide and infanticide in cases of severe postpartum depression or psychosis.
- Telephone calls and home visits are effective measures for extending comprehensive care into the home setting of the postpartal family at risk. Support groups in which child care is available also can be an invaluable community service by professional nurses.

PEARSON

EXPLORE **mynursingkit**™

MyNursingKit is your one stop for online chapter review materials and resources. Prepare for success with additional NCLEX®-style practice questions, interactive assignments and activities, web links, animations and videos, and more!

Register your access code from the front of your book at
www.mynursingkit.com

CHAPTER REFERENCES

American Academy of Pediatrics (AAP), Committee on Fetus and Newborn, & American College of Obstetricians and Gynecologists (ACOG), Committee on Obstetrics. (2007). *Guidelines for perinatal care* (6th ed.). Evanston, IL: Author.

American College of Obstetricians and Gynecologists. (2006). *Postpartum hemorrhage* (Practice Bulletin No. 76). Washington, DC: Author.

American Psychiatric Association (APA). (2000). *Diagnostic and statistical manual of mental disorders: DSM-IV-TR* (4th ed., text rev.). Washington, DC: Author.

Beck, C. T. (2002). Revision of the Postpartum Depression Predictors Inventory. *Journal of Obstetric, Gynecologic, and Neonatal Nursing, 31* (4), 394–402.

Beck, C. T. (2006). Postpartum depression: It isn't just the blues. *American Journal of Nursing, 106* (5), 40–51.

Beck, C. T. (2008). Postpartum mood and anxiety disorders: Case studies, research, and nursing

care. (Practice Bulletin) (2nd ed.). Washington, DC: Association of Women's Health, Obstetric and Neonatal Nurses.

Beck, C. T., & Driscoll, J. W. (2006). *Postpartum mood and anxiety disorders: A clinician's guide.* Sudbury, MA: Jones and Bartlett Publishers.

Beck, C. T., & Indman, P. (2005). The many faces of depression. *Journal of Obstetric, Gynecologic, and Neonatal Nursing, 34* (5), 569–576.

Chelmow, D., Aronson, M. P., & Wosu, U. (2007). Intraoperative and postoperative complications of gynecologic surgery. In A. H. DeCherney, L. Nathan, T. M. Goodwin, & N. Laufer (Eds.), *Current obstetric & gynecologic: Diagnosis & treatment* (10th ed., pp. 779–796). New York: Lange Medical Books/McGraw-Hill.

Corwin, E. J., Brownstead, J., Barton, N., Heckard, S., & Merin, K. (2005). The impact of fatigue on the development of postpartum depression. *Journal of Obstetric, Gynecologic, and Neonatal Nursing, 34* (5), 577–586.

Crowther, M., & McCourt, K. (2005). Venous thrombolism: A guide to prevention and

treatment. *The Nurse Practitioner, 30* (8), 26–29, 32–34, 45.

Cunningham, F. G., Gant, N. F., Leveno, K. J., Gilstrap, L. C., III, Hauth, J. C., & Wenstrom, K. D. (2005). *Williams obstetrics* (22nd ed.). New York: McGraw-Hill.

Davies, J. K., & Gibbs, R. S. (2008). Obstetrics and perinatal infections. In R. S. Gibbs, B. Y. Karlan, A. F. Haney, & Nygaard, I. (Eds.), *Danforth's obstetrics and gynecology* (10th ed., pp. 340–364). Philadelphia: Lippincott Williams & Wilkins.

Driscoll, J. W. (2008). Psychosocial adaptation to pregnancy and postpartum. In K. R. Simpson & P. A. Creehan, *AWHONN perinatal nursing* (3rd ed., pp. 78–87). Philadelphia, PA: Lippincott Williams & Wilkins.

Duff, P. (2007). Maternal and perinatal infection—Bacterial. In S. G. Gabbe, J. R. Niebyl, & J. L. Simpson (Eds.), *Obstetrics: Normal and problem pregnancies* (5th ed., pp. 1233–1248). Philadelphia, PA: Churchill Livingstone/Elsevier.

Gibbs, R. S., Sweet, R. L., & Duff, W. P. (2004). Maternal and fetal infectious disorders. In R. K. Creasy & R. Resnik (Eds.), *Maternal-fetal medicine: Principles and practice* (5th ed., pp. 741–800). Philadelphia: Saunders.

Gilbert, E. S. (2007). *Manual of high risk pregnancy and delivery* (4th ed.). St. Louis, MO: Mosby.

Goodman, J. H. (2004). Paternal postpartum depression, its relationship to maternal postpartum depression, and implications for family health. *Journal of Advanced Nursing, 45* (1), 26–35.

Haessler, A., & Rosenthal, M. B. (2007). Psychological aspects of obstetrics & gynecology. In A. H. DeCherney, L. Nathan, T. M. Goodwin, & N. Laufer (Eds.), *Current obstetric & gynecologic: Diagnosis & treatment* (10th ed., pp. 1003–1024). New York: Lange Medical Books/McGraw-Hill.

James, D. C. (2008). Postpartum care. In K. R. Simpson & P. A. Creehan, *AWHONN perinatal nursing* (3rd ed., pp. 473–526). Philadelphia, PA: Lippincott Williams & Wilkins.

Katz, V. L. (2007). Postpartum care. In S. G. Gabbe, J. R. Niebyl, & J. L. Simpson (Eds.), *Obstetrics: Normal and problem pregnancies* (5th ed., pp. 566–585). Philadelphia, PA: Churchill Livingstone/Elsevier.

Krakow, D. (2008). Medical and surgical complications of pregnancy. In R. S. Gibbs, B. Y. Karlan, A. F. Haney, & Nygaard, I. (Eds.), *Danforth's obstetrics and gynecology* (10th ed., pp. 276–312). Philadelphia: Lippincott Williams & Wilkins.

Mass, S. (2004). Breast pain: Engorgement, nipple pain and mastitis. *Clinical Obstetrics and Gynecology, 47* (3), 676–682.

Newton, E. R. (2007). Breastfeeding. In S. G. Gabbe, J. R. Niebyl, & J. L. Simpson (Eds.), *Obstetrics: Normal and problem pregnancies* (5th ed., pp. 586–615). Philadelphia, PA: Churchill Livingstone/Elsevier.

Pettker, C. M., & Lockwood, C. J. (2007). Thromboembolic disorders. In S. G. Gabbe, J. R. Niebyl, & J. L. Simpson (Eds.), *Obstetrics: Normal and problem pregnancies* (5th ed.,

pp. 1064–1080). Philadelphia, PA: Churchill Livingstone/Elsevier.

Poggi, S. B. H. (2007). Postpartum hemorrhage & the abnormal puerperium. In A. H. DeCherney, L. Nathan, T. M. Goodwin, & N. Laufer (Eds.), *Current obstetric & gynecologic: Diagnosis & treatment* (10th ed., pp. 477–497). New York: Lange Medical Books/McGraw-Hill.

Rebarker, A., & Roman, A. S. (2003, March). Seven ways to control postpartum hemorrhage. *Contemporary OB/GYN, 48* (3), 34–53.

Reid, G., & Bocking, A. (2003). The potential for probiotics to prevent bacterial vaginosis and preterm labor. *American Journal of Obstetrics & Gynecology, 189* (4), 1202–1208.

Wiener, S. (2006). Diagnosis and management of Candida of the nipple and breast. *Journal of Midwifery Womens Health, 51* (2), 125–128.

Yip, S. K., Shota, D., Pang, M. W., & Day, L. (2005). Postpartum urinary retention. *Obstetrics and Gynecology, 106* (3), 602–606.

Appendices

Appendix A

Common Abbreviations in Maternal-Newborn and Women's Health Nursing

AC	Abdominal circumference		**CRNP**	Certified registered nurse practitioner
accel	Acceleration of fetal heart rate		**C/S**	Cesarean section (or C-section)
AFAFP	Amniotic fluid alpha-fetoprotein		**CST**	Contraction stress test
AFI	Amniotic fluid index		**CT**	Chlamydia
AFP	Alpha-fetoprotein		**CVA**	Costovertebral angle
AFV	Amniotic fluid volume		**CVS**	Chorionic villus sampling
AGA	Average for gestational age		**D&C**	Dilatation and curettage
AI	Amnioinfusion		**D&E**	Dilatation and evacuation
AMOL	Active management of labor		**decels**	Deceleration of fetal heart rate
AOP	Apnea of prematurity *or* Anemia of prematurity		**DFMR**	Daily fetal movement response
			dil	Dilatation
ARBOW	Artificial rupture of bag of waters		**DTR**	Deep tendon reflexes
AROM	Artificial rupture of membranes		**DV**	Domestic violence
ART	Artificial reproductive technology		**EAB**	Elective abortion
BAT	Brown adipose tissue (brown fat)		**ECMO**	Extracorporeal membrane oxygenator
BBOW	Bulging bag of water		**EDB**	Estimated date of birth
BBT	Basal body temperature		**EDC**	Estimated date of confinement
ß-hCG	Beta-human chorionic gonadotropin		**EDD**	Estimated date of delivery
BL	Baseline (fetal heart rate baseline)		**EFM**	Electronic fetal monitoring
BOW	Bag of waters		**EFW**	Estimated fetal weight
BPD	Biparietal diameter *or* Bronchopulmonary dysplasia		**EIA**	Enzyme immunoassay
			ELF	Elective low forceps
BPP	Biophysical profile		**ELISA**	Enzyme-linked immunosorbent assay
BRB	Bright red bleeding *or* Breakthrough bleeding		**EP**	Ectopic pregnancy
BR CA	Breast cancer		**epis**	Episiotomy
BSE	Breast self-examination		**FAD**	Fetal activity diary
BSST	Breast self-stimulation test		**FAS**	Fetal alcohol syndrome
CC	Chest circumference *or* Cord compression		**FASD**	Fetal alcohol spectrum disorder
CEI	Continuous epidural infusion		**FBD**	Fibrocystic breast disease
C–H	Crown-to-heel length		**FBM**	Fetal breathing movements
CID	Cytomegalic inclusion disease		**FBS**	Fetal blood sample *or* Fasting blood sugar test
CLD	Chronic lung disease		**FCC**	Family-centered care
CM	Certified midwife		**FECG**	Fetal electrocardiogram
CMV	Cytomegalovirus		**FeSO₄**	Iron supplement
CNM	Certified nurse-midwife		**FHR**	Fetal heart rate
CNP	Certified nurse practitioner		**FHT**	Fetal heart tones
CNS	Clinical nurse specialist		**Fhx**	Family history
CP	Chest pain		**FL**	Femur length
CPAP	Continuous positive airway pressure		**FMC**	Fetal movement count
CPD	Cephalopelvic disproportion *or* Citrate-phosphate-dextrose		**FMR**	Fetal movement record
			FPG	Fasting plasma glucose test
CRL	Crown-rump length		**FSE**	Fetal scalp electrode

FSH	Follicle-stimulating hormone	**LOS**	Length of stay
FSHRH	Follicle-stimulating hormone-releasing hormone	**LOT**	Left-occiput-transverse
		L/S	Lecithin/sphingomyelin ratio
FSpO$_2$	Fetal arterial oxygen saturation	**LSA**	Left-sacrum-anterior
G or grav	Gravida	**LSP**	Left-sacrum-posterior
GC	Gonorrhea	**LST**	Left-sacrum-transverse
GDM	Gestational diabetes mellitus	**MAS**	Meconium aspiration syndrome
GIFT	Gamete intrafallopian transfer	**mec**	Meconium
GnRF	Gonadotropin-releasing factor	**mec st**	Meconium stain
GnRH	Gonadotropin-releasing hormone	**MLE**	Midline episiotomy
GTD	Gestational trophoblastic disease	**MSAFP**	Maternal serum alpha-fetoprotein
GTPAL	Gravida, term, preterm, abortion, living children; a system of recording maternity history	**MUGB**	4-methylumbelliferyl quanidinobenzoate
		multip	Multipara
HA	Head-abdominal ratio or headache	**NEC**	Necrotizing enterocolitis
HAI	Hemagglutination-inhibition test	**NGU**	Nongonococcal urethritis
HC	Head compression	**NP**	Nurse practitioner
hCG	Human chorionic gonadotropin	**NSCST**	Nipple stimulation contraction stress test
hCS	Human chorionic somatomammotropin (same as hPL)	**NST**	Nonstress test or Nonshivering thermogenesis
		NSVD	Normal sterile vaginal delivery
HIV	Human immunodeficiency virus	**NTD**	Neural tube defects
HMD	Hyaline membrane disease	**NTE**	Neutral thermal environment
hMG	Human menopausal gonadotropin	**OA**	Occiput anterior
hPL	Human placental lactogen	**OC**	Oral contraceptives
HPV	Human papilloma virus	**OCPs**	Oral contraceptive pills
HRT	Hormone replacement therapy	**OCT**	Oxytocin challenge test
HSV	Herpes simplex virus	**OF**	Occipitofrontal diameter of fetal head
ICSI	Intracytoplasmic sperm injection	**OFC**	Occipitofrontal circumference
IDM	Infant of a diabetic mother	**OGTT**	Oral glucose tolerance test
IPG	Impedance phlebography	**OM**	Occipitomental (diameter)
ISAM	Infant of a substance-abusing mother	**OP**	Occiput posterior
IU	International units	**p**	Para
IUD	Intrauterine device	**Pap smear**	Papanicolaou smear
IUFD	Intrauterine fetal death	**PCA**	Patient-controlled analgesia
IUGR	Intrauterine growth restriction	**PDA**	Patent ductus arteriosus
IUPC	Intrauterine pressure catheter	**PEEP**	Positive end-expiratory pressure
IUS	Intrauterine system	**PG**	Phosphatidylglycerol or Prostaglandin
IVF	In vitro fertilization	**PID**	Pelvic inflammatory disease
LADA	Left-acromion-dorsal-anterior	**Pit**	Pitocin
LADP	Left-acromion-dorsal-posterior	**PKU**	Phenylketonuria
LBC	Lamellar body count	**PMS**	Premenstrual syndrome
LBW	Low birth weight	**PNV**	Prenatal vitamins
LDR	Labor, delivery, and recovery room	**PPHN**	Persistent pulmonary hypertension
LGA	Large for gestational age	**Premie**	Premature infant
LH	Luteinizing hormone	**primip**	Primipara
LHRH	Luteinizing hormone-releasing hormone	**PROM**	Premature rupture of membranes
LMA	Left-mentum-anterior	**PSI**	Prostaglandin synthesis inhibitor
LML	Left mediolateral (episiotomy)	**PUBS**	Percutaneous umbilical blood sampling
LMP	Last menstrual period or Left-mentum-posterior	**RADA**	Right-acromion-dorsal-anterior
		RADP	Right-acromion-dorsal-posterior
LMT	Left-mentum-transverse	**RDS**	Respiratory distress syndrome
LOA	Left-occiput-anterior	**REM**	Rapid eye movements
LOF	Low outlet forceps	**RIA**	Radioimmunoassay
LOP	Left-occiput-posterior	**RLF**	Retrolental fibroplasia

RMA	Right-mentum-anterior	**TAB**	Therapeutic abortion
RMP	Right-mentum-posterior	**TC**	Thoracic circumference
RMT	Right-mentum-transverse	**TCM**	Transcutaneous monitoring
ROA	Right-occiput-anterior	**TDI or THI**	Therapeutic donor insemination (*H* designates
ROM	Rupture of membranes		mate is donor)
ROP	Right-occiput-posterior *or* Retinopathy	**TET**	Tubal embryo transfer
	of prematurity	**TOL**	Trail of labor
ROT	Right-occiput-transverse	**TORCH**	Toxoplasmosis, rubella, cytomegalovirus,
RRA	Radioreceptor assay		herpesvirus hominis type 2
RSA	Right-sacrum-anterior	**TSS**	Toxic shock syndrome
RSP	Right-sacrum-posterior	**Ū**	Umbilicus
RST	Right-sacrum-transverse	**UA**	Uterine activity
SAB	Spontaneous abortion	**UAC**	Umbilical artery catheter
SET	Surrogate embryo transfer	**UAU**	Uterine activity units
SGA	Small for gestational age	**UC**	Uterine contraction
SIDS	Sudden infant death syndrome	**UPI**	Uteroplacental insufficiency
SMB	Submentobregmatic diameter	**US**	Ultrasound
SOB	Suboccipitobregmatic diameter *or* Shortness	**VBAC**	Vaginal birth after cesarean
	of breath	**VDRL**	Venereal Disease Research Laboratories
SPA	Sperm penetration assay	**VIP**	Voluntary interruption of pregnancy
SRBOW	Spontaneous rupture of bag of waters	**VLBW**	Very low birth weight
SROM	Spontaneous rupture of membranes	**VVC**	Vulvovaginal *candidiasis*
STD	Sexually transmitted disease	**WIC**	Supplemental food program for Women,
STI	Sexually transmitted infection		Infants, and Children
STS	Serologic test for syphilis	**ZIFT**	Zygote intrafallopian transfer
SVE	Sterile vaginal exam		

Appendix B

Conversions and Equivalents

TEMPERATURE CONVERSION
(Fahrenheit temperature − 32) × 5/9 = Centigrade temperature
(Centigrade temperature × 9/5) + 32 = Fahrenheit temperature

SELECTED CONVERSION TO METRIC MEASURES

Known Value	Multiply by	To Find
inches	2.54	Centimeters
ounces	28	Grams
pounds	454	Grams
pounds	0.45	kilogram

SELECTED CONVERSION FROM METRIC MEASURES

Known Value	Multiply by	To Find
centimeters	0.4	inches
grams	0.035	ounces
grams	0.0022	pounds
kilograms	2.2	pounds

CONVERSION OF POUNDS AND OUNCES TO GRAMS

Pounds	Ounces 0	1	2	3	4	5	6	7	8	9	10	11	12	13	14	15
0	—	28	57	85	113	142	170	198	227	255	283	312	340	369	397	425
1	454	482	510	539	567	595	624	652	680	709	737	765	794	822	850	879
2	907	936	964	992	1021	1049	1077	1106	1134	1162	1191	1219	1247	1276	1304	1332
3	1361	1389	1417	1446	1474	1503	1531	1559	1588	1616	1644	1673	1701	1729	1758	1786
4	1814	1843	1871	1899	1928	1956	1984	2013	2041	2070	2098	2126	2155	2183	2211	2240
5	2268	2296	2325	2353	2381	2410	2438	2466	2495	2523	2551	2580	2608	2637	2665	2693
6	2722	2750	2778	2807	2835	2863	2892	2920	2948	2977	3005	3033	3062	3090	3118	3147
7	3175	3203	3232	3260	3289	3317	3345	3374	3402	3430	3459	3487	3515	3544	3572	3600
8	3629	3657	3685	3714	3742	3770	3799	3827	3856	3884	3912	3941	3969	3997	4026	4054
9	4082	4111	4139	4167	4196	4224	4252	4281	4309	4337	4366	4394	4423	4451	4479	4508
10	4536	4564	4593	4621	4649	4678	4706	4734	4763	4791	4819	4848	4876	4904	4933	4961
11	4990	5018	5046	5075	5103	5131	5160	5188	5216	5245	5273	5301	5330	5358	5386	5415
12	5443	5471	5500	5528	5557	5585	5613	5642	5670	5698	5727	5755	5783	5812	5840	5868
13	5897	5925	5953	5982	6010	6038	6067	6095	6123	6152	6180	6209	6237	6265	6294	6322
14	6350	6379	6407	6435	6464	6492	6520	6549	6577	6605	6634	6662	6690	6719	6747	6776
15	6804	6832	6860	6889	6917	6945	6973	7002	7030	7059	7087	7115	7144	7172	7201	7228
16	7257	7286	7313	7342	7371	7399	7427	7456	7484	7512	7541	7569	7597	7626	7654	7682
17	7711	7739	7768	7796	7824	7853	7881	7909	7938	7966	7994	8023	8051	8079	8108	8136
18	8165	8192	8221	8249	8278	8306	8335	8363	8391	8420	8448	8476	8504	8533	8561	8590
19	8618	8646	8675	8703	8731	8760	8788	8816	8845	8873	8902	8930	8958	8987	9015	9043
20	9072	9100	9128	9157	9185	9213	9242	9270	9298	9327	9355	9383	9412	9440	9469	9497
21	9525	9554	9582	9610	9639	9667	9695	9724	9752	9780	9809	9837	9865	9894	9922	9950
22	9979	10007	10036	10064	10092	10120	10149	10177	10206	10234	10262	10291	10319	10347	10376	10404

Appendix C

Guidelines for Working with Deaf Clients and Interpreters

1. First, remember that it requires trust on the part of the client to allow nonsigning caregivers and an interpreter into her life.
2. It is important to use a registered interpreter. Medical interpreters are registered with the Registry of Interpreters for the Deaf. Although family members and friends may offer to interpret, it is best to use registered medical interpreters because they are required to translate the clients' and nurses' words accurately without adding in any other opinion.
3. Greet the client and family with a handshake and body posture that indicates welcome. You may point to your name tag and use the American Sign Language (ASL) alphabet cards to spell out your name. The client may wish to select cards to indicate her name. It is especially important as you work together to make the effort to provide a greeting as you would with speaking clients; greetings help develop rapport.
4. Once the interpreter is present, continue to look at the client and speak directly to her. There will be a temptation to look at the interpreter, and it will help to remember that you are speaking to the client.
5. Avoid phrasing your words as if you are talking to the interpreter (e.g., "Can you tell her . . . ?"). Instead, phrase your questions as you do with speaking clients (e.g., "I'm going to ask you some questions now.").
6. Depend on the deaf client to ask questions.
7. Look at the client's face for signs of difficulty in understanding. Deaf clients have a behavior of "gesturing" that involves shaking their heads as if to indicate "yes" even when they do not understand. If the client is nodding "yes," ask her to repeat the directions you have just given.
8. Be as direct as possible. Keep to what you want to know or what you want to convey. Speak in short sentences, using nontechnical words. Avoid colloquial or slang words. Be sure to explain what you want to do before you do it. For instance, tell her you want to start an IV and explain the equipment. Then, with her permission, start the IV.
9. Be aware that deaf clients may have difficulty understanding when to take medications. It will be helpful to associate taking medications or completing some treatment or activity with meals. (For instance, while showing her the two capsules she is to take when she goes home, tell her to take the two capsules at breakfast and another two capsules at bedtime.) Avoid saying, "Take two capsules at 8:00 A.M., 2:00 P.M., and 12:00 A.M."
10. The difference in interpreting time may also affect obtaining a history. It is best to begin with a specific event in the past and work forward.

What to Do Until the Interpreter Arrives

1. Role-play as much as possible.
2. Demonstrate what you want the client to do or what you want to do.
3. Be resourceful.
4. Remember that some deaf clients can read lips. Some may read written language, but use care in assuming the client understands.

What to Do to Prepare for Working with a Deaf Client

1. Contact local agencies that work with deaf clients to see what resources are available. Ask about classes in ASL. Being able to use some basic signs will be very helpful while waiting for an interpreter to arrive.
2. Read to learn more about the deaf culture. Contact your local agency or the National Information Center on Deafness, Silver Springs, Maryland, to get suggestions on books you might read.
3. Investigate your health facility. What is available to assist you? Look for videos used for teaching in the maternal-child unit and note if they have captions. Remember that many deaf clients do not read written language, so it will be important to review the content of the video with an interpreter present.

Prepared with the kind assistance of Mr. Gerald Dement, Interpreter Coordinator, Pikes Peak Center on Deafness, Colorado Springs, Colorado.

Sign Language for Healthcare Professionals

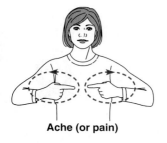

Ache (or pain)

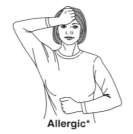

Allergic*

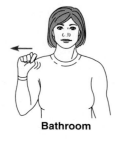

Bathroom

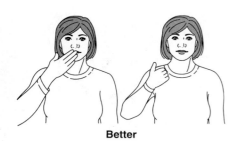

Better

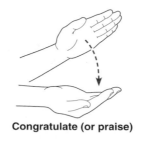

Congratulate (or praise)

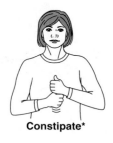

Constipate*

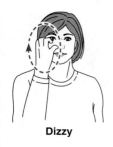

Dizzy

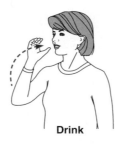

Drink

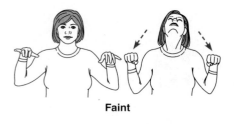

Faint

*Indicates signs that are in manually signed English. Those without an asterisk are in American Sign Language.

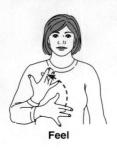

Feel

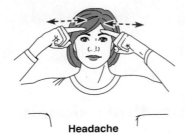

Headache

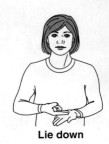

Lie down

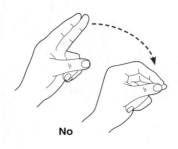

Medicine

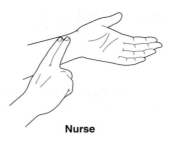

Name

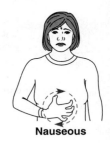

Nauseous

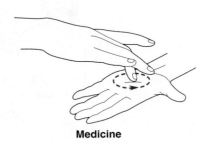

No

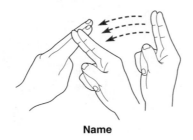

Nurse

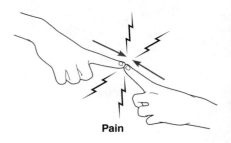

Pain

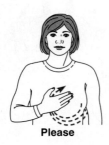

Please

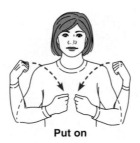

Put on

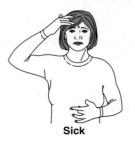

Sick

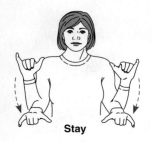

Stay

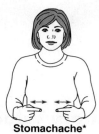

Stomachache*

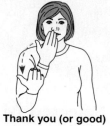

Thank you (or good)

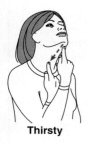

Thirsty

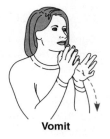

Vomit

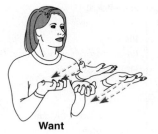

Want

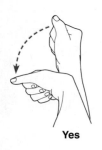

Yes

Appendix E

Selected Maternal-Newborn Laboratory Values

NORMAL MATERNAL LABORATORY VALUES

Test	Nonpregnant Values	Pregnant Values
Hematocrit	37% to 47%	32% to 42%
Hemoglobin	12 to 16 g/dL**	10 to 14 g/dL**
Platelets	150,000 to 350,000/mm³	Significant increase 3 to 5 days after birth (predisposes to thrombosis)
Partial thromboplastin time (PTT)	12 to 14 seconds	Slight decrease in pregnancy and again in labor (placental site clotting)
Fibrinogen	250 mg/dL	400 mg/dL
Serum glucose		
Fasting	70 to 80 mg/dL	65 mg/dL
2-hour postprandial	60 to 110 mg/dL	Less than 140 mg/dL
Total protein	6.7 to 8.3 g/dL	5.5 to 7.5 g/dL
White blood cell total	4500 to 10,000/mm³	5000 to 15,000/mm³
Polymorphonuclear cells	54% to 62%	60% to 85%
Lymphocytes	38% to 46%	15% to 40%

**At sea level

NORMAL TERM NEONATAL CORD BLOOD LABORATORY VALUES

Test	Normal Values
Hematocrit	43% to 63%*
Hemoglobin	14 to 20 g/dL
Platelets	150,000 to 350,000/mm³
Reticulocyte	3% to 7%
White blood cell total	10,000 to 30,000/mm³
White blood cell differential	
Polymorphonuclear (segs)	40% to 80%
Lymphocytes	20% to 40%
Monocytes	3% to 10%
Serum glucose	45 to 96 mg/dL*
Serum electrolytes	
Sodium	126 to 144 mEq/L*
Potassium	5.6 to 12.0 mEq/L*
Chloride	100 to 121 mEq/L*
Carbon dioxide	13 to 29 mmol/L
Bicarbonate	18 to 23 mEq/L
Calcium	8.2 to 11.1 mg/dL
Total protein	4.8 to 7.3 g/dL

Note: Adapted from Fanaroff, A. A., & Martin, R. J. (Eds.). (2006). *Neonatal-perinatal medicine* (8th ed.). Philadelphia, PA: Mosby.

*All laboratory values are approximate. Consult your local laboratory for guidelines as to normal values.

Suggested Answers to Critical Thinking Case Study Questions

Chapter 4 Conception and Fetal Development

She is correct that drugs may be teratogenic, but severe hyperthermia such as this (T 40°C [104°F]) is known to cause neural tube defects (spina bifida and anencephaly at this stage of gestation). Therefore, the healthcare provider must weigh the risk of teratogenicity of an antipyretic such as low-dose aspirin against the teratogenic potential of hyperthermia.

Chapter 5 Health Promotion for Women

Monique's concern about taking action beforehand eliminates the diaphragm, cervical cap, female condom, contraceptive sponge, and spermicides as options. Because she is interested in two men and little is known about their sexual histories, the IUD would not be a good choice even though it is reliable and its use is removed from the act of intercourse. Combined oral contraceptives (COCs) would be an excellent choice because Monique is a nonsmoker with no known contraindications. COCs remove contraception from coitus and are extremely reliable. Similarly, Monique might consider Lunelle® or Depo-Provera®, if she does not mind the injections.

Regardless of the method she chooses, it is important that you talk to Monique about requiring that any sexual partners use condoms. Condoms offer protection for both parties and are an important element in safe sex.

Chapter 6 Common Gynecologic Problems

The use of feminine hygiene products can result in vaginitis and actually promote sexually transmitted diseases, especially PID. Feminine hygiene products, especially douches, alter the acid-base balance of the vagina, allowing opportunistic organisms to replicate. Also, douching washes out the protective normal flora of the vagina, and the altered acid-base vaginal environment prevents the protective bacteria from growing. The action of douching can propel pathogenic organisms upward and promote an ascending infection such as PID. Ella should be told that douching is seldom necessary, and that cleansing daily with soap and water is an adequate hygienic measure. Ella should be told that she is at increased risk for PID because she has multiple sexual partners, uses an IUD, and douches. She should be counseled to consider other forms of contraceptives that are more protective against STIs and to consider limiting her sexual activity to a monogamous relationship.

Chapter 15 Pregnancy at Risk: Pregestational Problems

It is not unusual for women to be upset and frustrated with news that they may have newly diagnosed glucose intolerance during pregnancy. It has been described that women with gestational diabetes approach the new diagnosis as a crisis or anxiety-provoking situation. These women may experience more difficulty with coping and learning than do women with chronic diabetes who become pregnant.

It is important for the nurse to first assess the woman's knowledge about gestational diabetes before attempting to provide any teaching. The woman will benefit most from discussions that build on her current knowledge level. It will usually take several sessions to ensure that the new information is accurately understood and retained.

The nurse can reassure Mrs. Chang that the baby should be fine and can stress the importance of keeping her glucose levels in a normal range. Women with gestational diabetes may require treatment with diet therapy alone, or they may need insulin administration to control hyperglycemia.

It is believed that gestational diabetes does not cause birth defects because it occurs later in pregnancy, after the baby's organs are formed. The two most common risks to the baby are macrosomia, potentially causing a problem in labor and birth, and hypoglycemia.

Chapter 16 Pregnancy at Risk: Gestational Onset

This approach is not appropriate for Jena. Although it is unusual for a nonpregnant woman to develop pyelonephritis from a bladder infection, a significant number of pregnant women with bacteriuria develop cystitis or pyelonephritis unless their bladder infection is treated. This is related to the anatomic and physiologic changes of pregnancy, including decreased ureteral peristalsis, ureteral dilation, and increased bladder capacity. Because Jena is 6 months pregnant, she is probably being seen monthly for prenatal care. Because prompt treatment is essential, you should urge her to call her caregiver and discuss her symptoms.

Chapter 18 Intrapartal Nursing Assessment

We would encourage you to use creative ways to get the partner to leave the room, such as taking a child to the bathroom or getting some juice for the woman so you can interview her alone. It is best to first interview the woman by asking questions that are nonthreatening in nature, such as age, address, and basic demographic information, before moving to more personal information. Use this time to establish a trusting relationship and build rapport with the woman. Open communication using a nonjudgmental approach is essential in these types of situations. You could inform Lynn that domestic violence commonly occurs during pregnancy and that she is not to blame for her situation. Reinforce to her that all information she reveals is confidential. Reassure her that you are only asking to determine if she and her unborn baby are at additional risk.

Chapter 19 The Family in Childbirth: Needs and Care

Check the schedule to see if a female anesthesiologist will be available shortly. If not, advise the family that a male physician is the only anesthesiologist available at this time. Suggest that, if they decide to have the epidural, you will ensure Fatima is properly covered according to their instructions, and that you will avoid examinations while the male physician is in the room. Perform all assessments and procedures, such as urinary catheterization, Chux changes, and pericare before the male physician enters the room. Position Fatima appropriately for the procedure, draping her buttocks and ensuring she is properly covered. Allow her to put on a head covering if she prefers. Once the epidural has been placed, assist her in lying down, ensuring she is covered at all times. Allow Samir to remain in the room if he desires.

Chapter 20 Pharmacologic Management of Pain

We hope you would encourage her to take medication if she felt she needed it. There are many types of analgesic agents and many types of regional blocks that can help her if she decides she needs them. Sometimes, giving permission for someone to ask relieves her anxiety and decreases the need for interventions.

Chapter 22 Childbirth at Risk: Labor-Related Complications

Fetal head compression can occur as a result of advanced dilatation as the fetal head descends in the birth canal. It is also associated with decreased amniotic fluid which contributes to fetal head compression, which may result in the early FHR decelerations described. This type of deceleration is considered benign; no action is required. You may ask the woman if she is feeling rectal pressure and, if so, assess her for advanced dilatation by performing a vaginal examination. (As amniotic fluid levels decrease, the loss of fluid can also cause variable decelerations which require careful nursing assessment.)

Chapter 23 Birth-Related Procedures

Once uterine contractions reach the desired characteristics (frequency of every 2 to 3 minutes, duration of 40 to 60 seconds, and moderate to strong intensity), and cervical change is occurring, the infusion rate can be kept at the same rate. If hyperstimulation occurs (contractions occurring more than every 2 minutes without at least 1 minute of uterine relaxation in-between contractions), the rate should be decreased. If contractions become further apart with a decrease in intensity, frequency, or duration, the infusion rate should be increased.

Chapter 25 Nursing Assessment of the Newborn

The unique behavioral and temperamental characteristics of newborn infants should be discussed. Additionally, aspects of the Brazelton exam may be helpful to show Mrs. Reyes how her infant changes state with different stimuli and intervention. Teaching her how to console her newborn may also be helpful.

Chapter 26 Normal Newborn: Needs and Care

Though babies may make occasional cooing sounds, newborns tend to either cry or be silent. The nurse needs to immediately assess the situation as the "cute little noises" may be early signs of respiratory distress such as grunting.

Chapter 26 Normal Newborn: Needs and Care

Reassure Aisha that you will help her baby as you carry out the following activities.

- Position the infant with her head lowered and to the side.
- Bulb suction the nares and mouth repeatedly until the airway is cleared.
- Hold and comfort the infant when normal respirations are restored.
- Reassure Aisha and review this procedure with her.

Note: If bulb suctioning alone does not clear the airway, use DeLee wall suction and administer oxygen as needed to restore normal respirations.

Chapter 26 Normal Newborn: Needs and Care

We hope you would first examine the infant's genitalia and wipe between the labia to verify the source of bleeding. If there were no external lacerations, you would explain to the mother that a small amount of bleeding, called pseudomenstruation, sometimes occurs in newborn girls because of maternal hormone levels. This is considered normal and generally resolves in a few days. The tissue she observes is a vaginal skin tag, also a normal finding. It usually disappears in a few weeks.

Chapter 28 The Newborn at Risk: Conditions Present at Birth

We hope that you would tell her that nurses always wear gloves during the initial assessment of a newborn, during all admission procedures until the newborn has its first bath, and sometimes during diaper changes. You should also tell her that her baby will not be isolated from the other babies when in the nursery and that her baby can remain with her if she wishes. It is important to recognize the concern that Mrs. Corrigan may have about people knowing that her baby may have HIV and to assess her own feelings of social isolation.

Chapter 29 The Newborn at Risk: Birth-Related Stressors

It is important to give this mother clear, factual information regarding the type, cause, and usual course of the baby's respiratory problem. You see that Linn's laboratory tests, chest X-ray, and clinical course so far are indicative of transient tachypnea of the newborn. Respiratory distress syndrome is probably not the problem because Linn is not premature and did not have any asphyxia at birth. You recognize that prior experience with a premature newborn with respiratory distress and prolonged hospitalization will add to this mother's fear and anxiety regarding her new baby. Therefore, in addition to giving factual information regarding the baby's condition, it is important for you to see whether the mother can be brought to the nursery to see her baby or to have the mother receive a picture of the baby for reassurance. Before the mother visits the baby, clearly describe the oxygen and monitoring equipment that is helping Linn so that the mother will not be alarmed upon seeing her daughter.

Chapter 30 Postpartal Adaptation and Nursing Assessment

These findings are within the normal range. At 24 hours past the birth the fundus should be approximately one finger breadth below the umbilicus and located midline. A uterus that is deviated to the right may indicate that the bladder is full and Patty needs to urinate. You should determine whether she is having difficulty urinating and emptying her bladder; if so, you can try some nursing interventions to help her void. When the uterus is distended, the lochia will still be rubra, but the amount is excessive and may be related to a boggy uterus.

Chapter 31 The Postpartal Family: Needs and Care

Your best response would be, "You can only be discharged if both you and your practitioner feel you are ready. Federal law now states you can stay up to 4 days (96 hours) when you have had a cesarean birth."

Chapter 32 Home Care of the Postpartal Family

Acknowledge Ann's frustration and pain. Tell her you are glad she called and reassure her that this is a common occurrence and not an indication of breastfeeding failure. Let her express her feelings. Explain that her breasts are engorged, which is a problem many women encounter. It is not unusual for infants to refuse to nurse when the breast is hard and the nipple is difficult to grasp.

Identify methods to relieve engorgement:

a. Apply warm or cool soaks, whichever she prefers, for comfort and to stimulate letdown.

b. Instruct Ann on breast management to encourage letdown and to lessen the need for excessive suckling at the initiation of feedings.

c. Express a small amount of milk before latching the infant onto the breast.

d. Nurse the infant frequently.

e. Apply ice or intermittent cabbage leaves for a few minutes after feedings to decrease engorgement. (Do not leave cabbage leaves on for prolonged periods of time because this can dry up the milk.)

f. Use analgesics (if taken 20 to 30 minutes before feeding, the medication will have time to be effective).

Explain to Ann that her emotional state is probably because of the "baby blues" or "postpartum blues" and that these feelings usually subside in 24 to 72 hours. Instruct her to call her practitioner if the symptoms do not subside or if she develops symptoms of depression.

Ask Ann why she started supplemental feedings. Many women breastfeeding for the first time worry that their baby is not getting enough milk. If the mother's reply indicates a lack of information about breastfeeding, explain the following:

a. Breast milk digests faster than formula, so breastfeeding babies feed more frequently.

b. On average, babies nurse 8 to 12 times in 24 hours.

c. After lactation is well established, the baby will nurse less frequently. During growth spurts, however, all babies nurse more frequently for a few days.

Explain to Ann she may still breastfeed successfully, and if she desires to continue breastfeeding she should stop supplementing with formula.

Chapter 33 The Postpartal Family at Risk

You should have Wanda return to her room via wheelchair. Assess her leg for warmth, edema, redness, tenderness, and Homans' sign. Discuss with Wanda that she should not massage her leg or get out of bed until you consult with the primary provider concerning your findings. Notify her primary healthcare provider and document your assessment findings.

Glossary

Abdominal effleurage Gentle stroking used in massage.

Abortion Loss of pregnancy before the fetus is viable outside the uterus; miscarriage.

Abruptio placentae (ab-rŭp´shē-ō pla-sen´tē) Partial or total premature separation of a normally implanted placenta.

Abstinence Refraining voluntarily, especially from indulgence in food, alcoholic beverages, or sexual intercourse.

Acceleration Periodic increase in the baseline fetal heart rate.

Acculturation The process by which people adapt to a new cultural norm.

Acini cells Secretory cells in the human breast that create milk from nutrients in the bloodstream.

Acme Peak or highest point; time of greatest intensity (of a uterine contraction).

Acquaintance and date rape Rape in which the assailant is someone with whom the victim has had previous nonviolent interaction (acquaintance rape) or which occurs between a dating couple. Date rape is a form of acquaintance rape.

Acquired immunodeficiency syndrome (AIDS) An immunologic disorder caused by infection with the human immunodeficiency virus (HIV) and characterized by increasing susceptibility to opportunistic infections and rare cancers.

Acrocyanosis Cyanosis of the extremities.

Acrosomal reaction Breakdown of the hyaluronic acid in the corona radiata by enzymes from the heads of sperm; allows one spermatozoon to penetrate the ovum zona pellucida.

Active acquired immunity Formation of antibodies by the pregnant woman in response to illness or immunization.

Active alert state Alert state marked by an increase in facial and body movement, with periods of fussiness occurring. The infant in this state has increased sensitivity to disturbing stimuli.

Active management of labor (AMOL) Medical protocol for augmentation of labor that includes (1) a strict criterion for labor admission, (2) early amniotomy, (3) high-dose oxytocin infusion for inefficient labor contractions, and (4) a commitment to provision of continuous nursing care.

Active sleep See light sleep.

Acupressure (sometimes called *Chinese massage*) Therapy using pressure from the fingers and thumbs to stimulate pressure points.

Acupuncture Therapy using very fine (hairlike) stainless steel needles to stimulate specific acupuncture points depending on the client's medical assessment and condition.

Adequate intake (AI) A value cited for a nutrient when there are not sufficient data to calculate an estimated average requirement.

Adnexa Adjoining or accessory parts of a structure, such as the uterine adnexa: the ovaries and fallopian tubes.

Adolescence Period of human development initiated by puberty and ending with the attainment of young adulthood.

Afterbirth Placenta and membranes expelled after the birth of the infant, during the third stage of labor. Also called *secundines.*

Afterpains Cramplike pains due to contractions of the uterus that occur after childbirth. They are more common in multiparas, tend to be most severe during breastfeeding, and last 2 to 3 days.

Alcohol-related birth defect (ARBD) Birth defects and cognitive difficulties occurring in infants born to mothers who drink.

Alcohol related neurodevelopmental disorder (ARND) Occurs in children who have CNS neurodevelopmental abnormalities and complex behavior and cognitive abnormalities.

Alpha-fetoprotein (AFP) A fetal protein produced in the yolk sac for the first 6 weeks of gestation and then by the fetal liver.

Alternative therapy Any procedure or approach that is used in place of conventional medicine.

Alveoli Small units of the breast tissue in which milk is synthesized by the alveolar secretory epithelium.

Amenorrhea Suppression or absence of menstruation.

Amniocentesis Removal of amniotic fluid by insertion of a needle into the amniotic sac; amniotic fluid is used to assess fetal health or maturity.

Amnioinfusion Procedure used to infuse a sterile fluid (such as normal saline) through an intrauterine catheter into the uterus in an attempt to increase the fluid around the umbilical cord to decrease or prevent cord compression during labor contractions; also used to dilute thick meconium-stained amniotic fluid.

Amnion The inner of the two membranes that form the sac containing the fetus and the amniotic fluid.

Amnionitis Infection of the amniotic fluid.

Amniotic fluid The liquid surrounding the fetus in utero. It absorbs shocks, permits fetal movement, and prevents heat loss.

Amniotic fluid embolism Amniotic fluid that has leaked into the chorionic plate and entered the maternal circulation.

Amniotic fluid index (AFI) A method of reporting fluid volume. The AFI is calculated by dividing the maternal abdomen into four quadrants with the umbilicus as the reference point. Then the deepest vertical pocket is measured. These measurements are summed to calculate the AFI.

Amniotomy (am-nē-ot´ō-mē) The artificial rupturing of the amniotic membrane.

Ampulla The outer two-thirds of the fallopian tube; fertilization of the ovum by a spermatozoon usually occurs here.

Analgesic potentiators Can decrease anxiety and increase the effectiveness of analgesics when given simultaneously. Also known as *ataractic.*

Androgen Substance producing male characteristics, such as the male hormone testosterone.

Android pelvis Male-type pelvis.

Antepartum Time between conception and the onset of labor; usually used to describe the period during which a woman is pregnant.

Anterior fontanelle Diamond-shaped area between the two frontal and two parietal bones just above the newborn's forehead.

Anthropoid pelvis Pelvis in which the anteroposterior diameter is equal to or greater than the transverse diameter.

Apgar score A scoring system used to evaluate newborns at 1 minute and 5 minutes after birth. The total score is achieved by assessing five signs: heart rate, respiratory effort, muscle tone, reflex irritability, and color. Each of the signs is assigned a score of 0, 1, or 2. The highest possible score is 10.

Apnea A condition that occurs when respirations cease for more than 20 seconds, with generalized cyanosis.

Areola Pigmented ring surrounding the nipple of the breast.

Aromatherapy The use of certain essential oils, derived from plants, whose odor or aroma is believed to have a therapeutic effect.

Artificial rupture of membranes (AROM) Use of a device such as an amnihook or allis forceps to rupture the amniotic membranes.

Assimilation Phenomenon in which a minority group completely changes its cultural identity to become part of the majority culture.

Assisted reproductive technology (ART) Term used to describe the highly technologic approaches used to produce pregnancy.

Asynclitism Occurs when the sagittal suture is directed toward either the symphysis pubis or the sacral promontory and feels misaligned.

Attachment Enduring bonds or relationship of affection between persons.

Attachment theory A framework for understanding perinatal loss that begins with the basic premise that human beings are biologically predisposed to bond with emotionally significant persons in their lives.

Attitude In perinatal care, the relationship of the fetal parts to each other.

Autosome A chromosome that is not a sex chromosome.

Ayurveda The classical system of Hindu medicine. The term *ayurveda* means the knowledge of how to live a vital, healthful life.

Babinski reflex Reflex found normally in infants under 6 months of age in which the great toe dorsiflexes when the sole of the foot is stimulated.

Bacterial vaginosis A bacterial infection of the vagina, formerly called *Gardnerella vaginalis* or *Hemophilus vaginalis,* characterized by a foul-smelling, grayish vaginal discharge that exhibits a characteristic fishy odor when 10% potassium hydroxide (KOH) is added. Microscopic examination of a vaginal wet prep reveals the presence of "clue cells" (vaginal epithelial cells coated with gram-negative organisms).

Bag of waters (BOW) The membrane containing the amniotic fluid and the fetus.

Ballottement (băl-ŏt-mŏn´) A technique of palpation to detect or examine a floating object in the body. In obstetrics, the fetus, when pushed, floats away and then returns to touch the examiner's fingers.

Barlow maneuver A test designed to detect subluxation or dislocation of the hip. A dysplastic joint will be felt to be dislocated as the femur leaves the acetabulum.

Barr body Deeply staining chromatin mass located against the inner surface of the cell nucleus. It is found only in normal females. Also called *sex chromatin.*

Basal body temperature (BBT) The lowest waking temperature.

Baseline rate The average fetal heart rate observed during a 10-minute period of monitoring.

Baseline variability Changes in the fetal heart rate that result from the interplay between the sympathetic and the parasympathetic nervous systems.

Battledore placenta Placenta in which the umbilical cord is inserted on the periphery rather than centrally.

Bed sharing An infant sleeping in close social and/or physical contact with a committed caregiver (usually the mother). Also called *cosleeping.*

Bereavement To have suffered the *event* of loss.

Beta human chorionic gonadotropin (Beta hCG) A product of the trophoblast or placenta that is detected through serum testing and is a very accurate marker of the presence of pregnancy and placental health.

Bilirubin encephalopathy See *Kernicterus.*

Bimanual palpation Examination of the pelvic organs by placing one hand on the abdomen and one or two fingers of the other hand into the vagina.

Biofeedback The use of monitoring devices to help individuals learn to control their autonomic responses.

Biophysical profile (BPP) Assessment of five variables in the fetus that help to evaluate fetal risk: breathing movement, body movement, tone, amniotic fluid volume, and fetal heart rate reactivity.

Birth center A setting for labor and birth that emphasizes a family-centered approach rather than obstetric technology and treatment.

Birth defects Structural abnormalities present at birth.

Birthing room A room for labor and birth with a relaxed atmosphere.

Birth plan A written document prepared by the expectant parents that is used to identify available options in the birth setting.

Birth preference plan Decisions made by the expectant couple about aspects of the childbearing experience that are most important to them.

Birth rate Number of live births per 1000 population.

Bishop score A prelabor scoring system to assist in predicting whether an induction of labor may be successful. The total score is achieved by assessing five components: cervical dilatation, cervical effacement, cervical consistency, cervical position, and fetal station. Each of the components is assigned a score of 0 to 3, and the highest possible score is 13.

Blastocyst The inner solid mass of cells within the morula.

Bloody show Pink-tinged mucus secretions resulting from rupture of small capillaries as the cervix effaces and dilates.

Body stalk Future umbilical cord; structure that attaches the embryo to the yolk sac and contains blood vessels that extend into the chorionic villi.

Bogginess The softening of the uterus due to inadequate contraction of the muscle tissue.

Boggy uterus A term used to describe the uterine fundus when it is not firmly contracted after the birth of the baby and in the early postpartum period; excessive bleeding occurs from the placental site, and maternal hemorrhage may occur.

Bonding Process of parent-infant attachment occurring at or soon after birth.

Brachial palsy Partial or complete paralysis of portions of the arm resulting from trauma to the brachial plexus during a difficult birth.

Braxton Hicks contractions Intermittent painless contractions of the uterus that may occur every 10 to 20 minutes. They occur more frequently toward the end of pregnancy and are sometimes mistaken for true labor signs.

Brazleton's neonatal behavioral assessment A brief examination used to identify the infant's behavioral states and responses.

Breasts Mammary glands.

Breast self-examination (BSE) A manual examination conducted monthly by a woman to evaluate her own breasts for signs of masses, changes, nipple discharge, or evidence of abnormalities.

Breech presentation A birth in which the buttocks and/or feet are presented instead of the head.

Broad ligament The ligament extending from the lateral margins of the uterus to the pelvic wall; keeps the uterus centrally placed and provides stability within the pelvic cavity.

Bronchopulmonary dysplasia (BPD)/chronic lung disease of prematurity (CLD) Chronic pulmonary disease of multifactorial etiology characterized initially by alveolar and bronchial necrosis, which results in bronchial metaplasia and interstitial fibrosis. Appears in x-ray films as generalized small, radiolucent cysts within the lungs.

Brown adipose tissue (BAT) Fat deposits in newborns that provide greater heat-generating activity than ordinary fat. Found around the kidneys, adrenals, and neck; between the scapulas; and behind the sternum. Also called **brown fat.**

Calorie Amount of heat required to raise the temperature of 1 kg of water 1 degree centigrade.

Capacitation Removal of the plasma membrane overlying the spermatozoa's acrosomal area with the loss of seminal plasma proteins and the glycoprotein coat. If the glycoprotein coat is not removed, the sperm will not be able to penetrate the ovum.

Caput succedaneum (kap´ut suk-sĕ-dá-ne-um) Swelling or edema occurring in or under the fetal scalp during labor.

Cardinal ligaments The chief uterine supports, suspending the uterus from the side walls of the true pelvis.

Cardinal movements of labor The positional changes of the fetus as it moves through the birth canal during labor and birth. The positional changes are descent, flexion, internal rotation, extension, restitution, and external rotation.

Cardiopulmonary adaptation Adaptation of the newborn's cardiovascular and respiratory systems to life outside the womb.

Caring theory Consists of five attributes of the caregiver: (1) knowing, (2) being with, (3) doing for, (4) enabling, and (5) maintaining belief.

Cephalhematoma (sef´ăl-hé-mă-tōmă) Subcutaneous swelling containing blood found on the head of an infant several days after birth; it usually disappears within a few weeks to 2 months.

Cephalic presentation Birth in which the fetal head is presenting against the cervix.

Cephalopelvic disproportion (CPD) A condition in which the fetal head is of such a shape or size, or in such a position, that it cannot pass through the maternal pelvis.

Certified nurse specialist (CNS)

Certified nurse-midwife (CNM) An RN who has received special training and education in the care of the family during childbearing and the prenatal, labor and birth, and postpartal periods. After a period of formal education, the nurse-midwife takes a certification test to become a CNM.

Certified registered nurse (RNC) A registered nurse who has shown expertise in a specific field by passing a national certification examination.

Cervical cap A cup-shaped device placed over the cervix to prevent pregnancy.

Cervical dilatation Process in which the cervical os and the cervical canal widen from less than 1 cm to approximately 10 cm, allowing birth of the fetus.

Cervical funneling A cone-shaped indentation in the cervical os which is common in cases of cervical incompetence.

Cervical ripening Softening of the cervix; occurs normally as a physiologic process before labor or is stimulated to occur through the process of induction of labor.

Cervix The "neck" between the external os and the body of the uterus. The lower end of the cervix extends into the vagina.

Cesarean birth Birth of fetus accomplished by performing a surgical incision through the maternal abdomen and uterus.

Chadwick's sign Violet bluish color of the vaginal mucous membrane caused by increased vascularity; visible from about the fourth week of pregnancy.

Chemical conjunctivitis Irritation of the mucous membrane lining of the eyelid; may be due to instillation of silver nitrate ophthalmic drops.

Child abuse Nonaccidental physical or threatened harm, including mental or emotional injury, sexual abuse, and sexual exploitation.

Child neglect Failure by parents or other custodians to meet the medical, emotional, physical, or supervisory needs of a child.

Chiropractic Third largest independent health profession found in the United States. Uses spinal manipulation to address abnormal nerve transmission (subluxation) caused by misalignment of the spine.

Chlamydial infection Caused by **Chlamydia trachomatis,** this infection is the most common bacterial sexually transmitted infection in the United States.

Chloasma (klō-az´mă)(**melasma gravidarum**) Brownish pigmentation over the bridge of the nose and the cheeks during pregnancy and in some women who are taking oral contraceptives. Also called **mask of pregnancy.**

Chorioamnionitis (kō′rē-ō-am´nē-ō-ĭ´tis) An inflammation of the amniotic membranes stimulated by organisms in the amniotic fluid, which then becomes infiltrated with polymorphonuclear leukocytes.

Chorion The fetal membrane closest to the intrauterine wall that gives rise to the placenta and continues as the outer membrane surrounding the amnion.

Chorionic villus sampling (CVS) Procedure in which a specimen of the chorionic villi is obtained from the edge of the developing placenta at about 8 weeks' gestation. The sample can be used for chromosomal, enzyme, and DNA tests.

Chromosomes The threadlike structures within the nucleus of a cell that carry the genes.

Circumcision Surgical removal of the prepuce (foreskin) of the penis.

Circumoral cyanosis Bluish appearance around the mouth.

Circumvallate (ser-kŭm-val´āt) **placenta** A placenta with a thick, white fibrous ring around the edge.

Civil unions Legally recognized partnerships that involve rights and responsibilities comparable with those enjoyed by married couples. Often used by same-sex couples.

Cleavage Rapid mitotic division of the zygote; cells produced are called **blastomeres.**

Client Person seeking assistance from professionals who have the special skills and knowledge the individual lacks.

Client advocacy An approach to client care in which the nurse educates and supports the client and protects the client's rights.

Climacteric The period of time that marks the cessation of a woman's reproductive function; the "change of life," or menopause.

Clinical nurse specialist (CNS) A nurse possessing a master's degree and specialized knowledge and competence in a specific clinical area.

Clitoris Female organ homologous to the male penis; a small oval body of erectile tissue situated at the anterior junction of the vulva.

Coitus interruptus Method of contraception in which the male withdraws his penis from the vagina before ejaculation.

Cold stress Excessive heat loss resulting in compensatory mechanisms (increased respirations and nonshivering thermogenesis) to maintain core body temperature.

Colostrum (kō-los′trŭm) Secretion from the breast before the onset of true lactation; contains mainly serum and white blood corpuscles. It has a high protein content, provides some immune properties, and cleanses the newborn's intestinal tract of mucus and meconium.

Colposcopy The use of an instrument inserted into the vagina to examine the cervical and vaginal tissues by means of a magnifying lens.

Combined oral contraceptives (COCs) Commonly called birth control pills or "the pill," COCs are a form of contraception that uses a combination of a synthetic estrogen and a progestin.

Comparable worth The standard that the same wages should be paid for different types of work that require comparable skills, responsibility, education, and experience.

Complementary therapy Any procedure or product that is used together with conventional medical treatment.

Conception Union of male sperm and female ovum; fertilization.

Conceptional age The number of complete weeks since the moment of conception. Because the moment of conception is almost impossible to determine, conceptional age is estimated at 2 weeks less than gestational age.

Condom A rubber sheath that covers the penis to prevent conception or disease.

Conduction Loss of heat to a cooler surface by direct skin contact.

Condyloma (kon-di-lō′mă) Wartlike growth of skin, usually seen on the external genitals or anus. There are two types, a pointed variety and a broad, flat form usually found with syphilis.

Condylomata acuminata Known also as genital or venereal warts, they are a common sexually transmitted infection caused by the human papilloma virus (HPV).

Conjugate Important diameter of the pelvis, measured from the center of the promontory of the sacrum to the back of the symphysis pubis. The diagonal conjugate is measured and the true conjugate is estimated.

Conjugate vera The true conjugate, which extends from the middle of the sacral promontory to the middle of the pubic crest.

Continuous epidural infusion (CEI) Technique in which the epidural catheter is left in place following the cesarean birth and medication is continually administered via an electric pump.

Contraception The prevention of conception or impregnation.

Contraction Tightening and shortening of the uterine muscles during labor, causing effacement and dilatation of the cervix; contributes to the downward and outward descent of the fetus.

Contraction stress test (CST) A method of assessing the reaction of the fetus to the stress of uterine contractions. This test may be utilized when contractions are occurring spontaneously or when contractions are artificially induced by oxytocin challenge test (OCT) or breast self-stimulation test (BSST).

Convection Loss of heat from the warm body surface to cooler air currents.

Coombs' (kōōmz) **test** A test for antiglobulins in the red cells. The indirect test determines the presence of Rh-positive antibodies in maternal blood; the direct test determines the presence of maternal Rh-positive antibodies in fetal cord blood.

Cordocentesis Also called percutaneous umbilical blood sampling (PUBS), a technique used to obtain pure fetal blood from the umbilical cord while the fetus is in utero, which is used for diagnosis of hemophilias, hemoglobinopathies, fetal infections, chromosome abnormalities, nonimmune hydrops, and isoimmune hemolytic disorders, as well as assessment of fetal hemoglobin and hematocrit for calculation of transfusion requirements in the second and third trimesters.

Cornua The elongated portions of the uterus where the fallopian tubes open.

Corpus The upper two thirds of the uterus.

Corpus luteum A small yellow body that develops within a ruptured ovarian follicle; it secretes progesterone in the second half of the menstrual cycle and atrophies about 3 days before the beginning of menstrual flow. If pregnancy occurs, the corpus luteum continues to produce progesterone until the placenta takes over this function.

Cosleeping An infant sleeping in close social and/or physical contact with a committed caregiver (usually the mother).

Cotyledon (kot-i-lē′don) One of the rounded portions into which the placenta's uterine surface is divided, consisting of a mass of villi, fetal vessels, and an intervillous space.

Couplet care A family-centered approach for maternal-child nursing where both the mother and her baby are cared for by the same nurse, with the baby remaining at the mother's bedside. Also called mother-baby care.

Couvade (kū-vahd′) In some cultures, the male's observance of certain rituals and taboos to signify the transition to fatherhood.

Crack A form of freebase cocaine that is smoked.

Crisis intervention Actions taken by the nurse to help the client deal with an impending, potentially overwhelming crisis; regain his or her equilibrium; grow from the experience; and improve coping skills.

Critical thinking Intellectual processes that include separating fact from opinion, identifying prejudices and stereotypes that may influence interpretation of information, exploring differing ideas and views, and arriving at conclusions or insights.

Crowning Appearance of the presenting fetal part at the vaginal orifice during labor.

Crying state A state in the infant sleep/awake cycle in which the infant exhibits increased motor activity, grimaces, eyes that are tightly closed or open, and extreme responsiveness to stimuli.

Cultural beliefs Those beliefs that reflect the predominating values, attitudes, and practices accepted by a population, community, or ethnic group.

Cultural competency Referring to the skills and knowledge necessary to appreciate, understand, and work with individuals from different cultures.

Culture The beliefs, values, attitudes, and practices that are accepted by a population, community, or an individual.

Cycle of violence A theory that postulates that battering takes place in a cyclic fashion through three phases: the tension-building phase, the acute battering incident, and the tranquil phase (honeymoon period).

Cystocele The downward displacement of the bladder, which appears as a bulge in the anterior vaginal wall.

Date rape Occurs between a dating couple. In some cases an assailant uses alcohol or other drugs to sedate his intended victim *(drug-facilitated sexual assault)*. In date rape situations, the male is usually determined to have sex and will do whatever he feels necessary if denied.

Deceleration Periodic decrease in the baseline fetal heart rate.

Decidua (dē-sid´yūă) Endometrium or mucous membrane lining of the uterus in pregnancy that is shed after childbirth.

Decidua basalis The part of the decidua that unites with the chorion to form the placenta. It is shed in lochial discharge after childbirth.

Decidua capsularis The part of the decidua surrounding the chorionic sac.

Decidua vera (parietalis) Nonplacental decidua lining the uterus.

Decrement Decrease or stage of decline, as of a contraction.

Deep sleep State of sleep in which the infant will be nearly still except for occasional startles, twitches, and sucking.

Depo-Provera A long-acting, injectable progestin contraceptive.

Descriptive statistics Statistics that describe or summarize a set of data.

Desquamation (des-kwă-mā´shŭn) Shedding of the epithelial cells of the epidermis.

Diagonal conjugate Distance from the lower posterior border of the symphysis pubis to the sacral promontory; may be obtained by manual measurement.

Diaphragm A flexible disk that covers the cervix to prevent pregnancy.

Diastasis (dĭ-as´tă-sis) **recti** (rek´ti) **abdominis** Separation of the recti abdominis muscles along the median line. In women, it is seen with repeated childbirths or multiple gestations. In the newborn, it is usually caused by incomplete development.

Dietary reference intakes (DRIs) Specific allowances for pregnant and lactating women, DRIs are subdivided into the recommended dietary allowance (RDA) and adequate intake (AI).

Dilatation and curettage (D&C) Stretching of the cervical canal to permit passage of a curette, which is used to scrape the endometrium to empty the uterine contents or to obtain tissue for examination.

Dilatation of the cervix Expansion of the external os from an opening a few millimeters in size to an opening large enough to allow the passage of the infant.

Diploid number of chromosomes Containing a set of maternal and a set of paternal chromosomes; in humans, the diploid number of chromosomes is 46.

Disability Impairment in one or more of five function categories: cognition, communication, motor abilities, social abilities, or patterns of interactions.

Disassociation relaxation A pattern of active relaxation in which the woman learns to tighten one area of the body and then relax other areas simultaneously. This relaxation pattern is very effective for some women during labor.

Disenfranchised grief Grief that is not supported by the usual societal customs.

Domestic partnership A mechanism by which public and private employers can provide insurance coverage and pension-rights benefits to the partners of gay and lesbian employees.

Domestic violence Defined as the collective methods used to exert power and control by one individual over another in an adult intimate relationship. Forms of abuse typically fall into three categories: psychologic abuse, physical abuse, and sexual abuse.

Doula A supportive companion who accompanies a laboring woman to provide emotional, physical, and informational support and acts as an advocate for the woman and her family.

Down syndrome An abnormality resulting from the presence of an extra chromosome number 21 (trisomy 21); characteristics include mental retardation and altered physical appearance. Formerly called *mongolism.*

Drowsy awake state Awake state in which infants open and close their eyes although the eyes appear glazed and the face is often still. They may return to sleep or awaken further in response to stimuli.

Drowsy state A state in the infant sleep/awake cycle that occurs between light sleep and the quiet alert state. It is marked by infants opening and closing their eyes, but the eyes appear glazed and face is often still. They may return to sleep or awaken further in response to stimuli.

Drug-exposed infant The newborn of an alcoholic or drug-addicted woman.

Drug-facilitated sexual assault A sexual assault in which the perpetrator uses alcohol or other drugs to sedate his intended victim.

Dual process model A view of grief encompassing two competing facets: loss and restoration. The loss orientation is concerned with the individual's need to confront the reality of the loss, and the restoration orientation seeks to regain balance and temper the pain of grief.

Dubowitz tool A clinical gestational age assessment tool.

Ductus arteriosus A communication channel between the main pulmonary artery and the aorta of the fetus. It is obliterated after birth by rising PO_2 and changes in intravascular pressure in the presence of normal pulmonary functioning. It normally becomes a ligament after birth but sometimes remains patent (patent ductus arteriosus, a treatable condition).

Ductus venosus A fetal blood vessel that carries oxygenated blood between the umbilical vein and the inferior vena cava, bypassing the liver; it becomes a ligament after birth.

Duncan's mechanism Occurs when the maternal surface of the placenta rather than the shiny fetal surface presents upon birth.

Duration The time length of each contraction, measured from the beginning of the increment to the completion of the decrement.

Dysfunctional uterine bleeding (DUB) A condition characterized by anovulatory cycles with abnormal uterine bleeding that does not have a demonstrable organic cause.

Dysmenorrhea Painful menstruation.

Dyspareunia Painful intercourse.

Dystocia (dis-tō´sē-ă) Difficult labor due to mechanical factors produced by the fetus or the maternal pelvis or due to inadequate uterine or other muscular activity.

Early adolescence A term referring to adolescents who are age 14 and under.

Early decelerations Periodic change in fetal heart rate pattern caused by head compression; deceleration has a uniform appearance and early onset in relation to maternal contraction.

Early (primary) postpartal hemorrhage See *Postpartal hemorrhage.*

Eclampsia (ek-lamp´sē-ă) A major complication of pregnancy. Its cause is unknown; it occurs more often in the primigravida and is accompanied by elevated blood pressure, albuminuria, oliguria, tonic and clonic convulsions, and coma. It may occur during pregnancy (usually after the 20th week of gestation) or within 48 hours after childbirth.

Ectoderm Outer layer of cells in the developing embryo that gives rise to the skin, nails, and hair.

Ectopic pregnancy Implantation of the fertilized ovum outside the uterine cavity; common sites are the abdomen, fallopian tubes, and ovaries. Also called *oocyesis.*

Effacement Thinning and shortening of the cervix that occurs late in pregnancy or during labor.

Effleurage (e-fler-ahz´) A light stroking movement of the fingertips over the abdominal area during labor; used to provide distraction during labor contractions.

Ejaculation Expulsion of the seminal fluids from the penis.

Elder abuse Any deliberate action or lack of action that causes harm to an elderly person.

Electronic fetal monitoring (EFM) A method of placing a fetal monitor on the fetus in order to obtain a continuous tracing of the FHR, which allows many characteristics of the fetal heart rate to be observed and evaluated.

Emancipated minors Minors who are legally considered to have assumed the rights of an adult. An adolescent may be considered emancipated if he or she is self-supporting and living away from home, married, pregnant, a parent, or in the military.

Embryo The early stage of development of the young of any organism. In humans the embryonic period is from about 2 to 8 weeks' gestation and is characterized by cellular differentiation and predominantly hyperplastic growth.

Embryonic membranes The amnion and chorion.

Endoderm The inner layer of cells in the developing embryo that give rise to internal organs such as the intestines.

Endometrial biopsy Procedure providing information about the effects of progesterone produced by the corpus luteum after ovulation and endometrial receptivity.

Endometriosis Ectopic endometrium located outside the uterus in the pelvic cavity. Symptoms may include pelvic pain or pressure, dysmenorrhea, dispareunia, abnormal bleeding from the uterus or rectum, and sterility.

Endometritis (metritis) Infection of the endometrium.

Endometrium (en´dō-mē´trē-ŭm) The mucous membrane that lines the inner surface of the uterus.

En face An assumed position in which one person looks at another and maintains his or her face in the same vertical plane as that of the other.

Engagement The entrance of the fetal presenting part into the superior pelvic strait and the beginning of the descent through the pelvic canal.

Engorgement Vascular congestion or distention. In obstetrics, the swelling of breast tissue brought about by an increase in blood and lymph supply to the breast, preceding true lactation.

Engrossment Characteristic sense of absorption, preoccupation, and interest in the infant demonstrated by fathers during early contact with their infants.

Entrainment Phenomenon in which a newborn moves in rhythm to adult speech.

Environmental toxins Chemical compounds found in air, food, and water, whose bioaccumulation can lead to adverse health effects.

Epidural block Regional anesthesia effective through the first and second stages of labor.

Episiotomy (ĕ-piz-ē-ot´o-mē) Incision of the perineum to facilitate birth and to avoid laceration of the perineum.

Epstein's (ep´stīnz) **pearls** Small, white blebs found along the gum margins and at the junction of the hard and soft palates; commonly seen in the newborn as a normal manifestation.

Erb-Duchenne paralysis (Erb's palsy) Paralysis of the arm and chest wall as a result of a birth injury to the brachial plexus or a subsequent injury to the fifth and sixth cervical nerves.

Erythema toxicum Innocuous pink papular rash of unknown cause with superimposed vesicles; it appears within 24 to 48 hours after birth and resolves spontaneously within a few days.

Erythroblastosis fetalis Hemolytic disease of the newborn characterized by anemia, jaundice, enlargement of the liver and spleen, and generalized edema. Caused by isoimmunization due to Rh incompatibility or ABO incompatibility.

Essure Method of permanent sterilization that requires no surgical incision. Under hysteroscopy, a stainless steel micro-insert is placed into each proximal section of the fallopian tube.

Estimated date of birth (EDB) During a pregnancy, the approximate date when childbirth will occur; the "due date."

Estrogens The hormones estradiol and estrone, produced by the ovary.

Ethnicity A social identity that is associated with shared beliefs, behaviors, and patterns.

Ethnocentrism An individual's belief that the values and practices of his or her own culture are the best ones.

Euphemism A substituted word or expression with a more pleasant association than the one which, although more direct, is considered to be harsher.

Evaporation Loss of heat incurred when water on the skin surface is converted to a vapor.

Evidence-based practice An approach to problem solving and decision making based on the consideration of data from research, statistical analysis, quality measures, risk management measurements, and other sources of reliable information.

Exchange transfusion The replacement of 70% to 80% of circulating blood by withdrawing the recipient's blood and injecting a donor's blood in equal amounts, for the purpose of preventing the accumulation of bilirubin or other by-products of hemolysis in the blood.

External cephalic version (ECV) Procedure involving external manipulation of the maternal abdomen to change the presentation of the fetus from breech to cephalic.

External os The opening between the cervix and the vagina.

Fallopian tubes Tubes that extend from the lateral angle of the uterus and terminate near the ovary; they serve as a passageway for the ovum from the ovary to the uterus and for the spermatozoa from the uterus toward the ovary. Also called *oviducts* and *uterine tubes.*

False labor Contractions of the uterus, regular or irregular, that may be strong enough to be interpreted as true labor but do not dilate the cervix.

False pelvis The portion of the pelvis above the linea terminalis; its primary function is to support the weight of the enlarged pregnant uterus.

Family Two or more persons who are joined together by bonds of sharing and emotional closeness and who identify themselves as being part of a family.

Family assessment The process by which a nurse collects data regarding a family's current level of functioning, support systems, sociocultural influences, home and work environment, type of family, family structure, and needs.

Family-centered care An approach to health care based on the concept that a hospital can provide professional services to mothers, fathers, and infants in a homelike environment that would enhance the integrity of the family unit.

Family development The changes that families experience over time, including changes in relationships, communication patterns, roles, and interactions.

Family planning Actions an individual or a couple takes to avoid a pregnancy, to space future pregnancies for a specific reason, or to gain control over the number of children conceived.

Family power The individual who has either the potential or actual ability to change the behavior of other family members.

Family roles The specific roles of individuals within a family unit. Examples of roles include breadwinner, homemaker, mother, father, social planner, and family peacemaker.

Family values A system of ideas, attitudes, and beliefs about the worth of an entity or a concept that consciously or unconsciously bind together the members of the family in a common culture.

Fecundability The ability to become pregnant.

Female condom A thin, disposable polyurethane sheath with a flexible ring at each end that is placed inside the vagina and serves to prevent sperm from entering the cervix, thus preventing conception.

Female genital mutilation (FGM) Also known as *female genital cutting, female circumcision,* and *genital circumcision,* the practice of removing all or parts of a girl's or women's genitalia for cultural reasons.

Female reproductive cycle (FRC) The monthly rhythmic changes in sexually mature women.

Feminization of later life Worldwide trend for women to comprise a majority of the elderly population.

Feminization of poverty Term used to describe the fact that, in the United States, women comprise a majority of the adult poor.

Ferning capacity Formation of a palm-leaf pattern by the crystallization of cervical mucus as it dries at mid-menstrual cycle. The formation can be helpful in determining time of ovulation. Observed via microscopic examination of a thin layer of cervical mucus on a glass slide. This pattern is also observed when amniotic fluid is allowed to air dry on a slide and is a useful and quick test to determine whether amniotic membranes have ruptured.

Fertility awareness-based (FAB) methods Also known as natural family planning, fertility awareness-based methods are founded on an understanding of the changes that occur throughout a woman's ovulatory cycle. All these methods require periods of abstinence and recording of certain events throughout the cycle; cooperation of the partner is important.

Fertility rate Number of births per 1000 women aged 15 to 44 in a given population per year.

Fertilization Impregnation of an ovum by a spermatozoon; conception.

Fetal acoustic stimulation test (FAST) A fetal assessment test that uses sound from a speaker, bell, or artificial larynx to stimulate acceleration of the fetal heart; may be used in conjunction with the nonstress test.

Fetal activity diary (FAD) A method for tracking fetal activity taught to pregnant women.

Fetal alcohol effects (FAE) The less severe fetal manifestations of maternal alcohol ingestion, including mild to moderate cognitive problems and physical growth retardation.

Fetal alcohol spectrum disorder (FASD) Is current term that includes all categories of prenatal alcohol exposure, including FAS.

Fetal alcohol syndrome (FAS) Syndrome caused by maternal alcohol ingestion and characterized by microcephaly, intrauterine growth restriction, short palpebral fissures, and maxillary hypoplasia.

Fetal arterial oxygen saturation (FSpO₂) monitoring Approved by the Food and Drug Administration (FDA) in 2000 as a direct, real-time method to determine fetal oxygenation levels.

Fetal attitude Relationship of the fetal parts to one another. Normal fetal attitude is one of moderate flexion of the arms onto the chest and flexion of the legs onto the abdomen.

Fetal blood sampling Blood sample drawn from the fetal scalp (or from the fetus in breech position) to evaluate the acid-base status of the fetus.

Fetal bradycardia A fetal heart rate less than 120 beats per minute during a 10-minute period of continuous monitoring.

Fetal death Death of the developing fetus after 20 weeks' gestation. Also called *fetal demise.*

Fetal distress Evidence that the fetus is in jeopardy, such as a change in fetal activity or heart rate.

Fetal fibronectin (fFN) A glycoprotein that is produced by the trophoblast and fetal tissues whose presence between 20 and 34 weeks' gestation is a strong predictor of preterm birth associated with preterm spontaneous rupture of membranes.

Fetal heart rate (FHR) The number of times the fetal heart beats per minute; normal range is 120 to 160.

Fetal lie Relationship of the cephalocaudal axis (spinal column) of the fetus to the cephalocaudal axis (spinal column) of the woman. The fetus may be in a longitudinal or transverse lie.

Fetal movement record (FMR) See *Fetal activity diary (FAD).*

Fetal position Relationship of the landmark on the presenting fetal part to the front, sides, or back of the maternal pelvis.

Fetal presentation The fetal body part that enters the maternal pelvis first. The three possible presentations are cephalic, shoulder, and breech.

Fetal scalp blood sample A collection of fetal blood collected via the vagina from the fetal head by making a small nick with a scalpel and collecting a blood sample that is used to identify the fetal acid-base status and determine if hypoxia is occurring during labor.

Fetal tachycardia A fetal heart rate of 160 beats per minute or more during a 10-minute period of continuous monitoring.

Fetoscope An adaptation of a stethoscope that facilitates auscultation of the fetal heart rate.

Fetoscopy A technique for directly observing the fetus and obtaining a sample of fetal blood or skin.

Fetus The child in utero from about the seventh to ninth week of gestation until birth.

Fibrocystic breast changes Benign breast changes characterized by bilateral, cyclic breast pain and breast nodularities that may be unilateral or bilateral, and often in the upper outer quadrants of the breasts.

Fibrocystic breast disease Benign breast disorder characterized by a thickening of normal breast tissue and the formation of cysts.

Fimbria Any structure resembling a fringe; the fringelike extremity of the fallopian tubes.

First-trimester combined screening A comprehensive screening testing that includes the NTT and serum screening for pregnancy-associated plasma protein-A (PAPP-A) and free beta human chorionic gonadotropin (BHCG) to determine if a fetus is at risk for trisomies 13, 18, and 21.

Folic acid An important vitamin directly related to the outcome of pregnancy and to maternal and fetal health.

Follicle-stimulating hormone (FSH) Hormone produced by the anterior pituitary during the first half of the menstrual cycle, stimulating development of the graafian follicle.

Fontanelle (fon´tă nel´) In the fetus, an unossified space, or soft spot, consisting of a strong band of connective tissue lying between the cranial bones of the skull.

Foramen ovale Special opening between the atria of the fetal heart. Normally, the opening closes shortly after birth; if it remains open, it can be repaired surgically.

Forceps Obstetric instrument occasionally used to aid in childbirth.

Forceps-assisted birth A birth in which a set of instruments, known as forceps, are applied to the presenting part of the fetus to provide traction or to enable the fetal head to be rotated to an occiputanterior position. Forceps-assisted birth is also known as *instrumental delivery, operative delivery,* or *operative vaginal delivery.*

Forceps marks Reddened areas over the cheeks and jaws caused by the application of forceps. The red areas usually disappear within 1 to 2 days.

Foremilk Breast milk obtained at the beginning of the breast-feeding episode.

Fourth trimester First several postpartal weeks during which the woman returns to an essentially prepregnant state and becomes competent in caring for her newborn.

Frequency The time between the beginning of one contraction and the beginning of the next contraction.

Fundus The upper portion of the uterus between the fallopian tubes.

Funic presentation When the umbilical cord is interposed between the cervix and the presenting part. It can be located by clinical evaluation or by ultrasound

Galactorrhea Nipple discharge.

Gamete (gam´ēt) Female or male germ cell; contains a haploid number of chromosomes.

Gamete intrafallopian transfer (GIFT) Retrieval of oocytes by laparoscopy; immediately combining oocytes with washed, motile sperm in a catheter; and placement of the gametes into the fimbriated end of the fallopian tube.

Gametogenesis The process by which germ cells are produced.

General anesthesia A state of induced unconsciousness that may be achieved through intravenous injection, inhalation of anesthetic agents, or a combination of both methods.

Genotype The genetic composition of an individual.

Gestation (jes-tā´shŭn) Period of intrauterine development from conception through birth; pregnancy.

Gestational age The number of complete weeks of fetal development, calculated from the first day of the last normal menstrual cycle.

Gestational age assessment tools Systems used to evaluate the newborn's external physical characteristics and neurologic and/or neuromuscular development to accurately determine gestational age. These replace or supplement the traditional calculation from the woman's last menstrual period.

Gestational diabetes mellitus (GMD) A form of diabetes of variable severity with onset or first recognition during pregnancy.

Gestational trophoblastic disease (GTD) Disorder classified into two types: benign (hydatidiform mole) and malignant.

Gonadotropin-releasing hormone (GnRH) A hormone secreted by the hypothalamus that stimulates the anterior pituitary to secrete FSH and LH.

Gonadotropins Hormones that stimulate the gonads (ovaries in women or testes in men).

Gonorrhea A sexually transmitted infection caused by the bacterium *Neisseria gonorrhoeae.*

Goodell's sign Softening of the cervix that occurs during the second month of pregnancy.

Graafian follicle The ovarian cyst containing the ripe ovum; it secretes estrogens.

Grasping reflex Normal newborn reflex elicited by stimulating the palm with a finger or object, resulting in newborn firmly holding on to the finger or object.

Gravida (grav´i-dă) A pregnant woman.

Grief An individual's *reaction* to loss, including physical symptoms, thoughts, feelings, functional limitations, and spiritual responses.

Grief work The inner process of working through or managing the bereavement.

Guided imagery A state of intense, focused concentration used to create compelling mental images. It is sometimes considered a form of hypnosis.

Gynecoid pelvis Typical female pelvis in which the inlet is round instead of oval.

Habituation (ha-bit-chū-ā´shŭn) Infant's ability to diminish innate responses to specific repeated stimuli.

Haploid number of chromosomes Half the diploid number of chromosomes. In humans there are 23 chromosomes, the haploid number, in each germ cell.

Harlequin sign A rare color change that occurs between the longitudinal halves of the newborn's body, such that the dependent half is noticeably pinker than the superior half when the newborn is placed on one side; it is of no pathologic significance.

Hatha yoga The physical branch of yoga; in the United States, it is commonly practiced for wellness, illness prevention, and healing.

Hegar's sign A softening of the lower uterine segment found upon palpation in the second or third month of pregnancy.

HELLP syndrome A cluster of changes including *h*emolysis, *e*levated *l*iver enzymes, and *l*ow *p*latelet count; sometimes associated with severe preeclampsia.

Hemolytic disease of the newborn *Hyperbilirubinemia* secondary to Rh incompatibility.

Herpes genitalis A lifelong, recurrent sexually transmitted infection caused by the herpes simplex virus (HSV).

Heterozygous A genotypic situation in which two different alleles occur at a given locus on a pair of homologous chromosomes.

Hindmilk Breast milk released after initial let-down reflex; high in fat content.

Homeopathy Term derived from the Greek word *homos,* meaning "the same," and describing a healing system that uses as remedies minute dilutions of substances that, if ingested in larger amounts, would produce effects *similar* to the symptoms of the disorder being treated.

Homozygous A genotypic situation in which two similar genes occur at a given locus on homologous chromosomes.

Hormone replacement therapy (HRT) Administration of hormones, usually estrogen and a progestin, to alleviate the symptoms of menopause.

Hospital disposition The incineration at regular intervals of a dead fetus or infant's body, usually with other body parts.

Human chorionic gonadotropin (hCG) A hormone produced by the chorionic villi and found in the urine of pregnant women. Also called *prolan.*

Human immunodeficiency virus (HIV) A virus that causes a progressive disease that ultimately results in the development of acquired immunodeficiency syndrome (AIDS).

Human placental lactogen (hPL) A hormone synthesized by the syncytiotrophoblast that functions as an insulin antagonist and promotes lipolysis to increase the amounts of circulating free fatty acids available for maternal metabolic use.

Hydatidiform (hī-da-tid´i-form) **mole** Degenerative process in chorionic villi, giving rise to multiple cysts and rapid growth of the uterus, with hemorrhage.

Hydramnios (hī-dram´nē-os) An excess of amniotic fluid, leading to overdistention of the uterus. Frequently seen in diabetic pregnant women, even if there is no coexisting fetal anomaly. Also called *polyhydramnios.*

Hydrops fetalis See *Erythroblastosis fetalis.*

Hydrotherapy Type of therapy that makes use of hot or cold moisture in any form. Hydrotherapy is used to relax muscles, promote rest, decrease pain, reduce swelling, promote healing, cleanse wounds and burns, reduce fever, lessen cramps, and improve well-being.

Hyperbilirubinemia (hī-per-bil´i-rū-bi-nē´mē-ă) Excessive amount of bilirubin in the blood; indicative of hemolytic processes due to blood incompatibility, intrauterine infection, septicemia, neonatal renal infection, and other disorders.

Hyperemesis gravidarum Excessive vomiting during pregnancy, leading to dehydration and starvation.

Hyperventilation Rapid breathing that occurs over a prolonged period of time resulting in an imbalance of oxygen and carbon dioxide that can result in tingling or numbness in the tip of nose, lips, fingers, or toes; dizziness; spots before the eyes; or spasms of the hands or feet (carpal-pedal spasms).

Hypnosis Whether guided by a trained hypnotherapist or self-induced, a state of great mental and physical relaxation during which a person is very open to suggestions.

Hypoglycemia Abnormally low level of sugar in the blood.

Hysterectomy Surgical removal of the uterus.

Hysterosalpingogram Result of testing by instillation of radiopaque substance into the uterine cavity to visualize the uterus and fallopian tubes.

Hysterosalpingography (HSG) Testing by instillation of radiopaque substance into the uterine cavity to visualize the uterus and fallopian tubes.

Hysteroscopy Use of a special endoscope to examine the uterus.

Inborn error of metabolism A hereditary deficiency of a specific enzyme needed for normal metabolism of specific chemicals.

Incompetent cervix The premature dilatation of the cervix, usually in the second trimester of pregnancy.

Increment Increase or addition; to build up, as of a contraction.

Induction of labor The process of causing or initiating labor by use of medication or surgical rupture of membranes.

Infant A child under 1 year of age.

Infant mortality rate Number of deaths of infants under 1 year of age per 1000 live births in a given population per year.

Infant of diabetic mother (IDM) At-risk infant born to a woman previously diagnosed as diabetic or who develops symptoms of diabetes during pregnancy.

Infant of substance-abusing mother (ISAM) Formerly called infant of an addicted mother, an infant born to a mother who abuses or is addicted to drugs or alcohol.

Inferential statistics Statistics that allow an investigator to draw conclusions about what is happening between two or more variables in a population and to suggest or refute causal relationships between them.

Infertility Diminished ability to conceive.

Informed consent A legal concept that protects a person's rights to autonomy and self-determination by specifying that no action may be taken without that person's prior understanding and freely given consent.

Infundibulopelvic ligament Ligament that suspends and supports the ovaries.

Instrumental style of coping A style of coping by which persons generally use more cognitive skills to navigate loss and value care that includes an emphasis on problem solving.

Integrative medicine An approach that combines mainstream medical therapies with complementary therapies for which there is some high-quality scientific evidence of safety and effectiveness.

Intensity The strength of a uterine contraction during acme.

Internal os An inside mouth or opening; the opening between the cervix and the uterus.

Internal version Procedure used for the vaginal birth of a second twin. The obstetrician inserts a hand into the uterus, grasps the feet of the fetus, and changes the fetus from a transverse to a breech presentation.

Intimate partner violence See domestic violence.

Intrapartum The time from the onset of true labor until the birth of the infant and expulsion of the placenta.

Intrauterine device (IUD) Small metal or plastic form that is placed in the uterus to prevent implantation of a fertilized ovum.

Intrauterine drug-exposed infants Infants exposed while in the uterus to drugs of abuse taken by their mother.

Intrauterine fetal surgery Surgery performed on a fetus to correct anatomic lesions that are not compatible with life if left untreated.

Intrauterine growth restriction (IUGR) Fetal undergrowth due to any etiology, such as intrauterine infection, deficient nutrient supply, or congenital malformation. A term used to describe fetuses falling below the 10th percentile in ultrasonic estimation of weight at a given gestational age.

Intrauterine pressure catheter (IUPC) A catheter that can be placed through the cervix into the uterus to measure uterine pressure during labor. Some types of catheters may be inserted for the purpose of infusing warmed saline to add additional intrauterine fluid when oligohydramnios is present.

Intrauterine resuscitation Interventions initiated when nonreassuring fetal heart rate patterns are noted; they are directed at improving intrauterine blood flow.

Introitus Opening or entrance into a cavity or canal such as the vagina.

Intuitive style of coping A style of coping by which persons generally feel their way through loss and prefer care with an emphasis on emotional and psychosocial support.

In vitro fertilization (IVF) Procedure during which oocytes are removed from the ovary, mixed with spermatozoa, fertilized, and incubated in a glass petri dish; then up to four viable embryos are placed in the woman's uterus.

Involution Rolling or turning inward; the reduction in size of the uterus following childbirth.

Ischial spines Prominences that arise near the junction of the ilium and ischium and jut into the pelvic cavity; used as a reference point during labor to evaluate the descent of the fetal head into the birth canal.

Isthmus The straight, narrow part of the fallopian tube with a thick muscular wall and an opening (lumen) 2 to 3 mm in diameter; the site of tubal ligation. Also, a constriction in the uterus that is located above the cervix and below the corpus.

Jaundice Yellow pigmentation of body tissues caused by the presence of bile pigments. See also *Physiologic jaundice.*

Karyotype The set of chromosomes arranged in a standard order.

Kegel exercises Perineal muscle tightening that strengthens the pubococcygeus muscle and increases its tone.

Kernicterus (ker-nik´ter-ŭ s) An encephalopathy caused by deposition of unconjugated bilirubin in brain cells; may result in impaired brain function or death.

Kilocalorie (kcal) Equivalent to 1000 calories, it is the unit used to express the energy value of food.

Klinefelter syndrome A chromosomal abnormality caused by the presence of an extra X chromosome in the male. Characteristics include tall stature; sparse pubic and facial hair; gynecomastia; small, firm testes; and absence of spermatogenesis.

Labor The process by which the fetus is expelled from the maternal uterus. Also called *childbirth, confinement,* or *parturition.*

Labor augmentation The stimulation of uterine contractions when spontaneous contractions have failed to result in progressive cervical dilation or descent of the fetus.

Labor induction The stimulation of uterine contractions before the spontaneous onset of labor, with or without ruptured fetal membranes, for the purpose of accomplishing birth.

Lactase deficiency (lactose intolerance) A condition characterized by difficulty digesting milk and dairy products. Results from an inadequate amount of the enzyme lactase, which breaks down the milk sugar lactose into smaller digestible substances.

Lactation The process of producing and supplying breast milk.

Lacto-ovovegetarians Vegetarians who include milk, dairy products, and eggs in their diets and occasionally fish, poultry, and liver.

Lactose intolerance A condition in which an individual has difficulty digesting milk and milk products.

Lactovegetarians Vegetarians who include dairy products but no eggs in their diets.

La Leche League Organization that provides information on and assistance with breastfeeding.

Lamaze method A method of childbirth preparation.

Lanugo (lă-nū´gō) Fine, downy hair found on all body parts of the fetus, with the exception of the palms of the hands and the soles of the feet, after 20 weeks' gestation.

Laparoscopy Procedure that enables direct visualization of pelvic organs.

Large for gestational age (LGA) Excessive growth of a fetus in relation to the gestational time period.

Last menstrual period (LMP) The last normal menstrual period experienced by the woman before pregnancy; sometimes used to calculate the infant's gestational age.

Late adolescence A term referring to adolescents who are ages 18 to 19 years.

Late decelerations Symmetrical decrease in fetal heart rate beginning at or after the peak of the contraction and returning to baseline only after the contraction has ended, indicating possible uteroplacental insufficiency and potential that the fetus is not receiving adequate oxygenation.

Late preterm infant An infant born between 34 and 37 weeks of gestation.

Late (secondary) postpartal hemorrhage See *Postpartal hemorrhage.*

Lecithin/sphingomyelin (les´i-thin sfing´gō-mĭ´ĕ-lin) **(L/S) ratio** Lecithin and sphingomyelin are phospholipid components of surfactant; their ratio changes during gestation. When the L/S ratio reaches 2:1, the fetal lungs are thought to be mature and the fetus will have a low risk of respiratory distress syndrome (RDS) if born at that time.

Leiomyoma A benign tumor of the uterus, composed primarily of smooth muscle and connective tissue. Also referred to as a myoma or a fibroid.

Leopold's maneuvers A series of four maneuvers designed to provide a systematic approach whereby the examiner may determine fetal presentation and position.

Let-down reflex Pattern of stimulation, hormone release, and resulting muscle contraction that forces milk into the lactiferous ducts, making it available to the infant. Also called *milk ejection reflex.*

Leukorrhea Mucous discharge from the vagina or cervical canal that may be normal or pathologic, as in the presence of infection.

Lie Relationship of the long axis of the fetus and the long axis of the pregnant woman. The fetal lie may be longitudinal, transverse, or oblique.

Lightening Moving of the fetus and uterus downward into the pelvic cavity.

Light sleep State that makes up the highest proportion of newborn sleep and precedes awakening; characterized by some body movements, rapid eye movements (REM), and brief fussing or crying.

Linea nigra (lin´ē-ă ni´gră) The line of darker pigmentation extending from the umbilicus to the pubis noted in some women during the later months of pregnancy.

Local anesthesia Injection of an anesthetic agent into the subcutaneous tissue in a fanlike pattern.

Local infiltration anesthesia Accomplished by injecting an anesthetic agent into the intracutaneous, subcutaneous, and intramuscular areas of the perineum.

Lochia (lō´kē-ă) Maternal discharge of blood, mucus, and tissue from the uterus; may last for several weeks after birth.

Lochia alba White vaginal discharge that follows lochia serosa and that lasts from about the 10th to the 21st day after birth.

Lochia rubra Red, blood-tinged vaginal discharge that occurs following birth and lasts 2 to 4 days.

Lochia serosa Pink, serous, and blood-tinged vaginal discharge that follows lochia rubra and lasts until the 7th to 10th day after birth.

Luteinizing hormone (LH) Anterior pituitary hormone responsible for stimulating ovulation and for development of the corpus luteum.

Maceration The process of tissue breakdown that begins from the moment of death.

Macrosomia (mak-rō-sō´mē-ă) A condition seen in newborns of large body size and high birth weight (more than 4000 to 4500 g [8 lb, 13 oz to 9 lb, 14 oz]), such as those born of prediabetic and diabetic mothers.

Malposition An abnormal position of the fetus in the birth canal.

Malpresentation A presentation of the fetus into the birth canal that is not "normal"—that is, brow, face, shoulder, or breech presentation.

Mammogram A soft-tissue radiograph of the breast without the injection of a contrast medium.

Massage therapy Manipulation of the soft tissues of the body to reduce stress and tension, increase circulation, diminish pain, and promote a sense of well-being.

Mastitis Inflammation of the breast.

Maternal mortality rate The number of maternal deaths from any cause during the pregnancy cycle per 100,000 live births.

Maternal role attainment Process by which a woman learns mothering behaviors and becomes comfortable with her identity as a mother.

Maternal serum alpha-fetoprotein (MSAFP) Screening test performed between 16 and 22 gestational weeks that utilizes the multiple markers (the "triple screen") of alpha-fetoprotein (AFP), human chorionic growth hormone (hCG), and urine estriol (uE3) to screen pregnancies for neural tube defect, Down syndrome, and trisomy 18.

Mature milk Breast milk that contains 10% solids for energy and growth.

McDonald's sign A probable sign of pregnancy characterized by an ease in flexing the body of the uterus against the cervix.

Meaning reconstruction A framework for understanding perinatal loss that focuses on redefining ourselves and how we interact with the world after a significant loss. The goal of recovery, as related to meaning reconstruction, is a positive change in self-identity by assigning the loss a meaning, thereby allowing the individual to assimilate the loss into her or his world.

Meconium Dark green or black material present in the large intestine of a full-term infant; the first stools passed by the newborn.

Meconium aspiration syndrome (MAS) Respiratory disease of term, postterm, and SGA newborns caused by inhalation of meconium or meconium-stained amniotic fluid into the lungs; characterized by mild to severe respiratory distress, hyperexpansion of the chest, hyperinflated alveoli, and secondary atelectasis.

Meiosis The process of cell division that occurs in the maturation of sperm and ova that decreases their number of chromosomes by one half.

Melasma gravidarum See *Chloasma.*

Menarche (me-nar´kē) Beginning of menstrual and reproductive function in the female.

Mendelian inheritance A major category of inheritance whereby a trait is determined by a pair of genes on homologous chromosomes. Also called *single gene inheritance.*

Menopause The permanent cessation of menses.

Menorrhagia Excessive or profuse menstrual flow.

Menstrual cycle Cyclic buildup of the uterine lining, ovulation, and sloughing of the lining occurring approximately every 28 days in nonpregnant females.

Mentum The chin.

Mesoderm The intermediate layer of germ cells in the embryo that gives rise to connective tissue, bone marrow, muscles, blood, lymphoid tissue, and epithelial tissue.

Metrorrhagia Abnormal uterine bleeding occurring at irregular intervals.

Middle adolescence A term referring to adolescents who are ages 15 to 17 years.

Milia (mil´ē-ă) Tiny white papules appearing on the face of a newborn as a result of unopened sebaceous glands; they disappear spontaneously within a few weeks.

Milk/plasma ratio The comparison of the concentration of substances in the breast milk and the maternal blood serum.

Miscarriage See *Spontaneous abortion.*

Mitosis Process of cell division whereby both daughter cells have the same number and pattern of chromosomes as the original cell.

Molding Shaping of the fetal head by overlapping of the cranial bones to facilitate movement through the birth canal during labor.

Mongolian spot Dark, flat pigmentation of the lower back and buttocks noted at birth in some infants; usually disappears by the time the child reaches school age.

Moniliasis Yeastlike fungal infection caused by *Candida albicans.*

Monosomies A genetic condition that occurs when a normal gamete unites with a gamete that is missing a chromosome.

Mons pubis (monz pu´bis) Mound of subcutaneous fatty tissue covering the anterior portion of the symphysis pubis.

Morning sickness A term that refers to the nausea and vomiting that a woman may experience in early pregnancy. This lay term is sometimes used because these symptoms frequently occur in the early part of the day and disappear within a few hours.

Moro reflex Flexion of the newborn's thighs and knees accompanied by fingers that fan, then clench, as the arms are simultaneously thrown out and then brought together, as though embracing something. This reflex can be elicited by startling the newborn with a sudden noise or movement. Also called the *startle reflex.*

Morula Developmental stage of the fertilized ovum in which there is a solid mass of cells.

Mosaicism Condition of an individual who has at least two cell lines with differing karyotypes.

Mother-baby care Also called couplet care, a family-centered care approach in which the infant remains at the mother's bedside and both are cared for by the same nurse.

Mottling (mot´ling) Discoloration of the skin in irregular areas; may be seen with chilling, poor perfusion, or hypoxia.

Mourning The *process* by which individuals incorporate the loss experience into their lives, it is influenced by many factors including personality, gender, family dynamics, and social, religious, and cultural norms.

Mucous plug A collection of thick mucus that blocks the cervical canal during pregnancy. Also called *operculum.*

Multigravida (mŭl-tē-grav´i-dă) Woman who has been pregnant more than once.

Multipara (mŭl-tip´ă-ră) Woman who has had more than one pregnancy in which the fetus was viable.

Multiple pregnancy More than one fetus in the uterus at the same time.

Music therapy Form of sound therapy using one or more musical instruments and improvisations or musical compositions. *Sound therapy* is based on the premise that when the body is exposed to the correct sound frequency (including some very low and very high frequencies that humans cannot normally hear) the body restores itself.

Myometrium Uterine muscular structure.

Nägele's rule A method of determining the estimated date of birth (EDB): after obtaining the first day of the last menstrual period, subtract 3 months and add 7 days.

Naturopathy A healing system that employs various natural means of preventing and treating human disease, such as foods, herbs, rest, etc. (Also called *natural medicine.*)

Neonatal morbidity The risk of death during the newborn period—the first 28 days of life.

Neonatal mortality rate The number of cases per year of a disease, illness, or complication occurring in the neonatal period.

Neonatal mortality risk The chance of death within the newborn period.

Neonatal transition The first few hours of life, in which the newborn stabilizes his or her respiratory and circulatory functions.

Neonatology The specialty that focuses on the management of at-risk conditions of the newborn.

Neutral thermal environment (NTE) An environment that provides for minimal heat loss or expenditure.

Nevus (nē′vŭs) **flammeus** (flaem′iŭs) Large port-wine stain.

Nevus vasculosus "Strawberry mark": raised, clearly delineated, dark-red, rough-surfaced birthmark commonly found in the head region.

New Ballard score (NBS) A postnatal gestational age assessment tool, it is a refinement of a previous Ballard score tool with added criteria for more accurate assessment of the gestational age of newborns between 20 and 28 weeks' gestation and less than 1500 g.

Newborn Infant from birth through the first 28 days of life.

Newborn screening tests Tests that detect inborn errors of metabolism that, if left untreated, cause mental retardation and physical handicaps.

Newborns' and Mothers' Health Protection Act (NMHPA) Legislation which states that women who have given birth vaginally cannot be forcibly discharged from the hospital within 48 hours of the time of birth for insurance reasons. Cesarean birth mothers are covered by their insurance for 96 hours following the time of birth.

Nidation Implantation of a fertilized ovum in the endometrium.

Nipple A protrusion about 0.5 to 1.3 cm in diameter in the center of each mature breast.

Nipple preparation Prenatal activities designed to toughen the nipple in preparation for breastfeeding.

Nonmendelian (multifactorial) inheritance The occurrence of congenital disorders that result from an interaction of multiple genetic and environmental factors.

Nonstress test (NST) An assessment method by which the reaction (or response) of the fetal heart rate to fetal movement is evaluated.

Nuchal cord Term used to describe the umbilical cord when it is wrapped around the neck of the fetus.

Nuchal folds The accumulation of fluid between the posterior cervical spine and the overlying skin in the fetal neck identified during an ultrasound examination.

Nuchal translucency testing A combination of an ultrasound and maternal serum test that is used to screen fetuses between 11 weeks and 1 day and 13 weeks and 6 days to determine if a fetus is at risk for a chromosomal disorder, such as Down syndrome (trisomy 21) and trisomy 18.

Nulligravida (nŭl-i-grav′i-dă) A woman who has never been pregnant.

Nullipara A woman who has not given birth to a viable fetus.

Nurse practitioner A professional nurse who has received specialized education in either a master's degree program or a continuing education program and thus can function in an expanded role.

Nurse researcher A nurse with an advanced doctoral degree, typically a PhD, and assumes a leadership role in generating new research.

Obstetric conjugate Distance from the middle of the sacral promontory to an area approximately 1 cm below the pubic crest.

Oligohydramnios (ol′i-gō-hī-dram′nē-os) Decreased amount of amniotic fluid, which may indicate a fetal urinary tract defect.

Oocyte Early primitive ovum before it has completely developed.

Oogenesis Process during fetal life whereby the ovary produces oogonia, cells that become primitive ovarian eggs.

Oophoritis Infection of the ovaries.

Ophthalmia (of-thal′mē-ă) **neonatorum** Purulent infection of the eyes or conjunctiva of the newborn, usually caused by gonococci.

Oral contraceptives Birth control pills that work by inhibiting the release of an ovum and by maintaining a type of mucus that is hostile to sperm.

Orientation Infant's ability to respond to auditory and visual stimuli in the environment.

Ortolani maneuver A manual procedure performed to rule out the possibility of developmental dysplastic hip.

Osteoporosis A condition most common in postmenopausal women that is characterized by decreased bone strength related to diminished bone density and bone quality. It is thought to be associated with lowered estrogen and androgen levels. Osteoporosis puts an individual at increased risk for fractures of the hip, forearm, and vertebrae.

Ovarian ligaments Ligaments that anchor the lower pole of the ovary to the cornua of the uterus.

Ovary Female sex gland in which the ova are formed and in which estrogen and progesterone are produced. Normally there are two ovaries, located in the lower abdomen on each side of the uterus.

Ovulation Normal process of discharging a mature ovum from an ovary approximately 14 days before the onset of menses.

Ovum Female reproductive cell; egg.

Oxygen toxicity Excessive levels of oxygen therapy that result in pathologic changes in tissue.

Oxytocin Hormone normally produced by the posterior pituitary, responsible for stimulation of uterine contractions and the release of milk into the lactiferous ducts.

Oxytocin challenge test (OCT) See *Contraction stress test.*

Palpation The technique of assessing a uterine contraction by touch.

Pap smear Procedure to detect the presence of cancer of the uterus by microscopic examination of cells gently scraped from the cervix.

Para (par′ă) A woman who has borne offspring who reached the age of viability.

Parametritis Inflammation of the parametrial layer of the uterus.

Parent-newborn attachment Close affectional ties that develop between parent and child. See also *Attachment.*

Passive acquired immunity Transfer of antibodies (IgG) from the mother to the fetus in utero.

Patient-controlled analgesia (PCA) A method of pain control where anesthesia, usually morphine or meperidine, is initially administered by the anesthesiologist and subsequent doses are self-administered by pushing a button controlled by a special IV pump system.

Pedigree Graphic representation of a family tree.

Pelvic cavity Bony portion of the birth passages; a curved canal with a longer posterior than anterior wall.

Pelvic cellulitis (parametritis) Infection involving the connective tissue of the broad ligament or, in severe cases, the connective tissue of all the pelvic structures.

Pelvic diaphragm Part of the pelvic floor composed of deep fascia and the levator ani and the coccygeal muscles.

Pelvic floor Muscles and tissue that act as a buttress to the pelvic outlet.

Pelvic inflammatory disease (PID) An infection of the fallopian tubes that may or may not be accompanied by a pelvic abscess; may cause infertility secondary to tubal damage.

Pelvic inlet Upper border of the true pelvis.

Pelvic outlet Lower border of the true pelvis.

Pelvic tilt Also called *pelvic rocking;* exercise designed to reduce back strain and strengthen abdominal muscle tone.

Penis The male organ of copulation and reproduction.

Percutaneous umbilical blood sampling (PUBS) See *Cordocentesis.*

Perimenopause A term referring to the period of time before menopause during which the woman moves from normal ovulatory cycles to cessation of menses.

Perimetrium The outermost layer of the corpus of the uterus. Also known as the serosal layer.

Perinatal loss Death of a fetus or infant from the time of conception through the end of the newborn period 28 days after birth.

Perinatal mortality rate The number of neonatal and fetal deaths per 1000 live births.

Perinatology The medical specialty concerned with the diagnosis and treatment of high-risk conditions of the pregnant woman and her fetus.

Perineal (per´i-nē-ăl) **body** Wedge-shaped mass of fibromuscular tissue found between the lower part of the vagina and the anal canal.

Perineum (per´i-nē´ŭm) The area of tissue between the anus and scrotum in a man or between the anus and vagina in a woman.

Periodic breathing Sporadic episodes of apnea, not associated with cyanosis, that last for about 10 seconds and commonly occur in preterm infants.

Periods of reactivity Predictable patterns of newborn behavior during the first several hours after birth.

Peritonitis Infection involving the peritoneal cavity.

Persistent occiput-posterior (OP) position Malposition of the fetus in which the fetal occiput is posterior in the maternal pelvis.

Persistent pulmonary hypertension of the newborn (PPHN) Respiratory disease resulting from right-to-left shunting of blood away from the lungs and through the ductus arteriosus and patent foramen ovale.

Phenotype The whole physical, biochemical, and physiologic makeup of an individual as determined both genetically and environmentally.

Phenylketonuria (fen´il-kē´tō-nū´rē-ă) A common metabolic disease caused by an inborn error in the metabolism of the amino acid phenylalanine.

Phosphatidylglycerol (PG) (fos-fă-tī´dĭl-glis´er-ol) A phospholipid present in fetal surfactant after about 35 weeks' gestation.

Phototherapy The treatment of jaundice by exposure to light.

Physiologic anemia of infancy A harmless condition in which the hemoglobin level drops in the first 6 to 12 weeks after birth, then reverts to normal levels.

Physiologic anemia of pregnancy Apparent anemia that results because during pregnancy the plasma volume increases more than the erythrocytes increase.

Physiologic jaundice A harmless condition caused by the normal reduction of red blood cells, occurring 48 or more hours after birth, peaking at the 5th to 7th days, and disappearing between the 7th and 10th days.

Pica The eating of substances not ordinarily considered edible or to have nutritive value.

Placenta (plă-sen´tă) Specialized disk-shaped organ that connects the fetus to the uterine wall for gas and nutrient exchange. Also called *afterbirth.*

Placenta accreta Partial or complete absence of the decidua basalis and abnormal adherence of the placenta to the uterine wall.

Placenta increta A high-risk condition that occurs when the placenta attaches to the uterine wall and invades or attaches itself within the myometrium.

Placenta percreta A high-risk condition that occurs when the placenta penetrates the myometrium, sometimes attaching to peritoneal structures within the abdominal cavity, where the removal of the uterus (hysterectomy) is sometimes necessary.

Placenta previa Abnormal implantation of the placenta in the lower uterine segment. Classification of type is based on proximity to the cervical os: *total*—completely covers the os; *partial*—covers a portion of the os; *marginal*—is in close proximity to the os.

Platypelloid pelvis An unusually wide pelvis, having a flattened oval transverse shape and a shortened anteroposterior diameter.

Podalic version Type of version used to turn a second twin during a vaginal birth.

Polar body A small cell resulting from the meiotic division of the mature oocyte.

Polycystic ovarian syndrome (PCOS) The most common endocrine disorder affecting women of reproductive age, marked by menstrual dysfunction, androgen excess, obesity, hyperinsulinemia, and infertility.

Polycythemia An abnormal increase in the number of total red blood cells in the body's circulation.

Polydactyly (pol-ē-dak´ti-lē) A developmental anomaly characterized by more than five digits on the hands or feet.

Polypharmacy The act of taking multiple drugs to treat symptoms, when the etiology of the symptoms is actually a side effect from one or more prescribed medications.

Positive signs of pregnancy Indications that confirm the presence of pregnancy.

Postcoital emergency contraception (EC) A form of combined hormonal contraception that is used when a woman is worried about pregnancy because of unprotected intercourse, rape, or possible contraceptive failure (e.g., broken condom, slipped diaphragm, missed oral contraceptives, or too long a time between Depo-Provera injections).

Postcoital test (PCT) An examination that evaluates the cervical mucus, sperm motility, sperm-mucus interaction, and the sperm's ability to negotiate the cervical mucus barrier. Also called *Sims-Huhner test.*

Postconception age periods Period of time in embryonic/fetal development calculated from the time of fertilization of the ovum.

Postmature newborn See *Postterm newborn.*

Postmaturity See *Postterm newborn.*

Postpartal hemorrhage A loss of blood of greater than 500 mL following birth. The hemorrhage is classified as *early* if it occurs within the first 24 hours and *late* if it occurs after the first 24 hours.

Postpartal home care Home visits for postpartal families occurring in the home setting. This provides opportunities for expanding information and reinforcing self- and infant care techniques initially presented in the birth setting.

Postpartum After childbirth.

Postpartum blues A maternal adjustment reaction occurring in the first few postpartal days, characterized by mild depression, tearfulness, anxiety, headache, and irritability.

Postpartum depression (postpartum major mood disorder) Severe depression that occurs within the first year after giving birth with increased incidence at about the fourth week postpartum, just before resumption of menses, and upon weaning.

Postpartum psychosis Psychosis occurring within the first 3 months after birth.

Postterm labor Labor that occurs after 42 weeks' gestation.

Postterm newborn Any infant born after 42 weeks' gestation.

Postterm pregnancy Pregnancy that lasts beyond 42 weeks' gestation.

Post-traumatic stress disorder (PTSD) Intense psychologic distress resulting from a traumatic event and evidenced by recurrent, intrusive thoughts; flashbacks, persistent avoidance of stimuli associated with the trauma; a generalized feeling of "numbness"; and persistent signs of arousal.

Precipitous birth (1) Unduly rapid progression of labor. (2) A birth in which no physician is in attendance.

Precipitous labor Labor lasting less than 3 hours.

Preeclampsia (prē-ē-klamp´sē-ă) Toxemia of pregnancy, characterized by hypertension, albuminuria, and edema. See also *Eclampsia.*

Premature infant See *Preterm infant.*

Premature rupture of the membranes (PROM) See *Rupture of membranes (ROM).*

Premenstrual dysphoric disorder (PMDD) A disorder associated with the luteal phase of the menstrual cycle (2 weeks before onset of menses) in which a woman experiences five or more affective (emotional) or somatic (physical) symptoms, which are relieved with menstruation and have occurred during most cycles during the previous year.

Premenstrual syndrome (PMS) Cluster of symptoms experienced by some women, typically occurring from a few days up to 2 weeks before the onset of menses.

Prenatal education Programs offered to expectant families, adolescents, women, or partners to provide education regarding the pregnancy, labor, and birth experience.

Prep Shaving of the pubic area.

Presentation The fetal body part that enters the maternal pelvis first. The three possible presentations are cephalic, shoulder, and breech.

Presenting part The fetal part present in or on the cervical os.

Presumptive signs of pregnancy Symptoms that suggest but do not confirm pregnancy, such as cessation of menses, quickening, Chadwick's sign, and morning sickness.

Preterm infant Any infant born before 38 weeks' gestation.

Preterm labor Labor occurring between 20 and 38 weeks of pregnancy. Also called *premature labor.*

Primigravida (prī-mi-grav´i-dă) A woman who is pregnant for the first time.

Primipara (prī-mip´ă-ră) A woman who has given birth to her first child (past the point of viability), whether or not that child is living or was alive at birth.

Probable signs of pregnancy Manifestations that strongly suggest the likelihood of pregnancy, such as a positive pregnancy test, enlarging abdomen, and positive Goodell's, Hegar's, and Braxton Hicks signs.

Professional nurse A person who has graduated from an accredited basic program in nursing, has successfully completed the nursing licensure examination (NCLEX), and is currently licensed as a registered nurse (RN).

Progesterone A hormone produced by the corpus luteum, adrenal cortex, and placenta whose function is to stimulate proliferation of the endometrium to facilitate growth of the embryo.

Progressive relaxation A relaxation technique that involves relaxing first one portion of the body and then another portion, until total body relaxation is achieved; may be used during labor.

Prolactin A hormone secreted by the anterior pituitary that stimulates and sustains lactation in mammals.

Prolapsed umbilical cord Umbilical cord that becomes trapped in the vagina before the fetus is born.

Prolonged decelerations Decelerations in which the FHR decreases from the baseline for 2 to 10 minutes.

Prolonged labor Labor lasting more than 24 hours.

Prostaglandins Complex lipid compounds synthesized by many cells in the body.

Pseudomenstruation Blood-tinged mucus from the vagina in the newborn female infant; caused by withdrawal of maternal hormones that were present during pregnancy.

Psychologic disorders Abnormal mental or emotional conditions characterized by alterations in thinking, mood, or behavior.

Ptyalism Excessive salivation.

Puberty The developmental period between childhood and the attainment of adult sexual characteristics and functioning.

Pubic Pertaining to the pubes or pubis.

Pubis Pertaining to the pubes or pubic area.

Pudendal (pyū-den´dăl) **block** Injection of an anesthetizing agent at the pudendal nerve to produce numbness of the external genitals and the lower one third of the vagina to facilitate childbirth and permit episiotomy if necessary.

Puerperal infection Infection of the reproductive tract associated with childbirth and occurring any time up to 6 weeks postpartum.

Puerperal morbidity A maternal temperature of 38C (100.4F) or higher on any 2 of the first 10 postpartal days, excluding the first 24 hours. The temperature is to be taken by mouth at least four times per day.

Puerperium (pyū-er-pēr´ē-ŭm) The period after completion of the third stage of labor until involution of the uterus is complete, usually 6 weeks.

Quadruple screen The most widely used test to screen for Down syndrome (trisomy 21), trisomy 18, and neural tube defects (NTDs).

Quickening The first fetal movements felt by the pregnant woman, usually between 16 and 18 weeks' gestation.

Quiet alert state Alert state characterized by a brightening of the eyes and face. Infants are most attentive to their environment in this state and provide positive feedback to caregivers.

Quiet sleep See deep sleep.

Radiation Heat loss incurred when heat transfers to cooler surfaces and objects not in direct contact with the body.

Rape Sexual activity, often intercourse, against the will of the victim.

Rape trauma syndrome A term that refers to a variety of symptoms, clustered in phases, that a rape survivor experiences following an assault.

Reciprocal inhibition The principle that it is impossible to feel relaxed and tense at the same time; the basis for relaxation techniques.

Reciprocity An interactional cycle that occurs simultaneously between mother and infant. It involves mutual cuing behaviors, expectancy, rhythmicity, and synchrony.

Recommended dietary allowances (RDA) Government recommended allowances of various vitamins, minerals, and other nutrients.

Rectocele May develop when the posterior vaginal wall is weakened. The anterior wall of the rectum can then sag forward, ballooning into the vagina, pushing the weakened posterior wall of the vagina in front of it.

Reflexology Form of massage involving the application of pressure to designated points or reflexes on the client's feet, hands, or ears using the thumb and fingers.

Regional analgesia The temporary and reversible loss of sensation produced by injecting an anesthetic agent (called a local anesthetic) into an area that will bring the agent into direct contact with nervous tissue.

Regional anesthesia Injection of local anesthetic agents so that they come into direct contact with nervous tissue.

Reiki Tibetan-Japanese hand-mediated therapy designed to promote healing, reduce stress, and encourage relaxation. During Reiki sessions, practitioners place their hands on or above specific problem areas and transfer energy from themselves to their clients in order to restore the balance of the client's energy fields.

Relaxin A water-soluble protein secreted by the corpus luteum that causes relaxation of the symphysis and cervical dilatation.

Religion An institutionalized system that shares a common set of beliefs and practices.

Relinquishing mothers Those mothers who choose to give their infants up for adoption.

Respiratory distress syndrome (RDS) Respiratory disease of the newborn characterized by interference with ventilation at the alveolar level, thought to be caused by the presence of fibrinoid deposits lining the alveolar ducts. Formerly called *hyaline membrane disease.*

Responding model A set of guidelines for successful interactions with grieving families.

Retained placenta Retention of the placenta beyond 30 minutes after birth.

Retinopathy (ret-i-nop´ă-the) **of prematurity (ROP)** Formation of fibrotic tissue behind the lens; associated with retinal detachment and arrested eye growth, seen with hypoxemia in preterm infants.

Rh factor Antigens present on the surface of blood cells that make the blood cell incompatible with blood cells that do not have the antigen.

Rh immune globulin (RhoGAM) An anti-Rh *(D)* gamma globulin given after birth to an Rh-negative mother of an Rh-positive fetus or child. Prevents the development of permanent active immunity to the Rh antigen.

Rhythm method The timing of sexual intercourse to avoid the fertile time associated with ovulation.

Risk factors Any findings that suggest the pregnancy may have a negative outcome, for either the woman or her unborn child.

Roles Patterns of behavior normatively defined and expected of an occupant of a given social position.

Rooting reflex An infant's tendency to turn the head and open the lips to suck when one side of the mouth or cheek is touched.

Round ligaments Ligaments that arise from the side of the uterus near the fallopian tube insertion to help the broad ligament keep the uterus in place.

Rugae (ru´gē) Transverse ridges of mucous membranes lining the vagina that allow the vagina to stretch during the descent of the fetal head.

Rupture of membranes (ROM) Rupture may be PROM (premature), SROM (spontaneous), or AROM (artificial). Some clinicians may use the abbreviation RBOW (rupture of bag of waters).

Sacral promontory A projection into the pelvic cavity on the anterior upper portion of the sacrum; serves as an obstetric guide in determining pelvic measurements.

Salpingitis Infection of the fallopian tubes.

Saltatory pattern A fetal heart rate pattern of marked or excessive variability.

Scalp stimulation A test used during labor to assess fetal well-being by pressing a fingertip on the fetal scalp. A fetus not under excessive stress will respond to the digital stimulation with heart rate accelerations.

Scarf sign The position of the elbow when the hand of a supine infant is drawn across to the other shoulder until it meets resistance.

Schultze's mechanism Expulsion of the placenta with the shiny, or fetal, surface presenting first.

Secondary infertility Condition in which couples are unable to conceive after one or more successful pregnancies.

Self-quieting ability Infant's ability to use personal resources to quiet and console himself or herself.

Semen Thick whitish fluid ejaculated by the male during orgasm and containing the spermatozoa and their nutrients.

Sepsis neonatorum Infections experienced by a newborn during the first month of life.

Sex chromosomes The X and Y chromosomes, which are responsible for sex determination.

Sexual assault A broad term that refers to a variety of types of unwanted sexual touching or penetration without consent, from unwanted sexual contact or touching of an intimate part of another person to forced anal, oral, or genital penetration.

Sexually transmitted infection (STI) Refers to infections ordinarily transmitted by direct sexual contact with an infected individual. Also called *sexually transmitted disease.*

Shaken baby injuries Injuries acquired by an infant as a result of being shaken or hit.

Show A pinkish mucus discharge from the vagina that may occur a few hours to a few days before the onset of labor.

Simian line A single palmar crease frequently found in children with Down syndrome.

Sims-Huhner test See *Postcoital test (PCT).*

Sinusoidal baseline A fetal heart rate pattern consisting of a series of cycles that are extremely smooth and regular in amplitude and duration.

Situational contraceptives Contraceptive methods that involve no prior preparation (e.g., abstinence or coitus interruptus).

Skin turgor Elasticity of skin; provides information on hydration status.

Skin-to-skin contact Physical contact between the mother and baby whereby the naked baby is placed prone on the mother's chest during the first 24 hours.

Small for gestational age (SGA) Inadequate weight or growth for gestational age; birth weight below the 10th percentile.

Sonohysterography Transvaginal ultrasound during or after the introduction of sterile saline that defines the uterine cavity contour and readily demonstrates even small intrauterine lesions.

Spermatogenesis The process by which mature spermatozoa are formed, during which the number of chromosomes is halved.

Spermatozoa Mature sperm cells of the male animal, produced by the testes.

Spermicides A variety of creams, foams, jellies, and suppositories that, when inserted into the vagina before intercourse, destroy sperm or neutralize any vaginal secretions and thereby immobilize sperm.

Spinal block Injection of a local anesthetic agent directly into the spinal fluid in the spinal canal to provide anesthesia for vaginal and cesarean births.

Spinnbarkheit The elasticity of the cervical mucus that is present at ovulation.

Spirituality A belief in a transcendent power pertaining to the spirit or soul.

Spontaneous abortion Abortion that occurs naturally. Also called *miscarriage.*

Spontaneous rupture of membranes (SROM) The breaking of the "water" or membranes marked by the expulsion of amniotic fluid from the vagina.

Station Relationship of the presenting fetal part to an imaginary line drawn between the pelvic ischial spines.

Sterilization An inclusive term that refers to surgical procedures that permanently prevent pregnancy. In the male, sterilization is achieved through a procedure called a vasectomy. In the female, sterilization is done by tubal ligation.

Stillbirth The birth of a dead infant.

Striae (strī´ă) Stretch marks; shiny purplish lines that appear on the abdomen, breasts, thighs, and buttocks of pregnant women as a result of stretching the skin.

Subconjunctival hemorrhage (sŭb´kon-jŭnk-tī´văl hem´ō-rij) Hemorrhage on the sclera of a newborn's eye, usually caused by changes in vascular tension during birth.

Subdermal implants Capsules implanted in the woman's upper underarm that prevent ovulation in most women.

Subfertility A couple who has difficulty conceiving because both partners have reduced fertility.

Subinvolution (sŭb-in-vō-lū´shŭn) Failure of a part to return to its normal size after functional enlargement, such as failure of the uterus to return to normal size after pregnancy.

Sucking reflex Normal newborn reflex elicited by inserting a finger or nipple in the newborn's mouth, resulting in forceful, rhythmic sucking.

Sudden infant death syndrome (SIDS) The sudden death of an infant; the primary cause of infant death beyond the neonatal period in the United States.

Supine hypotensive syndrome (vena caval syndrome, aortocaval compression) A condition that can develop during pregnancy when the enlarging uterus puts pressure on the vena cava when the woman is supine. This pressure interferes with returning blood flow and produces a marked decrease in blood pressure with accompanying dizziness, pallor, and clamminess, which can be corrected by having the woman lie on her left side.

Surfactant (ser-fak´tănt) A substance composed of phospholipid, which stabilizes and lowers the surface tension of the alveoli during extrauterine respiratory exhalation, allowing a certain amount of air to remain in the alveoli during expiration.

Suture Fibrous connection of opposed joint surfaces, as in the skull.

Symphysis pubis Fibrocartilaginous joint between the pelvic bones in the midline.

Synclitism Condition in which the fetal sagittal suture is midway between the maternal symphysis pubis and the sacral promontory. Upon vaginal examination, the suture feels midline between two maternal landmarks.

Syndactyly (sin-dak´ti-lē) Malformation of the fingers or toes in which there may be webbing or complete fusion of two or more digits.

Syphilis A chronic, sexually transmitted infection caused by the spirochete *Treponema pallidum.*

Taboos Behaviors or objects that are avoided by individuals or groups.

Telangiectatic nevi (tel-an´jē-ek-tat´ik nē´vī) **(stork bites)** Small clusters of pink-red spots appearing on the nape of the neck and around the eyes of infants; localized areas of capillary dilatation.

Teratogens Nongenetic factors that can produce malformations of the fetus.

Term The normal duration of pregnancy.

Testes The male gonads, in which sperm and testosterone are produced.

Testosterone The male hormone; responsible for the development of secondary male characteristics.

Therapeutic abortion Medically induced termination of pregnancy when a malformed fetus is suspected or when the woman's health is in jeopardy.

Therapeutic insemination Procedure to produce a pregnancy in which sperm obtained from a woman's husband or from a donor is deposited in the woman's vagina.

Therapeutic touch Complementary therapy grounded in the belief that people are a system of energy with a self-healing potential. The therapeutic touch practitioner, often a nurse, unites his or her energy field with that of the client, directing it in a specific way to promote well-being and healing.

Thrombophlebitis Inflammation of a vein wall, resulting in thrombus.

Thrush A fungal infection of the oral mucous membranes caused by *Candida albicans.* Most often seen in infants; characterized by white plaques in the mouth.

Tocolysis Use of medications to arrest preterm labor.

Tonic neck reflex Postural reflex seen in the newborn. When the supine infant's head is turned to one side, the arm and leg on that side extend while the extremities on the opposite side flex. Also called the *fencing position.*

TORCH An acronym used to describe a group of infections that represent potentially severe problems during pregnancy. *TO,* toxoplasmosis; *R,* rubella; *C,* cytomegalovirus; *H,* herpesvirus.

Total serum bilirubin Sum of conjugated (direct) and unconjugated (indirect) bilirubin.

Touch relaxation A relaxation technique that involves relaxing an area of one's body as another person provides a "touch" cue to that specific area. Touch relaxation is very effective during labor contractions.

Toxic shock syndrome (TSS) Infection caused by *Staphylococcus aureus,* found primarily in women of reproductive age.

Traditional Chinese medicine System of medicine developed more than 3000 years ago in China that seeks to ensure the balance of energy, which is called *chi* or *qi* (pronounced "chee"). Chi is thought to maintain health and vitality and enable the body to carry out its physiologic functions.

Transitional milk Breast milk produced from the end of colostrum production until about 2 weeks postpartum.

Transvaginal ultrasound A follicular monitoring test that is used in women undergoing induction cycles, for timing ovulation for insemination and intercourse, for retrieving oocytes for in vitro fertilization, and for monitoring early pregnancy.

Transverse diameter The largest diameter of the pelvic inlet; helps determine the shape of the inlet.

Transverse lie A lie in which the fetus is positioned crosswise in the uterus.

Trichomonas vaginalis A parasitic protozoan that may cause inflammation of the vagina, characterized by itching and burning of vulvar tissue and by white, frothy discharge.

Trichomoniasis A sexually transmitted infection caused by ***Trichomonas vaginalis,*** a microscopic motile protozoan that thrives in an alkaline environment.

Trimester Three months, or one third of the gestational time for pregnancy.

Triple screen test Prenatal test of amniotic fluid or blood which assesses for appropriate levels of alpha-fetoprotein (AFB), human chorionic gonadotropin (hCG), and unconjugated estriol (UE3). The triple test is the most widely used test to screen for Down syndrome (trisomy 21), trisomy 18, and neural tube defects (NTDs).

Trisomy The presence of three homologous chromosomes rather than the normal two.

Trophoblast The outer layer of the blastoderm that will eventually establish the nutrient relationship with the uterine endometrium.

True pelvis The portion that lies below the linea terminalis, made up of the inlet, cavity, and outlet.

Trunk incurvation (Galant reflex) Reflex resulting from the stroking of the spine that causes the pelvis to turn to the stimulated side.

Tubal embryo transfer (TET) Procedure in which eggs are retrieved and incubated with the man's sperm then transferred back into the women's body at the embryo stage.

Tubal ligation Sterilization of a woman accomplished by transecting or occluding the fallopian tubes.

Tummy time Prone positioning while awake.

Turner syndrome A number of anomalies that occur when a woman has only one X chromosome. Characteristics include short stature; little sexual differentiation; webbing of the neck, with a low posterior hairline; and congenital cardiac anomalies.

Ultrasound High-frequency sound waves that may be directed, through the use of a transducer, into the maternal abdomen. The ultrasonic sound waves reflected by the underlying structures of varying densities allow identification of various maternal and fetal tissues, bones, and fluids.

Umbilical cord (ŭm-bil´i-kăl kōrd) The structure connecting the placenta to the umbilicus of the fetus and through which nutrients from the woman are exchanged for wastes from the fetus.

Umbilical velocimetry A noninvasive ultrasound test, measures blood flow changes that occur in maternal and fetal circulation in order to assess placental function.

Urinary tract infection (UTI) Significant ***bacteriuria*** in the presence of symptoms.

Uterine atony Relaxation of uterine muscle tone following birth.

Uterine inversion Prolapse of the uterine fundus through the cervix into the vagina; may occur just before or during expulsion of the placenta; associated with massive hemorrhage, requiring emergency treatment.

Uterosacral ligaments Ligaments that provide support for the uterus and cervix at the level of the ischial spines.

Uterus The hollow muscular organ in which the fertilized ovum is implanted and in which the developing fetus is nourished until birth.

Vacuum-assisted birth An obstetric procedure used to assist in the birth of a fetus by applying suction to the fetal head with a soft suction cup attached to a suction bottle (pump) by tubing and placing the device against the occiput of the fetal head.

Vagina The musculomembranous tube or passageway located between the external genitals and the uterus of a woman.

Vaginal birth after cesarean (VBAC) Practice of permitting a trial of labor and possible vaginal birth for women following a previous cesarean birth for nonrecurring causes such as fetal distress or placenta previa.

Variability Baseline fluctuations of two cycles per minute or greater in the FHR and classified by the visually quantified amplitude of peak-to-trough in beats per minute.

Variable deceleration Periodic change in fetal heart rate caused by umbilical cord compression; decelerations vary in onset, occurrence, and waveform.

Vasa previa Condition occurring when the fetal vessels course through membranes and are present at the cervical os. Although this is a rare cause of antepartum bleeding, it has a high rate of fetal death.

Vasectomy Surgical removal of a portion of the vas deferens (ductus deferens) to produce infertility.

Vegan A "pure" vegetarian; one who consumes no food from animal sources.

Vena caval syndrome Symptoms of dizziness, pallor, and clamminess that result from lowered blood pressure when a pregnant woman lies supine and the enlarged uterus presses on the vena cava. Also known as supine hypotensive syndrome.

Vernix caseosa (ver´niks kā´sē-ō-să) A protective, cheeselike, whitish substance made up of sebum and desquamated epithelial cells that is present on the fetal skin.

Version Turning of the fetus in utero.

Vertex The top or crown of the head.

Viability The potential for the pregnancy to result in a live birth.

Vibroacoustic stimulation (VAS) Application of device delivering 90 dB of sound and vibration for 1 to 3 seconds to the mother's abdomen to stimulate movement in the fetus, thereby accelerating the fetal heart rate. (Also called FAST for fetal acoustic stimulation test or VST for vibroacoustic stimulation test.)

Vicarious trauma (also called secondary trauma effect) A condition that can occur as a result of working with people who are trauma victims.

Visualization Complementary therapy in which a person goes into a relaxed state and focuses on or "visualizes" soothing or positive scenes such as a beach or a mountain glade. Visualization helps reduce stress and encourage relaxation.

Vulva The external structure of the female genitals, lying below the mons veneris.

Vulvovaginal candidiasis (VVC) Also called moniliasis or yeast infection, VVC is a genital infection most often caused by ***Candida albicans.***

Wandering baseline A smooth meandering unsteady baseline in the normal range without variability.

Weaning The process of discontinuing breastfeeding and accustoming an infant to another feeding method.

Wharton's (hwar'tunz) **jelly** Yellow-white gelatinous material surrounding the vessels of the umbilical cord.

Zona pellucida Transparent inner layer surrounding an ovum.

Zygote A fertilized egg.

Zygote intrafallopian transfer (ZIFT) Retrieval of oocytes under ultrasound guidance, followed by in vitro fertilization and laparoscopic replacement of fertilized eggs into the fimbriated end of the fallopian tube.

Index

Page numbers followed by *f* indicate figures and those followed by *t* indicate tables, boxes, or special features (e.g., Cultural Perspectives; Evidence-Based Practice).

A

AABR (automated auditory brain response) test, 717
Abdomen:
  exercises for childbirth preparation, 243
  newborn, 609–10, 623*t*
  postpartal assessment
    first 24 hours after birth, 812*t*, 816–18
    first home visit and anticipated progress at 6 weeks, 871*t*
  postpartal changes, 804, 804*f*
  prenatal assessment, 208–9*t*
  prenatal changes, 190, 208–9*t*
Abdominal distention, 847
Abdominal effleurage, 177–78, 178*f*
Abdominal reflex, 581*t*
ABO incompatibility, 363, 771
Aboriginal culture(s), treatment of cords and placentas, 568*t*
Abortion, 200, 339
  definition, 200
  habitual, 204*t*, 340
  induced
    controversies over, 93
    ethical issues, 9
    medical, 93–94
    nursing care management, 94–95
    surgical, 94
  spontaneous
    causes, 339–40
    classification, 340, 340*f*
    clinical therapy, 341–42
    Cultural Perspectives, 341*t*
    definition, 339
    nursing care management
      evaluation, 342
      nursing assessment and diagnosis, 341
      nursing plan and implementation, 341–42
Abrupt decelerations, fetal heart rate, 424
Abruptio placentae, 491
  clinical therapy, 493
  fetal-neonatal implications, 204*t*, 401*t*, 493
  grades, 491–92
  incidence, 491
  maternal implications, 204*t*, 401*t*, 492–93
  nursing care management, 493
  nursing care plan, 494–96*t*
    assessment, 494*t*
    client scenario, 494*t*
    critical thinking questions, 496*t*
    nursing diagnosis, 494*t*, 495*t*
    nursing interventions and rationales, 494–96*t*
  versus placenta previa, 492*t*
  signs and symptoms, 492*t*
  types, 491, 492*f*
Abscess, breast, 900
Abstinence:
  as contraceptive method, 85
  in prevention of adolescent pregnancy, 287

Accelerations, fetal heart rate, 423
Acceptance, in grief process, 526
Acculturation, 20
Accutane. *See* Isotretinoin
Acetabulum, 38
Acetaminophen:
  for breast engorgement, 877, 878*t*
  essential information, 838*t*
  for newborn, 865
Achondroplasia, 616*t*
Acid-base status, response to labor:
  fetal, 396
  maternal, 393
Acidosis:
  definition, 748
  in respiratory distress syndrome, 754
Acme, 381, 383*f*
ACOG. *See* American College of Obstetricians and Gynecologists
Acoustic stimulation test, fetal, 299
Acquaintance phase, in maternal-infant attachment, 810
Acquaintance rape, 107. *See also* Violence against women
Acquired immunodeficiency syndrome (AIDS), 324. *See also* Human immunodeficiency virus type 1
Acrocyanosis, 600, 600*f*, 617*t*
Acrosomal reaction, 54
Acrosome, 49*f*, 53
Active acquired immunity, 579
Active alert state, newborn, 865, 866*t*
Active awake state, newborn, 470
Active management of labor (AMOL), 507
Active phase of labor. *See also* First stage of labor
  characteristics, 388, 388*t*
  nursing care, 440
  psychologic characteristics and nursing support, 447*t*
Active sleep, newborn, 865
Active transport, 63
Activity, physical. *See* Exercise
Actonel. *See* Risedronate
Acupressure, 24
  in labor, 442*t*
  for nausea and vomiting of pregnancy, 232, 233*f*
Acupuncture, 24
  for infertility management, 146*t*
Acyclovir:
  for herpes genitalis, 121
  for herpes simplex virus infection during pregnancy, 368–69
  for neonatal sepsis, 786*t*
A&D ointment:
  for circumcision care, 862
  for diaper rash, 862
  for newborn dry skin, 862
  for nipple soreness, 876
Addicting drug use. *See* Infant of a substance-abusing mother; Substance-abusing mother
Adequate intake (AI), 256. *See also* Dietary reference intakes
Adjustment reaction with depressed mood (postpartum blues), 808, 907–8. *See also* Psychiatric disorders, postpartal

Admission procedures:
  maternal, 431, 435–37
  newborn, 634–35
Adolescence:
  contraceptive options, 287
  early, 277
  late, 277
  middle, 277
  physical changes, 277
  psychosocial development, 277
Adolescent mother. *See also* Adolescent pregnancy
  childbirth preparation classes, 173, 285–86, 286*f*
  hints for practice, 284*t*
  key facts to remember, 283*t*
  nursing care management
    community-based nursing care, 283
    evaluation, 286
    nursing assessment and diagnosis, 282–83
    nursing plan and implementation, 283–86
      confidentiality issues, 283
      development of relationship, 283–84
      facilitation of prenatal education, 285–86
      hospital-based nursing care, 286
      promotion of family adaptation, 285
      promotion of physical well-being, 284–85
      promotion of self-esteem, 284
  nutritional issues, 270–71. *See also* Maternal nutrition
  partner of, 280–82
  pelvic examination, 284*t*
  physiologic risks, 279
  postpartal nursing care, 849
  psychologic risks, 279
  reaction to pregnancy, 280*t*, 281*t*
  risks to child, 280
  sociologic risks, 279–80
  support during birth, 459–60, 460*f*
Adolescent pregnancy. *See also* Adolescent mother
  cultural perspectives, 278*t*
  factors contributing to
    high-risk behaviors, 278–79
    psychosocial, 279
    socioeconomic and cultural, 278
  family and support group reactions, 282
  incest in, 279
  incidence, 277
  prevention, 287–88
  psychosocial factors, 279
Adoption:
  by infertile couples, 149–50
  nursing care of birth mother, 849–50
Adrenal hyperplasia, 624*t*
Adrenals, changes in pregnancy, 187
AFI (amniotic fluid index), 295
AFP. *See* Alpha-fetoprotein
African American culture:
  cultural influences on pregnancy, 229*t*
  infant feeding practices, 689
  pregnancy beliefs and attitudes, 21
African Americans:
  adolescent birth rate, 278
  fetal alcohol syndrome incidence, 724
  newborn skin color, 600
  preterm birth rates, 708
  sole creases in newborn, 590
  umbilical hernia in, 610